KEY TO ESSENTIAL TERMINOLOGY

PATIENT ASSESSMENT DATA BASE

This provides an overview of the more commonly occurring etiologies and co-existing factors associated with a specific medical diagnosis, as well as the corresponding abnormal diagnostic findings and signs/symptoms.

NURSING PRIORITIES

This section establishes a general ranking of needs/concerns upon which the Nursing Diagnoses are ordered. In actual care plan construction, this ranking would be altered according to the individual patient situation.

NURSING DIAGNOSES

The general problem/concern (Diagnosis) is stated without the etiology and signs/symptoms, which would be added to create a patient problem statement when specific patient information is available. For example, when a patient develops chest pain and shortness of breath while walking, the nursing diagnosis of Activity Intolerance could be stated "Activity Intolerance related to imbalance between oxygen demand/supply as manifested by development of chest pain and dyspnea." In addition, diagnoses that have been identified within these care plan guides as actual or potential may be changed/deleted, or diagnoses may be added, depending on specific patient information.

SUPPORTING DATA/CONTRIBUTING FACTORS

This lists the usual/common reasons why a particular problem may occur and can be used to create the "related to" portion of the patient problem statement when the specific patient situation is known.

GENERAL PATIENT OUTCOME

These give direction to patient care as they identify what the patient/nurse hope to achieve. They are stated in general terms in this book to permit the practitioner to modify/individualize them by adding time lines and individual patient criteria so they become "measurable", e.g., "Patient able to walk length of hall and back without pain/dyspnea by discharge."

INTERVENTIONS

These are divided into independent and collaborative, and are ranked only by most to least common. When creating the individual care plan, these interventions would normally be re-ordered to reflect the patient's specific needs/situation. In addition, the division of independent/collaborative is arbitrary and depends on the individual nurse's capabilities and hospital/community standards.

CRITICAL CARE PLANS

Guidelines for Patient Care

Mary Frances Moorhouse, R.N., C.C.P., CCRN

Contract Practitioner
Critical Care
Colorado Springs, Colorado

Alice C. Geissler, R.N., CCRN

Rehabilitation Specialist
International Rehabilitation Associates
Colorado Springs, Colorado

Marilynn E. Doenges, B.S.N., M.A., R.N., C.S.

Clinical Specialist
Adult Psychiatric/Mental Health Nursing
Private Practice
Colorado Springs, Colorado

F.A. DAVIS COMPANY PHILADELPHIA

Printed in the United States of America.

The views expressed in this book are those of the authors and do not reflect the official policy or position of the Department of the Army, Department of Defense, or the US Government.

Library of Congress Cataloging-in-Publication Data

Moorhouse, Mary Frances, 1947–
Critical care plans.

Bibliography: p.
Includes index.
1. Intensive care nursing—Planning—Handbooks, manuals, etc. 2. Nursing care plans—Handbooks, manuals, etc. I. Geissler, Alice C., 1946– . II. Doenges, Marilynn E., 1922– . III. Title. [DNLM: 1. Critical Care—nurses' instruction. Wy 154 M825c]
RT120.I5M66 1987 610.73'61 87-6740
ISBN 0-8036-6311-0

This book is dedicated to our loved ones, Jan, Paul, and Jason Moorhouse; Bill Geissler; and Dean and Jim Doenges who have cooked their own meals, washed their own clothes, and taken care of us as well. Special thanks to Barbara Doenges for her assistance with the preparation of the bibliography and to David and John Doenges and Nancy Daigle who supported their mother with encouragement.

Also to Linda Nold and Bob Martone who were willing to aid us in any way we could imagine and who maintained a positive outlook as deadlines came and went and came again. To Ruth De George who tried to keep all the loose ends tied together.

Finally this book is dedicated to the students and practitioners who daily face the challenge of caring for the critically ill.

PREFACE

This care plan book serves as a guide for nurses who plan and promote health care for the critically ill patient. With the trends in health care of cost containment and shortened stays, patients in critical care units have higher acuity levels and stay for much shorter times than in the past. The average critical care nurse is forced to spend so much of the time coping with the technical aspects of the patient's care that the planning aspects tend to get shuffled to the background. The primary focus of this book is planning for holistic care in a setting where these life threatening conditions are the primary concern.

Chapter 1 examines current issues and their implications for the nurse caring for the critically ill patient and family/significant other(s). An overview of cultural, community, sociological, and ethical concepts impacting on the critical care nurse in the acute care setting is included. The need for cooperation and coordination with other health care professionals is an important concept that is integrated throughout the care plans.

The nursing process is used to identify patient needs and serves as the basis for nursing diagnosis and formulation of care plans with interventions based upon scientific rationale. Chapter 2 reviews the use of nursing process as it applies to the critical care setting. Nursing Diagnosis, as proposed by the North American Nursing Diagnosis Association (NANDA), is discussed to provide the nurse with an understanding of its application to the acute care setting. The use and adaptation of the care plan guides presented in this book are discussed and a sample history tool is included, reflecting a nursing approach of dividing information into Diagnostic Divisions as it is recorded, facilitating the choice of individual nursing diagnoses.

Chapters 3 through 12 are divided into systems with care plans formulated to apply the nursing process. The use of nursing diagnoses within this medical framework promotes health for the patient during the critical phase in the acute care setting. The patient assessment data base, which includes information gathered from the nursing history, physical, and laboratory findings, is used to formulate nursing priorities to guide the ranking of the patient problems.

A decision-making model is used to organize and prioritize nursing interventions based on the nurses acting independently/collaboratively within the health team. No attempt is made to indicate whether independent or collaborative actions come first as this must be dictated by the individual situation. Inclusion of rationale for the nursing actions will assist the nurse to decide whether the interventions are appropriate for an individual patient. With few exceptions, references are not included in order to conserve space. A bibliography is included to allow for further reference as needed.

In summary, this book is designed to be a ready reference for the practicing nurse as well as a catalyst for thought in planning, documenting, and evaluating care. Students will find the care plans helpful in identifying nursing diagnoses and interventions appropriate for planning care for the individual patient as they learn and develop skills in the critical care setting. This book is not intended to be a procedure manual and efforts have been made to avoid detailed descriptions of techniques/protocols that might be viewed as individual/regional in nature. Instead, the reader is referred to *AACN's Procedure Manual for Critical Care* for indepth direction for these concerns.

M.F.M.
A.C.G.
M.E.D.

CONTRIBUTORS

Karen Bell, R.N., M.S.N., C.E.N.
Major, Army Nurse Corps
Director, Practical Nurse Course
Fitzsimmons Army Medical Center
Aurora, Colorado

Kathleen Crocker, R.N., M.S.N., C.N.S.N.
Clinical Specialist, Nutrition Support Nursing
Director of Nursing
New England Critical Care, Inc.
Marlborough, Massachusetts
and formerly,
Clinical Specialist, Nutrition Support Nursing
Saint Vincent Charity Hospital and Health Center
Cleveland, Ohio

A. Gail Curry-Kane, B.S.N., R.N.
Nurse Epidemiologist
University of Health Sciences Center
Denver, Colorado

Pamela DeLoach, R.N., B.S.N.
Primary Nurse III
Neurotrauma Center
M.I.E.M.S.S.
Baltimore, Maryland

Marilynn E. Doenges, B.S.N., M.A., R.N., C.S.
Clinical Specialist
Adult Psychiatric/Mental Health Nursing
Private Practice
Colorado Springs, Colorado

Karen Dorman, R.N., B.S.N., CCRN
Research Associate
Department of Obstetrics and Gynecology
Baylor College of Medicine
Houston, Texas

Diane Dressler, R.N., M.S.N., CCRN
Clinical Nurse Specialist
Midwest Heart Surgery Institute, Ltd.
Milwaukee, Wisconsin

Kerry Fater, R.N., Ph.D.
Assistant Professor
Salve Regina College
School of Nursing
Newport, Rhode Island

Terry Mathew Foster, R.N., C.E.N., CCRN
Critical Care and Emergency Nursing Instructor
Our Lady of Mercy Hospital Anderson/Mariemont
Cincinnati, Ohio
and
Staff Nurse, Emergency Department
Saint Elizabeth Medical Center North Unit
Covington, Kentucky

Ruth Froyd, R.N., B.S.N., CCRN
Critical Care Staff Nurse
Austin, Texas

Alice C. Geissler, R.N., CCRN
Rehabilitation Specialist
International Rehabilitation Associates
Colorado Springs, Colorado

Irene Grossbach, R.N., M.S.N.
Pulmonary Nurse Specialist
Veterans Administration Medical Center
and
Assistant Professor
University of Minnesota
School of Nursing
Minneapolis, Minnesota

Betty Hagge, R.N., B.S.N.
Administrative Supervisor
Penrose Hospital
Colorado Springs, Colorado

Mary Fran Hazinski, R.N., M.S.N., C.S.
Pediatric Clinical Nurse Specialist
Pediatric Intensive Care Unit
Vanderbilt Hospital
Nashville, Tennessee

Mary F. Jeffries, LTC (Retired)
Tucson, Arizona

Ann M. Jansen, R.N., M.S., CCRN
Masters Candidate
Critical Care Clinician
Memorial Hospital
Colorado Springs, Colorado

Janet Kenty, R.N., M.S.N.
Perinatal Educational Coordinator/Staff Instructor
Nursing Education Department
Women and Infants' Hospital
Providence, Rhode Island

Merrily A. Mathewson, R.N., Ph.D., CCRN
President/Director of Education
Educational Services
Hamburg, New York

Cynthia McCall May, R.N., B.S.N., CCRN
Head Nurse, Adult Critical Care Unit
Memorial Hospital
Colorado Springs, Colorado

Linda S. Mayer, R.N., M.N.
Pulmonary Clinical Nurse Specialist
Division of Pulmonary Medicine
University of Kansas Medical Center
Kansas City, Kansas

Kathy McCord, R.N., M.S.N., CCRN
Head Nurse, Intensive Care Unit
Penrose Hospital
Colorado Springs, Colorado

Patricia Moloney-Harmon, R.N., M.S.N., CCRN
Head Nurse, Pediatric Intensive Care Unit
Johns Hopkins Hospital
Baltimore, Maryland

Mary Frances Moorhouse, R.N., C.C.P., CCRN
Contract Practitioner, Critical Care
Colorado Springs, Colorado

Linda J. Nielson, R.N., CCRN
Charge Nurse, Intensive Care Unit
St. Peter Hospital
Olympia, Washington

Karen J. Replogle, R.N., M.S., CCRN
Critical Care Nursing Consultant
Healthcare Education and Computing
Dayton, Ohio

Vicki Schreckengost, R.N., M.S.N., CCRN
Assistant Clinical Professor
Department of Physiological Nursing
University of California, San Francisco
and
Consultant, Critical Care
Educational Services, Inc.
Hamburg, New York

Sherry Smith, R.N., B.S.N., M.S.N., Ed.D.
Director and Professor
DePauw University
School of Nursing
Greencastle/Indianapolis, Indiana

Brenda Lebowitz Stoller, B.A., R.N., C.N.A.
Private Consultant for AIDS projects and programs
AMPC Fellow at New York University
Director of Nurses Network on AIDS
New York, New York

Rita Bolek Trofino, R.N., M.N.Ed.
Assistant Professor
Saint Francis College
Department of Nursing
Loretto, Pennsylvania

Connie Walleck, M.S., R.N., CCRN
Clinical Nurse Supervisor/Specialist
Neurotrauma Center
M.I.E.M.S.S.
Baltimore, Maryland

CONSULTANTS

Ursula Anderson, R.N., M.S.N., CCRN
Assistant Professor
The Catholic University of America
School of Nursing
Washington, D.C.

Betsy M. Barnes, B.S.N., M.S.N., CCRN
Assistant Professor
Lander College
Division of Nursing
Greenwood, South Carolina

Elizabeth W. Bayley, R.N., M.S.
Assistant Professor of Burn, Emergency and Trauma Nursing
Widener University
School of Nursing
Chester, Pennsylvania

Gerald Bennett, R.N., Ph.D.
Assistant Professor of Psychiatric/Mental Health Nursing
Medical College of Georgia
School of Nursing
Augusta, Georgia

Joea E. Bierchen, B.S.N., M.S.N., Ed.D.
Director of Nursing
New Mexico State University–Carlsbad
Carlsbad, New Mexico

Dorothy R. Blevins, R.N., B.S.N., M.S.N.
Associate Professor
Kent State University
School of Nursing
Kent, Ohio

Lynn Bond, R.N., Ph.D.
Assistant Professor of Physiological Nursing
University of Washington
School of Nursing
Seattle, Washington

Ellen K. Boyda, R.N., M.S., CCRN
Pulmonary Clinical Nurse Specialist
Pulmonary Rehabilitation Program Coordinator
Taylor Hospital
Ridley Park, Pennsylvania

Suzette Cardin, R.N., M.S., CCRN
Administrative Head Nurse, CCU/COU
UCLA Medical Center
Los Angeles, California

Jeanette K. Chambers, R.N., M.S., C.S.
Renal Clinical Nurse Specialist
Riverside Methodist Hospital
Columbus, Ohio

Sheryl A. Cleveland, R.N., M.S.N.
Assistant Professor
Midwestern State University
Department of Nursing
Wichita Falls, Texas

Rebecca E. Czarnik, R.N., M.S.N., CCRN
Trauma Nurse Coordinator
Mt. Carmel Medical Center
Columbus, Ohio

Joanne M. Farley, R.N., M.S.N., CCRN
Critical Care Nurse Specialist
Hahnemann University
Philadelphia, Pennsylvania

LuAnne M. Franco, R.N., M.S.N., CCRN
Neurosurgical Nurse Associate
Allen Neurosurgical Association
Allentown, Pennsylvania

Susan Jane Frye, R.N., M.S.N.
Critical Care Nurse Consultant
Iowa City, Iowa

Toni J. Galvan, R.N., M.S.N., CCRN
Assistant Professor

University of Texas, Tyler
Department of Nursing
Tyler, Texas

Susan L. Gelbard, R.N., M.S.N.
Assistant Professor
Barry University
School of Nursing
Miami Shores, Florida

Audrey G. Gift, R.N., Ph.D.
Assistant Professor
University of Maryland
School of Nursing
Baltimore, Maryland

Barbara Given, R.N., Ph.D., FAAN
Director of Graduate and Research Programs
Michigan State University
College of Nursing
East Lansing, Michigan

Sallie Page-Goertz, R.N.C., M.N.
Pediatric Clinical Nurse Specialist and Instructor of Pediatrics
The University of Kansas College of Health Sciences and Hospital
School of Medicine and Nursing
Kansas City, Kansas

Diana W. Gutherie, R.N., M.S.P.H., FAAN, C.
Diabetes Nurse Specialist and Associate Professor
Kansas Regional Diabetes Center, University of Kansas School of Medicine
Adjunct Professor
Wichita State University
Department of Nursing
Wichita, Kansas

Kathryn H. Haugh, R.N., M.S.N., CCRN
Assistant Professor
The University of Virginia
School of Nursing
Charlottesville, Virginia

Chris Hinds, R.N., S.N.P.N.
AIDS Project Coordinator
Evans Army Hospital
Ft. Carson, Colorado

Sheila M. Keller, R.N., M.S.N.
Instructor
Saint Agnes Medical Center
School of Nursing
Philadelphia, Pennsylvania

Karen M. Kleeman, R.N., Ph.D.
Assistant Professor of Psychophysiological Nursing
University of Maryland
School of Nursing
Baltimore, Maryland

Patricia Lounsbury, R.N., B.S.N., M.Ed., CCRN
Instructor of Arrhythmia Interpretation
Grand View College
Division of Nursing
Des Moines, Iowa

Judith H. Lower, R.N., CCRN, CNRN
Head Nurse of Neurosciences Critical Care Unit
Johns Hopkins Hospital
Baltimore, Maryland

Terry B. McGoldrick, R.N., M.S.N., CCRN, CNA
Information Systems Coordinator
Albert Einstein Medical Center–Northern Division
Philadelphia, Pennsylvania

Marilynn Mitchell, R.N., M.S.N., CCRN
Head Nurse of Neuro/ICC Units
Denver General Hospital
Denver, Colorado

Jill Morgan, R.N., M.S.N.
Director of Special Care Units
Memorial Hospital
Chattanooga, Tennessee

Colleen Norton, R.N., M.S.N., CCRN
Assistant Professor
The Catholic University of America
School of Nursing
Washington, D.C.

Kim Perry, R.N.
Critical Care Nurse
Crouse-Irving Memorial Hospital
Syracuse, New York

Rosemary Polomano, R.N., M.S.N., C.S.
Oncology Clinical Specialist
Hospital of the University of Pennsylvania
Philadelphia, Pennsylvania

Jan P. Price, R.N.
Trauma Nurse Coordinator
Grant Medical Center
Columbus, Ohio

Edie Randall, R.N., M.S., CCRN
Clinical Instructor
Arizona State University
School of Nursing
Tempe, Arizona

Lisa Robinson, R.N., Ph.D., FAAN, C.S.
Professor of Psychiatric Nursing
University of Maryland
School of Nursing
Baltimore, Maryland

Joanne S. Rokosky, R.N., B.S.N., M.N., C.S.
Respiratory Clinical Nurse Specialist
Visiting Nurse Service of Seattle–King County

Program Specialist
Washington State Nurses Association
Seattle, Washington

Meredith M. Rowe, R.N., M.S.N., C.S.
Adjunct Assistant Professor
Montana State University
College of Nursing
Great Falls, Montana

Mildred Mae Russin, R.N., M.S.N.
Instructor
University of Florida
College of Nursing
Gainesville, Florida

Alice Mary Ryan, R.N., B.S.N., CCRN
Instructor of Critical Care
The Medical College of Pennsylvania
Department of Nursing
Philadelphia, Pennsylvania

Anne Moraca-Sawicki, R.N., B.S.N., M.S.N.
Formerly Assistant Professor
D'Youville College
School of Nursing
Buffalo, New York

Connie Slay, R.N., B.S.N., M.S.N.
Cardiovascular Clinical Nurse Specialist
Bryn Mawr Hospital
Bryn Mawr, Pennsylvania

Sherry Smith, B.S.N., M.S.N., Ed.D.
Director and Professor
DePauw University
School of Nursing
Greencastle, Indiana

Catherine Spearing, R.N., M.S.N., C.S.
Pulmonary Clinical Nurse Specialist
University of Maryland Medical System
Division of Surgical Nursing
Baltimore, Maryland

June Stark, R.N., B.S.N., CCRN
Critical Care Instructor–Renal Nurse Consultant
New England Medical Center
Boston, Massachusetts

Cindy Stern, R.N., M.S.N.
Nursing Services
Jefferson University
Philadelphia, Pennsylvania

Chris Stewart-Amidei, R.N., M.S.N., CNRN, CCRN
Neurological Clinical Nurse Specialist
Loyola University Medical Center
Maywood, Illinois

April Hazard-Vallerand, R.N., M.S.N., CCRN
Instructor
University of Florida
College of Nursing
Gainesville, Florida

Betty K. Wajdowicz, R.N., B.S., M.A.
Professor
St. Petersburg Junior College
St. Petersburg, Florida

Barbara Wall, B.S.N., M.S.
Formerly, Assistant Professor
Barry University
School of Nursing
Miami Shores, Florida

Jeannette A. Waterman, B.S.N., M.S.N.
Instructor
Saint Agnes Medical Center
School of Nursing
Philadelphia, Pennsylvania

ABBREVIATIONS

ABGs: arterial blood gases
ADH: antidiuretic hormone
AF: atrial fibrillation
ARDS: adult respiratory distress syndrome
ARF: acute renal failure
ASHD: arteriosclerotic heart disease
ATN: acute tubular necrosis
AV: aortic valve, atrioventricular
BBB: bundle branch block
BEE: basal energy expenditure
B/P: blood pressure
BUN: blood urea nitrogen
Ca^{++}: calcium
CABG: coronary artery bypass graft
CAD: coronary artery disease
CAVH: continuous arteriovenous hemofiltration
CBC: complete blood count
Cl^{-}: chloride
cm: centimeter
CHF: congestive heart failure
CNS: central nervous system
CO: cardiac output
CO_2: carbon dioxide
COPD: chronic obstructive lung disease
CPK: creatinine phosphokinase
CPP: cerebral perfusion pressure
CPR: cardiopulmonary resuscitation
CPT: chest physiotherapy
Cr: creatinine
CRF: chronic renal failure
CSF: cerebral spinal fluid
CT: computerized axial tomography
CVA: cerebrovascular accident
CVP: central venous pressure
CXR: chest xray
DI: diabetes insipidus
DIC: disseminated intravascular coagulation
dl: deciliter
DM: diabetes mellitus
DKA: diabetic ketoacidosis
D5W: 5% dextrose in water
DTRS: deep tendon reflexes
DVT: deep vein thrombosis
ECF: extracellular fluid
ECG: electrocardiogram
ESR: erythrocyte sedimentation rate
ETT: endotracheal tube
FHR: fetal heart rate
FIO_2: fraction inspired oxygen
FFP: fresh frozen plasma
FRC: functional residual capacity
GFR: glomerular filtration rate
GI: gastrointestinal
HCO_3^{-}: bicarbonate
HCT: hematocrit
HGB: hemaglobin
HHNC: hyperosmolar hyperglycemic nonketotic coma
HOB: head of bed
HR: heart rate
IABP: intra-aortic balloon pump
ICF: intracellular fluid
IICP: increased intracranial pressure
IM: intramuscular
IMV: intermittent mechanical ventilation
IPPB: intermittent positive pressure breathing
IV: intravenous
JVD: jugular venous distention
K^{+}: potassium
L: liter
LAP: left atrial pressure
LDH: lactate dehydrogenase
LOC: level of consciousness
LVEDP: left ventricular end-diastolic pressure

LVF: left ventricular failure
MAP: mean arterial pressure
MDF: myocardial depressant factor
mEq: milliequivalent
Mg^{++}: magnesium
mg: milligram
MI: myocardial infarction
mmHg: millimeters of mercury
mOsm: milliosmal
MR: magnetic resonance
MV: mitral valve
Na^{+}: sodium
NG: nasogastric
NS: normal saline
NSR: normal sinus rhythm
O_2: oxygen
OTC: over-the-counter
P: pulse
PaO_2: partial pressure of oxygen in arterial blood
PAC: premature atrial contraction
$PaCO_2$: partial pressure of carbon dioxide in arterial blood
PAP: pulmonary artery pressure
PAT: paroxysmal atrial tachycardia
PCWP: pulmonary capillary wedge pressure
PE: pulmonary embolus
PEEP: positive end-expiratory pressure
pg: phostidylglycerol
PI: phosphotidylinositol
PJC: premature junctional contraction
PMI: point of maximal intensity
PO_4: phosphate
PT: protime
PTT: partial thromboplastin time
PVC: premature ventricular contraction
RAP: right atrial pressure
RBC: red blood cell
RVF: right ventricular failure
SB: sinus bradycardia
SC: subcutaneous
SCI: spinal cord injury
SGOT: serum glutamic oxaloacetic-acid-transaminase
SGPT: serum glutamic pyruvic transaminase
SIADH: syndrome of inappropriate antidiuretic hormone
SO: significant other
SR: sinus rhythm
ST: sinus tachycardia
SVO_2: systemic venous oxygen
SVR: systemic vascular resistance
TIA: transient ischemic attacks
TPN: total parenteral nutrition
UA: urinalysis
UO: urine output
UTI: urinary tract infection
VC: vital capacity
VF: ventricular fibrillation
V/Q: ventilation/perfusion
VS: vital signs
Vt: tidal volume
VT: ventricular tachycardia
WBC: white blood cells

CONTENTS

CHAPTER 1
ISSUES AND TRENDS IN CRITICAL CARE NURSING

The entire field of health care is changing; but nowhere are those changes occurring at a more rapid rate than in critical care, where the nurse offers direct assistance to both patients and families facing life-and-death dilemmas. This is an awesome and tremendously exacting responsibility. Intimately associated with "nursing" the patient and family is documentation of that care.

What lies ahead for critical care nursing and critical care planning? This chapter will examine some major trends that could have a lasting impact on critical care. These trends include

1. Scarcity of health care dollars, restructuring of hospitals
2. Quantification of nursing care costs
3. Decreased length of stay
4. Balance of high technology/high touch
5. Requirement for increased nursing knowledge
6. Need for collaboration and communication
7. Innovations in care planning through computerization

SCARCITY OF HEALTH CARE DOLLAR, RESTRUCTURING OF HOSPITALS

Major changes in payment mechanisms for hospital Medicare patients were introduced in 1983 in response to escalating costs for provision of health care within the United States. The government has indicated clearly that it is no longer willing to spend excessively for health care. Implementation of prospective reimbursement has impact on critical care nursing and has implications for patient care planning.

The focus of health care under prospective reimbursement is cost containment, requiring that nursing redefine the minimum standards of care while providing effective nursing care. As never before, the patient care plan must reflect a plan that best meets the patient's needs within the restrictions of time limitations and fewer resources.

Implementation of prospective reimbursement has led to decreased lengths of stay and increased levels of acuity for critical care patients. Hospitals, no longer compensated on a cost basis but reimbursed by patient episode, benefit financially because less technology per patient is used. Hospitals have responded to decreased dollars by reducing beds and staff. As a result of these changes, the critical care nurse must function more efficiently.

Hospitals are merging into existing or new corporations in order to spread the risks of operating in a tight economic environment. Health Maintenance Organizations and hospitals are sharing services for the benefit of patients as well as for cost containment. As a result, some services may be deleted or offered in only one facility. In addition, use of alternate health care providers, such as RediCare and outpatient services, may result in delays in admission and/or transfers to the critical care unit.

Rationing of health care dollars will occur as a result of prospective reimbursement. Hospitals cannot afford to prolong life without consideration of expense. As the health care dollar shrinks, many questions arise. How shall allocation of a fixed number of resources to many possible users be determined? Beyond that, who will decide who receives the benefits purchased with these scarce dollars? Whether decision is made by "ethics committees" or by some other less formal mechanism, the patient care plan will contribute to the decision-making process.

QUANTIFICATION OF NURSING CARE COSTS

In the wake of prospective reimbursement, fewer dollars, limited time, reduced beds and staff, attention is focused on the cost of providing nursing care to patients within the critical care unit. Quantification of nursing time requires identification of the intensity of nursing care required by patients. Clinically, intensity may be measured by a patient classification system or directly from the patient care plan. In addition, the care plan may be used for comparison from hospital to hospital for costs of nursing services and for documenting provision of minimal standards of care.

Quantification of nursing's contribution to patient care may lead to "costing" and "billing" for nursing care. Although only a few of the nation's 6000 hospitals currently "cost" and "bill" for nursing, a growing number of hospitals will adopt this practice as they are forced to monitor costs. In those hospitals already billing for nursing services, the patient care plan is an integral part of the quantification of nursing care costs.

DECREASED LENGTH OF STAY

Implementation of prospective reimbursement has profoundly affected hospital length of stays. Nurses are assuming a larger portion of responsibility for ensuring that patients are discharged on time according to their diagnosis-related group (DRG) classification. The provision of personalized care must be planned and provided with continuity as quantity of care time decreases. Efficient care planning can help the nurse identify those patients who can be transferred or discharged earlier. Aggressive discharge planning begins on admission to the critical care unit and incorporates knowledge of hospital and community resources available for the patient. Individualized care plans should reflect those resources identified by the nurse to ensure an early but safe discharge.

To facilitate early but safe discharge and to ensure continuity of care, the nurse may find traditional unit boundaries loosening (Edwardson, S., 1985). Nurses may follow patients from the intensive to general care units to achieve optimal outcomes. This "following" may be active planning of care as the patient convalesces or by the formation of a care plan early in the patient's stay that seeks to ensure optimal patient outcomes in the midst of decreased length of stay. Followup by intensive care unit (ICU) nurses also may be accomplished after discharge by phone contacts, home visits, and consultation with postdischarge care givers.

Many patients leaving the hospital earlier are still in need of health care. Hospitals are starting their own health care agencies, or hiring hospital-based coordinators to work with private home health care agencies. An effectively coordinated care plan can follow the patient home, ensuring continuity of care between the health care system and home.

BALANCE OF HIGH TECHNOLOGY/HIGH TOUCH

Long before John Naisbett's *Megatrends* (New York, Warner Books, 1982) became a bestseller and "high tech/high touch" became a trendy phrase, nurses expressed concern that the patient was in danger of being lost among the tubes, monitors, and machines as complex technology became an increasingly larger part of health care. This has led nurses to advocate recognition of patient individuality and the holistic concept of "Mind-Soul-Body" interaction by various means, such as adoption of the primary nurse format and heightened awareness of the "quality of life/right to die" dilemma. Inclusion of these concepts and consideration of the individual's cultural/socioeconomic background in the care plan can facilitate achieving balance between technologic wonders and human needs.

REQUIREMENT FOR INCREASED NURSING KNOWLEDGE

Increased patient acuity combined with shorter lengths of stay within the critical care environment require more intensive nursing interventions. The nurse needs greater clinical expertise, maturity, critical thinking ability, assertiveness, and patient management skills. Increased expertise presupposes increased productivity.

Nursing specialty certification programs share common goals: to provide consumer protection, to enhance nursing knowledge and competency, to increase nursing autonomy, and to strengthen collaboration. Certification recognizes the acquisition of additional knowledge and the attainment of predetermined standards established by the specialty group. Specialty certification will take on more importance in this cost-conscious era (Erikson, H., 1985) as managers seek to hire competent professionals.

Care planning serves as a means to increase nursing knowledge and practice. Standardized care plans establish priorities of care and define minimum standards of safe practice. Standardized care plans also serve as "memory joggers" to nurses caring for patients not usually seen in their area of clinical practice, providing information and promoting safe, effective practice.

NEED FOR COLLABORATION AND COMMUNICATION

As health care delivery becomes more complex and more economically centered, the need for communication and collaboration among health care professionals is intensified. Only through collaboration between departments/services/facilities can medical professionals deliver the most efficient and comprehensive care possible. The nurse, as the primary coordinator of overall patient care, strives to assure that the patient receives quality but cost-efficient care.

Interdepartment communication and collaboration may take form as a patient care conference. More commonly, the nurse works as a liason between health care providers. Information obtained from patient care conferences is incorporated into the overall plan of care for the patient. Thus, the care plan serves as the vehicle for/and documentation of ongoing communication among nurses and workers in other disciplines. Collaboration attempts to reduce the overall cost of hospitalization and to ensure adequate, safe patient care.

Patients and families, assuming responsibility for themselves (internal locus-of-control), are participating in more decisions determining the level and amount of health care they desire. The care plan should include moral/ethical concerns, such as "no code/living will" decisions, with date, time, and names of those participating. This provides legal and ethical documentation of the decision-making/communication process.

INNOVATIONS IN CARE PLANNING THROUGH COMPUTERIZATION

Many nurses believe that their limited time can be spent better at the bedside, giving patient care, rather than generating paperwork. Institutions using computerized care planning report increased numbers of care plans being generated and maintained than occurred previous to computerization (Lombard & Light, 1983). Computerization can decrease time spent in generating and maintaining care plans and may improve the quality of record keeping. In fact, computerized systems have had a favorable impact on the process, because nurses may quickly enter, display, update, evaluate, and print a care plan.

Most computerized systems use standardized patient care plans. Many use the nursing diagnoses accepted for testing by the North American Nursing Diagnosis Association (NANDA). Basic care plans reflect standards of care for particular patient problems and are designed to meet specific needs. Because the plans reflect a wealth of varied nursing experience, they allow even novice practitioners to formulate effective care strategies. These computerized care plans provide critical care nurses with an efficient means to develop comprehensive, continuous, individualized, and legible care plans for each patient.

CONCLUSION

The use of care plans reflecting only functional divisions of tasks/duties perpetuates the notion that care plans are "busy work," unrelated to care giving. Restructuring care plans using "nursing models" could increase usage and could provide succinct documentation/relevance, demonstrating the relationship between planning and documentation.

Efficient and effective use of the patient care plan can ensure that intensively ill patients receive individualized quality care in the midst of cost containment. It also provides documentation of the impact of nursing on patient care.

What lies ahead for critical care nursing and critical care planning? Definitely a tremendously exacting challenge!

CHAPTER 2
NURSING PROCESS, CARE PLANNING WITH NURSING DIAGNOSIS

There is a growing awareness that nursing care is a key factor in patient survival and in the maintenance, rehabilitative, and preventive aspects of health care. Publication of the American Nurses Association (ANA) Social Policy Statement (1980), defining nursing as the diagnosis and treatment of human responses to actual and potential health problems, and the ANA Standards of Practice have provided impetus and support for the use of nursing diagnosis in the practice setting. Prospective payment plans; movement out of the acute care (hospital) to other settings, for example, long-term/convalescent, rehabilitation, home health services; and other changes in the health care system are promoting the need for a common framework of communication and documentation. This assures continuity of care for the patient who moves from one area of the health care system to another. Evaluation and documentation of care are important parts of this process.

Nurses have visionary ideas for delivery of quality care to all patients. Turning those ideas into action often becomes a frustrating exercise in futility as what appears easy to do in theory becomes difficult in practice. In a hectic schedule, many nurses believe that time spent in writing care plans is time taken away from patient care. In reality, the delivery of quality care involves planning and coordination. It is our belief that as the nurse works with nursing diagnosis, learning the etiology/defining characteristics, goals will become apparent and interventions for attaining these goals will become clear. When properly written and utilized, care plans provide tools for patient care assessment, guidelines for documentation, and direction for continuity of care among nurses and other caregivers.

NURSING PROCESS

The term nursing process was introduced in the 1950s, but it has taken many years to develop national acceptance as an integral part of nursing care. It is adapted from the scientific approach to problem solving and requires the skills of (1) assessment (systematic collection of data relating to patients and their problems), (2) problem identification (analysis and interpretation of data), (3) planning (choice of solutions), (4) implementation (putting the plan into action), and (5) evaluation (assessing the effectiveness of the plan and changing the plan as indicated by the current needs). Although nurses use these terms separately, in reality they are interrelated and form a continuous circle of thought and action, providing an efficient method of organizing thought processes for clinical decision making. Nursing process is now included in the conceptual framework of most nursing curricula, and it is accepted in the legal definition of nursing in most nurse practice acts.

To utilize this process, the nurse must demonstrate fundamental abilities of knowledge, intelligence, creativity, interpersonal and technical skills. Some critical assumptions for the nurse to consider in the decision-making process are as follows.

- The patient is a human being with worth and dignity.
- There are basic human needs which must be met. When they are not, problems arise requiring interventions by another person until the individual can resume responsibility for self.

- The patient has a right to quality health and nursing care delivered with concern, compassion, and competence, focusing on wellness, prevention, and restoration.
- The therapeutic nurse-patient relationship is a critical element in this process.

NURSING DIAGNOSIS

Nurses have struggled for years to define nursing by identifying its parameters with a goal of attaining professional status. To this end, nurses have been meeting and conducting research to develop nursing diagnosis. Although there are differing definitions of nursing diagnosis, we have chosen to use Shoemaker's, taken from the *Classification of Nursing Diagnosis, Proceedings of the Fifth National Conference* (Kim, et al, 1984). "Nursing diagnosis is a clinical judgment about an individual, family, or community which is derived through a deliberate, systematic process of data collection and analysis. It provides the basis for prescriptions for definitive therapy for which the nurse is accountable. It is expressed concisely and it includes the etiology of the condition when known."

Nursing diagnosis (Table 2-1, p 9) provides a framework for using the nursing process. Although nursing practice is more than nursing diagnosis, it provides a common language for identifying patient problems, nursing interventions, and evaluation tools. This common language is important for several reasons. It promotes communication between nurses, shifts, units, and alternate care settings. It also provides a base for clinicians, educators, and researchers to document, validate, and/or alter the process. As nurses begin to use the diagnoses on a daily basis, they will become more familiar with their value in the communication process.

As the crux of the patient care plan, nursing diagnosis focuses attention on certain areas and is the prime determinant of the style of nursing care to be delivered. Nursing actions have been based on variables such as signs and symptoms, tests, and medical diagnosis. However, nursing diagnosis is now becoming a uniform way of identifying, focusing on, and dealing with specific problems/responses. The affective tone of the nursing diagnosis can shape expectations of the patient's response and influence the nurse's behavior toward the patient. For instance, if the nurse sees the patient as noncompliant, the nurse's attitudes and behavior may reflect anger and mistrust, and judgmental decisions may be made which do not accurately treat the patient's problem. Accurate diagnosis of a patient problem can become a standard for nursing practice, understood by all who are using the plan of care and leading to improved delivery of care.

DATA COLLECTION

The patient assessment is the foundation upon which identification of individual needs, responses, and problems is based. In order to facilitate these two steps of the Nursing Process (assessment and diagnosis), an Asssessment Tool (see p 13) has been constructed, using a nursing focus instead of the familiar medical approach of "review of systems." To achieve this nursing focus, the 72 NANDA nursing diagnoses have been grouped into related categories titled Diagnostic Divisions (Table 2-2, p 11), which reflect a blending of Maslow's Hierarchy of Needs and a self-care philosophy. These divisions serve as the outline for data collection which directs the nurse to the appropriate corresponding nursing diagnoses as the patient information is recorded.

Because these divisions are based on human responses and needs and are not specific "systems," information occasionally may be recorded in more than one area. For this reason, the nurse is encouraged to pursue all avenues and to collect as much data as possible before choosing the nursing diagnosis that best reflects the patient's situation. The nurse needs to be aware of biases which may interfere with reaching an accurate diagnosis. Keeping an open mind to numerous possibilities and not becoming stuck on a single symptom will facilitate this process. For example, when restlessness is identified, an inference may be made by the nurse that the patient is anxious. If the nurse believes that this is a psychologic symptom, the possibility that it may be a physiologically based symptom may be overlooked.

The nursing diagnosis, then, is as precise as the data will allow, communicating the patient's situation at the present time, reflecting changes as they occur, and providing direction for nursing care.

CARE PLANNING

Medicine, nursing, and other health disciplines are interrelated with implications for each other. This interrelationship should include the exchange of data, sharing of ideas or thoughts, and development of plans of care which include all data pertinent to the individual patient, family, and significant other(s).

The care plan documents patient care in areas of liability, accountability, and quality assurance. It provides a mechanism to assure continuity of care. The care plan should contain more than actions initiated by medical orders. It could provide the written coordination of care given by all disciplines. The nurse becomes the person responsible for coordinating these different activities into a functional plan, necessary to provide holistic care for the patient. Independent nursing actions are an integral part of this process. Interdependent, collaborative actions are based on the medical regimen as well as on suggestions and orders from other disciplines involved with the care of the patient. In this book, collaborative actions will be identified to assist the nurse in choosing appropriate interventions for the individual setting. The educational background/expertise of the nurse, established protocols/standards of care, and areas of practice (rural or urban, acute or community care settings) can influence whether an individual intervention is actually an independent nursing function or requires collaboration.

In the past, nurses believed that inasmuch as no two patients are identical, no two care plans could be alike. Therefore, care plans were formulated from scratch for each patient. An awareness evolved that this approach was not practical or cost effective because the information and interventions documented were frequently repeated from one care plan to the next. It is now recognized that although patients are individuals and have many differences, they also have many common characteristics, needs, and problems. Therefore, today's approach to the use of the nursing process is to consider similarities as well as differences among patients.

A standardized care plan is a method of responding to these similar problems and needs and can be modified to meet individual differences. The written care plan communicates the patient's past and present statuses and needs of the patient to all members of the health care team. It identifies problems resolved and those yet to be solved, approaches that have been successful, and patterns of patient responses.

CARE PLAN COMPONENTS

The format for each care plan consists of the Patient Assessment Data Base derived from information obtained during the History, Physical Examination, and Diagnostic Studies. Nursing Priorities are then determined. The priorities in this book are general ideas and may be reworded or reorganized according to individual situations. The Nursing Diagnosis then follows with Supporting Data/Contributing Factors, and General Patient Outcomes for each problem area/diagnosis and appropriate Independent/Collaborative Interventions with accompanying Rationale.

Care plan construction begins with the collection of data (assessment). The history consists of subjective and objective information encompassing the various concerns reflected in the 1986 list of Nursing Diagnoses (NANDA). Subjective data are those which are reported by the patient and/or significant other(s). It is important to accept what is reported because the patient is the "expert" in this area, but the nurse needs to note incongruencies which may indicate the interference of other factors, such as lack of knowledge, misconceptions, or fear.

Objective data are those which are observed or described (quantitatively or qualitatively) and verified by others. They include Diagnostic Studies and Physical Examination findings. Evaluation of both subjective and objective collected data leads to the identification of problems or areas of concern/need. These problems/needs are expressed as nursing diagnoses (see Table 2-1).

The key to accurate nursing diagnosis is problem identification, which focuses attention on an actual or potential physical or behavioral response that interferes with the quality of life the patient is used to or desires. It addresses concerns of the patient, significant other(s), and/or nurse which require nursing intervention and management. In this text the choice of individual nursing diagnosis is determined by the Supporting Data/Contributing Factors which reflect the etiology and defining characteristics most consistent with a specific medical situation.

Nurses feel at risk in committing themselves to documenting a nursing diagnosis. However, many references are currently available to aid in identifying and formulating the problem statement. Unlike medical diagnoses, nursing diagnoses change as the patient progresses through various stages of illness/maladaption to problem resolution. From the specific information obtained in the Patient Assessment Data Base, the etiology and symptoms can be identified and an individualized patient problem/diagnostic statement can be formulated, for example, "Activity Intolerance" related to imbalance between oxygen supply and demand manifested by severe dyspnea.

Goal statements (outcomes) must be formulated to give direction to nursing care. These General Patient Outcomes emerge from the diagnosis statement and are what the patient and nurse hope to achieve. They have been stated in general terms in this book to permit the practitioner to modify/individualize them by adding timelines, considerations of patient circumstances and needs, as well as other specifics. The terminology must be concise, realistic, measurable, and clear. Beginning the goal statement with an action verb (for example, "verbalizes") provides direction that is measurable. It is important that multidisciplinary goals do not conflict.

Interventions communicate actions which might be taken to achieve desired patient outcomes. The rationale for interventions needs to be sound and feasible with the intention of providing individualized care. Actions may be independent or collaborative and encompass orders from nursing, medicine, and other disciplines. Again, using an action verb, for example, "assess," provides direction to the nurse.

The nurse should plan care with the patient when possible, because both are accountable for that care and for achieving the desired goals. Written interventions that guide patient care need to be dated and signed to identify the person who is initiating and coordinating the care.

This book is intended to facilitate the application of the nursing process for the critical care patient and family/significant other(s). Each care plan is intended to be an informational guide so that the individual practitioner will be able to modify or extract only that information which is pertinent to the specific patient situation.

In summary, the authors believe that any nursing diagnosis can be actual or potential, and although this issue has not been resolved by the nursing diagnosis association (NANDA), it has been used in this manner in this book. Recognizing that the current NANDA list of diagnoses is not comprehensive, nurses need to use the diagnoses on a daily basis to become familiar with their parameters and to validate their usefulness. As noted, with few exceptions, we have presented NANDA's recommendations as formulated by the conferences. Brackets indicate additions or changes the authors have made to clarify the accepted nursing diagnoses; for example, [Learning Need]. Some diagnoses have been combined for convenience, indicating that two factors may be involved; for example, Fluid Volume, alteration in [fluctuation]. It is anticipated that the nurse will choose what is appropriate. Nurses can be creative as they work with the standardized format, redefining and sharing interventions as they are used with individual patients. We appreciate that not all diagnoses presented in these care plans may be appropriate for your patient or locale, and alternates should be chosen to meet individual patient needs.

We support the belief that practicing nurses and researchers need to study, to use, and to evaluate the diagnoses as presented. If the nursing profession can develop a central core of truly nursing material that can be used consistently in all areas of nursing education and practice, the profession will be immeasurably strengthened and the quality of patient care will be improved. As new nursing diagnoses are developed, it is important that the information they encompass are reflected in the data base. The nurse is encouraged to share insights and ideas with the Task Force of the National Group for Nursing Diagnoses, St. Louis University School of Nursing, 3525 Caroline Avenue, St. Louis, Missouri 63104.

TABLE 2-1. Nursing Diagnoses (through 7th NANDA Conference)

Activity Intolerance
Activity Intolerance, potential
Adjustment, impaired
Airway Clearance, ineffective
Anxiety

Body Temperature, potential, alteration in
Bowel Elimination, alteration in: constipation
Bowel Elimination, alteration in: diarrhea
Bowel Elimination, alteration in: incontinence
Breathing Pattern, ineffective

Cardiac, Output, alteration in: decreased
Comfort, alteration in: pain, acute
Comfort, alteration in: pain, chronic
Communication, impaired: verbal
Coping, family: potential for growth
Coping, ineffective family: compromised
Coping, ineffective family: disabled
Coping, ineffective individual

Diversional Activity, deficit

Family Process, alteration in
Fear
Fluid Volume, alteration in: excess
Fluid Volume, deficit, actual (1)
Fluid Volume, deficit, actual (2)
Fluid Volume, deficit, potential

Gas Exchange, impaired
Grieving, anticipatory
Grieving, dysfunctional
Growth and Development, altered

Health Maintenance, alteration in
Home Maintenance Management, impaired
Hopelessness
Hyperthermia
Hypothermia

Incontinence: functional
Incontinence: reflex
Incontinence: stress
Incontinence: total
Incontinence: urge
Infection, potential for
Injury: potential for: poisoning; suffocation; trauma

Knowledge Deficit (specify) *[Learning Need, (specify)]

Mobility, impaired, physical

Neglect, unilateral
Noncompliance, specify *[Compliance, alteration in, specify]
Nutrition, alteration in: less than body requirements
Nutrition, alteration in: more than body requirements
Nutrition, alteration in: potential for more than body requirements

TABLE 2-1. *continued*

Oral Mucous Membrane, alteration in

Parenting, alteration in: actual or potential
Post-trauma Response
Powerlessness

Rape Trauma Syndrome

Self-Care Deficit: feeding; bathing/hygiene; dressing/grooming; toileting
Self-Concept, disturbance in: body image; self-esteem; role performance, personal identity
Sensory-Perceptual Alteration: visual; auditory; kinesthetic; gustatory; tactile; olfactory
Sexual Dysfunction
Sexuality Patterns, altered
Skin Integrity, impairment of: actual
Skin Integrity, impairment of: potential
Sleep Pattern Disturbance
Social Interaction, impaired
Social Isolation
Spiritual Distress (distress of the human spirit)
Swallowing, impaired

Thermoregulation, ineffective
Thought Processes, alteration in
Tissue Integrity, impaired
Tissue Perfusion, alteration in: cerebral; cardiopulmonary; renal; gastrointestinal; peripheral

Urinary Elimination, alteration in patterns
Urinary Retention

Violence, potential for: self-directed or directed at others

---

*author recommendations

TABLE 2-2. Diagnostic Divisions

ACTIVITY/REST
- Activity Intolerance
- Activity Intolerance, potential
- Diversional Activity, deficit
- Sleep Pattern Disturbance

CIRCULATION
- Cardiac Output, alteration in: decreased
- Tissue Perfusion, alteration in (specify)

ELIMINATION
- Bowel Elimination, alteration in: constipation
- Bowel Elimination, alteration in: diarrhea
- Bowel Elimination, alteration in: incontinence
- Incontinence: functional
- Incontinence: reflex
- Incontinence: stress
- Incontinence: total
- Incontinence: urge
- Urinary Elimination, alteration in patterns
- Urinary Retention

EMOTIONAL REACTIONS
- Adjustment, impaired
- Anxiety
- Coping, ineffective individual
- Fear
- Grieving, anticipatory
- Grieving, dysfunctional
- Hopelessness
- Post-trauma Response
- Powerlessness
- Rape Trauma Syndrome
- Self-Concept, disturbance in: body image; self-esteem; role performance; personal identity
- Social Interaction, impaired
- Social Isolation
- Spiritual Distress (distress of the human spirit)
- Violence, potential for

FAMILY PATTERN ALTERATIONS
- Coping, family: potential for growth
- Coping, ineffective family: compromised
- Coping, ineffective family: disabling
- Family Process, alteration in
- Parenting, alteration in: actual or potential

FOOD/FLUID
- Fluid Volume, alteration in: excess
- Fluid Volume deficit, actual (1)
- Fluid Volume deficit, actual (2)
- Fluid Volume deficit, potential
- Nutrition, alteration in: less than body requirements
- Nutrition, alteration in: more than body requirements
- Nutrition, alteration in: potential for more than body requirements
- Oral Mucous Membranes, alteration in
- Swallowing, impaired

HYGIENE
- Self-Care Deficit: feeding; bathing/hygiene; dressing/grooming; toileting

TABLE 2.2 *continued*

NEUROLOGIC
Communication, impaired: verbal
Neglect, unilateral
Sensory-Perceptual Alteration
Thought Processes, alteration in
PAIN
Comfort, alteration in: pain, acute
Comfort, alteration in: pain, chronic
SAFETY
Body Temperature, potential alteration in
Hyperthermia
Hypothermia
Infection, potential for
Injury, potential for: poisoning; suffocation; trauma
Mobility, impaired physical
Skin Integrity, impairment of: actual
Skin Integrity, impairment of: potential
Thermoregulation, ineffective
Tissue Integrity, impaired
SEXUAL
Sexual Dysfunction
Sexuality Patterns, alteration in
TEACHING/LEARNING
Growth and Development, alteration in
Health Maintenance, alteration in
Home Maintenance Management, impaired
Knowledge Deficit (specify) [learning need (specify)]
Noncompliance (specify) [compliance, alteration in (specify)]
VENTILATION
Airway Clearance, ineffective
Breathing Pattern, ineffective
Gas Exchange, impaired

ASSESSMENT TOOL

This is a suggested guide to create a data base reflecting Diagnostic Divisions of Nursing Diagnoses. Although the divisions are alphabetized for ease of presentation, they can be arranged according to priority or to meet individual needs.

Name: ______

Age: ______ DOB: ______ Sex: ______ Race: ______

Admission Date: ______ Time: ______ From: ______

Source of Information: ______ Reliability (1–4): ______

ACTIVITY/REST

Subjective

Occupation: ______ Usual activities/Hobbies: ______

Limitations imposed by condition: ______

Sleep: Hours ______ Naps: ______ Aids: ______

Insomnia: ______ Related to: ______

Objective

Observed response to activity: Cardiovascular: ______

Respiratory: ______

Mental status (e.g., withdrawn/lethargic): ______

Neuromuscular assessment:

Muscle mass/tone: ______

Posture: ______ Tremors: ______

ROM: ______ Strength: ______

Deformity: ______ Other: ______

CIRCULATION

Subjective

History of: Hypertension: ______ Heart Trouble: ______

Rheumatic Fever: ______ Ankle/leg edema: ______

Phlebitis: ______ Slow healing: ______

Claudication: ______

Extremities: Numbness: ______ Tingling: ______

Cough/hemotysis: ______

Change in frequency/amount of urine: ______

Objective

B/P: R: Stand: ______ Sit: ______ Lying: ______

L: Stand: ______ Sit: ______ Lying: ______

Pulse pressure: ______ Ausculatory Gap: ______

Pulse (palpation): Carotid: ______ Temporal: ______

Jugular: ______ Radial: ______

Femoral: ______ Popliteal: ______

Posttibial: ______ Dorsalis pedis: ______

Cardiac (palpation): PMI: ______

Thrill: ______ Heaves: ______

Heart sounds: ______ Rate: ______

Rhythm: ______ Quality: ______

Friction rub: ______ Murmur: ______

Breath sounds: ______

Vascular bruit: (specify): ____

Jugular vein distention: ____

Extremities: Temperature: ____ Color: ____

Capillary refill: ____

Homan's sign: ____ Varicosities ____

Nails (describe abnormalities): ____

Distribution/quality of hair: ____

Color/cyanosis: Overall: ____ Mucous membranes: ____ Lips: ____

Nailbeds: ____ Conjunctiva: ____ Sclera: ____

ELIMINATION

Subjective

Usual bowel pattern: ____ Laxative use: ____

Character of stool: ____ Last BM: ____

History of bleeding: ____ Hemorrhoids: ____

Diarrhea: ____ Constipation: ____

Usual voiding pattern: ____ Incontinence: ____

Urgency: ____ Frequency: ____ Retention: ____

Character of urine: ____

Pain/burning/difficulty voiding: ____

History of kidney/bladder disease: ____

Objective

Abdomen tender: ____ Soft/Firm: ____

Palpable mass: ____ Size/Girth: ____

Bowel sounds: ____

Hemorrhoids (per rectal exam): Internal: ____ External: ____

Bladder palpable: ____ Overflow voiding: ____

EMOTIONAL REACTIONS

Subjective

Report of stress factors: ____

Financial concerns: ____

Relationship status: ____

Cultural factors: ____

Religion: ____

Objective

Emotional status (check those that apply):

Calm ____ Anxious ____ Angry ____

Withdrawn ____ Fearful ____ Irritable ____

Restive ____ Euphoric: ____ Other (specify) ____

Observed physiologic response(s):

FAMILY PATTERN ALTERATIONS

Subjective

Marital Status: ____ Years married: ____

Living with: ____

Extended family: ____

Other support person(s): ____

Role within family structure: ____

Report of problems: ____________________

Objective

Verbal/nonverbal communication with family/significant other(s): ____________________

____

Family interaction (behavioral) pattern: ____________________

FOOD/FLUID

Subjective

Usual diet (type): ____________________

Last meal/intake: ____________________

Loss of appetite: ____________________ Nausea/Vomiting: ____________________

Heartburn/indigestion: ____________ Related to: ____________ Relieved by: ____________

Allergy/food intolerance: ____________________

Mastication/swallowing problems: ____________________

Dentures: upper ____________________ lower: ____________________

Usual weight: ____________________ Changes in weight: ____________________

Use of diuretics: ____________________

Objective

Current weight: ____________ Height: ____________ Body build: ____________

Skin turgor: ____________________ Moist/dry: ____________________

Hernia/masses: ____________________

Edema: General: ____________________ Dependent: ____________________

Periorbital: ____________________ Ascites: ____________________

Jugular vein distention: ____________________

Thyroid enlarged: ____________________ Halitosis: ____________________

Condition of teeth/gums: ____________________

Appearance of Tongue: ____________________

Mucous membranes: ____________________

Bowel sounds (previously assessed): ____________________

Breath sounds (previously assessed): ____________________

Urine S/A or Chemstix: ____________________

HYGIENE

Subjective

Activities of daily living: Independent: ____________________

Dependent (specify): Mobility: ____________________ Feeding: ____________________

Hygiene: ____________________ Dressing: ____________________

Toileting: ____________________ Other: ____________________

Objective

General appearance: ____________________

Body odor: ____________________ Condition of scalp: ____________________

Presence of vermin: ____________________

NEUROLOGIC

Subjective

Fainting spells/dizziness: ____________________

Headaches: Location: ____________________ Frequency: ____________________

Tingling/numbness/weakness (location): ____________________

Stroke (residual effects): ______

Seizures: ______ How controlled: ______

Eyes: Vision loss: R ______ L ______

Ears: Hearing loss: R ______ L ______

Nose: Epistaxis: ______ Sense of smell: ______

Objective

Mental status (check those that apply):

Oriented/disoriented: Time: ______

Place: ______

Person: ______

Alert: ______ Drowsy: ______ Lethargic: ______

Stuporous: ______ Comatose: ______ Other: ______

Cooperative: ______ Combative: ______

Delusions: ______ Hallucinations: ______ Affect: ______

Memory: Recent: ______ Remote: ______

Glasses: ______ Contacts: ______ Hearing aids: ______

Pupil size/reaction: R ______ L ______

Facial droop: ______ Swallowing: ______

Handgrasp: R ______ L ______ Posturing: ______

Deep tendon reflexes: ______ Paralysis: ______

Speech: Clear: ______ Slurred: ______

Unintelligible: ______ Aphasic: ______

Unusual speech pattern/impairment: ______

Laryngectomy: ______ Speech aids: ______

PAIN

Subjective

Location: ______ Intensity (1–10): ______

Quality: ______ Duration: ______ Radiation: ______

Precipitating factors: ______

How relieved: ______

Objective

Facial grimacing: ______ Guarding affected area: ______

Emotional response ______ Narrowed focus: ______

SAFETY

Subjective

Allergies/sensitivity: ______ Reaction: ______

______ ______

History of sexually transmitted disease (date/type): ______

Blood transfusion: ______ When: ______

Reaction (describe): ______

Fractures/dislocations: ______

Arthritis/unstable joints: ______

Back problems: ______

Changes in moles: ______ Enlarged nodes: ______

Impaired: Vision ______ Hearing ______

Prosthesis: ______ Ambulatory devices: ______

Objective

Temperature: ______ Skin integrity: ______

Scars: ______ Rashes: ______

Lacerations: ______ Ulcerations: ______

Ecchymosis: ______ Blisters: ______

Burns, degree/percent: ______

General strength: ______

Muscle tone: ______

Gait: ______ ROM: ______

Paresthesia/paralysis: ______

SEXUAL

Female

Subjective

Age at menarche: ______ Length of cycle: ______ Duration: ______

Last menstrual period: ______ Menopause: ______

Vaginal discharge: ______ Bleeding between periods: ______

Practices breast self-examination: ______ Last PAP smear: ______

Complaints: ______

Objective

Breast examination: ______

Vaginal warts/lesions: ______

Male

Subjective

Penile discharge: ______ Prostate disorder: ______

Vasectomy: ______

Practices self-examination: Breast ______ Testicles: ______

Last proctoscopic exam: ______ Last prostate exam: ______

Complaints: ______

Objective

Examination: Breast: ______

Testicles: ______

TEACHING/LEARNING

Subjective

Dominant language (specify): ______

Education level: ______

Learning disabilities (specify): ______

Cognitive limitations (specify): ______

Familial risk factors (indicate relationship):

Diabetes ______ Tuberculosis ______

Heart disease ______ Strokes ______

High B/P ______ Epilepsy ______

Kidney disease ______ Cancer ______

Other (specify) ______

Prescribed medications: (circle last dose)

Drug:	Dose:	Times:	Take regularly:	Purpose:
______	______	______	______	______

Nonprescription drugs: OTC: ___

Street drugs: ___

Alcohol (amount/frequency): ___

Admitting diagnosis (physician): ___

Reason for hospitalization (patient): ___

History of current complaint: ___

Patient expectations of this hospitalization: ___

Previous illnesses and/or hospitalizations/surgeries: ___

Evidence of failure to improve: ___

Last complete physical examination: ___ By: ___

VENTILATION

Subjective

Dyspnea (related to): ___

Cough/sputum: ___

History of bronchitis: ___ Asthma: ___

Tuberculosis: ___ Emphysema: ___

Smoker: ___ Pk/day: ___ # of years: ___

Use of respiratory aids: ___ Oxygen: ___

Objective

Respiratory: Rate: ___ Depth: ___Symmetry: ___

Use of accessory muscles: ___ Nasal flaring: ___

Fremitis: ___

Breath sounds: ___

Egophony: ___

Cyanosis: ___ Clubbing of fingers: ___

Sputum characteristics: ___

Mentation/restlessness: ___

CHAPTER 3 CARDIOVASCULAR

CARDIAC SURGERY

PATIENT ASSESSMENT DATA BASE

HISTORY

Severe anatomic disease, for example, left main stenosis; symptomatic or asymptomatic triple vessel disease; clinically significant valvular stenosis or insufficiency.

Acute myocardial infarction: uncomplicated or with extension, hemodynamic impairment, or cardiogenic shock.

Atrial or ventricular septal defect with hemodynamic compromise.

Postcoronary artery bypass graft (CABG) surgery with recurrent angina, possible graft closure.

Left ventricular aneurysm resulting in congestive heart failure, intractable ventricular dysrhythmias, or systemic emboli.

Subjective

May complain of angina unresponsive to medical therapy, or unstable or variant angina.

PHYSICAL EXAMINATION

INSPECTION

Level of consciousness: should be arousable immediately postanesthesia; oriented to person, place, time, and responsive to significant other/family (later).

Respirations: rate, rhythm, and depth are variable dependent upon ventilator settings.

Pupils: usually constricted and equal, reflecting drug effect.

Skin color: general pallor often present.

Jugular veins: distention may be present in severe valvular disease/fluid overload.

Edema: (dependent/generalized) reflects intraoperative weight gain or preexisting edema formation.

Urine output: usually pale or dilute following diuretic administration.

Incision(s): serosanguinous oozing may be noted.

Electrocardiogram: initially extremely variable, reflecting cardiac irritability, electrolyte imbalance, and hormonal or drug effects.

Chest tubes: amount of bloody drainage varies.

Extremities: loss of movement may suggest intraoperative stroke.

Palpation

Peripheral pulses: should be present and equal in all extremities.

Skin: usually cool and dry; capillary refill may be slow.

Auscultation

Breath sounds: areas of decreased sounds may reflect atelectasis; rhonchi may be present.

Heart sounds: rate, rhythm, characteristics are variable in early postoperative period. Murmurs and rubs may develop.

Blood pressure: may be hypotensive, hypertensive, or normotensive.

Bowel sounds: initially absent.

DIAGNOSTIC STUDIES

Postoperative: to be compared with preoperative baseline data studies.

Hgb/Hct: determines oxygen-carrying capacity and need for blood replacement.

Electrolytes: imbalances may include hyperkalemia/hypokalemia, hypernatremia/hyponatremia, and hypocalcemia which may affect cardiac fluid balance.

Arterial blood gases: determines hypoxemia, hypocarbia/hypercarbia, and acid-base balance.

BUN/creatinine: reflects level of renal function.

Amylase: elevation is occasionally seen in high-risk patients and those with heart failure undergoing valve replacement.

Serum glucose: increased owing to mobilization of glycogen stores. Insulin concentrations may be decreased.

Cardiac isoenzymes: documents acute or perioperative myocardial infarction.

Chest x-ray examination: indicates cardiac size and position, pulmonary vasculature, and changes indicative of pulmonary complications (e.g., atelectasis/hemothorax); verifies endotracheal and chest tube placement, condition of sternal wires and valve prosthesis.

Electrocardiogram: identifies changes in electrical/mechanical function.

NURSING PRIORITIES

1. Maintain cardiac output and circulating volume.
2. Maximize tissue perfusion.
3. Promote adequate gas exchange.
4. Provide for emotional support of patient and significant other.
5. Minimize/prevent complications.

NURSING DIAGNOSIS:	**Cardiac Output, alterations in, decreased.**
SUPPORTING DATA/CONTRIBUTING FACTORS:	**Postoperatively, cardiac output may be diminished by decreased circulating fluid volume (preload); depressed myocardial contractility (pumping ability); changes in systemic vascular**

resistance (afterload); and alterations in electrical conduction.**

GENERAL PATIENT OUTCOMES: **Blood pressures; filling pressures; heart rate, rhythm, and conduction; cardiac output; peripheral pulses and urine output are within acceptable limits. Dysrhythmias are prevented or controlled; cardiac tamponade does not occur.**

INTERVENTIONS	RATIONALE
Independent	
Monitor and document trends in heart rate, mean arterial blood pressure (MAP), pulmonary artery pressure (PAP)/pulmonary capillary wedge pressure (PCWP), and left atrial pressure (LAP) continuously in immediate postoperative period. Decrease frequency as clinical status stabilizes.	Provides information concerning myocardial contractility, filling pressures, and function of valves. Reveals early trends so that appropriate interventions may be implemented. Postoperative hypertension and hypotension are common.
Measure/calculate cardiac output/cardiac index (CO/CI), and systemic vascular resistance (SVR).	Evaluates effectiveness of myocardial contractility and vascular response to sympathetic nervous stimulation, blood volume and viscosity, and circulating regulatory hormones. These parameters serve as a guide for determining titration of medications to maximize cardiac output.
Compare PCWP against left ventricular stroke work index to plot ventricular function curve, particularly following changes in drug therapy and during activity and position changes as indicated.	Improvement may occur in some hemodynamic parameters such as increased systolic pressure with administration of norepinephrine while graph actually demonstrates decreased ventricular function.
Monitor/document cardiac dysrhythmias (e.g., supraventricular tachycardias [SVT]/premature ventricular contractions [PVC]). Assess patient response to changes in cardiac output associated with dysrhythmia.	Hemodynamic compromise can occur with even slight variations of cardiac output created by dysrhythmias and may require intervention such as medication or pacing to maintain cardiac output.
Note dysrhythmias characteristic of potassium imbalance, for example, atrial dysrhythmias and PVCs (hypokalemia), bradycardia and conduction disturbances (hyperkalemia).	Although hypokalemia is the problem more frequently encountered in the immediate postoperative period, patients with low serum sodium, impaired renal function, or who have received large amounts of stored blood are at risk for hyperkalemia.
Note presence of pulsus alternans.	Indicator of left ventricular failure, and cardiac tamponade.
Record temperature and color of extremities and quality of peripherial pulses.	Warm extremities and strong pulses are indicators of adequate cardiac output.
Monitor body temperature and maintain within normal limits. Control environmental temperature, use blankets to maintain warmth.	Postoperative hypothermia increases vasoconstriction and may be manifested by labile blood pressure responses.
Note patient response to rewarming from surgically induced hypothermia.	Rapid warming may cause sudden peripheral vasodilation resulting in symptoms of hypovolemic shock, as the intravascular compartment size is increased, and circulating volume becomes inadequate.

INTERVENTIONS	RATIONALE
Independent	
Observe for development of signs/symptoms of cardiac tamponade: Note arterial hypotension accompanied by increased LA or PA diastolic pressure, jugular venous distention, muffled heart tones, decreased size of QRS complex, and sudden changes in amount of chest system drainage.	Tamponade is a pathologic condition of myocardial constriction resulting from accumulation of excess blood/fluid in the pericardium. Cardiac filling is impeded, creating venous congestion. Heart tones are diminished, and the chest becomes quiet. Tamponade can occur despite significant chest tube drainage; however, drainage is frequently decreased as cardiac output drops.
Assess for pulsus paradoxus.	Systolic pressure decrease of more than 10 mmHg during inspiration suggests cardiac tamponade. A reverse pulsus paradoxus (increase of more than 10 mmHg on inspiration) has been observed in mechanically ventilated hypovolemic patients with developing tamponade.
Compare right and left heart pressures.	Equalization of pressures (plateau pressures) is a late indicator of cardiac tamponade, as cardiac filling is impaired and cardiac output diminishes.
Note increasing pallor/cyanosis, altered sensorium, and decreased urine output.	Patient may be unresponsive or display other sequalae reflective of developing shock state.
Collaborative	
Titrate IV fluids as indicated.	Maintains circulating fluid volume and enhances cardiac output, especially in event of uncontrolled chest bleeding.
Administer ionotropic and vasoactive drugs as indicated; for example, epinephrine and sodium nitroprusside (Nipride) drip infusions.	Epinephrine stimulates myocardium and counteracts peripheral vasodilation. Sodium nitroprusside decreases peripheral resistance and improves myocardial function without increasing heart rate.
Monitor and replace potassium according to protocol.	Facilitates normal electrical conduction and efficient cardiac output. Potassium replacement is often dependent on periodic laboratory evaluation and should be modified when impaired renal function is present.
Administer oxygen via appropriate method. (Refer to Nursing Diagnosis: Gas Exchange, page 26.)	Maximizes oxygen delivery for myocardial uptake.
Treat dysrhythmias/cardiac arrest per protocol. (Refer to Care Plan: Myocardial Infarction; Nursing Diagnosis: Cardiac Output, page 65.)	Restores stable heart rhythm in order to maintain cardiac output.
Maintain surgically placed pacing wires (atrial/ventricular). Initiate pacing if indicated.	Supports cardiac output until more appropriate conduction is restored. Slows or accelerates impulse formation to correct conduction disturbances and overrides dysrhythmias which compromise ventricular function. Atrial and AV sequential pacing are most useful because they provide time for atrial emptying, enhancing "atrial kick."
Monitor intra-aortic balloon pump (IABP) if indicated. (Refer to Care Plan: Cardiogenic Shock; Nursing Diagnosis: Cardiac Output, page 35.)	Reduces the workload of the heart and increases myocardial perfusion by reducing preload and afterload.

INTERVENTIONS	RATIONALE
Collaborative	
Review serial electrocardiogram.	Most frequently done to follow evolution of acute or suspected perioperative myocardial infarctions.

NURSING DIAGNOSIS: **Fluid Volume Deficit, actual (2).**

SUPPORTING DATA/CONTRIBUTING FACTORS: **Blood and fluid loss is expected as a result of surgery and postoperative drainage from chest. Hypovolemia may be induced by any of several factors, for example, intraoperative bleeding with inadequate blood replacement; bleeding related to insufficient heparin reversal, fibrinolysis, or platelet destruction resulting from cardiopulmonary bypass pump; or volume depletion effects of intraoperative or postoperative diuretic therapy.**

GENERAL PATIENT OUTCOMES: **Blood loss from mediastinal or pleural tubes is within acceptable limits. Circulating volume is adequate to maintain hemodynamic stability. Complications of hemorrhage are minimized.**

INTERVENTIONS	RATIONALE
Independent	
Monitor vital signs and hemodynamic parameters (e.g., RAP or CVP, LAP, MAP).	Hypovolemia is reflected by decreases in right- and/or left-sided filling pressures and systemic arterial pressure.
Monitor and record chest drainage hourly. Note presence of constant or increasing drainage from chest/mediastinal tubes.	Acceptable drainage may be 100 to 200 ml an hour for several hours but should decrease appropriately thereafter. Excessive drainage may indicate impaired function of coagulation system or need for surgical re-exploration of chest.
Evaluate generalized oozing from incisions/puncture sites, and dressings.	Note: This type of bleeding is many times not confined to a specific blood vessel but rather to tissue bleeding.
Measure urine output, note specific gravity. Calculate 24-hour fluid balance.	Diuresis is promoted perioperatively to protect kidneys, as well as postoperatively to reduce total body water. This can result in hypovolemia and reduced renal perfusion, evidenced by falling urine output and increased specific gravity.

INTERVENTIONS	RATIONALE
Collaborative	
Administer blood products and IV solutions.	Colloids (blood, plasma, or albumin) or crystolloid solutions (lactated Ringer's, saline) may be used to maintain adequate circulating volume. Rapid temporary volume increase can be obtained with crystolloid solutions in emergency situations.
Monitor clotting studies: Activated clotting time (ACT),	Assesses heparin reversal post cardiopulmonary bypass. (The complex formed by heparin and protamine sulfate is unstable and may reverse itself even after seemingly adequate protamine has been administered).
platelet count,	May be reduced in number as a result of cardiopulmonary bypass. Thrombocytopenia (platelet count less than 30,000 to 50,000) may occur, requiring the transfusion of concentrated fresh platelets, dependent on the clinical situation and whether bleeding is present.
plasma fibrinogen level.	Surgical procedures may release plasminogen activator, resulting in fibrinolysis, premature clot destruction, and excessive bleeding.
Administer medications as indicated: protamine sulfate.	Reverses anticoagulation effects of heparin.

NURSING DIAGNOSIS:	**Tissue Perfusion, alteration in.**
SUPPORTING DATA/CONTRIBUTING FACTORS:	**Decreased cardiac output, hypovolemia, and hypotension are associated conditions which reduce blood flow to/perfusion of tissues and organs.**
GENERAL PATIENT OUTCOMES:	**Tissue perfusion/organ function is maintained, as evidenced by stable blood pressure, palpable peripheral pulses, skin warm and dry, usual mental status, adequate urine output, return of bowel function.**

INTERVENTIONS	RATIONALE
Independent	
Assess/record neurologic status as patient awakens from anesthesia. Note level of consciousness, pupil size/reaction, response to commands, recognition of significant others.	May suggest presence of complications; that is, cerebral hypoperfusion, hypoxemia, cerebral edema, emboli.

INTERVENTIONS	RATIONALE
Independent	
Monitor mean arterial pressure (MAP), and maintain within desired limits. Report hypertension (MAP >100) and hypotension (MAP < 60).	Myocardial perfusion is dependent on coronary blood flow, which is directly related to systemic blood pressure. Blood pressure elevations may be deleterious to graft anastomoses in CABG patients in the immediate postoperative phase. Hypotension causes hypoperfusion of myocardium.
Assess pulses in extremities, noting presence and quality.	Absence of pulse may indicate decreased tissue perfusion related to low cardiac output, or the presence of peripheral thrombosis or emboli obstructing flow.
Observe for change of skin color, quality of pulses, and sensory motor changes in vessel donor (CABG) and/or cannulated extremities.	Tissue perfusion in the operated extremity may be impaired by edema, improperly fitting antiembolic hose. Cannulated and restrained extremities are at risk owing to constriction or obstruction of blood flow.
Note changes indicative of thrombus formation, that is redness, swelling, warmth, pain.	Thromboembolic complications are uncommon but may be catastrophic if major body organs are affected such as brain, heart, lungs, and kidneys. (Refer to Care Plan: Pulmonary Embolism, page 95.)
Record hourly/24-hour urine output. (Refer to Nursing Diagnosis: Fluid Volume, deficit, actual (2), page 23.)	Decreased circulating volume/cardiac output can result in hypoperfusion of the kidneys and diminished urine output.
Assess gastrointestinal (GI) function: Monitor for gastric distention, nausea, vomiting, absence or loss of active bowel sounds. Guaiac secretions/excretions.	Nausea, vomiting, and decreased bowel sounds may indicate ileus formation. Although rare, gastric bleeding may occur secondary to ischemia (related to altered perfusion) and compounded by stress, altered gastric motility, and changes in level of acid production.
Note complaints of abdominal pain.	Abdominal complications (related to organ hypoperfusion during cardiopulmonary bypass) are infrequent, but they can be overwhelming when they occur. Among these complications are pancreatitis, gastrointestinal hemorrhage, and acute cholecystitis.
Monitor response to oral intake following removal of nasogastric (NG) tube.	Nausea, vomiting, and gastric distention may indicate inadequate GI function and need for nothing by mouth (NPO) status or replacement of NG tube.
Collaborative	
Apply antiembolic hose, elastic bandage wraps.	Promotes venous return by limiting venous stasis.
Administer heparin sodium as indicated.	May be used prophylactically to prevent microemboli formation on mechanical valve replacements.
Insert/maintain NG tube. Irrigate and reposition as necessary. Maintain adequate suction.	Intraoperative hypoperfusion usually results in loss of bowel function. Accumulation of gastric fluids or air causes gastric distension, which can result in regurgitation and aspiration or impedance of diaphragmatic excursion with respiratory dysfunction.
Advance oral feedings from fluids as tolerated to include low bulk, easily digested foods.	Nutritional support should be started as soon as possible to promote tissue healing.

INTERVENTIONS	RATIONALE
Collaborative	
Monitor lab values as indicated: Serum amylase,	Abnormal amylase levels may be one of the criteria for continuing nasogastric suction or NPO status.
BUN, creatinine.	Evaluates renal perfusion and function.

NURSING DIAGNOSIS:	**Gas Exchange, impaired [potential].**
SUPPORTING DATA/CONTRIBUTING FACTORS:	**Atelectasis occurs, which may be related to anesthesia, pain/splinting, interstitial edema, and immobility. Oxygen-carrying capacity may be diminished secondary to blood loss. Pneumothorax or hemothorax may occur related to inadequate function or premature discontinuation of chest tubes.**
GENERAL PATIENT OUTCOMES:	**Arterial blood gases are within patient's normal limits. Atelectasis is resolved. Lungs are reexpanded with absence of pneumothorax or hemothorax.**

INTERVENTIONS	RATIONALE
Independent	
Evaluate respiratory function: Note presence of spontaneous respirations while patient is on ventilator. Inspect chest for symmetrical movement. Monitor depth and rate of respirations. Auscultate breath sounds. Note presence of cyanosis or agitation. (Refer to Care Plan: Ventilatory Assistance, page 115.)	Patient responses are variable and may be affected by resolution of anesthesia, hypoxia, pain, fear, secretions, gastric distention, acidosis, carbon dioxide retention, or respiratory suppression from narcotics. Early recognition of abnormal ventilation may prevent complications.
Suction and reposition ventilated patient as indicated.	Gravity increases venous pressure in independent portions of the lung, creating congestion and impairing ventilation, which may lead to intrapulmonary shunting. Repositioning promotes ventilation of all areas of the lung and enhances drainage of secretions, which can then be removed by suctioning.
Enhance airway expansion postextubation by repositioning, assisting in coughing and deep breathing. Position for ease of breathing; elevate head of the bed.	Effective in preventing and resolving pulmonary congestion. Although atelectasis is common after surgery, pneumonia may develop if it persists.
Medicate for pain prior to respiratory treatment.	Reduces splinting related to incisional pain, allowing for easier chest movement, and may enhance patient participation in procedures.

INTERVENTIONS	RATIONALE
Independent	
Record response to respiratory treatment (e.g., breath sounds before/after therapy), and note amount and character of secretions produced.	Documents effectiveness of and/or need for changes in therapy.
Maintain chest tube patency and ordered level of suction.	Ensure that tubes are not clamped or blocked for any period of time, resulting in inadequate drainage, air leaks, or progressive collapse of the lungs.
Note signs of hemothorax or pneumothorax after chest tubes are removed, for example, respiratory distress, diminished breath sounds, hyperresonant or dull percussion, mediastinal shift to the contralateral side, severe agitation, drop in blood pressure, increasing CVP, subcutaneous emphysema (crepitus). (Refer to Care Plan: Hemothorax and Pneumothorax, page 88.)	A collapsed lung may be suspected when breath sounds diminish in an area or chest wall movement is reduced. Percussion of the chest may demonstrate hyperresonnance (pneumothorax) or dull percussion (hemothorax). Mediastinal shifts occur when a collection of air or blood compresses the lung and displaces mediastinal structures. Crepitus may be noted in the area of the air leak into tissues and may spread over the upper body if the problem is not resolved, especially in presence of mechanical ventilation.
Collaborative	
Monitor/graph serial ABGs. Correlate with fiberoptic readings and systemic mixed venous oxygen saturation (SVO_2) measurements and A-V shunt calculation.	Hypoxemia, respiratory acidosis, and A-V shunting owing to atelectasis may be noted, requiring therapy alterations. Metabolic acidosis is occasionally seen postoperatively as a result of poor perfusion or resucitation for cardiac arrest. Monitoring of SVO_2 provides early trend indicators of tissue oxygen extraction. Normal range is 60 to 80 percent. Lower levels suggest decreased oxygen delivery and increased tissue extraction.
Maintain patient on ventilator until patient is able to breathe independently.	Ventilator assistance is usually required for the first few hours postanesthesia to increase PO_2 and to decrease atelectasis.
Administer oxygen postextubation as indicated, per cannula or mask.	Adequate oxygenation should be maintained using method best tolerated by the patient.
Review serial chest x-ray examinations.	Monitors effectiveness of respiratory therapy and/or documents developing complications.
Assist with insertion of chest tubes or thorocentesis as indicated.	Relieves hemothorax or pneumothorax that can develop as a complication of an improperly functioning chest drainage system or continued blood/air accumulation after chest tube discontinuation.

NURSING DIAGNOSIS: **Knowledge Deficit [Learning Need].**

SUPPORTING DATA/CONTRIBUTING FACTORS: **Anxiety and fear may block or reduce retention of preoperative teaching. If procedure is done on an emergency basis, preoperative teaching may be omitted and teaching may be done as opportunity presents itself during the postoperative course.**

GENERAL PATIENT OUTCOMES:	**Verbalizes understanding of/ demonstrates adaptation to treatment regimen.**

INTERVENTIONS	RATIONALE
Independent	
Determine if preoperative instruction, including tour of the critical care unit, has been done.	Amount of preoperative preparation often has a direct correlation with adjustment during postoperative course. Determines learning needs.
Determine what patient/significant other(s) already knows or perceives about primary cardiac condition and surgery performed.	Preoperative communication between the patient, significant other(s), and care givers is an essential part of general preparation. Information regarding patient concerns and perceptions can be used in overall patient management.
Assess ability to understand and assimilate information.	Patient may be so ill or anxious that information may be misperceived or only partially understood.
Respect patient/significant other's need for and amount of information desired.	Some patients may deny seriousness of situation and prefer not hearing information. Within limits, this may serve as a protective mechanism. However, high-grade denial may result in the patient's taking risks that could compromise recovery.
Encourage and anticipate questions, and "Active Listen" responses.	Establishes rapport and provides opportunities to recognize concerns. Active Listening is a process that acknowledges meaning behind the words and conveys empathy for the patient.
Begin evaluation of discharge needs and initiate information giving with significant other(s) and patient. Repeat as opportunities arise.	Although specific discharge instructions may not be fully formulated, initial problems/concerns may be dealt with and preparations made for continuity of care and instruction.

NURSING DIAGNOSIS:	**Anxiety/Fear.**
SUPPORTING DATA/CONTRIBUTING FACTORS:	**There is a mystique about cardiac surgery that makes it more feared than other types of surgery. For many patients the heart represents the center of life, which may increase the perceived threat of surgery. Physiologic responses to anxiety and/or fear may compromise recovery.**
GENERAL PATIENT OUTCOMES:	**Verbalizes feelings and concerns. Demonstrates relaxed manner, reduced tension.**

INTERVENTIONS	RATIONALE
Independent	
Orient patient frequently when first awake from anesthesia and as needed thereafter.	Affirms that surgery is over and helps to keep the focus on the present.
Explain the need for restraints as the patient awakens from anesthesia.	Patient may be less anxious and more able to cooperate with maintaining invasive lines, ventilatory and drainage tubes.
Assess physiologic response to anxiety (e.g., B/P, heart rate).	Anxiety can cause elevations of these parameters.
Explain procedures prior to performing them.	Explanation can reduce anxiety and may elicit patient cooperation with uncomfortable procedures.
Provide patient with a method of communication while intubated for example, notepad and pencil, magic slate, picture board.	Minimizes feelings of frustration/fear that the patient may experience as a result of being unable to speak while intubated.
Encourage family/significant other(s) to visit.	Alleviates isolation and is helpful in reassuring family/significant other(s) about the condition of the patient, as well as reassuring patient that family/significant other(s) is coping.
Encourage patient and family to express feelings concerning surgery and recovery.	Expression of feelings can foster communication between the patient, family, and staff and create a more positive healing environment.
Assist in learning and performing relaxation exercises (e.g., distraction, deep breathing activities).	Provides a sense of having some control of the situation by giving the patient something to do, which can make a difference in the way the patient feels.
Recognize and acknowledge patient's desire for rapid return to independent activity.	Helps the patient maintain a positive self-image and may assist with successful return to activities of daily living.

NURSING DIAGNOSIS:	**Fluid Volume, excess [potential].**
SUPPORTING DATA/CONTRIBUTING FACTORS:	**Surgical stress elevates antidiuretic hormone and aldosterone levels, initiating sodium and water retention. Other factors contributing to fluid excess include bypass pump priming fluid; electrolyte and acid-base imbalances resulting from altered renal function; and choice and rate of fluid replacement.**
GENERAL PATIENT OUTCOMES:	**Urine output of 20 to 30 ml per hour or greater. Electrolyte values are within patient's normal parameters. Fluid output exceeds intake with a gradual drop in postoperative weight over 3 to 4 days.**

INTERVENTIONS	RATIONALE
Independent	
Monitor hemodynamic pressures, for example, CVP, PCWP, LAP.	Elevation of these parameters may indicate fluid volume excess.
Auscultate breath sounds, noting adventitious sounds (e.g., crackles). Note shortness of breath.	Presence of crackles and dyspnea may indicate developing pulmonary edema.
Monitor intake and output hourly for at least 24 hours. Measure specific gravity.	Permits early intervention in reversible fluid fluctuations. On the third or fourth day the patient should begin to mobilize extracellular fluid, with resulting spontaneous diuresis.
Document weight changes.	The patient's weight can be used as a guide in determining success in decreasing water retention.
Assess for presence of dependent edema. Note jugular vein distention. Listen for development of third heart sound.	Development of pulmonary congestion or edema formation reflects fluid overload.
Administer IV carefully via infusion pumps or microdrips.	Intravascular plasma volume may require support while interstitial water volume is reduced through diuresis.
Measure all sources of intake, including invasive flushes, and subtotal separately. Record changes in type and rate of infusions.	Fluids are monitored carefully to prevent elevated total body water levels, a hormonal response that favors sodium and water retention. Saline (infused with blood or invasive line flushes) may add to sodium imbalance. Subtotaling individual fluids focuses attention on excess or deficit components.
Provide appropriate oral beverage choices and assist patient in establishing intake schedule.	Provides patient some control and may enhance cooperation when sodium and/or fluid restrictions are imposed.
Collaborative	
Monitor electrolyte values.	Hypokalemia may result from increased total body water related to pump perfusion and IV therapy, or losses occurring from diuretic therapy and gastric secretion loss. Hyponatremia is almost always dilutional and can be corrected with fluid restrictions.
Administer drugs as indicated: diuretics, for example, furosemide (Lasix).	Reduces total body water and promotes urine flow to clear renal tubules of tissue breakdown products and free hemoglobin resulting from cardiopulmonary bypass procedure.
Observe sodium/fluid restriction if appropriate. Balance po/IV intake.	May be indicated to restore fluid balance. As oral intake increases, IV rates should be adjusted to prevent fluid overload.

NURSING DIAGNOSIS: **Infection, potential for.**

SUPPORTING DATA/CONTRIBUTING FACTORS: **Patient returns from the operating room with many invasive lines and**

	tubes and is at risk to develop infection, sepsis.
GENERAL PATIENT OUTCOMES:	**Patient is afebrile. Surgical wounds are free of purulent drainage and exudate.**

INTERVENTIONS	RATIONALE
Independent	
Wash hands frequently. Use strict asepsis in handling invasive lines and incisions.	Minimizes potential for nosocomial infection.
Monitor integrity of incisions, and invasive line sites. Note pain, erythema, edema. Document presence and character of drainage.	May indicate developing infection or failure to heal. Mediastinal infections, while rare, can be catastrophic.
Change line insertion dressings. Clean sites with antiseptic solution. Apply antibiotic dressings.	Limits entry of microorganisms into the body.
Change IV tubing/solutions as indicated.	Inhibits bacterial growth within tubing and solutions.
Provide mouth care routinely.	Helps maintain integrity of mucous membranes, limits bacterial growth, provides patient comfort.
Provide catheter and perineal care.	Inhibits entry of ascending bacteria and reduces possibility of sepsis.
Encourage patient to be out of bed as early as possible.	Aids in movement of secretions that predispose to pneumonia.
Note temperature elevation, increased heart rate, chills, diaphoresis.	May indicate developing sepsis.
Collaborative	
Obtain blood, urine, and drainage cultures as indicated.	Identifies infecting organisms(s) and guides antibiotic therapy.
Administer antibiotics as indicated.	Antibiotics may be given prophylactically and/or in response to results of cultures.

NURSING DIAGNOSIS:	**Sensory-Perceptual Alteration.**
SUPPORTING DATA/CONTRIBUTING FACTORS:	**Numerous factors coexist that may alter perception or interpretation of stimuli. The patient is initially in a restricted environment, confined to bed, unable to communicate. Sensory overload and sleep deprivation are environmental hazards. Pain and chemical alterations may impair sensory perception. Psychologic stress of heart**

	surgery/serious illness, or microembolization may contribute to disorientation or other alterations in behavior, e.g., post pump psychosis.
GENERAL PATIENT OUTCOMES:	**Sensory overload and deprivation is minimized. Patient reactions/ responses are appropriate to situation. Complications are prevented/ controlled.**

INTERVENTIONS	RATIONALE
Independent	
Maintain a calm and quiet atmosphere for the patient (i.e., provide periods of undisturbed rest, privacy; lower auditory alarms at bedside, alter lighting to simulate night/day pattern). (Refer to Nursing Diagnoses: Knowledge Deficit [Learning Need], page 27; Anxiety/ Fear, page 28; Care Plan: Psychosocial Aspects of Critical Care, page 379.	Sleep deprivation and sensory overload often occur because of patient's condition and constant monitoring. These can increase anxiety and can block coping behaviors.

NURSING DIAGNOSIS:	**Comfort, alteration in, pain, acute.**
SUPPORTING DATA/CONTRIBUTING FACTORS:	**Pain may be associated with mediasternotomy (direct trauma to chest wall), chest tubes, endotracheal tube, and donor site incisions (in CABG patients). During the perioperative phase the patient's arms are placed above the head, and the chest is retracted open. This position has the potential to cause stretch injuries to the brachial plexus, with pain reported in arms, shoulders, or hands.**
GENERAL PATIENT OUTCOMES:	**Verbalizes or demonstrates relief of pain. Patient is able to rest.**

INTERVENTIONS	RATIONALE
Independent	
Assess complaints of chest pain. Monitor vital signs (e.g., increased heart rate). Observe nonverbal clues (e.g., muscle guarding).	Pain is perceived/tolerated individually, and it is important to differentiate incisional pain from other types of chest pain, for example, angina or pericarditis.
Note unusual or vague complaints of discomfort.	May be warning sign of complications, such as thrombophlebitis, infection, gastrointestinal impairment.

INTERVENTIONS	RATIONALE
Independent	
Assess for pain and/or numbness in the ulnar area, fourth and fifth digits of the hand, and in arms or shoulders.	Indicates stretch injury of brachial plexus. Although no treatment is currently successful, the problem should resolve with time.
Provide comfort measures such as back rubs, position changes, therapeutic touch, diversional activities as indicated.	May promote relaxation, thereby reducing analgesic needs.
Collaborative	
Administer analgesics as indicated.	Morphine sulphate is usually drug of choice in early postoperative period because it does not depress the myocardium and therefore minimally affects cardiac output, but it can decrease systemic vascular resistance and lower blood pressure, particularly if the patient is hypovolemic. Giving drug on a regular time schedule maintains a steady blood level and is more effective in managing pain. Oral analgesics may be started after the patient is extubated and the nasogastric tube removed.

Cardiogenic Shock

PATIENT ASSESSMENT DATA BASE

HISTORY

Recent myocardial infarction or cardiovascular surgery with loss of left ventricular wall function.

History of chronic or progressing congestive heart failure.

Valvular dysfunction and cardiomyopathies.

Abnormalities in peripheral vascular regulation, i.e., malignant hypertension.

Subjective

May complain of chest pain, shortness of breath, or extreme weakness.

PHYSICAL EXAMINATION

Cardiogenic shock consists of sustained systemic arterial hypotension with evidence of inadequate perfusion to kidneys, brain, and skin. Physical findings are dependent on severity/duration of shock state but should include (*) manifestations:

Inspection

*Mentation: diminishing level of consciousness following restlessness, apprehension, and confusion.

*Skin: general pallor, progressing cyanosis of lips and mucous membranes.

*Urine output: decreased below obligatory levels or absent.

Respirations: usually tachypnic, increased work of breathing, use of accessory muscles, nasal flaring.

External jugular vein: distention present, elevation of pulse point.

Palpation

*Skin: cool, clammy.

Peripheral pulses: weak, thready, easily obliterated. Pulsus alternans or paradoxical pulsus may be noted.

Hepatojugular reflux: pressure on the liver elevates jugular venous pressure.

Auscultation

*Blood pressure: arterial systolic pressure of less than 80 mmHg, or a fall of greater than 30 mmHg in a hypertensive patient.

Heart: tachycardia, other dysrhythmias; extra heart sounds (e.g.; S_3/S_4 heart sounds, murmurs).

Breath sounds: crackles/wheezes may be present.

DIAGNOSTIC STUDIES

ABGs may initially demonstrate decreased $PaCO_2$, compensating for hypoxemia, and progressing metabolic acidosis. Later shock state presents both respiratory and metabolic acidosis owing to loss of compensatory mechanisms, rising lactic and pyruvic acid levels.

BUN/creatinine: elevations reflect alterations in renal function.

SGOT/SGPT: elevations seen in congestive heart/liver failure.

Electrolytes: imbalance may include hyperkalemia or hypokalemia, hypernatremia or hyponatremia owing to renal dysfunction, fluid imbalance, and/or drug therapies.

Serum lactacte may be elevated owing to metabolic acidosis.

Cardiac enzymes may be elevated in presence of acute or recent myocardial damage.

ECG: detects changes associated with myocardial ischemia/damage, ventricular hypertrophy, electrolyte imbalance, and changes characteristic of toxic effects of drugs.

Chest x-ray examination may demonstrate cardiomegaly and/or pulmonary vascular congestion.

Echocardiogram, coronary arteriography, left ventricular cineangiography may be done to determine status of coronary circulation and myocardial function.

NURSING PRIORITIES

1. Maximize cardiac output.
2. Promote adequate oxygenation and tissue perfusion.
3. Restore or maintain acid-base and electrolyte balances.
4. Alleviate or control pain.
5. Minimize or prevent complications.
6. Provide for emotional support of patient and significant other(s).

NURSING DIAGNOSIS:	**Cardiac Output, alteration in, decreased.**
SUPPORTING DATA/CONTRIBUTING FACTORS:	**Myocardial damage owing to infarction is the most common cause of cardiogenic shock. Other causes include persistent dysrhythmias, decompensated congestive heart failure, rupture of any heart structure, or recent cardiac surgery.**
GENERAL PATIENT OUTCOMES:	**Adequate cardiac output made evident by systolic BP greater than 90 mmHg (or within 30 mmHg of patient's usual pressure), cardiac index greater than 2.5, skin warm and dry, improved mentation, urine output greater than 20 ml/hour.**

INTERVENTIONS	RATIONALE
Independent	
Monitor heart sounds.	Abnormal heart sounds may include S_3 and S_4 associated with ischemia or rapid filling of noncompliant ventricle. Heart sounds may be muffled in presence of acute infarction or pulmonary congestion.

INTERVENTIONS	RATIONALE
Independent	
Document cardiac dysrhythmias.	Significant and continued dysrhythmias can occur as a result of depression of myocardial contractility, decreased coronary perfusion, ischemic or necrotic tissue, catecholamines, electrolyte imbalance, and toxic effects of drugs (e.g., Digoxin) or myocardial depressant drugs (e.g., Pronestyl).
Auscultate breath sounds.	Left ventricle (LV) failure results in pulmonary hypertension and congestion leading to fluid accumulation and bronchospasm made evident by presence of crackles, rhonchi, or wheezes.
Measure pulmonary artery pressure (PAP).	Elevation reflects pulmonary congestion which may lead to right heart failure.
Measure pulmonary capillary wedge pressure (PCWP) and pulmonary artery diastolic pressure (PADP).	PCWP and PADP are elevated in cardiogenic shock. PCWP less than 15 may be an indicator for increasing fluids, even in the presence of pulmonary congestion. However, a rapid or sustained elevation of PCWP (greater than 20 mmHg) following a minimal fluid challenge suggests pump failure rather than inadequate circulating volume.
Measure central venous pressure (CVP).	Elevation suggests volume overload, and/or heart failure (in the absence of volume overload).
Measure mean arterial pressure (MAP).	Circulating volume must be sufficient to maintain systolic BP at 80 to 90 mmHg, or no more than 30 mmHg below hypertensive patient's usual pressure. Decreased aortic pressure can cause hypoperfusion of the myocardium, resulting in ischemia and affecting myocardial contractility.
Measure/calculate cardiac output/index.	Measurement of cardiac function influenced by preload (circulating volume), afterload (vascular resistance), myocardial contractility, and heart rate. Cardiac index is a more specific determinant of cardiac output because body size is considered.
Note external jugular venous distention.	Increasing pressure in right atrium impedes entry of venous blood from vena cava. Inadequate venous drainage is manifested by distended neck veins. Note: Absence of neck vein distention is not necessarily indicative of absence of right heart failure.
Monitor body temperature.	Temperature elevations increase myocardial workload and oxygen consumption and potentially decrease cardiac output. Patient may feel cold owing to peripheral vasoconstriction. Rewarming may cause peripheral vasodilation, which increases the vascular bed, decreasing venous return and cardiac output.
Monitor peripheral and dependent edema.	Fluid shifts occur as a result of hypotension, decreased glomerular filtration, and capillary membrane changes in responses to circulating humoral agents associated with heart failure.

INTERVENTIONS	RATIONALE
Independent	
Monitor effects of IV fluid, blood and plasma expanders.	Decreased heart rate (work), stabilizing blood pressure, and increased urine output are objective signs of improved cardiac function and circulating volume.
Collaborative	
Monitor serial 12-lead ECG changes.	May show left ventricular hypertrophy and/or serial changes characteristic of myocardial ischemia/necrosis, electrolyte imbalance, drug therapy, and/or toxic drug effects.
Review serial chest x-rays.	Monitors progress/resolution of pulmonary congestion, verifies cardiac enlargement and placement of hemodynamic monitoring lines.
Monitor laboratory data; that is, ABGs,	Hypoxemia and acidosis negatively affect myocardial oxygenation and function.
Electrolytes,	Electrolyte imbalance contributes to dysrhythmias which may alter cardiac output.
Hgb and Hct,	Reflects fluid status and circulating volume and has an impact on oxygen-carrying capacity.
Drug levels.	Toxicity may occur owing to altered circulation, reduced organ perfusion, and metabolic function combined with narrow therapeutic ranges of some cardiac drugs (e.g., digoxin, nitroprusside).
Administer IV fluids, blood, plasma expanders.	Blood, plasma, colloid, and crystalloid solutions may be used to increase vascular volume and to improve cardiac output. Caution: Fluid needs must be carefully balanced against risk of volume overload and further myocardial compromise.
Assist with insertion of and maintain invasive monitoring lines (e.g., pulmonary artery thermodilution catheter).	Allows for measurement of ventricular function, cardiac output, pulmonary function, circulating volume.
Administer drugs as indicated: dopamine hydrochloride (Intropin),	Enhances cardiac output by increasing systemic vascular resistance (SVR) and exerting a positive inotropic effect on the heart, thereby improving stroke volume. Renal and mesenteric blood vessels are dilated, improving organ perfusion. Precautions: Peripheral effects include cyanosis of fingers and toes.
Dobutamine hydrochloride (Dobutrex),	Decreases peripheral vascular resistance, reducing afterload. Produces higher cardiac output and lower pulmonary wedge pressure when used concomitantly with nitroprusside. Precautions: It may increase ventricular ectopy, size of myocardial infarction, or be ineffective if beta blockers (Inderal) have been given. It may also increase insulin needs in diabetic patient.
Norepinephrine (Levophed),	May be used to support blood pressure by increasing vascular resistance (SVR) but has side effects of decreased renal and mesenteric perfusion so use must

INTERVENTIONS	RATIONALE
Collaborative	
	be balanced against potential risk of worsening shock state.
Nitroprusside sodium (Nipride),	Increases cardiac output by reducing afterload. Produces peripheral and systemic vasodilation by direct action on smooth muscle of blood vessels. Precautions: Severe hypotension occurs with inadvertent bolus. Although effects are usually reversible, seizures and cardiac arrest can occur.
Nitroglycerin IV (Nitrobid),	Reduces myocardial oxygen consumption, preload, and afterload. Reduces arterial blood pressure, PCWP, and systemic vascular resistance. Precautions: Special IV tubing is required to prevent absorption of drug by standard tubing. Drug effect is potentiated by other vasodilators.
Digoxin (Lanoxin),	Increases strength of myocardial contraction. Acts on automaticity, conduction, and refraction to produce a slower, stronger beat. Precautions: Potassium depletion increases risk of digitalis intoxication. Digitalis effect is potentiated by many other drugs. Digoxin is incompatible with calcium (may cause arrhythmias).
Lidocaine hydrochloride (Lidocaine),	Decreases ventricular excitability and dysrhythmias. Precautions: Give with caution in all forms of heart block, untreated bradycardia, hepatic failure. Overdose can precipitate cardiovascular collapse, convulsions, coma, and cardiac arrest.
Bretylium tosylate (Bretylol),	May be used to treat ventricular dysrhythmias if lidocaine is ineffective or contraindicated.
Potassium chloride,	Must be present within a narrow therapeutic range for normal functioning of excitable cells, such as heart, nerve, and muscle tissue. Precautions: Adequate kidney function is essential to maintain potassium balance. Observe for ECG changes characteristic of hyperkalemia and hypokalemia. (Refer to Appendix: Fluid and Electrolyte Imbalances, page 431.)
Corticosteroids.	Occasionally used to improve vascular tone, depress release of myocardial depressant factor, decrease capillary permeability, and reduce lactic acid accumulation associated with hypoxemia.
Assist with insertion of intra-aortic balloon pump (IABP) when used.	Augments circulating blood supply and diminishes oxygen demand, resulting in improved myocardial efficiency, that is, stroke volume and cardiac output.
Monitor IABP inflation and deflation indicators.	Adjustments are needed to correlate pump action with changes in heart rate/rhythm. Balloon should deflate immediately prior to systole, thus mechanically decreasing afterload. Balloon should inflate completely during early diastole to promote coronary and cerebral perfusion.

INTERVENTIONS	RATIONALE
Collaborative	
Assess effectiveness of IABP weaning as indicated.	Hemodynamic stability at 1:1 pumping usually indicates readiness to wean.
Assist with insertion of pacemaker, if indicated.	May be necessary to improve cardiac output in the presence of persistent dysrhythmias, which worsen ventricular muscle dysfunction.
Monitor ECG. Replace batteries, reposition patient, increase (MA).	Assesses packemaker function. Cardiac output can be affected by pacemaker malfunctions and requires immediate intervention. Battery failure is the most common cause of pacemaker malfunction; however, changing patient position and/or increasing MA may be necessary to correct loss of sensing/capture.

NURSING DIAGNOSIS:	**Tissue Perfusion, alteration in, decreased.**
SUPPORTING DATA/CONTRIBUTING FACTORS:	**Decreased cardiac output, hypoxia, and acidosis contribute to circulatory stagnation and inadequate tissue perfusion, affecting all systems.**
GENERAL PATIENT OUTCOMES:	**Adequate tissue perfusion is made evident by palpable peripheral pulses, warm and dry skin, improved mentation, and urinary output greater than 20 ml per hour.**

INTERVENTIONS	RATIONALE
Independent	
Note changes in mental status: listlessness, anxiety, confusion, lethargy, stupor, coma.	Changes in mentation and/or level of consciousness reflect cerebral blood flow and may be indication of alteration in systemic perfusion.
Assess for pallor, cyanosis, mottling, cool moist skin. Note presence and quality of peripheral pulses, capillary refill. Observe for increasing cyanosis in restrained or cannulated extremities.	Reflects vasoconstriction, a compensatory mechanism for sensed decrease in organ perfusion. Tissue perfusion may be further impeded by external factors (e.g., restraints, pressure dressings, improperly fitting antiembolic hose).
Auscultate bowel sounds; measure abdominal girth; note pain, nausea, vomiting; observe and guaiac nasogastric contents.	Reduced blood flow to mesentery may alter gastrointestinal function, producing mucosal irritation, ischemia, pain, loss of peristalsis, onset of ileus.
Monitor urinary output hourly, measure specific gravity.	Hypoperfusion of the kidneys can result in acute tubular necrosis (ATN), with urinary output below obligatory levels and loss of ability to concentrate urine. (Refer to Care Plan: Acute Renal Failure, page 207.)

INTERVENTIONS	RATIONALE
Collaborative	
Insert nasogastric tube.	Decompresses stomach, prevents vomiting, reduces hydrochloric acid secretion. Provides visual evidence if bleeding is present associated with gastric irritation, stress ulcers, coagulation disorders. (Refer to Care Plan: Upper GI/Esophageal Bleeding, page 197.)
Monitor BUN and creatinine, serum and urine electrolytes.	Improved electrolytes and appropriate response to diuretic therapy indicate improved renal perfusion. Failure of therapies may indicate need for dialysis. (Refer to Care Plan: Renal Dialysis, page 222.)
Administer drugs as indicated: cimetadine (Tagamet) or antacids,	Reduces production of and neutralizes hydrochloric acid, and thus may prevent stress-related gastric mucosa irritation or ulceration.
firosemide (Lasix).	Diuretics promote excretion of water, sodium, chlorides, and potassium, thereby reducing edema and pulmonary congestion.

NURSING DIAGNOSIS:	**Gas Exchange, impaired.**
SUPPORTING DATA/CONTRIBUTING FACTORS:	**Pulmonary congestion impedes gas diffusion within the lungs. In addition, decreased cardiac output and poor tissue perfusion enhance lactic acid accumulation, adversely affecting oxygen release at the cellular level.**
GENERAL PATIENT OUTCOMES:	**Improved ventilation and adequate oxygenation are evident by ABGs within patient's normal limits, absence of cyanosis and free of dyspnea.**

INTERVENTIONS	RATIONALE
Independent	
Maintain patent airway.	Suctioning may be required to clear secretions and to improve delivery of oxygen.
Monitor respiratory rate and effort, note use of accessory muscles.	Tachypnea or dyspnea may be the result of hypoxemia, acidosis, atelactasis, pulmonary edema, or pain.
Note peripheral or circumoral cyanosis.	Central cyanosis is a more sensitive indicator of hypoxemia, and peripheral cyanosis reflects vasoconstriction and, to a lesser degree, hypoxemia.
Maintain bedrest, provide self-care needs, schedule activities/procedures to provide maximal rest.	Reduces oxygen needs/consumption.

INTERVENTIONS	RATIONALE
Collaborative	
Monitor/graph serial ABGs. Calculate A-a gradient when possible.	Respiratory and metabolic acidosis may be present. Widening A-a gradient suggests worsening oxygen diffusion and warns of impending respiratory failure.
Provide supplemental oxygen as indicated, by means of nasal cannula, mask, high-flow rebreathing mask, or intubation and/or mechanical ventilation.	Necessary to correct failing respiratory effort, hypoxemia, and progressing acidosis. High-level oxygen delivery may be required for saturation of poorly circulating blood. Positive-end expiratory pressure (PEEP) may be used to improve alveolar ventilation, but should be used cautiously because of possibility of decreasing venous return and cardiac output. (Refer to Care Plan: Ventilatory Assistance, mechanical, page 115.)
Administer sodium bicarbonate as indicated.	May be used on occasion to correct acidosis and to improve oxygen release at cellular level.

NURSING DIAGNOSIS: **Comfort, alteration in, pain, acute.**

SUPPORTING DATA/CONTRIBUTING FACTORS: **Precipitating factors of cardiogenic shock (e.g., acute MI, cardiac surgery) are usually accompanied by pain. Discomfort also accompanies decreased tissue perfusion and therapeutic procedures.**

GENERAL PATIENT OUTCOMES: **Indicates alleviation of pain, demonstrates relaxed manner, and is able to rest.**

INTERVENTIONS	RATIONALE
Independent	
Observe physiologic changes that indicate pain, for example, increased heart or respiratory rate—with or without changes in blood pressure—unexplained changes in condition.	May provide clues indicating pain, especially when patient is unable to verbalize.
Note facial grimacing, panic look in eyes, muscle tension or guarding.	Objective signs of discomfort and apprehension.
Provide comfort measures, e.g. repositioning, pillow placement, touch (physical contact), Therapeutic Touch, and massage.	Stimulates circulation, reduces discomfort resulting from immobility, and provides reassurance which may assist the patient to rest.
Prevent oversedation.	Provides pain relief/rest balanced with time to be awake, interact with significant other(s).

INTERVENTIONS	RATIONALE
Collaborative	
Administer analgesics as indicated, for example, IV morphine sulphate.	Decreases preload, afterload, cardiac work, and oxygen consumption. Intravenous route is preferred because drug is not absorbed properly when administered intramuscularly (IM) in poorly perfused muscle. Small, frequent doses may produce adequate pain relief. Precautions: Nonventilated or synchronized intermittent maximal ventilation (SIMV) ventilated patients are at risk for respiratory failure if depression of central nervous system (CNS) respiratory centers occurs.

NURSING DIAGNOSIS:	**Fluid Volume, alteration [fluctuation].**
SUPPORTING DATA/CONTRIBUTING FACTORS:	**Potential exists for fluid excess owing to volume replacement in the presence of impaired circulation, sodium retention, and renal dysfunction. Inadequate circulating volume may result from fluid shifts out of vascular compartment, fluid restriction, and/or diuretic use.**
GENERAL PATIENT OUTCOMES:	**Adequate fluid volume is evident by central venous pressure (CVP) and vital signs within normal limits, balanced intake and output, stable weight, absence of edema, and clear breath sounds.**

INTERVENTIONS	RATIONALE
Independent	
Auscultate breath sounds.	Presence of adventitious breath sounds (e.g., crackles) indicates pulmonary congestion and may suggest fluid overload.
Monitor CVP. Note jugular vein distention.	Elevation suggests fluid excess.
Monitor hourly and 24-hour urine output and fluid balance.	Continued fluid administration may potentiate fluid overload, and use of diuretics and fluid restriction may deplete circulating volume.
Record total fluid intake. Include piggyback medications and cardiac output injectate.	In compromised myocardial function a small amount of fluid may precipitate decompensation.
Assess daily weight.	Weight increases may suggest volume overload, worsening cardiac failure, or developing renal failure.

INTERVENTIONS	RATIONALE
Independent	
Note presence and degree of peripheral or dependent edema.	Reflects fluid shifts out of the vascular compartment into the tissues.
Note effects of diuretics.	Increased urine output may indicate improvement in cardiac function and mobilization of extracellular fluid excesses.
Collaborative	
Monitor electrolytes, especially serum sodium and potassium. (Refer to Appendix: Fluid and Electrolyte Imbalances, page 431.)	Presence of hyponatremia may reflect dilutional effect of fluid excess requiring sodium and/or fluid restriction or actual sodium deficit, requiring IV replacement. Potassium excess may occur, associated with decreased renal function. "Low normal levels" actually may reflect total body hypokalemia as potassium shifts from the cell into the serum in response to acidosis.
Administer IV solutions as indicated.	Choice of fluid replacement is dependent upon patient needs. For example, hypertonic glucose or saline solutions may be given to meet cellular energy needs or to correct hyponatremia; sodium-restricted fluids may be used in the presence of fluid overload.
Administer and note effect of fluid challenges and volume-expanding solutions.	Differentiates volume deficit and cardiac failure, for example, improvement in hemodynamic parameters and urine output following a fluid challenge suggests the need for further fluid replacement. Colloid solutions pull fluid into intravascular space but remain in circulation; therefore crystalloid solutions may be preferred.

NURSING DIAGNOSIS:	**Nutrition, alteration in, less than body requirements.**
SUPPORTING DATA/CONTRIBUTING FACTORS:	**Available nutritional stores are depleted by shock state, patient's inability to ingest or digest food, and altered liver function.**
GENERAL PATIENT OUTCOMES:	**Nutritional intake is adequate to meet needs made evident by positive nitrogen balance, stable weight within patient's usual range.**

INTERVENTIONS	RATIONALE
Independent	
Assess GI function. (Refer to Nursing Diagnosis: Tissue Perfusion, page 53.)	Affects choice of route for nutritional support.

INTERVENTIONS	RATIONALE
Collaborative	
Administer nutrients as indicated:	
Dextrose solutions and multivitamin additives.	Provides glucose to meet cellular energy needs and replenishes depleted vitamin stores.
Hyperalimentation.	Supplies nutrients without need for digestion.
Tube feeding or supplements.	Initiate after GI function is assured.
(Refer to Care Plan: Nutritional Support, page 367.)	

NURSING DIAGNOSIS:	**Injury, potential for, poisoning.**
SUPPORTING DATA/CONTRIBUTING FACTORS:	**Potential exists for drug toxicity owing to impaired metabolism and clearance secondary to altered renal or liver perfusion and function. Inadequate perfusion of significant amounts of tissue results in higher concentrations of drugs in the bloodstream and perfused areas. In addition, infusion errors, such as boluses and incompatabilities, further compound risk of toxicity.**
GENERAL PATIENT OUTCOMES:	**Complications will be prevented/minimized.**

INTERVENTIONS	RATIONALE
Independent	
Monitor infusion pumps for proper function. Alarms must be on. Mark IV bottles and monitor fluid levels frequently.	Pumps can appear to be functioning without actually infusing fluids or drugs. Infusion pump cassettes may be dislodged, potentiating risk of large infusions of fluid and/or drugs.
Use microdrips or precision volume infusion sets in absence of infusion pumps.	Minimizes risk of accidental bolus and rapid infusion.
Color code/label IV lines near clamps and ports.	Ensures regulation of intended solution and identifies appropriate port(s) for intermittent drug administration.
Be aware of drug incompatibilities. Be alert for interactions, side effects, potentiations, inhibitions, allergic reactions. Clear line with small amounts of normal saline before and after boluses and piggyback administrations.	Many drugs necessary to the treatment of cardiogenic shock are incompatible with each other in solution, tubing, and syringe. Vasopressors, antihypertensives, and anticoagulants should not be given with any other drug. Many antibiotics also are incompatible with other drugs.
Infuse vasopressors, cardiac drugs, narcotics, and those drugs irritating to veins in central venous lines or large veins (such as anticubital) in the absence of cen-	Numerous cardiovascular drugs are extremely irritating to veins and tissues and may cause sloughing (e.g., dopamine, Levophed). Furthermore, infusion

INTERVENTIONS	RATIONALE
Independent	
tral lines. Observe for infiltration. Change sites as needed.	into peripheral veins may render medication ineffective owing to vascular constriction or slowed circulation and create possibility of rebound overdose if vasodilation occurs.
Collaborative	
Monitor drug effect (e.g., dopamine, Nipride, digoxin) and titrate as indicated.	Giving minimum amount to produce therapeutic response reduces hazards of toxicity.
Monitor serum drug levels of hepatic and nephrotoxic drugs.	Reduced organ function may prolong drug half-life and potentiate drug toxicity.

NURSING DIAGNOSIS:	**Injury, potential for, multiple factors.**
SUPPORTING DATA/CONTRIBUTING FACTORS:	**Potential exists for injury from numerous factors, including invasive lines and counterpulsation (IABP). Generalized weakness and therapeutic procedures contribute to problems associated with immobility. Various factors of the shock state (e.g., circulatory stagnation and acid-base imbalance) affect clotting factors and may result in DIC.**
GENERAL PATIENT OUTCOMES:	**Complications are prevented/minimized.**

INTERVENTIONS	RATIONALE
Independent	
Tape/protect continuity of invasive lines.	Prevents exsanguination and air embolus. Promotes accuracy of monitoring equipment.
Apply pressure dressing to insertion site of IABP.	Prevents arterial bleeding into surrounding tissue.
Maintain immobilization of cannulated leg.	Prevents catheter breakage resulting in artery or tissue damage.
Provide meticulous skin care. Reposition frequently as permitted by monitoring and special equipment. Apply lotion to and massage bony prominences; keep skin dry.	Reduces risk for skin breakdown while peripheral circulation is reduced and patient is immobile.
Provide footboard or boots, hand or trocanter roll, etc.	Maintains functional position of extremities.
Note peripheral erythema, edema, tenderness, presence of Homans' sign; sudden onset of pleural pain, increased dyspnea, hemoptysis, apprehension. (Refer to Care Plan: Pulmonary Embolism, page 95.)	Sluggish circulation, acid-base imbalances, increased platelet aggregation, reduced mobility, and presence of invasive lines potentiate risk of thrombophlebitis and embolus formation.

INTERVENTIONS	RATIONALE
Independent	
Provide soft limb restraints, side rails.	Patient may be disoriented and/or stuporous and needs protection from falls, self-extubation, disruption of vital treatments and invasive lines.
Observe for hematemesis, hemoptysis, hematuria, melena, purpura, ecchymosis. Check secretions and excretions for occult blood.	Objective signs of altered coagulation, possible developing DIC. (Refer to Care Plan: DIC, page 319.)
Collaborative	
Provide foam or flotation mattress.	Prevents skin breakdown when activity is restricted and peripheral perfusion is impaired.
Apply antiembolic hose/elastic leg wraps as indicated.	Reduces venous stasis; may improve venous return and muscle tone, thereby reducing risk of phlebitis.
Administer heparin or dextran as indicated.	May be used to prevent or to treat thromboemboli associated with counterpulsation, immobility, and venous stasis.
Monitor coagulation studies.	Necessary to assess therapeutic effects of heparin. Useful in diagnosing coagulopathias, such as DIC.

NURSING DIAGNOSIS:	**Infection, potential for.**
SUPPORTING DATA/CONTRIBUTING FACTORS:	**Presence of invasive lines/tubes, general debilitation, and alterations in immune response place patient at risk for development of nosocomial infections.**
GENERAL PATIENT OUTCOMES:	**Afebrile, absence of chills, lungs clear with sputum normal color and character, urine clear and odor free, incisions and insertion sites clean.**

INTERVENTIONS	RATIONALE
Independent	
Use proper handwashing technique.	First-line defense against nosocomial infection. Patients are at high risk for developing overwhelming infections.
Maintain aseptic technique when inserting invasive lines, administering IV solutions, changing IV bottles.	Break in aseptic technique may result in contamination.
Follow established protocol for incision and insertion site care. Change dressings as needed.	Minimizes bacterial growth as a result of contamination.
Encourage deep breathing, coughing, position changes. In intubated patient, use aseptic technique when suctioning and hyperinflate lungs with ambu bag.	Prevent stasis of secretions or introduction of contaminating agent with increased possibility of pulmonary infection.

INTERVENTIONS	RATIONALE
Independent	
Maintain aseptic technique when catheterizing. Administer periodic catheter and perineal care.	Minimizes urinary tract irritation and/or infection. (Prime factor in development of gram-negative infections.)
Note temperature elevation, diaphoresis, chills, presence of purulent drainage from wounds, cloudy or odiferous urine, changes in character of sputum.	Signs of infection which if untreated may progress to sepsis. (Refer to Care Plan: Sepsis/Septicemia/Septic Shock, page 329.)
Collaborative	
Monitor white blood count (WBC) and differential.	Elevations may reflect infectious process.
Obtain specimens as indicated (i.e., wound, urine, sputum, blood).	Confirms infection, identifying specific organism.
Administer antibiotics as indicated.	Treats/prevents infection.

NURSING DIAGNOSIS: **Anxiety/Fear.**

SUPPORTING DATA/CONTRIBUTING FACTORS: **Knowledge that the "heart is failing or not functioning adequately" produces a sense of impending doom. In addition, constant attention by caregivers and use of numerous machines, with their functioning noises/alarms, may potentiate anxiety and fear. Also, unresolved concerns may aggravate patient's condition, compromising chance for recovery, and/or resulting in ineffective coping by patient and significant other(s).**

GENERAL PATIENT OUTCOMES: **Patient and significant other(s) verbalize feelings. Significant other(s) is supported and able to support patient. Patient demonstrates reduction of anxiety and fear (e.g., is able to rest appropriately).**

INTERVENTIONS	RATIONALE
Independent	
Provide information that changes in audible rhythm of machinery—such as in ventilators, balloon pump—often reflect normal benign situations, such as sighing or minor heart rate changes. In addition, alarms provide patient protection, often indicating need for ad-	Patient and significant other(s) may be acutely aware of usual sounds of equipment and react with increased concern; information can provide reassurance.

INTERVENTIONS	RATIONALE
Independent	
justment in machinery or therapy (e.g., adding new IV fluid to pump, suctioning airway) rather than actual life-threatening situations.	
Promote liberal visitation, including during periods of rest as appropriate.	At a time when many procedures are required and lucid periods may be brief, the opportunity to spend time together, even quietly holding hands, may provide sense of comfort and reassurance.
Interact with significant other(s) away from patient's bedside. Answer questions honestly, encourage discussion of concerns/fears, support anticipatory grieving process.	Significant other(s) may have difficulty coping with threat of death. (Mortality is 80%+.) Helping them work through their feelings may enable them to provide support to the patient rather than increase patient's anxieties/fears.
Provide referral to clergy, hospital psychiatric nurse/social worker.	May benefit from assistance in dealing with critical illness, prospect of death, legal, financial, and spiritual concerns.

(Refer to Care Plans: Cardiac Surgery, page 19; Myocardial Infarction, page 62.)

Congestive Heart Failure

This care plan focuses on patients with acute or symptomatic congestive heart failure (functional classes II-IV). Patients with Stage II are symptomatic with minimal activity and may or may not be symptomatic at rest. Patients in Stage III have pulmonary involvement, and patients in Stage IV are symptomatic even at rest. Although pulmonary edema may be seen in a variety of settings, such as inhalation injury (smoke or chemical) and adult respiratory distress syndrome (ARDS), it is most often seen in association with left ventricular dysfunction and therefore is included in this care plan.

PATIENT ASSESSMENT DATA BASE

HISTORY

Conditions resulting in decreased myocardial contractility; that is, history of acute/severe myocardial infarction; cardiomyopathies; ruptured chordae tendineae; conduction disturbances; use of cardiosuppressive drugs, such as beta blockers, calcium channel blockers; systemic lupus erythematosus (SLE); scleroderma.

History of factors resulting in increased myocardial workload; that is, valvular heart disease, intracardiac shunting; anemia, high output states (thyrotoxicosis, septic shock), systemic and pulmonary hypertension.

Subjective

Dyspnea on exertion; may complain of orthopnea and paroxysmal nocturnal dyspnea (PND). May report sleeping sitting up or with one or two pillows.

Muscle aches, weakness, and poor exercise tolerance progressing throughout the day.

Dizziness or syncope, sleep pattern disturbances and fatigue.

Chest pain (chronic or acute anginal pain), right upper quadrant abdominal pain.

Lower extremity swelling, shoe tightness and discomfort.

Significant weight gain, pants and/or belt too tight.

Poor appetite, nausea, abdominal distention.

May note decreased urine output, nocturia, concentrated urine.

PHYSICAL EXAMINATION

Inspection

Respirations may be increased, dyspnea and changes in chest excursion may be noted.

Cough: may be dry and hacky; frothy, blood-tinged sputum may be produced.

Neck veins may be distended, reflecting elevated jugular venous pressure.

Skin: dusky, pale if vasoconstriction or low output state is present.

Edema may be seen in legs, feet, sacrum. Brawn edema (hard, discolored, fibrous subcutaneous reaction) may be present.

Abdomen: ascites may be noted.

Palpation

Heart: point of maximum intensity (PMI) may be displaced to the left and inferiorly due to ventricular dilatation or hypertrophy.

Peripheral pulses may be diminished owing to decreased stroke volume, peripheral vasoconstriction.

Liver may be palpable below the right rib margin owing to congestion.

Hepatojugular reflux: presence indicates elevated systemic venous pressure.

Edema may be pitting, graded from 0 to 4+.

Auscultation

Breath sounds: may be diminished; wheezing and/or crackles (often bibasilar in distribution) may be present owing to fluid in pulmonary tissues.

Heart sounds: S_1 and S_2 may be softened, owing to decreased force of myocardial contraction. S_3 may be heard when ventricular filling is excessively rapid or when the recipient ventricle is dilated and has increased residual volume. S_4 may also be present, caused by forceful atrial contraction into resistive/noncompliant ventricle. S_3 is diagnostic of heart failure, whereas the S_4 may be associated with other types of cardiovascular damage (e.g., hypertension, valve disease). Heart rate may be increased. Dysrhythmias may be present (e.g., atrial fibrillation, PVCs, bundle branch blocks). Diastolic and systolic murmurs, if present, may indicate mitral, tricuspid, or aortic valvular stenosis or regurgitation, intracardiac shunt defects, or excessive venous return.

Blood pressure may be low or elevated, depending on underlying mechanism, that is, myocardial damage or changes in systemic vascular resistance. Narrow pulse pressure reflects reduced stroke volume.

DIAGNOSTIC STUDIES

ECG: prominent P wave in I, III, and AVF may indicate increased right atrial filling pressure or enlargement. Dysrhythmias—for example tachycardia, atrial fibrillation, frequent PVCs—may be present.

Echocardiography: may reveal enlarged chamber dimensions, valve incompetence or stenosis, or areas of decreased ventricular wall motion.

Nuclear radiographic studies: pinpoints areas of decreased myocardial perfusion, measures ejection fraction, and estimates wall motion.

Cardiac catheterization: may be indicated to differentiate right versus left heart failure, and/or to assess patency of coronary arteries.

Chest x-ray examination: may show enlarged cardiac shadow, reflecting dilatation or hypertrophy, or changes in blood vessels, reflecting increased pulmonary venous pressure.

Myocardial enzymes: particularly CPK-MB bands, elevated in the presence of acute myocardial damage.

Liver enzymes: elevated in liver congestion or failure.

Electrolytes: may be altered owing to fluid shifts or decreased renal function, diuretic therapy.

Arterial blood gases: left ventricular failure is characterized by mild respiratory alkalosis (early); and hypoxemia with an increased PCO_2 (late).

BUN, creatinine: elevated BUN indicates decreased renal perfusion. Elevation of both BUN and creatinine is indicative of renal failure.

Serum albumin: may be decreased as a result of reduced protein intake or reduced protein synthesis in congested liver.

CBC: may reveal anemia, polycythemia, or demonstrate dilutional changes indicating water retention.

NURSING PRIORITIES

1. Decrease myocardial workload.
2. Improve myocardial contractility/systemic perfusion.
3. Assist with reduction of excess fluid volume.
4. Prevent complications.
5. Provide information about disease processes and therapy.

NURSING DIAGNOSIS:	**Cardiac Output, alteration in, decreased.**
SUPPORTING DATA/CONTRIBUTING FACTORS:	**Congestive heart failure occurs when damaged myocardium is unable to pump satisfactory amount of blood into systemic circulation to supply metabolic requirements of tissues.**
GENERAL PATIENT OUTCOMES:	**Cardiac rate, rhythm, and hemodynamic parameters within normal limits. Dysrhythmias are controlled or absent.**

INTERVENTIONS	RATIONALE
Independent	
Assess vital signs and hemodynamic indicators: heart rate, mean arterial pressure (MAP), pulmonary capillary wedge pressure (PCWP), cardiac output (CO).	Early in left ventricular failure (LVF), loss of ventricular compliance causes elevation of pressure at end of ventricular diastole (LVEDP). Heart rate increases in an attempt to compensate for decreased left ventricular (LV) contraction. LV filling time is shortened, less blood is ejected, cardiac output falls. Initially MAP may be maintained because of elevated systemic vascular resistance (SVR). Cardiac output can be within normal range accompanied by signs of congestion, that is, elevated PCWP in early, moderate, or chronic congestive heart failure (CHF). In advanced CHF, cardiac output will be severely diminished and systemic signs of congestion will be prominent.
Auscultate heart sounds.	Atrial gallup (S_4) or ventricular gallop (S_3) rhythms are common, reflecting noncompliance or distention of chambers.
Monitor electrocardiogram (ECG) changes.	ST segment depression and T wave flattening indicating ischemia can develop owing to increased myocardial oxygen demand, even if no coronary artery disease is present.
Document dysrhythmias, that is, sinus tachycardia, premature atrial contractions, paroxysmal atrial tachycardia, multifocal atrial tachycardia, premature ventricular contractions.	These dysrhythmias reduce ventricular filling time, decrease myocardial contractility, and increase myocardial oxygen demands, further compromising cardiac output.
Provide private room, bedrest, moderation in activities. (Refer to Nursing Diagnosis: Activity Intolerance, page 58.)	Bedrest should be maintained during acute or refractory CHF because physical rest decreases the production of catecholamines, which raises heart rate, myocardial oxygen demand, and blood pressure.
Collaborative	
Administer intravenous (IV) solutions, restricting total amount as indicated. Avoid saline solutions.	Stroke work is normally improved by increased volume (preload), but patients with LV failure usually have

INTERVENTIONS	RATIONALE
Collaborative	
	elevated LVEDP because of increased blood remaining in ventricles at the end of systole and therefore do not tolerate increased preload (precipitates pulmonary edema). CHF patients also tend to excrete less sodium, which acts to increase vascular volume and myocardial workload.
Monitor and replace electrolytes.	Fluid shifts and use of diuretics can alter electrolytes, especially potassium and chloride, affecting cardiac rhythm and contractility.
Administer drugs as indicated to increase stroke volume and to reduce congestion:	Accomplished by (1) reducing preload, (2) reducing afterload, and (3) improving contractility.
Diuretics, venodilators, for example, furosemide (Lasix), Bumetanide (Bumex), spironolactone (Aldactone), oral or topical nitrates (Nitro-Dur).	Preload reduction is most useful in treating patients with a relatively normal cardiac output (CO) and congestive symptoms. Venous return is reduced through vasodilatation with peripheral vascular pooling, thereby decreasing systemic and pulmonary venous pressures. Note: Excessive preload reduction may decrease CO by producing hypovolemia.
Arteriolar vasodilators, for example, hydralazine (Apresoline), nifedipine (Procardia).	Improves CO by decreasing SVR (afterload) with little or no change in systemic and pulmonary venous pressures. Most useful for patients with increased SVR and decreased CO.
Balanced arterial and venous dilators, for example, sodium nitroprusside (Nipride), captopril (Capoten).	Improves CO by dilating the vascular bed, reducing SVR and temporarily increasing venous pooling, thereby reducing venous return.
IV catacholamines, for example, dopamine hydrochloride (Intropin), dobutamine hydrochloride (Dobutrex),	Increases CO by enhancing cardiac contractility. Note: Dopamine increases MAP and causes little or no change in PCWP. Dobutamine decreases PCWP and causes little or no change in MAP.
Cardiac glycosides, for example, digoxin (Lanoxin),	Increases cardiac output by increasing force of myocardial contraction. Slows heart rate by decreasing conduction velocity and prolonging refractory period of the atrioventricular (AV) junction. (Refer to Nursing Diagnosis: Injury, potential for, poisoning, digitalis, page 59.)
Combined vasodilator and inotropic therapy, for example, Nipride and Intropin.	Produces more hemodynamic improvement when combined than when used alone. Most useful for patients with pulmonary congestion plus diminished CO. Note: Recent pharmocologically combined agents are now available (e.g., Amrinone).
Morphine sulfate.	Decreases vascular resistance, reducing venous return and decreasing myocardial workload. Allays anxiety and breaks the feedback cycle of anxiety/catecholamine release/anxiety.

NURSING DIAGNOSIS:	**Tissue Perfusion, alteration in.**
SUPPORTING DATA/CONTRIBUTING FACTORS:	**Decreased cardiac output, hypoxia, acidosis, and shock contribute to hypoperfusion of tissues and organs (including heart) and may result in damage or failure. Actual interruption of blood flow may occur owing to presence of thrombi or emboli centrally (cardiac) and/or peripherally, resulting in tissue damage.**
GENERAL PATIENT OUTCOMES:	**Hemodynamic stability is achieved with adequate tissue and organ perfusion, evident by palpable peripheral pulses, warm and dry skin, usual mentation, adequate urine output, and absence of respiratory distress.**

INTERVENTIONS	RATIONALE
Independent	
Assess for confusion, changes in mentation (e.g., personality); complaints of dizziness, syncope.	Cerebral perfusion is directly related to cardiac output and mentation may be a sensitive indicator of deterioration.
Monitor changes in blood pressure.	Hypertension is common in CHF, though postural hypotension may be present.
Note skin color, temperature.	Patients often demonstrate pallor associated with vasoconstriction, reduced cardiac output, anemia. Cyanosis may develop during severe episode of pulmonary edema or in refractory CHF. Dependent areas are often blue or mottled as venous congestion increases.
Assess presence and quality of peripheral pulses.	May be weak, thready, or difficult to obtain when CO decreased.
Assess bowel sounds. Note anorexia, nausea, abdominal distention, constipation.	Visceral congestion occurs in progressive CHF, altering gastric or intestinal function.
Provide small, frequent, easily digestible meals.	Reduced gastric motility may adversely affect digestion and absorption. Small frequent meals may enhance intake, while avoiding increased abdominal discomfort.
Monitor for hepatic congestion: Note right upper quadrant (RUQ) pain or tenderness, hepatomegaly, pulsations, jaundice.	Advancing heart failure leads to venous congestion, resulting in liver engorgement and altered organ function (e.g., impaired drug metabolism, prolonged drug half-life).

INTERVENTIONS	RATIONALE
Independent	
Monitor urine output and measure specific gravity.	Decreased renal perfusion compromises regulation of electrolytes and filtration of waste products and may be reflected by changes in urine output, altered serum and urine osmolality and specific gravity.
Elevate legs, avoid pressure under knee. Encourage active and passive exercises. Increase ambulation and activity as tolerated.	Decreases venous stasis and may reduce incidence of thrombus and embolus formation.
Check for calf tenderness (Homan's sign), swelling, redness.	Indicators of thrombophlebitis.
Monitor for symptoms of pulmonary embolus (PE): dyspnea, tachycardia, sudden arrhythmias, increased PAP, hypotension. (Refer to Care Plan: Pulmonary Embolism, page 95.)	Patients are at risk owing to venous stasis, peripheral vascular congestion, and chronic atrial dysrhythmias.
Collaborative	
Monitor laboratory values (BUN, creatinine),	Elevation of BUN, creatinine reflects kidney hypoperfusion or failure.
Liver function studies (SGOT, LDH),	May be elevated owing to liver congestion and indicates need for smaller dosages of medications, which are detoxified by the liver.
Coagulation studies, including PT, APTT.	Measures effectiveness of anticoagulant therapy.
Apply antiembolic stockings.	May help reduce venous stasis.
Administer drugs as indicated (e.g., heparin, warfarin sodium [Coumadin]).	Indicated for treatment and prevention of thromboembolic phenomena.

NURSING DIAGNOSIS:	**Fluid Volume, alteration in, excess.**
SUPPORTING DATA/CONTRIBUTING FACTORS:	**Decreased cardiac output reduces glomerular filtration rate, stimulating angiotensin and aldosterone production and sodium retention. Antidiuretic hormone (ADH) is increased and water retention occurs. Both mechanisms decrease urine output and increase plasma volume, which leads to elevated hydrostatic pressure and accumulation of interstitial edema.**
GENERAL PATIENT OUTCOMES:	**Blood pressures and heart and respiratory rates within patient's normal limits. Lung sounds are clearing. Absence of tissue edema. Balanced intake and output.**

INTERVENTIONS	RATIONALE
Independent	
Monitor CVP and PCWP, if available.	Elevation reflects increased vascular volume and may indicate developing pulmonary congestion, hypertension, worsening heart failure.
Auscultate breath sounds, noting adventitious sounds (i.e., crackles, wheezes).	Symptoms of pulmonary congestion which may persist for up to 48 hours after PCWP returns to normal range.
Assess for distended neck and peripheral vessels. Inspect dependent body areas for edema.	Excessive fluid retention may be demonstrated by venous engorgement, edema formation. Peripheral edema often begins in feet and ascends upward as failure worsens.
Measure abdominal girth.	When hydrostatic pressure exceeds colloid oncotic pressure, fluid begins to pass through capillary membranes to peritoneal space, resulting in ascites.
Establish fluid intake schedule, and note beverage preferences when possible.	Involves patient in therapy regimen which may enhance sense of control and cooperation with restrictions.
Monitor intake and output. Calculate 24-hour fluid balance.	Diuretic therapy resulting in sudden or excessive fluid reduction may cause hypovolemia, although ascites is still present.
Weigh daily.	Documents increase or decrease in congestion and edema in response to therapy. Gain of 5 pounds represents approximately 2 liters of fluid.
Maintain chair rest or bedrest.	Promotes diuresis by recumbency-induced increase of glomerular filtration and reduction of ADH production.
Elevate feet when sitting.	Enhances venous return and reduces dependent swelling.
Regulate IV fluids with microdrip or infusion pumps.	Prevents sudden expansion of vascular volume which could cause or increase cardiac decompensation.
Note increased lethargy, hypotension, muscle cramping.	Signs of hypokalemia and hyponatremia which may occur owing to fluid shifts and diuretic therapy.
Collaborative	
Monitor chest x-ray examination.	Reveals changes indicative of increase or resolution of congestion.
Administer drugs as indicated: diuretics, for example, furosemide (Lasix), bumetanide (Bumex),	Promotes excretion of fluid by inhibiting reabsorption of sodium and chloride in the renal tubules.
potassium.	Potassium wasting is a common side effect of diuretic therapy, which can adversely affect cardiac function.
Adhere to fluid and sodium restrictions.	May be necessary to reduce total body water to prevent fluid reaccumulation.
Consult with dietician to provide calories within diet restrictions.	Sodium restrictions are common, which may further depress appetite of anorexic patient.

NURSING DIAGNOSIS:	**Gas Exchange, impaired [potential].**
SUPPORTING DATA/CONTRIBUTING FACTORS:	**With myocardial decompensation, LVEDP elevation causes backward pressure in the pulmonary capillaries, forcing fluid into the perialveolar interstitial spaces. As this pressure rises, fluid enters the alveoli, which impairs gas exchange and creates symptoms of pulmonary congestion, edema.**
GENERAL PATIENT OUTCOMES:	**Free of symptoms of respiratory distress. Lung congestion is absent or decreased. ABGs are within patient's normal limits.**

INTERVENTIONS	RATIONALE
Independent	
Monitor respiratory function. Note dyspnea, tachypnea, use of accessory muscles, loud gurgling respirations, cough.	Baseline for documentation of disease progression or positive response to therapy. Irritating, hacky cough is a dominant symptom of congestion of bronchial mucosa.
Assess for symptoms of pulmonary edema, for example, sudden extreme dyspnea—that is, patient sits straight up and feels sensation of suffocation.	Differs from orthopnea and paroxysmal nocturnal dyspnea in that it develops much more rapidly because of extreme pulmonary capillary hypertension.
Auscultate breath sounds.	Rhonchi, wheezes, and moist crepitant crackles reflecting congestion may develop rapidly.
Note profuse sweating; cold, ashen, cyanotic skin.	Reflects sympathetic response to depression of cardiac function and reduced cardiac output, which is further compromised by work of breathing and hypoxia.
Note onset of production of pink, frothy sputum, apprehension, bulging neck veins, PCWP over 25 mmHg.	Pulmonary edema can occur insidiously with intra-alveolar edema or suddenly with elevation of LVEDP.
Elevate head of bed. Alter patient position q1-2h.	Facilitates diaphragmatic descent during inspiration and ventilation of basilar lung areas.
Instruct patient in effective coughing, deep breathing. Suction if indicated.	Clears airways and facilitates oxygen delivery.
Collaborative	
Monitor/graph ABGs.	May show severe hypoxemia during acute pulmonary edema or reveal compensatory changes in chronic CHF patient.
Monitor chest x-rays.	Provides information regarding increase or resolution of congestion. Note: Radiologic evidence of congestion can be delayed up to 24 hours after onset of symptoms.

INTERVENTIONS	RATIONALE
Collaborative	
Administer oxygen as indicated.	Increases alveolar oxygen concentration and may enhance arterial oxygenation to decrease tissue hypoxia. Note: Mechanical ventilation may be required if respiratory failure develops.
Administer drugs as indicated: diuretics, for example, furosemide (Lasix),	Furosemide reduces preload by rapid onset of diuresis (within 5 minutes). Its primary benefit in pulmonary edema is that it produces vasodilation prior to diuresis, which produces immediate preload and afterload reduction.
Vasodilators, for example, sodium nitroprusside (Nipride),	Decreases systemic vascular resistance (SVR), thereby reducing venous return (preload) and pulmonary congestion (lowers PCWP).
Bronchodilators, for example, Aminophylline.	Increases oxygen delivery by dilating small airways; produces mild venodilation, decreases ventricular filling pressure, and exerts mild diuretic effect.
Digitalis preparations, for example, digoxin (Lanoxin),	May reduce pulmonary congestion by enhancing myocardial contractility and cardiac output. Note: Narrow therapeutic range may actually precipitate or worsen pulmonary edema. (Refer to Nursing Diagnosis: Injury, potential for, poisoning, digitalis, page 59.)
Assist with cardioversion if indicated.	May be necessary when pulmonary edema is precipitated by tachydysrhythmias, which are refractory to drug therapy.
Assist with insertion of pacemaker, if indicated.	Bradydysrhythmias unresponsive to drug intervention may aggravate congestive failure or produce pulmonary edema.
Assist with rotating tourniquets, phlebotomy if indicated.	Although not frequently used, these treatments may be carried out to reduce venous return and circulating volume, especially in severe CHF with pulmonary edema refractory to other therapies.

NURSING DIAGNOSIS:	**Skin Integrity, impairment of, potential.**
SUPPORTING DATA/CONTRIBUTING FACTORS:	**Prolonged bedrest, edema, and decreased cardiac output impair circulation to skin.**
GENERAL PATIENT OUTCOMES:	**Skin is warm, dry, intact, free of ulcerations.**

INTERVENTIONS	RATIONALE
Independent	
Inspect skin, noting skeletal prominences, edema, areas of impaired circulation, obesity, emaciation.	Altered skin color in isolated areas may indicate damage caused by pressure or decreased circulation.

INTERVENTIONS	RATIONALE
Independent	
Reposition frequently.	Increases circulation and reduces time that weight deprives any one area of blood flow.
Give frequent skin care. Minimize contact with moisture and excretions.	Excessive dryness or moisture damages skin and hastens breakdown.
Massage reddened or blanched areas.	Massage improves blood flow, minimizing tissue hypoxia.
Avoid intramuscular medication.	May be poorly absorbed owing to tissue edema. Trauma predisposes patient to skin infection and tissue breakdown.
Collaborative	
Provide alternating pressure or egg crate mattress, sheep skin, elbow and heel protectors.	Reduces pressure to skin, may improve circulation.

NURSING DIAGNOSIS:	**Activity Intolerance, actual/potential.**
SUPPORTING DATA/CONTRIBUTING FACTORS:	**Reduced perfusion of skeletal muscles results in anaerobic metabolism, which produces weakness and fatigue.**
GENERAL PATIENT OUTCOMES:	**Achieves measurable increase in activity tolerance, evident by blood pressure, heart and respiratory rates within normal limits. Is free of pain and verbalizes reduction in fatigue.**

INTERVENTIONS	RATIONALE
Independent	
Document cardiovascular response to activity. Note tachycardia, other dysrhythmias, dyspnea, diaphoresis, pallor.	Compromised myocardium is unable to increase stroke volume during activity and may immediately increase heart rate and oxygen demands, thereby aggravating weakness and fatigue.
Check vital signs before and immediately after activity.	Orthostatic hypotension can occur with activity.
Evaluate accelerating activity intolerance.	May denote increasing cardiac decompensation rather than overactivity.
Assess for other causes of fatigue, for example, treatments, pain, medications.	Fatigue is a side effect of some medications (beta blockers, tranquilizers and sedatives). Pain and stressful regimens also extract energy and produce fatigue.
Restrict activity, space with rest periods.	Provides opportunity for myocardial recovery.
Encourage verbalization of feelings regarding limitations.	Expression of concerns may decrease anxiety, which is an energy drain that can contribute to feelings of fatigue.

INTERVENTIONS	RATIONALE
Collaborative	
Follow graded cardiac rehabilitation and activity program.	Gradual increase in activity avoids excessive increase in myocardial work load and oxygen consumption.

NURSING DIAGNOSIS: **Injury, potential for, poisoning, digitalis.**

SUPPORTING DATA/CONTRIBUTING FACTORS: **Digitalis half-life and therapeutic dose range are influenced by a number of diverse factors such as renal function, enterohepatic circulation, muscle mass, and electrolyte balance. In addition, interaction with other drugs (e.g., quinidine, verapamil, and some antibiotics) results in a potentially dangerous situation for patient receiving digitalis preparations.**

GENERAL PATIENT OUTCOMES: **GI distress, visual alterations are absent. Usual mentation is restored. Heart rate and conduction are stabilized.**

INTERVENTIONS	RATIONALE
Independent	
Assess for factors predisposing to toxicity; e.g., Stages III-IV CHF;	In the CHF patient, altered cardiac binding of digitalis may result in toxicity even with previously appropriate drug doses.
Acid-base imbalance, decreased potassium, decreased magnesium, hypoxemia;	These factors may be present in various stages of CHF and may cause a cumulative effect in digitalis level.
Age;	Elderly patients generally have decreased renal function and body weight (muscle mass) affecting digitalis metabolism.
Concomitant use of quinidine preparations, verapamil (Isoptin), antibiotics.	Quinidine usually doubles serum digitalis level. Verapamil frequently causes a 60% increase in digitalis level, and antibiotics can increase it 10-40%.
Assess factors that may alter drug absorption and excretion; that is, small bowel disease, impaired enterohepatic circulation, increased thyroid function, decreased calcium, concomitant use of neomycin sulfate (Neobiotic), magnesium, trisilicate (Trisomin), kaolin and pectin mixture (Kaopectate), cholestyramine (Questrin), sulfasalazine (Azulfidine).	Factors which affect digitalis absorption or decrease its half-life necessitate higher dosage of digitalis to achieve desired effect. If any of these factors are altered or removed (e.g., change in drug therapy) without alteration in digitalis dosage, toxicity can occur.

INTERVENTIONS	RATIONALE
Independent	
Monitor for and review signs/symptoms of toxicity with patient: GI: anorexia, N/V, diarrhea, abdominal discomfort.	Because these symptoms are caused by other pathologic states, including CHF, it may be difficult to diagnose digitalis toxicity.
Visual: altered color perception (especially red and green), flickering color forms, yellow halos.	Although the visual changes are quite characteristic and specific to digitalis toxicity, not all patients report visual disturbances.
Psychic: confusion, disorientation, restlessness, agitation, nightmares, psychosis.	Symptoms vary in individuals and can be difficult to relate to digitalis prior to confirmation of toxicity by laboratory values.
Monitor ECG, document developing conduction blocks, atrial/ventricular arrhythmias.	AV and sinus exit blocks, increasing atrial irritability, supraventricular/ventricular tachycardiacs, and premature beats may reflect digitalis effect. Note: Regularity of ventricular response in atrial fibrillation may indicate developing junctional rhythm secondary to increasing AV block.
Collaborative	
Monitor laboratory studies of organ function impacted by digitalis.	Renal and thyroid function studies, electrolytes, and ABG results may aid in determining response to drug dosage needs.
Monitor serum digitalis level when therapeutic effect is not present, renal function is impaired, or drug interaction or toxicity is suspected.	Useful when evaluated in conjunction with clinical picture and ECG. There is no constant relationship between serum levels and desired therapeutic effect because cardiac concentration of digitalis is several times greater than serum (with a highly variable ratio), and fluctuations in myocardial binding occur.
Obtain 12-lead ECG before and after digitalization.	Digitalis may produce ST wave changes that mimic ischemia.
Administer IV digitalis over several minutes.	Rapid administration may increase peripheral/coronary resistance resulting in adverse clinical effects. Intramuscular (IM) injections are absorbed erratically and may cause undermedication or overmedication.
Administer appropriate antiarrhythmics, for example, Atropine sulfate,	If digitalis toxicity occurs, these drugs may be needed to increase heart rate if bradycardia is present,
Lidocaine hydrochloride (Xylocaine),	Suppress ventricular ectopy,
Procainamide hydrochloride (Pronestyl),	Suppress ventricular ectopy and enhance AV conduction,
Propranolol hydrochloride (Inderal).	Treat ventricular ectopy. Note: This drug can result in worsening of CHF and AV block.
Assist with insertion of temporary pacemaker.	May overdrive high-grade block if drug therapy is unsuccessful.
Avoid cardioversion when toxicity is present unless phenytonin (Dilantin) is given prophylactically first.	May precipitate fatal ventricular dysrhythmias. Dilantin acts on the myocardium by selectively reducing cell's response to stimuli, thereby reducing incidence of dysrhythmias caused by digitalis toxicity and cardioversion.

NURSING DIAGNOSIS:	**Knowledge Deficit [Learning Need].**
SUPPORTING DATA/CONTRIBUTING FACTORS:	**Congestive heart failure is a life-threatening but controllable chronic disease requiring lifestyle adaptations.**
GENERAL PATIENT OUTCOMES:	**Verbalizes understanding of disease and treatment. Begins to participate in planning lifestyle changes.**

INTERVENTIONS	RATIONALE
Independent	
Review symptoms that require immediate medical attention, for example, rapid weight gain, edema, shortness of breath, increased fatigue.	When patient can identify symptoms requiring medical attention, may be more committed to following through with obtaining necessary medical treatment.
Reinforce treatment rationale.	Patient may alter regimen when feeling well and symptom-free, or when feeling "below par." Understanding of regimen, medications, and restrictions may augment cooperation.
Provide information and discuss patient's role in control of risk factors and precipitating or aggravating factors.	Adds to body of knowledge and permits patient to make decisions regarding control of condition.
Give instructions both verbally and in writing.	Anxiety may block comprehension of input or details. Patient may refer to written material at later date to refresh memory.
Provide opportunities for patient and/or family to ask questions, discuss concerns.	Allows for verification of understanding of information that has been given.

Myocardial Infarction

PATIENT ASSESSMENT DATA BASE

HISTORY

History of coronary artery disease (CAD), coronary artery spasm with or without CAD; aortic valve disease.

Associated risk factors, that is, hypertension, family history of heart disease, cigarette smoking, obesity, sedentary lifestyle, diabetes, age (more common after age 55), sex (men show greater incidence than women), tension, stress, type A personality, hyperlipidemia.

Myocardial infarction (MI) may be "silent," with clinical presentation of congestive heart failure, gall bladder attack, unexplained shock, syncopal episode, cerebral vascular incident, or jaw or "dental" problems.

Subjective

Reports pain different from angina in that it is constant (duration 30 minutes or more) and unrelieved by nitroglycerin or rest. Pain is usually substernal and may radiate to shoulders, arms, jaw, neck, epigastrium. May be described as burning, squeezing, aching, crushing, usually described as 10 on scale of 1-10, or the "worst pain ever experienced".

May complain of nausea, indigestion, palpitations.

May be extremely anxious.

PHYSICAL EXAMINATION

Inspection

Skin: pale, diaphoretic; pallor or cyanosis may be noted in nailbeds or around lips.

Respirations may be rapid, shallow, dyspneic.

Jugular vein: distention may be noted with head of bed elevated 45 degrees.

GI: vomiting, retching, belching may be noted.

Nonverbal clues of anxiety (e.g., lack of eye contact, restlessness) may be noted.

Palpation

Skin: cool, moist, clammy.

Pulses may be normal but more often reflect variations in heart rate and cardiac output.

Auscultation

Breath sounds may be normal initially, although adventitious sounds (e.g., crackles) may develop.

Heart sounds may reveal dysrhythmias, extra heart sounds, murmurs of valvular stenosis, insufficiency or papillary muscle dysfunction, friction rub.

Blood pressure: may be normal or hypertension or hypotension may be noted.

DIAGNOSTIC STUDIES

ECG: serial changes show evolution of infarction by T wave changes, ST elevation, and/or Q wave development in leads over the infarcted area. Determination of the age of the infarction may be made by ST and T changes. Chamber enlargements present characteristic changes in P waves (atrial) and R and S waves (ventricular).

Cardiac enzymes and isoenzymes: CPK-MB elevates within 4 to 12 hours and peaks in 24 hours. LDH elevates within 24 to 48 hours, peaks within 3 to 6 days, and may take as long as two weeks to return to normal. SGOT elevations (less reliable/specific) occur in 6 to 12 hours and peak in 36 hours.

WBC: leukocytosis (10,000 to 20,000) reflects inflammatory response to MI.

Electrolytes: imbalance may occur which alters conduction and can compromise contractility (e.g., hypokalemia or hyperkalemia).

Chemistry profiles may be abnormal, depending on acute or chronic abnormal organ function.

ABGs: hypoxemia may be present.

Chest x-ray examination may be normal or show cardiac enlargement.

Echocardiogram: identifies cardiac structure and function, for example, internal dimensions of ventricles, septal and ventricular wall motion, and valve configuration and function.

Scintiography: radionuclide blood pool imaging provides information regarding myocardial perfusion, permitting estimation of size and location of infarction if done within 2 to 6 days. Determines wall motion abnormalities and estimation of ejection fraction.

Coronary arteriography visualizes narrowing or occlusion of coronary arteries and is usually done in conjunction with measurements of chamber pressures and assessment of left ventricular function (ejection fraction). Procedure not usually done in acute phase of MI, unless angioplasty or emergency heart surgery is imminent.

NURSING PRIORITIES

1. Relieve pain, anxiety.
2. Reduce myocardial workload and oxygen demand.
3. Maintain hemodynamic stability.
4. Prevent/minimize complications.
5. Promote self-care and cardiac health.

NURSING DIAGNOSIS:	**Comfort, alteration in, pain, acute.**
SUPPORTING DATA/CONTRIBUTING FACTORS:	**Chest pain associated with acute myocardial infarction is variable, ranging from slight to unbearable. Characteristically, pain is intense and unrelieved by rest or nitroglycerin. Symptoms are produced by ischemia resulting from coronary artery occlusion with loss/restriction of blood flow to an area of the myocardium.**
GENERAL PATIENT OUTCOMES:	**Verbalizes relief/control of pain. Displays reduced tension/relaxed manner.**

INTERVENTIONS	RATIONALE
Independent	
Assess characteristics of pain, noting verbal complaints, nonverbal cues, and hemodynamic response; that is, moaning, crying, restlessness, diaphoresis, clutching chest, rapid breathing, blood pressure and heart rate changes.	Appearance and behavior of patients in pain may vary greatly, presenting a challenge in assessment. Most patients with an acute MI appear acutely ill, distracted, and focused on pain. Verbal history and deeper investigation of precipitating factors should be postponed until pain is relieved. Respirations may be increased as a result of pain and associated anxiety while release

INTERVENTIONS	RATIONALE
Independent	
	of stress-induced catecholamines will increase heart rate and blood pressure.
Obtain full description of pain from patient, including location, intensity (1-10), duration, quality (dull/crushing), and radiation.	Pain is a subjective experience and must be described by the patient. Assist patient to quantify pain by comparing it with other experiences with pain.
Review history of previous angina, anginal equivalent, or myocardial infarction pain, if applicable.	May differentiate preexisting and current pain patterns as well as identify complications such as extension of infarction, pulmonary embolus, or pericarditis.
Instruct patient to report pain immediately.	Delay in reporting pain may hinder pain relief and require increased amounts of medication. In addition, severe pain may induce shock by stimulating sympathetic nervous system.
Provide quiet environment.	Decreases external stimuli, which may aggravate anxiety and cardiac strain and limit coping abilities.
Instruct in relaxation techniques (e.g., abdominal breathing, distraction).	Helpful in decreasing perception of pain. Provides a sense of having some control over the situation.
Check vital signs before and after pain medication.	Hypotension/respiratory depression can occur as a result of narcotic administration.
Collaborative	
Administer IV analgesics (e.g., morphine) in small increments until pain is relieved or maximum dose is achieved.	Morphine is the usual drug of choice to reduce pain, provide sedation, and decrease myocardial workload. Respiratory depression is dose related and pain is usually relieved before respiratory effects are noted. Intramuscular injections can alter creatine phosphokinase (CPK) diagnostic indicator, are not well absorbed in underperfused tissue, and may contribute to drug toxicity when blood pressure returns to more normal levels.
Administer other medications as indicated: nitrates (nitroglycerin);	Nitrates are useful for pain control by coronary vasodilating effects, which increase coronary blood flow and myocardial perfusion. Peripheral vasodilation effects reduce the volume of blood returning to the heart (preload), thereby decreasing myocardial work and oxygen demand.
Beta blockers, for example, propranolol (Inderal);	Beta blockers are important second-line agents for pain control through effect of blocking sympathetic stimulation. They reduce heart rate, lower systolic blood pressure, and reduce myocardial oxygen demand. May be given alone or with nitrates. Note: Beta blockers may be contraindicated if myocardial contractility is severely impaired because of their negative inotropic properties, which further reduce contractility.
Calcium channel blockers, for example, nifidipine (Procardia).	These vasodilators are helpful in reducing pain caused by vasospasm of coronary arteries. They dilate coronary arteries, increase coronary blood flow, encourage collateral circulation, and reduce oxygen demands by inhibiting the influx of calcium through

INTERVENTIONS	RATIONALE
Collaborative	
	the muscle cell. Some of these agents also have antiarrhythmic properties.
Administer supplemental oxygen.	Enhances oxygen delivery to ischemic tissue and may reduce extent of infarction related to myocardial oxygen consumption.

NURSING DIAGNOSIS: **Cardiac Output, alteration in, decreased [potential].**

SUPPORTING DATA/CONTRIBUTING FACTORS: **Location and size of the infarction are critical to effects on ventricular contractility and function. Cardiac output may be impaired by electrical factors (dysrhythmias), mechanical factors altering preload and afterload (i.e., hypovolemia/changes in systemic vascular resistance), or structural defects related to the infarct (i.e., papillary muscle rupture, ventricular aneurysm).**

GENERAL PATIENT OUTCOMES: **Cardiac rate, rhythm, and hemodynamic parameters within normal limits. Dysrhythmias are controlled or absent. Absence of angina with activity.**

INTERVENTIONS	RATIONALE
Independent	
Auscultate blood pressures, compare both arms and lying, sitting, and standing pressures when able.	Hypotension may occur related to hypoperfusion, vagal stimulation, or ventricular dysfunction. However, hypertension is a common phenomenon and may be related to pain, anxiety, catecholamine release, or preexisting vascular problems. Note: Blood pressure tends to be 5 to 15 mmHg higher in right arm in many adults. Orthostatic hypotension may be present, associated with drug therapies or complications of infarct (e.g., congestive heart failure).
Measure hemodynamic pressures if available. Note mean arterial pressure (MAP), pulmonary arterial pressure (PAP), pulmonary capillary wedge pressure (PCWP), cardiac output and index, and systemic vascular resistance (SVR). Note effects of activity on hemodynamic parameters.	Precise determinations of intravascular responses and ventricular function by means of pulmonary and systemic arterial pressure monitoring is often helpful in the complicated MI for management of drug therapy, patient activity, and prevention or early detection of complications of infarction (e.g., extension of MI, heart failure, cardiogenic shock). (Refer to Care Plan: Cardiogenic Shock, page 34.)

INTERVENTIONS	RATIONALE
Independent	
Auscultate heart sounds. Note: splitting of S_1, S_2;	Heart sounds are frequently muffled during acute phase of MI and are more easily assessed during recovery phase. Pathologic splitting of S_1 may occur with premature ventricular contractions (PVCs) and/or right bundle branch blocks. Pathologic splitting of S_2 is related to angina, acute pulmonary embolus, right ventricular failure, PVCs, hypertension, atrial septal defects, and valve disorders.
Development of S_3, S_4;	Indicative of early cardiac decompensation and potential loss of cardiac output. S_3 is usually associated with CHF, but it may also be noted with mitral insufficiency (regurgitation) and left ventricular overload. S_4 may be associated with myocardial ischemia, ventricular stiffening, and pulmonary or systemic hypertension.
Presence, intensity of murmurs or rubs.	Indicates disturbances of normal blood flow within the heart, for example, incompetent valve, septal defect, or vibration of structures (papillary muscle, chordae tendinae). Presence of rub with an infarction is associated with pericardial effusion and pericarditis.
Auscultate breath sounds.	Crackles may develop, reflecting pulmonary congestion related to alterations in myocardial function.
Continuously monitor ECG, noting heart rate and rhythm.	Reveals early trends of developing complications that could compromise hemodynamic stability or increase ischemic damage.
Document dysrhythmias, that is, sinus tachycardia,	Tachycardia is a response to stress, pain, and hypoxia and is the result of decreased vagal tone or increased sympathetic nervous system activity and the release of catecholamines. Persistent tachycardia may worsen underlying pathology in patients with ischemic heart disease because of shortened diastolic filling time and increased oxygen demands.
Sinus bradycardia,	Common in patients with acute myocardial infarction (especially inferior), and the result of excessive parasympathetic activity or decrease in blood flow to the sinus node. Patients with severe heart disease may not be able to compensate for a slow rate by increasing stroke volume. Decreased cardiac output, congestive heart failure, or ventricular dysrhythmias may occur.
Atrial dysrhythmias,	Premature atrial contractions (PACs) occur as a response to ischemia and are normally harmless, but they can precede or precipitate atrial fibrillation. Acute and chronic atrial flutter and/or fibrillation may be seen with coronary artery or valvular disease, and may or may not be pathologic. Rapid atrial fibrillation reduces cardiac output owing to loss of atrial kick as well as insufficient ventricular filling time and increased oxygen demand.

INTERVENTIONS	RATIONALE
Independent	
Ventricular dysrhythmias,	PVCs are a common dysrhythmia reflecting cardiac irritability. When associated with myocardial infarction, PVCs may lead to serious complications. Frequent, multiple, or multifocal PVCs lead to decreased cardiac output and may terminate in ventricular tachycardia or fibrillation and sudden death.
Heart blocks.	Occur with delayed or altered transmission through normal conduction channels and may be result of infarction, reduced blood supply to SA and AV nodes, drug toxicity, cardiac surgery. Progressing heart block is associated with slow ventricular rates and decreased cardiac output and may lead to potentially lethal ventricular dysrhythmias or cardiac standstill.
Promote rest (bed or chair) and limit activity dependent on pain or hemodynamic response. Provide nonstress diversional activities.	Reduces myocardial workload and oxygen consumption, limiting risk of complications, that is, extension of MI, reduction of cardiac output.
Provide small and easily digested meals. Restrict caffeine intake (e.g., coffee, chocolate, cola).	Large meals may increase myocardial workload and cause vagal stimulation, resulting in bradycardia, ectopic beats. Caffeine is direct cardiac stimulant, increasing heart rate.
Collaborative	
Administer supplemental oxygen, as indicated.	Increases amount of oxygen available for myocardial uptake. In some patients supplemental oxygen can increase vascular resistance and reduce cardiac output and should therefore be used with caution.
Administer IV fluids cautiously via minidrip or infusion pump.	Patent access line is important for administration of emergency drugs and pain relief, but inadvertent bolus of large amounts of fluid may lead to pulmonary congestion, cardiac decompensation.
Assist with insertion of hemodynamic pressure monitoring lines (e.g., Swan-Ganz, arterial catheters).	Assists with determinations of cardiac function and response to drug therapies. Provides for early detection of complications such as deleterious effects of dysrhythmias or impending shock.
Review serial 12-lead ECGs.	Provides information regarding location, progression, and resolution of infarction, ventricular function, electrolyte imbalance, and effects of drug therapies.
Review serial chest x-ray examinations.	May reflect pulmonary edema related to ventricular dysfunction.
Monitor laboratory data: cardiac enzymes, ABGs, electrolytes.	Enzymes monitor resolution or extension of infarction. Presence of hypoxia indicates need for supplemental oxygen. Electrolyte imbalance (e.g., hypokalemia or hyperkalemia) adversely affects cardiac rhythm and contractility.
Administer appropriate medications, for example, dobutamine (Dobutrex), nitroglycerin (Nitrostat), furosemide (Lasix);	Cardiac output may be improved by combinations of (1) inotropic agents to increase ventricular contractility and output and reduce cardiac filling pressures;

INTERVENTIONS	RATIONALE
Collaborative	
	(2) vasodilators to decrease systemic vascular resistance, reducing hypertension and pulmonary congestion; and (3) diuretics to decrease preload (used cautiously to prevent decrease of cardiac output related to excessive diuresis).
Antidysrhythmic drugs as indicated:	Dysrhythmias are treated symptomatically except for prophylactic treatment of PVCs, which may be initiated on admission.
Group I: disopyramide (Norpace), procainamide (Pronestyl), quinidine (Quinaglute);	Useful for treatment of atrial and ventricular premature beats, repetitive dysrhythmias (e.g., tachycardias and atrial flutter or fibrillation), by altering both active and passive membrane properties to decrease conduction velocity, excitability, and automaticity. Note: Myocardial depressant/peripheral vasodilator effects may be potentiated when used in conjunction with any drugs possessing similar properties.
Group II: lidocaine (Xylocaine), phenytoin (Dilantin);	Effective for automatic and reentrant ventricular dysrhythmias and for digitalis-induced dysrhythmias. Action depends on the tissue affected and the level of extracellular potassium. Desired result is increased diastolic threshold potential and decreased action potential duration. Note: These drugs may aggravate myocardial depression.
Group III: propranolol (Inderal), nadolol (Corgard),	Beta-adrenergic blockers are effective in decreasing automaticity and abolishing reentrant dysrhythmias involving the AV junction, that is, supraventricular tachycardia, atrial flutter or fibrillation. Note: Negative inotropic or chronotropic effects may exacerbate sinus bradycardia, prolong AV conduction, and cause myocardial depression.
Group IV: bretylium tosylate (Bretylol),	Useful in terminating reentrant ventricular dysrhythmias by lengthening refractory period. Has an antiadrenergic effect of stabilizing sympathetic tone.
Group V: verapamil (Calan), nifedipine (Procardia), diltiazem (Cardiazem),	Calcium blockers alter "slow channel" conduction through junction to decrease ventricular response in supraventricular tachycardia, atrial flutter or fibrillation.
Others: atropine sulfate/isoproteranol hydrochloride (Isuprel).	Useful in treating bradydysrhythmias.
Assist with insertion/maintain pacemaker, when indicated.	Pacing may be a temporary support measure during acute phase or may be needed permanently if infarction severely damages conduction system. Indications for pacing include (1) severe persistent tachycardia or bradycardia with decreased cardiac output, (2) extensive septal damage as seen in anterior/anteroseptal MI with high degree of block progression, (3) inferior MI with transient AV block, or (4) persistent ectopy with hemodynamic compromise.

INTERVENTIONS	RATIONALE
Collaborative	
Prepare for emergency measures, that is, cardioversion, cardiopulmonary resuscitation (CPR), advanced life support, intra-aortic balloon pump, and emergency cardiac surgery.	Sudden coronary occlusion, lethal dysrhythmias, extension of infarct, and unrelenting pain are situations that may precipitate cardiac arrest and require immediate life-saving therapies.

NURSING DIAGNOSIS:	**Tissue Perfusion, alteration in, decreased.**
SUPPORTING DATA/CONTRIBUTING FACTORS:	**Actual interruption of blood flow may occur owing to presence of thrombi or emboli centrally (cardiac) and/or peripherally, resulting in tissue damage. Decreased cardiac output, hypoxia, acidosis, and shock contribute to hypoperfusion of tissues and organs (including heart) and may result in damage or failure.**
GENERAL PATIENT OUTCOMES:	**Hemodynamic stability is achieved, with adequate tissue and organ perfusion, evident by palpable peripheral pulses, warm and dry skin, usual mentation, adequate urine output, absence of respiratory distress.**

INTERVENTIONS	RATIONALE
Independent	
Note changes in mental status; that is, anxiety, confusion, lethargy, stupor, coma.	Cerebral perfusion is directly related to cardiac output and aortic perfusion pressure and is influenced by hypoxia and electrolyte and acid-base variations. Changes in sensorium also may indicate presence of systemic emboli.
Inspect for pallor, cyanosis, mottling, cool, clammy skin. Note changes in quality of peripheral pulse (especially in cannulated extremities).	Vasoconstriction results in decreased tissue perfusion. If uncorrected, the risks of cellular damage and acidosis increase. Localized occurrence of these signs may indicate presence of peripheral arterial embolus/thrombus.
Assess for Homan's sign (pain in calf on dorsiflexion), erythema, edema.	Indicators of thrombophlebitis.
Encourage active and/or passive leg exercises (avoid isometric exercises).	Enhances venous return. Isometric exercises may adversely affect cardiac output by increasing myocardial work and oxygen consumption.

INTERVENTIONS	RATIONALE
Independent	
Monitor respirations; note work of breathing.	Hypoxia and acidosis related to decreased cardiac output and cardiac tissue damage may be reflected by respiratory distress or may indicate pulmonary complications (e.g., atelectasis, embolus).
Assess gastrointestinal function; that is, decreased or absent bowel sounds, nausea, vomiting, abdominal distention, constipation.	Vasomotor response associated with reduced perfusion to mesentery can produce abdominal pain, nausea, and loss of peristalsis, resulting in development of ileus. Problems may be aggravated by use of narcotic analgesics and immobility.
Note changes in hourly and daily urine output. Record specific gravity.	Urinary output less than 20 to 30 ml per hour may reflect reduced renal perfusion, glomerular filtration, as a result of reduced cardiac output, hypotension, or loss of fluid into interstitial spaces. Specific gravity measurements reflect hydration status as well as renal function.
Collaborative	
Monitor laboratory data (e.g., ABGs, BUN, creatinine, electrolytes).	Reflects organ perfusion and function.
Administer thrombolytic agents, for example, streptokinase (Streptase), per protocol. Monitor for adverse reaction (e.g., bleeding, hematoma at site, bradycardia, allergic reactions).	In selected patients, intracoronary or peripheral infusion of streptokinase is given to lyse clots within coronary artery, thereby increasing blood flow to ischemic myocardial tissue.
Administer heparin/warfarin sodium (Coumadin) as indicated.	Low-dose heparin may be given prophylactically in high-risk patients (i.e., atrial fibrillation, obesity, ventricular aneurysm, or history of thrombophlebitis) to reduce risk of thrombophlebitis or mural thrombus formation. Heparin is used after streptokinase infusion to prevent recurrent thrombus formation. Coumadin is usually drug of choice for long-term, post-discharge anticoagulant therapy.
Provide preprocedure and postprocedure care for percutaneous transluminal coronary angioplasty (PTCA), including continuous ECG monitoring and evaluation of chest pain.	PTCA may be performed to increase coronary blood flow by compression of atheromatous lesions and dilatation of vessel lumen in an occluded coronary artery. Postprocedure care is similar to that of postcatheterization care, although this procedure is usually done for patients with impending or early myocardial ischemia that may progress to infarction.
Apply antiembolic hose.	Limits venous stasis, improves venous return, and reduces risk of thrombophlebitis in patient who is limited in activity.
Insert nasogastric tube if indicated.	Nausea and vomiting may subside with pain relief. However, if symptoms persist or progress, nasogastric tube may be indicated to decompress stomach.
Administer cimetadine (Tagamet), ranitidine (Zantac), antacids.	Reduces or neutralizes gastric acid, preventing discomfort and gastric irritation.

NURSING DIAGNOSIS:	**Activity Intolerance, actual/potential.**
SUPPORTING DATA/CONTRIBUTING FACTORS:	**Imbalance between myocardial oxygen supply and demand, as well as cardiac depressant effect of certain medications (beta blockers), may result in adverse physiologic responses to activity.**
GENERAL PATIENT OUTCOMES:	**Achieves measurable increase in tolerance for activity, evident by blood pressure, heart and respiratory rates within therapeutic limits. Absence of cyanosis, diaphoresis, and pain.**

INTERVENTIONS	RATIONALE
Independent	
Assess hemodynamic response to activity. (Refer to Nursing Diagnosis: Cardiac Output, page 65.)	Trends determine patient's response to increase in activity.
Monitor ECG and document dysrythmias. Correlate with complaints of pain or dyspnea.	Indicators of myocardial oxygen deprivation that may require decrease in activity, changes in medications, use of supplemental oxygen.
Implement and review programmed increases in levels of activity with gradual resumption of activities (e.g., walking, work, and sexual activity).	Gradual increase in activity increases strength and prevents overexertion, enhances collateral circulation, and restores normal lifestyle as much as possible.
Review symptoms requiring reduction in activity and notification of health care provider.	Pulse elevations beyond established patient limits and development of chest pain or dyspnea may indicate need for alterations in exercise regimen or medication changes.
Collaborative	
Refer to cardiac rehabilitation program.	Provides continued support/supervision postdischarge.

NURSING DIAGNOSIS:	**Fluid Volume, alteration in [fluctuation].**
SUPPORTING DATA/CONTRIBUTING FACTORS:	**Fluid excess may occur owing to myocardial failure (CHF) or renal dysfunction with sodium and/or water retention. Inadequate circulating volume may occur as a result of vasodilation (increased vascular bed), fluid shifts, excessive vomiting or diaphoresis, inadequate fluid replacement, or overdiuresis.**

GENERAL PATIENT OUTCOMES:	**Fluid balance is maintained as shown by blood pressure and heart rate within normal limits. Lungs are clear. Balanced intake and output, with absence of tissue edema.**

INTERVENTIONS	RATIONALE
Independent	
Measure hemodynamic pressures (e.g., CVP, PCWP, MAP). Compare with cuff blood pressures.	Provides information regarding fluid balance which may be apparent prior to clinical manifestations, that is, changes in urine output or weight.
Monitor blood pressures sitting, lying, standing, if possible.	Labile blood pressure or orthostatic hypotension often accompanies hypovolemia.
Auscultate breath sounds for presence of crackles.	May indicate cardiac decompensation with developing pulmonary edema.
Note jugular venous distention (JVD), development of dependent edema.	Signs of increasing cardiac decompensation. JVD is also noted in right ventricular infarction without CHF.
Monitor intake and output. Note 24-hour balance. Measure specific gravity.	Comparison of 24-hour totals identifies trends in fluid balance. Increasing specific gravity with decreasing output indicates dehydration or hypovolemia.
Record weight daily.	Weight increases with volume overload or CHF. Sudden drop may indicate excessive losses.
Collaborative	
Maintain total fluid intake at 2000 ml per 24 hours within cardiovascular tolerance.	Meets normal body fluid needs but may require alteration or restriction to avoid fluid excess.
Administer IV fluids per pump or microdrip.	Maintains patency of intravenous route while limiting fluid load.
Provide low-sodium diet, beverages.	Sodium enhances fluid retention and should therefore be restricted.
Administer diuretics, for example, furosemide (Lasix), spironolactone (Aldactone). Monitor potassium as indicated.	May be necessary to correct fluid overload. Drug choice is usually dependent on acute or chronic nature of symptoms. Note: Hypokalemia may result with use of potassium-depleting diuretics.

NURSING DIAGNOSIS:	**Anxiety/Fear.**
SUPPORTING DATA/CONTRIBUTING FACTORS:	**Patients experiencing an acute myocardial infarction display symptoms of extreme anxiety which may initially be associated with fear of dying and severe pain. Anxiety may precipitate or aggravate chest pain and associated symptoms of restlessness and tachycardia. Extreme anxi-**

	ety may adversely affect cardiac function, leading to complications (e.g., coronary spasm, dysrhythmias).
GENERAL PATIENT OUTCOMES:	**Anxiety/fear is reduced to manageable level. Demonstrates appropriate range of feelings and initial signs of effective coping, such as participation in treatment regimen.**

INTERVENTIONS	RATIONALE
Independent	
Identify and acknowledge patient's perception of situation. Do not deny feelings. Explain measures being taken to reduce pain. Maintain confident manner without false reassurance.	Coping with pain and emotional trauma of an MI is difficult. Patient may fear death and/or be anxious about immediate environment. Natural defense mechanisms of shock, denial, and anger will affect responses and ability to assimilate information. Patient and family also may be affected by anxiety or uneasiness displayed by health team members.
Accept, but do not reinforce, expressions of denial.	Denial may be beneficial in decreasing anxiety in acute phase of illness.
Orient patient and significant other(s) to procedures and expected activity. Repeat information frequently.	Patient is in unfamiliar surroundings and being subjected to numerous procedures while experiencing pain. Attention span is short, and time perception may be altered.
Answer questions factually; do not avoid questions. Provide consistent information.	Accurate information about the situation reduces fear, strengthens patient-nurse relationship, assists patient and significant other(s) to deal realistically with situation.
Reinforce idea that frequent assessments do not necessarily imply deterioration of condition.	Patient may feel reassured to know that frequent assessments may prevent development of more serious complications.
Encourage patient and significant other(s) to communicate.	Sharing information elicits support and comfort and can relieve tension of unexpressed worries.
Provide for rest periods and uninterrupted sleep time.	Enhances energy and coping mechanisms as well as reducing myocardial workload and oxygen consumption.
Collaborative	
Administer sedatives and hypnotics as indicated, e.g., diazepam (Valium), flurazepam hydrochloride (Dalmane), lorazepam (Ativan).	Anxiety associated with pain may disappear when pain is relieved. Ongoing anxiety related to concerns about impact of heart attack on future lifestyle, matters left unresolved, and effects of illness on family may be present in varying degrees for some time and may be manifested by symptoms of depression (insomnia, hostility, withdrawal) and/or denial (inappropriate affect or refusal to comply with medical regimen).

NURSING DIAGNOSIS:	**Bowel Elimination, alteration in, constipation [potential].**
SUPPORTING DATA/CONTRIBUTING FACTORS:	**Restricted activity, decreased fluid intake, alterations in dietary bulk, loss of privacy, and some medications contribute to loss of intestinal motility.**
GENERAL PATIENT OUTCOMES:	**Reestablish and maintain normal bowel functioning.**

INTERVENTIONS	RATIONALE
Independent	
Promote adequate fluid intake, including fruit juice.	Fluids, especially fruit juices, change the consistency of stool and improve movement through intestinal tract.
Encourage increased activity, within individual's restrictions.	Enhances intestinal motility.
Provide privacy and bedside commode or bathroom if possible.	Sitting down with feet on floor is most physiologically effective position for elimination and promotes psychologic comfort.
Instruct patient on importance of not straining at stool.	Valsalva maneuver, which requires holding breath and bearing down, causes bradycardia and temporarily decreases cardiac output. Rebound tachycardia, elevated blood pressure, cerebral infarct, and cardiac arrest are possible complications.
Collaborative	
Administer stool softeners as indicated.	Stool softeners decrease myocardial workload of straining at stool.

NURSING DIAGNOSIS:	**Knowledge Deficit [Learning Need].**
SUPPORTING DATA/CONTRIBUTING FACTORS:	**Many patients and significant others have a general lack of factual information regarding cardiac functioning and implications of heart disease and health status. This lack of knowledge limits ability to make informed choices regarding therapy and rehabilitation.**
GENERAL PATIENT OUTCOMES:	**Verbalizes understanding of disease process and treatment and begins to identify possible changes in lifestyle for discharge.**

INTERVENTIONS	RATIONALE
Independent	
Orient to unit, procedures, and equipment on an ongoing basis from admission.	Establishes expectation that this will be a "learning experience."
Assess patient's and significant other's level of knowledge and ability and desire to learn.	Necessary for creation of individual teaching plan.
Be alert to signs of avoidance, for example, changing subject away from information being presented or extremes of behavior (withdrawal, euphoria).	Denial of significance of situation can be a block to learning. Changing to a less formal or less structured style may be more effective until patient and significant other(s) are ready to accept current situation.
Present information in varied learning formats, for example, programmed books, audio-visual tapes, question-and-answer sessions.	Utilizing multiple learning methods enhances retention of material.
Review disease, risk factors, initial dietary and activity restrictions, medications, and symptoms requiring medical attention.	Information helpful in providing opportunity for patient to assume control and to participate in treatment regimen.
Encourage reduction of risk factors (e.g., smoking, alcohol consumption).	These behaviors and chemicals have direct adverse effects on cardiovascular function.
Warn against isometric activity, Valsalva maneuver, and activity requiring arms positioned above head.	These activities greatly increase cardiac work and myocardial oxygen consumption and may adversely affect myocardial contractility and output.
Identify alternate activities for "bad weather" days, such as walking in house or shopping mall.	Provides continuing daily activity program.
Document patient's and significant other's progress through teaching program, noting strengths and areas of weakness.	Permits other caregivers to continue program from shift to shift and after transfer to other units.
Stress importance of followup care and identify community resources and support groups (e.g., cardiac rehabilitation programs, "Coronary Clubs," smoking cessation clinics).	Emphasizes that this is a continuing health problem for which support and assistance is available postdischarge.

CHAPTER 4
RESPIRATORY

Adult Respiratory Distress Syndrome (ARDS)

ARDS may occur in previously healthy persons with a history of some event producing stress on the lung and resulting in lung insult/injury.

PATIENT ASSESSMENT DATA BASE

HISTORY

Commonly associated with the following conditions:

Trauma: thoracic or nonthoracic.

Sepsis.

Diffuse pulmonary infections: viral, bacterial, fungal.

Hematologic disorders: DIC, blood transfusions, cardiopulmonary bypass.

Immunologic response to host antigens: for example, Goodpasture's, SLE.

Metabolic disorders (e.g., pancreatitis).

Systemic reactions to processes initiated outside the lung, for example, shock, amniotic fluid or fat emboli.

Drug overdose: heroin, methadone, morphine.

Aspiration: gastric contents, water with near-drowning.

Inhaled toxins: smoke, chemicals, high concentration of oxygen.

Subjective

Sudden onset of dyspnea

PHYSICAL EXAMINATION

Physical findings vary, depending on the stage at which the diagnosis is made.

Early signs are often missed because abnormal physical findings are not evident until later stages.

ARDS has been described as presenting in four progressive stages: Stage 1: initial insult with successful resuscitation and mild respiratory alkalosis.

Stage 2: latent period with circulatory stabilization but developing respiratory difficulty.

Stage 3: worsening pulmonary insufficiency.

Stage 4: terminal hypoxia/hypercarbia.

Inspection

Respiratory pattern: rate greater than 30 breaths per minute, grunting respirations, increased work of breathing, use of accessory muscles, intercostal or suprasternal retractions, and nasal flaring.

Skin: pallor or cyanosis may be noted.

CNS effects: restlessness, anxiety, irritability, or obtundation (result of hypoxia and hypercarbia).

Palpation

Chest: possible unequal or decreased excursion. Increased fremitus may be noted associated with fluid-filled alveoli or consolidation.

Percussion

Chest: dullness over consolidated areas.

Ausculation

Blood pressure: adequate or elevated initially. Hypertension may occur as the cardiovascular system attempts to compensate for progressing hypoxemia. Hypotension occurs in later stages owing to shock.

Heart sounds may be normal in early stages. S_2 (pulmonic component) may develop as pulmonary hypertension occurs.

Breath sounds may be normal initially. Crackles, rhonchi, and bronchial breath sounds may develop.

DIAGNOSTIC STUDIES

Chest x-ray examination: unremarkable in initial stages or minimal scattered interstitial infiltrates or microatelectasis present. In later stages, diffuse bilateral interstitial and alveolar infiltrates become evident, eventually involving all five lobes.

ABGs: progressing hypoxemia (PaO_2 less than 55 mm Hg) occurs. Hypocapnia may be present in initial stages due to compensatory hyperventilation. Hypercapnia reflects deterioration. Respiratory alkalosis (pH greater than 7.45) may be noted in initial stages, but respiratory acidosis occurs in later stages because of increased deadspace and decreased alveolar ventilation. Metabolic acidosis may occur in later stages owing to rising lactate levels, resulting from anaerobic metabolism.

Pulmonary function tests: lung compliance and lung volumes are decreased, especially functional residual capacity (FRC); and increasing deadspace (V_D/V_T) is produced by areas where vasoconstriction and microemboli have occurred.

Shunt measurement ($\dot{Q}s/\dot{Q}t$): progressively increasing right-to-left shunt occurs (greater than 20 percent of cardiac output) as measured on 100 percent FIO_2.

Alveoloar-arterial gradient (A-a DO_2): increased in later stages, reflecting increasing difficulty with which oxygen crosses alveolar-capillary membrane.

Cardiac output: increased in initial stages owing to system compensating for hypoxia; decreased later owing to loss of compensating mechanisms, and/or shock.

Pulmonary capillary wedge pressure (PCWP): elevated if pulmonary hypertension and/or edema is present.

NURSING PRIORITIES

1. Promote optimal respiratory function and oxygenation.
2. Restore and maintain fluid balance, acid-base, and electrolytes.
3. Minimize/prevent complications.
4. Maintain adequate nutrition for healing and respiratory function.
5. Provide for emotional support of patient and family.

NURSING DIAGNOSIS:	**Airway Clearance, ineffective.**
SUPPORTING DATA/CONTRIBUTING FACTORS:	**During initial stage of adult respiratory distress syndrome (ARDS), an insult reduces perfusion of the cilia. This hypoperfusion, coupled with hypoventilation and hypoxia, limits the ability of the cilia to clear the airways. An increase in the amount and viscosity of pulmonary secretions further compounds this problem. As the syndrome progresses, airway resistance is increased by the premature closure of small airways secondary to developing interstitial edema.**
GENERAL PATIENT OUTCOMES:	**Patent airway is maintained. Secretions remain fluid and are readily expectorated.**

INTERVENTIONS	RATIONALE
Independent	
Note characteristics of breath sounds. (Refer to Nursing Diagnosis: Gas Exchange, impaired, page 80.)	Breath sounds reflect air flow through the tracheobronchial tree and are affected by the presence of fluid, mucus, or obstruction to air flow.
Maintain patent upper airways by proper positioning. use airway adjuncts as needed.	Altered levels of consciousness, sedation and maxiofacial trauma are some conditions that alter patient's ability to protect airway and to require intervention.
Provide pulmonary toilet (e.g., coughing, deep breathing, repositioning, and suctioning).	Improves drainage of pooled secretions, which decreases ventilation and predisposes to the development of atelectasis and possible pulmonary infections.
Collaborative	
Monitor and graph serial ABGs.	Evaluates oxygenation and ventilation status.
Administer humidified oxygen therapy.	Oxygen is administered to maintain the PaO_2 at 60 to 70 mm Hg. Humidity loosens secretions and moisturizes mucous membranes.

INTERVENTIONS	RATIONALE
Collaborative	
Provide aerosol therapy, ultrasonic nebulization, intermittent positive-pressure breathing (IPPB).	Treatments may be initiated to forcefully deliver oxygen bronchodilation, and humidity to alveoli and to mobilize secretions.
Administer chest physiotherapy, as indicated.	Gravity and percussion promote drainage of secretions from segmental bronchi into central bronchi where they may more readily be coughed or suctioned out.
Assist with broncoscopy if indicated.	Scope may be passed to visualize airways and to remove mucous plugs.

NURSING DIAGNOSIS: **Gas Exchange, impaired.**

SUPPORTING DATA/CONTRIBUTING FACTORS: **Alveolar-capillary injury results in increased capillary permeability which permits protein and fluid to leak into interstitial and alveolar spaces, impeding gas diffusion. Marked alveolar hypoventilation produces ventilation and perfusion mismatches, increasing deadspace and intrapulmonary shunting. Damage to Type II pneumocytes inactivates surfactant or reduces surfactant production, which increases alveolar surface tension, causing alveolar collapse and decreased lung compliance. In addition, pulmonary vasoconstriction may occur as a result of humoral substances and hypoxemia. At the cellular level, release of oxygen is impeded in Stages 1 and 2 owing to a shift of the oxyhemoglobin curve secondary to respiratory alkalosis and decreased $PaCO_2$. In Stages 3 and 4, oxygen release is still impeded as decreasing PaO_2 alters the pressure gradient required for oxygen to pass from the blood to interstitial fluid and cells and results in further tissue hypoxia.**

GENERAL PATIENT OUTCOMES: **Adequate oxygenation and ventilation is shown by ABGs, A-a gradient, and shunt measurement within patient's normal limits. Signs of respiratory distress are absent.**

INTERVENTIONS	RATIONALE
Independent	
Assess respiratory status frequently:	Detects early signs of respiratory deterioration.
Note increased respiratory rate, and effort or changes in breathing pattern.	Tachypnea is a compensatory mechanism for hypoxia. Intercostal retractions and nasal flaring reflect increased respiratory effort.
Note decrease in chest excursion and increase in fremitus.	Chest excursion may be unequal or limited because of accumulation of fluid, edema, and secretions in lung segments. Palpation may reveal increased fremitus, indicating fluid-filled areas.
Note presence of adventitious sounds, e.g., crackles, wheezes, pleural friction rub.	Crackles are evidence of increased fluid in tissue spaces as a result of increased alveolar-capillary membrane permeability. Wheezes may be evidence of bronchoconstriction and/or airway narrowing owing to mucus or edema. Friction rub reflects an area of pleural inflammation as may be seen in pneumonia, pulmonary infarction, or pleurisy.
Assess for presence of cyanosis.	Usually a significant drop in oxygenation is required before cyanosis appears. Central cyanosis of tongue and lips is most indicative for systemic hypoxemia. Peripheral cyanosis of extremities is associated with vasoconstriction.
Monitor cardiac rhythm, document dysrythmias.	Hypoxemia often causes irritability of the myocardium, producing a variety of dysrythmias, both atrial and ventricular in origin. Sympathetic stimulation triggered by hypoxemia may lead to tachydysrythmias. Acidosis may depress myocardial automaticity and produce bradydysrythmias.
Monitor intake and output, note effects of fluid administration and diuresis. (Refer to Nursing Diagnosis: Fluid Volume, alteration in [fluctuation], page 82.)	Balance is needed between decreasing total lung water to enhance ventilation and perfusion, while maintaining intravascular volume so as not to jeopardize perfusion of vital organs.
Monitor bronchodilator (e.g., Sus-Phrine, Aminophylline) administration and watch for side effects: nausea, vomiting, tachycardia, hypertension, tremor, insomnia.	Given to improve ventilation and to aid in removal of secretions. Drugs may be sympathomimetics or xanthines, which potentiate or are potentiated by numerous other drugs. Rapid infusion may cause severe side effects.
Collaborative	
Assist with intubation.	Due to the progressive nature of ARDS, early intubation is advised because it allows more control of the pulmonary parameters. The endotracheal tube should have an adequate internal diameter to facilitate suctioning and to decrease resistance to airflow.
Maintain mechanical ventilation. (Refer to Care Plan: Ventilatory Assistance, mechanical, page 115.)	Ventilatory support is suggested when the PaO_2 is less than 60 mm Hg despite FIO_2s greater than 0.5. High tidal volumes are required to prevent further atelectasis and to reduce hypoxemia (10 to 15 ml per kg of body weight). High inspiratory and end-expiratory pressures (PEEP) are often needed to improve gas exchange and to allow use of lower FIO_2s.

INTERVENTIONS	RATIONALE
Collaborative	
Monitor hemodynamic indices of pulmonary function e.g., mixed venous PO_2, pulmonary artery pressure (PAP), pulmonary capillary wedge pressure (PCWP).	Mixed venous PO_2, arterial blood gases, PAP, and PCWP provide data for calculating intrapulmonary shunting. When these measurements are combined with cardiac output (CO), they provide information for regulating PEEP in order to enhance oxygenation without compromising CO and tissue perfusion.
Review serial chest x-ray examinations.	May show pulmonary congestion, cardiac enlargement, pneumothorax. Verifies placement of hemodynamic monitoring lines and endotracheal tube.
Monitor serial ABGs.	Reflects ventilation, oxygenation status. Used as basis for changes in ventilator and other therapies.
Administer medications as indicated: Aerosol therapy: Bronchodilators and beta stimulators, e.g., metaproterenol sulfate (Alupent), isoetharine hydrochloride (Bronkosol),	Bronchodilators given with saline per aerosol enhance mucociliary drainage of secretions and smooth muscle relaxation.
Diuretics, for example, furosemide (Lasix),	Given for elevated pulmonary pressures or volume overload. Reduces interstitial edema by decreasing intravascular volume and hydrostatic pressure.
Sodium bicarbonate,	Used with caution to correct acidosis. Note: May interfere with oxygen release at the cellular level and thus actually increase tissue hypoxia.
Steroids, for example, methylprednisolone (Medrol),	May be of benefit in reducing inflammation by decreasing total peripheral resistance; decreasing alveolar and capillary permeability; increasing RBC 2, 3, DPG (enhances oxygen delivery); and promoting surfactant production.
Antibiotics,	Retard bacterial growth and may prevent the development of sepsis.
Anticoagulants, such as low-dose heparin.	May be used to prevent pulmonary emboli for patient at risk.
Administer intravenous (IV) fluids, as indicated, for example, crystalloids, packed red cells.	Maintains hydrostatic pressure and improves oncotic pressure to prevent or reduce pulmonary edema and reduce hypoxemia.

NURSING DIAGNOSIS:	**Fluid Volume, alteration in [fluctuation].**
SUPPORTING DATA/CONTRIBUTING FACTORS:	**With ARDS, fluid regulation is a delicate balance. Diuretics are used to reduce intravascular hydrostatic pressure and pulmonary edema. This reduction in vascular volume coupled with the possible compromise of cardiac output from PEEP, may jeopardize the perfusion of vital organs and tissues. However, overhydration can**

	worsen pulmonary edema and induce cardiogenic pulmonary edema.
GENERAL PATIENT OUTCOMES:	**Blood pressure, pulse, hemodynamic pressures, weight, and urine output are within patient's normal limits. Lung sounds are clearing.**

INTERVENTIONS	RATIONALE
Independent	
Note signs and symptoms of decreased cardiac output: elevated pulse, decreased blood pressure (BP), changes in mentation, decreased urine output.	Movement of fluid from intravascular to interstitial space can lead to decreased cardiac output and tissue perfusion.
Assess for signs of fluid overload and edema: increased crackles, respiratory distress, dependent and/or periorbital edema.	Early detection of overhydration may prevent cardiac decompensation, pulmonary edema.
Monitor hourly and daily total intake and output.	Evaluates fluid balance and renal perfusion. Desirable urine output is at least 20 to 30 ml per hour.
Weigh daily.	Monitors retention of fluids and effectiveness of diuretic therapy.
Monitor hemodynamic parameters: mean arterial pressure (MAP),	Indicator of cardiac and systemic vascular response to fluid volume, vasoactive drugs, and effects of PEEP.
Pulmonary artery pressure (PAP),	Tissue edema, fluid collection, and the increased airway pressure associated with decreased lung compliance causes pulmonary hypertension which is reflected by elevated pulmonary artery pressures.
Pulmonary capillary wedge pressure (PCWP),	Reflects left ventricular function and is useful in determining response to fluids, diuretics, vasopressors, and vasodilators. PCWP may be severely elevated in cardiogenic pulmonary edema owing to left ventricular failure.
Cardiac output, cardiac index (CO/CI).	CO reflects efficiency of the pump and may be used to indicate fluid needs and to monitor effects of replacement therapy. CI corrects for body size and is therefore a more specific indicator of cardiac function.
Collaborative	
Administer IV fluids as indicated.	Restores circulatory volume and osmotic pressure. Use of colloid solutions is controversial because they are thought by some to increase extravascular lung water. Crystolloids are less expensive than colloids and may be just as effective.
Monitor/replace electrolytes as indicated.	Sodium and potassium may be depleted as a result of diuretic therapy.
Assist with insertion of pulmonary artery catheter.	Allows monitoring of PAP, PCWP, CO/CI. (Refer to Care Plan: Cardiogenic Shock, page 34.)

NURSING DIAGNOSIS:	**Tissue Perfusion, alteration in (specify).**
SUPPORTING DATA/CONTRIBUTING FACTORS:	**Multiple factors affecting tissue perfusion may be present. Venous return and cardiac output may be reduced by increased intrathoracic pressure and use of PEEP, vascular pooling associated with shock state, and the use of diuretic therapy to reduce pulmonary edema.**
GENERAL PATIENT OUTCOMES:	**Tissue perfusion is maintained as shown by alert mental status, warm and dry skin, absence of dysrythmias, and adequate urine output.**

INTERVENTIONS	RATIONALE
Independent	
Monitor hemodynamic status as noted previously in Nursing Diagnosis: Fluid Volume, alteration in [fluctuations], page 82.	Numerical indicators of systemic perfusion.
Note findings related to decreased perfusion, for example, cool and moist skin, pallor, peripheral cyanosis.	Reflects compensatory peripheral vasoconstriction which permits oxygenated blood to be shunted to vital organs.
Note changes in mental status, (e.g., listlessness, restlessness, anxiety).	Hypotension and respiratory failure may lead to cerebral hypoxia and alterations in level of consciousness.
Monitor cardiac rhythm, note dysrhythmias.	Systemic hypotension or reduced oxygen delivery to the myocardium can produce a variety of ectopics and dysrythmias.
Assess bowel sounds, abdominal girth, nausea, vomiting, constipation, presence of blood in gastric contents.	Sympathetic stimulation produces vasoconstriction and decreased peristalsis of the gastrointestinal (GI) tract and can result in ischemia of the mucosa of the stomach and/or bowel.
Monitor hourly urine output. Note specific gravity.	Hourly output less than 20 to 30 ml per hour may indicate decreased renal perfusion. Renal tubular ischemia and/or (SIADH) may result if hypoxemia and vasoconstriction are prolonged.
Collaborative	
Administer IV fluids, blood products.	Fluids and blood products reverse effects of hypovolemia and hypotension and increase blood flow to tissues, thereby improving tissue oxygenation.
Administer drugs as indicated:	
dopamine hydrochloride (Intropin),	Enhances tissue perfusion by constricting peripheral

INTERVENTIONS	RATIONALE
Collaborative	
	vessels to increase venous return and cardiac output, dilates renal and mesenteric vessels, and increases systolic blood pressure.
Vasodilators: for example, nitroglycerin (Nitrostat IV), and nitroprusside sodium (Nipride),	May be used to enhance peripheral perfusion but require caution because they can increase right-to-left shunt through dilation of pulmonary vasculature.
Cimetidine (Tagamet),	Histamine H_2 antagonist. Reduces hydrochloric acid (produced in response to stress) and possibility of GI bleed.
Antacids.	Neutralizes hydrochloric acid.
Monitor serum lactate levels and pH.	Decreased tissue perfusion results in anaerobic metabolism, raising lactate levels and producing metabolic acidosis.
Monitor BUN, creatinine, and serum/urine electrolytes.	Decreased perfusion of the kidneys reduces filtration and excretion, causing elevation of BUN and creatinine levels and producing electrolyte imbalance.
Insert/maintain nasogastric tube.	Decreases production/prevents accumulation of hydrochloric acid and pancreatic stimulation or release of enzymes.

NURSING DIAGNOSIS:	**Nutrition, alteration in, less than body requirements.**
SUPPORTING DATA/CONTRIBUTING FACTORS:	**At a time when patient experiences altered ability to ingest/properly digest food, increased calories/protein are needed to meet the energy requirements induced by stress, healing, and weaning from the ventilator.**
GENERAL PATIENT OUTCOMES:	**Nutritional intake is adequate to meet metabolic needs as shown by positive nitrogen balance and weight maintained within patient's usual range.**

INTERVENTIONS	RATIONALE
Independent	
Assess GI function. (Refer to Nursing Diagnosis: Tissue Perfusion, page 84.)	Affects choice of route for nutritional support.
Collaborative	
Administer dextrose solutions/multivitamin additions.	Intravenous source of glucose and vitamins which have been depleted. Note: Carbohydrate content

INTERVENTIONS	RATIONALE
Collaborative	
	must be considered so as not to increase CO_2 production, especially when weaning from ventilator.
Provide hyperalimentation, tube feedings. (Refer to Care Plan: Nutritional Support, page 367.)	Supplements nutritional needs.

NURSING DIAGNOSIS:	**Anxiety/Fear.**
SUPPORTING DATA/CONTRIBUTING FACTORS:	**ARDS has a sudden and unexpected onset, usually in a previously healthy individual, and prognosis for survival is only about 50 percent. The resulting respiratory distress in combination with many other factors associated with the critical care environment (sensory deprivation or overload, sleep deprivation, concerns about the unknown, and powerlessness in the situation) may eventually lead to loss of effective coping behaviors.**
GENERAL PATIENT OUTCOMES:	**Remains oriented and alert. Depression/psychotic behavior is prevented or minimized. Verbalizes/indicates awareness of feelings. Demonstrates appropriate range of feelings, decreased tension/relaxed manner.**

(Refer to Care Plan: Psychosocial Aspects of Critical Care, page 379.)

NURSING DIAGNOSIS:	**Injury, potential for, multiple factors.**
SUPPORTING DATA/CONTRIBUTING FACTORS:	**Potential exists for injury from many factors, including complications of ARDS or its treatment modalities, that is, nosocomial pulmonary infections, pulmonary emboli, barotrauma, sepsis, DIC, GI hemorrhage, ileus, and renal failure. Other factors that provide a potential for injury are malnutrition, immobility, intravessel lines, and nephrotoxic drugs.**
GENERAL PATIENT OUTCOMES:	**Complications are prevented.**

INTERVENTIONS	RATIONALE
Independent	
Suction only when necessary, using intermittent suction when withdrawing catheter, and limiting amount of negative pressure.	Vigorous or frequent suctioning can cause trauma to trachea.
Observe for signs of barotrauma, for example, subcutaneous emphysema, pneumothorax, asymmetrical chest movements, diminished or absent breath sounds on affected side, displacement of trachea away from the affected side, tachycardia, cyanosis, hypotension. (Refer to Care Plan: Ventilatory Assistance (mechanical), page 115.)	High inspiratory pressure and the use of PEEP make the possibility of barotrauma more likely in the patient with ARDS. May require chest tube placement.
Monitor for GI bleeding, ileus. (Refer to Nursing Diagnosis: Tissue Perfusion, page 84.)	Alteration in perfusion or peristalsis may result in complications.
Monitor for renal failure. (Refer to Care Plan: Acute Renal Failure, page 207.)	Alteration in renal perfusion/use of nephrotoxic drugs may result in failure.
Use proper handwashing and sterile technique.	Inhibits bacterial contamination.
Provide meticulous skin care.	Patient who is immobilized for many days is prone to skin breakdown.
Provide soft limb restraints, keep siderails up.	May be disoriented or stuporuous and attempt to extubate self.
Collaborative	
Monitor serum drug levels.	Give minimum amount to produce therapeutic response and thereby reduce hazard of toxicity.
Monitor coagulation studies.	Used to regulate anticoagulant therapy. Alterations may indicate development of DIC. (Refer to Care Plan: Disseminated Intravascular Coagulation, page 319.)
Administer antibiotics, as indicated by culture, sensitivities.	Prevents, treats infection.
Administer low-dose heparin.	May prevent thrombus formation, pulmonary emboli.
Provide special devices to reduce skin pressure (e.g., "egg crate" mattress, alternating pressure beds).	Enhances circulation, aids in prevention of skin breakdown.
Maintain continuity of invasive lines. (Refer to Care Plan: Cardiogenic Shock; Nursing Diagnosis: Injury, potential for, page 44.)	Disconnection may result in hemorrhage, emboli, bacterial contamination.

Hemothorax and Pneumothorax

The lung may collapse partially or completely owing to collection of air (pneumothorax), blood (hemothorax), or other fluid (pleural effusion) in the pleural potential/space. The intrathoracic pressure changes induced by increased pleural space volumes can affect the entire chest. Lung capacity is reduced, causing respiratory distress. With increases in pressure, tension is produced on mediastinal structures. Blood flow may be impeded and venous return decreased, compromising cardiac output.

PATIENT ASSESSMENT DATA BASE

History and physical findings will vary, depending on the amount of air and/or fluid accumulation, rate of accumulation, and the patient's underlying lung function.

HISTORY

Chest surgery or pleural/medastinal trauma.

Placement of central lines.

Empyema and effusion resulting from inflammation or infection of the underlying lung.

Malignant effusions resulting from obstruction of venous return by tumor, pleural implants, or malignant cells in the pleural space.

Rupture of emphysematous bulla, subpleural bleb, or complication of positive pressure mechanical ventilator/ PEEP therapy.

Subjective

Complains of pain, difficulty breathing.

PHYSICAL EXAMINATION

Inspection

Respiratory pattern: may note increased work of breathing, "air hunger," increased rate, use of accessory muscles, intercostal retractions, forced abdominal expirations. Alarm notification of unexplained increase in peak inspiratory and static pressure in ventilator dependent patient.

Thoracic excursion: reduced on the affected side, paradoxical chest movement. Deviation of trachea to unaffected side.

Skin: cyanosis or pallor and diaphoresis may be present.

Venous congestion: manifested by elevation of central venous pressure, distended neck veins.

Consciousness, mentation: may be anxious, restless, confused, stuporous, comatose.

Palpation

Trachea: deviation to unaffected side.

Heart: PMI displaced in presence of mediastinal shift.

Pulses: rapid and/or irregular, weak, thready.

Skin: crepitation in areas of air leak may be noted.

Percussion

Lungs: Hyperresonant over air-filled area. Dull over fluid-filled area.

Auscultation

Breath sounds: diminished or absent sounds may be noted in affected area.

Heart: rate may be rapid, irregular. Hamman's sign (crunching sound correlating with heartbeat), reflecting air in mediastinum could be noted.

Blood pressure: hypertension or hypotension may be present.

DIAGNOSTIC STUDIES

Chest x-ray examination: reveals air and/or fluid accumulation; shift of mediastinal structures.

ABGs: variable, depending on the degree of compromised lung function, altered breathing mechanics and ability to compensate. $PaCO_2$ usually elevated. PaO_2 may be normal or decreased.

NURSING PRIORITIES

1. Promote/maintain lung reexpansion for adequate oxygenation, ventilation.
2. Minimize/prevent complications.
3. Reduce discomfort/pain.

NURSING DIAGNOSIS:	**Breathing pattern, ineffective.**
SUPPORTING DATA/CONTRIBUTING FACTORS:	**Air/fluid accumulation in the chest affects respiratory muscle mechanics and ability to inflate the lungs. Decreased lung expansion and increased work of breathing contribute to gas exchange abnormalities.**
GENERAL PATIENT OUTCOMES:	**Adequate ventilation/gas exchange as shown by respiratory parameters within patient's normal range and reestablishment of usual breathing pattern.**

INTERVENTIONS	RATIONALE
Independent	
Monitor development of signs and symptoms outlined in physical examination.	Early detection and intervention in developing hemothorax or pneumothorax can minimize or prevent complications.
Maintain position of comfort, usually with head of bed elevated.	Maximizes lung expansion and enhances ventilation.
Maintain calm, confident, reassuring approach. Stay with patient.	Minimizes anxiety, which can increase respiratory rate, metabolic demands.
Prepare thoracic catheter and drainage system for insertion or reinsertion as indicated.	Prompt placement of a thoracic catheter and reestablishing negative intrapleural pressures permit reexpansion of the lung, improve breathing, and promote healing of the parenchymal leak.

INTERVENTIONS	RATIONALE
Independent	
ONCE CHEST TUBE INSERTED: Check suction control chamber for correct amount of suction (water level or regulator at correct setting, continuous bubbling in water-filled chamber, depending on type of chest drainage unit). Add water as necessary or dial in correct negative pressure level on regulator.	Maintains prescribed intrapleural negativity, which promotes optimum lung expansion and/or fluid drainage.
Check fluid level in water seal chamber or bottle and maintain at prescribed level.	Water in the water seal chamber serves as a barrier which prevents atmospheric air from entering the pleural space should the suction source be disconnected and aids in evaluating whether the chest drainage system is functioning appropriately. Note: The greater the fluid level in water seal chamber, or the further the glass connector tube extends below the fluid level in the water seal bottle, the more positive pressure is required to push air out of drainage unit, which makes breathing more difficult.
Drape tubing in a straight line from bed to drainage container. Coil extra tubing on bed. Check to make sure tubing has no dependent loops and is not kinked. Drain accumulated fluid as necessary.	Improper draping or fluid accumulation impedes negative suction and may prevent air/fluid evacuation, thereby increasing size of pneumothorax or hemothorax.
Assess underwater seal chamber for air leak as indicated by bubbling in water seal chamber.	Underwater seal bubbling during expiration reflects venting of pneumothorax.
Determine location of inappropriate air leak (e.g., patient or system).	Continuous bubbling when suction is applied indicates a persistent air leak which may occur at thoracic catheter insertion site, connections, or the chest drainage unit.
Clamp thoracic catheter just distal to exit from chest.	If bubbling stops, leak is patient centered (insertion site or in patient).
Place vaseline gauze and/or antibiotic ointment around insertion site and reapply sterile 4 × 4 gauze and tape in an occlusive manner, if indicated.	May correct patient-centered air leak.
If leak continues, clamp tubing in stepwise fashion beyond next connection site toward the drainage unit.	Isolates location of system centered air leak.
Band connection sites securely.	Prevents/corrects air leaks resulting from improperly sealed connectors.
Monitor changes in air leak and bubbling in water seal chamber.	Bubbling usually decreases as the lung reexpands and air leak subsides. Bubbling may occur only during expiration or coughing as pleural space diminishes. Absence of bubbling during pleural drainage may indicate complete lung reexpansion or complications, for example, obstruction in the line.
Monitor water seal chamber for "tidaling" (fluctuations) of fluid level.	The water seal chamber serves as an intrapleural manometer and is a gauge of intrapleural pressure, for example, pressure differences between inspiration and expiration affect the extent of tidaling. Fluctuations of 2 to 6 cm during inspirations generally indicates that

INTERVENTIONS	RATIONALE
Independent	
	the thoracic catheter and collection tube is patent. Tidaling is greater during gravity drainage than when suction is applied.
Note abnormal differences between inspiratory and expiratory tidaling.	Fluctuations are accentuated when volume increases or when the chest cavity is forced to create greater intrapleural pressures, for example, during coughing, when a large pneumothorax is present, or when airway obstruction causes increased breathing difficulty.
Evaluate integrity of system if tidaling ceases and correct problems as indicated (e.g., tube kinking or obstruction).	May indicate actual reexpansion of the lung or obstruction caused by clots or kinking of the thoracic catheter or collection tube, or displacement of the thoracic catheter outside the pleural space.
Evaluate need for tube stripping or "milking." Note type and volume or change in volume of drainage.	Stripping may be necessary to maintain drainage or to dislodge clots. Tube obstruction owing to drainage is not a problem if a pneumothorax is being resolved. It is also unlikely that serous/serosanguinous drainage will obstruct tubes. However, fresh blood may form clots in tube, especially if thoracic catheter has a narrow diameter.
Strip tubes carefully (and only when indicated) per protocol in a manner which minimizes excess negative pressure buildup that is, compressing and releasing tubing in short sections.	Chest tube stripping can create transient negative suction as great as 400 cm H_2O. High negative suction may invaginate tissue into catheter eyelets and cause rupture of small blood vessels. The system becomes static when tissues collapse around thoracic catheter. This results in less efficient drainage and/or delayed resolution of pleural air leaks.
Vent drainage system when negative pressure increases above prescribed levels (as indicated by reading on separate chamber/manometer, or by elevation of water in narrow tube of the water seal chamber).	Increased negativity in the system can occur when the chest cavity is not vented to the atmosphere. Venting involves opening the closed drainage system to the atmosphere, rapidly reducing excess negative pressure to prescribed levels.
Encourage deep breathing, coughing, and position changes.	Prevents and reexpands atelectatic areas and promotes mobilization of secretions.
Collaborative	
Review serial chest x-rays.	Monitors progress of resolving hemothorax and pneumothorax and re-expansion of lung.
Monitor/graph serial ABGs.	Assesses adequacy of respiratory function and/or need for alterations in therapy.
Administer oxygen as indicated.	Provides additional oxygen in presence of altered ventilation.
Encourage use of respiratory aids (e.g., incentive spirometer).	Aids in resolving atelectasis.
Assist with bronchoscopy as dictated.	May be performed to clear secretions or mucous plugs and may reexpand atelectatic areas.

NURSING DIAGNOSIS:	**Injury, potential for, multifactors.**
SUPPORTING DATA/CONTRIBUTING FACTORS:	**The patient with a hemothorax or pneumothorax is at risk for complications associated with insertion and maintenance of a chest drainage system. Maintenance of intrapleural negativity is essential in order to prevent complications of hemothorax or pneumothorax. Various situations may occur that impair optimum elimination of fluid/air, or may cause atmospheric air to enter the pleural space. Occasionally empyema (also a predisposing factor) may result from invasion of microorganisms after chest tube insertion. Injury/surgical trauma or arterial rupture may result in hypovolemia or shock.**
GENERAL PATIENT OUTCOMES:	**Complications are prevented/minimized.**

INTERVENTIONS	RATIONALE
Independent	
Review reason for chest tube placement/location of thoracic catheter.	Assists in interpretation of patient/system data as well as determination of priorities in management.
Anchor thoracic catheter to chest wall and provide for extra length of tubing before turning or moving patient.	Prevents thoracic catheter dislodgment and tubing disconnection and reduces discomfort associated with pulling or jarring motion.
Secure tubing connection sites with bands or tape.	Prevents tubing disconnection.
Pad banding sites with gauze or tape.	Protects skin from irritation and pressure.
Secure drainage unit in stand or cart, or attach to side rails. Place in low traffic area.	Maintains upright position, reducing risk of accidental tipping or breakage of unit.
Provide safe transportation if patient needs to be sent to procedures outside the unit. Before transporting:	Promotes continuation of optimum evacuation of fluid/air from the pleural cavity.
Check water seal chamber to verify fluid is at correct level and to assess leaks. Disconnect from suction source and transport patient, or maintain on continuous suction and have procedure performed at the bedside.	If patient is draining large amount of fluid/air, chest tube should not be disconnected or clamped because prolonged interruption of suction may result in reaccumulation of fluid/air, compromising respiratory status.
Observe insertion site, noting skin condition, presence/odor of drainage from thoracic catheter. Change sterile occlusive dressing as indicated.	Provides for early recognition and treatment of developing skin or tissue infection.
Obtain drainage samples for analysis by allowing fluid to collect in dependent loop of tubing and inserting	Maintains continuous negative intrapleural pressure and prevents infection, which may result from opening

INTERVENTIONS	RATIONALE
Independent	
small gauge needle which is attached to a syringe.	system.
Observe for unusual change or increase in bloody drainage. Monitor vital signs.	Sudden/excessive hemorrhage may require surgical intervention and/or fluid replacement. Significant decrease in drainage may indicate tube obstruction.
Observe for signs of respiratory distress if thoracic catheter becomes disconnected from drainage unit or dislodged from chest. Reconnect thoracic catheter to suction, if possible. Cover insertion site immediately with dressing and apply firm pressure, if thoracic catheter is dislodged from chest.	Pneumothorax may (re)occur when pleural cavity open to air. Reestablishing intrapleural negative pressure or preventing atmospheric air from entering pleural cavity limits development of pneumothorax.
After thoracic catheter is removed: Observe for signs that may indicate reoccurrence of pneumothorax. Maintain sterile occlusive dressing. Evaluate drainage from insertion site.	Early detection of developing pneumothorax or infection is essential to preventing/minimizing complications.
Collaborative	
Administer: IV fluids, blood products.	Fluid/blood replacement may be required to prevent complications of hypovolemia or shock.
Administer antibiotics, as indicated.	Treats and prevents infection.

NURSING DIAGNOSIS:	**Comfort, alteration in, pain, acute.**
SUPPORTING DATA/CONTRIBUTING FACTORS:	**Placement of tube within pleural/potential space is irritating to nerve endings.**
GENERAL PATIENT OUTCOMES:	**Verbalizes/demonstrates decrease of pain.**

INTERVENTIONS	RATIONALE
Independent	
Evaluate changes in or development of sudden chest pain.	May indicate increasing hemothorax or pneumothorax or presence of tension pneumothorax.
Assist with position changes, providing extra length of tubing. Place padding around insertion site when turned on side.	Minimizes discomfort associated with pulling of chest tube or skin pressure at connection site.
Encourage patient to support thoracic catheter insertion with pillows when coughing.	Splinting decreases pain and improves cough effort.
Demonstrate and assist with active/passive exercises.	Reduces joint stiffness and muscle discomfort resulting from immobility.
Medicate before planned activities as indicated.	Reduces discomfort and may enhance participation in care.

INTERVENTIONS	RATIONALE
Independent	
Review purpose and safety factors of chest drainage system with patient and family.	Reduces anxiety related to perception that problems with tubes and bottles might result in serious injury or death.
Collaborative	
Administer narcotics or sedatives.	Promotes relaxation and relief of pain.

Pulmonary Embolism (Massive)

Pulmonary embolism (PE) is a term used to describe a blockage of a portion of the pulmonary arterial system, usually by a blood clot arising from deep systemic veins (e.g., pelvis or legs. Its causes also may include fat, air, or tumor tissue. It may be the most common pulmonary complication in hospitalized patients. However, unless the embolism is large, signs and symptoms may be nonspecific, making diagnosis difficult. Although submassive PE is referred to in this care plan, the main focus is the patient suffering massive embolic phenomena. (Refer to Care Plan: Fractures/Multiple Trauma, page 269.)

PATIENT ASSESSMENT DATA BASE

HISTORY

History or presence of conditions predisposing to thrombus formation (Virchow's triad):

Hypercoagulability of blood: exists during pregnancy, in postoperative period, in certain malignancies, with use of oral contraceptives, and after discontinuation of anticoagulants.

Vessel endothelial wall damage resulting from trauma (i.e., injury to iliac and pelvic veins, sepsis, previous venous disease, burns).

Venous stasis from prolonged immobility (i.e., surgery, bedrest, muscular weakness, lengthy periods of reduced cardiac output, obesity, deep vein thrombus).

Conditions that increase blood viscosity (e.g., polycythemia vera, dehydration, COPD).

History of chronic atrial fibrillation, transmural myocardial infarction, or subendocardial infarction involving right ventricle.

Subjective

Complains of sudden dyspnea, diffuse discomfort, wheezing, hemoptysis, feelings of impending doom/restlessness.

PHYSICAL EXAMINATION

Inspection

Respirations: tachypnea, increased work of breathing (dyspnea), or gasping respirations may be present. (May be only symptom present in submassive PE.)

Cough may be dry or productive and is frequently irritating, hacking.

Sputum may be blood tinged or frankly bloody.

Color: pallor or cyanosis may be present. Circumoral cyanosis (central) can be present in massive PE.

Neck veins: distended external jugular veins may be noted in massive obstruction (cor pulmonale).

Mentation: restless, anxious, lethargic.

Fever: elevation of 1 to 2 degrees Fahrenheit is common.

Extremities: erythema, localized edema (phlebitis) may be noted.

Percussion

Lungs may be dull, indicating consolidation.

Palpation

Pulses may be normal, weak, thready (as in shock), or strong, bounding (as in polycythemia vera).

Heart: right ventricular heave may be noted in massive obstruction.

Extremities: phlebotic veins, increased skin temperature, and/or tense muscle tissue may be palpated if thrombophlebitis is present. Homan's sign may be noted.

Auscultation

Breath sounds may be decreased or absent in involved area. Adventitious breath sounds (e.g., wheezing or crackles) may be noted.

Heart sounds may be normal, but extra heart sounds may be present in massive PE. Loud pulmonic S_2 may be heard in cor pulmonale (60 to 70 percent obstruction).

DIAGNOSTIC STUDIES

ABGs: may show hypoxemia (decreased PaO_2), hypocarbia (decreased PCO_2). Severe respiratory alkalosis may be present in massive PE.

Wide difference in A/V PO_2 (increased anatomic dead space) and shunting (usually present in severe PE) resulting in hypoxemia with PaO_2 less than 80 mm Hg.

Blood chemistries: triad frequently seen is increased LDH/bilirubin; normal SGOT/WBC; and elevated FS (fibrin split) products. (WBC may be increased if infection or pulmonary infarction present.)

Chest x-ray examination: frequently normal, may demonstrate difference in diameter of previously equal blood vessels; abrupt cessation of a vessel; shadow of a clot with no distal blood flow; diaphragmatic elevation on affected side.

ECG may be normal, or demonstrate changes indicative of right ventricular strain (e.g., tall, peaked T waves/ RBBB pattern). Tachycardia and other dysrhythmias may be present, associated with hypoxemia and electrolyte imbalance.

Ventilation and perfusion scan may demonstrate abnormal perfusion pattern conforming to segment or lobe, with ventilation in excess of perfusion (ventilation/perfusion mismatch). Absence of ventilation in a nonperfused area confirms likelihood of PE.

Pulmonary angiography—most specific study for PE. Presence of filling defect or artery "cutoff" confirms diagnosis.

NURSING PRIORITIES

1. Maintain adequate oxygenation and ventilation.
2. Minimize potential for complications.
3. Relieve pain and anxiety.

NURSING DIAGNOSIS:	**Gas Exchange, impaired.**
SUPPORTING DATA/CONTRIBUTING FACTORS:	**Pathologic changes that impede ventilation or perfusion may include obstruction of alveoli, focal atelectasis, congestion of capillaries, and surfactant deficiencies. Intrapulmonary shunting and ventilation and perfusion mismatching may involve ventilation of unperfused alveoli with alveolar shrinking, increased airway**

	resistance, and increased work of breathing.
GENERAL PATIENT OUTCOMES:	**Adequate oxygenation and ventilation as evidenced by ABGs within patient's normal limits, lungs clear, free of signs of respiratory distress.**

INTERVENTIONS	RATIONALE
Independent	
Monitor respiratory rate, depth, and chest expansion. Note respiratory effort, including use of accessory muscles and/or nasal flaring.	Rate is usually increased. Dyspnea ("air hunger") and increased work of breathing is usually present. Depth of respirations varies, depending on degree of respiratory failure. Chest expansion may be limited if pleuritic chest pain is present.
Note characteristics of breath sounds (e.g., decreased or absent and presence of adventitious sounds such as crackles, wheezes, pleural rub).	May be decreased or absent if airway obstruction exists owing to bleeding or atelectasis or consolidation. Rhonchi and wheezing accompany respiratory failure. Crackles are associated with increased hydrostatic forces in the pulmonary vascular system, which promote fluid movement into interstitial spaces.
Observe cough pattern, character of secretions.	Massive embolism leads to tissue destruction (pulmonary infarctions) and bleeding. Alveolar congestion may manifest as a dry or irritated cough or may produce bloody sputum (hemoptysis). Concomitant anticoagulant therapy may increase free bleeding, jeopardizing airway clearance and further impair gas exchange.
Position in semi or high fowler's position with frequent change of position from side to side.	Upright position favors lung expansion, facilitates respiratory effort. Turning enhances aeration of different lung segments, thereby improving gas diffusion.
Encourage deep breathing. Suction nasotracheally and endotracheally as required.	Patients have increased secretions that impair ventilation and so are at risk for pulmonary complications (e.g., pneumonia, atelectasis). Effective pulmonary toilet facilitates ventilation and gas distribution as well as easing respiratory distress.
Monitor effects of sedation/analgesics and encourage frequent sighing and deep breathing.	Medication helps reduce anxiety and oxygen consumption but may reduce frequency of natural sighing or may depress respiratory effort.
Schedule nursing care to provide rest. Refrain from performing nonessential procedures.	Patient may be overwhelmed by anxiety, which is associated with severe respiratory distress and may be compounded by intensive care environment and procedures. Rest enhances coping mechanisms and decreases oxygen consumption associated with activity.
Instruct patient to avoid straining at stool or during procedures and position changes.	Changes in rate of blood flow and intra-abdominal pressures (such as those that occur with Valsalva's maneuver) may dislodge thrombus, as well as increase oxygen consumption and/or myocardial workload.

INTERVENTIONS	RATIONALE
Independent	
Observe for signs and symptoms of ARDS. (Refer to Care Plan: ARDS, page 77.)	Pulmonary embolus is a precipitating factor in the development of ARDS.
Collaborative	
Monitor and graph serial ABGs.	Determines effectiveness of and/or need for alteration in treatment of hypoxemia.
Administer humidified oxygen by cannula, mask, or ventilator.	Corrects hypoxemia. Humidification keeps mucus membranes moist and mobilizes secretions to facilitate airway clearance. Intubation and mechanical ventilation may be required if shock is present, lung compliance is decreased, or pulmonary hypertension is evident. (Refer to Care Plan: Ventilatory Assistance (Mechanical), page 115.)
Assist with chest physiotherapy (e.g., postural drainage and percussion).	Promotes drainage of secretions from lung segments into bronchi where they more readily may be removed by coughing and suctioning.
Administer drugs as indicated:	
Bronchodilators, for example, Aminophylline;	Decreases bronchoconstriction resulting from hypocarbia and improves alveolar ventilation.
Analgesics and sedatives, for example, morphine sulfate;	May be given to relieve pain, reduce work of breathing, and/or minimize anxiety.
Dextran (low molecular weight).	Appears to increase pulmonary blood flow to previously underperfused segments, increase oxygen saturation, and enhance anticoagulation.
Administer fluids, intravenously (IV) or by mouth.	Maintains/restores fluid balance and liquifies secretions; however, care must be exercised to avoid fluid overload, thereby increasing pulmonary congestion.

NURSING DIAGNOSIS: **Tissue Perfusion, alteration in.**

SUPPORTING DATA/CONTRIBUTING FACTORS: **Pulmonary vascular resistance increases as a primary consequence of obstructed blood flow and is manifested by increased pulmonary artery pressures. If pulmonary hypertension is severe, right ventricular failure may result. Other hemodynamic changes and alterations in tissue and organ perfusion depend on the extent of pulmonary blood flow obstruction, as well as patient's prior cardiopulmonary status.**

GENERAL PATIENT OUTCOMES:	**Pulmonary artery pressure is within patient's normal range. Systemic tissue perfusion is adequate as shown by usual mentation, warm and dry skin, urine output greater than 20 ml per hour.**

INTERVENTIONS	RATIONALE
Independent	
Measure pulmonary artery pressure (PAP), blood pressure, mean arterial pressure (MAP).	Pulmonary artery hypertension may be present in varying degrees, depending on the amount of obstruction and effects on cardiac function. Systemic hypotension or shock may be result of several problems, such as right ventricular failure (in massive pulmonary obstruction), or decreased cardiac output related to impaired venous return.
Monitor electrocardiogram, (ECG) noting heart rate and rhythm.	Tachycardia is usually present as result of hypoxia, in a compensatory effort to increase blood flow and tissue perfusion. Rhythm alterations are related to hypoxemia, electrolyte imbalance, and increased right heart strain. Intractable dysrhythmias may be present in massive pulmonary embolus.
Auscultate heart sounds.	Extra heart sounds (e.g., S_3, S_4) and increased S_2 pulmonic components may be noted as cardiac workload increases.
Assess level of consciousness.	Hypoxia and accompanying acidosis decrease mental acuity, resulting in restlessness, confusion, obtundation, and/or sensory and motor changes. Cerebrovascular accident (CVA) also can occur from emboli that originate from the left side of the heart.
Note skin and mucous membrane color and temperature and capillary refill.	Pallor or cyanosis of skin, nailbeds, buccal membranes; and cool, mottled skin, with poor capillary refill are indicative of peripheral vasoconstriction and/or impaired systemic blood flow.
Measure urine output. Note specific gravity. Monitor weight.	Indicates adequacy of renal function, which may be altered by reduced cardiac output or decreased perfusion of the kidneys. Changes in weight reflect general hydration and developing or resolution of edema and renal insufficiency.
Note gastrointestinal function that is, bowel sounds, abdominal distention, nausea, vomiting, changes in stool.	Reduced blood flow or tissue oxygenation slows peristalsis and may result in ileus. Nausea and/or vomiting may require insertion of nasogastric tube, medication, and alternate feeding methods. (Refer to Care Plan: Nutritional Support, page 367.)
Assess extremities for presence and quality of pulses, calf tenderness or swelling, positive Homan's sign.	Pulmonary embolus is frequently precipitated by thrombus arising from deep veins (pelvis or legs) which may or may not be readily apparent.

INTERVENTIONS	RATIONALE
Independent	
Elevate legs or foot portion of bed as indicated. Avoid use of knee gatch and sitting in chair for prolonged periods of time.	Enhances venous return, reduces stasis. Use of knee gatch and sitting in chair places pressure on popliteal area and pools blood in pelvic veins.
Monitor use of antiembolic hose and remove periodically for brief periods of time.	Controversial therapeutic aid which may limit venous stasis but may also result in edema formation in legs secondary to constriction.
Collaborative	
Administer fluids IV or by mouth as indicated.	Reduces hyperviscosity of blood, which potentiates thrombus formation. Fluids may be required to support circulating volume and/or tissue perfusion in presence of shock state.
Assist with insertion of arterial and pulmonary artery pressure lines when indicated. Observe safety protocols. (Refer to Care Plan: Cardiogenic Shock, Nursing Diagnosis: Injury, potential for, multiple factors, page 45.)	Monitors pulmonary pressures, cardiac function, systemic blood pressure, and the effects of fluid and drug therapy.
Monitor laboratory studies, that is, electrolytes, BUN, creatinine, ABGs.	Notes changes in organ function that may require alterations in treatment.
Administer drugs as indicated:	
Heparin (intermittent or continuous IV infusion).	Heparin prevents further thrombosis by preventing clot propagation. IV route is preferred because subcutaneous absorption may be impaired. Continuous infusion is preferred to prevent peak and ebb levels, which may increase coagulation imbalances. Heparin dosage is gradually reduced with concomitant administration of oral anticoagulants (Coumadin) for long-term therapy.
Warfarin sodium (Coumadin).	Oral agent preferred for long-term therapy after initial anticoagulation is achieved. Therapy is started concomitant with heparin owing to slower onset and less precise control and therapeutic effect of Coumadin.
Streptokinase (Streptase) or urikinase (Breakinase).	These thrombolytic agents appear to lyse pulmonary emboli, increase pulmonary capillary perfusion, and decrease hemodynamic abnormalities. May be indicated with massive PE to achieve earlier reduction of the degree of obstruction with more rapid restoration of hemodynamic stability.
Sodium nitroprusside (Nipride) and/or dopamine hydrochloride (Intropin).	Vasodilators may be used with or without vasopressors to decrease pulmonary hypertension while supporting cardiac function (especially when massive emboli have produced a shock state).
Prepare for surgery as indicated, for example, pulmonary embolectomy, or	Pulmonary embolectomy is usually reserved for patients with massive pulmonary embolus (50 percent or more obstruction) who do not respond to anticoagulant therapy or who exhibit life-threatening cardiopulmonary compromise.

INTERVENTIONS	RATIONALE
Collaborative	
Vena caval ligation, intracaval umbrella.	Usually indicated with recurrent emboli despite adequate anticoagulation, when anticoagulants are contraindicated, or when septic emboli arising from below renal veins do not respond to treatment.

NURSING DIAGNOSIS: **Injury, potential for, altered clotting factors.**

SUPPORTING DATA/CONTRIBUTING FACTORS: **Usual treatment of PE is aimed at interrupting the clotting process. This places the patient at risk for bleeding/hemorrhage.**

GENERAL PATIENT OUTCOMES: **Bleeding is prevented/minimized.**

INTERVENTIONS	RATIONALE
Independent	
Inspect for bleeding from mucous membranes, bruising after minimal trauma, oozing from puncture sites, presence of petechiae. Hematest excretions or secretions.	Signs of excessive prolongation of clotting time, which may indicate need for reduction or cessation of anticoagulant therapy.
Apply pressure dressings to venipuncture sites. Avoid massaging subcutaneous injection sites.	Helps prevent local hematoma formation.
Instruct patient in appropriate safety factors (e.g., use of electric razor, gentle brushing and swabbing of teeth and gums; avoidance of forceful blowing of nose and scratching skin.	Enhances patient understanding/cooperation in avoiding trauma-induced bleeding.
Emphasize need for patient to report any signs of bleeding.	Early detection and intervention may prevent serious hemorrhage.
Follow safety protocols during administration of thrombolytic therapy (e.g., bedrest, padded side rails, limited frequency of cuff blood pressures, avoidance of venipunctures and IM injections).	Streptokinase produces greater alteration in hemostasis than heparin with greater risk of hemorrhage.
Collaborative	
Monitor PT and PTT (coagulation profile).	It is usually desirable to maintain PT and PTT approximately two times normal (control) to achieve therapeutic results.
Avoid use of medication containing salicylates.	May potentiate bleeding.
Administer antidotes as indicated:	
Protamine sulfate,	Heparin antagonist. 1 mg of protamine neutralizes up to 100 U of heparin in event of overdose or severe bleeding.

INTERVENTIONS	RATIONALE
Collaborative	
Aminocaproic acid (Amicar),	Antidote for thrombolytic therapy which enhances clotting by inhibiting plasminogen activator substances.
Administer blood, plasma, clotting factors as indicated.	May be necessary for replacement of excessive blood loss.

Radical Neck Surgery/Laryngectomy: Cancer

This therapeutic procedure for cancer of the neck and/or vocal cords also may be indicated for primary lesions of the lip and/or tongue or nasopharnyx when metastasis to lymph chain has occurred.

Partial Laryngectomy

Partial laryngectomy may be performed when tumor has not involved surrounding muscles and cord is intact. Patient will have a temporary tracheostomy tube and may have return of some voice after healing.

Total Laryngectomy

Total laryngectomy requires removal of epiglottis, thyroid cartilage, hyoid bone, and 2 to 3 rings of trachea. Pharyngeal opening of trachea is closed, and the remaining trachea is brought out to neck wound and sutured to skin, forming a permanent stoma. Laryngeal tube (somewhat longer than tracheostomy tube) remains in place until wound is healed.

PATIENT ASSESSMENT DATA BASE

HISTORY

History of tobacco chewing or smoking, alcohol consumption, inhalation of hardwood sawdust, exposure to toxic chemicals, heavy metals, or radiation, heavy exposure to sunlight.

May have concurrent chronic lung disease associated with long history of heavy cigarette smoking.

Males affected more than females (10 to 1 ratio), with average age more than 50 years.

Subjective

Complaints vary depending on the area(s) affected and can include: Difficulty or pain on swallowing.
Hoarseness or voice change.
Persistent sore throat aggravated by talking.
Cold sore on lip that didn't heal.
Pain referred to side of head or neck.
Dyspnea with or without cough.
Chronic halitosis.

PHYSICAL EXAMINATION

Postoperative physical findings vary tremendously, depending on operative procedures and structural changes.

Inspection

Edema: involving part of or entire face, minimal or pronounced.

Anterior tongue: enlarged if venous or lymphatic drainage is obstructed.

Cranial nerve involvement may result in loss of gag or cough reflex, facial paralysis, inability to close eyelid or to blink, loss of sense of taste and/or smell.

Skin color: operative areas should be pink or similar to surrounding tissue. Wide skin defects may be covered by skin flaps from deltoid area or grafts from other sites.

Palpation

Skin: should be warm and dry. Poor turgor or tenting may be noted if patient is malnourished or dehydrated.

Edema: present in surgical areas, mild to extensive.

Auscultation

Breath sounds: diminished sounds may reflect hypoventilation or atelectasis. Secretions may be noted in major airways.

Bowel sounds: diminished to absent.

DIAGNOSTIC STUDIES

Once diagnosis is made, baseline preoperative studies may be normal or abnormal, depending on severity of cancer, prior treatments, or secondary pathology, and may include

CBC.
Immunologic surveys.
Biochemical profile.
Coagulation studies, PT/APTT.
Liver function studies.
Endocrine studies, T_3, T_4.
ABGs.
Pulmonary function studies.
Chest x-ray examination.

NURSING PRIORITIES

1. Maintain patent airway.
2. Provide means of communication.
3. Protect skin integrity.
4. Control pain.
5. Maintain adequate nutrition.
6. Provide emotional support.
7. Prevent or minimize complications.

NURSING DIAGNOSIS:	**Airway Clearance, ineffective.**
SUPPORTING DATA/CONTRIBUTING FACTORS:	**Surgery involving structures of the head and neck creates numerous problems which may affect the airway. The laryngectomy procedure renders the patient a partial or total neck breather. Structural changes may alter ability to swallow or cough. Edema from operative procedures as well as lymphatic accumulation can mechanically obstruct airway. Secretions are usually copious, and aspiration is a constant possibility. Secretions may become thick, obstructing airways with mucous plugs. Bleeding from eroded blood vessels can create life-threatening hazard.**
GENERAL PATIENT OUTCOMES:	**Patent airway is maintained. Aspiration is prevented. Secretions remain**

fluid and are readily cleared. Complications are prevented and/or recognized and treated promptly.

INTERVENTIONS	RATIONALE
Independent	
Elevate head of bed 30 to 45 degrees.	Facilitates drainage of secretions, work of breathing, and lung expansion. May help reduce facial edema.
Encourage swallowing, if able.	Reduces pooling of oral secretions.
Encourage coughing and deep breathing.	Mobilizes secretions to clear airway and helps prevent respiratory complications.
Maintain proper position of tracheostomy or laryngectomy tube. Document operative position, placement.	As edema develops or subsides, tube may be displaced, affecting airway patency.
Check and/or adjust, ties.	Should be snug but not constrictive to tissue or major blood vessels.
Observe surrounding tissue for bleeding. Change position to check for pooling of blood behind patient's neck or on posterior dressings.	Small amount oozing may be present immediately postoperatively. Continued bleeding or sudden eruption of uncontained hemorrhage presents a sudden and very real possibility.
Suction tracheostomy tube, oral and nasal cavities using sterile technique. Note amount, color, consistency of secretions.	Prevents airway obstruction by secretions which can lead to respiratory complications. Swallowing ability may be limited or altered; patient cannot blow nose.
If patient has been taught procedure for self-suction, begin as soon as possible.	Preoperative preparation on self-suctioning is often done to assist patient to exercise some control in postoperative care and to reduce anxiety associated with difficult breathing.
Cleanse tracheostomy tube/inner cannula as indicated.	Prevents accumulation of secretions and thickening mucus which can obstruct airways.
Have spare sterile tracheostomy tube on hand at patient's bedside.	In event of contamination of inner cannula or other problem, proper equipment is readily available.
Monitor for signs of respiratory distress such as increased rate of respirations, restlessness, dyspnea, cyanosis, abnormal breath sounds.	Airway obstruction can lead to ineffective breathing or impaired gas exchange, resulting in complications, for example, atelectasis, pneumonia, or respiratory arrest.
Collaborative	
Provide supplemental humidification by:	Normal physiologic means of filtering/humidifying air is bypassed.
Oxygen mist collar, room humidifier, increase fluid intake (IV in initial postoperative period).	Decreases mucus crusting and airway obstruction and facilitates coughing and suctioning of secretions through stoma. Note: Thick mucous plugs are a common cause of respiratory distress or arrest in later postoperative period.
Monitor/graph serial ABGs; chest x-ray examinations.	Recognize changes that might require alteration in therapy.

NURSING DIAGNOSIS:	**Communication, impaired, verbal.**
SUPPORTING DATA/CONTRIBUTING FACTORS:	**Surgical intervention in throat/neck cancers may involve removal of larynx with immediate, permanent loss of the voice (total laryngectomy).**
GENERAL PATIENT OUTCOMES:	**Will be able to communicate needs, reducing fear and anxiety during acute phase.**

INTERVENTIONS	RATIONALE
Independent	
Provide immediate and continual means to summon nurse (e.g., call light, bell), and let the patient know they will be answered immediately. Stop by to check on patient without being summoned.	Patient needs assurance that nurse is vigilant and will respond to the summons. The patient will be reassured by the knowledge that the nurse cares enough to come at times other than when summoned.
Provide alternate means of communication, such as pad and pencil, magic slate.	Asists patient in establishing a way to express needs, wants, ideas, questions.
Anticipate needs. Validate meaning of nonverbal communication. Keep communication simple. Maintain eye contact.	Establishes therapeutic relationship and reduces frustration created by misunderstanding what patient is communicating.
Provide reality orientation, such as clock, radio, window bed.	Gives basic "life information" without patient having to ask.
Collaborative	
Refer to appropriate therapists and agencies for followup treatment, rehabilitation (e.g., laryngectomee clubs), alternate speech methods—esophogeal speech, electrical devices—social and rehabilitative services.	Even the patient and family who are well prepared in advance by proper instruction and advice experience a sense of loss when the ability to speak is permanently altered. Rehabilitation time may be lengthy and involve a number of resources.

NURSING DIAGNOSIS:	**Skin Integrity, impairment of, actual.**
SUPPORTING DATA/CONTRIBUTING FACTORS:	**Surgery of head and neck presents suture lines in various locations. Healing may be impaired by course of cancer, poor nutritional state, and/or previous therapeutic measures such as radiation and immunosuppressive drugs. Suture line and graft integrity are threatened by swelling and drainage of secretions. Skin grafts may fail, owing to inadequate blood supply, resulting in compromised integrity or tissue necrosis.**

GENERAL PATIENT OUTCOMES:	**Wounds remain infection free and healing begins. Complications are prevented or minimized.**

INTERVENTIONS	RATIONALE
Independent	
Assess skin color, temperature, and capillary refill of operative area, skin flap.	Color of skin flaps should be pink or similar to color of skin surrounding donor site. Flap should be warm when gentle finger pressure is applied and should blanch, with return of color within seconds. Cyanosis and slow refill may indicate venous congestion which can lead to tissue ischemia and necrosis.
Keep head of bed elevated 30 to 45 degrees. Monitor facial edema (usually peaks by third to fifth day postoperatively).	Reduces edema related to excision of lymph channels and post operative tissue congestion.
Protect skin flap, suture lines, from tension and pressure.	Pressure from oxygen tubings, tracheostomy tapes, feeding tubes, hemovacs can cause tissue injury as a result of compression of blood vessels.
Note drainage from surgical sites, suture lines, drains.	Bloody drainage should decrease steadily after first 24 hours. Steady oozing or frank bleeding indicates problem requiring medical intervention.
Measure hemovac drainage (if used).	Used to facilitate drainage and to keep the surgical area clean and dry.
Change dressings as indicated.	Surgical site may or may not be covered. Pressure dressings are contraindicated over skin flaps because blood supply is easily compromised.
Cleanse incisions with sterile saline and peroxide (mixed 1:1) after dressings have been removed.	Prevents crust formation which can trap purulent drainage thus destroying skin edges and increasing width of wound. Peroxide should not be used full strength because it may cauterize wound edges and impair wound healing.
Monitor donor site if skin graft performed: Check dressings as indicated.	May be adjacent to operative site or elsewhere (thigh). Pressure dressings may be used initially to absorb serum and blood and are usually removed within 24 to 48 hours.
Monitor for signs of wound infection (e.g., redness, increasing edema, pain, exudates, and temperature elevation).	Impedes healing, which may already be slow because of changes induced by chemotherapy, radiation therapy and/or malnutrition.
Collaborative	
Administer IV fluids as indicated.	Maintains circulating fluid volume and tissue perfusion.
Administer IV and topical antibiotics as indicated.	Prevents and controls infection.
Cover donor site with vaseline gauze or moisture impermeable dressing. Keep bed linen and clothing off site.	Nonadherent dressing covers exposed sensory nerve endings and protects site from contamination. Areas need to be protected from painful pressure.

NURSING DIAGNOSIS:	**Oral Mucous Membrane, alteration in (actual/potential).**
SUPPORTING DATA/CONTRIBUTING FACTORS:	**Although oral cavity may be site of cancerous growth, many other factors also may affect integrity of mucous membranes. Drying may occur owing to decrease in saliva production (xerostomia) secondary to surgical procedure or cytotoxic injury by antineoplastic agents and/or radiation therapy. History of poor oral hygiene, chronic membrane irritation, and xerostomia may cause mucositis. In addition, nutritional deficits retard healing and rebuilding of healthy tissues, especially in patient with compromised immune system.**
GENERAL PATIENT OUTCOMES:	**Oral mucous membranes are maintained in or restored to optimum condition, are moist and free of crusts or exudate.**

INTERVENTIONS	RATIONALE
Independent	
Inspect mouth, teeth, lips, membranes. Note changes in	
Saliva,	May become thick and mucoid if patient dehydrated. Damage to salivary glands may decrease production of saliva (xerostomia). Dysphagia may compromise patient's ability to swallow, resulting in pooling/drooling of saliva.
Tongue,	May be dry, coated. If surgery has included partial resection of tongue, soft palate, and pharynx, patient will have decreased sensation and tongue movement, difficulty swallowing, and increased risk of aspiration.
Lips,	May be dry, crusty, red, inflamed. If surgery has removed part of lip, uncontrollable drooling may occur.
Teeth and/or gums,	Teeth may not be intact (surgical) or may be in poor condition owing to malnutrition, chemical agents. Gums also may be surgically altered or inflamed owing to prior therapies, poor hygiene, smoking.
Mucous membranes,	Mucous membranes may be dry, ulcerated, erythematous, edematous (mucositis).

INTERVENTIONS	RATIONALE
Independent	
Suction oral cavity gently and frequently.	Prevents pooling of secretions around suture lines. Saliva contains digestive enzymes erosive to exposed tissue. Because drooling may be constant (if patient unable to swallow), patient can promote own comfort and decrease aspiration by self-suctioning.
Irrigate mouth at frequent intervals with hydrogen peroxide and saline solution (1:1).	Promotes hydration, reduces infecting agents, promotes tissue healing and comfort.

NURSING DIAGNOSIS: **Comfort, alteration in, pain, acute.**

SUPPORTING DATA/CONTRIBUTING FACTORS: **Surgical incisions, swelling, and/or nasogastric tube can contribute significantly to dysphagia and pain.**

GENERAL PATIENT OUTCOMES: **Verbalizes or displays relief of pain, reduced tension, relaxed manner.**

INTERVENTIONS	RATIONALE
Independent	
Check mouth, throat suture line for trauma.	Tissues are inflamed and may be easily traumatized by suction catheter or feeding tube.
Encourage patient to expectorate saliva or suction gently if unable to swallow.	Swallowing causes muscle activity that may be painful because of edema or strain on suture lines. Swelling and surgical removal of certain portions of tongue and/or pharynx may prevent swallowing.
Provide oral irrigations, anesthetic gargles and sprays.	Reduces bacterial growth and halitosis; provides comfort. Use of commercial mouthwashes is usually limited or avoided because they may contain phenol and alcohol, which are drying to mucous membranes. Note: Gargling may be contraindicated if patient is unable to handle secretions.
Support head/neck with pillows. Teach patient to support neck during activity.	Muscle weakness results from muscle/nerve resection. Lack of support may strain suture line, resulting in pain and possible injury or hemorrhage.
Provide diversional activities (e.g., television, radio, reading).	Gives patient something else to focus on besides discomfort and pain.
Collaborative	
Administer analgesics as indicated.	Degree of pain is related to extent and psychologic impact of surgery as well as to general body condition.

NURSING DIAGNOSIS:	**Nutrition, alteration in, less than body requirements.**
SUPPORTING DATA/CONTRIBUTING FACTORS:	**Surgery temporarily or permanently alters mode of food intake. Taste and smell feedback mechanisms may be altered because of chemotherapy, radiation, surgical or structural changes. Patient may be anorexic or experience nausea, vomiting, and/or malabsorption related to cancer and/or therapies. Tissue healing requires increased nutrients during a time when patient is unable to eat and least desires food.**
GENERAL PATIENT OUTCOMES:	**Nutritional intake is adequate to meet metabolic needs as shown by positive nitrogen balance, stable or appropriate weight gain, and beginning of healing of surgical incisions.**

INTERVENTIONS	RATIONALE
Independent	
Ascultate bowel sounds.	Return of bowel sounds postoperatively indicates readiness to begin tube feeding.
Maintain feeding tube, that is, check for tube placement; flush with water if indicated.	Tube is usually inserted in surgery and may be attached to suction initially to reduce nausea and vomiting.
Monitor intake and output and weight as indicated.	Provides information regarding nutritional needs/effectiveness of therapy. Note: Rapid weight gain may reflect edema formation.
Review importance of nutrition in tissue healing. Explain that patient will later learn to blenderize and give own feedings if required.	Can help promote positive attitude and feeling of contributing to progress of healing and self-care.
Collaborative	
Consult with dietician to determine caloric needs for body size, healing.	Provides direction for diet modifications (e.g., increased protein, carbohydrates).
Administer nutritionally balanced tube feedings: for example, blenderized regular food or commercial preparations as indicated by physician or dietician preference.	Provides nutrients when swallowing is not possible. Variation can be made to add or limit certain factors such as fat, sugars. (Refer to Care Plan: Nutritional Support, page 367.)
Begin with small feedings, advance as tolerated. Note signs of gastric fullness, regurgitation, diarrhea.	High-calorie, high-protein content may result in GI intolerance, requiring change in rate and type of enteric formula, or, in some cases, a switch to IV support.

INTERVENTIONS	RATIONALE
Collaborative	
Administer alternate nutrition, if indicated that is, hyperalimentation.	Supplies nutrients during time patient is unable to eat. (Refer to Care Plan: Nutritional Support, page 367.)
Provide adequate fluid intake by IV, feeding tube, or orally if patient can swallow.	Keeps patient hydrated to offset insensible losses and drainage from surgical areas. Meets free water needs associated with enteral feeding.
Monitor laboratory studies (e.g., BUN, glucose, liver function, protein, electrolytes).	Indicators of utilization of nutrients as well as of organ function.

NURSING DIAGNOSIS: **Self-Concept, disturbance in, body image; self-esteem; role performance; personal identity (potential).**

SUPPORTING DATA/CONTRIBUTING FACTORS: **The head and neck is a highly important region in terms of body image. Anatomic contour of the face and neck may be severely disrupted, and physiologic functions, such as voice production and deglutination, may be permanently impaired by radical surgery. The patient who has sustained drastic disfigurement and/or severe functional impairment is likely to experience tremendous anxiety while attempting to incorporate these changes into self-concept. May have fears about how job will be affected, financial matters, and self-care.**

GENERAL PATIENT OUTCOMES: **Demonstrates initial adaptation to body changes; begins to develop plans for altered lifestyle.**

INTERVENTIONS	RATIONALE
Independent	
Establish therapeutic nurse-patient relationship.	Maintaining calm, reassuring manner will help allay patient's fear of mutilation and/or dying.
Alert staff that facial expressions need to convey acceptance of patient's appearance.	Patient may be watching for expressions of revulsion. Staff acceptance will enhance dignity and courage.
Note nonverbal body language (e.g., keeping eyes closed).	Patient may be fearful of family and staff reactions or of revealing own feelings.
Acknowledge and accept feelings of grief, hostility.	Patient and family need reassurance that feelings and reactions are normal.

INTERVENTIONS	RATIONALE
Independent	
Encourage patient and significant other(s) to communicate feelings to each other.	All those involved may have difficulty in this area but should understand that they may gain courage from one another.
Assess level of patient's prior knowledge of and anxiety related to diagnosis and surgery.	Information can provide clue to patient's postoperative reactions.
Discuss inaccuracies in perception of disease process and therapies with patient and significant other(s).	Overwhelming stressors are present and may be coupled with limited knowledge. Misconceptions are inevitable and can prevent progress, resulting in failure to improve. Simple reteaching may quickly reduce anxiety.
Note emotional changes, for example, signs of grieving, anger. Accept patient's decision about viewing self.	May experience immediate depression and/or shock after surgery, especially upon first looking at self in mirror.
Allow patient to progress at own rate.	Acceptance/resolution cannot be forced.
Maintain positive attitude toward patient, encouraging patient to exercise control. Accept patient's choice to not participate in self-care, continue to provide opportunities.	Allowing patient to make some decisions regarding nursing care, and encouraging self-care efforts involves patient in directing own wellness.
Provide patient with information available to improve self-esteem.	Written information, visits from laryngectomees, or speech therapist may help patient feel hopeful about future.
Provide and repeat explanations at patient's level of acceptance.	Initial information needs to be very basic, geared toward immediate physical care needs. Do not assume that patient remembers last explanation. Provide additional information as condition improves and patient's readiness to learn progresses.
Provide specific, accurate information about life-threatening situations and assist patient and significant other(s) to acknowledge and integrate learning into lifestyle.	Patient is a neck breather, must wear a medical alert tag or bracelet providing information on proper way to resuscitate should respiratory arrest occur. Significant other(s) should be instructed in cardiopulmonary resuscitation (CPR). Patient cannot swim and must protect stoma against dust and inhaled contamination.
Collaborative	
Discuss and refer questions patient may have about effects of surgery and disability on future job and self-care capabilities.	Vocational and occupational therapists will become involved in care as patient progresses.
Refer to social services and/or pastoral care. (Refer to Care Plan: Psychosocial Aspects of Critical Care, page 379.)	Some patients may not have family or support system (other than hospital staff) to assist with emotional support, lifestyle adaptations, or financial needs. Intact family will also benefit from support and information.

NURSING DIAGNOSIS: **Injury, potential for, chylus fistula formation/hemorrhage.**

SUPPORTING DATA/CONTRIBUTING FACTORS:	**Inadvertent disruption of left thoracic duct can occur during surgery leading to leaking of chyle (products of digestion) or development of a chylus fistula with potential for tissue destruction as well as serious depletion of protein and fluids. There is potential for bleeding in immediate postoperative period because of vascularity of head and neck. A more ominous type of hemorrhage can occur later in postoperative period in patients who have had radical neck surgery with extensive loss of muscle and/or protective skin layers. Common carotid artery rupture ("blowout") can occur in these patients as a result of fistula formation, skin necrosis or infection.**
GENERAL PATIENT OUTCOMES:	**Complications prevented or recognized early and appropriate measures initiated.**

INTERVENTIONS	RATIONALE
Independent	
Assess amount of lymph drainage: Note sudden or advancing subclavicular swelling or continued leaking from suture lines, skin tissues.	Lymph normally drains into lymphatic duct (right) and thoracic duct (left). Thoracic duct is more prone to trauma during surgery because it may loop as far as 6 cm into neck before returning to chest and entering subclavian vein. Duct is ligated during surgery if disruption is detected. Inadvertant trauma may be manifested postoperatively by local tissue swelling and/or persistent or copious drainage.
Observe color and character of drainage.	Thoracic duct drainage is milky, opaque, because it contains chyle, a product of intestinal digestion.
Assess bleeding from tracheostomy/laryngectomy site, and tracheal secretions.	Bleeding should be minimal and decrease within few hours postoperatively.
Monitor vital signs, dressings, drainage tubes, skin flap sites for hemorrhage.	Patient may need to be returned to surgery to have active bleeders ligated.
Assess/monitor for risk of carotid rupture. Observe for tissue crusting or sloughing in carotid area.	Although any patient is at risk, patient who has had previous radiation to neck area and has lost 10 to 15 percent of body weight prior to surgery is at very high risk. Once carotid artery is exposed, it is susceptible to drying, crust formation, and rupture.
Collaborative	
Control leaking chyle, as indicated: that is, apply	Skin and surrounding tissues need to be protected

INTERVENTIONS	RATIONALE
Collaborative	
dressings or collecting bag to keep skin areas dry. Assist with aspiration and prepare for surgical intervention.	from tissue destruction by digestive enzymes. Lymphatic vessels may seal in a few days or require surgical intervention if chylus fistula develops.
Administer fluids, electrolytes, and serum albumin as indicated.	Replacement may be required if chylus drainage is copius or prolonged.
Place on "carotid precautions," that is, close observation with surgical packing and resuscitation supplies nearby.	Be prepared for life-threatening situation. Patient and family will be extremely frightened and require information and support.
Prepare for surgical intervention, if indicated.	The chances of surviving carotid rupture are slim, therefore early recognition of developing tissue sloughing in carotid area is essential to any life-saving intervention.

Ventilatory Assistance (Mechanical)

Mechanical ventilation is required whenever a patient can no longer adequately oxygenate or ventilate to provide sufficient gas exchange to meet tissue demands for oxygen. A variety of conditions produce ventilatory failure, reflected in a $PaCO_2$ greater than 50, and/or PaO_2 less than 60. Positive pressure ventilators are the most common types of ventilators used in critical care areas. New developments include high-frequency positive pressure ventilators (HFPPV) or high-frequency jet ventilators (HFJV), which deliver 60 to 2400 breaths per minute with small tidal volumes.

PATIENT ASSESSMENT DATA BASE

HISTORY

Extrapulmonary Causes

Diseases of pleura and chest wall: pneumothorax, pleural effusion, thoracic wall deformities, chest trauma, flail chest.

Neuromuscular disorders: myasthenia gravis, muscular dystrophy, polio, botulism.

Peripheral nerve and spinal cord disorders: polio, Guillian-Barre, amyotrophic lateral sclerosis (ALS), multiple sclerosis, tetanus.

Central nervous system disorders: sedative or narcotic overdose, head/spinal cord trauma, cerebrovascular accident, Pickwickian syndrome.

Cardiovascular disorders: congestive heart failure, myocardial infarction, cardiogenic shock.

Renal insufficiency.

Intrinsic Lung and Airway Disease Causes

Large airway obstruction: foreign body, tumor.

Parenchymal disease: emphysema, pulmonary fibrosis, pulmonary edema, pneumonia, acute respiratory distress syndrome (ARDS).

Bronchial disease: bronchitis, asthma.

Subjective

If able, patient may complain of severe dyspnea, apprehension, feelings of impending doom.

PHYSICAL EXAMINATION

Note: Specifics in the Physical Examination and Diagnostic Studies will reflect the underlying disorder.

Inspection

Respiratory rate: absent, decreased, or rapid (greater than 30 per minute).

Respiratory pattern: use of accessory muscles, sternal retraction, nasal flaring.

Mental status: may be anxious or restless, confused or disoriented.

Skin: may note cyanosis, pallor, diaphoresis.

Palpation

Pulse: may be weak or thready or reflect dysrhythmias.

Auscultation

Breath sounds: absent or decreased, crackles, rhonchi, wheezes.

Heart rate: tachycardia (early), bradycardia, or other dysrhythmias.

Blood pressure: hypertension, hypotension may be noted.

DIAGNOSTIC STUDIES

PaO_2: related to, but distinct from, ability to ventilate: hypoxemia may indicate need for oxygen, but may or may not indicate need for mechanical ventilation.

$PaCO_2$: usually greater than 50 mm Hg.

pH: reflects respiratory hypoxemia, acidosis, alkalosis.

Vital capacity (VC) less than 15 to 20 ml per kg and maximum inspiratory force (MIF) less than -25 cm H_2O reflects respiratory muscle weakness.

Tidal volume (V_T) less than 5 ml per Kg and vital capacity (VC) less than 15 ml per Kg reflect inability to inflate lungs.

V_D/V_T (ratio of deadspace to tidal volume) equal to or greater than 0.6 reflects excessive work of breathing.

$\dot{V}_E$ (minute ventilation) decrease reflects inability to maintain adequate ventilation over a minute's time.

NURSING PRIORITIES

1. Promote adequate oxygenation, ventilation.
2. Control or minimize discomfort and dyssynchronization of breathing with ventilator.
3. Minimize complications.
4. Provide for patient and family support and the reduction of anxiety.

NURSING DIAGNOSIS:	**Breathing Pattern, ineffective.**
SUPPORTING DATA/CONTRIBUTING FACTORS:	**Depending on the specific precipitating disorder, the patient's pattern of breathing is altered or inadequate due to respiratory muscle weakness, depression of respiratory center, or an increase of deadspace; resulting in increased work of breathing, cessation of respirations, or inability to inflate the lungs.**
GENERAL PATIENT OUTCOMES:	**Adequate ventilation and gas exchange as evidenced by ABGs within patient's normal limits; lungs fully expanded, breath sounds clearing with absence of retractions and use of accessory muscles.**

INTERVENTIONS	RATIONALE
Independent	
Maintain patent airway. (Refer to Nursing Diagnosis: Airway Clearance, ineffective, page 119.)	Airway obstruction is one of the most frequent causes of breathing difficulty.

INTERVENTIONS	RATIONALE
Independent	
Inflate tracheostomy/endotracheal tube cuff using the minimal leak or occlusive technique. Check cuff inflation every 4 to 8 hours and whenever cuff is deflated or reinflated.	The cuff must be properly inflated to insure adequate ventilation and delivery of desired V_T. Underinflation may allow aspiration of gastric contents or respiratory secretions. Overinflation may damage the trachea.
Evaluate respiratory status periodically, noting bilateral breath sounds, symmetry of chest movement, adventitious breath sounds.	Auscultation provides information regarding airflow through the tracheobronchial tree and the presence of fluid, mucus, or obstruction. Note: Frequent crackles or wheezes indicate developing complications secondary to retained secretions, hypoventilation.
Count patient's respirations for one full minute and compare with ventilator set rate.	Varies with individual, ventilator flow rate, and ventilator mode (e.g., control assist or SIMV). Rapid rates can produce respiratory alkalosis. Hypoventilation will allow increased $PaCO_2$ and acidosis to persist, requiring increased tidal volume and rate to correct.
Verify that patient's respiratory rate is "in phase" with ventilator.	If patient is not "in phase" with ventilator, adjustments may be required in tidal volume, rate, and/or deadspace.
Ventilate manually with bag, as indicated.	Necessary to provide or restore adequate ventilation when patient or equipment problems require that the patient be temporarily removed from the ventilator.
Monitor ordered ventilatory settings: routinely throughout each shift; frequently on unstable patients; when ventilator settings changed; when ABGs drawn.	Settings are adjusted according to patient's primary disease and results of ABGs, to maintain parameters within appropriate limits.
Note oxygen concentration (FIO_2). Verify machine setting, oxygen outlet. Monitor in-line oxygen analyzer.	Adjusted according to arterial oxygen levels and saturation to maintain PaO_2 acceptable for patient's condition, usually greater than 60 mmHg. Because machine dials are not always accurate, analyzer determines whether patient is receiving desired concentration of oxygen.
Be aware of FIO_2 levels greater than 0.6.	Hypoxemia treatment is a more important consideration initially than oxygen toxicity. However, capillary changes related to toxicity and leading to fibrosis may begin within 48 hours. FIO_2 levels should be decreased as soon as possible. Addition of positive end-exploratory pressure (PEEP) may be required to accomplish this.
Maintain optimal PEEP. Avoid routine suctioning, use PEEP valve if available. Hyperinflate lungs with bag when necessary to remove from ventilator.	PEEP promotes alveolar expansion; increases functional residual capacity; allows use of lowest possible FIO_2. Each time the ventilator tubing is disconnected, PEEP is broken and may take up to 30 minutes to reestablish. Minimizing suctioning or suctioning through PEEP valve may be helpful in maintaining desired PEEP level.
Assess tidal volume (10 to 15 ml Kg). Verify proper function of spirometer, bellows, or computer readout. Note alterations from desired volume delivered.	Monitors amount of air inspired and expired. Changes may indicate alteration in lung compliance or leakage through machine or around cuff.
Note airway pressure.	Once the tidal volume has been established, the airway pressure should remain relatively constant. An in-

INTERVENTIONS	RATIONALE
Independent	crease in the pressure reading reflects an increase in airway resistance, as may occur with bronchospasm and retained secretions; and/or decreases in lung compliance, as may occur with pneumothorax, pulmonary edema, atelectasis, ARDS, and obstruction of the endotracheal tube.
Monitor flow rate and note inspiratory-expiratory ratio.	Adjusted so that inspiratory volume is completed in the time allowed, based on the desired RR and I:E ratio. Slower flow rates are preferred for optimal gas distribution. Expiratory phase is usually twice the length of the inspiratory phase but may be longer to improve gas exchange and to prevent air trapping as seen in chronic obstructive pulmonary disease (COPD).
Assess sigh rate, (5 to 10 minute intervals) and volume (about 1½ to 2 times V_T).	Hyperinflation (sighing) ventilates alveoli, promotes movement of secretions, and helps reduce or prevent atelectasis.
Note inspired humidity and temperature.	Usual warming and humidifying of the nasopharynx is bypassed with intubation. Note: The temperature of inspired air should be maintained at about body temperature because overheating may result in damage to cilia or hyperthermia.
Monitor tubings for kinking or accumulation of water. Drain as indicated.	Kinking prevents adequate volume delivery. Water prevents proper gas distribution and predisposes to bacterial growth in tubing.
Use automatic "reset button" to temporarily bypass alarm systems. Never turn off alarms, even for suctioning.	Ventilators have a series of visual and audible alarms, for example, oxygen, low or high pressure, I:E ratios. Failure to reset alarms places patient at risk for unobserved ventilator failure, respiratory distress or arrest.
Note readiness to wean as evidenced by: Patient awake and oriented, emotionally ready, if possible, with stable vital signs; requires less than 5 cm PEEP and FIO_2 less than 50 percent. After 30-minute trial period, resting minute ventilation at least 10 liters and can double with maximum voluntary effort, vital capacity greater than 10 ml per Kg, static compliance greater than 30.	Provides gradual, controlled return to respiratory independence while enhancing respiratory muscle tone, reducing exhaustion and possibility of recurrent respiratory failure. Weaning method chosen may be T-tube or IMV. IMV allows own breathing pattern with intermittent breaths by the ventilator.
During and after weaning: Discuss procedure and stay with patient during initial periods off ventilator. Assess for respiratory distress: dyspnea, tachypnea, use of accessory muscles, apprehension, fatigue, hemodynamic changes, increasing PCO_2.	Patient may have developed a physiologic or psychologic dependence on the ventilator and may feel uncomfortable being alone. Early detection of respiratory distress and prompt intervention may avoid return to the ventilator.
Collaborative	
Monitor/graph serial ABGs. Calculate alveolar-arterial (A-a) gradients, shunt measurements. Note end-expiratory pressure, compliance.	Used for adjustment of ventilator settings and to assess effectiveness of ventilation and readiness for weaning.
Obtain ABGs 15 to 30 minutes after ventilator adjustments.	Assesses patient response to ventilator changes.

INTERVENTIONS	RATIONALE
Collaborative	
Monitor serial chest x-ray examinations.	Assures proper position of the endotracheal tube with tip 3 cm above the carina. Detects development of complications (e.g., atelectasis, pulmonary edema).
Administer medications as indicated:	
Morphine sulfate.	Provides pain relief, sedation, with reduced adverse effects in well-ventilated, well-oxygenated patient. Central nervous system (CNS) depressant effects may be reversed with Narcan if necessary for weaning.
Pancuronium bromide (Pavulon). Use smallest dose possible to achieve desired result, and in conjunction with sedation.	Paralysis alleviates the problem of "fighting the ventilator" but renders the patient completely dependent on the ventilator. Sedation produces sleep and may reduce fear associated with being paralyzed, apneic. Note: Drug effect can be potentiated by electrolyte and acid-base imbalance.

NURSING DIAGNOSIS: **Airway Clearance, ineffective.**

SUPPORTING DATA/CONTRIBUTING FACTORS: **The introduction of an artificial airway into the trachea acts as a foreign body and stimulates production of secretions. An endotracheal tube passes through the larynx, preventing approximation of the vocal cords, which is required for coughing. The patient's underlying pathology may also compromise the airway and/or create bronchoconstriction.**

GENERAL PATIENT OUTCOMES: **Airways clear of secretions, free of bronchoconstriction as shown by absence of ronchi and wheezing on auscultation.**

INTERVENTIONS	RATIONALE
Independent	
Assess airway patency.	Airway obstruction can be caused by secretion, hemorrhage, COPD, bronchospasm, and/or problems with tracheostomy or endotracheal tubes.
Assess for bilateral symmetrical chest excursion and equal breath sounds.	Symmetrical chest movement with breath sounds throughout lung fields indicates proper tube placement. Lower airway obstruction (e.g., pneumonia/ secretions) produces changes in breath sounds such as rhonchi and wheezes.

INTERVENTIONS	RATIONALE
Independent	
Monitor endotracheal tube placement. Note tube number at lips and secure with tape or tube holder.	The endotracheal tube may slip into the right mainstem bronchus owing to anatomic structure of the bronchi, thereby obstructing airflow to the left lung.
Insert oral airway or bite block if patient biting endotracheal tube.	Prevents obstruction of airflow.
Monitor for symptoms that may indicate need for suctioning: dyspnea, excessive coughing, pressure alarm sounding on ventilator, visible secretions in tube and/or increased rhonchi.	Intubated patient has ineffective cough reflex or inability to expectorate secretions and is dependent on alternate means to remove secretions.
Suction as needed. Instill 2 to 5 ml of sterile normal saline. Hyperventilate with bag or ventilator sigh with 100 percent oxygen presuctioning and postsuctioning. Choose appropriate suction catheter and limit duration of suction to 15 seconds or less.	Suctioning should not be routine because it may irritate trachea and interfere with PEEP if used. Normal saline may be used to loosen secretions, thereby enhancing airway clearance. Suction catheter diameter (greater than 50 percent of the internal diameter of endotracheal or tracheotomy tube) and/or prolonged suctioning may result in hypoxia.
Monitor ECG for dysrhythmias during suctioning.	Hypoxia is common cause of dysrhythmias.
Reposition frequently.	Promotes drainage of secretion and ventilation of all lung segments.
Collaborative	
Administer chest physiotherapy as indicated (e.g., postural drainage, clapping, percussion).	Promotes ventilation of all lung segments and aids drainage of secretions.
Administer IV and aerosol bronchodilators, as indicated; for example, Aminophylline, metaproterenal sulfate (Alupent), idoetharine hydrochloride (Bronkosol).	Promotes ventilation and removal of secretions by relaxation of bronchial smooth muscle, bronchospasm.
Assist with fiberoptic bronchoscopy, if indicated.	May be performed to remove secretions or mucus plugs and to visualize airways.

NURSING DIAGNOSIS:	**Communication, impaired verbal.**
SUPPORTING DATA/CONTRIBUTING FACTORS:	**Intubation prevents approximation of vocal cords and vocalization.**
GENERAL PATIENT OUTCOMES:	**Able to communicate needs and wants.**

INTERVENTIONS	RATIONALE
Independent	
Establish means of communication: Ask "yes or no" questions; provide magic slate, paper and pencil, picture board, flash cards. Maintain eye contact. Validate	Provides a variety of communication possibilities. Patient may be able to move head and feels comfortable with simple gestures. Eye contact assures patient of

INTERVENTIONS	RATIONALE
Independent	
meaning of attempted verbal and nonverbal expressions.	nurse's interest in understanding. If unable to understand patient attempts at communication, family and other caregivers may be able to provide insight or interpretation and thereby minimize patient's frustration and anxiety.
Place call light within reach. Anticipate needs. Tell patient that the nurse is immediately available should assistance be needed.	May be able to relax, feel safe, and breathe with ventilator, knowing nurse is vigilant and needs will be met.
Encourage significant other(s) to talk with patient, providing information about family and daily happenings.	Even though patient cannot speak, this can be important in maintaining contact with reality and enabling patient to feel part of family unit.
Explain that patient will be able to speak after extubation (if true) although voice may be hoarse for a period of time.	Provides reassurance that speech loss is not permanent.
Collaborative	
Refer to speech therapist, specialist.	Helpful in evaluating ability to use sign language, artificial larynx, or speaking trachs for long-term/permanent loss of voice.

NURSING DIAGNOSIS:	**Oral Mucous Membrane, alteration in, actual/potential.**
SUPPORTING DATA/CONTRIBUTING FACTORS:	**With oral intubation, patient is not able to swallow oral fluids to hydrate mucous membranes. Mouth is in open position and endotracheal tube may cause pressure ulcers in mouth.**
GENERAL PATIENT OUTCOMES:	**Oral mucous membranes remain moist and without ulceration.**

INTERVENTIONS	RATIONALE
Independent	
Administer mouth care routinely as needed. Cleanse mouth with water, saline, or preferred mouthwashes. Brush teeth with soft toothbrush or swab. Apply lip lubrication.	Prevents drying and ulceration of mucous membranes and reduces medium for bacterial growth. Promotes comfort.
Alternate tube position in mouth.	Reduces risk of lip and mouth ulceration.
Collaborative	
Maintain enteral/parenteral hydration.	Keeps mucous membranes moist.

NURSING DIAGNOSIS:	**Anxiety/Fear.**
SUPPORTING DATA/CONTRIBUTING FACTORS:	**Intubation and the introduction of mechanical ventilation is usually done under emergency circumstances. This raises anxiety and accentuates fears about death. Severe anxiety may compromise patient's breathing.**
GENERAL PATIENT OUTCOMES:	**Demonstrates reduction in anxiety/fear as shown by relaxed manner, able to sleep or rest between procedures, breathing with ventilator.**

INTERVENTIONS	RATIONALE
Independent	
Give information about reason for ventilation or planned therapies. Include significant other(s) in explanations.	Provides reality orientation to patient who cannot voice specific concerns and may diminish feelings of panic and fear.

(Refer to Care Plan: Psychosocial Aspects of Critical Care, page 379.)

NURSING DIAGNOSIS:	**Nutrition, alteration in, less than body requirements.**
SUPPORTING DATA/CONTRIBUTING FACTORS:	**At a time when patient experiences altered ability to ingest and properly digest food, an increase in calories and protein is needed to meet the increased energy requirements produced by stress, the healing process, and weaning from the ventilator.**
GENERAL PATIENT OUTCOMES:	**Nutrition intake adequate to meet metabolic needs as shown by positive nitrogen balance and stable weight.**

INTERVENTIONS	RATIONALE
Independent	
Assess gastrointestinal (GI) function: presence and quality of bowel sounds, changes in abdominal girth, presence of anorexia, nausea, vomiting, constipation, or gastric bleeding.	Information necessary to identify appropriate route for nutritional support.

Collaborative

INTERVENTIONS	RATIONALE
Administer:	
Dextrose solutions and/or multivitamin additives.	Source of glucose and depleted vitamins. Carbohydrate content must be considered so as not to increase carbon dioxide production, especially during weaning from ventilator.
Hyperalimentation.	Supplies nutrition without using GI system.
Tube feedings.	Use when GI function assured.

(Refer to Care Plan: Nutritional Support, page 367.)

NURSING DIAGNOSIS:	**Infection, potential for.**
SUPPORTING DATA/CONTRIBUTING FACTORS:	**Intubation bypasses nasopharyngeal filtration structures and provides direct access to tracheal bronchial tree, increasing risk of infection.**
GENERAL PATIENT OUTCOMES:	**Free of infection, afebrile, lungs clear, sputum nonpurulent.**

INTERVENTIONS	RATIONALE
Independent	
Monitor for signs of infection; for example, temperature elevation, purulent sputum, drainage from endotracheal tube or tracheostomy stoma, elevated white blood count (WBC), changes in chest x-ray examination.	Early detection and internvention may reduce severity of infection.
Use proper handwashing technique.	Most important defense against nosocomial infections.
Maintain aseptic technique when suctioning, caring for endotracheal tube or tracheostomy.	Break in technique causes contamination and promotes development of infection or sepsis.
Cleanse tracheostomy insertion site routinely. Provide dry dressing, antibiotic ointment.	Reduces skin inflammation, risk of infection.
Encourage and assist with deep breathing, coughing, turning.	Promotes mobilization and clearance of secretions.
Collaborative	
Obtain appropriate specimens for culture and sensitivity (e.g., blood, sputum).	Results determine choice of antibiotic therapy.
Administer antibiotics, as indicated.	Treats or prevents infection.
Monitor plasma drug levels and/or "peak" and "trough" levels, as indicated (e.g., antibiotics, amino-	Assesses dose adequacy and renal and liver clearance rates in order to maintain therapeutic levels,

INTERVENTIONS	RATIONALE
Collaborative	
phylline, as indicated).	thereby avoiding toxicity and dangerous drug interactions.

NURSING DIAGNOSIS:	**Injury, potential for, multiple factors.**
SUPPORTING DATA/CONTRIBUTING FACTORS:	**The use of positive pressure ventilation and PEEP can cause barotrauma (pneumothorax). Oxygen toxicity is a potential hazard of prolonged use of high concentrations of oxygen. Administration of many drugs leads to the possibility of toxicity or dangerous interactions. Positive pressure ventilation increases intrathoracic pressure, which can reduce venous return and cardiac output.**
GENERAL PATIENT OUTCOMES:	**Absence of complications with vital signs within normal limits, symmetrical chest movement, breath sounds clear, skin intact.**

INTERVENTIONS	RATIONALE
Independent	
Trauma	
Monitor for signs of barotrauma: asymmetrical chest movement, diminished breath sounds on affected side, displacement of trachea to unaffected side, tachycardia, cyanosis, hypotension, accumulation of air under skin, crackling with palpation (crepitus).	Pressure generated by positive pressure ventilation and/or PEEP may cause rupture of alveoli and air leak into pleural space, mediastinum, or subcutaneous tissues. Pressure shifts the trachea away from the affected side. The lung collapses and great vessels in mediastinum may be compressed, thereby compromising cardiac output.
Use minimal leak or occlusive inflation technique with low pressure cuffed tube. Check cuff pressures routinely and whenever cuff is deflated or reinflated.	Cuff must be adequately inflated to insure ventilation and to prevent aspiration. Overinflation may cause tracheal damage, such as stenosis or tracheal-esophageal fistula.
Tape or tie tube securely.	Maintains proper tube alignment to prevent tracheal erosion or accidental extubation.
Decreased Cardiac Output	
Measure vital signs/hemodynamic pressures, for example, cardiac output (CO)/pulmonary capillary wedge pressure (PCWP) after initiating or altering PEEP.	Increased thoracic pressures are expected with use of PEEP. Excessive reduction in venous return or cardiac output may lead to serious complications.

INTERVENTIONS	RATIONALE
Independent	
Other	
Provide meticulous skin care by means of frequent position changes, massage, dry and wrinkle free linen.	Minimizes effects of immobility; protects bony prominences and prevents decubitus formation.
Assist with passive and/or active range of motion exercises and get patient up in chair as soon as able.	Preserves muscle tone and strength, promotes circulation, and improves ventilation and airway clearance.
Provide soft limb restraints, if indicated.	May be disoriented and attempt to extubate self.
Collaborative	
Trauma	
Use lowest possible ventilating pressures and levels of PEEP.	Minimizes risk of barotrauma.
Assist with change of endotracheal or tracheostomy tube.	Frequency of tube change varies with institutional policy and individual circumstances. Regular changing ensures tube (cuff) function and may decrease bacterial contamination. However, frequent changes can increase trauma and formation of granulation tissue that may increase airway obstruction.
Assist with chest tube insertion, if indicated.	Relieves pneumothorax, reexpands lung. (Refer to Care Plan: Hemothorax and Pneumothorax, page 88.)
Decreased Cardiac Output	
Administer intravenous (IV) fluids as indicated.	May improve hypotension, resulting from marginal or low flow states, so that use of PEEP may be continued.
Monitor ABGs in presence of decreasing cardiac output.	Cardiac output can be altered by factors other than PEEP. Respiratory and ventilator problems may be detected by alterations in blood gas, indicating hypoxia or hypoventilation as a cause for decreased CO.
Administer medications as indicated, for example, dopamine hydrochloride (Intropin).	Improves CO by increasing systemic vascular resistance, thereby increasing systolic blood pressure.

NURSING DIAGNOSIS: **Fluid Volume, alteration in [fluctuations].**

SUPPORTING DATA/CONTRIBUTING FACTORS: **Fluid volume deficit results from use of diuretics to reduce pulmonary fluid, actual loss from hemorrhage, or inadequate free water replacement with nutritional support. Renal failure associated with hypoxia or acidosis and excess secretion of ADH (SIADH) may result in fluid volume excess.**

GENERAL PATIENT OUTCOMES:	**Fluid balance is maintained with vital signs and urine output within normal limits, breath sounds clear, absence of tissue edema, weight stable.**

INTERVENTIONS	RATIONALE
Independent	
Monitor blood pressure, CVP, PCWP, PAP, CO.	Reflects changes associated with fluid fluctuations.
Assess breath sounds for crackles and wheezes.	Retention of inspired water vapor may cause or increase pulmonary interstitial edema, reducing oxygen diffusion.
Monitor urine output.	Hourly outputs less than 20 to 30 ml per hour require intervention as may indicate fluid volume deficit, renal insufficiency, or inappropriate antidiuretic hormone (ADH) secretion.
Calculate 24-hour fluid balance. Note daily weight fluctuation.	Fluids enhance circulating volume and tissue perfusion; however, fluid restriction may be required if overload is indicated by continued positive fluid balance and weight gain, or if SIADH occurs.
Test stools, emesis, nasogastric drainage for blood.	Ventilated patients are sometimes prone to develop bleeding complications (e.g., stress ulcer).
Collaborative	
Administer and restrict fluids as indicated.	Replaces and reduces total body water.
Monitor BUN, creatinine, electrolytes.	Decreased kidney perfusion, filtration, and excretion causes an elevation in BUN, creatinine, and other electrolyte imbalances.
Administer diuretics, as indicated.	Reduces total body water, and thereby reduces lung water, decreasing pulmonary edema.
Administer demeclocycline hydrochloride (Declomycin), if indicated.	Controls SIADH if other measures are unsuccessful, that is, water restriction, administration of diuretics, hypertonic saline and potassium.

CHAPTER 5 NEUROLOGIC

Brain Injury/Increased Intracranial Pressure

PATIENT ASSESSMENT DATA BASE

HISTORY

History of loss of consciousness, neurologic disease, infection, metabolic disorders (e.g., diabetes), head trauma, drug/alcohol abuse, seizures.

History of heart disease, blood dyscrasias, vascular disease, embolic disease, hypertension, obesity, cigarette smoking, cardiac arrest.

Recent anticoagulant therapy.

Presence of factors that exert pressure against brain surfaces, for example, epidural or subdural hematomas or meningiomas, intracerebral or intracerebellar hematomas or hemorrhages such as occur with aneurysms, A-V malformation, brain lesions.

Head trauma with brain injury, swelling, and/or vasogenic edema.

Infectious processes (e.g., encephalitis).

Hydrocephalus with altered production or absorption of cerebrospinal fluid.

Metabolic disorders resulting in defective osmo-regulation, producing cytotoxic edema and intracellular fluid accumulation.

Subjective

May be reported by significant other or emergency medical caregivers if patient unconscious:

Report of behavioral changes: confusion, lethargy, agitation, forgetfulness, subtle personality changes may be first sign noticed by significant other(s).

Headache of variable intensity; diplopia (double vision), photophobia, or other visual deficits; vertigo or syncope; loss of ability to read or write.

Nausea, vomiting (projectile or unexpected).

Motor function changes: unsteady gait, temporary paresthesias, hemiparesis, paralysis of extremities.

PHYSICAL EXAMINATION

Inspection

LEVEL OF CONSCIOUSNESS

Vebal response: note best response; for example, slurred, incomprehensible, confused, repetitive, or no response.

Mentation/sensorium: observe orientation to person, place, time.

MOTOR FUNCTION

Integration of consciousness: note response to simple commands; for example, grasping and releasing hand, or holding up two fingers.

Muscle strength: note ability to resist; for example, push against your hand, or to extend arms without pronation and downward drift. Note flaccid response.

Symmetry: note movement of all extremities, absence of spontaneous movement, or favoring one side.

Posturing: note decorticate or decerebrate response to painful or noxious stimuli.

Seizure: involuntary movements, rigidity, and general seizure activity may occur.

OTHER

Eyes: note pupil equality, size and reaction to light. Observe for ptosis of eyelid. Note positive or negative doll's eyes response, and papilledema which is a reliable sign of increased intracranial pressure (IICP), but typically occurs late.

Respirations: note altered rate, depth, and regularity, for example, periods of apnea alternating with hyperventilation.

Cough/gag reflex may be impaired as manifested by coughing, drooling, lack of swallowing, and respiratory distress.

Cerebrospinal fluid (CSF) drainage: frequent swallowing may be noted, or drainage from nose (rhinorrhea) or ears (otorrhea).

Skin: may have head/facial bruising, lacerations, abrasions (new or old), discoloration around eyes (raccoon) or ears (Battle's sign) indicating head trauma.

Auscultation

Heart rate: dysrhythmias, for example, bradycardia or alternating tachycardia and bradycardia may occur.

Blood pressure (BP) may be normal, although variations are possible, depending on neurologic status and other underlying conditions or disease states. Increased systolic, with normal or decreased diastolic, causes a widening pulse pressure, which is a late sign of increased intracranial pressure.

Breath sounds may be normal; areas of decreased or absent breath sounds or airway congestion may be noted.

Palpation

Tactile/painful stimulation: if verbal response is absent, note reaction to light touch, pin prick, shoulder shaking, pinching biceps, and suborbital pressure. Appropriate response would be eye opening, facial grimacing, or purposeful withdrawal from the stimuli.

Temperature may be hyperthermic as a result of increased pressure on the hypothalamus or presence of infection.

DIAGNOSTIC STUDIES

CAT scan (with or without contrast): identifies space-occupying lesions, hemorrhage, neoplasms, abcesses, ventricular size, brain tissue shift.

Magnetic resonance imager (MRI): uses similar to those of CAT scan without radioactivity.

Cerebral angiograms pinpoint hemorrhage sites, demonstrate abnormal vascular patterns, or shifts secondary to IICP.

Cerebral blood flow studies determine existing blood flow and blockage(s) in the brain.

Brain scan detects damaged brain tissue or tumors.

Skull film detects changes in bony structure, shifts of midline structures, changes consistent with chronic increased intracranial pressure.

Nonemergent studies that may be done:
- Digital subtraction angiogram (DSA): radiographic visualization of intracranial and extracranial circulation.
- Evoked potentials (BAER'S): Electrical neurometrics determine levels of cortical and brainstem function.
- Position emission transaxial tomography (PETT) detects changes in metabolic function in the brain.
- Lumbar puncture: not done if IICP suspected. May be diagnostic for suspected subarachnoid hemorrhage or to rule out meningitis, vasculitis, or neoplasm.

Arterial blood gas: determines presence of ventilation or oxygenation problems which may exacerbate IICP.

Serum chemistry and electrolyte levels may be useful in determining metabolic cause of coma or may reveal imbalances that may contribute to IICP.

Toxicology screen detects drugs as possible cause of unconsciousness.

Serum anticonvulsant level may be done to insure that patient is adequately "loaded" to prevent seizures.

ECG: dysrhythmias, ST segment abnormalities may be generated by intracranial pressure changes.

NURSING PRIORITIES

1. Monitor/limit elevation of intracranial pressure.
2. Maintain/enhance cerebral perfusion.
3. Provide comfort and emotional support.
4. Minimize/prevent complications.

NURSING DIAGNOSIS:	**Tissue Perfusion, alteration in, cerebral.**
SUPPORTING DATA/CONTRIBUTING FACTORS:	**Cerebral perfusion may be compromised by intracranial pressure changes caused by (1) space-occupying lesions (e.g., tumor, hemorrhage, hematoma, or aneurysm); (2) cerebral edema, which may be a local or generalized response to injury, metabolic responses, or drugs or ETOH ingestion; (3) decreased systemic blood pressure and hypoxia; or (4) direct interruption of flow by thrombus or embolus, which produces tissue ischemia or infarction.**
GENERAL PATIENT OUTCOMES:	**Intracranial pressure (ICP) remains within normal limits (less than 25 mmHg). Cerebral perfusion pressure (CPP) is maintained at minimum of 50,**

	preferably 70 to 90, mmHg. Usual or improved level of consciousness and motor and sensory function. Appropriate pupil size, reactivity, and ocular movement. Absence of headache and vomiting. Stable vital signs.

INTERVENTIONS	RATIONALE
Independent	
Monitor neurologic status closely and compare with baseline, such as Glasgow Coma Scale:	Assesses trends in level of consciousness (LOC) and potential for increased intracranial pressure (IICP), through best motor, verbal, pupillary and oculomotor responses, and is useful in determining location, extent, and progression of central nervous system (CNS) damage.
Assess level of consciousness by verbal or tactile/painful stimuli: note if patient is awake and alert; oriented to person, place, time; drowsy, difficult to arouse, stuporous, comatose.	Responses reflect amount of brain impairment and help localize area of involvement. If minimal damage has occurred in the cerebral cortex, the patient may be aroused by verbal stimuli but may appear drowsy or uncooperative. More extensive damage to the cerebral cortex may be displayed by slow response to commands, lapsing into sleep when not stimulated, disorientation, and stupor. Damage to the midbrain, pons, and medulla are evident by lack of appropriate response to stimuli.
Note: If patient has been placed in barbiturate coma, do not stimulate with pain to test.	Pentobarbital given at levels to induce coma will cause cessation of body movement; corneal, pupil, and gag responses. Serum drug levels, increasing blood pressure or agitation, are better indicators of effectiveness of drug therapy than use of painful stimuli.
Assess motor function: note integration of consciousness and voluntary movement. Look for purposeful and nonpurposeful movement. Assess muscle strength; observe for symmetrical spontaneous movement. Note nuchal rigidity or twitching, increased restlessness or irritability.	Consciousness and involuntary movement are integrated if the patient can both grasp and release the tester's hand or hold up two fingers on command. Purposeful movement can be grimacing or withdrawing from a painful stimuli, or movements that the patient desires, such as sitting up. Other movements (e.g., posturing and abnormal flexion), usually indicate diffuse cortical damage. Absence of spontaneous movement on one side of the body indicates damage to the motor tracts in the opposite cerebral hemispheres. Nuchal rigidity and purposeless activity may reflect developing seizure activity, which can cause or increase ICP.
Record position of eyes (e.g., deviated, dysconjugated).	Early sign of IICP is impaired abduction of eyes, indicating injury to the abducens (VI) nerve.
Assess pupillary changes: note size, shape, equality, light reactivity (e.g., direct/consensual).	Pupil reactions are regulated by the third cranial nerve in the midbrain and are therefore useful in determining if the brainstem is intact. Pupil size indicates balance between parasympathetic and sympathetic innervations. Response to light reflects combined function of

INTERVENTIONS	RATIONALE
Independent	
	optic (II) and oculomotor (III) cranial nerves. Unilaterally dilated, fixed pupil (loss of ciliospinal reflex) reflects IICP from an ipsilateral intracranial lesion that is stretching or compressing the oculomotor nerve and suggests imminent uncal/transtentorial herniation. Bilateral pinpoint pupils without reaction may indicate damage to pons.
Assess for loss of doll's eyes (oculocephalic reflex) and oculovestibular reflex via caloric irrigation test.	Assesses cranial nerves VIII-III-VI and thus integrity of brainstem.
Monitor vital signs:	
Blood pressure,	Normally autoregulation maintains constant cerebral blood flow despite fluctuations in systemic blood pressure, by dilation or constriction of cerebral arteries. Loss of autoregulation may follow local or diffuse vascular damage. As a result, cerebral blood flow fluctuates with systemic blood pressure (e.g., systemic hypertension can increase cerebral blood flow and thus IICP). A late and ominous manifestation of IICP is an elevated systolic BP with widening pulse pressure (difference between systolic and diastolic BP), decreased pulse, and respiratory rate (Cushing's reflex).
Hemodynamic pressures (e.g., MAP, CO, PAWP),	Systemic conditions/shock may compromise cardiac output, systemic pressure and thus cerebral perfusion pressure (CPP). In addition, the vasodilatory effect of therapy may reduce venous return with the same end results.
Pulse and continuous ECG.	Changes in rate and rhythm (most often bradycardia), presence of dysrhythmias, and nonspecific ST/T wave changes may develop, reflecting brainstem pressure or injury in the absence of underlying cardiac disease.
Respirations, noting pattern and rhythm, such as post-hyperventilation apnea, Cheyne-Stokes, central neurogenic hyperventilation, apneustic, ataxic (Biot's), and cluster breathing.	Six different patterns of irregular breathing correlate with lesions at various levels, for example, posthyperventilation apnea may occur with metabolic or structural forebrain disease; Cheyne-Stokes is associated with bilateral lesions of cerebral hemispheres, midbrain, and upper pons; central neurogenic hyperventilation accompanies lesions in the lower midbrain and upper pons; apneustic breathing indicates injury in mid and lower pons; cluster breathing may occur with involvement of the lower pons and upper medulla; and ataxic breathing is associated with lesions of the medulla. These respiratory dysrhythmias negatively affect $PaCO_2/PaO_2$ and directly alter cerebral blood flow (CBF) and ICP.
Assess reflexes (e.g., blink, cough, gag, Babinski).	Although not specific in terms of measuring degree or severity of IICP, alterations in reflexes reflect injury at level of mid brain or brainstem and have direct implications for patient safety. Loss of corneal reflex (cranial nerves V and VIII) suggests damage to the pons and medulla. Absence of cough and gag reflexes (cranial

INTERVENTIONS	RATIONALE
Independent	
	nerves IX and X) reflects damage to medulla. Presence of positive Babinski reflex indicates injury along the pyramidal pathway.
Monitor intracranial pressure and waveforms.	Although not available in all critical care units, direct monitoring of ICP is used to detect increasing pressure and need for initiation of interventions to reduce cerebral hypoxia and irreversible neurologic damage. Numeric readings are used to calculate CPP, and both pressure readings and waveforms are evaluated for specific fluctuations in the patient's intracranial pressure (e.g., response to nursing measures and activities).
Calculate and monitor cerebral perfusion pressure (CPP = MAP − ICP).	CPP is the amount of pressure required in the cerebral vasculature to provide oxygen and nutrients to brain tissue. Desired range of CPP to maintain adequate cerebral blood flow (CBF), is between 70 and 90 mm Hg. CPP less than 50 mm Hg leads to decrease in CBF, resulting in cerebral ischemia.
Maintain integrity of invasive ICP monitoring device.	Prevents break in system which could result in inaccurate ICP readings and/or result in loss of CSF, leading to ventricular collapse or infection.
Carry out nursing measures to reduce or minimize fluctuations of ICP:	
Maintain head/neck in midline/neutral position.	Hyperextension and hyperflexion or turning head to one side compresses the jugular veins and can inhibit venous return, thereby increasing ICP.
Avoid or limit activity that increases intrathoracic and intraabdominal pressures such as coughing, vomiting (Valsalva maneuver). Avoid extreme flexion of hips and knees.	Creates backward pressure reflected to jugular veins which impairs venous return and may increase ICP. Note: Use of PEEP (especially greater than 10 cm) in mechanically ventilated patients may produce same effect.
Promote comfort measures (e.g., back massage, soft voice, Therapeutic Touch). (Refer to Nursing Diagnosis: Comfort, alteration in, pain, acute, page 137.)	Pain and anxiety may be present, causing increased ICP, even if patient appears unresponsive.
Provide quiet, comforting atmosphere; dim lights; and limit extraneous conversation by staff.	Promotes rest and decreases sensory stimulation and overload, which can increase ICP.
Provide rest periods between care activities. Limit duration of procedures.	Continual activity has a cumulative effect demonstrated by elevations of ICP.
Encourage family and significant other(s) to talk to patient if appropriate.	Appears to have a relaxing effect on many patients, manifested by reduced ICP.
Monitor temperature and regulate environmental temperature as indicated; for example, limit use of blankets and bedclothes, or administer tepid sponge bath in presence of temperature elevation.	Fever may reflect damage to hypothalamus and increase metabolic needs and oxygen consumption. Environmental regulation is a nontraumatic aid to control hyperthermia.
Wrap extremities in blankets when hypothermia blanket is being used.	Maintains peripheral circulation and prevents or reduces shivering, which can increase metabolic needs and ICP.

INTERVENTIONS	RATIONALE
Independent	
Limit duration of tracheal suctioning to 15 seconds and hyperoxygenate before and after procedure.	Prevents hypoxia during procedure, which may cause cerebral vasodilation or vascular congestion, thereby increasing ICP.
Maintain patency of indwelling catheter if used, or bladder for distention.	Bladder distention may trigger autonomic responses, which may increase ICP.
Use restraints with caution and only if patient is in danger of injuring/extubating self.	Restraints may cause patient to "fight" harder, thereby increasing ICP.
Collaborative	
Elevate head of bed 15 to 45 degrees as tolerated or ordered.	Promotes venous drainage from head, thereby decreasing ICP.
Administer intravenous (IV) fluids per microdrip or infusion pump.	Careful control of infusion rate and prevention of inadvertent fluid bolus minimizes fluctuations in vascular load and ICP. Fluid restriction may be used to lower total body water and thereby reduce cerebral edema.
Hyperventilate (when mechanically ventilated) to keep $PaCO_2$ between 25 and 30 mmHg during initial 48 to 72 hours.	Elevated $PaCO_2$ will increase intracranial blood flow and volume because of its vasodilating effects, ultimately increasing ICP. Lower $PaCO_2$ causes cerebral vasoconstriction, thereby reducing CBF volume and decreasing ICP, but must be balanced against the potential for increasing cerebral ischemia.
Administer medications to reduce ICP as indicated:	
Manitol (Osmitrol);	Osmotic diuretic that pulls water from the brain cells, thereby temporarily reducing the size of the cerebrum and thus decreasing ICP. Precautions: Serum osmolality should be closely monitored, because an increased osmolality (e.g., greather than 310) may disrupt the blood-brain barrier, actually increasing edema. Monitor for systemic hypotension, which can decrease CPP. Watch for rebound increase in ICP, which may occur 8 to 12 hours after osmotic diuresis.
Furosemide (Lasix);	May be used to reduce total body water and thus cerebral edema.
Steroids, for example, dexamethasone (Decadron), methylprednisolone (Medrol);	May reduce capillary permeability to limit cerebral edema formation. Also may reduce risk of "rebound" phenomenon when mannitol is used.
Pancuronium bromide (Pavulon);	May be used to reduce agitation and associated IICP in the agitated or combative patient on the ventilator.
Sedatives, for example, fentanyl (Sublimaze);	Produce immediate analgesia and sedation, thereby lowering metabolic rate (e.g., heart and respiratory rates and blood pressure). Should be given IV and when the patient is intubated and mechanically ventilated to offset side effect of respiratory depression. Precautions: These can produce hyperexcitability, leading to seizure activity. Should be used cautiously in patients with liver and kidney dysfunction.

INTERVENTIONS	RATIONALE
Collaborative	
Chlorpromazine (Thorazine);	Drug of choice in treating posturing and shivering, which can increase ICP. Precautions: This drug can lower the seizure threshold or precipitate Dilantin toxicity by interfering with Dilantin metabolism.
Barbiturates, for example, pentobarbital (Nembutal), thiopental (Pentothal sodium);	Drug-induced coma may be desirable for reducing cerebral metabolism and blood flow when conventional measures fail to reduce intracranial hypertension. Precautions: Pulmonary artery catheter may be desired to monitor for myocardial depression.
Phenytoin (Dilantin);	Drug of choice for treatment and prevention of seizure activity.
Acetiminophen (Tylenol).	Treats hyperthermia, lowering metabolic needs and deleterious CNS effects.
Monitor serum and urine electrolytes and osmolality as indicated.	Intracranial hypertension, use of barbiturate therapy, PEEP, or hypotonic solutions may lead to fluid and electrolyte imbalances, further affecting ICP. Example: A decrease in serum osmolality stimulates antidiuretic hormone (ADH) release, which may lead to syndrome of inappropriate antidiuretic hormone (SIADH), manifested by low serum sodium, high urine osmolality, fluid retention (low urine output, positive fluid balance) resulting in IICP.
Apply hypothermia blanket, observing operational and safety factors.	May be used to maintain normothermia. Caution required to prevent complications, for example, temperature drift below desired levels.
Maintain intracranial pressure monitoring device; for example, subarachnoid bolt, epidural or subdural sensor, or intraventricular catheter. Balance and calibrate as needed.	Subarachnoid bolt allows for direct measurement of intracranial pressure through CSF and can be quickly placed without penetrating the cerebrum. Epidural monitor (reflects pressure changes only) can be easily placed and cannot become occluded. Intraventricular catheter is used to measure volume/pressure response and allows for drainage of CSF to reduce pressure.
Remove CSF to reduce ICP as specifically indicated, noting failure of nursing measures to reduce ICP; and document frequency of drainage, time interval for drainage, color, clarity, consistency, and amount of fluid drained.	Intraventricular catheters are placed to prevent ventricular dilation caused by intraventricular hemorrhage or to prevent blockage of cerebrospinal flow as might occur with cerebral swelling.

NURSING DIAGNOSIS:	**Breathing Pattern, ineffective/Gas Exchange, impaired.**
SUPPORTING DATA/CONTRIBUTING FACTORS:	**Compression/injury to respiratory center alters breathing patterns, resulting in hypoventilation or hyperventilation, with fluctuations in $PaO_2/PaCO_2$. Disruption in muscle innervation and**

tone may jeopardize airway by relaxation of the tongue or inability to generate effective cough to clear secretions. Sympathetic stimulation causes peripheral vasoconstriction and increasing vascular resistance which shunts blood into the pulmonary vasculature, potentiating risk of neurogenic pulmonary edema. Any of these factors may adversely affect ICP.

GENERAL PATIENT OUTCOMES:	**Patent airway is maintained. Effective breathing pattern is established and maintained. Breath sounds are clear. Signs of hypoxia and hypercarbia are absent.**

INTERVENTIONS	RATIONALE
Independent	
Assess patency of airway.	Occlusion of airway (even partially) can increase intrathoracic pressure, increase $PaCO_2$, decrease PaO_2, and thus increase ICP.
Insert soft nasopharyngeal airway if possible. Avoid taping oral airway in place, and remove airway as soon as able.	Soft nasopharyngeal airways may be preferred because hard oropharyngeal airway (taped in place) prevents the patient from pushing airway from back of throat, thereby stimulating gag reflex which produces a Valsalva maneuver, and elevates ICP. Note: Nasopharyngeal airway is contraindicated in presence of rhinorrhea, which may reflect break in integrity of skull and potentiate risk of direct brain trauma or infection.
Note competence of gag and swallow reflexes.	Ability to mobilize or clear secretions is important to maintain airway. Loss of reflex may indicate need for intubation.
Describe and document respirations, skin color, chest expansion, symptoms of distress (e.g., nasal flaring, use of accessory muscles).	May indicate developing pulmonary complications or reflect change in ICP.
Auscultate breath sounds. Note areas of hypoventilation, presence of adventitious sounds (crackles, rhonchi, wheezes).	Identifies pulmonary problems such as atelectasis, congestion, or airway obstruction, which may impede gas diffusion, jeopardize cerebral oxygenation, and increase ICP.
Elevate head of bed and reposition as indicated.	Enhances lung expansion and reduces pulmonary congestion.
Hyperoxygenate before and after suctioning (suction no longer than 10 to 15 seconds). Note character, color, odor of secretions.	Tracheal suctioning can cause or aggravate hypoxia, which produces vasoconstriction, adversely effecting cerebral perfusion.
Monitor use of respiratory depressant drugs (e.g., sedatives, barbiturates).	Depressing natural respiratory functions may increase risk of respiratory complications.

Collaborative

Monitor and graph serial ABGs.	$PaCO_2$ greater than 42, PaO_2 less than 50, and acidosis may increase cerebral vasodilation and result in increased cerebral blood volume and sustained increase in ICP.
Monitor serial chest x-ray examinations.	Reveals ventilatory state and signs of developing complications (e.g., atelectasis, pneumonia).
Provide oxygen therapy and maintain mechanical ventilation as indicated. (Refer to Care Plan: Ventilatory Assistance mechanical, page 115.)	Supplemental oxygen maximizes arterial PO_2 and aids in prevention of hypoxia. If respiratory centers are depressed, mechanical support may be required.
Assist with chest physiotherapy if indicated.	Mobilizes secretions to clear lung fields and reduce infiltrates. Note: May be contraindicated in patients with acute IICP.

NURSING DIAGNOSIS:	**Fluid Volume Deficit, potential.**
SUPPORTING DATA/CONTRIBUTING FACTORS:	**Increased metabolic needs (e.g., stress, fever); use of diuretics to reduce ICP; development of metabolic and/or endocrine complications, e.g., diabetes insipidus (DI); vomiting and excessive diaphoresis may cause fluid deficit.**
GENERAL PATIENT OUTCOMES:	**Fluid and electrolyte balance is maintained as shown by balanced intake and output, moist mucous membranes, good skin turgor, and appropriate urine output.**

INTERVENTIONS	RATIONALE
Independent	
Measure intake and output, noting negative fluid balance (output greater than intake) and specific gravity. Weigh as indicated.	Useful in assessing fluid status and early detection of complications (e.g., DI). Weights may be required daily for close regulation of fluid needs.
Note presence of nausea and vomiting.	May indicate direct stimulation of emetic center in medulla or reflex action to dehydrate body in presence of increased ICP.
Maintain normothermia.	Decreases insensible fluid loss through excessive diaphoresis.
Monitor symptoms of DI; for example, high urine output (as much as 15 to 16 liters per day) low specific gravity (1.000 to 1.005), excessive thirst, poor skin turgor, negative fluid balance.	May have CNS (post head trauma) or renal cause. Copious diuresis and low ADH secretion cause dehydration and may lead to shock.

Collaborative

Monitor laboratory results; for example, urine and serum sodium, potassium, osmolality.	Provides information regarding CNS effects on renal function. Rapid depletion of potassium and elevation of serum sodium (greather than 150 mEq per liter) may occur as a result of DI.
Replace fluids and electrolytes.	Intake must at least equal output to maintain circulating fluid volume and cerebral perfusion pressure. Rapid fluid replacement in combination with drug therapy may result in fluid overload, leading to cerebral edema and convulsions.
Administer medications as indicated:	
Antiemetics.	Inhibits stimulation of vomiting center.
Vasopressin (Pitressin) IV or subcutaneously, or desmopressin acetate (DDAVP) intranasal spray.	Antidiuretic hormone effect promotes water reabsorption and more appropriate urine output.

NURSING DIAGNOSIS: **Comfort, alteration in, pain, acute.**

SUPPORTING DATA/CONTRIBUTING FACTORS: **Discomfort may occur as a result of direct trauma (head or other coexisting injuries) and/or increased ICP, resulting in headache.**

GENERAL PATIENT OUTCOMES: **Pain, discomfort, are minimized.**

INTERVENTIONS	RATIONALE
Independent	
Note description of pain; for example, dull, sharp, throbbing, constant, intermittent. Note nonverbal behaviors, for example, facial grimacing, putting hand to head, restlessness, and agitation.	Aids in localizing pain in order to provide appropriate interventions. Headaches may be treated with sedatives or analgesics if severe or associated with agitation.
Explain treatments and procedures, even if the patient is unconscious. Attempt to limit or avoid painful procedures, or premedicate if indicated.	The patient may react to external stimuli even while appearing unresponsive.
Provide comfort measures (e.g., position changes, massage, Therapeutic Touch).	Helps reduce pain and associated anxiety or restlessness, and conveys a sense of warmth and caring.
Collaborative	
Administer analgesics (e.g., codeine).	Provides pain relief and comfort. Opiates are usually avoided because they mask neurologic signs.

NURSING DIAGNOSIS: **Sensory-Perceptual Alteration.**

SUPPORTING DATA/CONTRIBUTING FACTORS: **Cerebral insult may produce altered sensory reception, transmission, and/**

	or integration in which the accustomed stimuli are not experienced or recognized/interpreted accurately. Brain dysfunction or physical or chemical alterations, including ETOH intoxication, may further compound this problem.
GENERAL PATIENT OUTCOMES:	**Level of consciousness/orientation is improved and maintained. Irritability and agitation are decreased.**

INTERVENTIONS	RATIONALE
Independent	
Monitor orientation, mood/affect, sensorium, thought process.	Upper cerebral functions are often the first to be affected by altered circulation, oxygenation.
Compare current responses with past behaviors with significant others.	Presence of hallucinations or alteration in interpretation of stimuli may have occurred independent of current condition, or be part of developing sequelae.
Speak in calm, quiet voice, use short simple phrases, maintain eye contact.	Establishes rapport, communication. Patient may have limited attention span and understanding during acute and recovery stages.
Restrict bedside discussions (e.g., of patient's condition or extraneous conversations unrelated to the patient).	Avoids misinterpretation of statements and may decrease patient's fear and anxiety.
Provide quiet environment. Use meaningful tactile stimulation (e.g., touch, hand holding) and auditory stimulus (tapes, radio, visitors).	Decreases sensory overload. Carefully selected sensory stimulation may promote reduction in anxiety and agitation, reduce ICP, and enhance orientation.
Involve family in patient care.	Patient may respond more to loved ones. Family may benefit from active participation in care. Note: Significant other(s) may have difficulty accepting and dealing with patient's aberrant behavior and may require assistance in coping with situation.
Collaborative	
Provide for speech therapy, physical therapy, occupational therapy consultation.	May have useful devices for communication and will be needed for ongoing rehabilitation needs.

NURSING DIAGNOSIS:	**Injury, potential for, complications of altered mobility.**
SUPPORTING DATA/CONTRIBUTING FACTORS:	**Altered mobility resulting from decreased consciousness and cognitive impairment potentiates the risk of complications such as skin breakdown, loss of muscle and joint func-**

	tions, and development of peripheral thrombosis.
GENERAL PATIENT OUTCOMES:	**Skin integrity is restored and maintained. Musculoskeletal function is maintained. Thrombophlebitis is prevented.**

INTERVENTIONS	RATIONALE
Independent	
Develop repositioning schedule; turn with care.	Promotes circulation and tissue perfusion. Note: Rapid turning may cause orthostatic hypotension or sudden increase in blood pressure and ICP (Valsalva effect).
Provide range of motion (passive and/or active) exercises with caution.	Maintains joint and muscle mobility and limits venous stasis.
Provide frequent skin care, massage skin and bony prominences. Use protective padding, (e.g., sheepskin, lamb's wool). Maintain dry, wrinkle-free sheets.	Promotes tissue perfusion and aids in preventing skin breakdown.
Monitor symptoms of skin breakdown (e.g., changes in skin color, reduced capillary refill).	Skin integrity may be impaired by multitrauma, nutritional deficits, posturing movements, or flaccid paralysis; skin breakdown occurs rapidly if preventive care is not taken.
Inspect incision, abrasion and suture lines, noting drainage color, odor, amount.	Alterations in circulation and developing infections may retard tissue healing.
Pad side rails, provide hand coverings (e.g., "boxing gloves").	Limits injury to restless or combative patient.
Limit use of restraints, provide for general limb movement.	Restraints permitting general movement limit possibility of self-inflicted injury without producing Valsalva maneuver or IICP induced by fighting against tight restraints.
Provide splints, hightop shoes or booties, hand rolls.	Maintains functional body alignment to prevent or limit contractures.
Take calf and thigh measurements. Monitor extremities for warmth and redness, assess tenderness, presence of Homan's sign.	Venous stasis may lead to thrombophlebitis.
Collaborative	
Provide foam or alternating air mattress, special flotation bed.	Minimizes pressure to skin area, enhances circulation, thereby reducing risk of ulceration.
Provide eye care (e.g., artificial tears, patching as needed).	Maintains lubrication of eye, reduces mucus buildup, and prevents corneal abrasions in the event of loss of blink reflex.
Apply antiembolic stockings as indicated.	Improves venous return and limits stasis by providing muscle and venous wall support.
Obtain consultations, such as physical and occupational therapies.	Begin mobilizing patient, when feasible, to improve strength and muscle tone and to begin work on activities of daily living.

NURSING DIAGNOSIS:	Infection, potential for.
SUPPORTING DATA/CONTRIBUTING FACTORS:	CSF leaks, use of invasive monitoring devices, or complications from trauma or surgery may lead to infection or meningitis.
GENERAL PATIENT OUTCOMES:	Patient is afebrile, CNS infection is minimized or prevented.

INTERVENTIONS	RATIONALE
Independent	
Observe strict sterile technique when assisting with insertion or maintaining invasive ICP monitoring device. Maintain integrity of closed system.	Inhibits introduction of pathologic microorganisms.
Maintain dry, sterile dressing around cranial insertion site. Change dressings per protocol.	Inhibits growth of pathologic microorganisms. Note: Occlusive dressings may be used when an intraventricular catheter is in place and may be changed by the neurosurgeon to evaluate source of drainage.
Monitor and record any leakage of fluid from nose (rhinorrhea), ears (otorrhea), head dressings, or around ICP monitoring site.	May indicate CSF loss. Note: Clear drainage with a yellow ring, or sanguinous drainage with a clear ring, positive for glucose is usually CSF.
Monitor symptoms of meningitis (e.g., change in level of consciousness, increased white blood count, temperature elevation, nuchal rigidity, photophobia, positive Kernig's sign).	Possible complication of brain injury or monitoring device.
Collaborative	
Obtain CSF culture as indicated.	Identifies organisms of infection in order to provide appropriate therapy.
Administer antibiotics as indicated.	May be prophylactic or specific for identified pathologic organisms.

NURSING DIAGNOSIS:	Bowel Elimination, alteration in, constipation.
SUPPORTING DATA/CONTRIBUTING FACTORS:	Immobility, decreased peristalsis and nutritional status contribute to problems of elimination.
GENERAL PATIENT OUTCOMES:	Patient is free of impaction and has a routine bowel movement.

INTERVENTIONS	RATIONALE
Independent	
Ausculate bowel sounds.	Hypoactive or absent bowel sounds indicate depressed gastrointestinal (GI) function.
Check for impaction. Avoid prolonged rectal stimulation.	Decreases chance of autonomic reflex responses. Prolonged stimulation may cause Valsalva response or increased ICP.
Collaborative	
Initiate bowel regimen using suppositories and stool softeners such as Ducolax and Pericolace.	Prevents constipation and resulting effects of autonomic responses (e.g., hypertension, bradycardia).

NURSING DIAGNOSIS: **Nutrition, alteration in, less than body requirements [potential].**

SUPPORTING DATA/CONTRIBUTING FACTORS: **Decreased level of consciousness, vomiting, or mechanical ventilation disturbs normal food intake. Gastric bleeding (Cushing's ulcers) is a complication that alters GI function and reduces nutrient absorption. Increased metabolic needs are present secondary to cerebral trauma or tissue injury.**

GENERAL PATIENT OUTCOMES: **Caloric intake is adequate to maintain weight and promote healing.**

INTERVENTIONS	RATIONALE
Independent	
Maintain nothing-by-mouth (NPO) status as indicated.	Cerebral injuries or edema may cause projectile vomiting, potentiating risk of aspiration.
Auscutate bowel sounds.	GI function (peristalsis) is necessary for adequate gastric emptying and utilization of nutrients.
Assess gag and swallow reflexes.	Oral feeding cannot be safely resumed until adequate swallow reflex is present.
Elevate head of bed during and after oral or gastric feeding.	Reduces risk of aspiration and aids in gastric emptying.
Provide adequate free water daily as indicated.	Use of high-protein feedings may produce osmotic diuresis or dehydration unless adequate fluid is provided.
Check gastric secretions for pH and occult blood if feeding tube in place.	Gastric bleeding, ulcers, are common complications. Irritation or bleeding may occur if pH is less than 5. (Refer to Care Plan: Upper GI/Esophageal Bleeding, page 197.)

Independent

Weigh as indicated.	Monitors adequacy of caloric intake.

Collaborative

Administer nutritional feedings by appropriate methods, for example, parenteral, enteral, or oral routes using prepared or commercial feedings, semisolids or liquids, or regular food. (Refer to Care Plan: Nutritional Support, page 367.)	Ensure adequate caloric intake. Protein may be restricted during cerebral edema phase because alterations in vascular membrane permeability allow protein shifts to occur, enhancing edema formation. Note: Placement of nasogastric tube should be avoided when CSF leak is present (indicates basilar skull fractures) because risk of infections or sinusitis is very high. Dobhoff tube may be preferred.
Monitor laboratory studies (e.g., iron, BUN, glucose, liver function tests, protein, amylase).	Indicates nutritional needs, effectiveness of therapy and organ function.

Guillain-Barre Syndrome (Polyradiculitis)

PATIENT ASSESSMENT DATA BASE

HISTORY

An acute illness or other immune-inciting event may have occurred 1 to 3 weeks prior to the onset of Guillian-Barre syndrome, although some patients do not seem to have any precipitating factors. Some of the following factors have been associated with the syndrome: viral illness (e.g., gastroenteritis, upper respiratory infection), surgery, trauma, innoculation for smallpox, influenza, tetanus, measles, and lymphoproliferative neoplasms.

Subjective

Complains of paresthesia (numbness, tingling) beginning in the toes or fingers and ascending upward (stocking or glove distribution).

Notes progressive motor weakness beginning in the feet or hands and ascending upward (e.g., unsteady gait, tripping, falling, or loss of fine motor control of hands).

May complain of neuropathic or radicular pain or muscle tenderness.

May complain of shortness of breath, difficulty breathing, difficulty in swallowing, chewing, and/or speaking.

PHYSICAL EXAMINATION

Inspection

Extremities: symmetrical weakness, impaired senses of position and vibration, diminished or absent deep tendon reflexes, loss of muscle tone may be noted.

Respirations: shallow, labored breathing with decreased ventilatory capacity may occur as early as 4th-5th day from onset of symptoms.

Other

Autonomic nervous system dysfunction may result in dysrhythmias, hypertension or hypotension, and/or loss of sweating.

Fever is usually absent, except with infection.

DIAGNOSTIC STUDIES

Serial lumber puncture: demonstrates classic phenomenon of normal pressure and normal number of white cells, with elevating protein levels that peak in 4 to 6 weeks. Because protein elevation may not appear in first 4 or 5 days, serial lumbar punctures may be indicated in 1 to 2 weeks.

Electromyelography (EMG): results depend on stage and progression of syndrome. Nerve conduction velocity may be slowed. Fibrillations (repetitive firing of the same motor unit) are more common in later stage.

Chest x-ray examinations may demonstrate progressive signs of respiratory involvement (e.g., infections owing to hypoventilation and immobility).

Respiratory function tests demonstrate decreased vital capacity, tidal volume, and inspiratory force.

NURSING PRIORITIES

1. Maintain/support respiratory function.
2. Minimize/prevent complications.
3. Control/eliminate pain.

4. Provide fluid and nutritional support.
5. Provide emotional support for patient, family members, significant others.

NURSING DIAGNOSIS:	**Breathing Pattern, ineffective.**
SUPPORTING DATA/CONTRIBUTING FACTORS:	**Progression of weakness and paralysis can include intracostal or diaphragm muscles, causing decreased respiratory vital capacity, ineffective airway clearance and/or impaired gas exchange. When cranial nerves are involved, there may be loss of gag and swallow reflexes with risk of tracheobronchial obstruction, owing to inability to effectively clear airway.**
GENERAL PATIENT OUTCOMES:	**Ventilation is adequate as shown by ABGs within normal limits, breath sounds clear, absence of cyanosis and signs of respiratory distress.**

INTERVENTIONS	RATIONALE
Independent	
Maintain patent airway. Note loss of gag, swallow, cough reflexes. Suction oral secretions and keep NPO, if necessary.	Loss of muscle strength and function may result in inability to maintain and/or clear airway, preventing adequate ventilation. Note: Once muscles of head and neck are involved, frequent evaluation of gag, swallow, and cough reflexes must be carried out to prevent aspiration and respiratory failure.
Monitor respiratory rate and tidal volume,	Increased respiratory distress and decreased tidal volume may indicate advancing muscular weakness and/or paralysis, which can result in respiratory failure.
Auscultate breath sounds, noting loss of breath sounds and/or development of adventitious sounds such as rhonchi, wheezes.	Increased airway resistance and/or accumulation of secretions will impede gas diffusion and lead to pulmonary complications (e.g., pneumonia).
Elevate head of bed, or place patient in supported sitting position.	Enhances lung expansion and cough efforts, decreases work of breathing, and limits risk of aspiration of secretions and gastric reflux.
Maintain calm, supportive approach. (Refer to Nursing Diagnosis: Anxiety, page 153.)	Aids in reducing anxiety related to progression of disease and loss of ability to breathe.
Collaborative	
Monitor and graph serial vital capacity, tidal volume, inspiratory force.	Detects worsening of muscle paralysis and declining respiratory effort.
Monitor and graph serial ABGs.	Determines effectiveness of current ventilation and need for and effectiveness of interventions.

INTERVENTIONS	RATIONALE
Collaborative	
Review serial chest x-ray examinations.	Reveals changes indicative of pulmonary congestion, pneumonia, and/or atelectasis.
Administer oxygen and humidification as indicated, using appropriate route (e.g., cannula, mask, mechanical ventilation).	Treats hyoxemia. Humidity may help loosen secretions and keep mucous membranes moist, thereby reducing irritation in airways.
Assist with intubation, maintain mechanical ventilation. (Refer to Care Plan: Ventilatory Assistance, mechanical, page 115.)	Required when the patient's vital capacity, tidal volume, and inspiratory force are reduced by 30 to 50 percent, PCO_2 is increased, PO_2 is decreased, or patient is unable to clear secretions.
Administer or assist with pulmonary hygiene measures; for example, breathing exercises, chest percussion, vibration, and postural drainage.	Improves ventilation and reduces atelectasis by loosening and mobilizing secretions and enhancing expansion of alveoli.
Assist with kinetic therapy (e.g., RotoRest bed), as indicated.	May be used to enhance circulation and oxygenation of lung segments and to promote mobilization of secretions, thereby reducing risk of atelectasis, pneumonia, and/or pulmonary emboli.

NURSING DIAGNOSIS: **Tissue Perfusion, alteration in [potential].**

SUPPORTING DATA/CONTRIBUTING FACTORS: **Changes in vascular tone with associated venous stasis and reduced cardiac output may alter systemic tissue or organ function. These changes may be aggravated by autonomic nervous system dysfunction, manifested by severe hypertension or hypotension and serious cardiac dysrhythmias. Loss of peripheral vascular tone and immobility potentiate thromboembolic phenomena.**

GENERAL PATIENT OUTCOMES: **Blood pressure and cardiac output within normal limits. Serious dysrhythmias do not occur or are controlled. Complications of venous stasis are minimized or absent.**

INTERVENTIONS	RATIONALE
Independent	
Monitor blood pressure, noting wide fluctuations. Reposition carefully, observing for signs of postural hypotension.	Changes in blood pressure can occur because of loss of sympathetic outflow to maintain peripheral vascular tone. Profound hypotension is related to loss of periph-

INTERVENTIONS	RATIONALE
Independent	
	eral vascular resistance, with resulting vasodilation and venous pooling, which create impaired venous return and reduce cardiac output. Labile blood pressures with severe hypertension or hypotension may occur owing to autonomic dysfunction. Reflexes to adjust blood pressure during position changes may be impaired, causing severe hypotension when patient position is changed (even side to side).
Monitor and record cardiac rate and rhythm. Note dysrhythmias that occur with suctioning, and limit suction duration if dysrhythmias occur.	Cardiac rate may be slowed because of impaired sympathetic innervation or unopposed vagal stimulation. Bradycardia (exaggerated by suctioning) can lead to asystole. Other dysrhythmias may occur owing to hypoxemia and reduced cardiac output.
Monitor temperature. Provide comfortable environmental temperature. Add or remove blankets and use room fans as indicated.	Difficulties with temperature regulation are related to loss of peripheral vascular constriction, dilation. Patient usually takes on temperature of environment. Warming and cooling should be done cautiously to prevent hot or cold injury, inasmuch as the patient may have impaired sensation.
Document intake and output.	Relaxation of vascular tone, fluid shifts, and reduced fluid intake predispose patient to compromised circulating volume, which may require replacement fluids to maintain adequate blood pressure and urine output.
Monitor for symptoms of thrombophlebitis (redness, swelling, or increased calf and thigh measurements, or pulmonary embolus—sudden dyspnea and tachycardia. (Refer to Care Plan: Pulmonary Embolism (Massive), page 95.)	Clot formation is a hazard with increasing immobility, loss of peripheral vascular tone, and tendency for venous stasis. Deep venous thrombosis (may go unrecognized in patient unable to sense discomfort) may lead to pulmonary emboli if not detected and promptly treated.
Collaborative	
Insert and maintain hemodynamic pressure monitoring lines if indicated (e.g., CVP, pulmonary arterial line).	Assists in assessing effects of fluid management and drug therapies.
Administer intravenous (IV) fluids, volume expanders.	Corrects or prevents hypovolemia and hypotension. Volume expanders should be used cautiously in order to prevent fluid overload, because patient with impaired vascular tone may be sensitive to even small increases in volume.
Provide thermal blanket, if indicated.	May be required to maintain more normal core temperatures, if fluctuations are extreme.
Apply antiembolic stockings.	Promote venous return and thus may prevent venous stasis and lessen chance of thrombus formation.
Administer heparin, if indicated, following safety protocols for assuring accurate dose, (e.g., infusion pump).	Heparin is sometimes used prophylactically or in response to signs and symptoms of thrombus formation.

NURSING DIAGNOSIS:	**Bowel Elimination, alterations in [potential].**
SUPPORTING DATA/CONTRIBUTING FACTORS:	**Neuromuscular impairment results in abdominal muscle weakness, loss of anal sensation and reflexes, and altered gastric motility, resulting in changes in usual pattern of elimination.**
GENERAL PATIENT OUTCOMES:	**Bowel elimination pattern is reestablished, producing soft, formed stool, free of impaction.**

INTERVENTIONS	RATIONALE
Independent	
Auscultate bowel sounds, noting presence, absence, or change.	Decreased or absent sounds may indicate onset of ileus owing to loss of intestinal motility and/or electrolyte imbalance. Hyperactive bowel sounds may be noted if diarrhea occurs (e.g., intolerance to tube feeding or side effect of kinetic therapy).
Monitor for signs of ileus (e.g., nausea, vomiting, diarrhea, cessation of stools).	Rate of progression to complete ileus is variable but expected, even before onset of nausea and vomiting.
Assess for abdominal tenderness, distention. Measure abdominal girth if indicated.	May indicate development of ileus, bowel obstruction, or fecal impaction owing to impaired intestinal function.
Monitor and evaluate hydration status. If able to swallow, encourage patient to take at least 2000 ml per day. Provide fluids frequently, encourage fruit juices.	Adequate hydration promotes softer stool, thereby enhancing elimination.
Record bowel movements, noting adequacy and consistency.	Assesses effectiveness of bowel program and identifies need for changes in therapy.
Check rectum for impaction.	Gentle manual removal of stool may be necessary, along with other interventions to establish elimination.
Provide privacy and optimal positioning at scheduled times.	Enhances defecation efforts.
Collaborative	
Insert, maintain nasogastric tube.	Reduces nausea and vomiting and decompresses abdominal distention associated with loss of peristalsis, presence of ileus.
Increase dietary fiber and bulk when feedings are resumed, or change type and rate of tube feedings.	Aids in regulating fecal consistency and reduces complications (e.g., diarrhea, constipation).
Administer stool softeners, suppositories, and/or laxatives as needed.	Prevents impaction and assists in regulation of bowel function.

NURSING DIAGNOSIS:	Urinary Elimination, alteration in pattern [potential].
SUPPORTING DATA/CONTRIBUTING FACTORS:	Neuromuscular impairment, autonomic dysfunction (resulting in loss of sensation), and immobility may lead to bladder dysfunction, urinary retention.
GENERAL PATIENT OUTCOMES:	Bladder empties adequately with urine clear, free of foul odor.

INTERVENTIONS	RATIONALE
Independent	
Record frequency and amount of voidings.	Provides information for assessment of bladder functioning.
Palpate bladder for distention.	If sphincter reflex is absent, the bladder will fill and distend.
Encourage adequate fluid intake (up to 2000 ml), including acidifying (cranberry) juices.	Maintains glomerular filtration rate and reduces risk of infection and formation of urinary stones.
Collaborative	
Catheterize for residual urine.	Monitors effectiveness of bladder emptying.
Insert indwelling catheter.	May be needed if urinary retention occurs or if frequent urinary output measurements are desired.

NURSING DIAGNOSIS:	Mobility, impaired, physical.
SUPPORTING DATA/CONTRIBUTING FACTORS:	Neuromuscular impairment results in loss of coordination, decreased muscle strength, and partial or complete paralysis.
GENERAL PATIENT OUTCOMES:	Deformities are prevented; complications are minimized. Activities are resumed.

INTERVENTIONS	RATIONALE
Independent	
Support extremities and joints with pillows, rolls, foot boards. Maintain extremities in functional position.	Prevents contractures and loss of joint function.

INTERVENTIONS	RATIONALE
Independent	
Perform range of motion exercises.	Stimulates circulation, improves muscle tone, and promotes joint mobility.
Avoid active exercise during the acute phase.	Vigorous exercise may precipitate autonomic dysfunction or lead to exacerbation of disease symptoms, causing physiologic and emotional regression.
Coordinate care to allow adequate rest periods.	Overtaxing muscles can increase time needed for remyelination, thereby prolonging recovery time.

(Refer to Nursing Diagnosis: Skin Integrity, impaired, potential, below.)

Collaborative	
Obtain physical and occupational therapies consultation.	Plan for assistance during lengthy recovery period.

NURSING DIAGNOSIS:	**Skin Integrity, impaired, potential.**
SUPPORTING DATA/CONTRIBUTING FACTORS:	**Immobility or paralysis places the skin at great risk for breakdown owing to loss of sensation, sympathetic tone, and reflexes.**
GENERAL PATIENT OUTCOMES:	**Skin breakdown is prevented.**

INTERVENTIONS	RATIONALE
Independent	
Observe skin for signs of irritation.	Early discovery and preventive action can avoid progression of skin irritation to ulceration.
Use mild soap and apply nonalcohol lotions.	Soap and numerous alcohol-containing lotions have a drying effect, which may increase risk of breakdown.
Change position frequently. Massage skin over bony prominences.	Prevents decubiti, improves circulation, alleviates pressure points and possible nerve injury related to pressure on impaired tissue and skin.
Monitor temperature of bath water, heating devices.	Patient may not be able to sense heat and could experience burns.
Collaborative	
Provide alternating pressure mattress, flotation system or kinetic therapy.	Reduces pressure on bony prominences and enhances circulation.

(Refer to Nursing Diagnosis: Mobility, impaired, page 148.)

NURSING DIAGNOSIS:	**Infection, potential for.**
SUPPORTING DATA/CONTRIBUTING FACTORS:	**Immobility, loss of pain sensation, use of respiratory equipment and invasive lines potentiate risk of infections.**
GENERAL PATIENT OUTCOMES:	**Patient is afebrile. Lungs are clear. Skin and mucous membranes are intact. Urine is clear, odor free.**

INTERVENTIONS	RATIONALE
Independent	
Check IV sites per protocol, with special care given to total parenteral nutrition (TPN) lines and dressings.	Sources of local and systemic infections. Patient may be unaware of pain or swelling owing to decreased or absent pain sensation.
Monitor changes in temperature, vital signs. Note fever, chills, diaphoresis, color changes, odor of urine and drainage.	Identifies onset of infection in order that diagnostic and therapeutic interventions may be initiated promptly to prevent sepsis.
Pay strict attention to eye cleanliness and lubrication.	Provides protection necessary to prevent corneal abrasions, eye infections.
Change IV and ventilator tubing per protocol.	Decreases potential for bacterial growth.
Provide peri/catheter care as indicated.	Ascending urinary tract infections are common in presence of decreased muscle or sphincter tone and use of indwelling catheters.
Use sterile technique when suctioning endotracheal or tracheostomy tube.	Prevents introduction of microorganisms which could produce life-threatening infection in an already compromised respiratory system.
Monitor visitors and caregivers for respiratory infections.	Patient with compromised or stressed immune system is more susceptible to secondary infections.
Collaborative	
Obtain sputum, urine, and blood specimens for culture as necessary.	Identifies infecting organism and guides antibiotic therapy.
Administer antibiotics as indicated.	Treat aggressively if infection occurs to prevent sepsis.

NURSING DIAGNOSIS:	**Comfort, alteration in, pain, acute.**
SUPPORTING DATA/CONTRIBUTING FACTORS:	**As paresthesia progresses, it is accompanied by muscle pain, tenderness, and aching, which are most severe in the shoulders, pelvis, thighs, back, and buttocks.**
GENERAL PATIENT OUTCOMES:	**Comfort is attained, pain relieved.**

INTERVENTIONS	RATIONALE
Independent	
Provide comfort through touch, Therapeutic Touch, heat or cold applications, and judicious use of vibration, massage.	Warmth and sense of caring by caregivers serves to help patient gain control over the constant discomfort caused by the paresthesias.
Reposition frequently. Provide support by means of pillows, foam inserts, blankets.	Alleviate cramping and pain of remaining in one position. Note: Some patients prefer to lie on their backs in a "frog leg" position.
Collaborative	
Provide moist heat packs, warm tub bath.	May provide relief from aching muscles.
Initiate hydrotherapy program, if indicated.	Provides pain relief and an opportunity to exercise in an environment with reduced gravitational resistance.
Administer analgesics, as indicated.	Narcotics (except codeine, which has a lesser effect) should be avoided if possible because of their respiratory depressant effect and gastrointestinal side effects.
Refer to physiotherapy.	Ultrasound, diathermy, and transcutaneous electrical nerve stimulation (TENS) may be used to help relieve discomfort.

NURSING DIAGNOSIS:	**Nutrition, alteration in, less than body requirements.**
SUPPORTING DATA/CONTRIBUTING FACTORS:	**Muscle weakness, with impaired ability to chew and swallow, can lead to nutritional deficit and weight loss.**
GENERAL PATIENT OUTCOMES:	**Nutrient intake is adequate to meet nutritional needs as shown by positive nitrogen balance and weight maintained at desired level.**

INTERVENTIONS	RATIONALE
Independent	
Assess ability to chew and swallow on an ongoing basis.	Increasing muscle weakness may indicate need for alternative methods of feeding (i.e., TPN, nasogastric tube feedings).
Auscultate bowel sounds. Note abdominal distension.	Disturbance of gastric function may require alteration of dietary therapy.
Record caloric intake.	Identifies nutrient deficiencies and needs.
Note patient's likes and dislikes and involve in dietary choices.	Promotes sense of control and may enhance intake efforts.
Encourage self-feeding if possible. Allow patient time to finish self-directed efforts. Feed patient as needed.	Degree of loss of motor control will affect ability to feed self. Self-esteem and sense of control may be en-

INTERVENTIONS	RATIONALE
Independent	
	hanced by self-directed efforts, even when very limited.
Encourage S.O.(s) to participate at mealtime (e.g., assist with feeding, bringing food from home, etc.).	Provides socialization time with family and significant other(s), which may promote patient's food intake.
Provide calorie-containing fluids in place of plain water (e.g., add polycase or honey to beverages).	Enhances caloric intake without increasing physical effort.
Weigh daily.	Assesses effectiveness of dietary regimen.
Collaborative	
Insert and maintain feeding tube.	May be necessary if patient cannot swallow or if gag and cough reflexes are impaired.
Administer parenteral, enteral feedings. Give dietary supplements as indicated (e.g., Ensure).	Assures proper electrolyte, nutrient, and caloric intake.
Monitor laboratory studies as indicated. (Refer to Care Plan: Nutritional Support, page 367.)	Assess needs and effectiveness of nutritional support.

NURSING DIAGNOSIS:	**Sensory-Perceptual Alteration (specify).**
SUPPORTING DATA/CONTRIBUTING FACTORS:	**Patients with Guillain-Barre syndrome suffer alterations in sensory perception related to multiple factors. Environmental factors include intensive care environment, with confinement to bedrest, sleep deprivation, and social isolation. The nature of the disease is a factor, with altered perception of stimuli or impaired ability to communicate or respond to stimuli. Chemical alterations are possible owing to electrolyte imbalance and hypoxia. Extreme psychologic distress or anxiety may create a narrowed perception.**
GENERAL PATIENT OUTCOMES:	**Sensory impairments are recognized and minimized. Communication is established and maintained. Complications are prevented.**

INTERVENTIONS	RATIONALE
Independent	
Monitor changes in neurologic status at regular intervals. Record serial findings on flow sheets (e.g., assess ability to speak, responses to simple commands and painful stimuli, awareness of hot and cold, dull and sharp).	Progression and regression of symptoms may vary greatly. Progression may be quite rapid, but recovery usually takes a long period of time. Flow charts are helpful in understanding possible responses and absence of responses, and they alert the nurse to impending complications.
Provide alternate means of communication if patient cannot speak. Establish "blink method" if needed.	If process develops slowly, patient can be instructed in alternate method of communication, which may help reduce anxiety and panic associated with loss of speech. If process is sudden (a few hours), constant, consistent effort on the part of the staff may be required to establish effective communication.
Provide safe environment (e.g., side rails, protection from thermal injury). Note perceptual deficits on chart in room to alert all caregivers (e.g., "Patient cannot speak").	Loss of sensation, as well as of motor control, leaves patient at the mercy of all caregivers, who must maintain a therapeutic environment and prevent injury.
Patch eyes on a rotating basis if ptosis is present.	Prevents corneal abrasions without total loss of visual input.
Orient and reorient patient to environment and staff.	Helps reduce anxiety and is especially helpful if patient is unable to keep eyes open.
Provide explanations of care; plan care with patient, involving significant others when possible.	Understanding can improve cooperation in needed activities. Involving patient and family in care planning restores some sense of control over life, which enhances self-esteem.
Limit procedures and activities to allow for undisturbed periods of rest and diversional activities.	Provides appropriate rest and reduces excess stimuli, which can increase anxiety and diminish coping mechanisms.
Provide sensory stimulation, including familiar sounds (music), clocks (time), television (news items), conversation.	Patient is usually conscious and may feel completely isolated as paralysis progresses, unless orientation is provided.
Encourage significant other(s) to talk to and touch patient frequently and keep abreast of family events.	Helps family and significant other(s) to feel involved in patient's life and may reduce patient's anxiety regarding family when separated.
(Refer to Nursing Diagnosis: Anxiety, below.)	
Collaborative	
Refer to resources for assistance, that is, physical and occupational therapists, pastoral care, social service departments, rehabilitation specialists.	As acute phase ends and recovery begins, all services and departments may be coordinating efforts to promote wellness.

NURSING DIAGNOSIS:	**Anxiety.**
SUPPORTING DATA/CONTRIBUTING FACTORS:	**Paralysis, pain and loss of independence are very frightening. Feelings of anxiety, depression, powerlessness,**

	and poor self-esteem can occur owing to slow recovery and unknown outcomes of disease process.
GENERAL PATIENT OUTCOMES:	**Anxiety is decreased to a manageable level as shown by relaxed manner, resting and sleeping appropriately, verbalizing feelings of reduced anxiety.**

INTERVENTIONS	RATIONALE
Independent	
Assess level of anxiety and interactions with significant others.	Provides a baseline for interventions and referrals.
Encourage patient to vent emotions in own way while providing constant assurance and support.	Acceptance of individual reactions and nonjudgmental care by the staff help establish therapeutic environment for the patient to begin to attain some sense of self-esteem and self-control.
Provide information about the disease and treatment.	Patient and family need to know that recovery is slow and that treatment is aimed at preventing and minimizing complications. Information will help patient and significant others recognize progress that is being made.
Assess functional capacity constantly. Place needed, familiar objects within sight and reach.	Increasing weakness or paralysis limits independence and increases anxiety. Familiar objects provide sense of security.
Establish ways of contacting and communicating with staff.	Patient whose ability to communicate is impaired may feel isolated and can become panic-stricken.
Assist patient to take part in planning care as much as possible.	Allows some control over environment and may diminish feelings of despair, anger, and frustration.
Note dependent, overdemanding behavior, refusal to participate in care or make decisions.	Extreme dependence on others can lead to anxiety, regression, anger, depression.
Collaborative	
Refer to other sources as needed (e.g., social worker, psychiatric therapist, pastor, family therapist).	Emotional impact may be severe and require support services of numerous professionals for both patient and family members during lengthy illness and/or rehabilitation.

Spinal Cord Injury: Acute Phase

PATIENT ASSESSMENT DATA BASE

HISTORY

History of recent trauma to the spinal cord and vertebral column including blunt trauma resulting in contusion (bruising), shearing (tearing), or shattering (breaking) of structures; penetrating trauma resulting in transection of the spinal cord; or fracture of bony structures with resultant damage to and possible transection of the spinal cord.

Falls, motor vehicle accidents, sports injuries, gunshot wounds or stab wounds resulting in bony dislocation, fracture fragments, rupture of ligaments and intravertebral disks or disruption of blood supply are responsible for spinal compression or contusion injuries and/or transection of the spinal cord.

Spinal cord damage can be caused by flexion, hyperextension, compression, or rotation of the vertebral column.

Disease processes with acute loss of cord function include tumors, ruptured arteriovenous malformations, infectious processes, and hematomas.

Subjective

May complain of lack of sensation/movement of affected extremities.

PHYSICAL EXAMINATION

Spinal cord lesions are categorized as complete or incomplete: Complete spinal cord injury results in a total loss of sensation and voluntary motor function below the level of the lesion. Incomplete spinal cord injury presents a mixed loss of sensation and voluntary motor activity below the level of the lesion.

Physical findings will vary dependent on the level of injury and degree of spinal shock:
- C1-4: Quadriplegia with total loss of respiratory function.
- C4-5: Quadriplegia with possible phrenic nerve involvement and possible loss of respiratory function.
- C5-6: Quadriplegia with gross arm movements; possible diaphragmatic breathing.
- C6-7: Quadriplegia with biceps muscles intact; diaphragmatic breathing.
- C7-8: Quadriplegia with triceps and biceps intact; diaphragmatic breathing.
- T1-L2: Paraplegia with varying function of intercostal and abdominal muscles.
- Below L2 (cauda equina injury): Mixed motor-sensory loss, bowel and bladder dysfunction.

Spinal shock (usually develops within 30 to 60 minutes after trauma), causes total or nearly total suppression of all reflexes at spinal segments below the level of the lesion, rendering the patient areflexic with flaccid paralysis. This phenomenon is more profound in patients with cervical injuries and includes a classic triad of symptoms: hypotension; bradycardia; and warm, dry extremities.

Because of spinal shock, initial evaluation of loss of motor function and sensation may not be an accurate assessment of eventual neurologic status.

DIAGNOSTIC STUDIES

Spinal series locates level and type of bony injury (fractures, dislocation), alignment and reduction after application of traction.

CAT scan of spine locates injury, evaluates structural alterations or edema.

Myelogram may be done to visualize spinal column if pathology is unclear or occlusion of spinal subarachnoid space is suspected, but is not usually done after penetrating injuries.

Chest x-ray demonstrates pulmonary status (e.g., atelectasis, changes in level of diaphragm).

Tidal volume/vital capacity: measures maximum volume of inspiration and expiration and is especially critical in patients with cervical lesions with possible phrenic nerve involvement, as indicator that ventilatory assistance is required.

ABGs: indicates effectiveness of gas exchange and ventilatory effort.

NURSING PRIORITIES

1. Maximize respiratory function.
2. Prevent further injury to spinal column.
3. Support cardiovascular function.
4. Prevent or minimize complications.
5. Support special psychologic adjustments of patient and significant other(s).

NURSING DIAGNOSIS:	**Breathing Pattern, ineffective [potential].**
SUPPORTING DATA/CONTRIBUTING FACTORS:	**Impairment of innervation of the diaphragm owing to lesions at C4 or above, or lesions at or above T1 with loss of intercostal muscle function can lead to hypoventilation, carbon dioxide retention, hypoxia, atelectasis, and retention of secretions. Reflexic abdominal spasms and gastric distention can further impair function of the diaphragm, interfering with lung expansion and breathing ability.**
GENERAL PATIENT OUTCOMES:	**Adequate ventilation is maintained as shown by ABGs within normal limits. Free of signs of respiratory distress. Respiratory complications are prevented or controlled.**

INTERVENTIONS	RATIONALE
Independent	
Maintain patent airway; use adjuncts as indicated.	May be indicated in patient with high cervical injury and impaired gag and cough reflexes.
Assess respiratory function: note presence or absence of spontaneous effort and quality of respirations (i.e., labored, or use of accessory muscles).	C1-C4 injuries result in complete loss of respiratory function. Injuries at C4-C5 can result in variable loss of respiratory function owing to phrenic nerve involvement and loss of diaphragmatic function. Injuries below C6-C7 level spare phrenic nerve, and diaphragmatic breathing is possible; however, loss of intercostal muscles results in loss of effective cough, sigh, deep breathing.
Assess strength of cough. Assist with coughing by placing hands below diaphragm and pushing upward as patient exhales.	Level of injury determines function of intercostal muscles and ability to cough spontaneously to move secretions. "Quad coughing" is performed to assist paralyzed abdominal muscles and add volume to cough.
Suction as necessary. Document quality and quantity of secretions. Limit suction duration to less than 15 seconds.	If cough is ineffective, suctioning may be needed to remove secretions, lowering risk of aspiration, enhance gas distribution, and prevent respiratory infec-

INTERVENTIONS	RATIONALE
Independent	
	tion. Prolonged suctioning increases hypoxia, which adversely affects central nervous system (CNS) function and may worsen bradycardia owing to vagal stimulation.
Auscultate breath sounds. Note areas of absent or decreased breath sounds or development of adventitious sounds (e.g., rhonchi).	Hypoventilation is common and leads to accumulation of secretions, atelectasis, and possible complications (e.g., pneumonia).
Note skin color for developing cyanosis, duskiness.	May appear to be breathing adequately, but compromised blood supply and disrupted tissue metabolism increases oxygen demand and may result in hypoxemia.
Assess for abdominal distention, muscle spasms.	May impede diaphragmatic excursion, reducing lung expansion, respiratory function.
Collaborative	
Measure and graph vital capacity, tidal volume, inspiratory force.	Determines level of respiratory muscle function. Serial vital capacity measurements are the most accurate method of predicting impending respiratory failure, requiring intubation or mechanical ventilation.
Monitor and graph serial ABGs.	Identifies respiratory problems; for example, hypoventilation (low PaO_2/elevated $PaCO_2$) and/or response to therapies. Hypoxemia is most commonly caused by retained secretions but also may be indicative of other pulmonary complications (e.g., emboli).
Administer oxygen by appropriate method, that is, nasal prongs, intubation, ventilator. (Refer to Care Plan: Ventilatory Assistance, mechanical, page 115.)	Method is determined by level of injury and degree of respiratory insufficiency. A high arterial PO_2 is desired to minimize hypoxic effects, which worsen neurologic deficits.
Assist with aggressive chest physiotherapy; for example, chest percussion and use of respiratory adjuncts (e.g., incentive spirometer).	Preventing retained secretions is essential to enhance gas exchange and reduce risk of infection, pneumonia.

NURSING DIAGNOSIS:	**Mobility, impaired physical.**
SUPPORTING DATA/CONTRIBUTING FACTORS:	**Instability of the vertebral column dictates that the patient be immobilized by halo or tongs and traction to prevent further spinal injury. Complications of immobility impacted by neurogenic dysfunction (flaccid paralysis) vary from patient to patient and may include pneumonia, muscle atrophy or contractures, skin irritation or breakdown, and thrombophlebitis.**

GENERAL PATIENT OUTCOMES:	**Further damage to spinal cord is prevented. Complications are minimized or prevented.**

INTERVENTIONS	RATIONALE
Independent	
Check traction to assure that frames are secure, pulleys are aligned, weights are hanging free.	Necessary for maintenance of traction needed for proper spinal alignment and prevention of further spinal cord injury.
Check weights for ordered traction (usually 10 to 20 pounds).	Depends on patient's size and amount of cervical reduction needed for the vertebrae to be maintained in appropriate position.
Elevate head of frame or electric bed 6 inches.	Creates counter balance to traction, maintaining both patient position and traction pull.
Promote pulmonary hygiene (e.g., deep breathe, cough, suction). (Refer to Nursing Diagnosis: Breathing Pattern, ineffective, page 134.)	Aids in clearing secretions to reduce risk of atelectasis and pneumonia.
Provide turn sheets and adequate assistance for position changes.	Necessary to maintain proper alignment and prevent injury during repositioning or turning.
Reposition, using foam wedges, rolls, support pillows.	Maintains proper body alignment and functional position, reduces pressure areas. (Refer to Nursing Diagnosis: Skin Integrity, impaired, potential, page 164.)
Position arms at 90 degree angle several times daily.	Prevents frozen shoulder contractures.
Perform full range of motion exercises on all extremities and joints using slow, smooth movements.	Enhances venous blood flow, maintains muscle tone and joint mobility, and prevents contractures.
Measure blood pressure before and after activity.	Orthostatic hypotension may occur as a result of venous pooling secondary to loss of vascular tone. Movement from side to side or elevations of head of bed may aggravate hypotension and produce syncope.
Assess motor function by requesting patient to shrug shoulders, spread fingers, squeeze examiner's hands, move toes, or whatever is appropriate for level of injury.	As spinal shock and edema resolve, deep tendon reflexes and restoration of some motor function may occur.
Assess for deep vein thrombosis, noting redness, swelling, muscle tension. Record daily calf and thigh measurements, if indicated.	A high percentage of patients with cervical cord injury develop thrombi owing to immobilization, altered peripheral circulation, and flaccid paralysis.
Note sudden onset of dyspnea, cyanosis, and/or other signs of respiratory distress. (Refer to Care Plan: Pulmonary Embolism (Massive), page 95.)	Development of pulmonary emboli may be "silent," because pain reception is altered and deep vein thrombosis may not be previously recognized.
Collaborative	
Maintain cervical alignment by means of skeletal traction: tongs, calipers; halo/vest as indicated.	Reduces fracture or dislocation and maintains alignment of cervical spine.
Place patient in kinetic therapy bed when appropriate.	Effectively immobilizes unstable spinal column during all phases of acute care and is thought to decrease

INTERVENTIONS	RATIONALE
Collaborative	
	complications associated with immobility by improving systemic circulation.
Apply antiembolic hose or Jobst leotard.	Limits pooling of blood in lower extremities or abdomen, thus improving vasomotor tone and reducing incidence of thrombus formation and pulmonary emboli.
Monitor and graph serial ABGs.	Hypoxia unrelated to retained secretions or atelectasis suggests possibility of pulmonary emboli from deep vein thrombosis.
Administer medications as indicated:	
Dexamethasone (Decadron), Medrol (Solu Medrol),	Anti-inflammatory agents may be given to reduce spinal cord edema, improving spinal cord perfusion and thereby reducing effects of ischemia.
Mannitol (Osmitrol),	Hyperosmolar diuretic with rapid onset which may be used to reduce spinal cord edema while supporting renal function.
Heparin.	May be given prophylactically or as treatment for documented pulmonary emboli/thrombophlebitis.
Prepare for surgery, that is, spinal laminectomy or fusion if indicated.	May be performed for spinal decompression or removal of bone fragments.
Assist with therapies as indicated; for example, hyperbaric oxygenation, hypothermia (spinal cord cooling).	Currently under study, these procedures are being used to enhance oxygen delivery or to reduce edema formation to minimize nerve damage.

NURSING DIAGNOSIS:	**Cardiac Output, alteration in, decreased [potential].**
SUPPORTING DATA/CONTRIBUTING FACTORS:	**The majority of visceral innervation is from sympathetic outflow via the thoracolumbar tracts. Therefore, lesions of the thoracic or cervical cord will alter cardiovascular function owing to imbalance of sympathetic or parasympathetic innervation.**
GENERAL PATIENT OUTCOMES:	**Adequate cardiac output or tissue perfusion is maintained as shown by stable blood pressure, absence of syncope. Complications are prevented or controlled.**

INTERVENTIONS	RATIONALE
Independent	
Monitor cardiac rhythm and rate. Document dysrhythmias.	Bradycardia and asystole are common complications in acute cervical injuries. Presence of bradycardia with or without junctional rhythm and escape beats probably indicates sympathetic blockade. Hypothermia may aggravate bradycardias. Preinjury heart rate should be considered; for example, young person with usual rate of 60 may now have heart rate of 30 to 40 owing to unopposed vagal influence. Cardiac arrest (if it occurs) is most commonly a result of vagal stimulation or hypoxia.
Monitor blood pressure. Note hypotension or hypertension and changes in blood pressure related to position.	Hypotension is common during spinal shock owing to sympathetic blockade, resulting in vasodilatation, venous pooling, and decreased venous return and cardiac output. Hypertension is a common manifestation of autonomic dysreflexia (rare in spinal shock or acute phase), which occurs in patients with spinal cord lesions at or above T6 and is due to exaggerated autonomic responses below the level of injury. Note: Severe hypertension that accompanies autonomic dysreflexia is a medical emergency. Orthostatic hypotension (owing to lack of vasomotor tone in the lower extremities) is a continuing problem for the quadriplegic or paraplegic patient.
Collaborative	
Administer intravenous (IV) solutions (e.g., lactated Ringer's, D5 1/2 normal saline).	Maintains hydration, circulating volume, and blood pressure. Note: It is imortant to avoid even mild dehydration, which may compromise spinal circulation unless dictated by concomitant brain injury or cerebral edema.
Administer plasma volume expanders (e.g., Dextran) as indicated.	May be used to improve or support capillary blood flow to spinal cord.
Administer medications as indicated:	
Atropine,	Cholinergic blocker that relieves bradycardia induced by unopposed parasympathetic stimulation.
Dopamine hydrochloride (Intropin) or dobutamine hydrochloride (Dobutrex),	Vasopressors may be indicated in unresolved or severe hypotension related to compromised sympathetic outflow.
Diazoxide (Hyperstat); hydralazine (Apresoline).	Antihypertensives may be used to treat the severe hypertension associated with autonomic dysreflexia which may become a problem as spinal shock resolves.

NURSING DIAGNOSIS: **Sensory-Perceptual Alteration.**

SUPPORTING DATA/CONTRIBUTING FACTORS: **Injury of the spinal cord and presence of spinal shock, alters sensory reception, transmission, and integration,**

	which places the patient at risk for bodily injury and can contribute to anxiety, disorientation, bizarre thinking, and exaggerated emotional responses.
GENERAL PATIENT OUTCOMES:	**Patient is oriented to person, place, time. Verbalizes/demonstrates reduced anxiety. Bodily injury is prevented.**

INTERVENTIONS	RATIONALE
Independent	
Provide means to summon help such as special sensitive call light.	Enables the patient to have a sense of control and reduces fear of being left alone. Note: Quadriplegic on ventilator requires continuous observation.
Protect from bodily harm (e.g., falls, positioning on arm or object, burns).	Patient may not sense pain or be aware of body position and heat.
Obtain assistance when changing patient position on turning frame or kinetic bed, secure patient with safety belts.	Maintains spinal alignment while preventing injury of patient and/or caregivers.
Monitor body and environmental temperature. Maintain constant room temperature, eliminate drafts. Add or remove blankets as needed.	Patients with cervical cord injury are subject to disturbances of internal temperature regulation and are affected by surrounding environment. Sweating is lost below the level of injury, which further alters patient's temperature regulation, but may be profuse above the level of injury, especially during episodes of autonomic dysreflexia.
Assist the patient to recognize normal alterations in sensation and perception.	May help reduce anxiety associated with heightened awareness of sensation; for example, sound may be amplified through skeletal tongs, or dizziness does accompany position changes.
Explain procedures prior to and during care, identifying the body part involved.	Maintains perception of body as a whole.
Provide tactile stimulation, touching patient in intact sensory areas (e.g., shoulders, face, head).	Touching conveys caring and fulfills a normal physiologic and psychologic need.
Position patient to see surroundings and activities. Provide prism glasses if on turning frame. Talk to patient frequently.	Provides sensory input which may be severely limited, especially when patient is prone on turning frame.
Provide diversional activities such as television, radio, talking books, liberal visitation, use of clock, calendar.	Aids in maintaining reality orientation and provides some sense of normalcy and passage of time.
Encourage rest periods; simulate day and night rest patterns by altering lighting and reducing auditory stimuli.	Limits sensory input to aid in reestablishing circadian rhythm and natural sleep patterns.
Assess and record sensory function or deficit by means of touch, proprioception, and pin prick, progressing from area of deficit to neurologically intact area.	Changes may not occur during spinal shock phase but as it resolves documentation should be recorded by dermatome charts or anatomic landmarks, such as, "2 inches above nipple line."

NURSING DIAGNOSIS:	**Urinary Elimination, alteration in pattern.**
SUPPORTING DATA/CONTRIBUTING FACTORS:	**Urinary retention occurs owing to bladder atony and contraction of urinary sphincter during spinal shock and is manifested by bladder distention, which may lead to urinary reflux, infections, stone formation, and renal deterioration. Bladder distention after spinal shock phase may be a precipitator of autonomic dysreflexia.**
GENERAL PATIENT OUTCOMES:	**Urinary retention is prevented, shown by absence of suprapubic distention and balanced intake and output. Urine is clear and odor free.**

INTERVENTIONS	RATIONALE
Independent	
Palpate bladder for distention.	Spinal injury above L2 results in bladder dysfunction owing to loss of bladder contraction and ability to relax urinary sphincter.
Encourage fluid intake (2 to 4 liters per day), including acid ash juices, such as cranberry.	Helps maintain renal function, prevents infection and formation of urinary stones. Note: Fluid may be restricted when intermittent catheterization program is initiated.
Monitor hourly and 24-hour intake and output, noting specific gravity.	Indicators of fluid balance (over or under hydration).
Observe for cloudy or bloody urine, foul odor.	Signs of urinary or kidney infection, which has potential complications of sepsis, autonomic dysreflexia.
Collaborative	
Keep bladder deflated by means of indwelling catheter initially. Institute intermittent catheterization when appropriate.	Indwelling catheter may be desired during acute phase to monitor output more carefully and to prevent urinary retention. Bladder training is initiated to approximate physiologic function by intermittent emptying and to reduce complications usually seen with indwelling catheters (e.g., infection).
Monitor BUN, creatinine, white blood count (WBC).	Reflects renal function, development of infection.

NURSING DIAGNOSIS:	**Bowel Elimination, alteration in [pattern].**
SUPPORTING DATA/CONTRIBUTING FACTORS:	**Innervation of the bowel and rectum is disrupted, resulting in loss of ability**

	to evacuate the bowel voluntarily. Gastric dilatation and ileus frequently accompany spinal shock. In addition, altered dietary and fluid intake affect consistency of the stool.
GENERAL PATIENT OUTCOMES:	**Gastrointestinal function is restored or maintained. Bowel evacuation program is established.**

INTERVENTIONS	RATIONALE
Independent	
Auscultate bowel sounds, noting location and characteristics.	May be absent initially during spinal shock. High tinkling sounds may be present with ileus.
Monitor abdominal distention if bowel sounds are discreased or absent.	Loss of peristalsis (related to impaired innervation) paralyzes the bowel, creating ileus and bowel distention. Overdistention of the bowel may be a precipitator of autonomic dysreflexia.
Note nausea and vomiting. Check gastric secretions and stools for occult blood.	GI bleeding may occur as a side effect of therapy (e.g., steroids or anticoagulants) or in response to stress of injury (Cushing's ulcer). (Refer to Care Plan: Upper GI/Esophageal Bleeding, page 197.)
Check for presence of impaction.	Early detection necessary in order to treat effectively. Note: Impaction may potentiate autonomic dysreflexia when spinal shock abates.
Promote increased fluid intake, including fruit juices.	Improves consistency of stool for transit through the bowel.
Collaborative	
Insert and maintain nasogastric tube and attach to suction if appropriate.	Initially may be used to reduce gastric distention and prevent vomiting, thereby lowering risk of aspiration.
Consult with dietician to provide appropriate diet when hemodynamaically stable.	Immediately postinjury, patient may be kept nothing by mouth (NPO) with parenteral fluids only. Adverse conditions may require tube feedings or total parenteral nutrition (TPN) when intake is reestablished; that is, multiple trauma, intubation, or swallowing problems associated with being immobilized in supine position. (Refer to Care Plan: Nutritional Support, page 367.)
Administer stool softeners and suppositories as indicated.	Permanent bowel dysfunction occurs with spinal injury above L2. Constipation and incontinence can be avoided by routine bowel evacuation.
Use rectal tube as needed.	Reduce bowel distention, which may impede respiratory function or precipitate autonomic responses.
Administer antacids/cimetidine (Tagamet) or ranitidine (Zantac).	Reduces and neutralizes gastric acid, may prevent gastric irritation.

NURSING DIAGNOSIS:	**Skin Integrity, impaired (potential).**
SUPPORTING DATA/CONTRIBUTING FACTORS:	**Inadequate peripheral circulation associated with spinal shock, immobility, nutritional deficits, or direct injury (multiple trauma) place the skin at risk for irritation and ulceration.**
GENERAL PATIENT OUTCOMES:	**Decubiti are prevented.**

INTERVENTIONS	RATIONALE
Independent	
Inspect all skin areas, note capillary filling (e.g., blanching, redness, swelling). Note: Skin under halo frame or vest and areas where skin continuously touches (e.g., between legs, under breasts).	Skin is prone to breakdown because of changes in peripheral circulation, pressure, and altered temperature regulation.
Observe halo and tongs insertion sites. Note swelling, redness, skin breakdown. Cleanse routinely and apply antibiotic ointment per protocol.	Sites are prone to inflammation and infection and provide route for pathologic microorganisms to enter cranial cavity.
Massage and protect pressure points by use of lamb's wool, foam padding, egg crate mattress, and skin hardening and protective agents (e.g., tincture of benzoin, Karaya, Sween cream).	Enhances circulation and protects skin surfaces, reducing risk of ulceration. Quadriplegic and paraplegic patients will require life-long protection from decubuti formation, which can cause extensive tissue necrosis and sepsis.
Reposition frequently by means of turning frame or kinetic bed. Place patient in prone position periodically.	Improves skin circulation and reduces pressure time on bony prominences.
Wash and dry skin, especially in high moisture areas, such as perineum.	Clean dry skin is less prone to breakdown.
Collaborative	
Provide kinetic therapy or electric bed, alternating pressure mattress.	Improves systemic and peripheral circulation and reduces skin disruption due to pressure.

NURSING DIAGNOSIS:	**Self-Concept, disturbance in, body image; self-esteem; role performance; personal identity.**
SUPPORTING DATA/CONTRIBUTING FACTORS:	**Drastic changes in physical function and lifestyle are produced by spinal cord injury which affect the patient's view of self and ability to perform desired activities. Spinal cord injury provokes a cycle of emotional stages (grief process), including denial and despair. In addition, the patient may**

be overwhelmed by a sense of powerlessness, producing feelings and reactions of anger.

GENERAL PATIENT OUTCOMES: **Patient and significant other(s) focus on the here and now and begin to develop strategies for coping with anticipated changes.**

INTERVENTIONS	RATIONALE
Independent	
Acknowledge difficulty in determining degree of functional incapacity and/or chance of functional improvement.	During acute phase of injury, long-term effects are unknown, which delays the patient's ability to integrate situation into self-concept.
Listen to patient's comments and responses to situation.	Provides clues to view of self, role changes, and needs and is useful for providing information at patient's level of acceptance.
Assess dynamics of patient, family, and significant other(s) (e.g., patient's role in family, cultural factors).	Patient's previous role in family unit is usually disrupted or altered by injury, adding to difficulty in integrating self-concept.
Encourage family and significant other to treat patient as normally as possible (e.g., discussing home situations, family news).	Involving patient in family unit reduces feelings of social isolation, helplessness, and uselessness.
Provide accurate information. Discuss concerns honestly about prognosis and treatment at patient's level of acceptance.	Focus of information should be on present and immediate needs, and information should be repeated until patient has assimilated or integrated information.
Discuss meaning of loss or change with patient and family. Assess interactions between patient and family.	Actual change in body image may be different from that perceived by patient. Distortions may be unconsciously reinforced by family.
Accept patient, show concern for individual as a person. Encourage patient, identify strengths, give positive reinforcement for progress noted.	Establishes therapeutic atmosphere for patient to begin self-acceptance.
Include patient, family, and significant other(s) in care, allowing patient to make decisions and to participate in self-care activities as possible.	Recognizes that patient is still responsible for own life and provides some sense of control over situation. Sets stage for future lifestyle pattern and interaction required in daily care. Note: Patient may reject all help or may be completely dependent during this phase.
Arrange visit by similarly affected person if patient desires and/or situation allows.	May be helpful to patient by providing hope for the future.

NURSING DIAGNOSIS: **Grieving, anticipatory.**

SUPPORTING DATA/CONTRIBUTING FACTORS: **Grieving is a normal response to perceived and actual loss of physiopsychosocial well-being and may be mani-**

	fested by a wide range of emotional responses, including guilt, fear, sadness, and denial of potential loss of function.
GENERAL PATIENT OUTCOMES:	**Patient is expressing feelings and beginning to progress through recognized stages of grief, focusing on one day at a time.**

INTERVENTIONS	RATIONALE
Independent	
Identify signs of grieving, (e.g., shock, denial, anger, depression).	Patient experiences many emotional reactions to the injury and its impact on life. These stages are not static, and the rate at which the patient progresses through them is variable.
Shock	
Note lack of communication or emotional response, absence of questions.	Shock is the initial reaction associated with overwhelming injury. Primary concern is to maintain life, and patient is probably too ill to express feelings.
Provide simple, accurate information to patient and significant other(s) regarding diagnosis and care. Be honest—do not give false information, while providing emotional support.	The patient's awareness of surroundings and activity may be blocked initially, and attention span may be limited. Little is actually known about the final outcome of the patient's injuries during acute phase, and limited knowledge may add to frustration and grief of family. Therefore, early focus of emotional support may be on family and significant other(s).
Encourage expressions of sadness, grief, guilt, and fear between patient, family, and significant other(s).	Knowledge that these are appropriate feelings which should be expressed may be very supportive to patient and family.
Incorporate family and significant other(s) into problem solving and planning for patient's care.	Assists in establishing therapeutic nurse-patient-family relationships.
Denial	
Assist patient and significant other(s) to verbalize feelings about situation, avoiding judgment about what is expressed.	Important beginning step to deal with what has happened. Helpful in identifying patient's coping mechanisms.
Note comments indicating that patient expects to walk shortly and/or is making a bargain with God. Do not confront these comments.	Patient may not deny entire disability but may deny its permanency. Situation is compounded by actual uncertainty of outcome, and denial may be useful for coping at this time.
Focus on present needs (e.g., range of motion exercises, skin care).	Attention on "here and now" reduces frustration and hopelessness of uncertain future and may make dealing with today's problems more manageable.
Anger	
Identify use of manipulative behavior and reactions to caregivers.	Patient may express anger verbally or physically (e.g., spitting, biting). Patient may say that nothing is done

INTERVENTIONS	RATIONALE
Independent	
	right by caregivers and family or may pit one caregiver against another.
Encourage patient to take control when possible; for example, establishing care routines, dietary choices, diversional activities.	Helps reduce anger associated with powerlessness and provides patient with some sense of control and expectation of responsibility for own behavior.
Accept expressions of anger and hopelessness. Avoid arguing. Show concern for the patient.	Patient is acknowledged as a worthwhile individual, and nonjudgmental care is provided.
Set limits on acting-out and unacceptable behavior when necessary (e.g., abusive language, sexually agressive or suggestive behavior).	Although it is important to express negative feelings, patient and staff need to be protected from violence and embarrassment. This phase is traumatic for all involved. Family support is essential.
Depression	
Note loss of interest in living, sleep disturbance, suicidal thoughts, hopelessness. Listen to but do not confront these expressions. Let patient know nurse is available for support.	Phase may last weeks, months, or even years. Acceptance of these feelings and consistent support during this phase is important to a satisfactory resolution.
Collaborative	
Refer to pastoral care.	Patient may suffer great spiritual distress, including feelings of guilt, deprivation of peace, and anger at God.
Refer to psychiatric nurse, social worker, or psychiatrist to assist patient, family, and significant other(s). Patient will need assistance to work through feelings of alienation, guilt, and resentment concerning lifestyle and role changes.	Family is required to make adaptive changes to a member who may be permanently "different," which may require supportive in-depth and long-term assistance psychotherapy to cope with these changes and the future.

CHAPTER 6 GASTROENTEROLOGY

Cirrhosis

Cirrhosis is a chronic liver disease characterized by diffuse destruction and abnormal regeneration of liver cells. Ensuing fibrotic changes impair liver function and can obstruct hepatic circulation. Cirrhotic patients are most often seen in the critical care unit because of complications, such as bleeding esophogeal varices, renal failure, and hepatic encephalopathy.

PATIENT ASSESSMENT DATA BASE

HISTORY

History of alcohol abuse, alcoholic liver disease; biliary disease, hepatitis, or exposure to hepatitis, toxins, or chemicals; liver trauma; upper gastrointestinal bleeding; episodes of bleeding varices; drug/medication use, especially those known to affect liver function; congestive heart failure, pericarditis, rheumatic heart disease; cancer, which may cause liver malfunction leading to chronic liver failure.

Subjective

Complains of abdominal pain, anorexia, weight loss, or weight gain (from fluid), weakness, fatigue, diarrhea/constipation, dark urine, itchy skin.

PHYSICAL EXAMINATION

Inspection

Respirations: dyspnea/limited thoracic expansion owing to ascites.

Mental status: may note depressed mentation, personality changes, lethargy, slurred speech.

Reflexes: asterixis may be noted (an uncontrolled, continuous flapping of hands), which indicates onset of hepatic encephalopathy.

Skin: many manifestations may be present; for example, dry with poor turgor, jaundice, pruritis (deposition of bile salts), bruising (altered clotting factors), spider hemangiomata/palmar erythema/telangiectasis, and abdominal striae. Muscle wasting/decreased tricep-skin fold measurement.

Edema: may be generalized in tissues as fluid retention occurs in response to increased antidiuretic hormone (ADH) and aldosterone levels.

Sexual manifestations: testicular atrophy, gynecomastia, loss of hair (on chest, underarms, and pubic area), and/or menstrual disorders may reflect estrogen-androgen imbalance.

Urine: oliguria (decreased output) and dark-colored urine are due to increased excretion of conjugated bilirubin and increased ADH.

Auscultation

Lungs: adventitious sounds in presence of pleural effusion/congestive failure.

Palpation

Hepato-jugular reflex: Jugular vein: distention/elevation of pulse point may be noted when liver palpated.

Abdomen: hepatomegaly, splenomegaly, ascites, and distended abdominal veins may be noted.

DIAGNOSTIC STUDIES

Serum bilirubin: elevated owing to cellular disruption, inability of liver to conjugate, or biliary obstruction.

SGOT/SGPT: increased owing to cellular damage and release of enzymes.

Alkaline phosphatase: elevated owing to reduced excretion.

Serum albumin: decreased owing to depressed synthesis of albumin.

Globulins: (IgA and IgG immunoglobulin) elevated owing to increased synthesis.

CBC: Hgb/Hct and RBCs may be decreased owing to bleeding. Increased RBC destruction is seen with hypersplenism and iron deficiency. Leukopenia may be present as a result of hypersplenism.

Prothrombin time: prolonged owing to decreased synthesis of prothrombin.

Fibrinogen level is decreased, reflecting reduced production.

BUN: elevation indicates breakdown of blood/protein.

Serum ammonia: elevated owing to inability to convert ammonia to urea.

Serum glucose: hypoglycemia may be present owing to impaired gluconeogenesis.

Urine urobilinogen: increase indicates interference with normal deposit of urobilinogen.

Electrolytes: hypokalemia/hypernatremia may be present owing to increased aldosterone.

Calcium: may be decreased owing to impaired absorption of vitamin D.

Liver biopsy: detects fatty infiltrates, fibrosis, destruction/regeneration of hepatic tissues.

Paracentesis: total protein may be decreased (ascites).

NURSING PRIORITIES

1. Restore/maintain fluid/electrolyte balance.
2. Prevent injury/minimize complications.
3. Restore/maintain nutritional status.
4. Provide support for patient/family.

NURSING DIAGNOSIS:	**Fluid Volume, alteration in, excess.**
SUPPORTING DATA/CONTRIBUTING FACTORS:	**As liver cell damage progresses, hydrostatic pressure is increased (portal hy-**

pertension) and colloid osmotic pressure is decreased (low serum albumin), which promotes loss of fluid into the peritoneal space, producing ascites and hypovolemia. Hypovolemia stimulates the secretion of ADH and aldosterone, which promotes water and sodium retention.

GENERAL PATIENT OUTCOMES:	**Fluid volume is restored to/maintained at optimal level manifested by blood pressure, pulse, central venous pressure within patient's normal limits. Lungs are clear; edema and ascites are absent. Electrolytes are within normal range.**

INTERVENTIONS	RATIONALE
Independent	
Monitor blood pressure and hemodynamic parameters if available; for example, central venous pressure (CVP), pulmonary capillary wedge pressure (PCWP).	Elevations are usually associated with fluid volume excess but may not be present owing to fluid shifts out of the vascular space.
Assess respiratory status; for example, increased respiratory rate, dyspnea.	Indicative of pulmonary congestion/edema.
Auscultate lungs, noting diminshed/absent breath sounds and developing adventitious sounds (e.g., crackles).	Increasing pulmonary congestion may result in consolidation and complications; for example, pulmonary edema leading to impaired gas exchange.
Monitor ECG for dysrhythmias. Auscultate heart sounds for development of S_3/S_4 gallop rhythm.	May be caused by congestive heart failure, decreased coronary artery perfusion, and electrolyte imbalance.
Note distention of external jugular veins.	Associated with vascular congestion.
Measure abdominal girth.	Reflects accumulation of ascites resulting from loss of plasma proteins/fluid into peritoneal space.
Assess degree of peripheral/dependent edema.	Fluids shift into tissues as a result of sodium and water retention, decreased albumin, and increased ADH.
Measure intake/output (I/O), noting positive balance (intake in excess of output). Weigh daily and note gain greater than 0.5 kg per day.	Comparison of I/O with weight reflects circulating volume needs, developing/resolution of fluid shifts, and effects of therapy. Positive balance reflects continuing fluid retention. Note: Decreased circulating volume owing to fluid shifts may directly affect renal perfusion/function resulting in hepatorenal syndrome. (Refer to Care Plans: Acute Renal Failure, page 207, and Renal Dialysis, page 222.)
Encourage bed rest when ascites is present.	May promote diuresis, especially if drug therapy is ineffective.

INTERVENTIONS	RATIONALE
Collaborative	
Monitor electrolytes, particularly potassium and sodium and serum albumin.	Decreased renal blood flow accompanied by elevated ADH and aldosterone levels, decreased albumin, and the use of diuretics to reduce total body water may cause various electrolyte imbalances. (Refer to Appendix: Fluid/Electrolyte Imbalances, page 431.)
Monitor serial chest x-ray examinations.	Increased frequency of vascular congestion, pulmonary edema, and pleural effusions occur in liver dysfunction.
Restrict sodium and fluids as indicated.	Sodium may be restricted to minimize fluid retention in extravascular spaces. Fluid restriction may be necessary to correct/prevent dilutional hyponatremia.
Administer salt-free albumin/plasma expanders as indicated.	Albumin may be used to increase the colloid osmotic pressure in vascular compartment to pull fluid into vascular space, thereby increasing effective circulating volume and decreasing ascitic formation.
Administer medications as indicated:	
Diuretics; for example, spironolactone (Aldactone),	Blocks effect of aldosterone and increases water excretion while sparing potassium.
Potassium,	Serum and cellular potassium is usually depleted in liver disease.
Positive inotropic drugs and arterial vasodilators.	Given to increase cardiac output/improve renal blood flow/function, thereby reducing excess fluid.

NURSING DIAGNOSIS: **Injury, potential for hemorrhage/altered clotting factors.**

SUPPORTING DATA/CONTRIBUTING FACTORS: **In cirrhosis, blood flow from the liver may be obstructed, increasing pressure in the portal vein, resulting in the development of collateral circulatory channels within the gastrointestinal (GI) tract. These fragile, dilated vessels (most commonly esophageal varices) may rupture as portal hypertension increases with advanced cirrhosis. These vessels receive a significant amount of blood so that an uncontrolled variceal bleed can be fatal. In addition, clotting factors are diminished in liver disease because of decreased production of prothrombin, fibrinogen, and clotting factors VII, IX, and X, as well as impaired vitamin K absorption and release of thromboplastin.**

GENERAL PATIENT OUTCOMES:	**Hemorrhage is prevented, recognized/treated promptly.**

INTERVENTIONS	RATIONALE
Independent	
Assess for signs/symptoms of GI bleed; for example, check all secretions for frank or occult blood. Observe color and consistency of stools and vomitus.	The GI tract (esophageal varices and hemorrhoids) is the most usual source of bleeding owing to mucosal fragility and alterations in hemostasis associated with liver dysfunction. (Refer to Care Plan: Upper GI/Esophageal Bleeding, page 197.)
Monitor for presence of petechiae, ecchymosis, bleeding from one or more sites.	Subacute disseminated intravascular coagulation (DIC) may develop secondary to altered clotting factors. (Refer to Care Plan: Disseminated Intravascular Coagulation, page 319.)
Monitor pulse, blood pressure (BP), hemodynamic pressures (e.g., CO, PCWP, CVP), as indicated.	An increased pulse with decreased BP, CO, PCWP, and CVP can indicate a decreased circulating blood volume requiring further evaluation.
Note changes in mentation/level of consciousness.	Changes may indicate decreased cerebral perfusion secondary to fluid shifts/hypovolemia.
Avoid rectal temperatures; be gentle with GI tube insertions.	The rectal and esophageal vessels are most vulnerable to rupture.
Collaborative	
Monitor hemoglobin (hgb), hematocrit (Hct), and clotting factors.	Indicators of anemia, active bleeding, or impending complications (e.g., DIC).
Administer blood, packed red blood cells (RBCs), fresh frozen plasma, and platelets, as indicated.	Used to expand circulating volume, to improve oxygen-carrying capacity of blood, and to replace clotting factors.
Assist with insertion/maintenance of GI/esophageal tube (e.g., Sengstaken-Blakemore tube).	Temporarily controls bleeding of esophageal varices when control by other means (e.g., lavage) and hemodynamic stability cannot be achieved. (Refer to Care Plan: Upper GI/Esophageal Bleeding, page 197.)
Provide gastric lavage with room temperature/cool saline solution as indicated.	Evacuation of blood from GI tract decreases ammonia production and risk of hepatic encephalopathy.
Administer supplemental vitamins (e.g., vitamins K, C), as indicated.	Promotes prothrombin synthesis and coagulation if liver functional. Vitamin C deficiencies increase susceptibility of GI system to irritation/bleeding.

NURSING DIAGNOSIS:	**Nutrition, alteration in, less than body requirements.**
SUPPORTING DATA/CONTRIBUTING FACTORS:	**Patients may be malnourished owing to previous poor eating habits, or anorexia, nausea/vomiting associated with cirrhosis. Loss of functional liver**

	tissue results in impaired metabolism of carbohydrates and storage of nutrients, as well as malabsorption of fats/fat, soluble vitamins owing to decreased bile production.
GENERAL PATIENT OUTCOMES:	**Nutritional intake adequate to meet metabolic needs as evidenced by appropriate positive nitrogen balance, stable muscle mass, appropriate weight loss or gain for situation.**

INTERVENTIONS	RATIONALE
Independent	
Encourage patient to eat all meals/supplementary feedings, when oral feeding is resumed.	Patient is often reluctant to eat owing to anorexia, loss of interest in food.
Serve small frequent meals.	Poor tolerance to larger meals may be due to increased intra-abdominal pressure/ascites.
Note food intolerance/aversions. Encourage patient selection of foods whenever possible.	Patient may be more likely to eat if food is to patient's liking.
Provide mouth care frequently and prior to meals.	Patient is prone to sore and/or bleeding gums and bad taste in mouth, which add to anorexia.
Weigh as indicated. Compare changes in fluid status, recent weight history, tricep-skin fold measurement.	It may be difficult to use weight as a direct indicator of nutritional status in view of edema/ascites. Tricep-skin fold test is useful in assessing changes in muscle mass and subcutaneous fat reserves.
Promote undisturbed rest periods.	Reduces metabolic demands and promotes cellular regeneration.
Collaborative	
Monitor laboratory studies, for example, serum glucose, albumin, total protein. (Refer to Care Plan: Nutritional Support, page 367.)	Glucose may be decreased because of impaired gluconeogenesis, depleted glycogen stores, or inadequate intake. Protein may be low due to impaired metabolism, decreased hepatic synthesis, or loss into the peritoneal cavity.
Maintain nothing-by-mouth (NPO) status when indicated.	Initially GI rest may be required to reduce demands on the liver and GI production of ammonia/urea.
Consult with dietician to provide diet that is high in calories and simple carbohydrates, low in fat, and moderate to high in protein; sodium and fluid may be restricted.	High-calorie foods are desired inasmuch as patients intake is usually limited. Simple carbohydrates provide readily available energy. Fats are poorly absorbed owing to liver dysfunction. Proteins are needed to improve serum protein levels and to promote liver cell regeneration. Note: Protein is restricted if ammonia level is elevated or if patient has clinical signs of hepatic encephalopathy. (Refer to Nursing Diagnosis: Thought Processes, alteration in, page 178.) Sodium/fluid may be restricted to reduce fluid retention.

INTERVENTIONS	RATIONALE
Collaborative	
Administer vitamin supplements as indicated; for example, A, D, E, K, and B complex.	Patient has poor tolerance of fat, which reduces absorption of fat-soluble vitamins from the GI tract. In addition, liver is unable to store vitamins. Initially vitamins may be given parenterally, with oral supplements continued once intake is resumed.
Administer digestive enzymes; for example, pancreatin (Viokase), as indicated.	Promotes digestion of fats and may reduce steatorrhea/diarrhea.
Administer tube feedings/hyperalimentation/lipids, as indicated.	May be required to supplement diet or to provide nutrients when patient is unable to eat. Special tube feedings are available that provide essential amino acids yet are low in protein and sodium. Intravenous (IV) support may be necessary if patient is unable to tolerate GI route. (Refer to Care Plan: Nutritional Support, page 367.)

NURSING DIAGNOSIS: **Breathing Pattern, ineffective [potential].**

SUPPORTING DATA/CONTRIBUTING FACTORS: **Decreased lung expansion may be present owing to intra-abdominal fluid collection/ascites. Pulmonary infections may develop owing to immune system depression, immobility, decreased lung expansion, and accumulation of secretions. Respirations may be ineffective if level of consciousness is severely impaired (e.g., advancing hepatic coma).**

GENERAL PATIENT OUTCOMES: **Respiratory rate, rhythm/depth, and arterial blood gases (ABGs) are within patient's normal range. Signs of respiratory distress/infection are absent.**

INTERVENTIONS	RATIONALE
Independent	
Monitor respiratory rate and effort.	Rapid, shallow respirations/dyspnea may be present owing to hypoxia and fluid accumulation/ascites.
Auscultate breath sounds, noting adventitious sounds; for example, crackles, wheezes, rhonchi.	Presence of crackles/rhonchi reflects accumulation of fluid/secretions and indicates developing complications.
Investigate changes in level of consciousness.	Changes in mentation may reflect hypoxemia and respiratory failure which often accompany hepatic coma.

INTERVENTIONS	RATIONALE
Independent	
Keep head of bed elevated and position patient on side, when possible.	Facilitates breathing by reducing pressure on the diaphragm. Minimizes risk of aspiration of secretions.
Encourage deep breathing/coughing and position changes. Assist patient with respiratory adjuncts (e.g., incentive spirometer).	Aids in lung expansion and assists in mobilizing secretions.
Monitor temperature. Note chills, increased coughing, changes in color/character of sputum.	Indicators of developing respiratory infection.
Collaborative	
Monitor serial ABGs/chest x-rays examinations.	Reveals change in respiratory status, developing pulmonary complications. Note: Use of IV solutions containing lactate may potentiate development of lactic acidosis, inasmuch as the liver is unable to metabolize lactate.
Administer supplemental oxygen, as indicated.	May be necessary to treat/prevent hypoxia. If respirations/oxygenation is inadequate, mechanical ventilation may be required.
Assist with paracentesis.	Occasionally done to remove fluid when respiratory embarrassment is not corrected by other measures.

NURSING DIAGNOSIS:	**Skin Integrity, impairment of, potential.**
SUPPORTING DATA/CONTRIBUTING FACTORS:	**Skin integrity can be compromised by several factors. Edema of tissues decreases circulation to skin, and ascites increases weight on supporting tissues. In addition, mobility is often impaired by decreased level of consciousness and/or discomfort caused by ascites. Pruritis can occur as a result of bile salts accumulation, and consequent scratching can add to skin breakdown.**
GENERAL PATIENT OUTCOMES:	**Skin integrity is maintained, dermal trauma is prevented.**

INTERVENTIONS	RATIONALE
Independent	
Reposition frequently. Observe for and massage stressed skin and pressure points.	Early recognition/intervention prevents skin breakdown.

INTERVENTIONS	RATIONALE
Independent	
Use nondrying soap for bathing; apply lotion to avoid dryness.	Dry, rough skin increases pruritis, resulting in scratching and skin excoriation.
Keep bedclothes dry and free of wrinkles.	Decreases skin irritation.
Cut/file fingernails short. Provide gloves during sleep if necessary.	Reduces risk of dermal injury from scratching.
Encourage active/perform passive range of motion.	Improves circulation to skin, improves muscle tone and joint mobility.
Collaborative	
Provide sheepskin, padding, eggcrate/alternating pressure mattresses, as indicated.	Reduces prolonged pressure on any skin area, thereby reducing risk of decubiti.
Apply calamine lotion with 1 percent phenol.	Relieves discomfort of pruritis and may reduce scratching.
Administer cholestyramine (Questran) with fruit juice if indicated.	Reduces accumulation of bile pigments in the skin. Note: This may alter vitamin K absorption and contribute to alteration in clotting/homeostasis.

NURSING DIAGNOSIS: **Fear.**

SUPPORTING DATA/CONTRIBUTING FACTORS: **Progression of incurable debilitating disease is accompanied by changes in body image/role functions and produces feelings of fear, anxiety, and powerlessness related to uncertainty of prognosis and a real threat of death.**

GENERAL PATIENT OUTCOMES: **Verbalizes/demonstrates appropriate range of feelings. Receives support from caregivers and significant others.**

INTERVENTIONS	RATIONALE
Independent	
Discuss situation/encourage verbalization of fears. Explain relationship between nature of disease and symptoms.	The cirrhosis patient is very sensitive to body changes and may also experience feelings of guilt when cause is related to alcohol (80 percent) or drug use.
Support and encourage patient; provide care with a positive friendly attitude.	Caregivers sometimes allow judgmental feelings to affect the care of the patient, and they need to make every effort to help the patient feel valued as a person.
Encourage family/significant other(s) to verbalize feelings, visit/participate in care.	Family members may feel guilty about the patient's condition and fearful of impending death. They need nonjudgmental emotional support and free access to

INTERVENTIONS	RATIONALE
Independent	
	patient. Participation in care helps them feel useful and promotes trust between staff, patient, and family/significant other(s).
Collaborative	
Refer to other support services; for example, counselors, psychiatric resources, social service, and/or clergy.	Increased vulnerability/concerns associated with this critical illness may require services of professional counselors.

NURSING DIAGNOSIS:	**Thought Processes, alteration in.**
SUPPORTING DATA/CONTRIBUTING FACTORS:	**Numerous factors such as infection, gastric bleeding, azotemia, shock, and high-protein diet can increase levels of serum ammonia owing to the liver's inability to convert ammonia to urea for excretion. In addition, if renal insufficiency is present, reduced clearance will result in increased blood urea levels. Elevated ammonia and urea accompanied by hypoxemia (resulting from acidosis) produces changes in mental function.**
GENERAL PATIENT OUTCOMES:	**Oriented with thought processes within patient's norm.**

INTERVENTIONS	RATIONALE
Independent	
Observe/document changes in mentation; for example, confusion, slowing/slurred speech, hallucinations.	Decreased level of consciousness may reflect hypoxia, hypovolemia/hypotension, or alcohol withdrawal or indicate progression of liver dysfunction leading to hepatic encephalopathy. (Refer to Care Plan: Chemical Dependency: Alcohol Toxicity/Withdrawal, page 343.)
Arouse patient at intervals; orient to time, place, person.	Symptoms fluctuate, and observation of subtle changes can be difficult unless well documented.
Investigate temperature elevations. Monitor for signs of infection.	Infection may precipitate hepatic encephalopathy owing to tissue catabolism and release of nitrogen.
Protect from injury (e.g., observe closely, use side rails).	Confusion and belligerent behavior may develop.

INTERVENTIONS	RATIONALE
Collaborative	
Monitor laboratory studies; for example,	
Electrolytes/pH,	Hypokalemia and metabolic alkalosis increase production/ resorption of ammonia and potentiate transfer of ammonia across blood-brain barrier.
Ammonia, BUN,	Accumulation of nitrogenous substances potentiates development of encephalopathy.
Glucose,	Hypoglycemia may contribute to changes in mentation.
Hgb/Hct.	Alterations in oxygen-carying capacity contribute to hypoxemia.
Administer medications to reduce intestinal ammonia as indicated; for example,	
Neomycin sulfate (Neobiotic),	Nonabsorbable antibiotic that suppresses urea-splitting bacteria and results in decreased protein degradation and ammonia production.
Lactulose (Cephulac).	Laxative effect promotes excretion of protein and blood from intestines, thereby reducing production of ammonia.
Restrict hepatotoxic drugs, such as sedatives, narcotics, and barbiturates.	Drug metabolism is decreased and may result in toxic levels, inasmuch as the liver is unable to clear drug(s) from system.
Administer oxazepam (Serax) by mouth or small IV dose of diazepam (Valium) as indicated.	Cautious use of sedation may be beneficial if severe agitation creates potential risk of injury for patient.
Restrict protein intake as indicated. Encourage use of fruit juices in place of water when possible.	Protein is broken down in the intestine, producing ammonia. Dietary/fluid restrictions resulting in retention of intestinal contents (constipation) increases intestinal bacterial action and ammonia production. Use of fruit juices may enhance bowel activity.
Provide supplemental oxygen.	Mentation is affected by oxygen concentration and utilization in hepatic encephalopathy. Although supplemental oxygen may not improve the abnormal utilization, hypoxemia may improve.
Administer glucose solutions.	Provides energy source for cellular functioning when hypoglycemia present.

Acute Pancreatitis

PATIENT ASSESSMENT DATA BASE

HISTORY

History of recent excessive alcohol intake.

History of gallstones with partial or complete common bile duct obstruction, gastritis, duodenal ulcer, diverticulitis.

Family history of pancreatitis.

History of external abdominal trauma or surgery, for example, procedures on the pancreas, biliary tract, stomach, or duodenum.

Onset of bacterial infection; for example, mumps, scarlet fever.

History of erosive connective tissue disease, for example, Crohn's disease.

History of malignant tumors.

Current pregnancy (third trimester), with shifting of abdominal contents and compression of biliary duct.

Use of prescribed medications such as antihypertensives, opiates, thiazides, steroids, some antibiotics, and estrogen side effects.

Subjective

Unrelenting abdominal pain, usually located in the epigastrium and periumbilical regions and often radiating to the chest and back. Vomiting, retching, and dry heaves. May report anorexia, weakness, diarrhea, weight loss, and fever.

PHYSICAL EXAMINATION

Inspection

Position: patient may curl up with both arms over abdomen to relieve pain.

Mental status: mental confusion, agitation, restlessness, distress, and apprehension are common.

Respirations: tachypnea with/without dyspnea may accompany pain.

Skin: may be pale, cold, mottled, and moist owing to vasoconstriction, fluid shifts (ascites), and edema. Jaundice (caused by inflammation/obstruction of the common duct) may be mild/pronounced. Turner's sign (blue-green-brown discoloration in the flanks from blood accumulation) or Cullen's sign (similar discoloration around the umbilicus) may be seen 3 to 6 days after onset of hemorrhagic pancreatitis.

Extremities: coarse tremors may be noted, caused by hypocalcemia.

Urine: may be dark amber/brown/foamy, reflecting presence of bile.

Stool: usually frothy, foul-smelling, grayish, greasy, and frequently nonformed.

Palpation

Abdomen: upper abdominal guarding, distention, and rebound tenderness are usually noted. Rigidity may or may not be present.

Auscultation

Bowel sounds: may be decreased or absent owing to reduced peristalis/ileus.

Vital signs: hypertension may be present during acute pain. Tachycardia and hypotension with weak/inaudible blood pressure may be noted, owing to hypovolemic shock or toxemia from circulating toxins.

Breath sounds: basilar crackles may be present due to pleural effusion associated with insufficient alveolar inflation of lower lobes because of abdominal pain and increased abdominal size (pressure).

Other

Temperature: elevations are usually low grade. Persistent elevation suggests complications (e.g., pancreatic abscess, peritonitis).

DIAGNOSTIC STUDIES

Serum amylase: increased due to obstruction of normal outflow of pancreatic enzymes because of parenchymal damage. Level rises 2 to 12 hours after onset of symptoms and usually returns to normal in 3 to 5 days (normal result does not rule out disease).

Urine amylase: increased due to parenchymal damage. Level rises within 2 to 3 days after onset of attack.

Serum lipase: usually elevates along with amylase but remains elevated much longer.

Serum bilirubin: increases are common and may be caused by alcoholic liver disease or extrinsic compression of the common bile duct.

Alkaline phosphatase: usually elevated if pancreatitis is accompanied by biliary disease.

Serum albumin and protein: may be decreased owing to colloid loss secondary to increased capillary permeability and transudation of fluid into extracellular space.

Serum calcium: hypocalcemia, which may appear 2 to 3 days after onset of the disease, usually indicates fat necrosis and may accompany pancreatic necrosis.

Serum potassium: hypokalemia may be present owing to gastric losses, and hyperkalemia may develop secondary to tissue necrosis, acidosis, and renal insufficiency.

Triglycerides: levels may exceed 1700 mg/dl and may be the causative agent in acute pancreatitis.

LDH/SGOT: may be elevated up to 15 times above normal limit owing to biliary and liver involvement.

CBC: WBC of 10,000 to 25,000 is present in 80 percent of patients. Hematocrit is usually elevated owing to hemoconcentration associated with vomiting or from effusion of fluid into pancreas or retroperitoneal area.

Serum glucose: transient elevations are common, especially during initial acute attacks. Sustained glucose level greater than 200 reflects widespread beta cell damage and pancreatic necrosis and is a poor prognostic sign.

Prothrombin time: prolonged due to liver involvement and fat necrosis.

Urine: hematuria and proteinuria may be present, reflecting glomerular damage.

Stool: increased fat content (steatorrhea) is indicative of insufficient digestion of fats and protein.

ABGs: hypoxemia and hypercapnea may be present, reflecting associated respiratory insufficiency.

CAT scan/ultrasound of abdomen: may be used to identify pancreatic inflammation, carcinoma, or obstruction of the biliary tract.

Endoscopy: fiberoptic visualization of the pancreatic ducts is useful to diagnose fistulas, obstructive biliary disease, and pancreatic duct strictures/anomolies. Note: This procedure is contraindicated during acute phase.

X-ray examination of abdomen: may demonstrate presence of dilated loop of small bowel adjacent to pancreas or may identify intra-abdominal precipitator or complication, for example, presence of free intraperitoneal air caused by perforation, abscess formation, or pancreatic calcification.

Upper GI series: frequently exhibits evidence of pancreatic enlargement/inflammation.

Chest x-ray examination: pleural effusion may be noted.

NURSING PRIORITIES

1. Restore/maintain hemodynamic stability.
2. Promote comfort.
3. Restore/maintain adequate nutrition.
4. Prevent/minimize complications.

NURSING DIAGNOSIS:	**Fluid Volume Deficit, potential.**
SUPPORTING DATA/CONTRIBUTING FACTORS:	**Fluid losses may occur due to vomiting/gastric suctioning, third spacing, ascites, and gastrointestinal or pancreatic bleeding.**
GENERAL PATIENT OUTCOMES:	**Adequate circulating volume as evidenced by BP and pulse within patient normals, skin warm/dry with palpable peripheral pulses, urine output greater than 20 to 30 ml per hour.**

INTERVENTIONS	RATIONALE
Independent	
Monitor blood pressure (BP). Measure central venous pressure (CVP), PAP/PCWP, if available.	Fluid shifts into third space, bleeding, and release of vasodilators (kinins) may result in severe hypotension. Reduced cardiac output/poor organ perfusion secondary to a hypotensive episode can precipitate widespread systemic complications.
Calculate 24-hour fluid balance. Measure/estimate all fluid losses, including vomiting/gastric aspirate, diarrhea.	Useful in evaluating fluid replacement/electrolyte needs.
Note decrease in urine output (less than 400 ml in 24 hours).	Oliguria may occur, signaling renal impairment/acute tubular necrosis (ATN), related to increase in renal vascular resistance, reduction or alteration in renal blood flow.
Weigh as indicated. Correlate with calculated fluid balance.	Provides an additional perameter for evaluating fluid status. Weight loss may suggest hypovolemia related to increased metabolic rate. However, edema/fluid retention and ascites may be reflected by increased weight.
Note signs of poor skin turgor, dry skin/mucous membranes, thirst.	Further physiologic indicators of dehydration.
Observe/record peripheral and dependent edema. Measure abdominal girth if ascites present.	Edema/fluid shifts occur as a result of increased vascular permeability, sodium retention, and decreased colloid osmotic pressure in the intravascular compartment. Note: Fluid loss (sequestration) of greater than 6 liters in 48 hours is considered a poor prognostic sign.

INTERVENTIONS	RATIONALE
Independent	
Investigate changes in sensorium (e.g., confusion, slowed response).	Changes may be related in hypovolemia, hypoxia, electrolyte imbalance, or impending delerium tremens (in the patient with acute pancreatitis secondary to excessive alcohol intake). Severe pancreatic disease may cause toxic psychosis.
Monitor cardiac rate/rhythm. Document changes in electrocardiogram (ECG), such as tall peaked T-waves/depressed ST segment, prolonged PR interval/widening QRS complex and dysrhythmias.	Cardiac changes/dysrythmias may reflect hypovolemia or electrolyte imbalance, commonly hypokalemia/hypocalcemia. Hyperkalemia may occur related to tissue necrosis, acidosis, and renal insufficiency and may precipitate lethal dysrhythmias if uncorrected.
Observe/report signs of calcium deficit; for example, tetany, twitching, positive Chvostek's or Trousseau's sign.	Symptoms of calcium imbalance. Calcium binds with free fats in the intestine and is lost by excretion in the stool.
Assess amount/color/character of gastric drainage.	Fluid loss by gastric secretions may be more than 2 liters per day, potentiating hypovolemia/electrolyte imbalance.
Collaborative	
Administer fluid replacement as indicated (e.g., saline solutions, albumin, blood/blood products, dextran).	The choice of replacement solution may be less important than rapidity and adequacy of volume restoration. Saline solutions and albumin may be used to promote mobilization of fluid back into vascular space. Low molecular weight dextran (dextran 40) is sometimes used to reduce the risk of renal dysfunction and pulmonary edema associated with pancreatitis.
Insert/maintain urinary catheter.	Provides more accurate measurement of output, reflecting hydration/renal perfusion.
Monitor laboratory results; for example, hemoglobin (Hgb), hematocrit (Hct), serum protein/albumin, electrolytes.	Identifies deficits, therapy needs, and progression of disease process as outlined in Patient Assessment Data Base, Diagnostic Studies, page 181.
Replace electrolytes (e.g., sodium/potassium, chloride/calcium), as indicated.	Decreased intake and excessive losses greatly affect electrolyte/acid base balance which is necessary to maintain optimal cellular/organ function.
Monitor renal function studies: blood urea nitrogen (BUN), creatinine, urine osmolarity, and urine sodium and potassium.	Acute tubular necrosis may develop owing to prolonged hypovolemia/shock, damaged capillary endothelium (by circulating humoral agents; for example, bradykinin and seratonin), or glomerular damage (necrosis from enzyme activity). (Refer to Care Plan: Acute Renal Failure, page 207.)
Prepare for/assist with peritoneal lavage/hemoperitoneal dialysis.	Removes toxic chemicals/pancreatic enzymes and allows for more rapid correction of metabolic abnormalities in severe unresponsive cases of acute pancreatitis. May be indicated when ATN is not responsive to usual therapies; for example, correction of fluid volume/hypotension, acidosis, and hyperkalemia. Note: High risk of sepsis must be weighed against possible advantages of peritoneal lavage.

NURSING DIAGNOSIS:	**Comfort, alteration in, pain [acute].**
SUPPORTING DATA/CONTRIBUTING FACTORS:	**Obstruction of the pancreatic/biliary ducts, contamination of peritoneal surfaces by pancreatic exudate ("chemical burn"), autodigestion of the pancreas, and extension of inflammation to the retroperitoneal nerve plexis results in pain of varying severity. Other factors such as nausea/vomiting and distention can contribute to the patient's discomfort.**
GENERAL PATIENT OUTCOMES:	**Verbalizes reduction of pain and demonstrates relaxed facial expression/body posture.**

INTERVENTIONS	RATIONALE
Independent	
Assess verbal complaints of pain. Ask patient to be specific about location and intensity of pain. Note factors that aggravate/relieve pain.	Pain is often diffuse, severe, and unrelenting. Localized pain may indicate development of pseudocysts/abcesses.
Maintain bedrest. Provide quiet, restful environment.	Decreases metabolic rate and gastrointestinal stimulation/secretions, thereby reducing pancreatic activity.
Promote position of comfort (e.g., on one side with knees flexed).	May allow some measure of comfort/pain relief by reducing abdominal pressure/tension.
Use other comfort measures; for example, back rubs/massage, Therapeutic Touch, relaxation techniques.	Assists relaxation and enables patient to focus on something other than pain.
Withhold food/fluid, as indicated, and keep environment free of food odors.	Food/fluid intake or sensory stimulation can activate pancreatic enzymes, increasing pain.
Administer analgesics in a timely manner (smaller, more frequent doses).	Severe/prolonged pain can aggravate shock and is more difficult to relieve, requiring larger doses of medication which can mask underlying problems/complications, and which may contribute to respiratory depression.
Collaborative	
Administer medications as indicated:	
Narcotic analgesics; for example, meperidine (Demerol),	Meperidine is effective in relieving pain and may be preferred over morphine, which can display side effect of biliary-pancreatic duct spasm. Note: Patients who have recurrent pancreatitis episodes may be difficult to manage because they may be addicted to the narcotics given for pain relief.

INTERVENTIONS	RATIONALE
Collaborative	
Sedatives; for example, diazepam (Valium); antispasmodics; for example, atropine,	Potentiates action of narcotic to promote rest and to reduce muscular/ductal spasm, thereby reducing metabolic needs/enzyme secretions.
Antacids; for example, Mylanta,	Neutralizes gastric acid to reduce production of pancreatic enzymes and to reduce incidence of gastric ulcers and upper gastrointestinal (GI) bleed.
Cimetidine (Tagamet)/ranitidine, (Zantac).	Decreasing secretion of hydrochloric acid (HCl) reduces stimulation of the pancreas and associated pain.
Maintain gastric suction.	Prevents accumulation of gastric secretions, which can stimulate pancreatic enzyme activity.

NURSING DIAGNOSIS: **Nutrition, alteration in, less than body requirements.**

SUPPORTING DATA/CONTRIBUTING FACTORS: **Nutrients are lost because of vomiting, decreased oral intake associated with anorexia, and prescribed dietary restrictions. Loss of digestive enzymes and insulin (related to pancreatic outflow obstruction or necrosis/autodigestion) directly affects the digestion and utilization of nutrients. Increased metabolic needs associated with the inflammatory process occurs at a time when the patient is unable to ingest/utilize nutrients.**

GENERAL PATIENT OUTCOMES: **Adequate nutrition is re-established/maintained, evidenced by positive nitrogen balance and weight within patient's normal limits.**

INTERVENTIONS	RATIONALE
Independent	
Assess presence/character of bowel sounds.	Gastric distention and intestinal atony are frequently present resulting in reduced/absent bowel sounds. Return of bowel sounds/relief of symptoms signals readiness for discontinuence of nasogastric suctioning, usually within following 24 to 48 hours.
Assist patient in selecting food/fluids that meet nutritional needs/restrictions when diet resumed.	Previous dietary habits may be unsatisfactory in meeting current needs for tissue regeneration/healing. Use of gastric stimulants (e.g., caffeine), gas-producing

INTERVENTIONS	RATIONALE
Independent	
	foods, alcohol, or ingestion of large meals may result in excessive stimulation of the pancreas/recurrence of symptoms.
Observe color/consistency/amount of stools. Note frothy consistency/foul odor.	Steatorrhea (fatty stools) may develop from incomplete digestion of fats.
Note signs of increased thirst/urination, changes in mentation/visual acuity.	May warn of developing hyperglycemia associated with increased release of glucagon (damage to alpha cells) or decreased release of insulin (damge to beta cells).
Test urine for sugar/acetone.	Early detection of inadequate glucose utilization may prevent development of ketoacidosis.
Collaborative	
Maintain nothing-by-mouth (NPO) status and institute nasogastric suctioning in acute phase.	Prevents stimulation/release of pancreatic enzymes (secretin) released when chyme and HCl acid enter the duodenum.
Monitor blood glucose levels.	Hypergylcemia is frequently present but not usually in levels high enough to produce ketoacidosis.
Administer hyperalimentation/lipids, if indicated. (Refer to Care Plan: Nutritional Support, page 367.)	Intravenous (IV) administration of calories, lipids, and amino acids should be instituted before nutrient/ nitrogen depletion becomes advanced.
Resume oral intake with clear liquids and advance diet slowly to provide high-protein/high-carbohydrate, low-fat diet, as indicated.	Oral feedings given too early in the course of illness may exacerbate symptoms. Loss of pancreatic function/reduced insulin production may require initiation of American Diabetes Association (ADA) diet.
Administer medications as indicated:	
Regular insulin;	Corrects persistent hyperglycemia caused by injury to beta cells and increased release of glucocorticoids. Usually short-term therapy unless permanent damage occurs.
Vitamins (e.g., A, D, E, K);	Replacement required as fat metabolism is altered, reducing absorption/storage of fat-soluble vitamins.

NURSING DIAGNOSIS: **Gas Exchange, impaired [potential].**

SUPPORTING DATA/CONTRIBUTING FACTORS: **Pulmonary complications of acute pancreatitis are many and varied owing to effects of toxins released by the inflamed pancreas. One such complication, Adult Respiratory Distress Syndrome (ARDS), is thought to be related to the effect of circulating pancreatic enzymes/free fatty acids on pulmonary surfactant production, which**

	can damage the alveolar-capillary membrane. In addition, hypoventilation (abdominal pain), elevation of diaphragm (ascites), or hyperventilation (anxiety/acidosis) may alter gas diffusion.
GENERAL PATIENT OUTCOMES:	**Normal respiratory function is restored/maintained as evidenced by normal rate/depth of respiration, free of cyanosis/dyspnea. Arterial blood gases are within patient's normal range.**

INTERVENTIONS	RATIONALE
Independent	
Monitor/assess respiratory rate/quality/effort. Auscultate breath sounds, noting presence of adventitious sounds (e.g., crackles, wheezes).	Increased respiratory rate, difficulty breathing, and sounds of congestion may indicate respiratory insufficiency, fluid overload, and/or pleural effusion.
Encourage deep breathing/coughing and position changes frequently.	Enhances ventilation of all lung segments, mobilizes secretions, and reduces pulmonary atelectasis/congestion.
Place in semi/high Fowler's position.	Facilitates lung expansion, improves diaphragmatic excursion.
Investigate complaints of sudden sharp chest pain, development of tachypnea/tachycardia, presence of cyanosis.	Signs/symptoms suggestive of pulmonary embolus.
Collaborative	
Monitor/graph serial arterial blood gases (ABGs).	Arterial hypoxemia may reflect hypoventilation or more serious complications such as respiratory acidosis, pneumonia, emboli, developing ARDS. (Refer to Care Plans: Adult Respiratory Distress Syndrome, page 77, Pulmonary Embolism (Massive), page 95.)
Monitor serial chest x-ray examinations.	May identify developing complications; for example, atelectasis, pulmonary interstitial edema, pleural effusion, and microemboli.
Provide supplemental oxygen as indicated, by prongs/mask or mechanical ventilator. (Refer to Care Plan: Ventilatory Assistance (Mechanical), page 115.)	Improves circulating oxygen to meet tissue/organ needs.
Assist with use of respiratory adjuncts; for example, incentive spirometer.	Promotes maximal inflation of lungs and may prevent atelectasis/other respiratory complications.
Administer albumin and diuretics as indicated.	Pulmonary congestion caused by the inflammatory process, and/or vigorous fluid administration may be alleviated by use of plasma expander and diuretics to correct fluid imbalances.

INTERVENTIONS	RATIONALE
Collaborative	
Assist with thoracentesis/paracentesis.	May be beneficial when pleural effusions or ascites compromises respiratory status.

NURSING DIAGNOSIS: **Injury, potential for, multiple complications.**

SUPPORTING DATA/CONTRIBUTING FACTORS: **Complications fall into two groups: those occurring immediately or within the first 72 hours, which involve organ systems that are affected either by the release of pancreatic enzymes or by associated hypotension and metabolic abnormalities (for example, circulatory collapse/cardiovascular complications) and later complications relating to intrapancreatic events (e.g., development of a pseudocyst, abscess, or peritonitis).**

GENERAL PATIENT OUTCOMES: **Complications are prevented/minimized.**

INTERVENTIONS	RATIONALE
Independent	
Monitor cardiac rate/rhythm continuously. Auscultate heart sounds and note presence of gallops or rubs.	Cardiovascular complications are common and include myocardial infarction, pericarditis, and pericardial effusion with/without tamponade. S_3 gallop in conjunction with jugular vein distention and crackles suggests right heart failure/pulmonary edema.
Note increased abdominal pain, rigidity/rebound tenderness, diminished/absent bowel sounds.	Suggestive of peritonitis. (Refer to Care Plan: Peritonitis, page 191.)
Monitor for presence of abscess; for example, increased abdominal pain/tenderness, recurrent fever (greater than 101 degrees), leukocytosis (white blood count greater than 10,000), hypotension, tachycardia, and chills.	Abscesses should be suspected whenever a patient is deteriorating steadily despite all supportive measures. Abscesses can occur 2 or more weeks after the onset of pancreatitis, and mortality can exceed 50 percent.
Assess for development of pancreatic pseudocysts (e.g., patient unable to tolerate feeding, persistent fever, renewed amylase elevation, worsening abdominal pain, or symptoms of bowel obstruction).	Pseudocysts are a collection of pancreatic tissues, fluid, and debris which build gradually over several weeks and ultimately encapsulate. If small, they may be treated with diet therapy (low fat and no alcohol), but larger ones may require surgical interventions.
Inspect skin for petechiae, hematomas, and unusual wound or venipuncture bleeding. Note hematuria,	Disseminated intravascular coagulation (DIC) may be initiated by release of active pancreatic proteases into

INTERVENTIONS	RATIONALE
Independent	
mucous membrane bleeding, and bloody gastric contents. (Refer to Care Plan: Disseminated Intravascular Coagulation, page 319.)	the circulation. The most frequently affected organs are the kidneys, skin, and lungs.
Collaborative	
Monitor serial 12-lead electrocardiograms (ECGs), as indicated.	Cardiac complications are treated according to type and severity. In presence of shock the myocardium may be severely compromised. Cardiac output is decreased and blood pressure remains low despite adequate replacement fluids. Pericardial tap may be required if severe pericardial effusion develops.
Monitor clotting studies: prothrombin time (PT)/partial thromboplastin time (PTT), platelet count, fibrinogen degradation products, and so forth.	Mild forms of DIC detectable only by serial laboratory studies may account for the early hypoxia and renal function impairment of acute pancreatitis.
Administer heparin.	Prevents the activation of factor X, inhibiting platelet aggregation. Usually reserved for those patients whose organ failure is due to thrombosis.
Prepare for surgical intervention as necessary.	Abscesses may be surgically drained with resection of necrotic tissue. Pseudocysts persisting for more than 5 weeks should be drained because the risk and incidence of infection/rupture rise rapidly after that time.

NURSING DIAGNOSIS:	**Infection, potential for [sepsis].**
SUPPORTING DATA/CONTRIBUTING FACTORS:	**Sepsis is a primary cause of death in more than 20 percent of cases of acute pancreatitis owing to multiorgan involvement and nutritional deficiencies which compromise the patient's immune system.**
GENERAL PATIENT OUTCOMES:	**Afebrile, free of signs of infection, blood cultures are negative.**

INTERVENTIONS	RATIONALE
Independent	
Observe for signs and symptoms of infection (e.g., fever) and respiratory distress in conjunction with jaundice.	Cholestatic jaundice and decreased pulmonary function may be the first signs of sepsis involving gram-negative organisms.
Use strict aseptic technique when changing surgical dressings or working with invasive lines, indwelling catheter, or tubes/drains. Change IV/hyperalimentation tubing per protocol. Change soiled dressings	Limits sources of infection which can lead to sepsis in severely compromised patient.

INTERVENTIONS	RATIONALE
Independent	
promptly. Provide urinary catheter care on a routine basis.	
Collaborative	
Obtain culture specimens (e.g., blood, wound, urine, sputum, or pancreatic aspirate).	Identifies presence of infection and causative organism.
Administer antibiotic therapy as indicated.	Cephalosporins plus aminoglycosides (gentamicin/tobramycin) are generally recommended for sepsis. Therapy will be based on the sensitivities of the specific organisms cultured.

Peritonitis

Peritonitis is an inflammation of the membranous lining of the abdominal cavity and viscera. Primary peritonitis results from a blood-borne or lymph-borne organism and most commonly occurs in patients with chronic debilitating diseases who experience compromised immunity. Secondary peritonitis occurs as a result of contamination from adjoining structures such as a ruptured organ, a defect in the visceral wall, or inflammatory processes of the abdominal/pelvic organs. In the acute phase the likelihood of sepsis is high, and prognosis for recovery is guarded.

PATIENT ASSESSMENT DATA BASE

HISTORY

Primary: History of cirrhosis with ascites, chronic liver disease, kidney disease (e.g., uremia, nephrotic syndrome in children).

Secondary: History of surgery of stomach, intestines, or biliary tract (postoperative peritonitis); perforation of any part of gastrointestinal tract; for example, peptic ulcer, ruptured appendix/gallbladder, ulcerative colitis; trauma: gunshot/stab wound, motor vehicle accident; acute/recurrent/chronic inflammatory processes: for example, pancreatitis, appendicitis, salpingitis/pelvic inflammatory disease.

Subjective

Complains of persistent, severe abdominal pain, which may be sharp/localized (parietal peritonitis), diffuse throughout abdomen (visceral peritonitis), or referred to either shoulder (diaphragmatic/phrenic nerve stimulation). Pain is intensified by movement and breathing.

May complain of nausea, vomiting, inability to pass stool or flatus, thirst, loss of appetite, and weakness.

PHYSICAL EXAMINATION

Inspection

Abdomen: distention may be noted; hiccups may be present if diaphragmatic peritoneum is irritated. Drainage may be noted from abdominal wounds or surgically placed drains.

Respirations: usually shallow and rapid.

Skin: jaundice, pallor, and diaphoresis may be present. Cyanosis may be noted if shock state exists.

Fever: elevation of body temperature to 103 degrees F (39.5 degrees C) or above is not uncommon.

Auscultation

Vital signs: tachycardia and hypotension may be noted owing to increased epinephrine and norepinephrine as a secondary effect of peritoneal injury.

Bowel sounds: usually absent or hypoactive (ileus). Frequent/loud/rushing sounds may be noted if intestinal obstruction occurs.

Palpation

Abdomen: muscle rigidity, guarding, and rebound tenderness may be present.

Percussion

Abdomen: hyperresonance/tympany may be noted, especially if paralytic ileus present. Loss of dullness over liver may indicate free air in abdomen.

DIAGNOSTIC STUDIES

CBC: WBCs elevated, sometimes greater than 20,000. Red blood cell count may be increased, indicating hemoconcentration.

Serum protein/albumin: may be decreased owing to fluid shifts.

Serum amylase: usually elevated.

ABGs: respiratory alkalosis and metabolic acidosis may be noted.

Cultures: causative organism may be identified from blood, exudate/secretions, or ascitic fluid.

Abdominal x-ray examination: may reveal gas distention of bowel/ileus. If a perforated viscera is the etiology, free air will be found in the abdomen.

Paracentesis: peritoneal fluid samples may contain blood, pus/exudate, amylase, bile, and creatinine.

NURSING PRIORITIES

1. Control infection.
2. Restore/maintain circulating volume.
3. Promote comfort.
4. Maintain nutrition.

NURSING DIAGNOSIS:	**Infection, potential for [septicemia].**
SUPPORTING DATA/CONTRIBUTING FACTORS:	**Infecting organisms which enter the peritoneal cavity increase capillary permeability and absorption of bacteria/toxins into the bloodstream, which can lead to septicemia.**
GENERAL PATIENT OUTCOMES:	**Blood cultures are negative. Patient is afebrile.**

INTERVENTIONS	RATIONALE
Independent	
Assess vital signs frequently. Measure hemodynamic parameters; for example, central venous pressure (CVP), pulmonary artery pressure (PAP), cardiac output (CO), if available.	Unresolved or progressing hypotension, decreased pulse pressure, tachycardia, fever, and tachypnea are signs of impending septic shock. Cardiac output may be somewhat elevated initially, owing to an increased systemic vascular resistance (SVR). Eventually circulating endotoxins produce vasodilatation and a low cardiac output state. (Refer to Care Plan: Sepsis/Septicemia/Septic Shock, page 329.)
Note changes in mental status (e.g., confusion, stupor).	Hypoxemia, reduced cerebral blood flow associated with hypotension, and acidosis result in deteriorating mental status.
Note skin color/temperature/moisture.	Warm, flushed, dry skin is an early sign of septicemia. Later manifestations include cool, clammy, pale skin

INTERVENTIONS	RATIONALE
Independent	
	and cyanosis as shock becomes refractory.
Monitor urine output.	Oliguria develops as a result of hypotension, decreased renal perfusion, and circulating toxins as septic shock ensues.
Maintain strict aseptic techniques in care of abdominal drains/open wounds and invasive sites. Change dressings as indicated.	Limits cross contamination/spread of infecting organisms. After surgical intervention, some patients may have open wounds and/or multiple drains.
Collaborative	
Obtain specimens/monitor results of serial blood, urine, wound cultures.	Identifies causative microorganisms and assesses effectiveness of antibiotic regimen.
Administer antibiotics; for example, gentamicin (Garamycin), amikacin (Amikin), clindamycin (Cleocin) via intravenous/peritoneal infusion as indicated.	Antibiotic therapy is directed at anaerobic bacteria and aerobic gram-negative bacilli. Route of administration may be intravenous and/or via peritoneal catheters.
Assist with peritoneal aspiration, if indicated.	May occasionally be done to determine infecting organism so that appropriate antibiotics may be ordered.
Prepare for surgical interventions after patient status stabilized.	May be performed to plicate ulcer, to resect bowel, to remove ruptured appendix/gallbladder, to drain localized abscess, or to remove peritoneal exudates.

NURSING DIAGNOSIS: **Fluid Volume Deficit, actual (2).**

SUPPORTING DATA/CONTRIBUTING FACTORS: **The peritoneum is a semipermeable membrane with a bidirectional flow of fluids and electrolytes. When inflammation occurs, the normally transparent membrane becomes opaque and vascular dilatation causes congestion, edema, and fluid shifts from the extracellular, intravascular, and interstitial compartments into the peritoneal space. The extent of fluid shift depends on the amount of peritoneum involved and may reach 4 to 6 liters in 24 hours. Fluid loss is increased by vomiting which occurs in response to bacterial toxins and fluid/gas accumulation within the intestine. Resulting loss of circulating volume produces hypotension, reduced venous return/cardiac output, and decreased tissue perfusion.**

GENERAL PATIENT OUTCOMES:	**Fluid volume is restored/maintained as evidenced by hemodynamic parameters, urine output, and weight within patient's normal limits.**

INTERVENTIONS	RATIONALE
Independent	
Monitor vital signs/hemodynamic pressure (e.g., blood pressure, pulse, CVP/PCWP).	Assesses needs/effectiveness of fluid replacement therapy and response to medications.
Maintain accurate intake/output and correlate with daily weights. Include measured/estimated gastric and drainage losses.	Reflects overall hydration status. Urine output may be diminished owing to hypovolemia and decreased renal perfusion, but weight may still increase, reflecting edema/ascites accumulation.
Measure urine specific gravity.	Reflects hydration status and changes in renal function which may warn of developing failure. Note: Many antibiotics have nephrotoxic effects which may further compromsie fluid volume status. (Refer to Care Plan: Acute Renal Failure, page 207.)
Observe skin/mucous membrane dryness. Note peripheral/sacral edema.	Hypovolemia and fluid shifts contribute to poor skin turgor, taut edematous tissues.
Provide frequent oral care.	Nothing-by-mouth (NPO) status, hypovolemia, and vomiting contribute to breakdown of oral mucous membrane and discomfort.
Eliminate noxious sights/smells from the environment.	Reduces stimulation of vomiting center.
Collaborative	
Monitor serum electrolytes, albumin, blood urea nitrogen (BUN), creatinine.	Varied fluctuations in potassium, sodium, and protein are possible consequences of fluid shifts and hypovolemia. Work of kidneys is increased by circulating toxins, pigments, and necrotic tissue products. Decreased cardiac output and renal perfusion affect kidney's ability to excrete toxins.
Administer plasma, fluids, electrolytes, diuretics as indicated.	Replenishes/maintains circulating volume and electrolyte balance. Colloids help move water back into the intravascular compartment by increasing osmotic gradient. Diuretics may be used to assist in excretion of toxins, thereby enhancing renal function.

NURSING DIAGNOSIS:	**Comfort, alteration in, pain [acute].**
SUPPORTING DATA/CONTRIBUTING FACTORS:	**Stimulation of the parietal peritoneum (containing somatic nerves) lining the abdominal and pelvic cavities produces pain which is intensified by respirations, body movement, and abdominal distention.**

GENERAL PATIENT OUTCOMES:	Patient verbalizes diminished pain; exhibits fewer pain indicators (e.g., relaxed facial expression).

INTERVENTIONS	RATIONALE
Independent	
Assess pain complaints frequently/before administration of analgesics.	Changes in location/intensity are not uncommon but may reflect developing complications. Pain tends to become constant, more intense, and diffuse over the entire abdomen as inflammatory process accelerates, or pain may localize if an abscess develops.
Maintain semi-Fowler's position, as indicated.	Facilitates fluid/wound drainage by gravity, reducing diaphragmatic irritation/abdominal tension and thereby reducing pain.
Move patient slowly and delibately, splinting painful area.	Reduces muscle tension/guarding, which may help minimize pain of movement.
Provide alternate comfort measures; for example, massage, back rubs, breathing/relaxation exercises.	Promotes relaxation and may enhance patient's general coping abilities by changing focus of attention.
Provide frequent oral care, elimination of noxious environmental stimuli.	Reduces nausea/vomiting, which can increase intra-abdominal pressure/pain.
Collaborative	
Administer medications as indicated:	
Analgesics/narcotics,	Reduces metabolic rate and intestinal irritation associated with circulating/local toxins, which aids in pain relief and promotes healing. Note: Pain is usually severe and may require narcotic for pain control.
Antiemetics; for example, hydroxyzine (Vistaril), promethazine (Phenergan).	Prevents vomiting, which can increase abdominal pain.

NURSING DIAGNOSIS:	Nutrition, alteration in, less than body requirements.
SUPPORTING DATA/CONTRIBUTING FACTORS:	Nausea/vomiting, intestinal dysfunction, metabolic abnormalities, and use of gastric suction reduce availability and absorption of nutrients and can lead to a rapid progressive catabolism secondary to increased metabolic demands.
GENERAL PATIENT OUTCOMES:	Intake is adequate to meet nutrition needs as evidenced by positive nitrogen balance. Weight loss is minimized/appropriate muscle mass maintained.

INTERVENTIONS	RATIONALE
Independent	
Assess bowel sounds, noting absent/hyperactive sounds.	Although bowel sounds are frequently absent, inflammation/irritation of the intestine may be accompanied by intestinal hyperactivity, diminished water absorption, and diarrhea.
Promote bowel rest (e.g., food/oral fluid restriction, bedrest).	Reduces hyperactivity of bowel.
Eliminate noxious sights/smells from environment.	Peritoneal irritation stimulates the vagal afferents that pass directly to the vomiting centers. Elimination of noxious environmental stimuli may further reduce stimulation of the bilateral vomiting centers in dorsal portions of the lateral reticular formation of the medulla.
Measure abdominal girth.	Provides quantitative indication of increases/decreases in gastric/intestinal distention, and/or ascites.
Assess abdomen frequently for return to softness, reappearance of normal bowel sounds, and passage of flatus.	Indicates return of normal bowel function and ability to resume oral intake.
Administer Total Parenteral Nutrition (TPN) as prescribed. (Refer to Care Plan: Nutritional Support, page 367.)	Promotes nutrient utilization and positive nitrogen balance in patients unable to assimilate nutrients in a normal fashion.
Monitor BUN, protein, albumin, glucose as indicated.	Reflects nutritional status/needs.

Upper Gastrointestinal/Esophageal Bleeding

Bleeding duodenal ulcer is the most frequent cause of massive upper gastrointestinal (GI) hemorrhage, but bleeding also may occur owing to gastric ulcers, gastritis, and esophageal varices. Rupture of esophageal varices can occur from portal hypertension reflected backward through the lesser splanchnic venous system, resulting in spontaneous hemorrhage. Severe vomiting can precipitate gastric bleeding owing to tear of the mucosa at the gastroesophageal junction (Mallory-Weiss syndrome). Stress ulcer can result from severe burns, major trauma/surgery, or severe systemic disease and may cause sudden, massive GI bleeding. Esophagitis, esophageal/gastric carcinoma, hiatal hernia, hemophilia, leukemia, and disseminated intravascular coagulation (DIC) are less common causes of upper GI bleeding.

PATIENT ASSESSMENT DATA BASE

HISTORY

History of previous ulcer or GI bleeding/melena.

History of chronic, recent, and/or excessive alcohol use; heavy tobacco use.

Recent physiologic stress such as burns, trauma, surgery, major medical illness.

Recent psychologic stress, such as change in marital relationship/status, job-related or financial stress.

Use of over the counter (OTC) drugs containing aspirin or prescription drugs such as corticosteroids/anticoagulants, which can affect the gastric mucosal barrier.

Recent travel out of country, with ensuing onset of flulike symptoms (e.g., forceful vomiting/diarrhea).

Subjective

May complain of stomach/epigastric pain or burning sensation (usually accompanies duodenal and gastric ulcers); vomiting of blood, changes in bowel pattern, weakness, lightheadedness and/or confusion.

PHYSICAL EXAMINATION

Inspection

Hematemesis: vomitus may be bright red or coffeeground in appearance.

Melena/hematochezia: stools are usually black/tarry but may be dark red, bright red, or "currant jelly" in appearance owing to massive bleeding from esophagus, stomach, or small intestine.

Mentation: restlessness, disorientation, anxiety may be noted.

Respirations: tachypnea/hyperventilation may be present.

Skin: pallor may be noted, with or without diaphoresis. If bleeding is due to gastric or esophageal varices/portal hypertension, the following manifestations indicative of liver disease may also be present: gynecomastia, jaundice, spider angiomas. Bruising or petechiae might indicate a coagulation disorder.

Urine output: less than 20 ml/hour may reflect hypovolemia and decreased renal perfusion.

Auscultation

Cardiac: tachycardia may be noted, compensating for hypovolemia/reduced cardiac output; dysrhythmias may occur secondary to electrolyte imbalance and hypoxemia.

Bowel sounds: may be hyperactive, reflecting increased motility owing to the presence of blood in the intestines.

Blood pressure: hypotension may be present.

Palpation

Pulse may be weak, thready.

Other

Temperature may be elevated (38.4° to 39° C; 101° to 102°F).

DIAGNOSTIC STUDIES

Endoscopy: esophagogastroduodenoscopy is the key diagnostic test for upper GI bleeding; it visualizes site of bleeding and degree of tissue injury.

Angiography: GI vasculature may be reviewed if endoscopy is inconclusive or impractical.

Barium swallow with x-ray examination may be done for differential diagnosis following endoscopy or angiography.

Hgb/Hct: decreased levels occur within 6 to 24 hours after bleed.

WBC may be elevated, reflecting body's response to injury.

BUN elevates within 24 to 48 hours as blood proteins are broken down in the gastrointestinal tract, and/or kidney perfusion is decreased.

Creatinine levels usually are not elevated if renal perfusion is maintained.

Ammonia may be elevated if severe liver dysfunction disrupts the metabolism and proper excretion of urea. Massive whole blood transfusions also increase ammonia level.

Coagulation profile: increased platelets and decreased clotting times may be noted, reflecting body's attempt to restore hemostasis. Severe abnormalities may reveal coagulopathy (e.g., DIC as cause of bleed).

ABGs may reveal initial respiratory alkalosis compensating for diminished blood flow through lungs. Later, metabolic acidosis develops in response to sluggish liver flow/accumulation of metabolic waste products.

Sodium may be elevated as a hormonal compensation for lost fluid.

Potassium initially may be depleted owing to massive gastric emptying or bloody diarrhea. Elevated potassium levels may occur after massive transfusions of stored blood, or with acute renal impairment.

NURSING PRIORITIES

1. Control hemorrhage.
2. Achieve/maintain hemodynamic stability.
3. Assist patient/family to develop awareness of measures to prevent recurrence.

NURSING DIAGNOSIS:	**Fluid Volume Deficit, actual (2).**
SUPPORTING DATA/CONTRIBUTING FACTORS:	**Upper GI bleeding depletes circulating blood volume, disturbs fluid/electrolyte balance, and places the patient at risk for hypovolemic/hemorrhagic shock and death.**
GENERAL PATIENT OUTCOMES:	**Vital signs are within patient's normal limits. Urine output is greater than 20 to 30 ml per hour. Gastric lavage re-**

	turns clear or only pink tinged and free of clots.

INTERVENTIONS	RATIONALE
Independent	
Monitor vital signs, compare with patient's normal/previous readings when lying/sitting.	Changes in blood pressure (BP) and pulse may be used for rough estimate of blood loss, that is, BP lower than 90 mmHg and pulse less than 110 reflects a 25 percent decrease in volume—approximately 1000 ml. BP 70 to 90 mmHg and pulse 110 to 130 suggests a blood loss of 25 to 40 percent. BP lower than 70 with pulse greater than 130 indicates severe shock state. Note: Postural hypotension (drop of systolic blood pressure when raised from recumbent position) of greater than 10 mmHg and/or pulse increase greater than 20 per minute reflects a 20 to 25 percent decrease in circulating volume.
Note patient's individual physiologic response to bleed: for example, changes in mentation, weakness, restlessness, anxiety; pallor, diaphoresis; tachypnea; temperature elevation.	Symptomatology may be useful in gauging severity/length of bleeding episode. Worsening of symptoms may reflect continued bleeding or inadequate fluid replacement.
Measure hemodynamic parameters; for example, central venous pressure (CVP), PAP/PCWP, cardiac output (CO):	Reflects circulating volume/cardiac response to bleeding and fluid replacement; for example, CVP values between 5 and 10 cm H_2O usually reflect adequate volume. A pulmonary artery catheter may be inserted to measure cardiac output and to provide a reflection of ventricular response in the critically ill bleeder.
Investigate complaints of chest pain with or without electrocardiogram (ECG) changes.	May reflect cardiac ischemia related to decreased perfusion or side effect of vasopressin therapy. Note: Impaired oxygenation status resulting from blood loss can bring on myocardial infarction (MI) in patient with cardiac disease.
Measure intake and output, correlate weight changes. Include fluid losses via emesis, gastric suction/lavage, and stools.	Provides guidelines for fluid replacement. Note: Urinary output may not increase as anticipated in spite of adequate fluid replacement when vasopressin is used, owing to its potential side effect of sodium/water retention.
Keep accurate record of subtotals of solutions/blood during replacement therapy.	Potential exists for overtransfusion of fluids, especially when volume expanders are given before blood transfusions.
Maintain bedrest, avoid exertion (e.g., vomiting/straining at stool).	Activity/vomiting increases intra-abdominal pressure, predisposing to further bleeding.
Observe for secondary bleeding; for example, nose/gums, oozing from puncture sites, appearance of ecchymotic areas following minimal trauma.	Loss of/inadequate replacement of clotting factors may precipitate development of DIC. (Refer to Care Plan: Disseminated Intravascular Coagulation, page 319.)

INTERVENTIONS	RATIONALE
Collaborative	
Administer fluids/blood via large-bore intravenous (IV)/central lines.	Allows for rapid infusion of replacement fluids/blood to combat shock. Volume expanders may be infused until type and crossmatch can be completed and transfusions begun. Approximately 80 to 90 percent of gastric bleeding is controlled by fluid resuscitation and medical management.
Insert/maintain large-bore nasogastric tube.	Removes irritating gastric secretions, blood, and clots to reduce nausea/vomiting and to facilitate diagnostic endoscopy. Note: Blood remaining in the stomach/intestines will be broken down into ammonia, which can produce a toxic central nervous system (CNS) effect (e.g., encephalopathy).
Perform gastric lavage with cold or room temperature saline until aspirate is light pink or clear, and free of clots.	Removes clots and may reduce bleeding by local vasoconstriction. Facilitates visualization by endoscopy to locate bleeding source. Occasionally medication (Levophed) may be added to lavage solution to achieve better local vasoconstriction. Indications for Levophed use must be balanced against possible effect of mucosal ischemia. Note: Some research suggests that iced saline may not be any more effective than room temperature solution in controlling bleed and may actually damage gastric mucosa.
Assist with insertion/maintain esophageal/gastric balloon tamponade in presence of esophageal bleeding.	For those with esophogeal varices, a double or triple lumen tube with esophageal and gastric balloons may be inserted to exert pressure on varices. This treatment is successful in reducing hemorrhage in 50 to 75 percent of patients with variceal bleed.
Administer fresh whole blood/packed red cells,	Fresh whole blood is indicated for acute bleed with shock, because stored blood may be deficient in clotting factors. Packed cells may be adequate for stable patients with subacute/chronic bleed and is required for patients with CHF, to prevent fluid overload.
Fresh frozen plasma (FFP) and/or platelets.	Clotting factors/components are depleted by two mechanisms: hemorrhagic loss and the clotting process at the site of the bleed. Fresh frozen plasma is an excellent source of clotting factors. Platelet replacement may potentiate formation of platelet plug and clotting at injury sites.
Administer medications, as indicated:	
Cimetidine (Tagamet), ranitidine (Zantac);	Histamine H_2 blockers reduce gastric acid production to aid in increasing gastric pH and to reduce irritation of gastric mucosa.
Amphojel, Maalox, Mylanta, Riopan;	Antacids administered orally by gavage work with cimetidine to maintain gastric pH level at 4.5 or higher to reduce risk of rebleed. Note: Head of bed should be raised during antacid gavage to prevent gastric reflux, because aspiration of antacids can cause serious pulmonary complications.

INTERVENTIONS	RATIONALE
Collaborative	
Vasopressin, intra-arterial/IV;	Produces vasoconstriction of preportal splanchnic arterioles which decreases blood flow to abdominal organs, thereby reducing portal blood flow/pressure and hemorrhage. Selective arterial infusion may be indicated for the bleeding patient with advanced liver disease who is considered a poor surgical risk. Note: Cardiac output and diuresis may be reduced by this drug. In addition, generalized increase of systemic vascular resistance (SVR)/afterload may precipitate angina/MI.
Sodium nitroprusside, (Nipride)/nitroglycerin.	May be effective in improving cardiac output/hepatic blood flow to offset vasoconstrictive side effects of vasopressin therapy.
Monitor hemoglobin (Hgb)/hematocrit (Hct) levels.	Aids in establishing blood replacement needs and monitoring effectiveness of therapy; for example, 1 unit of whole blood should raise Hct 2 to 3 percent.
Note blood urea nitrogen (BUN) creatinine levels.	Blood urea nitrogen greater than 40, with normal creatinine level indicates a major bleed. Blood urea nitrogen should return to patient's normal level approximately 12 hours after bleed has ceased.
Assist with/prepare for:	
Endoscopy, angiography;	Endoscopy may be done to locate source of upper GI bleeding; angiography may be needed if source of bleeding can not be identified.
Sclerotherapy;	Injection of an irritating (sclerosing) agent into esophogeal varices to create thrombosis may be useful to prevent recurrence after initial bleed is controlled.
Electrocoagulation or photocoagulation (laser) therapy;	Provides direct coagulation of bleeding sites.
Surgical intervention.	Total/partial gastrectomy, pyloroplasty, and/or vagotomy may be required to control/prevent future gastric bleed. Shunt procedures may be done to divert blood flow and to reduce pressure within esophogeal vessels when other measures fail.

NURSING DIAGNOSIS:	**Tissue Perfusion, alteration in.**
SUPPORTING DATA/CONTRIBUTING FACTORS:	**Gastrointestinal bleeding results in a reduction of oxygen-carrying hemoglobin, and increased oxygen extraction. Sluggish blood flow to viscera and kidneys contributes to lactic and metabolic acidosis, which further diminishes tissue perfusion.**

GENERAL PATIENT OUTCOMES:	**Tissue perfusion is maintained/improved as evidenced by stabilized vital signs, warm skin, palpable peripheral pulses, and arterial blood gases (ABGs) within patient norms, urine output greater than 20 to 30 ml per hour.**

INTERVENTIONS	RATIONALE
Independent	
Maintain bedrest during active bleeding. Schedule activities/provide undisturbed rest periods.	Aids in cessation of bleeding, because it decreases hypertension, reduces oxygen demands, and decreases gastrointestinal activity.
Note complaints of abdominal pain, especially sudden, severe pain or pain radiating to shoulder.	Pain caused by gastric ulcer is often relieved after acute bleed, owing to buffering effects of blood. Continued severe or sudden pain may reflect ischemia caused by vasoconstrictive therapy, bleeding into biliary tract (hematobilia), or may indicate perforation/onset of peritonitis. (Refer to Care Plan: Peritonitis, page 191.)
Investigate changes in level of consciousness, complaints of dizziness/headache.	Changes may reflect inadequate cerebral perfusion as a result of reduced arterial blood pressure. Note: Changes in sensorium may also reflect elevated ammonia levels/hepatic encephalopathy in patient with liver disease. (Refer to Care Plan: Cirrhosis, page 169.)
Monitor ECG, cardiac rate/rhythm.	Dysrhythmias and ischemic changes can occur as a result of hypotension, hypoxia, acidosis, electrolyte imbalance, or cooling near the heart if cold saline lavage is used to control bleeding.
Assess skin for coolness, pallor, diaphoresis, delayed capillary refill; and weak, thready peripheral pulses.	Vasoconstriction is a sympathetic response to lowered circulating volume and/or may occur as side effect of vasopressin administration.
Observe skin blanching, redness; massage with lotion. Change position frequently.	Compromised peripheral circulation increases risk of skin breakdown.
Note urinary output and specific gravity.	Decreased systemic perfusion may cause kidney ischemia/failure manifested by decreased urine output. Acute tubular necrosis (ATN) may develop if hypovolemic state is prolonged. (Refer to Care Plan: Acute Renal Failure, page 207.)
Auscultate bowel sounds.	May be hyperactive indicating presence of blood in intestines.
Collaborative	
Provide supplemental oxygen.	Diminished perfusion increases oxygen extraction by peripheral tissues, increasing risk of hypoxemia and lactic acidosis.

INTERVENTIONS	RATIONALE
Collaborative	
Monitor/graph serial ABGs.	Identify hypoxemia, effectiveness of therapy.
Administer IV fluids as indicated.	Maintains circulating volume and perfusion. Note: Use of Ringer's lactate may be contraindicated in presence of hepatic failure, because metabolism of lactate is impaired and lactic acidosis may develop.

NURSING DIAGNOSIS: **Injury, potential for, suffocation/trauma.**

SUPPORTING DATA/CONTRIBUTING FACTORS: **Single (Linton), double (Sengstaken-Blakemore), or triple (Nachlas-Linton) lumen tubes used to stop bleeding by compression of vessel/varices may cause complications; for example, airway obstruction, aspiration, and/or esophageal necrosis/rupture.**

GENERAL PATIENT OUTCOMES: **Complications are prevented.**

INTERVENTIONS	RATIONALE
Independent	
Elevate head of bed 30 degrees/place bed on 6 to 8-inch blocks during variceal bleed, as indicated.	Reduces portal blood flow, permitting more effective compression of varices, and enhances respiratory function/lung expansion.
Maintain patency of esophageal drainage tube. Aspirate esophagus proximal to balloons as needed.	Patient cannot swallow, and secretions collect in esophagus proximal to balloon, which increases risk of aspiration.
Label all lumens of tube.	Proper identification should prevent inadvertent irrigation of gastric/esophageal balloons, or inflation of stomach with air.
Keep scissors at bedside at all times. Cut tube/remove immediately if signs of respiratory distress/obstruction occur.	Although rare, gastric balloon can rupture or migrate toward laryngopharnyx, thereby obstructing airway and potentiating risk of aspiration.
Assess/report complaints of sudden back/upper abdominal pain with drop in blood pressure, increase in pulse.	May indicate esophageal rupture, requiring immediate medical intervention.
Provide frequent mouth care.	Patient receives nothing by mouth and is unable to swallow, which produces mucositis, halitosis, and discomfort.
Restrain patient as indicated.	Confused/combative patient may disrupt tube function or placement, thereby compromising airway.

INTERVENTIONS	RATIONALE
Collaborative	
Assist with tube placement:	
Obtain portable x-ray film of tube placement PRIOR TO INFLATION of the gastric balloon.	Verification of placement of the gastric balloon in the cardia of the stomach and NOT IN THE ESOPHAGUS is crucial to preventing esophageal rupture during inflation.
Maintain all balloons at specified pressures; release as indicated.	The pressure in esophageal balloon compresses varices to stop bleeding but should be released intermittently to reduce complications of esophageal edema/ulceration. Note: Patient may report substernal pressure when esophageal balloon is inflated.
Insert drainage tube into esophagus above inflated balloon if multilumen tube does not have esophageal drainage port.	Reduces risk of aspiration by draining oral secretions that collect in esophagus and cannot be swallowed.
Apply gentle tension/traction to the tube by inserting sponge under patient's nose, or securing to mouth guard of football helmet, etc.	Maintains position of gastric balloon against the cardioesophogeal junction, reducing risk of balloon migration as well as pressure on the nares.

NURSING DIAGNOSIS:	**Fear/Anxiety.**
SUPPORTING DATA/CONTRIBUTING FACTORS:	**The appearance of frank bleeding or vomiting of blood produces apprehension/anxiety and fear of dying, unless shock state limits awareness of gravity of situation.**
GENERAL PATIENT OUTCOMES:	**Verbalizes appropriate range of feelings and demonstrates lessened fear by relaxed facial expression/body posture.**

INTERVENTIONS	RATIONALE
Independent	
Note behavioral clues; for example, restlessness, irritability, lack of eye contact, combativeness/attack behavior.	Indicators of degree of fear patient is experiencing; for example, patient may feel out of control of the situation or reach a state of panic.
Acknowledge that this is a fearful situation and that others have expressed similar fears. Assist patient in expressing feelings by Active Listening.	When patient is expressing own fear, the validation that these feelings are normal can help patient feel less isolated. Active Listening is a skill in which the underlying feeling message is acknowledged by the nurse. It also communicates empathy and confidence in the individual's ability to deal with the situation.
Stay with patient/make arrangements for family/significant other(s) to be with patient. Use touch and eye contact as appropriate.	Helps reduce fear of going through a frightening experience alone.

INTERVENTIONS	RATIONALE
Independent	
Monitor physiologic responses; for example, tachypnea, palpitations, dizziness, headache, tingling sensations.	May be indicative of the degree of fear patient is experiencing but also may be related to physical condition/shock state.
Provide accurate, concrete information about what is being done (e.g., sensations to expect, usual procedures undertaken).	Involves patient in plan of care and decreases unnecessary anxiety about unknowns.
Help identify/initiate positive coping behaviors used successfully in past.	Successful behaviors can be fostered in dealing with current fear, enhancing patient's sense of self-control and providing reassurance.
Collaborative	
Refer to psychiatric nurse/social services/spiritual advisor.	May need additional assistance during recovery to deal with consequences of emergency situation/adjustments to required/desired changes in lifestyle.

NURSING DIAGNOSIS:	**Knowledge Deficit [Learning Need].**
SUPPORTING DATA/CONTRIBUTING FACTORS:	**Once acute episode of bleeding has been controlled, a change in lifestyle is often mandatory to minimize recurrence. The crisis of this episode can provide an opportunity for the patient to think/make decisions about these changes.**
GENERAL PATIENT OUTCOMES:	**Verbalizes understanding of cause of own bleeding episode (if known) and treatment modalities used. Begins to discuss own role in preventing a recurrence.**

INTERVENTIONS	RATIONALE
Independent	
Determine patient perception of cause of bleeding.	Establishes knowledge base and provides some insight into how the teaching plan needs to be constructed for this individual.
Provide/review information regarding etiology of the bleeding and ways to reduce risk/contributing factors. Encourage questions.	Opportunities are available to provide information which will assist the individual to think about decisions that will need to be made for the future.
Review significance of signs/symptoms such as coffee-ground emesis, tarry stools, abdominal distention, severe epigastric/abdominal pain radiating to shoulder/back.	These symptoms are indicators for immediate medical evaluation/intervention.

INTERVENTIONS	RATIONALE
Independent	
Discuss/review dietary changes/restrictions which may be necessary.	Extremely hot/cold foods, raw fruits/vegetables, and spicy foods increase production of gastric acid, which may result in mucosal irritation. Milk is not a strong acid buffer, and the protein/calcium content actually promotes acid secretion. Chocolate and coffee, or ingestion of food and/or fluids before bedtime, may contribute to gastric reflux, leading to esophagitis/irritation of varices.
Discuss use/choice of antacids.	Liquid form is generally more effective than tablets. Alternating two different antacids may reduce side effects of constipation/diarrhea if they occur.
Stress importance of reading labels on OTC drugs and avoid drugs containing aspirin.	Aspirin damages the protective mucosa, by allowing hydrogen ions to diffuse backward across the gastric mucosal barrier, permitting gastric erosion, ulceration, and bleeding to occur.
Collaborative	
Refer to support groups/counseling for lifestyle/behavior changes/reduction of associated risk factors (e.g., substance abuse/stop-smoking clinics).	Alcohol users have a higher incidence of gastritis/esophageal varices, and cigarette smoking is associated with peptic ulcers and delayed healing.

CHAPTER 7
UROLOGY

Acute Renal Failure

This care plan focuses on the patient during the oliguric/diuretic phase of intrarenal/parenchymal renal failure following damge to glomerulus, tubular system, and/or renal vasculature which is commonly associated with an altered hemodynamic state and complicated by altered tissue perfusion, acidosis, tissue injury.

PATIENT ASSESSMENT DATA BASE

HISTORY

History of malignant hypertension, diabetes mellitus, gout, systemic lupus erythematosus (SLE), glomerulonephritis, polycystic disease, streptococcal disease (especially in young children), renal artery occlusion (thrombosis, embolism), vasculitis (polyarteritis nodosa).

Vascular failure, vasogenic shock, neurogenic shock with pooling of blood. Excessive fluid losses from hemorrhage, large wounds, burns, or gastric drainage with negative fluid balance/hypovolemia.

Postoperative cardiac/thoracic surgery with use of bypass pump. Surgery/anesthesia causing perioperative or postoperative hypotension with vasoconstriction and release of antidiuretic hormone (ADH). Surgery of major blood vessels (e.g., aorta, renal vessels). Extensive surgery in the elderly.

Recent trauma to kidney; for example, motor vehicle accident, injury to flank area. Extensive burns.

History of multiple transfusions or transfusion reactions.

History of massive infection/sepsis.

Exposure to nephrotoxic drugs; environmental poisons. Current/recent use of antibiotics/aminoglycosides (gentomicin, tobramycin, amikacin).

History of diagnostic procedures using contrast media or radiation to abdomen.

Family history of polycystic disease, heriditary nephritis, urinary calculus, malignancy, and cardiovascular disease.

Subjective

Reported change in urination pattern: increased frequency, polyuria, nocturia (early failure), or oliguria/anuria (later phase); dysuria, hesitancy, urgency, and retention owing to inflammation/infection of the urinary tract.

Reported change in urine color such as deep yellow, red, brown, cloudy.

May complain of flank pain, heartburn, nausea, anorexia, vomiting, diarrhea, abdominal bloating, prickling sensations in lower extremities.

PHYSICAL EXAMINATIONS

Signs and clinical manifestations vary, depending on cause and duration of renal failure and coexisting disease/conditions.

Inspection

Level of consciousness: decreased attention span/ability to concentrate, loss of memory, confusion, drowsiness, and decreasing levels of consciousness/coma may occur owing to hypoxemia, electrolyte/acid base imbalance, azotemia, and/or cerebral edema.

Respirations: increased rate, dyspnea may be noted. Presence of Kussmaul's respirations indicates metabolic acidosis.

Cough: may be productive of pink-tinged sputum in presence of pulmonary edema/cardiac failure.

Neuromuscular: twitching, fasciculations, myoclonic jerks, tremors, muscle cramps may be noted owing to calcium imbalance. "Restless leg" syndrome may be present.

Neck veins: jugular venous distension may be noted at 45 degrees in presence of hypervolemia.

Edema: may note generalized tissue (including periorbital) or dependent edema (e.g., ankles, sacrum).

Skin: petechiae/ecchymotic areas associated with platelet/bleeding disorders; pallor suggests anemia.

Palpation

Pulses may be weak/thready (dehydration), full/bounding (hypervolemia), and/or irregular (dysrhythmia).

Abdomen: liver tenderness may be noted with CHF/hypervolemia.

Bladder should not be palpable unless retention present.

Auscultation

Breath sounds: rhonchi/crackles may be present.

BP: orthostatic hypotension suggests dehydration, although hypertension is common.

Heart sounds: irregularities may be indicative of electrolyte imbalance. S_3/gallop rhythm may indicate early CHF.

Other

Temperature may be elevated, reflecting dehydration or sepsis.

DIAGNOSTIC STUDIES

Urine:

Volume: usually less than 400 ml per 24 hours, reflecting oliguric phase of acute renal failure (ARF) which occurs within 24 to 48 hours after renal insult.

Specific gravity: approximately 1.010, reflecting intrinsic damage.

Osmolality: less than 350 mOsm/kg is indicative of tubular damage, and urine/serum ration is often 1:1.

Creatinine clearance may be significantly decreased before blood urea nitrogen (BUN) and serum creatinine show significant elevation.

Sodium: greater than 40 mEq/liter because kidney is not able to reabsorb sodium.

HCO_3: elevated if acidosis present.

RBCs: may be present because of infection, stones, trauma, tumor mass, or alterations in glomerular filtration.

Protein: high-grade proteinuria (3 to 4 +) strongly indicates glomerular damage when RBCs and casts are also present. Low-grade proteinuria (1 to 2 +) and WBCs may be indicative of infection or interstitial nephritis. In acute tubular necrosis (ATN), there is usually minimal proteinuria.

Casts: usually signal renal disease or infection. Cellular casts with brownish pigments and numerous renal tubular epithelial cells is diagnostic of ATN. Red casts suggest acute glomerular nephritis.

Blood:

Hct: decreased in presence of anemia (usually occurs during first week of oliguria).

RBCs: often decreased owing to increased fragility/decreased survival.

pH: metabolic acidosis may develop owing to decreased renal ability to excrete hydrogen and end-products of metabolism.

BUN/creatinine usually rise in proportion with a ratio of 10:1.

Serum osmolality: greater than 285 mOsm/Kg, often equal to urine.

Potassium: elevated related to retention as well as cellular shifts (acidosis) or tissue release (red cell hemolysis).

Protein: decreased serum level may reflect protein loss via urine/fluid shifts, decreased protein intake, or decreased synthesis owing to lack of essential amino acids.

Radiographic studies may reveal calicectasis, hydronephrosis, narrowing and delayed filling or emptying as a cause of ARF.

KUB demonstrates size of kidneys and presence of stones.

Retrograde pyelogram outlines abnormalities of renal pelvis and ureters.

Renal arteriogram assesses renal circulation and identifies extravascularities, masses.

Voiding cystourethrogram shows bladder size, reflux into ureters, retention.

Renal ultrasound determines kidney/bladder size, masses, cysts, obstruction.

ECG may be abnormal, reflecting electrolyte and acid/base imbalances.

NURSING PRIORITIES

1. Reestablish/maintain fluid and electrolyte balance.
2. Prevent/minimize secondary complications.
3. Provide emotional/psychologic support for patient/significant other(s).

NURSING DIAGNOSIS: **Fluid Volume, alteration in, excess.**

SUPPORTING DATA/CONTRIBUTING FACTORS: **During the oliguric phase of ARF, fluid is retained and urine output is usually less than 400 ml 24 hours. This phase can last 10 to 14 days but may last for several weeks. During this time protein is lost, owing to increased permeability of the glomerular membrane. In addition, dilutional effects of increased extracellular fluid (ECF) and**

	decreased intravascular colloidal osmotic pressure permits fluid and protein to diffuse into interstitial tissues. The resulting fluid overload/shifts and associated electrolyte imbalance affects other organ systems adversely.
GENERAL PATIENT OUTCOMES:	**Urine output and specific gravity are within patient's normal limits. Edema is absent/reduced, and weight is stabilized. Breath sounds clear.**

INTERVENTIONS	RATIONALE
Independent	
Monitor vital signs: blood pressure (BP), pulse; and hemodynamic parameters as indicated; for example, central venous pressure (CVP), PAP.	Failure of the kidneys to excrete urine, compounded by excessive fluid resuscitation during efforts to treat underlying cause or convert oliguric phase, as well as alterations in the renin-angiotensin system, may result in hypertension and tachycardia.
Auscultate heart/breath sounds.	Fluid overload may lead to CHF and pulmonary edema as evidenced by development of extra heart sounds, (e.g., S_3 reflecting rapid ventricular filling and decreased ventricular compliance). Adventitious breath sounds (e.g., crackles or wheezes) are indicative of pulmonary congestion. (Refer to Care Plan: Congestive Heart Failure, page 49.)
Record accurate intake and output. Include pressure line flushes, injectate, antibiotic additives in total fluid intake, as well as fluid losses through gastrointestinal (GI) tract and wounds. Estimate insensible losses through diaphoresis.	Necessary to determine fluid replacement needs and to reduce risk of fluid overload.
Monitor urine specific gravity.	Measures the kidney's ability to concentrate urine. In intrarenal failure, specific gravity is usually equal to/less than 1.010, indicating kidney has lost the ability to concentrate the urine.
Plan oral fluid replacement with patient, within multiple restrictions. Space desired beverages throughout 24 hours. Vary offerings—hot/cold/frozen.	Helps avoid periods without fluids, minimizing boredom of limited choices and reducing sense of deprivation/thirst. Some fluids, such as water, cranberry juice, Kool Ade, have no protein, potassium, or sodium and need to be considered only in the light of fluid restriction. Other beverages, for example, grape and apple juice, contain sodium and potassium.
Weigh daily on same scale with same equipment and clothing.	Daily body weight is best monitor of fluid status. A weight gain of more than 0.5 kg per day suggests fluid retention.
Assess skin, face, dependent areas for edema. Evaluate edema using scale of +1 to +4.	Edema occurs primarily in dependent tissues of the body, such as hands, feet, lumbosacral area. Patient

INTERVENTIONS	RATIONALE
Independent	
	can gain up to 10 pounds (4.5 kg) of fluid before pitting edema is detected. Periorbital edema may be a presenting sign of this fluid shift, because these fragile tissues are easily distended by even minimal fluid accumulation.
Collaborative	
Monitor laboratory data:	
Serum sodium,	Dilutional hyponatremia may result from fluid overload or inability of kidney to conserve sodium. Elevated serum sodium indicates deficit of total body water, as well as shift of sodium into cells in acidosis.
Urine sodium and creatinine,	In ATN, tubular functional integrity is lost and sodium reabsorption is impaired, resulting in elevation of urine sodium. Urine creatine is usually decreased as serum creatinine elevates.
Serum potassium,	Renal retention of potassium allows it to accumulate. Acidosis increases potassium retention (as the kidney selectively retains it in order to excrete excess hydrogen ions) and potentiates shifts from intracellular to the serum.
Hematocrit (Hct),	Decreased values usually indicate anemia, but other possible causes, such as hypovolemia or occult hemorrhage, should be evaluated.
Monitor serial chest x-ray examinations.	Findings of increased cardiac size, prominent pulmonary vascular markings, pleural effusion/infiltrates/congestion indicate fluid overload.
Administer medications, as indicated; for example,	
Diuretics: furosemide (Lasix), mannitol (Osmitrol);	Given early in oliguric phase in an effort to convert to nonoliguric phase/to increase urine flow to flush the tubular lumen of debris and to enhance urine output.
Antihypertensives: clonidine (Catapres), methyldopa (Aldomet).	May be given to treat hypertension by counteracting effects of vasoconstriction secondary to reninangiotensin cycle, and/or circulating volume overload.
Restrict sodium and water as indicated.	Prevents/minimizes fluid overload by controlling volume intake and decreasing serum sodium (mainly responsible for the osmotic pressure of the extracellular fluid). Fluid restriction is also a method of treating hyponatremia.
Insert/maintain indwelling catheter, as indicated.	Provides means of accurate monitoring of urine output during acute phase. However, catheterization may not be desired because of increased risk of infection.
Prepare for dialysis as indicated. (Refer to Care Plan: Renal Dialysis, page 222.)	Done to decrease fluid overload, correct electrolyte imbalances and remove toxins.

NURSING DIAGNOSIS:	**Nutrition, alteration in, less than body requirements.**
SUPPORTING DATA/CONTRIBUTING FACTORS:	**Uremia and electrolyte imbalances produce anorexia, nausea/vomiting, and ulcerations of oral mucosa. Protein catabolism and dietary restrictions increase loss of body stores/muscle mass.**
GENERAL PATIENT OUTCOMES:	**Nutritional intake is sufficient to meet metabolic needs/to prevent catabolism as evidenced by positive nitrogen balance and weight loss less than 0.2 to 0.5 kg per day.**

INTERVENTIONS	RATIONALE
Independent	
Assess/document dietary intake. Estimate caloric value.	General physical condition, multiple dietary restrictions, and uremic symptoms (e.g., nausea, anorexia, altered taste) affect food intake. Careful monitoring is required to identify deficiencies/supplemental needs.
Provide patient/significant other(s) with a list of permitted foods/fluids and encourage involvement in menu planning.	Provides patient a measure of control and may increase cooperation with dietary restrictions. Food from home may enhance appetite and provide patient some measure of control within the dietary restrictions.
Provide foods in small servings.	Facilitates gastric emptying and minimizes anorexia/nausea associated with uremic state/diminished peristalsis.
Eliminate noxious environmental odors. Recommend ingestion of dry foods slowly, avoidance of gastric irritants (e.g., spicy/caffeine-containing foods/fluids) and fluids with meals.	May reduce nausea/gastric distress, improving dietary intake.
Offer frequent mouth care; rinse with 0.25 percent acetic acid; provide gum, hard candy, breath mints.	Mucous membranes may become dry and cracked. Mouth care soothes, lubricates, and helps freshen mouth taste, which is often unpleasant owing to uremia and restricted oral intake. Rinsing with acetic acid helps neutralize ammonium formed by conversion of urea. Use of mints/gum helps improve mouth taste.
Weigh daily.	The fasting/catabolic patient will normally lose 0.2 to 0.5 kg per day.
Collaborative	
Consult with dietician.	Determines dietary needs/restrictions and possible need for modifications; for example, supplements, tube feedings, hyperalimentation.

INTERVENTIONS	RATIONALE
Collaborative	
Restrict potassium intake as indicated.	Urine flow provides for the major excretion of potassium. During oliguric phase of ARF, potassium retention may occur rapidly. In addition, breakdown of tissues in catabolic state releases intracellular stores of potassium.
Provide/restrict protein as necessary. Include essential amino acids.	Approximately 0.5 gms of protein per kilogram of body weight is needed to maintain positive nitrogen balance. Patients in renal failure use nitrogen from urea; therefore, the amount of needed exogenous protein is less than normal. Essential amino acids improve nitrogen balance and provide relief of uremic symptoms.
Provide carbohydrate/glucose sources to meet caloric needs. Avoid concentrated sugar sources.	Carbohydrates (CHO) and fats produce carbon dioxide (CO_2), water (H_2O), and energy and therefore do not increase kidney workload. Carbohydrate calories help prevent ketoacid formation from protein and fat oxidation. Note: CHO intolerance mimicking diabetes mellitus may occur in severe renal failure.
Administer hyperalimentation or high-carbohydrate/low-protein tube feeding.	Beneficial to patients who cannot take sufficient oral nutrition. Acute renal failure patients in a hypercatabolic state may recover faster and have fewer complications when receiving supplemental nutritional support.
Administer medications as indicated; for example,	
Iron preparations,	Iron deficiency may occur if protein is restricted. Iron may be given intramuscularly (IM) if oral medication not well tolerated.
Calcium supplements,	Improves blood clotting, bone metabolism, neuromuscular function.
Phosphorus,	Important in bone, glucose/fat metabolism, and acid base balance. Although hyperphosphatemia is often present in renal failure, use of hyperalimentation/high-glucose loads may result in phosphorus deficit, requiring replacement.
Vitamin D,	Replacement corrects deficiency owing to loss of renal ability to metabolize vitamin D, which is necessary for absorption of calcium from the GI tract.
B complex vitamins,	Vital as coenzyme in cell growth and actions. Intake is decreased owing to protein restrictions.
Antiemetics; for example, prochlorperazine maleate (Compazine), trimethobenzamide hydrochloride (Tigan).	Given to relieve nausea/vomiting.

NURSING DIAGNOSIS:	**Infection, potential for.**
SUPPORTING DATA/CONTRIBUTING FACTORS:	**Serious infections (especially respiratory), occur in 30 to 70 percent of ARF**

	patients owing to depression of immunologic defenses and are the most common cause of death. Indwelling urinary catheter and other invasive lines provide access for bacteria. Protein catabolism and uremia retard wound healing and tissue repair.
GENERAL PATIENT OUTCOMES:	**Patient is afebrile. Signs of infection are absent.**

INTERVENTIONS	RATIONALE
Independent	
Monitor vital signs.	Fever with increased pulse and respirations is typical of increased metabolic rate resulting from bacterial/viral invasion.
Encourage deep breathing, coughing, frequent position changes.	Prevents atelectasis and mobilizes secretions.
Auscultate lungs, noting adventitious breath sounds.	Pulmonary secretions/developing congestion may be indicative of pulmonary infection (e.g., pneumonia).
Use aseptic technique when caring for intravenous sites/invasive line insertion sites. Change site/dressings/tubing per protocol. Note edema, erythema, purulent drainage.	Limits introduction of bacteria into body. Early detection/treatment of developing infection may prevent sepsis.
Provide catheter care each shift and as necessary.	Prevention of superimposed urinary tract infection is vital.
Monitor urine for unusual odor/cloudiness.	May indicate developing infection.
Assess skin integrity. (Refer to Nursing Diagnosis: Skin Integrity, impairment of, potential, page 219.)	Excoriations from scratching may become secondarily infected.
Collaborative	
Note elevation of white blood count (WBC).	Although elevated WBC may indicate infection, leukocytosis is commonly seen in ARF and may reflect inflammatory injury within the kidney.
Obtain specimen(s) for culture and sensitivity.	Identifies invading organism and effectiveness of various antibiotics.
Assist with use of respiratory adjuncts; for example, incentive spirometer/intermittent positive-pressure breathing (IPPB).	May be helpful in preventing atelectasis and mobilizing secretions to prevent pneumonia.

NURSING DIAGNOSIS:	**Injury, potential for, abnormal blood profile (e.g., decreased Hct and clotting factors).**

SUPPORTING DATA/CONTRIBUTING FACTORS:	**Uremia suppresses erythropoietin production/secretion, and decreases RBC production. This, coupled with decreased RBC survival and increased RBC fragility often leads to anemia. In addition, clotting alterations can occur with decreased platelet aggregation, and increased capillary fragility enhancing the risk of hemorrhage/worsening the anemia.**
GENERAL PATIENT OUTCOMES:	**Free of hypoxic symptoms related to anemia. Absence of bleeding.**

INTERVENTIONS	RATIONALE
Independent	
Note complaints of increasing fatigue/weakness, pallor, dyspnea, chest pain.	May reflect developing anemia.
Monitor level of consciousness.	Anemia reduces oxygen-carrying capacity of the blood which may cause cerebral hypoxia manifested by altered consciousness, behavioral changes, and confusion.
Observe for bleeding from mucous membranes/venopuncture sites following slight trauma. (Refer to Care Plan: Disseminated Intravascular Coagulation, page 319.)	May occur easily, owing to capillary fragility and altered clotting function.
Monitor heart sounds.	S_2 may be more prominent, reflecting cardiac strain owing to increased workload of heart to circulate oxygen.
Hematest GI secretions/stools for blood.	Stress and hemostatic abnormalities result in GI hemorrhage in 10 to 30 percent of patients with ARF. Gastrointestinal bleeding can usually be controlled with conservative therapy, but it may be the cause of death in critically ill patients.
Collaborative	
Monitor laboratory studies:	
Hemoglobin (Hgb)/hematocrit (Hct),	Uremia decreases production of erythropoietin, depressing red blood cell (RBC) production and RBC life. Dehydration can increase Hgb/Hct levels because of hemoconcentration.
Platelet count, clotting factors.	Generally, platelet counts of less than 50,000 are associated with spontaneous bleeding.
Administer whole blood/packed cells as indicated.	Blood transfusions are often necessary, owing to the inability of the kidney to produce erythropoetin, which facilitates the manufacture of RBCs. Washed RBCs may be given if potassium is elevated.

INTERVENTIONS	RATIONALE
Collaborative	
Administer medications as indicated; for example,	
Cimetadine (Tagamet), ranitidine (Zantac), antacids.	May be given prophylactically to reduce/neutralize gastric acid and thereby reduce the risk of GI hemorrhage.

NURSING DIAGNOSIS: **Fluid Volume Deficit, potential.**

SUPPORTING DATA/CONTRIBUTING FACTORS: **The diuretic phase of ARF is characterized by a steadily rising urinary volume as glomerular filtration improves. Delayed return of tubular function/reabsorption capabilities results in excessive urine loss (polyuria), which may contribute to fluid volume deficit.**

GENERAL PATIENT OUTCOMES: **Intake/output near balance, good skin turgor, moist mucous membranes, peripheral pulses palpable, electrolytes within normal limits.**

INTERVENTIONS	RATIONALE
Independent	
Note signs/symptoms of dehydration; for example, dry mucous membranes, thirst, dulled sensorium, peripheral vasoconstriction.	In diuretic phase of renal failure, urine output can exceed 3 liters per day (polyuria). Extracellular fluid (ECF) volume depletion activates the thirst center. Sodium depletion causes persistent thirst unrelieved by drinking water. Continued fluid losses/inadequate replacement may lead to hypovolemic state.
Measure intake and output accurately. Weigh daily. Calculate insensible fluid losses.	Helps estimate fluid replacement needs. Fluid intake should approximate losses through urine, nasogastric/wound drainage, and insensible losses (e.g., diaphoressis and metabolism. Weight change helps assess fluid fluctuations. Note: Some sources believe fluid replacement should not exceed two thirds of the previous day's output to prevent prolonging the diuresis.
Monitor vital signs; compare lying, sitting, standing blood pressure and HR. Monitor hemodynamic pressures if available.	Drop of 20 mmHg in systolic blood pressure (orthostatic hypotension) and increased heart rate (greater than 20 beats per minute) when raised from recumbent position reflects hypovolemia. Central venous pressure and PCWP are a more accurate measure of fluid status, but use of invasive lines must be balanced against increased risk of infection.
Monitor electrocardiogram (ECG) continuously. (Refer to Nursing Diagnosis: Cardiac Output, alteration in, decreased, page 217.)	Sudden shifts in electrolytes may occur with plasma losses, which can affect electromechanical function of the heart.

INTERVENTIONS	RATIONALE
Independent	
Provide scheduled fluids throughout 24-hour period.	Diuretic phase of ARF may revert to oliguric if fluid intake is not maintained, or nocturnal dehydration occurs.
Control environmental temperature, limit bed linens as indicated.	Cool environment may reduce diaphoresis, which contributes to overall fluid losses.
Collaborative	
Monitor laboratory studies:	
Serum potassium,	Hypokalemia may develop during diuretic phase owing to delayed/incomplete return of tubular function.
Serum/urine sodium.	In nonoliguric ARF or diuretic phase of ARF, daily urine output plus insensible losses may easily exceed three liters per day, resulting in sodium wasting. Fluid/electrolyte restriction may lead to sodium deficits. Sodium level of 120 mEq/liter or less must be corrected promptly.
Give intravenous (IV) fluids (e.g., D5W, N.S., D5 1/4 NS, D5 1/2 NS, lactated Ringer's). Correct fluid deficit gradually.	Fluid intake calculated to replace two thirds or more of previous day's losses with replacement of sodium losses to prevent hyponatremia.
Administer medications as indicated:	
Sodium bicarbonate,	Used to correct acidosis when plasma bicarbonate is decreased. Note: If hypocalcemia is present, correction of acidosis may cause tetany, because calcium does not ionize well in alkalotic states.
Diphenoxylate hydrochloride with atropine (Lomotil).	May decrease excessive diarrhea, which can contribute to water loss/dehydration.

NURSING DIAGNOSIS: **Cardiac Output, alteration in, decreased [potential].**

SUPPORTING DATA/CONTRIBUTING FACTORS: **With fluid overload, cardiac output may fall, owing to cardiac failure. Electrolyte imbalance affecting cardiac rhythm can reduce cardiac output. In addition, fluid shifts or excess fluid losses (during diuretic phase of ARF) can reduce venous return/cardiac output.**

GENERAL PATIENT OUTCOMES: **Cardiac output is maintained as evidenced by BP and heart rate within patient's normals, palpable peripheral pulses, and adequate capillary refill.**

INTERVENTIONS	RATIONALE
Independent	
Monitor BP and pulse. Measure cardiac output if available.	Fluid volume excess combined with hypertension (which often occurs in ARF), as well as the effects of anemia, increases cardiac workload and can lead to cardiac stress/failure.
Assess color of skin, mucous membranes, and nailbeds. Note capillary refill time.	Pallor may reflect peripheral vasoconstriction or anemia, and cyanosis is related to decreased hemoglobin oxygen saturation and may reflect pulmonary congestion, cardiac failure, and/or anemia. Delayed capillary refill time may reflect decreased cardiac output/hypovolemia.
Monitor ECG continuously for changes that may be associated with potassium and calcium imbalance.	Peaked T wave, widened QRS, prolonged PR, flattened/absent P waves, depressed ST segment occur in response to elevated potassium levels and can progress to atrial/ventricular standstill. Hypokalemia may develop during diuretic phase, evidenced by peaked P waves, flat T waves, ST depression, and appearance of U waves. Prolonged QT interval may reflect calcium deficit.
Note occurrence of bradycardia, hypotension, vasodilation, flushing, nausea/vomiting, central nervous system (CNS) depression. Review medication regimen for magnesium-containing antacids/laxatives.	Signs of hypermagnesmia, which can lead to respiratory/cardiac arrest, occurs if patient is taking drugs containing magnesium.
Note complaints of muscle cramps, hyperreflexia, numbness/tingling of fingers, positive Chvostek's/Trousseaus's sign.	Neuromuscular indicators of hypocalcemia, which can affect cardiac contractility/function.
Encourage adequate rest, spacing of/assistance with self-care activities.	Reduces oxygen consumption/cardiac workload.
Collaborative	
Monitor laboratory studies:	
Serum potassium,	Potassium is elevated as a result of release from cells (acidosis) and decreased renal excretion. High serum levels suggest tissue destruction or exogenous source of intake. Serum levels of 7 mEq or greater or any value associated with ECG changes constitute a medical emergency.
Serum calcium,	In addition to its own cardiac effects, calcium deficit enhances the toxic effects of potassium.
Serum magnesium.	Dialysis or calcium administration may be necessary to combat the CNS depressive effects of elevated magnesium.
Reduce/maintain circulating volume as indicated. (Refer to Nursing Diagnosis: Fluid Volume, alteration in, excess, page 209; Fluid Volume Deficit, potential, page 216.)	Cardiac output is dependent on circulating volume and myocardial function. Decreased cardiac output may reflect cardiac failure or hypovolemia.

INTERVENTIONS	RATIONALE
Collaborative	
Provide supplemental oxygen.	May reduce hypoxemia and associated tachycardia, decreasing cardiac workload.
Administer medications as indicated:	
Digoxin (Lanoxin),	May be given to improve cardiac output by increasing myocardial contractility and stroke volume. Dosage is dependent on renal function and potassium balance to obtain therapeutic effect without toxicity.
Calcium gluconate,	Calcium can offset the effects of hyperkalemia, because it modifies cardiac irritability, even though the plasma potassium concentration is not changed. Note: Increased calcium enhances digitalis effect, which may lead to digitalis toxicity.
Aluminum hydroxide gels (Amphojel),	Decrease phosphate levels, which may occur as a result of failure of glomerular filtration. Phosphate-binding gels may cause constipation, nausea, and vomiting. On occasion, excessive use may cause phosphate depletion and resultant hypercalcemia.
Glucose/insulin solution,	Temporary measure to lower serum potassium by driving potassium into cells.
Sodium bicarbonate,	May be given to correct acidosis or hyperkalemia because it buffers excess hydrogen (associated with metabolic acidosis), allowing hydrogen to exchange with potassium. Useful if patient is acidotic and not fluid overloaded.
Sodium polystyrene sulfonate (Kayexalate) with/without sorbitol.	Exchange resin, which trades sodium for potassium in the gastrointestinal tract. Sorbitol may be included to cause osmotic diarrhea to help excrete potassium.

NURSING DIAGNOSIS:	**Skin Integrity, impairment of, potential.**
SUPPORTING DATA/CONTRIBUTING FACTORS:	**Effects of fluid excess (edema), deficit (dehydration), reduced mobility, and uremic pruritis may result in skin irritation/breakdown. Note: With treatment options (dialysis), skin effects associated with severe uremia (e.g., uremic frost) are not usually present.**
GENERAL PATIENT OUTCOMES:	**Skin integrity is maintained.**

INTERVENTIONS	RATIONALE
Independent	
Inspect skin for redness, excoriation.	Indicates areas of poor circulation/breakdown, which may lead to decubitus/infection.
Change position frequently; move patient carefully; pad bony prominences. Elevate edematous extremities.	Decreases pressure damage, because circulation to skin may be impaired. Promotes venous return, reducing edema formation.
Provide soothing skin care. Restrict use of soaps.	Baking soda, oatmeal, cornstarch baths/soaks decrease itching and are less drying than soaps. Lotions, ointments relieve dry, cracked skin.
Keep fingernails short. Recommend applying firm pressure to puritic areas instead of scratching. Provide gloves during sleep.	Reduces injury to skin surfaces created by scratching.
Collaborative	
Provide foam/flotation mattress.	Reduces skin breakdown from prolonged pressure on tissues.

NURSING DIAGNOSIS:	**Anxiety/Fear.**
SUPPORTING DATA/CONTRIBUTING FACTORS:	**Severity of condition/prognosis, fear of death, potentiate feelings of anxiety. In addition, effects of azotemia, acidosis, hypoxia, and electrolyte imbalances may result in confusion/alteration in thought processes, which can be very frightening for the patient/significant other(s).**
GENERAL PATIENT OUTCOMES:	**Verbalizes reduction of anxiety/fears. Appears relaxed, is able to sleep/rest appropriately.**

INTERVENTIONS	RATIONALE
Independent	
Assess patient/family knowledge of renal failure and effects of current condition. Encourage questions.	Identifies needs/concerns to be addressed.
Emphasize what patient can do for self, and encourage participation in plan of care within limits of fatigue.	Highlights positive versus negative consequences and helps family avoid overprotectiveness. Promotes sense of control/involvement in care.
Provide simple explanations of procedures.	Reduces degree of "unknown" and associated anxiety.
Reorient to person/place/time as necessary. Tell patient/significant other(s) that as BUN/edema re-	Azotemia/cerebral edema may alter memory/ability to concentrate. When patient/significant other(s) are

INTERVENTIONS	RATIONALE
Independent	
solves, thought processes should clear and neuromuscular symptoms abate.	aware of these problems, reorientation/information can reduce anxiety/fear.
Reduce extraneous environmental stimuli.	Sensory overload potentiates confusion/anxiety.
Encourage use of relaxation techniques/adequate rest periods.	Reduces fatigue associated with anemia/illness and may enhance coping mechanisms.
Discuss parameters that may necessitate dialysis (e.g., signs of progressive renal disease).	Prepares patient for dialysis if it becomes necessary, allows time to ask questions.
Collaborative	
Refer to supportive resources; for example, psychiatric nurse, social services, clergy.	Patient/significant other(s) may need additional help in dealing with stress of illness/prognosis.

Renal Dialysis

Dialysis is a process that functionally substitutes for impaired renal function by removing excess fluid and/or accumulated endogenous or exogenous toxins. This care plan focuses on the care of patients undergoing acute/temporary renal dialysis; for example, peritoneal dialysis, hemodialysis, or continuous arteriovenous hemofiltration (CAVH). This care plan is organized to present the concerns/nursing care common to either form of diagnoses under general considerations beginning on this page, with specifics of peritoneal dialysis care on page 229 and hemodialysis on page 236.

PATIENT ASSESSMENT DATA BASE

History

Clinical evidence of acute renal failure (ARF) with the accumulation of endogenous or exogenous wastes/toxins (e.g., BUN, uric acid, creatinine, hyperkalemia, hyperphosphatemia; severe acidosis) and/or fluid volume excess.

History of acute poisoning/drug overdose (e.g., iron, lead, zinc, mercury, aspirin, arsenic, barbiturates, amphetamines, heroin, digitalis preparations).

History of acute trauma with severe crush injuries or burns; severe frostbite; transfusion reactions; hepatic coma.

Subjective

May report decreased/absent urinary output, increased weight, nausea/vomiting, fatigue, shortened memory span, anorexia, metallic taste.

PHYSICAL EXAMINATION

Refer to Care Plan: Acute Renal Failure, page 207.

DIAGNOSTIC STUDIES

Procedures and results are variable, depending on cause (e.g., removal of fluid/toxins with/without renal impairment or presence of prerenal/intrarenal/postrenal failure) and phase (oliguric or diuretic) of renal failure.

Refer to Care Plan: Acute Renal Failure, page 207.

NURSING PRIORITIES

1. Promote removal of toxic products and restoration of fluid/electrolyte balance.
2. Maintain patient comfort.
3. Minimize potential for complications.
4. Promote adequate nutrition.
5. Provide information and support to the patient/family.

GENERAL CONSIDERATIONS

This section addresses the general nursing management issues of the patient receiving some form of dialysis.

NURSING DIAGNOSIS:	**Nutrition, alteration in, less than body requirements.**
SUPPORTING DATA/CONTRIBUTING FACTORS:	**Anorexia, nausea/vomiting, and oral stomatitis may be present, interfering with intake of essential nutrients nec-**

	essary to prevent tissue catabolism. In addition, protein can cross the semipermeable membrane/peritoneum and be lost during dialysis.
GENERAL PATIENT OUTCOMES:	**Nutritional intake is sufficient to achieve a positive nitrogen balance. Weight is stable. Muscle mass is increased/maintained.**

INTERVENTIONS	RATIONALE
Independent	
Monitor food/fluid ingested and calculate daily caloric intake.	Identifies nutritional deficits/therapy needs.
Measure muscle mass via tricep-skin fold.	Assesses adequacy of nutrient utilization by measuring changes in fat deposits, which may suggest presence/absence of tissue catabolism.
Note presence of nausea/anorexia.	Symptoms accompany accumulation of endogenous toxins and may alter/reduce intake.
Provide frequent mouth care.	Reduces risk of oral stomatitis/clears mouth of undesirable tastes, which can interfere with food intake.
Serve small, frequent meals. Schedule meals according to dialysis needs.	Smaller portions may enhance intake. Type of dialysis influences meal patterns; for example, patients receiving hemodialysis might not be fed directly before/during procedure, inasmuch as this can alter fluid removal, and patients undergoing peritoneal dialysis may be unable to ingest food while abdomen is distended with dialysate.
Encourage patient to participate in menu planning.	May enhance oral intake and promotes sense of control/responsibility.
Promote visits by significant other(s) during meals.	Provides diversion and promotes social aspects of eating.
Collaborative	
Monitor serum protein/albumin levels.	Indicator of protein needs. Note: Peritoneal dialysis is associated with significant protein loss.
Provide a high-carbohydrate diet that includes ordered amount of high-quality protein and essential amino acids with restriction of sodium/potassium as indicated.	Provides sufficient nutrients to maintain positive nitrogen balance, prevent muscle wasting, promote healing and electrolyte balance.
Administer multivitamins, including ascorbic acid, folic acid, vitamin D, and iron supplements as indicated.	Replaces vitamins lost because of malnutrition/anemia or during dialysis.
Administer parenteral supplements as indicated. (Refer to Care Plan: Nutritional Support, page 367.)	Hyperalimentation may be needed to enhance renal tubular regeneration/resolution of underlying disease process, or to provide nutrients if oral/enteral feeding is contraindicated.

Administer antiemetics (e.g., prochlorperazine maleate (Compazine).	Reduces stimulation of the vomiting center.
Insert/maintain nasogastric tube if indicated.	May be necessary if persistent vomiting occurs or if enteric feeding is desired.

NURSING DIAGNOSIS: **Mobility, Impaired physical.**

SUPPORTING DATA/CONTRIBUTING FACTORS: **The patient is unable to move about during lengthy dialysis procedure because of fear of/real danger of dislodging dialysis lines/catheter. In addition, general condition (fatigue) of the patient contributes to inactivity and increases the risk of complications associated with immobility.**

GENERAL PATIENT OUTCOMES: **Maintains optimal mobility/function and is free of associated complications.**

INTERVENTIONS	RATIONALE
Independent	
Assess activity limitations. With patient's input, institute a planned activity program.	Identifies need for interventions. Increases patient's sense of well-being/control.
Change position frequently, as patient tolerates. Provide skin massage and perform range of motion exercises. Utilize sheepskin elbow//heel pads as indicated.	Decreases discomfort, maintains muscle strength/joint mobility, enhances circulation and prevents skin breakdown.
Encourage deep breathing and coughing. Elevate head of bed as allowed. Turn side to side.	Mobilizes secretions, improves lung expansion, and reduces risk of respiratory complications (e.g., atelectasis, pneumonia).
Provide diversion as appropriate to patient's condition, (e.g., visitors, radio/TV, books).	Decreases boredom, promotes relaxation.
Collaborative	
Provide flotation mattress/bed.	Reduces pressure areas and may enhance circulation, thereby reducing risk of skin breakdown.

NURSING DIAGNOSIS: **Self-Care Deficit.**

SUPPORTING DATA/CONTRIBUTING FACTORS: **Malaise/general weakness, pain, neurologic deficits (owing to accumulated toxins), and/or anxiety may make it difficult for the patient to carry out activities of daily living such as bathing, feeding, and so forth.**

GENERAL PATIENT OUTCOMES:	**Participates in activities of daily living within the constraints of the illness.**

INTERVENTIONS	RATIONALE
Independent	
Determine patient's ability to participate in self-care activities.	Underlying condition will dictate level of deficit/needs.
Assist as necessary with activities of daily living, such as bathing and feeding.	Meet hygiene/dietary/elimination needs while supporting patient's participation and independence.
Schedule activities allowing patient sufficient time to accomplish tasks to fullest extent of ability.	Conserves patient's energy while promoting optimal participation in activities/self-care.

NURSING DIAGNOSIS:	**Bowel Elimination, alteration in, constipation.**
SUPPORTING DATA/CONTRIBUTING FACTORS:	**Decreased fluid intake, altered dietary pattern, decreased mobility, and electrolyte imbalances affect gastric motility and alter consistency of stool, thereby potentiating constipation.**
GENERAL PATIENT OUTCOMES:	**Normal patterns of bowel function are restored/maintained.**

INTERVENTIONS	RATIONALE
Independent	
Auscultate bowel sounds. Note consistancy/frequency of bowel movements, presence of abdominal distention.	Decreased peristalsis, hard formed/dry stools suggest constipation and require intervention.
Measure nasogastric aspirates when tube in place.	Large output suggests ileus (common early complication of peritoneal dialysis), accumulation of gas and intestinal fluid which cannot be passed rectally.
Encourage ambulation if able.	Activity will promote return to normal bowel activity.
Provide privacy at bedside commode/bathroom.	Promotes psychologic comfort needed for elimination.
Collaborative	
Provide fresh fruits/vegetables and high-fiber diet if oral intake tolerated.	Provides bulk, which improves stool consistency.
Administer stool softeners/suppositories, enemas as indicated.	Promotes bowel evacuation.
Keep patient NPO (nothing by mouth) and/or insert nasogastric tube as indicated.	Decompresses stomach and prevents further abdominal distention if ileus occurs.

NURSING DIAGNOSIS:	**Thought Processes, alteration in.**
SUPPORTING DATA/CONTRIBUTING FACTORS:	**Presence of toxins, electrolyte imbalance, hypervolemia/fluid shifts, or hyperglycemia (from infusion of a dialysate with a high glucose concentration) may result in lethargy, confusion, dementia.**
GENERAL PATIENT OUTCOMES:	**Patient is alert/oriented, level of toxins reduced, and blood sugar is within normal limits.**

INTERVENTIONS	RATIONALE
Independent	
Assess for behavioral change/change in level of consciousness (e.g., orientation to time, place and person).	Indicates developing complication/need for further assessment.
Keep explanations simple, reorient frequently. Provide "normal" day/night lighting patterns, clock, calendar.	Improves reality orientation.
Provide a safe environment, restrain as indicated, pad siderails.	Prevents patient trauma and/or inadvertant removal of dialysis lines/catheter.
Drain peritoneal dialysate promptly at end of specified equilibration period.	Prompt outflow will decrease risk of hyperglycemia/hyperosmolar fluid shifts affecting cerebral function.
Note development of headache, nausea/vomiting, confusion/agitation, hypertension, seizure activity.	May reflect development of disequilibrium syndrome, which can occur near completion of/following hemodialysis. This is thought to be caused by ultrafiltration or by the too rapid removal of urea from the bloodstream when not accompanied by equivalent removal from brain tissue. The hypertonic cerebrospinal fluid causes a fluid shift into the brain, resulting in cerebral edema.
Monitor changes in speech pattern, development of dementia, myoclonus activity during hemodialysis.	Occasionally, accumulation of aluminum may cause dialysis dementia progressing to death if untreated.
Collaborative	
Monitor serum glucose, alternate/change dialysate concentrations or add insulin if indicated.	Hyperglycemia may develop secondary to glucose crossing peritoneal membrane and entering circulation. May require initiation of insulin therapy.
Obtain aluminum level as indicated.	Elevation may warn of impending cerebral involvement/dialysis dementia.
Administer medication, as indicated (e.g., Dilantin).	If disequilibrium syndrome occurs during dialysis, medication may be needed to control seizures as well as a change in dialysis prescription, or discontinuation of therapy.

NURSING DIAGNOSIS:	**Knowledge Deficit [Learning Need].**
SUPPORTING DATA/CONTRIBUTING FACTORS:	**Acute renal failure may occur suddenly, and the patient without previous kidney disease may not understand the disease process or dialysis treatment.**
GENERAL PATIENT OUTCOMES:	**Verbalizes understanding of the illness and the need for dialysis treatment.**

INTERVENTIONS	RATIONALE
Independent	
Note level of anxiety/fear, and alteration of thought processes.	These factors have direct impact on ability to participate/access and use knowledge.
Assess level of knowledge/learning needs of patient/significant other(s).	Better understanding and acceptance may result when the "teaching" plan is developed considering these parameters.
Explain patient's disease process, procedures and purpose of dialysis in terms understandable to the patient. Repeat explanations. Provide assurance that certain responses are normal during dialysis.	Providing information at the level of the patient/family's understanding will reduce anxiety and misconceptions about what the patient is experiencing.
Encourage and provide opportunity for questions.	Enhances learning process and reduces anxiety associated with the unknown.

NURSING DIAGNOSIS:	**Anxiety/Fear.**
SUPPORTING DATA/CONTRIBUTING FACTORS:	**In addition to the stressful environment of the critical care unit, the patient/family may have little previous experience or knowledge of dialysis. Patient may be too ill to enquire about care, family may experience frustration/concern regarding outcome/prognosis.**
GENERAL PATIENT OUTCOMES:	**Verbalizes/exhibits behaviors that indicate reduced fear.**

INTERVENTIONS	RATIONALE
Independent	
Assess level of fear of patient and family/significant	Helps determine the kind of intervention required.

INTERVENTIONS	RATIONALE
Independent	
other(s). Note signs of denial/depression, narrowed focus of attention.	
Explain procedures/care as delivered. Repeat explanations frequently/as needed.	Fear of unknown is lessened by information/knowledge and may enhance acceptance of dialysis. Alteration in thought processes and high levels of anxiety/fear may reduce comprehension, requiring repetition of important information.
Acknowledge normalcy of feelings of anxiety in this situation.	Knowing feelings are normal can allay fear that they are losing control.
Encourage and provide opportunities for patient/family to ask questions and to verbalize concerns.	Creates feeling of openness and cooperation and provides information that will assist in problem/need identification.
Encourage family/significant other(s) to participate in care, as indicated.	Involvement in care promotes sense of sharing, strengthens feelings of usefulness, and may lessen fear of the unknown.
Acknowledge concerns of patient/significant other(s). (Refer to Care Plan: Psychosocial Aspects of Critical Care, page 379.)	Prognosis/possibility of need for long-term dialysis and resultant lifestyle changes are a major concern for this patient and those who may be involved in future care.

PERITONEAL DIALYSIS

The peritoneum serves as the semipermeable membrane permitting transfer of nitrogenous wastes/toxins and fluid from the blood into a dialysate solution. Peritoneal dialysis is sometimes preferred because it uses a simpler technique and provides more gradual physiologic changes than hemodialysis.

NURSING DIAGNOSIS:	**Fluid Volume, alteration in, excess [potential].**
SUPPORTING DATA/CONTRIBUTING FACTORS:	**Dialysate may not provide the proper osmotic gradient to remove fluid from body tissues. Drainage may be impeded by malpositioned/kinked catheter, body position, fibrin clots in the catheter, or bowel distention resulting in retention of dialysate. In addition, excessive oral/IV intake may cause fluid overload.**
GENERAL PATIENT OUTCOMES:	**Amount of peritoneal outflow approximates infusion. Free of signs of edema, pulmonary congestion.**

INTERVENTIONS	RATIONALE
Independent	
Assess patency of catheter, noting difficulty in drainage. Note presence of fibrin strings/plugs.	Slowing of flow rate/presence of fibrin suggests partial catheter occlusion, requiring further evaluation/intervention.
Check tubing for kinks, note placement of bottles/bags. Anchor catheter so that good inflow/outflow is achieved.	Improper functioning of dialysis equipment may result in decreased outflow of effluent.
Turn from side to side; elevate the head of the bed; apply gentle pressure to the abdomen.	Position change/gentle pressure may enhance outflow of fluid.
Maintain a record of inflow/outflow volumes and cumulative fluid balance.	In most cases, the amount drained should equal or exceed the amount instilled. A positive balance indicates need of further evaluation.
Record serial weights, compare with intake/output balance. Weigh patient when abdomen is empty of dialysate (consistent reference point).	Serial body weights are an accurate assessment of fluid volume status. A positive fluid balance with an increase in weight indicates fluid retention.
Note decrease in bowel sounds, changes in stool consistency, complaints of constipation.	Bowel distention/constipation may impede outflow of effluent. (Refer to Nursing Diagnosis: Bowel Elimination, alteration in, constipation, page 225.)
Monitor blood pressure (BP), pulse; measure central venous pressure (CVP)/pulmonary artery pressure (PAP), if available. Note presence of neck vein distention.	Elevations indicate hypervolemia.

INTERVENTIONS	RATIONALE
Independent	
Assess heart and breath sounds, noting S_3 and/or crackles, rhonchi.	Fluid overload may potentiate CHF/pulmonary edema.
Evaluate development of dyspnea/increased respiratory effort.	Abdominal distention/diaphragmatic defect with leakage of dialysate into thoracic cavity may cause respiratory distress.
Assess for headache, muscle cramps, mental confusion, disorientation.	Symptoms suggest hyponatremia or water intoxication.
Collaborative	
Monitor serum sodium.	Hyponatremia may result as dilutional effect of fluid volume overload.
Add heparin to initial dialysis runs, assist with irrigation of catheter with heparinized saline.	May be useful in preventing fibrin,clot formation, which can obstruct peritoneal catheter.
Alter dialysate regimen as indicated.	Changes may be needed in the glucose/sodium concentration to facilitate efficient dialysis and fluid loss.
Maintain fluid restriction as indicated.	In the presence of renal failure, fluid intake may be restricted to decrease fluid volume overload.

NURSING DIAGNOSIS:	**Fluid Volume, deficit, potential.**
SUPPORTING DATA/CONTRIBUTING FACTORS:	**Dialysate is a hypertonic solution that provides an osmotic gradient sufficient to allow the passage of intravascular fluid through the peritoneal membrane into the dialysate. Rapid removal of fluid from the intravascular space may result in a circulating volume deficit because movement of water from tissues to vascular bed occurs at a slower rate.**
GENERAL PATIENT OUTCOMES:	**Desired alteration in fluid volume is achieved. Weight and blood pressure are within patient's normal range. Electrolyte levels are within acceptable range.**

INTERVENTIONS	RATIONALE
Independent	
Maintain record of inflow/outflow volumes and individual/cumulative fluid balance.	Provides information about the status of the patient's loss or gain at the end of each exchange.

INTERVENTIONS	RATIONALE
Independent	
Adhere to schedule for draining dialysate from abdomen.	Prolonged dwell times, especially when 4.5 percent glucose solution is used, may cause excess fluid loss.
Assess weight when abdomen is empty, following initial 6 to 10 runs, then daily as indicated.	Detects rate of fluid removal by comparison with baseline body weights.
Monitor BP (lying and sitting) and pulse. Monitor CVP and PAP if available.	Decreased BP, postural hypotension, and increased pulse are early signs of hypovolemia. Serial readings can detect early changes in fluid volume status so that corrections can be made.
Note complaints of dizziness, nausea, increasing thirst.	May indicate hyperosmolar syndrome/hypovolemia.
Collaborative	
Monitor serum sodium and glucose levels.	Hypertonic solutions may cause hypernatremia by removing more water than sodium. In addition, dextrose may be absorbed from the dialysate, thereby elevating serum glucose.
Monitor serum potassium levels.	Hypokalemia may occur with dialysis and can cause cardiac arrhythmias.

NURSING DIAGNOSIS: **Injury, potential for [trauma].**

SUPPORTING DATA/CONTRIBUTING FACTORS: **The catheter is inserted via a trocar into the peritoneal cavity through a small midline stab, 3 to 5 cm below the umbilicus. The site is near the bowel/bladder with potential for perforation during insertion or by manipulation of the catheter.**

GENERAL PATIENT OUTCOMES: **Injury does not occur to bowel or bladder.**

INTERVENTIONS	RATIONALE
Independent	
Have patient empty bladder prior to peritoneal catheter insertion if indwelling catheter not present.	An empty bladder is more distant from insertion site and reduces likelihood of being punctured during catheter insertion.
Anchor catheter/tubing with tape. Stress importance of patient avoiding pulling/pushing on catheter. Restrain hands if indicated.	Reduces risk of trauma by manipulation of the catheter.
Note presence of fecal material in dialysate effluent, or strong urge to defecate, accompanied by severe, watery diarrhea.	Suggests bowel perforation with mixing of dialysate and bowel contents.

INTERVENTIONS	RATIONALE
Independent	
Note complaints of intense urge to void, or large urine output following initiation of dialysis run. Test urine for sugar as indicated.	Suggests bladder perforation with dialysate leaking into bladder. Dialysate contains glucose, and if it is leaking into the bladder, the urine and dialysate will have the same glucose concentration.
Stop dialysis if there is evidence of bowel/bladder perforation, leaving peritoneal catheter in place.	Prompt action will prevent further injury. Immediate surgical repair may be required. Leaving catheter in place facilitates diagnosing/locating the perforation.

NURSING DIAGNOSIS:	**Comfort, alteration in, pain [acute].**
SUPPORTING DATA/CONTRIBUTING FACTORS:	**Sources of discomfort/pain include insertion of catheter through abdominal wall, catheter irritation within the peritoneal cavity, improper catheter placement, infusion of cold or acidic dialysate, abdominal distention, and/or intraperitoneal infection.**
GENERAL PATIENT OUTCOMES:	**Verbalizes decrease of pain/discomfort. Demonstrates relaxed posture/facial expression, able to sleep/rest appropriately.**

INTERVENTIONS	RATIONALE
Independent	
Investigate patient's complaints of pain; note quality, location, and precipitating factors. Identify measures that alleviate the pain/discomfort.	Knowing the nature and location will assist in identification of source of pain and appropriate interventions.
Explain that initial discomfort usually subsides after the first few exchanges.	Explanation may reduce anxiety and promote relaxation during procedure.
Monitor for pain that begins during inflow and continues during equilibration phase.	Pain will occur at these times if acidic dialysate chemical causes irritation of peritoneal membrane.
Note discomfort that is most pronounced near the end of inflow.	Likely the result of abdominal distention from dialysate. Amount of infusion may have to be decreased initially.
Note complaint of pain in area of shoulder blade. Prevent introduction of air into system when initiating runs/during bag changes.	Inadvertent introduction of air into the abdomen irritates the diaphragm and results in referred pain to shoulder blade. This type of discomfort also may be reported during initiation of therapy and usually is related to stretching/irritation of the diaphragm with abdominal distention. Smaller exchange volumes may be required until patient adjusts.

INTERVENTIONS	RATIONALE
Independent	
Elevate head of bed at intervals. Turn patient from side to side. Provide back care and tissue massage.	Position changes may relieve abdominal discomfort.
Warm dialysate to body temperature before infusing.	Warming the solution increases the rate of urea removal by dilating peritoneal vessels. Cold dialysate causes vasoconstriction, which can cause discomfort. Note: Cold dialysate can also lower the core body temperature and precipitate cardiac arrest.
Monitor for severe/continuous abdominal pain and temperature elevation (especially after dialysis has been discontinued).	May indicate developing peritonitis. (Refer to Nursing Diagnosis: Infection, potential for, peritonitis, below.)
Collaborative	
Administer analgesics.	Relieves pain and discomfort.
Add sodium hydroxide to dialysate, if indicated.	Occasionally used to alter pH if patient is not tolerating acidic dialylsate.

NURSING DIAGNOSIS:	**Infection, potential for [peritonitis].**
SUPPORTING DATA/CONTRIBUTING FACTORS:	**Peritonitis is a serious complication of peritoneal dialysis. Sources of infection include contamination of the catheter during insertion, when changing the tubings/bottles/bags, or skin contaminates at the catheter insertion site. Sterile peritonitis (an inflammatory process) also may occur as a response to the composition of dialysate.**
GENERAL PATIENT OUTCOMES:	**Free of signs/symptoms of infection.**

INTERVENTIONS	RATIONALE
Independent	
Observe meticulous aseptic techniques and wear masks during catheter insertion, dressing changes, and whenever the system is opened. Change tubings per protocol.	Prevents the introduction of organisms and airborne contamination, which may cause infection.
Change dressings as indicated, being careful not to dislodge the catheter. Note character, color, odor of drainage from around insertion site.	Moist environment promotes bacterial growth. Purulent drainage at insertion site suggests presence of local infection.
Observe color and clarity of fluent.	Cloudy effluent is suggestive of peritoneal infection.

INTERVENTIONS	RATIONALE
Independent	
Monitor for nausea/vomiting, abdominal pain, rebound tenderness, fever, and leukocytosis.	Signs/symptoms of peritonitis.
Apply Betadine barrier in distal, clamped portion of catheter when intermittent dialysis therapy used.	Reduces risk of bacterial entry through catheter between dialysis treatments when catheter is disconnected from closed system.
Collaborative	
Monitor white blood cell (WBC) count of effluent.	Presence of WBCs initially may reflect normal response to a foreign substance, however continued/new elevation suggests developing infection.
Obtain specimens of blood, effluent, and/or drainage from insertion site as indicated for culture/sensitivity.	Identifies type of organism(s) present.
Monitor renal clearance/blood urea nitrogen (BUN), creatinine.	Choice and dosage of antibiotics will be influenced by renal function; for example, if function is inadequate, medication dosage is often reduced.
Administer antibiotics systemically or in dialysate as indicated.	Treats infection, prevents sepsis.

NURSING DIAGNOSIS: **Breathing Pattern, ineffective [potential].**

SUPPORTING DATA/CONTRIBUTING FACTORS: **Decreased lung expansion may occur owing to abdominal pressure and restricted diaphragmatic excursion, which may result in respiratory distress and increased risk of pulmonary complications (e.g., atelectasis/pneumonia).**

GENERAL PATIENT OUTCOMES: **Arterial blood gases (ABGs)/respiratory rate within patient's normal limits, breath sounds are clear, and patient is free of dyspnea/cyanosis. cyanosis.**

INTERVENTIONS	RATIONALE
Independent	
Monitor respiratory rate/effort.	Tachypnea, dyspnea, shortness of breath, and shallow breathing suggest increased respiratory effort/developing complications.
Auscultate lungs, noting decreased, absent, or adven-	Decreased areas of ventilation suggest presence of

INTERVENTIONS	RATIONALE
Independent	
titious breath sounds (e.g., crackles/wheezes/rhonchi).	atelectasis, and adventitious sounds may suggest fluid overload, retained secretions, or infection.
Note character, amount, and color of secretions.	Patient is susceptible to pulmonary infections as a result of depressed cough reflex and respiratory effort and increased viscosity of secretions.
Elevate head of bed. Promote deep breathing exercises and coughing.	Facilitates ventilation and mobilization of secretions.
Collaborative	
Review ABGs and serial chest x-ray examinations.	Appearance of changes in PaO_2/$PaCO_2$ and infiltrates/congestion on chest x-ray film suggests developing pulmonary problems.
Administer supplemental oxygen by cannula, mask/mechanical ventilation.	May be needed to maintain adequate oxygenation. Mechanical ventilatory support may be required if respiratory insufficiency/failure occurs. (Refer to Care Plan: Ventilatory Assistance, Mechanical, page 115.)

ACUTE HEMODIALYSIS

Blood is shunted through an artificial kidney (dializer) to remove toxins/excess fluid and then is returned to the venous circulation. Hemodialysis is a faster and more efficient method than peritoneal dialysis for removing urea and other toxic products.

NURSING DIAGNOSIS:	**Injury, potential for [loss of vascular access].**
SUPPORTING DATA/CONTRIBUTING FACTORS:	**Hemodialysis requires vascular access by means of femoral/subclavian catheters, external AV shunt (in the absence of internal AV fistulas). These lines are prone to clotting, hemorrhage related to accidental disconnection, and infection.**
GENERAL PATIENT OUTCOMES:	**Vascular access is maintained/ complications are prevented.**

INTERVENTIONS	RATIONALE
Independent	
CLOTTING	
Monitor for AV shunt patency at frequent intervals:	
Palpate for distal thrill,	Thrill is caused by turbulence created by high-pressure arterial blood flow entering low-pressure venous system and should be palpable above venous exit site.
Auscultate for a bruit,	Bruit is the sound caused by the turbulence created by arterial blood entering venous system and may be audible by stethoscope, although it may be very faint in external AV shunts.
Note color of blood,	Change of color from uniform medium red color to dark purplish red color suggests sluggish blood flow/ early clotting. Separation within tubing is indicative of clotting. Very dark reddish black blood next to clear yellow fluid indicates full clot formation.
Palpate shunt for warmth.	Diminished blood flow will result in "coolness" of shunt.
If there is evidence of loss of shunt patency, notify physician and/or initiate declotting procedure.	Rapid intervention may save vascular access.
Avoid trauma to shunt; for example, handle tubing gently, maintain cannulae alignment. Limit activity of extremity. Avoid taking BP or drawing blood samples in shunt extremity. Instruct patient not to sleep on affected extremity.	Decreases risk of clotting/disconnection.

INTERVENTIONS	RATIONALE
Independent	
Assess skin color, temperature, pulses of limb distal to access.	Altered/decreased blood flow may manifest as tissue ischemia.
HEMORRHAGE	
Attach two cannula clamps to shunt dressing. Have tourniquet available. If cannulae separates, clamp first the arterial cannula, then venous cannula. If tubing comes out of vessel, clamp cannula that is still in place and apply direct pressure to bleeding site. Place tourniquet above site or inflate BP cuff to pressure just above patient's systolic blood pressure.	Prevents massive blood loss if cannulae separates or shunt is dislodged.
INFECTION	
Avoid contamination of access site. Use aseptic technique when giving shunt care, applying/changing dressings, and when starting/completing dialysis process.	Prevents introduction of organisms that can cause infection.
Keep dressings dry. Check for drainage. Inspect site for redness and edema. Palpate site for warmth.	Signs of local infection which can progress to sepsis if untreated.
Monitor temperature. Note presence of fever, chills, hypotension.	Signs of infection/sepsis.
Collaborative	
Culture the site/obtain blood samples as indicated.	Determines presence of and identifies pathogens.
Administer medications as indicated, for example,	
Anticoagulants: low-dose heparin,	Infused on arterial side of continuous arteriovenous filter to prevent clotting in the filter without systemic side effects.
Antibiotics, systemic and/or topical.	Prompt treatment of infection may save access, prevent sepsis.

NURSING DIAGNOSIS: **Fluid Volume Deficit, potential.**

SUPPORTING DATA/CONTRIBUTING FACTORS: **Ultrafiltration is the process of removing water from the circulation by manipulating transmembrane hydrostatic pressures. If excessive fluid shifts occur, fluid volume deficit may develop. In addition, hypovolemia may occur as a result of diuretic therapy or fluid restrictions. Actual blood loss related to systemic heparinization or disconnection of the shunt can further deplete the circulating volume.**

GENERAL PATIENT OUTCOMES:	**Fluid balance is maintained as evidenced by stable/appropriate weight and vital signs, good skin turgor, moist mucous membranes, absence of bleeding.**

INTERVENTIONS	RATIONALE
Independent	
Monitor blood pressure, pulse, CVP, PAP, PCWP if available during dialysis.	Hypotension, tachycardia, falling hemodynamic pressures suggest volume depletion.
Place patient in a more horizontal position as necessary.	Maximizes venous return when hypotension occurs.
Note/ascertain if diuretics and/or antihypertensives are to be withheld.	Diuretics may enhance fluid loss; antihypertensives prevent normal vascular response to volume changes potentiating hypotension.
Assess shunt/access catheter to verify continuity.	Disconnected shunt/open access will permit exsanguination.
Monitor hourly outputs (filtrate) during CAVH and compare with total intake to calculate net fluid balance.	Excess/rapid fluid removal may result in hypotension/hypovolemia.
Weigh daily before/after dialysis run, using a bed scale.	Weight loss over precisely measured time is an indicator of ultrafiltration and fluid removal.
Assess for oozing or frank bleeding at access site, mucous membranes, incisions/wounds. Hematest/guaiac, gastric drainage, stools.	Systemic heparinization during dialysis will increase clotting times and place patient at risk for bleeding. Excessive blood loss will result in hypovolemia/decreased cardiac output.
Apply external shunt dressing. Permit no puncture of shunt.	Minimizes stress on cannula insertion site to reduce inadvertent dislodging and bleeding from site.
Collaborative	
Administer IV solutions (e.g., normal saline) or volume expanders (e.g., albumin), during dialysis as indicated.	Volume expanders may be required during/following hemodialysis if sudden/marked hypotension occurs. Filter replacement fluid (FRF) consisting of saline/dextrose solutions, electrolytes, and sodium bicarbonate may be infused in the venous side of CAV hemofilter when high ultrafiltration rates are used to remove extracellular fluid and toxic solutes.
Administer blood/packed red cells as indicated.	Destruction of red blood cells (hemolysis) by mechanical dialysis, hemorrhagic losses, alteration in red cell production may result in increased anemia.
Reduce rate of ultrafiltration during dialysis as indicated.	Decreasing the rate of blood flow reduces the amount of water being removed and may correct hypotension/hypovolemia.
Monitor Hgb and Hct.	May be reduced because of anemia, hemodilution, or actual blood loss.
Monitor clotting times; for example, ACT, PT/PTT, and	Use of heparin to prevent clotting in blood lines and

INTERVENTIONS	RATIONALE
Independent	
platelet count.	hemofilter alters coagulation and may potentiate bleeding.
Administer protamine sulfate, if indicated.	Acts as a heparin antagonist which may be needed to return clotting times to normal, or if heparin rebound occurs (up to 16 hours after hemodialysis).
Monitor serum electrolytes and pH.	Imbalances may require changes in the dialysate solution or supplemental replacement to achieve balance.

NURSING DIAGNOSIS: **Fluid Volume, alteration in, excess [potential].**

SUPPORTING DATA/CONTRIBUTING FACTORS: **Ultrafiltration may be negatively affected by variable factors; for example, BP/cardiac output, equipment constraints, composition/timing of oral intake resulting in fluid retention.**

GENERAL PATIENT OUTCOMES: **"Dry weight" is within patient's normal range, free of edema, breath sounds clear, and serum sodium levels within normal limits.**

INTERVENTIONS	RATIONALE
Independent	
Monitor BP, pulse, and weight.	Hypertension and tachycardia between hemodialysis runs may result from fluid overload. Weight gain between treatments should not exceed 0.5 kg per day.
Note presence of peripheral/sacral edema, respiratory crackles, dyspnea, orthopnea, distended neck veins, ECG changes indicative of ventricular hypertrophy. (Refer to Care Plan: Congestive Heart Failure, page 49.)	Fluid volume excess because of inefficient dialysis or repeated hypervolemia between dialysis treatments may cause heart failure, as indicated by signs/symptoms of respiratory and/or systemic venous congestion.
Note changes in mentation. (Refer to Nursing Diagnosis: Thought Processes, alteration in, page 226.)	Fluid overload/hypervolemia may potentiate cerebral edema/disequilbrium syndrome.
Collaborative	
Monitor serum sodium levels. Restrict sodium intake as indicated.	High sodium levels are associated with fluid overload edema, hypertension, and cardiac complications.
Restrict oral/IV fluid intake as indicated, spacing allowed fluids through 24-hour period.	The intermittent nature of hemodialysis results in fluid retention/overload between procedures, requiring fluid restriction. Spacing fluids helps reduce thirst.

CHAPTER 8
ENDOCRINOLOGY

Diabetic Ketoacidosis

PATIENT ASSESSMENT DATA BASE

HISTORY

Presence of precipitating factors; for example, inadequate secretion of endogenous insulin, insufficient exogenous insulin, and/or increased requirements for insulin, precipitating a relative or absolute insulin deficiency.

Presence of signs/symptoms in a previously undiagnosed diabetic patient with or without family history of diabetes.

Insulin-dependent diabetic (Type I) who reduced insulin dosage, omitted one or more doses. Failure to increase insulin to compensate for increased insulin need (e.g., acute infection, pregnancy, growth spurts, trauma, surgery, and/or emotional stress).

Recent/current bacterial/viral infection with resultant dehydration, nausea, vomiting, and diarrhea.

Change in diet; for example, increased/reduced intake.

History of hyperthyroidism resulting in increased nutritional intake/metabolic demands.

Use of/increased dosage of medications that interfere with insulin secretion and/or action, such as Dilantin, thiazide diuretics, or steroids.

Subjective

Symptoms may develop over several weeks or in just a few hours (as in a young juvenile diabetic), affecting complaints/subjective symptoms.

May complain of polydipsia, polyuria, muscle cramps/weakness, fatigue, headache, nausea/vomiting, weight loss, abdominal pain.

PHYSICAL EXAMINATION

Inspection

Level of consciousness: confusion/stupor progressing to coma.

Respirations: tachypnea and Kussmaul's respirations are present owing to acidosis.

Urine: polyuria is an early sign, but oliguria or anuria may be present if severe dehydration has occurred.

Neuromuscular: motor weakness and decreased deep tendon reflexes may be noted.

Skin: warm and dry; dry mucous membranes, poor skin turgor, cracked lips, flushed face.

Abdomen: rigidity, gastric dilatation, and vomiting may be noted.

Auscultation

Blood pressure: hypotension/postural hypotension may be present in varying degrees, depending on the severity of diuresis, dehydration, and hypovolemia.

Palpation

Pulses: peripheral pulses may be weak, thready, and easily obliterated owing to hypovolemia and vasoconstriction.

Abdomen: rigidity and gastric dilatation may be present.

DIAGNOSTIC STUDIES

Serum glucose: increased greater than 300, usually less than 800 mg/dl, but may be higher.

Plasma acetone (ketones): strongly positive.

Free fatty acids: greater than 1500 mEq/liter.

Serum osmolality: usually less than 330 mOsm/liter.

Electrolytes: sodium may be normal, elevated, or decreased. Potassium is normal or falsely elevated initially, then decreased. Phosphorus is frequently decreased.

ABGs: pH/HCO_3 reflecting metabolic acidosis. PCO_2 decreased in attempt to compensate for acidosis.

CBC: Hct may be elevated in presence of dehydration; leukocytosis suggests hemoconcentration/stress, though possibility of infection must be evaluated.

BUN: may be normal or elevated, reflecting dehydration/decreased renal perfusion.

Serum amylase: elevation may indicate acute pancreatitis as a cause of diabetic ketoacidosis (DKA).

Serum insulin levels may be decreased, indicating insulin insufficiency (endogenous/exogenous).

Urine: strongly positive for sugar and acetone. Specific gravity may be elevated.

Culture and sensitivities may reveal urinary, respiratory, or wound infections as precipitating factor.

NURSING PRIORITIES

1. Restore fluid/electrolyte balance.
2. Correct/reverse metabolic abnormalities.
3. Identify/assist with management of underlying cause/disease.
4. Prevent/control complications.

NURSING DIAGNOSIS: **Fluid Volume Deficit, actual (1).**

SUPPORTING DATA/CONTRIBUTING FACTORS: **Glucose is normally filtered in the kidney glomerulus and reabsorbed. When the renal threshold for reabsorption of glucose is reached (nor-**

mally about 180 mg/dl), it is excreted in the urine. Glucose remaining in glomerular filtrate inhibits water reabsorption, and osmotic diuresis ensues, carrying large amounts of water, sodium, potassium, and phosphates out of the body. In addition, the presence of ketones potentiates the diuresis. Continued losses/insufficient replacement may lead to hypovolemic shock state.**

GENERAL PATIENT OUTCOMES: **Blood pressure/pulse are within normal range. Blood sugar/electrolytes are within acceptable limits. Intake/output are balanced.**

INTERVENTIONS	RATIONALE
Independent	
Obtain history from patient/significant other(s) of intensity/duration of present symptoms (e.g., hyperglycemia, vomiting, excessive urination).	Assists in estimation of total volume depletion. Fluid losses will continue throughout first few hours of therapy, before metabolic control is achieved, and volume replacement estimation must be based on preexisting deficits as well as on ongoing deficits.
Monitor blood pressure and hemodynamic pressures (e.g., CVP and MAP, if available). Note postural hypotension, decreased pulse pressure.	Hypovolemia is invariably associated with hyperglycemia and may cause severe hypotension. Estimates of severity of hypovolemia may be made when patient's systolic blood pressure drops more than 10 mmHg on position change from recumbent to sitting and standing positions. Continued hypotension may indicate insufficient fluid replacement/or cardiac complication (e.g., acute myocardial infarction).
Note signs of dehydration; for example, poor skin turgor, dry mucous membranes, thirst, tachycardia, weak/thready/easily obliterated pulses, delayed capillary refill, decreased urine output.	Presence/combination of symptoms assists in estimation of fluid deficit/replacement needs.
Record hourly intake/output and specific gravity during acute phase.	Provides ongoing estimates of volume replacement needs and evaluates ability of kidney to concentrate urine.
Weigh daily.	Provides best assessment of current fluid status and adequacy of fluid replacement.
Note complaints of nausea, abdominal pain; presence of vomiting, gastric dilatation.	Dehydration/electrolyte deficits alter gastric motility/function, frequently resulting in vomiting and potentiating the fluid/electrolyte losses.
Collaborative	
Assist with insertion of intravenous (IV)/pressure moni-	Facilitates fluid volume management. Central line or

INTERVENTIONS	RATIONALE
Collaborative	
toring lines.	large peripheral vein is preferred for rapid infusion of large amounts of fluid.
Administer fluids as indicated:	
0.9 percent normal saline, 0.45 percent normal saline, 0.45 percent normal saline with 5 percent dextrose.	Large amounts of fluids are given initially to restore/to maintain intravascular volume and renal blood flow and to reduce serum osmolality. Rapid infusion of at least one liter within the first hour replaces approximately one third of extracellular deficit in the average adult patient. Normal saline is usually given initially to reverse hyperosmolar state. Thereafter, choice of fluids depends on patient's changing needs.
Albumin, plasma, dextran.	Plasma expanders occasionally may be needed in the presence of severe fluid depletion/shock if blood pressure does not respond to crystalloid fluid restoration.
Insert indwelling catheter.	Provides method for accurate, ongoing measurement of output during acute phase. Note: Lengthy use of the catheter is undesirable because of risk of infection.
Monitor laboratory studies; for example,	
Hematocrit (Hct),	Hematocrit is often very elevated owing to the hemoconcentration that occurs with dehydration.
Blood urea nitrogen (BUN)/creatinine,	Elevated BUN may reflect cellular breakdown from dehydration or point to the onset of kidney failure. The creatinine will be elevated in both instances.
Serum osmolality,	Remains elevated owing to hyperglycemia and dehydration.
Sodium,	May be low, reflecting urinary sodium loss occurring with osmotic diuresis, or dilution secondary to hyperglycemia. High sodium values reflect decreased glomerular filtration, resulting from severe fluid loss/dehydration, and sodium reabsorption in response to aldosterone secretion (response to dehydration).
Potassium.	Loss of intracellular potassium (owing to acidosis) in conjunction with increased urinary losses results in an overall deficit which may not be apparent until fluid resuscitation reverses potassium shifts. (Refer to Nursing Diagnosis: Cardiac Output, page 246.)
Insert nasogastric tube and connect to suction as indicated.	Decompresses stomach/abdominal distention and relieves vomiting.

NURSING DIAGNOSIS:	**Nutrition, alteration in, less than body requirements.**
SUPPORTING DATA/CONTRIBUTING FACTORS:	**Insulin deficiency is the prime precipitating factor in DKA, coupled with an**

excess of counterregulatory hormones (e.g., epinephrine, cortisol, growth hormones). If insulin is not available in sufficient amounts, glucose cannot be transported across cell membranes and therefore remains in the blood. The body begins to break down fat (lipolysis) to obtain energy for metabolic needs and accelerates because insulin is insufficient to inhibit it. These processes result in depletion of cellular protein/fat stores/liver glycogen. In addition, gastrointestinal (GI) symptoms such as anorexia, nausea/vomiting, inhibit intake.

GENERAL PATIENT OUTCOMES:	**Glucose/insulin balance is restored with serum glucose within/approaching normal range and serum acetone negative. Fat and protein catabolism (ketosis) is reversed and acidosis corrected as evidenced by pH/HCO_3 within normal limits.**

INTERVENTIONS	RATIONALE
Independent	
Auscultate bowel sounds. Note complaints of nausea, abdominal pain, presence of vomiting. Maintain nothing-by-mouth (NPO) status as indicated.	Hyperglycemia and fluid/electrolyte imbalances often decrease gastric motility/function, resulting in distention/ileus formation.
Provide liquids containing carbohydrates and electrolytes as soon as patient can retain/tolerate oral fluids.	When patient is alert and bowel function restored, beverages containing carbohydrates and potassium may be given to assist in reduction of IV rate and correction of electrolyte deficit.
Monitor urine sugar.	It is expected that urine sugar will remain elevated while blood sugar is decreasing; however, urine sugar of less than 1% may indicate hypoglycemia and the need for evaluation of serum glucose.
Monitor urine ketones.	Indicator of fat/protein breakdown. Decreasing ketone levels reflect reestablishment of carbohydrate metabolism.
Observed for signs of hypoglycemia; for example, changes in level of consciousness, dilated pupils, yawning, cool/clammy skin, circumoral pallor, rapid strong pulse. If patient responsive, may note behavioral changes, irritability/anxiety; complaints of headache, lightheadedness, visual disturbance; trembling hands/shakiness.	Once carbohydrate metabolism is reestablished, reduction of blood glucose levels may accelerate, resulting in hypoglycemia. If patient is comatose, this change may occur without notable change in level of consciousness. In addition, if clinical signs suggest hypoglycemia in spite of reported blood glucose elevation, Somogyi effect should be considered.

INTERVENTIONS	RATIONALE
Collaboratives	
Perform finger-stick glucose monitoring.	Bedside analysis of serum glucose levels is more accurate than urine sugar analysis which is a reflection of a previous blood glucose level.
Monitor/graph serial laboratory studies; for example,	
Serum glucose,	Blood sugar should decrease slowly with fluid and insulin administration.
Insulin,	Levels will rise if therapy is effective and insulin-resistant diabetes is not present.
Serum acetone, pH, HCO_3.	With the administration of sufficient insulin to utilize glucose instead of fat for cellular energy, the release of free fatty acids ceases, and acetone decreases/acidosis is corrected.
Administer insulin by continuous or intermittent IV infusion.	Regular insulin has a rapid onset and quickly promotes transport of glucose into cells. Intravenous method is preferred because absorption may be erratic by subcutaneous method if volume depletion/peripheral vasoconstriction is present. Insulin drip is usually discontinued when serum glucose nears 200 in order to prevent hypoglycemia.
Administer glucose solutions (e.g., 5 percent dextrose/0.45 normal saline).	Glucose solutions are added after insulin and fluid therapy lower blood sugar to approximately 250 mg/dl. As carbohydrate metabolism accelerates, care must be exercised to avoid hypoglycemia.
Administer sodium bicarbonate IV as indicated.	Usually not required unless acidosis is severe/life-threatening, necessitating more rapid correction than by fluid replacement/insulin administration.
Refer to dietician when intake is resumed.	Facilitates calculation of current/replacement nutritional needs, including use of hyperalimentation if condition warrants. (Refer to Care Plan: Nutritional Support, page 367.)

NURSING DIAGNOSIS:	**Cardiac Output, alteration in, decreased [potential].**
SUPPORTING DATA/CONTRIBUTING FACTORS:	**Fluid losses/shifts decrease circulating volume (preload), hypoxia (in combination with acidosis) alters systemic vascular resistance, lowering venous return (preload/afterload). Potassium imbalance negatively affects cardiac conduction/function. Any or all of these may decrease cardiac output (CO) and tissue perfusion.**

GENERAL PATIENT OUTCOMES:	Vital signs and CO within patient normals. Peripheral pulses palpable, of good quality; appropriate capillary refill. Dysrhythmias are controlled/prevented.

INTERVENTIONS	RATIONALE
Independent	
Monitor vital signs and hemodynamic parameters as indicated (e.g., PAP, PWCP, CO).	Heart rate will elevate initially to compensate for decreased CO. Severity of symptoms may warrant invasive monitoring to assess cardiac function/response to therapy.
Note skin color/temperature, capillary refill. Palpate peripheral pulses.	Pallor, cool/clammy skin; delayed capillary refill; weak/thready peripheral pulses suggest decreased CO/peripheral perfusion.
Monitor cardiac rhythm continuously.	Early detection/treatment of dysrhythmias associated with potassium imbalance may prevent compromised cardiac function/cardiac arrest. Presence of peaked T waves, loss of P wave, widened QRS, tachycardia changing to bradycardia are indicative of hyperkalemia. Inverted or flattened T waves, prolonged Q-T interval, presence of U waves suggest hypokalemia. Note: These changes can be exaggerated on a cardiac monitor and may be better evaluated on a 12-lead ECG.
Monitor hourly urine output, note color/specific gravity.	Although polyuria/osmotic diuresis is usual, falling output/concentrated urine suggests decrease in renal perfusion/cardiac output.
Collaborative	
Administer IV fluids as indicated.	Restoring circulating volume usually improves CO. (Refer to Nursing Diagnosis: Fluid Volume Deficit, actual (1), page 242.)
Monitor/replace serum potassium (e.g., KPO_4, KCl).	Levels may appear elevated initially as potassium shifts out of the cell owing to dehydration and acidosis. Urinary loss of potassium occurs with osmotic diuresis. As patient is rehydrated, adequate insulin provided, and acidosis corrected, potassium reenters the cell and serum deficit is evident. Replacement therapy should commence upon restoration/verification of renal function. Note: Potassium phosphate (KPO_4) may be drug of choice to prevent chloride excess when sodium chloride is used for fluid replacement.

NURSING DIAGNOSIS:	Breathing Pattern, ineffective (potential).

SUPPORTING DATA/CONTRIBUTING FACTORS:	**Respiratory compensation for metabolic acidosis is rapid/deep/labored respirations (Kussmaul's). Respiratory pattern also can be altered by general weakness/muscle paralysis secondary to electrolyte imbalances (e.g., hypokalemia) affecting ventilation and airway clearance. These changes in pattern potentiate the risks of atelectasis, hypoxia, and respiratory failure.**
GENERAL PATIENT OUTCOMES:	**Respiratory rate within patient norm; free of dyspnea/cyanosis, with arterial blood gases (ABGs) within normal limits.**

INTERVENTIONS	RATIONALE
Independent	
Note Kussmaul breathing and "acetone breath." Monitor for periods of apnea.	Lungs remove carbonic acid by venting carbon dioxide, producing a compensatory respiratory alkalosis (Kussmaul breathing). Fruity odor (acetone breath) is due to spontaneous breakdown of acetoacetic acid and should disappear as ketotic state is corrected. Note: Regular periods of apnea may develop with Kussmaul breathing.
Monitor respiratory rate/character. Note use of accessory muscles, presence of cyanosis.	Correction of elevated glucose levels and acidosis will be manifested by a return to more normal breathing pattern. However, increased work of breathing, shallow/rapid respirations, and presence of cyanosis may indicate worsening acidosis/impending respiratory failure.
Auscultate breath sounds, note rhonchi/crackles.	Rhonchi suggests accumulation of secretions and may reflect pneumonia (a precipitating factor/complication of DKA). Pulmonary edema may result from rapid fluid replacement/cardiac decompensation.
Reposition and encourage cough at least every 2 hours.	Aids in ventilating all lung segments and mobilization/clearing of secretions.
Assess mentation/sensorium.	Changes in level of consciousness can be due to multiple factors (e.g., hyperglycemia with fluid shifts, acidosis, decreased perfusion) and therefore may not be "diagnostic" for hypoxia. However, presence of stupor/coma increases risk of aspiration/compromised airway.
Suction airway as indicated.	Patient may be unable to clear airway adequately of thickened secretions.

INTERVENTIONS	RATIONALE
Collaborative	
Monitor/graph serial ABGs.	Useful in assessing therapy needs/effectiveness and developing complications.
Administer supplemental oxygen. Assist with intubation/ventilation as indicated.	Supplemental oxygen is useful for treatment of hypoxia while awaiting correction of metabolic acidosis. Mechanical ventilation is usually not required if acute acidosis and electrolyte imbalances are corrected but may be necessary in severe respiratory depression.
Administer sodium bicarbonate, if indicated.	May be required to correct severe acidosis, thus reducing respiratory effort.

NURSING DIAGNOSIS: **Infection, potential for.**

SUPPORTING DATA/CONTRIBUTING FACTORS: **Frequently, DKA may be precipitated by infection. If the infection is not identified and/or treated appropriately, sepsis may develop. In addition, high glucose levels, decreased leukocyte function, and alterations in circulation potentiate risk of nosocomial infections.**

GENERAL PATIENT OUTCOMES: **Free of chills/fever. Absence of purulent drainage/discharge and signs of inflammation. Urine is clear.**

INTERVENTIONS	RATIONALE
Independent	
Observe for signs of infection/inflammation (e.g., fever, purulent sputum, or cloudy, odorous urine).	Patient may be admitted with infection that was not identified/treated previously (precipitating ketoacidotic state). Patients also may develop a nasocomial infection due to increased susceptibility secondary to disease process.
Maintain aseptic technique for inserting/administering IV solutions/medications and providing site care.	High glucose content of blood presents a rich growth medium for infecting organisms.
Provide periodic catheter/perineal care.	Minimizes risk of urinary tract infection in catheterized patient. Note: Comatose patient already may be at risk if urinary retention occurred prior to admission.
Change positions frequently. Encourage/assist with coughing, deep breathing if patient is alert. Suction with sterile technique as indicated.	Prevents stasis of secretions with increased risk of infection.
Provide meticulous skin care. Massage/pad bony prominences. Keep skin dry. Reposition frequently. Use "egg crate" mattress, sheepskin.	Peripheral circulation may be impaired, placing patient at risk for skin irritation/breakdown.

INTERVENTIONS	RATIONALE
Collaborative	
Obtain specimens for culture/sensitivity.	Identifies infecting agent and appropriate drug therapy.
Administer antibiotics as indicated.	Early treatment may prevent spread of infection/development of sepsis. (Refer to Care Plan: Sepsis/Septicemia/Septic Shock, page 329.)

Hyperglycemic Hyperosmolar Nonketotic Coma (HHNC)

Coma/near-coma state due to marked hyperglycemia, hyperosmolarity, hypernatremia and dehydration. Differentiated from DKA by absence of ketosis and related acidosis.

PATIENT ASSESSMENT DATA BASE

HISTORY

Patient is typically age 50 or over, is a Type II, noninsulin dependent diabetic (NIDDM), and may have underlying cardiovascular or renal disease. However, HHNC can occur in patients with no previous diagnosis of diabetes.

Patient usually has major concomitant illness/precipitating factor; for example, gram-negative sepsis, myocardial infarction, pneumonia, gastrointestinal (GI) bleed, pylonephritis, pancreatitis.

Trauma and fluid loss, such as occur with burns or major surgery, may cause previously undiagnosed diabetic to become hyperglycemic and hyperosmolar.

Peritoneal dialysis with hypertonic glucose solution or hyperalimentation may place patient at risk for glucose overload.

Drugs: immunosuppressive drugs, thiazide diuretics, Dilantin, Inderal, and cimetidine are among those thought to either impair or to reduce the release of endogenous insulin.

Subjective

Historian may report that patient complained of polydipsia, polyuria, increasing confusion, loss of ability to care for self preceding onset of coma.

PHYSICAL EXAMINATION

Inspection

Mentation: may range from confusion and lethargy to stupor, coma.

Neuromuscular: hyperreflexia, hemiparesis, focal seizures.

Skin may be dry with poor turgor. Mucous membranes often dry, cracked, and coated.

Capillary refill: delayed.

Cardiac dysrhythmias may be seen on monitor, reflecting electrolyte imbalance or underlying cardiac disease.

Respiration: tachypnea usually present without Kussmaul respirations. Acetone odor on breath is absent. (Notable difference between HHNC and DKA.)

Urine output: polyuria is an early sign; however, oliguria may be present as a result of dehydration.

Auscultation

Blood pressure: hypotension/postural hypotension usually present.

Bowel sounds are diminished in approximately one half of patients, reflecting decreased motility/ileus.

Palpation

Pulse is usually rapid, with weak, easily obliterated peripheral pulses, owing to hypovolemia.

Abdomen: tenderness may be noted.

DIAGNOSTIC STUDIES

Glucose: commonly greater than 900 mg/ml (higher levels than normally seen in DKA).

Serum osmolality: greater than 350 mOsm/kg.

Sodium may be normal, decreased, but more commonly elevated; related to hyperosmolality/hyperglycemia and affects of diuresis.

Potassium may be normal or elevated, although elevation actually reflects intracellular depletion.

CBC: Hematocrit level (Hct) elevated secondary to hemoconcentration. Leukocytosis may be marked.

BUN/creatinine may be elevated, with BUN disproportionately higher than creatinine reflecting prerenal azotemia.

Arterial blood gas (ABG): slight metabolic acidosis may be present with HCO_3 greater than 19 mEq/liter.

Plasma and urine ketones: absent or mild (notable difference between DKA and HHNC).

Urine sugar: elevated up to 5 percent.

NURSING PRIORITIES

1. Restore/maintain circulating volume/perfusion.
2. Correct metabolic abnormality.
3. Prevent/minimize complications.

NURSING DIAGNOSIS:	**Fluid Volume Deficit, actual (1).**
SUPPORTING DATA/CONTRIBUTING FACTORS:	**Although the precise mechanisms initiating the process are unclear, a major component in HHNC is a relative lack of insulin, which occurs because of either impaired release of insulin or reduced peripheral effectiveness of insulin. Either mechanism produces and perpetuates hyperglycemia. The excessive numbers of glucose molecules circulating in the blood create an osmotic gradient which pulls water from cells and interstitial spaces and prevents water reabsorption in the kidney tubules. An osmotic diuresis occurs with intense polyuria and glycosuria. Ensuing hypovolemia decreases renal blood flow, severely hampering the kidney's excretion of glucose. The result is worsening hyperglycemia and severe dehydration which become self-perpetuating and can lead to hypovolemic shock/death.**
GENERAL PATIENT OUTCOMES:	**Blood pressure/CVP within patient's normal limits. Urine output greater**

than 20 to 30 ml per hour with specific gravity, serum osmolality/electrolytes within normal range.

INTERVENTIONS	RATIONALE
Independent	
Note signs of dehydration: pale, cool/dry skin, poor skin turgor, delayed capillary refill, weak/thready pulse.	Manifestations of severe dehydration with depletion of total body water.
Monitor blood pressure, hemodynamic pressures, and heart rate. Note postural hypotension, decreased pulse pressure.	Assists in approximation of fluid depletion/replacement needs.
Measure hemodynamic pressures as available; for example, CVP, PAP, CO.	More accurate evaluation of fluid deficit/replacement needs and response to therapy (especially in the elderly patient).
Observe changes in sensorium. Note progress/regression of seizure activity.	Intracellular dehydration in the brain and high serum osmolality are thought to create central nervous system (CNS) dysfunction. Neurologic abnormalities are common and may be manifested by confusion, stupor, coma, focal/grand mal seizures, hemiparesis, positive Babinski signs, and muscle fasciculations. The patient can be mistakenly thought to be having a cerebral vascular accident (CVA). Note: Rapid administration of fluids can lead to water intoxication and cerebral edema.
Measure hourly intake and output; urine specific gravity.	Restoration of circulating volume precedes return of normal kidney function.
Weigh daily.	Body weight is an accurate indication of both intracellular and extracellular fluid depletion and fluid replacement needs. Weight loss from dehydration will stabilize with fluid replacement. Excessive weight gain thereafter should alert the nurse to possibility of fluid overload, cardiac/kidney failure.
Auscultate breath sounds.	Preexisting cardiovascular and/or pulmonary disease may be exacerbated by rapid administration of fluids, resulting in pulmonary congestion, pulmonary edema, and congestive heart failure.
Administer frequent mouth care. Give water if patient can swallow.	Relieves discomfort of dry mucous membranes.
Turn/reposition frequently. Massage skin, pad bony prominences.	With severe dehydration, skin and tissue ischemia can develop quickly.
Observe for abdominal pain/rigidity. Auscultate bowel sounds.	Gastric distention/ileus are associated with electrolyte deficits/dehydration and may cause vomiting, increasing fluid/electrolyte losses.
Encourage oral fluids as soon as patient can tolerate intake.	Improvement in level of consciousness and return of bowel function are indicators of readiness to begin oral intake.

INTERVENTIONS	RATIONALE
Collaborative	
Monitor laboratory studies as indicated, for example,	Reflects level of hydration and kidney function.
Hct,	Hematocrit is usually elevated, owing to hemoconcentration/severe dehydration.
Blood urea nitrogen (BUN)/creatinine,	Elevated BUN may reflect cellular breakdown from dehydration or point to the onset of kidney failure. The creatinine will be elevated in both instances.
Serum osmolality,	Remains elevated owing to hyperglycemia and dehydration.
Serum sodium.	May be low, reflecting urinary sodium loss occurring with osmotic diuresis or dilution secondary to hyperglycemia. High sodium values reflect decreased glomerular filtration of sodium, resulting from severe fluid loss/dehydration and sodium reabsorption in response to aldosterone secretion (response to dehydration).
Administer intravenous (IV) solutions, for example, 0.45 percent normal saline,	Quantity of fluid needed for replacement is obviously variable, but the patient may have lost 20 to 25 percent of total body water. After water deficit has been estimated, half of this amount is frequently administered over first 12 hours (may be as much as 5 to 6 liters) and the remainder over next 24 hours.
Dextrose and water solutions,	When serum glucose nears 250 to 300 mg or osmolality nears 300 mOsm/kg, glucose is added to prevent hypoglycemia.
Albumin, plasma.	Volume expanders may be needed if blood pressure does not respond to fluid restoration.
Insert/maintain indwelling urinary catheter.	Provides accurate measurement of output.

NURSING DIAGNOSIS:	**Cardiac Output, alteration in, decreased.**
SUPPORTING DATA/CONTRIBUTING FACTORS:	**Severe dehydration/hypovolemia results in reduced CO. Cardiac dysrhythmias can occur secondary to acid-base and electrolyte imbalance, which may also be life-threatening.**
GENERAL PATIENT OUTCOMES:	**Vital signs, hemodynamic measurements within patient norms. Absence of dysrhythmias.**

INTERVENTIONS	RATIONALE
Independent	
Monitor hemodynamic pressures, for example, MAP, CVP, PAP, CO.	Evaluates circulating volume/cardiac response to fluid replacement.
Assess peripheral perfusion, note presence of pale, cool/clammy skin, delayed capillary refill, reduced peripheral pulses.	Vasconstriction is a compensatory mechanism to maintain perfusion of essential organs when CO is decreased and may warn of impending hypovolemic shock.
Monitor electrocardiogram (ECG)/document dysrhythmias.	Dysrhythmias may compromise CO, cause cardiac arrest.
Note ECG pattern changes; for example, peaked T waves, loss of P wave, and widened QRS.	Changes indicative of hyperkalemia. Potassium moves out of cells in response to acidosis, which elevates serum levels and may be seen in early stages of HHNC.
Inverted or flattened T waves, peaked P waves, prolonged Q-T interval, development of U waves.	Changes indicative of hypokalemia. Potassium level falls owing to osmotic diuresis, hemodilution as fluids are administered, and correction of acidosis.
Note urinary output/specific gravity.	Renal perfusion/urinary output is sacrificed until CO improves.
Collaborative	
Administer volume expanders; for example, dextran, albumin, isotonic saline.	Restores CO by rapid reexpansion of circulating volume in profound dehydration/shock. Note: Overzealous use may cause cerebral edema.
Monitor potassium levels frequently.	May at first appear elevated as potassium shifts into the vascular compartment during cellular dehydration and catabolism. Urinary losses of potassium occur during the osmotic diuresis. A net serum loss of potassium becomes apparent when the patient is rehydrated and potassium reenters the cells.
Administer potassium replacement (e.g., KCl).	Administration of supplements should begin as soon as urine output is established (at least 30 ml per hour), especially if serum levels are low or "normal."

NURSING DIAGNOSIS:	**Nutrition, alteration in, less than body requirements.**
SUPPORTING DATA/CONTRIBUTING FACTORS:	**Insulin production is not adequate for cellular utilization of the glucose load but is sufficient to inhibit lipolysis. Peripheral utilization of glucose declines while the liver increases release of glucagon in an attempt to meet energy needs. As a result, marked hyperglycemia develops without the accompany-**

	ing ketosis seen in diabetic ketoacidosis (DKA).
GENERAL PATIENT OUTCOMES:	**Blood sugar returns to normal range.**

INTERVENTIONS	RATIONALE
Independent	
Observe for signs/symptoms of hypoglycemia during rehydration; for example, no improvement/ deterioration in level of consciousness, dilated pupils, yawning, cool/clammy skin, rapid pulse, tremors. If patient is responsive, may note behavioral changes, irritability/anxiety; c/o headache, light-headedness, visual disturbance, tremors.	Patients tend to be sensitive to administration of exogenous insulin and may progress rapidly into hypoglycemia without noticeable change in sensorium.
Monitor urine sugar/ketones.	Urine sugar may remain elevated while blood sugar is decreasing; however, urine sugar of 1 percent or less may indicate developing hypoglycemia. Ketones should remain trace or negative inasmuch as this is a nonketoacidotic state.
Provide oral food/fluids as appropriate.	When patient is alert and bowel function is restored, feedings may begin.
Collaborative	
Monitor serial blood sugar/insulin levels. Perform finger-stick glucose checks.	Glucose levels may decrease rapidly with rehydration and use of insulin, requiring reduction/alteration in therapy to prevent hypoglycemia and cerebral edema. Bedside blood glucose monitoring is a relatively simple technique that provides a more accurate measurement of the current glucose level than does urine testing, which reflects previous blood sugar levels.
Administer short-acting, regular insulin, via intermittent/continuous IV infusion.	Insulin should be given judiciously because patients have some endogenous production and may be quite sensitive to exogenous insulin. Subcutaneous administration is not recommended initially because tissue perfusion/absorption may be reduced. After rehydration, insulin therapy may not be essential if patient has adequate endogenous insulin production and is not insulin-resistent.
Administer IV glucose solutions as indicated.	As serum glucose nears 250 mg/dl, glucose is added to prevent development of hypoglycemia.
Consult dietician/nutritional support team for review of caloric needs of patients with hypermetabolic state/ nutritional support and effectiveness of current diet therapy.	Patients with preexisting conditions that are debilitating to the body (e.g., burns, severe infections, recent surgery) may already be on high-calorie diets/total parenteral nutrition (precipitator of HHNC). Alterations in therapy may be required. (Refer to Care Plan: Nutritional Support, page 367.)

NURSING DIAGNOSIS:	**Sensory-Perceptual Alteration [potential].**
SUPPORTING DATA/CONTRIBUTING FACTORS:	**Cerebral impairment is believed to be the result of intracellular dehydration of the brain. Disturbances in electrolyte balance and oxygen delivery also may account for altered sensorium. Cerebral edema can occur with too rapid a fall in serum osmolality, causing fluid to shift into the brain intracellularly and resulting in swelling and neurologic abnormalities.**
GENERAL PATIENT OUTCOMES:	**Level of consciousness is improved/ maintained.**

INTERVENTIONS	RATIONALE
Independent	
Assess changes in level of consciousness; for example, response to stimuli, pupil reaction, and movement of extremities. Note transient improvement in mental status with relapse to coma.	Rapidly declining glucose levels may result in change from hyperglycemia coma to hypoglycemic state without notable difference/permanent improvement in level of consciousness.
Monitor for seizure activity; provide safety measures (e.g., side rails, soft restraints) as required.	Seizures may occur owing to cerebral dehydration secondary to elevated glucose levels, cerebral edema during rapid rehydration, and cellular deprivation of glucose in the presence of hypoglycemia.
Provide for airway protection using adjuncts as needed; suction secretions as necessary, keep head of bed elevated.	Patient is at risk for aspiration of secretions/ pneumonia.
Explain procedures; orient to time, place, events; provide tactile stimulation as care is given.	Hearing may be intact in coma. Sensory stimulation (e.g., talk, touch) provides reassurance needed by patient. As level of consciousness improves, these measures may reduce anxiety/confusion.
Collaborative	
Monitor fluid administration, blood sugar, electrolytes, serum osmolality.	Cerebral edema may be avoided by attention to rate of fluid replacement, slow reduction of hyperglycemia and serum osmolality.

Thyroid Crisis/Storm

A state in which the strain of hyperthyroidism results in a life-threatening situation.

PATIENT ASSESSMENT DATA BASE

HISTORY

Family history of hyperthyroid states. Women more susceptible than men.

History of hypothyroidism with thyroid hormone replacement or antithyroid therapy with premature withdrawal of drugs. Overtreatment or overdose of thyroid drugs.

Diagnosed nodular toxic goiter, pituitary tumor, or adrenocortical insufficiency.

Recent thyroidectomy for nodules, cancer, toxic adenomas; past irradiation thyroiditis.

Recent stressful situation, such as trauma (emotional/physical).

Less common precipitators of thyrotoxicosis are pregnancy/childbirth/cesarean section, infection (especially pulmonary), prolonged exposure to cold, recent x-ray contrast studies, cardiac disorders, pulmonary embolus, and cerebral vascular accident (CVA).

Diabetic ketoacidosis will enhance danger from, but not susceptibility to, thyroid storm.

Subjective

May note palpations, chest pain, dyspnea, and fatigue/weakness.

Report weight loss despite well-maintained or increased appetite.

May complain of nausea/vomiting; large, frequent stools; polyuria.

May report menstrual disturbances (e.g., amenorrhea).

Complaints of nervousness, emotional lability, insomnia, weakness are common.

May report heat intolerance, excessive sweating, unexplained temperature elevations.

May report accelerated mental activity with loss of control of thoughts/ideas, presence of visual/auditory hallucinations, and fears of insanity.

PHYSICAL EXAMINATION

Clinical manifestations vary, depending on severity of present hyperthyroid activity, patient's age, and/or underlying disease/precipitating factors. Associated deterioration of cardiovascular, central venous, and gastrointestinal systems may lead to coma/circulatory collapse.

Inspection

Mental status: wide range of response; for example, agitation, hyperactive behavior (e.g., nervous picking at clothing/bedding, restless/thrashing about) or lethargy, stupor, and coma.

Speech: may be rapid, high-pitched, excitable. Hoarseness may be noted if vocal cords are compressed by enlarged thyroid.

Eyes: may demonstrate exophthalmia; for example, characteristic wide-eyed stare, infrequent blink, lid lag, difficulty in gazing upward, and/or papilledema.

Skin: usually smooth, warm, and flushed, with excessive sweating. Excessive pigmentation may be noted in areas of edema. Poor skin tugor and dry mucous membranes may be noted.

Nails: typically soft/friable. Clubbing of fingers/toes may be noted.

Hair: usually fine and silky. Temporal hair loss may be noted.

Muscles: fine rhythmic tremors of fingers/hands, tongue, eyelids may be noted.

Respirations: tachynea may be present owing to hypermetabolic activity.

Temperature: usually elevated to 101°F/30°C—and abrupt fluctuations are common.

Palpation

Pulse: may be full/bounding, or weak/thready. Tachycardia at rest is indicative of hypermetabolic state.

Edema: localized/nonpitting edema is usually seen in legs/feet.

Reflexes: hyperreactive.

Thyroid gland: may/may not be enlarged but should not be palpated at this time owing to risk of increasing release of hormones.

Auscultation

Blood pressure: usually elevated with wide pulse pressure; may be decreased in presence of extreme vasodilation/ shock.

Heart sounds: Pronounced S_1; gallop rhythms, systolic murmurs, tachycardia, and dysrhythmias may be noted (e.g., atrial fibrillation).

Breath sounds may be clear, or rhonchi/crackles may be present, owing to cardiac failure related to hypermetabolic state.

DIAGNOSTIC STUDIES

Results of thyroid studies may be affected by numerous factors and must be correlated with clinical presentations; for example, acute hepatitis releases hepatic-bound thyroid hormone. Values may be altered by other factors as well; for example, recent isotope scan or lack of iodine in diet.

Serum thyroxine (T_4), and triiodothyronine (T_3) are usually increased. T_3 is commonly increased proportionately more than T_4.

Thyroid RAI uptake: increase reflects increase of thyroid iodide clearance. Low value RAIU (in association with signs/symptoms of thyrotoxicosis) may signal presence of thyroditis/ectopic thyroid tissue.

Calcium, phosphorus, alkaline phosphatase may be elevated.

Electrolytes: hyponatremia may reflect dilutional effect of increased water intake. Hypokalemia may be noted, owing to gastrointestinal (GI) losses and diuresis.

Glucose: hyperglycemia may result from decreased serum insulin levels and increased glycogenolysis.

Chest x-ray examination may reveal cardiac enlargement, pulmonary congestion.

NURSING DIAGNOSIS

1. Minimize/control hypermetabolic symptoms.
2. Promote comfort.
3. Minimize complications.
4. Provide emotional support.

NURSING DIAGNOSIS:	**Cardiac Output, alteration in, decreased [potential].**

SUPPORTING DATA/CONTRIBUTING FACTORS:	**A hypermetabolic state and associated marked increase in heat production increases circulatory demands. This stressor, combined with the pseudocatecholamine effects of thyroid hormone on the myocardium, can elevate cardiac output (CO) as much as twice normal levels, leading to a high-output failure state. In addition, decreased circulating volume may occur, owing to vomiting, diarrhea, and severe diaphoresis, which reduces venous return and compromises CO.**
GENERAL PATIENT OUTCOMES:	**Vital signs and hemodynamic pressures are within patient norms. Peripheral pulses palpable and of good quality. Breath sounds clear.**

INTERVENTIONS	RATIONALE
Independent	
Monitor blood pressure (BP) lying/sitting and standing, if able. Note widened pulse pressure.	General/orthostatic hypotension may occur as a result of excessive peripheral vasodilation and decreased circulating volume. Widened pulse pressure reflects increased stroke volume and decreased systemic vascular resistance (SVR).
Monitor hemodynamic parameters as available CVP/PAP, PCWP, CO, SVR.	Provides information regarding cardiac function and response to drug therapy and identifies developing complications (e.g., cardiac failure). Note: In some patients, use of beta-blocking agents may limit adrenergic stimulation necessary for optimal cardiac function, potentiating cardiac failure.
Investigate complaints of chest pain/angina.	May reflect increased myocardial oxygen demands/ischemia.
Auscultate heart sounds, noting changes in S_1, development of S_3-S_4/gallops and systolic murmurs.	Prominent S_1 and murmurs are associated with increased flow state, and development of S_3 may warn of impending cardiac failure.
Monitor electrocardiogram (ECG): note rate/rhythm. Document dysrhythmias.	Tachycardia (greater than normally expected with fever/increased circulatory demand) may reflect direct myocardial stimulation by thyroid hormone. Atrial dysrhythmias and heart blocks often occur and may compromise cardiac function/output.
Auscultate breath sounds, noting adventitious sounds (e.g., crackles).	Early sign of developing cardiac failure.
Monitor temperature; provide cool environment; limit bed linens/clothes; administer tepid sponge baths.	Fever (may exceed 104°F) results in increased peripheral vasodilation, which causes venous pooling/

INTERVENTIONS	RATIONALE
Independent	
	hypotension and may aggravate diuresis and dehydration.
Observe signs/symptoms of dehydration: severe thirst, dry mucous membranes, weak/thready pulse, poor capillary refill, decreased urine output, and hypotension.	Rapid dehydration can occur, which reduces circulating volume and compromises cardiac output.
Record intake/output. Note urine specific gravity. Weigh daily.	May lose significant amounts of fluid through vomiting, diarrhea, diuresis, diaphoresis. Urine concentration and weight loss are indicators of dehydration.
Encourage chair rest/bedrest, limit nonessential activity.	Activity increases metabolic/circulatory demands, which may potentiate cardiac failure.
Note history of asthma/bronchoconstrictive disease, pregnancy, sinus bradycardia/heart blocks, advanced heart failure.	Presence of these conditions contraindicate use of beta-adrenergic blocking agents.
Observe for adverse side effects of adrenergic antagonists; for example, severe decrease in pulse, BP; developing CHF; cardiac arrest.	Indicates need for reduction/discontinuation of therapy.
Collaborative	
Administer intravenous (IV) fluids as indicated.	Rapid fluid replacement may be necessary to improve circulating volume but must be balanced against signs of cardiac failure/need for inotropic support.
Administer medications as indicated:	
Beta blockers, for example, propranolol (Inderal), atenolol (Tenormin), nadolol (Corgard);	First drug of choice for acute storm. Useful in decreasing heart rate/cardiac work by blocking beta-adrenergic receptor sites and blocking conversion of T_4 to T_3. Note: If severe bradycardia develops, atropine may be required.
Thyroid hormone antagonists, for example, Prophylthiouracil (PTU),	Blocks thyroid hormone synthesis and inhibits peripheral conversion of T_4 to T_3. Effect is slow, so may not relieve the thyroid storm. Note: Once PTU therapy is begun, abrupt withdrawal may precipitate thyroid crisis.
Sodium iodine IV or super-saturated potassium iodide (SSKI) by mouth,	Inhibits thyroid hormone release, reduces vascularity, and enhances involution of thyroid gland. Should be started 1 to 3 hours after initiation of antithyroid drug therapy to minimize hormone formation from the iodine.
Methimazole (Tapazole);	Inhibits thyroid hormone synthesis. Note: Both PTU and Tapazole may be given by nasogastric tube if patient is unable to swallow/cooperate.
Corticosteroids; for example, dexamethazone (Decadron);	Provides glucocorticol support. Decreases hyperthermia, relieves relative adrenal insufficiency, inhibits calcium absorption, and reduces peripheral conversion of T_3 from T_4.

INTERVENTIONS	RATIONALE
Collaborative	
Digoxin (Lanoxin);	Digitalization may be required in congestive failure patients before beta-adrenergic blocking therapy can be considered/safely initiated.
Furosemide (Lasix);	Diuresis may be necessary if congestive failure occurs. Note: It also may be effective in reducing calcium level if neuromuscular function is impaired.
Acetaminophen (Tylenol);	Drug of choice to reduce temperature and associated metabolic demands. Salicylates are contraindicated because they actually increase level of circulating thyroid hormones by blocking binding of T_3-T_4 with thyroid-binding proteins.
Sedatives, barbiturates;	Promotes rest, thereby reducing metabolic demands.
Muscle relaxants.	Reduce shivering associated with hyperthermia, which can increase metabolic demands.
Monitor serum potassium, replace as indicated.	Hypokalemia resulting from intestinal losses, altered intake, or diuretic therapy may cause dysrhythmias, which compromise cardiac function/output.
Monitor serum calcium.	Elevation may alter cardiac contractility.
Review serial ECGs.	May demonstrate effects of electrolyte imbalance or ischemic changes reflecting inadequate myocardial oxygen supply in presence of increased metabolic demands.
Monitor chest x-ray examinations.	Cardiac enlargement may occur in response to increased circulatory demands. Pulmonary congestion may be noted with cardiac decompensation.
Provide supplemental oxygen as indicated.	May be necessary to meet increased metabolic demands/oxygen consumption.
Provide hypothermia blanket as indicated.	May be necessary to lower body temperature (104°F and above) to reduce metabolic demands/oxygen consumption.
Administer/assist with transfusions/plasmapheresis, dialysis as indicated. (Refer to Care Plan: Renal Dialysis, page 222.)	May be done to achieve rapid depletion of extrathyroidal hormone pool in desperately ill/comatose patient.

NURSING DIAGNOSIS: **Nutrition, alteration in, less than body requirements.**

SUPPORTING DATA/CONTRIBUTING FACTORS: **Hypermetabolism increases basic nutritional needs at a time when protein catabolism exceeds the rate of protein synthesis. This causes a negative nitrogen balance with weight/muscle mass loss. In addition, GI symptoms**

	may reduce oral intake while increased gastric motility alters absorption of nutrients.
GENERAL PATIENT OUTCOMES:	**Intake adequate to meet nutritional needs as evidenced by positive nitrogen balance, weight stabilized.**

INTERVENTIONS	RATIONALE
Independent	
Auscultate bowel sounds.	Hyperactive bowel sounds reflect increased gastric motility, which can reduce/alter absorption.
Note signs of gastric involvement; for example, nausea/vomiting, diarrhea, abdominal pain/tenderness.	May affect choice of dietary support.
Observe/record food intake. Calculate calorie count.	Although appetite is usually increased, intake is still not adequate to meet needs. Anorexia may develop as condition worsens.
Provide small/frequent feedings of easily digestible foods. Avoid caffeine and highly seasoned/fibrous foods.	Reduces gastric side effects related to hypermotility/anorexia.
Weigh daily.	Sudden weight gain/loss may reflect fluid imbalance while steady loss indicates imbalance between nutritional needs/intake.
Assess for signs/symptoms of hyperglycemia; for example, polyuria, polydipsia, nocturia, depression, lethargy, fatigue/weakness, blurring of vision, pruritis.	Increased glycogenolysis and reduced serum insulin levels occur in response to excessive thyroid hormones.
Monitor urine sugar/acetone.	Although diabetic ketoacidosis (DKA) may precipitate crisis, hyperglycemia may occur in nondiabetic patient, owing to increased level of thyroid hormones. In addition, presence of ketones suggests inadequate intake for hypermetabolic state.
Collaborative	
Provide diet high in calories/protein. Include supplemental feedings/vitamins.	Maximizes intake to meet metabolic needs. Vitamin absorption may be impaired because of increased gastric motility, and deficiencies may result.
Administer IV glucose solutions; hyperalimentation; vitamin supplements, especially B complex. (Refer to Care Plan: Nutritional Support, page 367.)	Pancreatic fatigue/hyperglycemia may occur with use of hyperalimentation solutions. However, if the patient cannot eat, IV dextrose/total parenteral nutrition provides necessaray calories. Vitamins are rapidly depleted in hypermetabolic state. B complex vitamins are essential for proper function of nervous system.
Monitor serum glucose.	Hyperglycemia may occur in response to increased glycogneolysis and decreased serum insulin levels. Symptoms of hypoglycemia may be masked by the use of beta blockers.

INTERVENTIONS	RATIONALE
Collaborative	
Administer insulin as indicated.	May be necessary to control hyperglycemia.

NURSING DIAGNOSIS:	**Breathing Pattern, ineffective [potential].**
SUPPORTING DATA/CONTRIBUTING FACTORS:	**Generalized weakness and/or actual muscle mass loss/atrophy decreases vital capacity and alters ability to maintain airway. In addition, increased oxygen consumption and carbon dioxide production results in increased respiratory rate. As the respiratory system is maximally stressed, deterioration/failure can occur.**
GENERAL PATIENT OUTCOMES:	**Respiratory rate/effort are within patient's normals. Absence of dyspnea/cyanosis. Breath sounds clear.**

INTERVENTIONS	RATIONALE
Independent	
Assess respiratory rate/depth use of accessory muscles.	Tachypnea accompanies hypermetabolic state. As oxygen needs increase, hypoxia may occur accompanied by respiratory distress.
Auscultate lungs, noting rhonchi/crackles.	May indicate pooling of secretions, congestive heart failure/fluid overload.
Note central cyanosis of lips, tongue, ear lobes.	Indicator of systemic oxygen deficit.
Encourage semi-Fowler's position.	Maximizes chest expansion and may be position of comfort if patient is dyspneic.
Reduce/limit activity. (Refer to Nursing Diagnosis: Activity Intolerance, below.)	Reduce oxygen demand/consumption.
Collaborative	
Monitor/graph serial ABGs.	Identifies oxygen needs, effectiveness of therapy.
Provide supplemental oxygen.	Provides additional oxygen to meet increased metabolic demands.

NURSING DIAGNOSIS:	**Activity Intolerance [potential].**

SUPPORTING DATA/CONTRIBUTING FACTORS:	**Hypermetabolic state and altered nutritional intake result in generalized weakness, muscle atrophy, and reduced energy levels. In addition, imbalance between oxygen demand and supply may reduce energy level/cardiopulmonary reserves.**
GENERAL PATIENT OUTCOMES:	**Verbalizes/demonstrates measurable increase in activity tolerance.**

INTERVENTIONS	RATIONALE
Independent	
Monitor physiologic response to activity; for example, BP, pulse, respiratory rate, hemodynamic pressures.	Marked alterations from baseline vital signs indicate need for reduction in activity.
Schedule activities, provide frequent rest periods.	May be chronically tired yet unable to sleep owing to hyperactive state.
Assist with self-care activities. Avoid prolonged/overlapping activities.	Conserves energy, avoids fatigue.
Provide diversional activities that are calming.	Permits constructive use of nervous energy while reducing metabolic demands.

NURSING DIAGNOSIS:	**Anxiety.**
SUPPORTING DATA/CONTRIBUTING FACTORS:	**Hypermetabolic state includes central nervous system (CNS) stimulation related to psuedocatecholamine effect of thyroid hormones. Patient may experience external symptoms (e.g., dry mouth, shakiness) as well as increased feelings of apprehension, loss of control, panic, changes in cognition which distort environmental stimuli.**
GENERAL PATIENT OUTCOMES:	**Verbalizes reduction of anxiety, understanding of etiology of emotional reaction and expected resolution.**

INTERVENTIONS	RATIONALE
Independent	
Monitor physical responses: palpitations, repetitive movements, hyperventilation, insomnia.	Increased number of beta-adrenergic receptor sites coupled with effects of excess thyroid hormones produces clinical manifestations of catecholamine excess

INTERVENTIONS	RATIONALE
Independent	
	in face of normal levels of norepinephrine/epinephrine.
Observe behavior indicative of level of anxiety.	Mild anxiety may be displayed by irritability and insomnia. Severe anxiety progressing to panic state may produce feelings of impending doom, terror, inability to speak or move, and/or shouting/swearing.
Stay with patient, maintaining calm manner. Acknowledge fear and allow patient's behavior to belong to the patient.	Affirms to patient/significant other(s), that although patient feels out of control, the environment is safe. Don't express personal responses to inappropriate remarks/actions.
Describe/explain procedures, environment or noises that may be heard by the patient.	Provides accurate information which reduces distortions, misinterpretations which can contribute to anxiety/fear reactions.
Speak in brief statements, using simple words.	Attention span may be shortened, concentration is reduced, limiting ability to comprehend/learn new information. Note: Teaching should be delayed until crisis situation is resolved.
Reduce external stimuli:	
Place in quiet room; provide soft, soothing music; reduce bright lights; reduce number of people contacting patient.	Creates a therapeutic environment, recognizing that critical care unit activity/personnel may increase patient's anxiety.
Discuss with patient/significant other(s) reasons for emotional lability/psychotic reaction. (Refer to Nursing Diagnosis: Thought Processes, below.)	Understanding that behavior is physically based can allow for different responses/approaches.
Reinforce expectation that emotional control should return as drug therapy progresses.	Provides information and reassures patient that the situation is temporary and will improve with treatment.
Collaborative	
Administer antianxiety medications (tranquilizers, sedatives) as ordered. Monitor effects.	May be used in conjunction with medical regimen to reduce hyperthyroid secretion.
Refer to support systems as needed (e.g., counseling, social services, pastoral care).	Ongoing therapy support may be desired/required by patient/significant others if crisis precipitates lifestyle alterations.

NURSING DIAGNOSIS:	**Thought Processes, alteration in [potential].**
SUPPORTING DATA/CONTRIBUTING FACTORS:	**Increased CNS stimulation/accelerated mental activity and altered sleep patterns may interfere with the patient's ability to think clearly/accurately, to interpret environment.**

GENERAL PATIENT OUTCOMES:	Adverse changes in mentation are prevented/minimized, patient alert/oriented within own norms.

INTERVENTIONS	RATIONALE
Independent	
Assess thinking processes, for example, memory, attention span, orientation to person/place/time.	Determines extent of interference with sensory processing.
Note changes in behavior.	May be hypervigilant, restless, extremely sensitive or crying, or develop frank psychosis.
Assess level of anxiety. (Refer to Nursing Diagnosis: Anxiety, page 265.)	Anxiety may alter thought processes.
Provide quiet environment: decreased stimuli, cool room, dim lights. Limit procedures/personnel.	Reduction of external stimuli may decrease hyperactivity/reflexia, CNS irritability, emotional lability, auditory/visual hallucinations.
Reorient to person/place/time. Present reality concisely and briefly without challenging illogical thinking.	Helps to establish and to maintain awareness of reality/environment. Limits defensive reaction.
Provide clock, calendar, room with outside window or alter level of lighting to simulate day/night.	Provides continual orientation cues to assist patient in maintaining sense of normalcy.
Provide safety measures; for example, padded side rails, soft restraints, close supervision.	Prevents injury to patient who may be hallucinating/disoriented.
Encourage visits by family/significant other(s). Provide support as needed.	Provides socialization and orientation. Note: Patient's agitation/psychotic behavior may precipitate family quarrels/conflicts.
Collaborative	
Administer sedatives/tranquilizers/antipsychotic medications as indicated.	Promotes relaxation, reduces CNS hyperactivity/agitation.

CHAPTER 9 ORTHOPEDIC

Fractures/Multiple Trauma

Trauma patients most likely to be cared for in the critical care setting are those with multiple system injuries, including fractures, burns, head/spinal trauma, chest injuries with cardiac/pulmonary involvement, and/or grossly contaminated wounds. This care plan addresses the patient with fractures and related complications. The nurse will be referred to related care plans for more in-depth discussion as appropriate.

PATIENT ASSESSMENT DATA BASE

HISTORY

History of traumatic event; note mechanism of injury.

History of malnutrition, previous fractures, or bone/endocrine disease which may predispose a patient to fractures.

Subjective

Pain: sudden severe pain at the time of injury may be localized to the area of tissue/skeletal damage. After immobilization of the affected part, pain may be resolved, or patient may experience muscle spasms/cramping. Severe pain after immobilization frequently indicates complications. If there is severe nerve damage, the patient may have no pain at all. Paresthesia (numbness, tingling) is commonly present.

Function: loss of function of affected part may be immediate owing to the fracture(s), or immobilization and tissue swelling.

PHYSICAL EXAMINATION

Symptoms vary and depend on site, severity, and type of fracture, as well as on damage to other structures (e.g., tissues/blood vessels/internal organs).

Inspection

Mentation: agitation may be related to pain/anxiety; confusion/disorientation may reflect decreased oxygenation/cerebral perfusion or effects of drugs/alcohol; coma is suggestive of concomitant head injury. (Refer to Care Plan: Brain Injury/Increased Intracranial Pressure, page 127.)

Respirations: tachypnea with increased work of breathing/dyspnea, asymmetrical chest movement, and presence of pallor/cyanosis suggest presence of chest trauma. (Refer to Care Plan: Hemothorax and Pneumothorax, page 88.)

Abdomen: contusions/abrasions, and occasionally distention, may suggest internal organ damage requiring further evaluation/observation.

Renal: presence of hematuria/anuria may indicate injury to bladder/kidney.

Neuromuscular: complete loss of motion/sensation may suggest spinal cord injury. (Refer to Care Plan: Spinal Cord Injury: Acute Phase, page 155.) Local deformities; for example, abnormal angulation, shortening, rotation, crepitation (grating sound), muscle spasms, visible weakness/loss of function, indicate fracture.

Skin: lacerations, tissue avulsion, bleeding may be present. Color changes, (e.g., pallor, bruising, and slow capillary refill) may be noted.

Edema: localized swelling is usually present and may increase gradually or suddenly.

Auscultation

Blood pressure may be normal; presence of hypotension may be related to blood loss; hypertension is occasionally seen as a response to pain/anxiety.

Heart sounds: tachycardia may reflect stress response or may suggest hypovolemia; dysrhythmias may occur because of myocardial injury, or ischemia related to shock state.

Breath sounds: areas of inequality/absence may reflect direct injury/loss of respiratory integrity.

Bowel sounds: diminished/absence suggests intra-abdominal injury.

Palpation

Pulse may be reduced/absent distal to local injury. General weak or thready pulses reflect hypovolemia.

Edema: tissue swelling, hematoma mass may/may not be noted at site(s) of injury.

Abdomen: tension/tenderness suggests internal involvement.

DIAGNOSTIC STUDIES

CBC: Hct may be increased (hemoconcentration) or decreased (anemia), signifying hemorrhage at the fracture site or distant organs (in multiple trauma). Increased WBC is a normal response following trauma.

Creatinine: muscle trauma increases load of creatinine for renal clearance.

Electrolytes: dilutional alterations may occur owing to blood loss with rapid fluid resuscitation.

ABGs: changes in blood gases and pH must be evaluated in the light of overall assessment and may be a response to stress, or reflect respiratory system injury/compromise.

Coagulation profile: alterations may occur owing to blood loss, multiple transfusions, or liver injury.

X-ray examinations: determine location/extent of fractures/trauma.

Bone scans visualize fractures/loss of bone.

Arteriograms may be done if vascular damage is suspected.

NURSING PRIORITIES

Nursing priorities in the multiple trauma patient will be dependent on the extent of systemic injuries, which are addressed in related care plans. These priorities focus on orthopedic trauma.

1. Prevent further bone/tissue injury.
2. Relieve/prevent pain.
3. Minimize complications and promote healing.

NURSING DIAGNOSIS:	**Injury, potential for trauma [additional].**
SUPPORTING DATA/CONTRIBUTING FACTORS:	**Loss of skeletal integrity (fractures) places patient at risk for further vascular, nerve, and soft-tissue damage. Instability of the fracture also may result in misalignment, delayed healing or nonunion of bone.**
GENERAL PATIENT OUTCOMES:	**Fracture is stabilized and alignment maintained. Further injury is avoided.**

INTERVENTIONS	RATIONALE
Independent: Skeletal Traction	
Maintain position/integrity of traction (e.g., Hoffman's, Buck's, Dunlop, Pearson).	Skeletal traction is used in fractures of the major long bones because it permits use of greater weight for traction pull than can be applied to skin tissues. A Steinman pin or Kirschner wire may be used as the traction source, depending on the bone that is fractured, the severity of the fracture, and the amount of displacement.
Ascertain that all clamps are functional. Lubricate pulleys, and check ropes for fraying. Secure and wrap knots with adhesive tape.	Assures that traction set-up is functioning properly to avoid interruption of fracture approximation.
Keep ropes nonobstructed and weights hanging free. Avoid lifting/releasing weights.	Optimal amount of traction weight is maintained. Note: Assisting with free movement of weights during repositioning of patient avoids excess pull on fracture with associated pain and muscle spasm.
Assist with placement of lifts under bed wheels if indicated.	Helps maintain proper patient position, aids the function of the traction by providing counter balance.
Position the patient so that appropriate pull is maintained on the *long axis* of the bone.	Promotes bone alignment and reduces complications (e.g., nonunion, delayed healing).
Monitor position/location of supporting ring of splints/ sling.	Traction apparatus can cause pressure on vessels/ nerves, particularly in the axilla and groin, resulting in ischemia and possible permanent nerve damage.
Assist with application/maintain skin traction device, if used (e.g., adhesive/elastic bandage wrap). Assess all skin surfaces to be placed in traction. Cleanse skin and pad appropriately.	Maintains position of traction apparatus without altering skin and soft-tissue integrity. Clean dry surface is necessary for proper application of traction. Padding may be needed in areas of skin abrasions/open wounds.
Independent: Casts/Splints	
Support fracture site with pillows/folded blankets. Maintain neutral position of affected part with trochanter roll, sandbags, splints, footboard.	Prevents unnecessary movement and promotes proper alignment/healing.

INTERVENTIONS	RATIONALE
Independent	
Evaluate splinted extremity for resolution of edema.	Coaptation splint (e.g., Jones/Sugar Tong) may be used to provide immobilization of fracture while excessive tissue swelling is present. As edema subsides, increased mobility may occur, requiring readjustment of splint or application of plaster cast.

NURSING DIAGNOSIS:	**Comfort, alteration in, pain [acute].**
SUPPORTING DATA/CONTRIBUTING FACTORS:	**Movement of bone fragments, edema, and injury to the soft tissue may cause severe pain. Other factors that may hamper a patient's comfort include stress, anxiety, traction/immobility, complications.**
GENERAL PATIENT OUTCOMES:	**Verbalizes relief of pain, demonstrates relaxed manner, able to sleep/rest appropriately.**

INTERVENTIONS	RATIONALE
Independent	
Elevate injured extremity, support with pillows. Avoid use of plastic sheets/pillows under casted limbs.	Promotes venous return, decreases edema, and may reduce pain. Plastic pads/covered pillows can increase discomfort by enhancing heat production in the drying cast.
Apply cold/ice pack first 24 hours and as necessary.	Reduces edema/hematoma formation, decreases pain sensation.
Investigate complaints of pain/discomfort. Observe skin areas under cast edges/traction apparatus. Pad areas as indicated.	Pain may indicate improper position/fitting of cast/traction, or tissue irritation related to presence of debris, wrinkles, and so forth in cast or traction padding.
Provide massage, back rub, position changes.	Improves general circulation, reduces areas of local pressure and muscle fatigue.
Perform and supervise active/passive range of motion exercises.	Maintains strength/mobility of unaffected muscles and facilitates resolution of inflammation in injured tissues.
Instruct in/encourage use of trapeze and "post" position.	Facilitates movement during hygiene/skin care, linen changes, and so forth and reduces discomfort of remaining flat in bed. Post position involves placing the uninjured foot flat on the bed with the knee bent while grasping the trapeze and lifting body off the bed.
Explain procedures prior to beginning them.	Allows patient to prepare mentally for activity as well as to participate in controlling level of discomfort.

INTERVENTIONS	RATIONALE
Independent	
Investigate/document any complaints of different/sudden pain or unrelieved pressure.	May signal a developing complication; for example, infection, tissue ischemia, compartmental syndrome. (Refer to Nursing Diagnosis: Tissue Perfusion, page 275.)
Collaborative	
Maintain immobilization of affected part by means of bedrest, cast, splint, traction. (Refer to Nursing Diagnosis: Injury, potential for trauma [additional], page 271; Skin Integrity, impairment of [actual/potential], page 281.)	Relieves pain and prevents bone displacement/extension of tissue injury.
Administer analgesics/muscle relaxants, especially before procedures/care activities.	Given to reduce pain and/or muscle spasms if the patient did not sustain a concomitant head injury. Note: Narcotic analgesics (e.g., codeine, Demerol, morphine) may be given around the clock for several days to maintain blood level of analgesia. Hydroxyzine pamoate (Vistaril) may be used to potentiate effects of narcotics to improve/to prolong pain relief.

NURSING DIAGNOSIS: **Fluid Volume Deficit, potential.**

SUPPORTING DATA/CONTRIBUTING FACTORS: **Blood loss from fracture(s), direct vascular injury, soft-tissue trauma, intra-abdominal organ trauma, and/or gastric hemorrhage (stress ulcer) may result in hypovolemia significant enough to cause a shock state. In addition, activation of clotting cycle, or repeated transfusions of blood depleted of clotting factors, may result in coagulopathy (DIC), which further compromises circulating volume.**

GENERAL PATIENT OUTCOMES: **Circulating volume is maintained as evidenced by blood pressure, pulse within normal range, urine output adequate for individual situation.**

INTERVENTIONS	RATIONALE
Independent	
Assess heart/respiratory rate, blood pressure, and skin color/temperature frequently.	In the otherwise healthy adult trauma victim, tachycardia and tachypnea may be the only signs of shock until just prior to decompensation. Hypotension with narrowing pulse pressure, tachycardia, weak/thready

INTERVENTIONS	RATIONALE
Independent	
	pulse, and peripheral vasoconstriction are indicative of severe hypovolemia and impending shock.
Measure hemodynamic pressures if available; for example, CVP, PAP, MAP, CO.	Documents trends in fluid balance and response to therapy.
Measure intake/output. Note urine color and specific gravity.	Renal function may be decreased as a result of trauma or may reflect a compensatory stress response to hemorrhage. Dark amber, concentrated urine of less than 20 to 30 ml per hour with elevated specific gravity reflects dehydration/hypovolemia. Bright red blood in the urine may suggest trauma to urinary system (early) or developing coagulapathy (later).
Observe urine for presence of myoglobin (e.g., brownish red to black color).	Increased fluid/glomerular filtration is necessary to prevent renal parenchymal damage (ATN) when myoglobin is released as a result of massive tissue trauma. (Refer to Care Plan: Acute Renal Failure, page 207.)
Monitor bleeding from open wounds. Mark area of bleeding/drainage on cast, if indicated.	Continuing blood loss suggests underlying vascular injury.
Measure injured extremity and compare with uninjured extremity. Note appearance, spread of hematoma.	Circumference of injured extremity is an indicator of tissue swelling/edema or may indicate hemorrhage into the tissues; for example, 1 inch increase in adult thigh can equal approximately 1 unit of sequestered blood.
Note abdominal tenderness, distention, worsening signs of hypovolemia/impending shock which occur in spite of adequate fluid replacement.	May indicate major intra-abdominal hemorrhage (e.g., ruptured spleen).
Guaiac stools/gastric aspirant.	High incidence of stress ulcer/gastric bleeding accompanies fractures/trauma. (Refer to Care Plan: Upper Gastrointestinal/Esophageal Bleeding, page 197.)
Note continued bleeding at trauma site(s), oozing from mucous membranes, or blood in urine.	Signs suggestive of clotting disorder requiring further investigation. (Refer to Care Plan: Disseminated Intravascular Coagulation, page 319.)
Monitor for signs of transfusion reaction/incompatibility; for example, fever, chills, flank/back/shoulder pain, chest tightness, nausea/vomiting (immediate reactions); reduced urinary output, hives, rash, itching (secondary reactions).	Reactions can occur anytime during or post transfusion and require intervention per hospital protocol.
Collaborative	
Administer intravenous (IV) solutions (usually lactated Ringer's/saline solutions), blood/blood products (whole blood, packed cells, platelets/fresh frozen plasma).	Restores circulating blood volume. Note: Rapid/multiple unit administration of cold blood may cause generalized hypothermia, cardiac dysrhythmias/standstill, and disseminated intravascular coagulation (DIC).
Monitor laboratory studies:	
Hemoglobin (Hgb)/hematocrit (Hct),	Assists in calculation of blood loss, replacement needs, and effectiveness of therapy.

INTERVENTIONS	RATIONALE
Collaborative	
Clotting studies/profile,	Multiple transfusions of banked blood may result in deficient proteins/clotting factors necessary to promote coagulation. Prolongation of clotting times and presence of fibrin split products indicates developing coagulopathy/DIC.
Serum potassium,	Hyperkalemia may result from multiple transfusion of stored blood, especially in presence of altered renal function owing to hypovolemic state.
Serum bilirubin.	Multiple transfusions may cause elevation of serum bilirubin (and occurrence of jaundice). Up to 10 percent of transfused blood is hemolized during initial 24 hours following administration, which may result in production of bilirubin in excess of the liver's ability to excrete it.
Assist with gastric or peritoneal lavage, as indicated.	May be done to diagnose gastric or intra-abdominal hemorrhage.

NURSING DIAGNOSIS: **Tissue Perfusion, alteration in, decreased [potential].**

SUPPORTING DATA/CONTRIBUTING FACTORS: **Excessive tissue trauma with edema, and/or direct vascular injury with bleeding into a "closed compartment," directly affects circulation within an injured extremity. Excessive blood loss also can affect systemic tissue perfusion and organ function and reduce local tissue perfusion.**

GENERAL PATIENT OUTCOMES: **Tissue perfusion is maintained as evidenced by palpable pulses, skin warm/dry, sensorium appropriate for patient, adequate urine output for individual situation.**

INTERVENTIONS	RATIONALE
Independent: Local	
Maintain elevation of injured extremity(ies) unless contraindicated.	Promotes venous drainage/decreases edema. Note: In presence of increased compartment pressure, elevation of extremity actually impedes arterial flow, decreasing perfusion.
Assess peripheral pulse distal to injury via palpation/Doppler; compare with normal limb.	Decreased/absent pulse may reflect vascular injury. Note: Occasionally a pulse may be palpated when actual circulation is blocked by a soft clot through which

INTERVENTIONS	RATIONALE
Independent: Local	
	pulsations may be felt. In addition, perfusion through larger arteries may continue even though increased compartment pressure has collapsed arteriole/venule circulation.
Palpate temperature of extremities; observe color, capillary refill.	Localized cool skin, presence of cyanosis or mottling, and delay of capillary refill are indicators of circulatory impairment and tissue hypoxia. Note: Systemic occurrence of these signs/symptoms may reflect hypovolemia. (Refer to Nursing Diagnosis: Fluid Volume Deficit, potential, page 273.)
Perform/record neurovascular assessments, noting changes in motor/sensory function. Assess position of splint/sling. Ask patient to localize the presence of pain/discomfort.	Muscle/soft-tissue injury with edema, hemorrhage into a closed compartment (extremity), or malpositioned traction apparatus may cause undue pressure on vessels/nerves, resulting in decreased perfusion, numbness/tingling.
Test sensation of peroneal nerve by pinch/pinprick in the dorsal web between first and second toe and assess ability to dorsiflex toes if indicated.	Length and position of peroneal nerve increases risk of injury in presence of leg fracture, edema/compartmental syndrome, or malposition of traction apparatus.
Assess entire length of injured extremity for swelling/edema formation. Note complaints of increasing pain on passive movement of extremity, development of paresthesia, muscle tenseness/tenderness with erythemia.	Continued bleeding/edema formation within a muscle enclosed by tight fascia can result in interrupted blood flow and ischemic myositis/compartmental syndrome, necessitating emergency interventions to relieve pressure/restore circulation.
Note sudden signs of limb ischemia; for example, decreased skin temperature, pallor, increased pain.	Fracture dislocations of joints (especially the knee) may cause damage to adjacent arteries with resulting loss of distal blood flow after localized swelling occurs.
Encourage patient to exercise digits/joints distal to injury.	Maintains movement/flexibility and enhances circulation.
Independent: Systemic	
Monitor vital signs/hemodynamic pressures when available. Note signs of general pallor/cyanosis, cool skin, changes in mentation. (Refer to Nursing Diagnosis: Fluid Volume Deficit, potential, page 273.)	Inadequate circulating volume will compromise systemic tissue perfusion.
Monitor cardiac rate/rhythm continuously.	Dysrhythmias decreasing cardiac output and altering tissue perfusion may develop owing to increased circulatory demands/decreased oxygen-carrying capacity of blood.
Use caution when providing external warmth/rewarming hypothermic patient.	Retain body heat without stimulating excessive vasodilation which can increase size of vascular bed, compromising circulating blood volume and tissue perfusion.
Position patient in low Fowler's position, back-lying position, or with head of bed flat and feet elevated as indicated.	Increases venous return during hypotension, improving cerebral/systemic perfusion. Note: Avoid use of full Trendelenburg position, which may compromise respiratory function.

INTERVENTIONS	RATIONALE
Collaborative: Local	
Assist with cast splitting/bivalve procedure as indicated.	May be required to relieve restriction of circulation resulting from edema formation in injured extremity.
Apply/remove Military Antishock Trousers (MAST) per protocol.	May be indicated to increase peripheral vascular resistance, cardiac output, and systemic perfusion. Note: Improper deflation may result in acute compartmental syndrome of the legs.
Prepare for arteriography as indicated.	Assesses vessel patency, documents need for surgical intervention when circulation of extremity is compromised.
Assist with measurement of intracompartmental pressures as indicated.	Intermittent/continuous measurement of intramuscular/interstitial pressures in injured extremity may be useful in assessing perfusion pressure and the diagnosis/management of compartmental syndrome.
Prepare for surgical intervention (e.g., fibulectomy/fasciotomy) as indicated.	Failure to relieve pressure/to correct compartmental syndrome within 4 to 6 hours of onset can result in severe contractures/loss of function and disfigurement of extremity distal to injury, or even necessitate amputation.

NURSING DIAGNOSIS:	**Gas Exchange, impaired (potential).**
SUPPORTING DATA/CONTRIBUTING FACTORS:	**Patients with multiple/long-bone fractures may develop fat emboli which can occlude pulmonary circulation, resulting in pulmonary hypertension, hypoxia, parenchymal damage, airway constriction, and respiratory insufficiency. Immobility may potentiate thrombus/emboli formation with similar results. Either complication increases risk of the development of adult respiratory distress syndrome (ARDS). In addition, chest wall injuries may result in hemothorax/pneumothorax, compromising respiratory function.**
GENERAL PATIENT OUTCOMES:	**Respiratory function is maintained as evidenced by absence of dyspnea/cyanosis, respiratory rate and ABGs within patient's normal limits.**

INTERVENTIONS	RATIONALE
Independent: Systemic	
Auscultate breath sounds; for example, dull, distant, unequal, hyperresonant; presence of crackles, rhonchi, wheezes. Note inspiratory crowing/croupy sounds.	Changes in/presence of adventitious breath sounds reflects developing respiratory complications, such as atelectasis, pneumonia, pulmonary edema/emboli, ARDS, or hemothorax pneumothorax. Inspiratory crowing reflects upper airway edema and is suggestive of fat emboli. Note: Signs of pulmonary edema are frequently noncardiac in nature and may be due to excessive fluid replacement.
Monitor respiratory rate and effort. Note stridorous breathing, use of accessory muscles, retractions, development of central cyanosis.	Tachypnea, dyspnea and changes in mentation are early signs of respiratory insufficiency and may be only indicator of developing emboli in the early stage. Remaining signs/symptoms reflect advanced respiratory distress/impending failure. Presence of fat emboli in pulmonary vascular bed compromises gas diffusion and may lead to ARDS. (Refer to Care Plan: Adult Respiratory Distress Syndrome, page 77.)
Assess chest movement (e.g., equality/symmetry). Note tracheal position. Palpate for subcutaneous emphysema (crepitus).	Chest wall injuries may result in hemo/pneumothorax, seriously impairing respiratory function/gas exchange. (Refer to Care Plan: Hemothorax and Pneumothorax, page 88.)
Handle injured tissues/bones gently, especially during first several days.	This may prevent the development of fat emboli (usually seen in first 12 to 72 hours), which are closely associated with fractures, especially of long bone and pelvis.
Instruct and assist with deep breathing and coughing exercises. Reposition frequently.	Promotes alveolar ventilation and perfusion. Repositioning promotes drainage of secretions and decreases congestion in dependent lung areas.
Note increasing restlessness, confusion, lethargy, stupor.	Impaired gas exchange/presence of pulmonary emboli can cause deterioration in the patient's level of consciousness as hypoxemia/acidosis develops.
Observe sputum for signs of blood.	Hemoptysis may occur with pulmonary thromboemboli.
Monitor cardiac rate/rhythm. Note ECG signs of cardiac strain/congestive heart failure. Assess for development of hypertension.	Catecholamine release and hypoxia (related to presence of pulmonary emboli) have direct effect on the myocardium, causing tachycardia/dysrhythmias. Furthermore, fat emboli within the myocardial vasculature can cause vasculitis, reducing coronary circulation and causing ischemia. In addition, pulmonary emboli/obstruction may produce signs of cardiac failure. (Refer to Care Plans: Pulmonary Embolism, page 95; Congestive Heart Failure, page 49.)
Inspect skin for petechia above nipple line, in axilla spreading to abdomen/trunk; buccal mucosa, hard palate, conjunctival sacs, and retina.	Petechia may appear within 2 to 3 days after injury and are the most characteristic sign of fat emboli. They are the result of intravascular thrombosis.
Note tenderness, swelling, pain on dorsiflexion of foot (positive Homan's sign).	There is an increased potential for thrombophlebitis, resulting in pulmonary emboli in patients immobile for 5 or more days. (Refer to Care Plan: Pulmonary Embolism, page 95.)

INTERVENTIONS	RATIONALE
Independent: Systemic	
Encourage ankle exercises.	Increases muscle tone and reduces venous stasis in lower extremities, which may reduce incidence of thrombus formation.
Collaborative	
Administer supplemental oxygen via cannula, mask, ventilator. (Refer to Care Plan: Ventilatory Assistance [Mechanical], page 115.)	Increases available oxygen for optimal tissue oxygenation. Note: Mechanical ventilation/use of positive end-expiratory pressure (PEEP) may be required if more than 50 percent oxygen is required to raise the patient's PaO_2 to 80 mmHg.
Monitor laboratory studies as indicated:	
Serial ABGs,	Decreased PaO_2 and increased $PaCO_2$ indicate impaired gas exchange/developing failure.
Hgb, calcium, sedimentation rate (ESR), serum lipase, fat screen, platelets.	Anemia, hypocalcemia, elevated ESR and lipase levels, fat globules in blood/urine/sputum, and decreased platelet count (thrombocytopenia) are often associated with fat emboli.
Review chest x-ray examinations.	Presence of diffuse/"snowstorm" pattern of multiple infiltrates suggests fat/multiple thromboemboli. Congestion also may indicate pulmonary edema/ developing pneumonia.
Assist with/prepare for lung scan as indicated.	May be necessary to diagnose presence of emboli/ pulmonary vasculature obstruction.
Administer medications as indicated:	
Corticosteroids,	Steroids have been used with some success to prevent/to treat fat embolus. Anti-inflammatory effects are thought to reduce local tissue injury and risk of fat emboli by blocking chemical inflammation caused by free fatty acids, and/or by reducing capillary endothelial damage.
Low-dose heparin,	May clear lipemic plasma and may inhibit lipase activity in presence of fat emboli to reduce effects of vasculitis with resultant platelet-fibrin thrombosis.
Continuous heparin infusion,	Blocks the clotting cycle and prevents clot propagation in presence of thrombophlebitis.
Low-molecular dextran,	Alters platelets and decreases intimal adhesions, which may be of benefit in reduction of fat or thromboemboli. Also appears to increase pulmonary blood flow to previously underperfused lung segments.
Intravenous (IV) alcohol,	Occasionally used for treatment of fat emboli because of its lipase inhibiting activity.
Diuretics, for example, furosemide (Lasix).	Useful in reversing pulmonary edema often associated with fat emboli.
Apply antiembolic hose.	In the absence of phlebitis, decreases venous pooling and may enhance venous return, thereby reducing risk of thrombus formation.

NURSING DIAGNOSIS:	**Mobility, impaired, physical.**
SUPPORTING DATA/CONTRIBUTING FACTORS:	**Initially, range of motion/mobility is restricted because of fracture/pain and therapies (e.g., cast/traction, surgical reduction). Secondarily, psychologic immobility may limit movement further, with potential for development of complications associated with immobility; for example, contractures, pneumonia, phlebitis, depression.**
GENERAL PATIENT OUTCOMES:	**Mobility is maintained at the highest possible level, and complications are prevented/minimized.**

INTERVENTIONS	RATIONALE
Independent	
Assess degree of immobility produced by injury and note patient's perception of immobility.	Patient may be restricted by self-view/self-perception out of proportion with actual physical limitations, requiring information/intervention to promote progress toward wellness.
Encourage patient to discuss problems related to injuries.	Helps alleviate anxiety. Patient may feel need to relive the accident experience.
Maintain stimulating environment; for example, radio, television, newspapers, personal possessions, pictures, clock, calendar, visits from family/friends.	Reduces isolation, promotes reality orientation, and provides some normal life activity.
Encourage participation in diversional/recreational activities.	Provides opportunity for movement/release of energy, refocuses attention, enhances patient's sense of self-control/self-worth, and aids in reducing social isolation.
Instruct/assist with active, passive, isometric exercises of affected and unaffected extremities.	Improves muscle tone, maintains joint mobility, prevents contractures, and improves circulation. Note: Exercises are contraindicated while acute bleeding/edema present.
Provide footboard, wrist splints, trochantor/hand rolls as appropriate.	Useful in maintaining functional position of extremities, hands/feet and preventing complications (e.g., contractures/foot drop).
Assist with/encourage self-care, hygiene (e.g., bathing, shaving).	Improves muscle strength and circulation, enhances patient control in situation, and promotes self-directed wellness.
Reposition, aid in coughing and deep breathing.	Prevents/reduces incidence of skin/respiratory complications (e.g., ducubiti, atelectasis, pneumonia).
Monitor elimination habits and provide for regular bowel routine. Place on bedside commode, if feasible. Provide privacy.	Bedrest, use of analgesics, and changes in dietary habits produce constipation, which may require intervention (e.g., use of bowel softeners).

INTERVENTIONS	RATIONALE
Independent	
Encourage fluids, including fruit juices.	Keeping the body well hydrated decreases risk of renal calculi/stone formation and constipation.
Provide/assist with mobility by means of wheelchair, walker, and canes as soon as possible. Instruct in safe use of mobility aids.	Early mobility reduces complications of bedrest (e.g., phlebitis) and promotes healing.
Monitor blood pressure with resumption of activity. Note complaints of dizziness.	Postural hypotension is a common problem and may require interventions (e.g., tilt table with gradual elevation to upright position).
Collaborative	
Provide diet high in proteins, carbohydrates, vitamins, and minerals via appropriate route. (Refer to Care Plan: Nutritional Support, page 367.)	In the presence of musculoskeletal injuries, nutrients required for healing are rapidly depleted, resulting in a weight loss of as much as 20 to 30 pounds during skeletal traction. Choice of diet and route of administration are dependent on nature of injuries and level of gastric functioning.
Refer to/consult with physical therapist/rehabilitation specialist.	Patient may require long-term assistance with movement, strengthening, and weight-bearing activities, as well as adjuncts such as walkers, crutches, canes.
Refer to psychiatric nurse/therapist as indicated.	Patient and significant other(s) may require more intensive treatment to deal with reality of current condition/prognosis.

NURSING DIAGNOSIS:	**Skin Integrity, impairment of, actual/potential.**
SUPPORTING DATA/CONTRIBUTING FACTORS:	**A compound fracture or surgical repair involves a significant interruption of the integrity of the skin, presenting individual considerations for care. The skin area under a cast or surrounding traction pins is at risk for injury, ulceration, infection, and necrosis.**
GENERAL PATIENT OUTCOMES:	**Wounds are healed. Pressure sores are prevented/minimized.**

INTERVENTIONS	RATIONALE
Independent	
Inspect skin, noting bleeding, discoloration, duskiness, blanching, and capillary refill.	Provides information regarding skin circulation and possible areas of decreased circulation caused by restriction by cast/splint, or edema formation.
Assess position of splint ring of traction device.	Improper positioning may cause tissue injury/breakdown.

INTERVENTIONS	RATIONALE
Independent	
Provide cast care:	
When cast is wet, use palm of hand to move. Support on pillows.	Prevents indentations/flattening over bony prominences and weight-bearing areas (e.g., back of heels), which would cause abrasions/tissue trauma.
Promote cast drying by removing bed linen, exposing to circulating air.	Prevents skin breakdown caused by prolonged moisture trapped under cast.
Observe for pressure areas, especially at the edges of and under the splint/cast.	Pressure areas can cause ulcerations, necrosis, and/or nerve palsies.
Pad (petal) the edges of the cast.	Prevents excoriation/tissue trauma.
Protect cast and skin in perineal area. Provide frequent pericare.	Prevents tissue breakdown and infection by fecal contamination.
Instruct patient/significant other(s) to avoid inserting objects inside casts.	"Scratching an itch" may cause tissue injury.
Massage skin and bony prominences. Keep the bed dry and free of wrinkles. Provide elbow/heel pads as indicated.	Promotes circulation, reduces risk of abrasions/skin breakdown.
Resposition frequently. Encourage use of trapeze if possible.	Lessens constant pressure on same areas and minimizes risk of skin breakdown. Use of trapeze may reduce risk of abrasions to elbows/heels.
Clean and inspect skeletal pin sites per protocol. Tape or cork pin/wire ends.	Prevents infection at the pin site. Reduces risk of skin injury/linen snagging on points of wires.
Collaborative	
Provide alternating pressure mattresses, eggcrate/foam pads.	Reduces pressure/improves circulation, aiding in prevention of decubiti.

NURSING DIAGNOSIS:	**Infection, potential for.**
SUPPORTING DATA/CONTRIBUTING FACTORS:	**Loss of skin integrity by trauma, including compound fractures/wounds (which may be contaminated by bacteria), surgical incisions, insertion of wires/external fixation device into bone, and presence of invasive lines/monitoring devices increase the risk of developing infection/sepsis.**
GENERAL PATIENT OUTCOMES:	**Infection prevented or minimized. Wounds healing free of purulent drainage. Afebrile.**

INTERVENTIONS	RATIONALE
Independent	
Assess pin sites/skin areas (especially beneath casts), noting complaints of increased pain/burning sensation or presence of edema, erythema, foul odor/drainage.	Indicates onset of local infection.
Provide sterile pin/wound care.	Utilizing aseptic technique and meticulous handwashing during care may prevent cross contamination and infection.
Observe wounds for bullae formation, crepitation, bronze discoloration of skin, frothy/fruity-smelling drainage.	Signs suggestive of gas gangrene.
Assess muscle tone, deep tendon reflexes, and ability to speak.	Muscle rigidity, tonic spasms of jaw muscles, dysphagia reflect development of tetanus.
Monitor vital signs. Note presence of chills, malaise, changes in mentation.	Hypotension, confusion may be seen with gas gangrene; tachycardia and chills/fever reflect developing sepsis.
Investigate abrupt onset of pain/limitation of movement with localized edema/erythema in injured extremity.	May indicate development of osteomyelitis.
Collaborative	
Monitor laboratory studies as indicated; for example,	
Complete blood count (CBC),	Anemia may be noted with osteomyelitis, and leukocytosis is present with any infective process.
ESR,	Elevated in osteomyelitis.
Cultures of wound/serum/bone,	Diagnose/identify infective organism.
Radioisotope scans,	Hot spots signify increased areas of vascularity, indicative of osteomyelitis.
Administer IV/topical antibiotics as indicated.	Wide-spectrum antibiotics may be used prophylactically, or antibiotic therapy may be geared toward specific identified microorganisms.
Administer tetanus toxoid prophylatically, if indicated.	Possibility of tetanus increases when injury/wound(s) occur in outdoor/rural areas.
Provide wound irrigations, application of warm/moist soaks as indicated.	Local debridement/cleansing of wounds reduces microorganisms and incidence of systemic infection.
Assist with procedures; for example, incision/drainage, placement of drains, hyperbaric oxygen therapy.	Numerous procedures may be carried out in treatment of local infections, osteomyelitis, gas gangrene.

NURSING DIAGNOSIS:	**Anxiety/Fear.**
SUPPORTING DATA/CONTRIBUTING FACTORS:	**The sudden change in status that occurs with this type of trauma thrusts the patient into a dependent situation**

	and creates financial concern owing to inability to work. Separation from one's family, change(s) in body image, and uncertainty about outcome create a situation in which anxiety/fear can be a significant factor. If the patient is a survivor of a catastrophic event in which others died, feelings of relief and guilt may contribute to anxiety.
GENERAL PATIENT OUTCOMES:	**Verbalizes awareness of feelings of anxiety and begins to discuss concerns/fears.**

INTERVENTIONS	RATIONALE
Independent	
Assess patient's perception of events.	Important to assessment of degree of anxiety. Impaired interpretation of reality, dissociation/amnesia, vagueness about event may reflect developing post-trauma response.
Active Listen to patient's expression of concerns.	Listening to the patient's feelings as well as to the words helps the patient sort out feelings and identify concerns. Active listening also conveys a sense of trust in the patient's ability to deal with what has happened.
Note occurence of repetitive dreams/nightmares, expressions of guilt regarding event/survival.	Indicators that patient is having difficulty resolving/integrating feelings and may need professional assistance as recovery progresses.
Provide support and encouragement to patient significant other(s).	Helpful in dealing with the situation as it exists.
Explain procedures/special equipment as much as possible.	Providing clear information can allay fear of the unknown.

(Refer to Care Plan: Psychosocial Aspects of Critical Care, page 379.)

CHAPTER 10 INTEGUMENTARY

Burns: Thermal/Chemical/Electrical (Acute Phase)

PATIENT ASSESSMENT DATA BASE

HISTORY

Obtain history of circumstances surrounding burn injury and approximate duration of contact with injuring agent if known.

Thermal burns: note if injuring agent was flame, hot liquid, or object. If flame burn, ascertain if patient was in a closed space and note source of smoke (certain chemical by-products may potentiate inhalation injury).

Chemical burns: note type/content of injuring agent, as well as concentration and temperature of agent.

Electrical burns: note type/voltage of current. Current generates heat in proportion to resistance offered and travels the pathway of least resistance (i.e., nerves offer the least resistance and bones the greatest resistance). Underlying injury will be more severe than visible injury.

Age of client is necessary in estimating extent, percentage, and seriousness of injury.

Note initial first aid rendered.

Determine date of last tetanus immunization.

Subjective

Complaints of pain vary; for example, first-degree burns are extremely sensitive to touch, pressure, air movement, and temperature changes; second-degree moderate thickness burns are very painful, but pain response in second-degree deep thickness burns is dependent upon intactness of nerve endings; third degree burns are painless.

PHYSICAL EXAMINATION

Inspection

Face/neck: *Flame burns:* note singed nasal hairs; dry, red mucosa of nose and mouth; blisters on posterior pharynx; circumoral and/or circumnasal edema; hoarseness; wheezy cough; carbonaceous particles in sputum; drooling/inability to swallow oral secretions; and cyanosis indicative of inhalation injury.

Thoracic excursion may be limited in presence of circumferential chest burns.

Skin: *General:* exact depth of tissue destruction may not be evident for 3 to 5 days, owing to the process of microvascular thromboses in some wounds. Unburned skin areas may be cool/clammy, pale, with slow capillary refill in presence of decreased cardiac output caused by fluid loss/shock state.

Flame injury: there may be areas of mixed depth of injury, owing to varied intensity of heat produced by burning clothing.

Superficial partial-thickness burns (first-degree): involve only the epidermis. Wounds appear bright pink to red, with minimal edema and no blisters. The skin blanches with pressure and is often warm/dry.

Moderate partial-thickness burns (second-degree): involve the epidermis and dermis. Wounds appear red to pink, with moderate edema and moist, weeping blisters.

Deep partial-thickness burns (second-degree): involve the deep dermis. Wounds appear pink to pale ivory, with moderate edema and blisters. These wounds are dryer than the moderate partial-thickness burns.

Full-thickness burns (third-degree): involve the subcutaneous tissue and may involve the muscle and bone. Wound appearance varies from white, cherry red, to brown or black, with blistering uncommon. These wounds have a dry, leathery texture.

Chemical injury: appearance of wound varies according to causative agent. Skin may be yellowish brown with soft leather-like texture; blisters, ulcers, necrosis, or thick eschar may be present. Injuries are generally deeper than they appear cutaneously, and tissue destruction can continue for up to 72 hours after injury.

Electrical injury: the external cutaneous injury is usually much less than the underlying necrosis. Appearance of wounds varies and may include entry/exit wounds of current, arc burns from current moving in close proximity to body, and thermal burns caused by ignition of clothing.

Musculoskeletal: fractures may occur owing to trauma; for example, falls, explosions, motor-vehicular accidents, or following contact with electrical current, which causes strong tetanic muscle contractions. (Refer to Care Plan: Fractures/Multiple Trauma, page 269.)

Urine output: may be decreased/absent. Color may be reddish-black if myoglobin present, indicating deep muscle damage.

Auscultation

Upper airway: stridor/wheezes suggest obstruction caused by laryngospasm, laryngeal edema, and/or profuse airway secretions (rhonchi).

Blood pressure: hypotension may be noted if shock present.

Peripheral pulses: may be diminished distal to extremity injury.

Breath sounds: crackles indicate pulmonary edema.

Bowel sounds: often decreased/absent in cutaneous burns of greater than 20 percent because stress reduces gastric motility/peristalsis.

Palpation

Pulse: may be rapid in presence of shock/anxiety/pain; or irregular if dysrhythmias are present (such as may follow electrical shock).

DIAGNOSTIC STUDIES

CBC: initial increased Hct suggests hemoconcentration caused by fluid shift/loss. Later, decreased Hct and RBCs may occur, owing to heat damage to vascular endothelium.

WBC: leukocytosis can occur owing to loss of cells at wound site and inflammatory response to injury.

ABGs: baseline especially important with suspicion of inhalation injury. Reduced PaO_2/increased $PaCO_2$ may be seen with carbon monoxide retention. Acidosis may occur owing to reduced renal function and loss of compensatory respiratory mechanisms.

COHbg (carboxyhemoglobin): elevation of greater than 15 percent indicates carbon monoxide poisoning/inhalation injury.

Serum electrolytes: potassium initially may be elevated owing to loss from injured tissues/red blood cell destruction and decreased renal function; serum calcium/magnesium may be decreased. Sodium may be decreased with body water losses.

Alkaline phosphatase: elevated owing to interstitial fluid shifts/impairment of sodium pump.

Serum glucose: elevation reflects stress response.

Serum albumin: albumin/globulin ratio may be reversed, owing to loss of protein in edema fluid.

BUN: elevation reflects decreased renal perfusion/function.

Urine: presence of albumin, hemoglobin, and myoglobin indicates deep tissue damage and protein loss (especially seen with serious electrical burns). Reddish-black color of urine is due to presence of myoglobin.

Wound cultures may be obtained for baseline data.

Chest x-ray examination may appear normal in early postburn period even with inhalation injury.

Fiberoptic bronchoscopy: useful in diagnosing extent of inhalation injury; findings can include edema, hemorrhage, and/or ulceration of upper respiratory tract.

Flow volume loop: provides noninvasive assessment of effects/extent of inhalation injury.

Xenon lung scan may be done to determine extent of inhalation injury as evidenced by delayed washout of xenon and asymmetric, localized areas of retention.

ECG: signs of myocardial ischemia/dysrhythmias may occur with electrical burns.

Photographs of burns: provides documentation/baseline comparison for later burn wound healing.

NURSING PRIORITIES

1. Maintain patent airway/respiratory function.
2. Restore hemodynamic stability/circulating volume.
3. Control/minimize pain.
4. Minimize/prevent complications.
5. Provide emotional support for patient/significant other(s).

NURSING DIAGNOSIS:	**Airway Clearance, ineffective [potential].**
SUPPORTING DATA/CONTRIBUTING FACTORS:	**Smoke inhalation can cause mucosal edema and loss of ciliary action, leading to congestion and atelectasis. The upper airway can be injured by flame, steam, hot air, and chemicals/gases, which cause inflammation, edema, and airway obstruction. Circumferential full-thickness burns of the neck, thorax, and chest can occlude the airway by compressing the airway or by**

	limiting chest excursion. Fluid shifts may result in pulmonary edema, decreased lung compliance, and respiratory distress syndrome.
GENERAL PATIENT OUTCOMES:	**Clear breath sounds, respiratory rate within normal range, free of dyspnea/ cyanosis.**

INTERVENTIONS	RATIONALE
Independent	
Elevate head of bed.	Promotes optimal lung expansion/respiratory function.
Encourage coughing/deep breathing exercises and frequent position changes.	Promotes lung expansion, mobilization and drainage of secretions.
Suction (if necessary) with extreme care, maintaining sterile technique.	Helps maintain clear airway, but should be done cautiously because of mucosal edema and inflammation. Sterile technique reduces risk of infection.
Promote voice rest but assess ability to speak and/or swallow oral secretions.	Increasing hoarseness/decreased ability to swallow suggests increasing tracheal edema and may indicate need for prompt intubation.
Monitor respiratory rate, rhythm, depth; note presence of pallor/cyanosis and carbonaceous or pink-tinged sputum.	Tachypnea, use of accessory muscles, presence of cyanosis, and changes in sputum reflect developing respiratory distress/pulmonary edema. Note: Full-thickness circumferential chest burns increase the risk of respiratory insufficiency/distress as tight eschar restricts chest movement and reduces vital capacity.
Auscultate lungs, noting stridor, wheezing/crackles, diminished breath sounds, brassy cough.	Airway obstruction/respiratory distress can occur very quickly or may not appear until 48 hours postburn. Children less than 2 years of age are especially at risk because of airway size and proximity of anatomic structures.
Investigate changes in behavior/mentation (e.g., restlessness, agitation, confusion).	Although often related to pain, changes in consciousness may reflect developing/worsening hypoxia.
Note presence of cherry-red color of uninjured skin.	Suggests presence of carbon monoxide.
Monitor 24-hour fluid balance, noting variations/ changes.	Fluid shifts or excess fluid replacement increases risk of pulmonary edema. Inhalation injury increases fluid demands as much as 35 percent or more, owing to obligatory edema.
Monitor invasive hemodynamic parameters if available; for example, (PAP)/(PCWP).	Elevation of pulmonary pressures may indicate developing pulmonary edema before other symptoms (such as adventious breath sounds) are present.
Collaborative	
Administer humidified oxygen via appropriate mode (e.g., face mask, endotracheal tube/mechanical ventilation).	Oxygen corrects hypoxemia/acidosis. Humidity decreases drying of respiratory tract and reduces viscosity of sputum. Intubation/mechanical support may be

INTERVENTIONS	RATIONALE
Collaborative	
	required if airway edema or circumferential burn injury interferes with respiratory function/oxygenation.
Monitor/graph serial arterial blood gases (ABGs), COHgb levels. Calculate A-a gradient.	Baseline is essential for further assessment of respiratory status and guide to treatment. Decreased PaO_2, increased $PaCO_2$, and widening A-a gradient suggest inhalation injury/developing respiratory distress. Elevation of carboxyhemoglobin (COHgb) levels reflects carbon monoxide poisoning. Carbon monoxide has a greater affinity for hemoglobin and thus competes with oxygen for binding sites producing hypoxemia.
Review serial chest x-ray examinations.	Changes reflecting atelectasis, pulmonary edema, may not occur for 2 to 3 days postburn.
Provide/assist with chest physiotherapy/incentive spirometry.	Chest physiotherapy drains dependent areas of the lung. Incentive spirometry may be done to improve lung expansion, thereby promoting respiratory function and reducing atelectasis.
Administer bronchodilators; for example, theophylline (aminophyllin), as indicated.	Dilates airways by relaxing bronchial muscles.
Assist with fiberoptic bronchoscopy.	Useful in establishing presence/degree of injury, and to clear debris from bronchial tree.
Assist with escharotomy as necessary.	May be needed to relieve pressure on airways caused by constricting edema from circumferential chest/neck burns, thereby permitting proper chest excursion and lung expansion, and increasing tidal volume.

NURSING DIAGNOSIS:	**Fluid Volume Deficit, potential.**
SUPPORTING DATA/CONTRIBUTING FACTORS:	**Partial and full-thickness burn injuries can result in massive losses of sodium and water (especially during first 24 to 72 hours) as a result of increased capillary permeability, protein shifts, inflammatory process, and evaporation. These fluid losses can result in hypovolemic shock, electrolyte imbalances, and metabolic acidosis. Later, hemorrhagic losses secondary to development of Curling's ulcer also may lead to hypovolemia.**
GENERAL PATIENT OUTCOMES:	**Fluid volume maintained as evidenced by stable vital signs, urine output adequate for specific circumstance (0.5 to 1.0 ml per kg).**

INTERVENTIONS	RATIONALE
Independent	
Monitor vital signs and hemodynamic pressures; for example, central venous pressure (CVP), PCWP and cardiac output (CO) as available.	Serves as a guide to fluid resuscitation needs. Invasive monitoring is indicated for patients with major burns, smoke inhalation, or patients with preexisting cardiac disease.
Monitor hourly intake and output. Measure specific gravity. Observe color of urine and hematest urine as indicated.	Generally, fluid replacement should be titrated to ensure urinary output of 50 ml per hour in the adult and 0.5 ml per kilogram per hour in the child. If gross myoglobinuria is present, adult minimum urine output is 75 to 100 ml per hour to prevent tubular damage/necrosis. Urine can appear red to black with massive muscle destruction owing to presence of blood and release of myoglobin.
Investigate changes in mentation.	Deterioration in the level of consciousness may indicate inadequate circulating volume/reduced cerebral perfusion.
Maintain integrity and function of indwelling urinary catheter.	Prevents stasis or reflux of urine. Retention of urine with its by-products of tissue cell destruction can lead to renal problems such as infection.
Weigh daily.	Fluid replacement formulas partly depend on weight. A 15 to 20 percent weight gain in the first 72 hours during fluid replacement can be anticipated, with return to preburn weight approximately 10 days postburn.
Measure circumference of burned extremities daily as indicated.	May be helpful in estimating extent of edema formation in tissues.
Observe signs and symptoms of stress ulcer (Curling's ulcer); for example, gastric distention, hematemesis, tarry stools. Guaiac nasogastric drainage and stools periodically.	Curling's ulcer occurs in up to one-half of all severely burned patients. (Refer to Care Plan: Upper Gastrointestinal/Esophageal Bleeding, page 197.)
Collaborative	
Insert/maintain large bore intravenous (IV) catheter(s).	To accommodate rapid infusion of fluids.
Maintain/calculate IV replacement of fluids, electrolytes, plasma, albumin, according to extent of injury and daily weight. Administer crystalloid IV formula (such as 5 percent dextrose and Ringer's lactate with added amino acids) during the resuscitation period.	Fluid resuscitation replaces lost fluids/electrolytes and helps prevent complications (e.g., shock, acute tubular necrosis). Replacement formulas vary (e.g., Brooke, Evans, Parkland), but most experts encourage infusion of one half of initial 24-hour total during the first 8 hours following injury, when fluid loss is greatest. Note: Glucose solutions may be withheld initially if blood sugar is markedly elevated in response to stress.
Administer colloids (e.g., salt-poor albumin) as indicated.	Colloids are not routinely used in the first 24 hours postburn because capillary changes permit leakage of protein-rich fluids into interstitial spaces, thereby contributing to edema formation. During second 24 hours, capillary membrane begins to stabilize, and colloids may replenish circulating volume. Note: Use of salt-poor albumin reduces potential for sodium excess.

Monitor laboratory studies; for example, studies hemoglobin (Hgb)/hematocrit (Hct), serum/urine potassium	After first 48 hours, red cell and potassium losses may require replacement based on laboratory results.
Administer drugs as indicated; for example, Mannitol (Osmitrol),	In the presence of gross myoglobin, mannitol may be indicated to enhance urine output and to clear tubules of debris/to prevent necrosis.
Potassium (KCl),	Although hyperkalemia may occur during first 24 to 48 hours, subsequent replacement may be necessary because of large urinary losses.
Antacids: calcium carbonate (Titralac), magaldrate (Riopan); histamine inhibitors: cimetidine (Tagamet), ranitidine (Zantac).	Curling's ulcer can develop in severely burned patients. Antacids may reduce gastric acidity, and cimetidine and ranitidine decrease production of hydrochloric acid to reduce risk of gastric irritation/bleeding.
Add electrolytes to water used for wound debridement.	Washing solution that approximates tissue fluids may minimize osmotic fluid shifts.

NURSING DIAGNOSIS:	**Cardiac Output, alteration in, decreased.**
SUPPORTING DATA/CONTRIBUTING FACTORS:	**The fluid shift accompanying burns decreases the circulating blood volume. In addition, electrolyte imbalances (producing cardiac dysrhythmias) or myocardial damage/alteration of conductivity (owing to electrical injuries) further reduces cardiac output. Lastly, release of myocardial depressant factor (MDF) may limit the heart's ability to respond to/compensate for the stress state.**
GENERAL PATIENT OUTCOMES:	**Vital signs, sensorium, and urinary output within patient's normal range.**

INTERVENTIONS	RATIONALE
Independent	
Monitor blood pressure and hemodynamic pressures; for example, central venous pressure (CVP) and cardiac output (CO), if available.	Indicators of circulating volume and myocardial function and may warn of impending shock.
Investigate changes in sensorium.	Cerebral perfusion is dependent on CO. A decrease in output often results in mental cloudiness/confusion.
Monitor/document cardiac rhythm.	Dysrhythmias can occur as a result of electrical injury/electrolyte shifts, which require appropriate intervention to prevent compromised CO/tissue perfusion.
Monitor urine output and specific gravity.	Decreased output and changes in specific gravity may indicate reduced CO and/or renal hypoperfusion.

INTERVENTIONS	RATIONALE
Collaborative	
Maintain fluid replacement per protocol. (Refer to Nursing Diagnosis: Fluid Volume Deficit, potential, page 289.)	Maximizes circulating volume and tissue perfusion.
Monitor electrolytes, especially sodium, potassium, calcium. Administer replacement therapy as indicated.	Losses/shifts of sodium, potassium, and calcium affect cellular membrane potential/excitability, thereby altering myocardial conductivity and potentiating risk of dysrhythmias.

NURSING DIAGNOSIS:	**Tissue Perfusion, alteration in.**
SUPPORTING DATA/CONTRIBUTING FACTORS:	**Circumferential burns of extremities with resultant edema impedes peripheral circulation.**
GENERAL PATIENT OUTCOMES:	**Peripheral pulses are present/equal. Capillary refill and skin color are normal in uninjured areas.**

INTERVENTIONS	RATIONALE
Independent	
Elevate affected extremities. Remove jewelry/arm band. Avoid taping around a burned extremity/digit. Remove blood pressure (BP) cuff after each reading.	Promotes circulation/venous return and may decrease edema. If BP readings must be obtained on an injured extremity, leaving the cuff in place may increase edema formation/reduce perfusion and convert partial thickness burn to a more serious injury.
Assess color, sensation, movement, peripheral pulses (via Doppler) and capillary refill on extremities with circumferential burns.	Edema formation can readily compress blood vessels, thereby impeding circulation and increasing venous stasis/edema.
Investigate complaints of deep/throbbing ache, numbness.	Indicators of decreased perfusion.
Encourage active range of motion exercises.	Promotes circulation and venous return.
Collaborative	
Measure intracompartmental pressures as indicated. (Refer to Care Plan: Fractures/Multiple Trauma; Nursing Diagnosis: Tissue Perfusion, alteration in, page 275.)	Ischemic myositis may develop owing to decreased perfusion.
Assist with escharotomy/fasciotomy, as indicated.	Enhances circulation by relieving constriction caused by edema formation.

NURSING DIAGNOSIS:	**Comfort, alteration in, pain, acute.**

SUPPORTING DATA/CONTRIBUTING FACTORS:	**Most burns have mixed areas of destruction, so pain is usually present. As wound debridement is initiated and the healing process begins, pain may increase in severity.**
GENERAL PATIENT OUTCOMES:	**Verbalizes reduction of pain, demonstrates relaxed facial expressions/body posture.**

INTERVENTIONS	RATIONALE
Independent	
Cover wounds as soon as possible.	Temperature changes and air movement can cause great pain to exposed nerve endings.
Elevate burned extremities.	Reduces edema and associated discomfort.
Provide bed cradle as indicated.	Elevation of linens off wounds may help reduce pain.
Wrap digits/extremities in position of function (avoiding flexed position of affected joints) and elevate, using splints and footboards as necessary; encourage active range of motion as indicated; change position frequently.	Position of function reduces deformities/contractures and promotes comfort. Although flexed position of injured joints may feel more comfortable, it can lead to flexion contractures. Note: Exercising of injured/affected joints is dependent on degree/extent of injury.
Maintain comfortable environmental temperature.	Temperature regulation may be lost with major burns. External heat sources may be necessary to prevent chilling.
Assess complaints of pain, noting location, character, and intensity, using a 0 to 10 scale.	Changes in location, character, and intensity of pain may indicate developing complications (e.g., limb ischemia) or herald improvement/return of nerve function/sensation. Note: Pain is usually most severe during dressing changes and debridement.
Evaluate individual response to pain.	Pain perception is influenced by many factors, such as duration/severity of pain, past experiences, cultural/spiritual beliefs, and coping mechanisms.
Encourage therapeutic discussion of pain and negative emotions.	Verbalization of feelings allows outlet for emotions and may enhance coping mechanisms.
Provide frequent information/explanations of procedures as appropriate, especially during wound debridement.	Accepting the level at which the patient is functioning and providing empathic support can do much to alleviate pain and to promote relaxation by reducing degree of unknowns.
Provide instruction/encourage use of nonpharmacologic methods to lessen pain, such as visual imagery and breathing techniques.	Enhances patient's sense of control and increases ability to deal with pain/discomfort. Reduces pharmacologic dependency.
Provide diversional activities appropriate for age and condition.	Helps to lessen concentration of pain experience and refocuses attention.
Provide uninterrupted sleep periods.	Sleep deprivation can increase perception of pain, reduce coping abilities.

INTERVENTIONS	RATIONALE
Collaborative	
Administer small doses of narcotics IV (e.g., morphine sulfate) at frequent intervals and at least 20 minutes prior to beginning of wound care procedures.	Narcotics help reduce the severe physical and psychologic pain associated with dressing changes and debridement. Intravenous method is used because of poor peripheral absorption.
Avoid withholding analgesics unless respiratory effort is compromised.	Concerns of patient addiction or doubts regarding degree of pain experienced are not valid during this phase of care.
Provide/instruct in use of pain cocktails, self-administered anesthetics such as 50 percent nitrous oxide/50 percent oxygen mixtures, and IV-administered anesthetics such as ketamine.	Alternate methods of pain relief provide patient a sense of control, but they must be used with caution inasmuch as they initially may mask changes in condition.

NURSING DIAGNOSIS:	**Nutrition, alteration in, less than body requirements.**
SUPPORTING DATA/CONTRIBUTING FACTORS:	**Catecholamines (released incidental to the injury) cause a hypermetabolic state proportional to the severity of injury that can be as much as 50 to 60 percent greater than normal. In addition, protein is lost as fluids shift into the interstitial spaces. Both of these factors potentiate protein catabolism, resulting in muscle mass/total body weight decreases and development of negative nitrogen balance.**
GENERAL PATIENT OUTCOMES:	**Nutritional intake is adequate to meet metabolic needs as evidenced by stable weight/muscle mass, positive nitrogen balance, and tissue regeneration.**

INTERVENTIONS	RATIONALE
Independent	
Ascultate bowel sounds, noting hypoactive/absence of sound.	Ileus is often associated with postburn period but usually subsides within 36 to 48 hours, at which time oral feedings can be initiated.
Maintain strict caloric count. Weigh client daily. Reassess percent of open body surface area/wounds weekly.	Appropriate guides to proper caloric intake. As burn wound heals, percentage of burned areas is reevaluated to calculate prescribed dietary formulas, and appropriate adjustments are made.

INTERVENTIONS	RATIONALE
Independent	
Monitor triceps-skin fold/arm muscle circumference as indicated.	May be useful in estimating muscle mass/subcutaneous fat reserves if upper extremity not burned.
Provide small, frequent meals.	Helps prevent gastric distention/discomfort and encourages intake.
Encourage patient to view diet as a treatment or medicine and to make food/beverage choices high in calories/protein. Stress need to avoid use of plain water.	Critically ill patients seldom have desire to eat but need to gain understanding of role of nutrients in healing. Calories and proteins are needed to maintain weight, to meet metabolic needs, and to promote wound healing. Ingestion of water that has not been fortified with sucrose/caloric supplements is filling without providing any nutrient value.
Assess food likes/dislikes. Encourage family significant other(s) to bring in food from home, as appropriate.	Enhances sense of control/participation in care and may improve intake.
Encourage patient to sit up for meals and to visit with family member and significant other(s).	Sitting helps prevent aspiration and aids in proper digestion of food. Socialization promotes relaxation and may enhance intake.
Provide oral hygiene before meals.	Helps promote a good appetite.
Perform clinitest/acetest as indicated.	Monitors for development of hyperglycemia related to hormonal changes/demands, or use of hyperalimentation to meet caloric needs.
Collaborative	
Refer to dietician/nutritional support team to establish nutritional needs.	Several formulas (e.g., Curreri, Wilmore, Davies/Liljedahl) are available to estimate patient nutritional needs based on weight, body surface area, and percent of body surface injury.
Initiate oral feedings when appropriate, providing diet high in calories/protein with vitamin supplements.	Oral route is most preferable. Calories (as many as 5000 per day), proteins, and vitamins are needed to meet metabolic needs, to maintain weight, and to encourage proper wound healing.
Insert/maintain small feeding tube for enteric feedings/supplements.	Provides continuous/supplemental feedings when patient is unable to consume total daily calorie requirements orally.
Administer parenteral hyperalimentation as indicated. (Refer to Care Plan: Nutritional Support, page 367.)	If patient develops severe complications or sustains esophageal/gastric injuries that do not permit enteral feedings, hyperalimentation will maintain nutritional intake/meet metabolic needs.
Monitor laboratory studies as indicated: serum albumin, creatinine, transferrin, urine urea nitrogen, and so forth. (Refer to Care Plan: Nutritional Support, page 367.)	Indicators of nutritional needs and adequacy of diet/therapy.
Monitor/graph serial arterial blood gases (ABGs).	Patients receiving high-carbohydrate diets may have increased carbon dioxide (CO_2) levels from carbohydrate metabolism, which alters acid/base balance.

INTERVENTIONS	RATIONALE
Collaborative	
Administer insulin as indicated.	Elevated serum glucose levels may develop owing to high caloric intake/pancreatic fatigue.

NURSING DIAGNOSIS:	**Infection, potential for.**
SUPPORTING DATA/CONTRIBUTING FACTORS:	**The loss of skin removes a mechanical barrier to infection. The patient can experience autocontamination from the oropharynx, unburned skin, and fecal flora; or cross-contamination from the air, staff, and visitors. Systemic changes that occur with a major burn lowers resistance to infection. Infection beginning in the burn wound can readily be transferred to the bloodstream.**
GENERAL PATIENT OUTCOMES:	**Afebrile with wounds healing and free of purulent exudate.**

INTERVENTIONS	RATIONALE
Independent	
Maintain isolation as indicated.	Dependent on type/extent of wounds; isolation may range from simple wound/skin to complete/reverse.
Use strict aseptic technique with wound care, and provide sterile or freshly laundered bed linens/gowns.	Nosocomial bacterial flora will be reduced. Cross-contamination is prevented.
Shave/clip all hair from around burned areas to include a 1-inch border. Do not shave the eyebrows.	Hair is a good medium for bacterial growth.
Monitor/limit visitors, if necessary. Explain isolation procedure to visitors, if utilized.	Prevents cross-contamination from visitors.
Provide special care for eyes (e.g., use eye covers and tear formulas, as appropriate).	Eyes may be swollen shut and/or become infected by drainage from surrounding burns. If lids are burned, eye covers may be needed to prevent corneal damage.
Prevent skin-to-skin surface contact (e.g., wrap each burned finger/toe separately, do not allow burned ear to touch scalp).	Prevents adherence to surface it may be touching and encourages proper healing. Note: Ear cartilage has limited circulation and is prone to pressure necrosis.
Remove dressings and cleanse burned areas in a hydrotherapy/whirlpool tub or in a shower stall with hand-held shower head. Maintain temperature of water at 100°F (37.8°C). Wash areas with a mild cleansing agent or surgical soap, such as Betadine.	Water softens and aids in removal of eschar (slough layer of dead skin or tissue) and dressings. Sources vary as to whether bath or shower is best. Bath has advantage of water providing support for exercising extremities but may promote cross-contamination of

INTERVENTIONS	RATIONALE
Independent	
	wounds. Showering enhances wound inspection and prevents contamination from floating debris/excrement.
Debride necrotic/loose tissue with scissors and forceps. Do not disturb intact blisters if they are smaller than 2 to 3 cm; do not interfere with joint function; and do not appear infected.	Promotes healing. Prevents autocontamination. Small, intact blisters help protect skin unless the burn injury is the result of chemicals (in which case fluid contained in blisters may continue to cause tissue destruction).
Examine wounds daily; note/document changes in appearance, odor, or quantity of drainage.	Early detection of burn wound infection allows for prompt treatment.
Monitor for clinical signs of sepsis: fever, increased respiratory rate/depth, hyperglycemia with glycosuria, decreased platelet count, and changes in sensorium.	Allows for early detection and prompt intervention.
Collaborative	
Maintain reverse isolation as indicated.	Cross-contamination is prevented, and the patient's exposure to multiple bacterial flora will be reduced.
Obtain routine cultures and sensitivities of wounds. Assist with excisional biopsies when infection is suspected, noting quantitative microbial counts of 10^5 or greater per gram of tissue as well as increased white blood cell (WBC) count.	Allows specific and early treatment of wound infection. Bacteria can colonize the wound surface without invading the underlying tissue; therefore, biopsies may be obtained to diagnose infection. In addition, biopsies provide better qualitative and quantitative counts than do cultures.
Photograph wound initially and at frequent intervals.	Provides baseline and documentation of healing process.
Administer topical antibiotics as appropriate for specific burn wound infection:	Helps prevent/control wound infections and prevent drying of wound, which can cause further tissue destruction.
Silver sulfadiazine (Silvadene),	Wide-spectrum antimicrobial agent that is relatively painless but has less eschar penetration than Sulfamylon and may cause rash or depression of WBCs.
Mafenide acetate (Sulfamylon),	Antibiotic of choice with confirmed invasive burn wound sepsis. Useful against gram-negative/gram-positive organisms. Does cause burning/pain on application and for 30 minutes following. May cause rash, metabolic acidosis, and decreased $PaCO_2$.
Silver nitrate,	Effective against staphylococcus aureus, escherichia coli, and pseudomonas aeruginosa, but has poor eschar penetration, is painful, and may cause electrolyte imbalance. Dressings must be constantly saturated. Stains skin surfaces black.
Povidone-iodine (Betadine),	Broad-spectrum antimicrobial agent but is painful on application and may cause metabolic acidosis/increased iodine absorption.
Subeschar clysis/systemic antibiotics specific to pathogenic organism,	Local and systemic antibiotics are given to control pathogens identified by culture/sensitivity. Subeschar clysis has been found effective against pathogens to

INTERVENTIONS	RATIONALE
Collaborative	
	prevent sepsis in granulated tissues at the line of demarcation between viable/nonviable tissue.
Tetanus immunization as appropriate.	Tissue destruction and altered defense mechanisms increase risk of developing tetanus. In addition, deep burns such as those caused by electricity have an increased risk of developing gas gangrene.

NURSING DIAGNOSIS:	**Fear/Anxiety.**
SUPPORTING DATA/CONTRIBUTING FACTORS:	**The memory of the trauma experience and fear about the possibility of death and/or disfigurement contribute to fear/anxiety for this patient. The gowns, caps, and masks worn by personnel as well as the isolation procedures may appear intimidating/frightening. Restricted/limited contact with others may potentiate feelings of aloneness, which may increase anxiety. In addition, many procedures may need to be done quickly (to prevent further complications) and may result in a sense of a loss of individuality. Lastly, fears/concerns of family/significant other(s) may be communicated to the patient. There is often time for only cursory explanations.**
GENERAL PATIENT OUTCOMES:	**Verbalizes fears/anxiety and discusses concerns about treatment/outcome.**

INTERVENTIONS	RATIONALE
Independent	
Provide constant explanations and information about care.	Allows patient and significant other(s) to understand progression of care, and clarifies misconceptions. Knowing what to expect usually reduces fear and anxiety and promotes cooperation.
Show slides or pictures of burn care/other patient outcomes, being selective in what is shown as appropriate to the individual situation.	Allows patient/significant other(s) to be realistic in expectations. Also assists in demonstration of importance of certain devices and procedures.
Demonstrate willingness to listen and to talk to patient when free of painful procedures.	Helps patient/significant other(s) know that support is available and that caregiver is interested in the person, not just care of the burn.

INTERVENTIONS	RATIONALE
Independent	
Assist the family to express their feelings of grief and guilt.	The family may initially be most concerned about the patient's dying and begin to grieve. They also may feel guilty, believing that in some way they could have prevented the incident.
Be nonjudgmental in dealing with the patient and family.	Family relationships are disrupted. Financial, lifestyle/role changes make this a difficult time for those involved with the patient, and they may react in many different ways.
Collaborative	
Involve entire burn team in care from admission to discharge.	Provides a wider support system and promotes coordination of activities. Continuity of care allows the patient to see that goals are being achieved, thereby reducing fear and anxiety.

NURSING DIAGNOSIS:	**Thought Processes, impaired.**
SUPPORTING DATA/CONTRIBUTING FACTORS:	**During the initial period following the burn, the patient may exhibit primitive defenses of denial and repression, which serve a protective purpose. This may be followed by anxiety, agitation, and alteration in the level of consciousness. If delirium occurs, it is important to rule out physiologic causes before assuming it is psychologically based.**
GENERAL PATIENT OUTCOMES:	**Verbalizes awareness of situation and begins to develop coping skills appropriate to what is happening.**

INTERVENTIONS	RATIONALE
Independent	
Assess mental status, including mood/affect, comprehension of events, and content of thoughts (e.g., illusions or manifestations of terror/panic).	Initially the patient may use denial and repression to reduce and to filter information that might be overwhelming. Some patients display calm manner and alert mental status, representing a dissociation from reality, which is also a protective mechanism.
Monitor level of consciousness and behavior continuously. Note the presence of delirium, which may be manifested by hypervigilance, hypovigilance, hallucinations, nightmares, agitation, apathy, disorientation,	After the initial shock phase, mentation may be altered, depending on the severity of the condition and medications being given. Extreme anxiety may be exhibited by fear, confusion, sleep disturbances, and de-

INTERVENTIONS	RATIONALE
Independent	
labile affect—all of which may vary from moment to moment.	lirium. (The patient is literally fighting for life.) Delirium also can be the result of life-threatening physiologic causes, such as shock or sepsis.
Provide constant and consistent orientation, explaining what has happened and reason for treatments and procedures.	Helps the patient stay in touch with surroundings and reality.
Encourage the patient to talk about the burn circumstances when ready.	Patient may want to tell the story of what happened over and over in order to make some sense out of what is a terrifying situation.
Encourage family/significant other(s) to visit and discuss family happenings. Remind patient of past and future events.	Maintains contact with a familiar reality, creating a sense of attachment and continuity of life.
Provide opportunity for questions and give open, honest answers.	Patients may worry about the outcome and ask about dying, disfigurement. Compassionate statements reflecting the reality of the situation can help the patient/significant other(s) acknowledge that reality and begin to deal with what has happened.
Encourage family/significant other(s) to ventilate concerns/frustrations regarding patient's fluctuating mental status.	Although condition is usually only temporary, deviations in thought processes (delirium) may be very frightening and result in confrontation or avoidance by the family/significant other(s).
Collaborative	
Treat underlying causes of delirium (e.g., shock, sepsis, hypoxia) as determined by tests.	Physiologic conditions must be treated or ruled out, as well as psychologic problems.
Administer medications as indicated; for example,	
Haloperidol (Haldol), Lorazepam (Ativan).	May be needed to calm patient when severely agitated.

CHAPTER 11
SYSTEMIC CONDITIONS

Acquired Immune Deficiency Syndrome (AIDS)

Current literature recommends that the term AIDS should be reserved for a person with at least one life-threatening opportunistic infection or Kaposi's sarcoma, who has no other identifiable reason for profound immunodeficiency, and who has a positive Western Blot test. This care plan focuses on the patient who is acutely ill with opportunistic infection(s)/multiorgan involvement.

PATIENT ASSESSMENT DATA BASE

HISTORY

The syndrome is most likely to occur in a person belonging to one of the following six known categories, however, it may occur outside of these groups.

1. Homosexual men
2. Bisexual men
3. Intravenous drug user
4. Recipient of infected blood or blood products
5. Sexual partners of a person from an aforementioned risk group
6. Children born to an infected mother

Subjective

May complain of fever, chills, night sweats, anorexia, unexplained weight loss, extreme fatigue/malaise, constant or copious diarrhea, dry or productive cough, dyspnea, unexplained bruising, and/or change in mental status, all of unknown origin.

PHYSICAL EXAMINATION

Findings will vary and are dependent on clinical manifestations (e.g., opportunistic infections), stage of the disease(s), and the involved organs/body tissues.

Inspection

Skin: skin turgor may be poor, owing to malnutrition and dehydration (wasting syndrome). Generalized tissue edema may be noted (is associated with and often precedes Kaposi's sarcoma lesions). May present with pallor or cyanosis, multiple petechiae, eccymosis, ulcers, vesicles, rashes, and purple-brown raised lesions. Lesions present are usually due to herpes simplex, herpes zoster, Kaposi's sarcoma, or other various forms of dermatitis.

Oral cavity: white cheesy patches (oral candidiasis) or other lesions may be noted; for example, Kaposi's sarcoma may be present on the tongue/interior of the mouth.

Respirations: shortness of breath, dyspnea on exertion, use of accessory muscles may be noted. Productive or nonproductive cough may be present.

Mentation: a broad continuum of responses from headaches and confusion to profound dementia may be present, depending on the degree of central nervous system (CNS) involvement and the accompanying opportunistic infections.

Musculoskeletal: varying degrees of muscle wasting/weakness and focal motor deficits/seizures associated with subacute or progressive encephalopathy may be present.

Gastrointestinal: may present with intolerance to foods; copious, frequent diarrhea; vomiting. Rectal/perianal abscesses may be present.

Genitalia: mucotaneous manifestations are often present (e.g., herpes).

Auscultation

Breath sounds: may be normal, but adventitious sounds/areas of decreased ventilation often present, reflecting respiratory complications.

Palpation

Lymph glands: enlargement often noted behind ears, in neck, under chin, collarbone or armpits, next to elbow, and in the groin.

Other

Temperature: low-grade fever and/or intermittent temperature spikes usually present.

DIAGNOSTIC STUDIES

CBC/WBC: lymphopenia is present in most cases, differential shift to the left suggests infectious process.

Anergy panel: cutaneous anergy (lack of reactivity to antigens patient has been exposed to previously) is a common indicator of depressed cell-mediated immunity.

Antibody titers: positivity or elevation may be indicative of exposure to infectious agent.

Serologic:

Serum antibody test: Human immunodeficiency virus (HIV, formerly HTLVIII/LAV) screen enzyme-linked immunosorbent assay (ELISA) positive test is indicative of exposure to HIV virus.

Western Blot Test: positive test confirms presence of AIDS.

T4: immune system indicator: type of white cell that orders B cells to produce antibodies (helper cells), T8 (cytopathic cells): alteration in function, numbers, and ratio is noted (reverse of normal 2:1 ratio indicates immune suppression).

Quantitative Ig levels: greater than 2000 mg/dl IgG, and greater than 350 mg/dl IgA, with normal to near normal IgM is an indicator of the ability of the body to show whether infectious processing is intact.

Cultures: urine, blood, lesions, sputum, and secretions may be cultured to identify the opportunistic infection. Some of the most commonly identified are the following:

Protozoa and helminthic infections: Pneumocystis carinii pneumonia (PCP), Cryptosporidium, disseminated meningitis, and encephalitis.

Fungal infections: Candida albicans (candidiasis), Cryptococcus neoformans (cryptococcosis).

Bacterial infections: Mycobacterium avium-intercelluare, Shigella (Shigellosis), Salmonella (Salmonellosis).

Viral infections: Cytomegalovirus (CMV), herpes simplex, herpes zoster.

Radiologic Studies:

Chest x-ray examination may initially be normal or may reveal progressive interstitial infiltrates from PCP (most common opportunistic disease) or other pulmonary complications.

Gallium scan: diffuse pulmonary uptake occurs in PCP and other forms of pneumonia.

Biopsies/tracheobronchial washings may be done for differential diagnosis of pneumonias, Kaposi's sarcoma, or other neoplasms.

Broncoscopy may be done with biopsy when PCP or lung malignancies are suspected.

Endoscopy: disseminated candida may be present, especially in esophagus. Kaposi's sarcoma may be present in gastrointestinal (GI) system.

NURSING PRIORITIES

1. Protect patient from life-threatening infections/complications.
2. Promote/enhance quality of life.
3. Provide information/emotional support for patient/significant other(s).

NURSING DIAGNOSIS:	**Infection, potential for progression to sepsis/onset of new opportunistic infection).**
SUPPORTING DATA/CONTRIBUTING FACTORS:	**Depression of the immune system in combination with malnutrition and in the presence of multi-infectious processes/microorganisms potentiates patient's risk of developing sepsis and/or new opportunistic infections. In addition, use of antimicrobial agents directly alters usual flora, potentiating risk of infection.**
GENERAL PATIENT OUTCOMES:	**Infection prevented/minimized. Patient afebrile, pulse within normal range, breath sounds clear, absence of purulent drainage/localized erythema, urine clear.**

INTERVENTIONS	RATIONALE
Independent	
Wash hands before and after all care contacts. Instruct patient/significant other(s) to wash hands as indicated.	Reduces risk of cross-contamination.
Provide a clean, well-ventilated environment. Maintain isolation/monitor visitors as indicated.	Reduces possibility of patient contracting an iatrogenic infection.

INTERVENTIONS	RATIONALE
Independent	
Clean up spills of body fluids/blood with bleach solution (1:10).	Controls microorganisms on hard surfaces.
Instruct patient and significant other(s) about signs/symptoms of infection, extent and rationale for isolation precautions and maintenance of personal hygiene.	Assists in reducing transmission of infections and reduces unwarranted fear of social contact with patient.
Monitor temperature.	Provides information for baseline data and alerts to frequency of elevations.
Note increased respiratory distress; cough; production of copious amounts of thick, odorous sputum; and congested lungs. (Refer to Nursing Diagnosis: Gas Exchange, impaired, page 306.)	May indicate developing pneumocystis carinii pneumonia (PCP), the most common opportunistic disease occurring in the AIDS patient. However, other fungal, viral, and bacterial infections that compromise the respiratory system may occur.
Investigate complaints of headache, alterations in vision. Note changes in mentation and behavior. Monitor for nuchal rigidity/seizure activity.	Central nervous system (CNS) infections (encephalitis/meningitis) may occur caused by protozoa and helminthic organisms (e.g., strongyloidosis, toxoplasmosis), or fungus (e.g., cryptococcus). Symptoms may vary from subtle changes in mood/sensorium (personality changes or depression) to hallucinations, memory loss, severe dementias, seizures, and loss of vision.
Examine skin/oral mucous membranes for white patches/lesions. (Refer to Nursing Diagnosis: Skin Integrity, impairment of, potential/actual, page 311.)	Oral candidiasis, Kaposi's sarcoma, and herpes are common opportunistic diseases affecting the cutaneous membranes.
Monitor complaints of heartburn, dysphagia, retrosternal pain on swallowing, increased abdominal cramping, profuse diarrhea.	Esophagitis may occur secondary to oral candidiasis or herpes. Cryptosporidosis is a parasitic infection responsible for watery diarrhea (often greater than 15 liters per day). (Refer to Nursing Diagnosis: Fluid Volume Deficit, potential, page 305.)
Inspect wounds/site of invasive devices, noting signs of local inflammation/infection.	Early identification/treatment of secondary infection may prevent sepsis. (Refer to Care Plan: Sepsis/Septicemia/Septic Shock, page 329.)
Wear gloves and gowns during direct contact with secretions/excretions or anytime there is a break in skin of caregivers hands. Wear mask and protective eyewear to protect nose, mouth, and eyes from secretions during procedures such as suctioning, intubation/extubation, or splattering excretions.	Caregivers do not routinely require usage of masks, gowns, or gloves, except when direct contact is anticipated with body fluids (blood, serum), secretions (saliva, sputum, mucous), or excretions (urine, feces, semen, wound drainage, and vomitus).
Dispose of needles/sharps in rigid, puncture-resistant containers.	Prevents accidental innoculation of caregivers. Use of needle cutters and recapping is not recommended. Note: Accidental innoculations/punctures should be reported immediately and followup evaluations done per protocol.
Label blood bags, body fluid containers, soiled dressings/linens and package appropriately for disposal per isolation protocol.	Alerts appropriate personnel/departments to exercise their own isolation procedures.

INTERVENTIONS	RATIONALE
Collaborative	
Monitor laboratory studies; for example, complete blood count (CBC) with differential.	Shifts in the differential and increased white blood count (WBC) indicate infectious process.
Collect specimens of lesions, blood, urine, and sputum for culture/sensitivity as indicated.	May be done to identify cause of fever, diagnose infecting organisms/appropriate course of treatment.
Administer antibiotic, antifungal/antimicrobial agents; for example, co-trimoxazole (Bactrim, Septra), nystatin (Mycostatin), pentamidine (Pentam 300); or experimental drugs such as azidothymidime (AZT) and DHPG.	Combats infectious process. Some drugs are targeted for specific organisms/affected system. Other drugs are targeted to improve immune function. Although no cure is currently available, experimental agents such as AZT are aimed at blocking the enzyme that enables the virus to begin reproducing, thereby retarding the progression of the disease. DHPG is used when CMV is present to prevent blindness/life threatening dissemination. Note: AZT may potentiate acute stage, so usage is currently limited.

NURSING DIAGNOSIS: **Fluid Volume Deficit, potential.**

SUPPORTING DATA/CONTRIBUTING FACTORS: **Copious diarrhea, malnutrition, fever, profuse sweating, and vomiting result in excessive fluid/electrolyte depletion.**

GENERAL PATIENT OUTCOMES: **Hydration is maintained as evidenced by moist mucous membranes, good skin turgor, stable BP, adequate urine output.**

INTERVENTIONS	RATIONALE
Independent	
Monitor for decreased skin turgor, dry mucous membranes, thirst, postural hypotension, tachycardia, low urine output.	Fluid volume may be depleted as a result of diarrhea, lack of oral fluid intake, or fluid shifts associated with disease process, (e.g., sepsis).
Note temperature elevation, duration of febrile episode.	Excessive diaphoresis and increased metabolic demands associated with fever result in increased insensible fluid losses.
Measure hemodynamic pressures if available; for example, central venous pressure (CVP).	Direct assessment of circulating fluid volume.
Measure intake and output; note urine specific gravity. Quantify amount of diarrheal loss. Weigh as indicated.	Increased specific gravity/decreased output reflects altered renal perfusion/circulating volume. Note: Monitoring fluid balance in AIDS is difficult owing to excessive gastrointestinal/insensible losses. In addition, weight loss may reflect muscle wasting as well as state of hydration.

INTERVENTIONS	RATIONALE
Independent	
Encourage oral fluid intake at minimum of 2500 ml per day. Make fluids easily accessible to patient; use fluids that are tolerable to the patient and that replace needed electrolytes (e.g., Gatorade, broth).	Restores fluid balance, reduces thirst, and moisturizes mucous membranes. Certain fluids may be too painful to consume (e.g. acidic juices) because of mouth lesions. If nausea prevents oral intake, fluids may be replaced by feeding tube or parenteral route.
Provide foods high in bulk. Avoid foods potentiating diarrhea (e.g., nuts, cabbage, milk products).	Bulk improves consistency of stool, and avoidance of foods that are irritating to GI tract may reduce diarrhea.
Collaborative	
Administer intravenous (IV) fluids/electrolytes.	May be necessary to support/to augment circulating volume, especially if oral intake is inadequate.
Monitor laboratory studies, as indicated; for example, hemoglobin (Hgb)/hematocrit, (Hct).	Dilutional changes useful in estimating fluid needs.
Serum/urine electrolytes,	Alerts to possible electrolyte disturbances and determines replacement needs.
Blood urea nitrogen (BUN) creatinine.	Evaluates renal perfusion/function.
Administer antiemetics; for example, prochlorperazine maleate (Compazine), trimethobenzamide hydrochloride (Tigan), metoclopramide hydrochloride (Reglan).	Reduces incidence of vomiting to reduce further loss of fluids/electrolytes.
Administer antidiarrheals; for example, diphenoxylate (Lomotil), ioperamide (Imodium), camphorated tincture of opium (paregoric), or antispasmodics, mepenzolate bromide (Cantil).	Decreases the amount and fluidity of stool; may reduce intestinal spasm and perstalsis. Note: Antibiotics also may be used to treat diarrhea if its cause is infection.

NURSING DIAGNOSIS:	**Gas Exchange, impaired (potential).**
SUPPORTING DATA/CONTRIBUTING FACTORS:	**Development of opportunistic infections owing to immunosuppression/malignancies may seriously affect gas exchange/respiratory function. Generalized weakness and wasting of respiratory musculature result in ineffective breathing patterns, retained secretions, and impaired gas exchange.**
GENERAL PATIENT OUTCOMES:	**Respiratory rate and arterial blood gases (ABGs) within patient's normal limits. Free of dyspnea/cyanosis. Breath sounds and chest x-ray examination clear or improving.**

INTERVENTIONS	RATIONALE
Independent	
Auscultate breath sounds, noting areas of decreased/absent ventilation and presence of adventitious sounds (e.g., crackles, wheezes, rhonchi).	Suggests developing pulmonary complication/infection (e.g., atelectasis/pneumonia).
Note onset of cyanosis, tachypnea, dyspnea, anxiety, use of accessory muscles and increased work of breathing.	Reflects respiratory distress and need for increased surveillance and treatment.
Assist patient in assuming position that facilitates respirations and coughing. Turn, assist in coughing and deep breathing as indicated.	Promotes optimal pulmonary function, and reduces incidence of aspiration or infection caused by atelectasis.
Suction as indicated, using sterile technique and observing safety precautions (e.g., mask, protective eyewear).	Assists in clearing the ventilatory passages, thereby facilitating gas exchange.
Assess changes in level of consciousness.	Hypoxemia can result in changes ranging from anxiety and confusion to unresponsiveness.
Investigate complaints of chest pain.	Pleuritic chest pain may reflect nonspecific pneumonitis or pleural effusions associated with malignancies.
Collaborative	
Monitor/graph serial ABGs.	Reflects the oxygenation and ventilation status of the patient and therapy needs.
Review serial chest x-ray examinations.	Presence of diffuse infiltrates may suggest pneumonia, PCP, and areas of congestion/consolidation may reflect other pulmonary complications; for example, atelectasis or Kaposi's sarcoma lesions.
Instruct in use of incentive spirometer. Provide chest physiotherapy (e.g., percussion, vibration, and postural drainage).	Encourages proper breathing technique and improves lung expansion. Chest physiotherapy loosens secretions, dislodges mucous plugs to promote airway clearance. Note: In the event of multiple skin lesions, this therapy may be discontinued.
Provide humidified supplemental oxygen by cannula, mask, intubation/mechanical ventilation. (Refer to Care Plan: Ventilatory Assistance (Mechanical), page 115.)	Maintains effective ventilation/oxygenation during respiratory crisis.
Administer medications as indicated:	
Antimicrobials; for example, co-trimoxazole (Bactrim, Septra);	These two drugs are useful in treating PCP; however, choice of therapy is dependent on individual situation/infecting organism(s).
Bronchodilators/cough expectorant/depressants.	May be needed to improve/maintain airway patency or to help clear secretions.

NURSING DIAGNOSIS: **Injury, potential for, altered clotting factors.**

SUPPORTING DATA/CONTRIBUTING FACTORS:	**Decreased vitamin K absorption, alteration in hepatic function, presence of autoimmune antiplatelet antibodies, malignancies (Kaposi's sarcoma), and/or circulating endotoxins (sepsis) may alter coagulation and potentiate risk of bleeding.**
GENERAL PATIENT OUTCOMES:	**Bleeding is prevented/controlled.**

INTERVENTIONS	RATIONALE
Independent	
Hematest body fluids for occult blood (e.g., urine, stool, sputum, vomitus).	Prompt detection of bleeding/initiation of therapy may prevent critical hemorrhage. (Refer to Care Plan: Upper Gastrointestinal/Esophageal Bleeding, page 197.)
Observe for epistaxis, hemoptysis, hematuria, nonmenstrual vaginal bleeding, or oozing from lesions/body orifices, IV insertion sites.	Spontaneous bleeding may indicate development of disseminated intravascular coagulation (DIC). (Refer to Care Plan: Disseminated Intravascular Coagulation (DIC), page 319.)
Monitor for changes in vital signs and skin color; for example, blood pressure (BP), pulse, respirations, skin pallor/discoloration.	Presence of bleeding/hemorrhage may lead to circulatory failure/shock.
Monitor for change in level of consciousness and visual disturbances.	Change may reflect cerebral bleeding.
Avoid intramuscular (IM) injections, rectal temperatures/suppositories, rectal tubes.	Protects patient from procedure-related causes of bleeding. Insertion of thermometers or rectal tubes can damage or tear rectal mucosa.
Maintain a safe environment; for example, keep all necessary objects and call bell within patient's reach, keep bed in low position and bedrest (for platelets less than 10,000). Avoid use of aspirin products.	Reduces accidental injury, which could result in bleeding.
Collaborative	
Review laboratory studies; for example, prothrombin time (PT), partial thromboplastin time (PTT), clotting time, platelets, Hgb/Hct.	Detects alterations in clotting capability, identifies therapy needs.
Administer blood or clotting factors as indicated.	Transfusions may be required in the event of massive spontaneous bleeding.

NURSING DIAGNOSIS:	**Nutrition, alteration in, less than body requirements.**
SUPPORTING DATA/CONTRIBUTING FACTORS:	**Nausea and vomiting, intestinal disturbances, drug toxicity, and hyperactive gag reflex (resulting from pres-**

ence of lesions in the mouth and throat) limit the patient's desire and ability to eat. Diarrhea may lead to excessive GI losses and malabsorption. In addition, presence of fever/infection increases metabolic activity/nutritional needs at a time when the patient is unable/least desires to eat.

GENERAL PATIENT OUTCOMES: **Nutritional intake is adequate for needs as evidenced by positive nitrogen balance, weight stabilized/gain recorded, and improvement in activity tolerance. Nausea/vomiting is alleviated.**

INTERVENTIONS	RATIONALE
Independent	
Assess ability to chew, to taste, and to swallow.	Lesions of the mouth, throat, and esophagus may cause dysphagia and limit patient's ability to chew, reduce desire to eat.
Auscultate bowel sounds.	Hypermotility of intestinal tract is common and is associated with vomiting and diarrhea.
Remove existing noxious environmental stimuli or conditions that aggravate gag reflex.	Reduces stimulus of the vomiting center in the medulla.
Provide frequent mouth care, observing secretion precautions. Avoid alcohol-containing mouth washes.	Promotes patient comfort by reducing discomfort associated with nausea/vomiting, oral lesions, mucosal dryness, and halitosis.
Weigh as indicated.	Weight loss is an indicator of adequacy of nutritional intake.
Plan diet with patient/significant other(s), using small meals, nonacidic foods and beverages, with choice of foods palatable to patient. Encourage "foods from home" if appropriate.	Limit food(s) that induce nausea/vomiting or that are poorly tolerated by the patient. Including patient in planning gives patient sense of control of environment and may enhance intake. Fulfilling cravings for noninstitutional food also may improve intake.
Record caloric intake.	Identifies need for supplements or alternate feeding methods.
Collaborative	
Review laboratory studies (e.g., BUN, glucose, liver function studies, electrolytes, protein, and albumin).	Indicates nutritional status and organ function and identifies replacement needs.
Maintain nothing-by mouth (NPO) status when appropriate.	May be needed to reduce vomiting.
Insert/maintain nasogastric tube if indicated.	May be needed to reduce nausea/vomiting or to administer tube feedings. Note: Esophageal irritation from existing infection (Candida/Herpes or K.S.) may

INTERVENTIONS	RATIONALE
Collaborative	
	provide site for secondary infections/trauma and therefore should be used with caution.
Consult with dietician to provide dietary modifications. (Refer to Care Plan: Nutritional Support, page 367.)	If patient is eating, intake may be enhanced by individualized menus to meet specific needs/desires.
Administer total parenteral nutrition (TPN) (hyperalimentation/intralipids) as indicated.	Parenteral nutrients may be required if oral/enteral feedings are not tolerated.
Administer antiemetics; for example, metoclopramide hydrochloride (Reglan).	Reduces incidence of vomiting, promotes gastric function.
Administer parenteral vitamin supplements as indicated.	Vitamins are deficient as a result of decreased food intake and/or disorders of digestion and absorption in the GI system. When oral intake resumed/tolerated, vitamins may be administered orally.

NURSING DIAGNOSIS:	**Comfort, alteration in, pain acute/chronic.**
SUPPORTING DATA/CONTRIBUTING FACTORS:	**Discomfort and/or pain may be present, associated with presence of malignancies or opportunistic infections which may cause internal/external cutaneous lesions, headaches, chest pain, night sweats, and tissue necrosis. Abdominal cramping and rectal pain/excoriation is associated with diarrhea.**
GENERAL PATIENT OUTCOMES:	**Verbalizes relief of pain, demonstrates relaxed posture/facial expression, and is able to sleep/rest appropriately.**

INTERVENTIONS	RATIONALE
Independent	
Assess pain, noting patient's description of location, intensity/degree, frequency, and time of onset. Note nonverbal clues (e.g., restlessness, tachycardia, grimacing).	Useful for noting development/resolution of complications and identifies interventions needed.
Encourage verbalization of feelings.	Can reduce anxiety and fear and thereby reduce perception of itensity of pain.
Provide distractions (e.g., conversation, television).	Diverting concentration may alleviate some degree of pain.
Use palliative measure (e.g., repositioning, massage).	Promotes relaxation/decreases muscle tension.

INTERVENTIONS	RATIONALE
Independent	
Apply warm/moist packs to pentamidine (Pentam 300) injection sites for 20 minutes after administration.	These injections are known to cause sterile abscesses and pain.
Provide cold compresses/sponge with tepid water.	Reduces fever without increasing discomfort of skin lesions. Note: Mottled skin/vasomotor changes indicate severe drop in skin temperature, and bath should be halted immediately.
Instruct patient in use of guided imagery, relaxation techniques.	May decrease the need of narcotic analgesics (CNS depressants) when there is already a neuromotor, degenerative process involved.
Provide oral care. (Refer to Nursing Diagnosis: Oral Mucous Membranes, alteration in, page 312.)	Oral ulcerations/lesions may cause severe discomfort.
Collaborative	
Administer analgesics/antipyretics: acetaminophen (Tylenol), narcotic analgesics.	Provides relief of pain/discomfort, reduces fever.

NURSING DIAGNOSIS:	**Skin Integrity, impairment of, potential/actual.**
SUPPORTING DATA/CONTRIBUTING FACTORS:	**AIDS-related dermatitis, bacterial and fungal infections (e.g., herpes, candida), opportunistic disease processes (e.g., Kaposi's sarcoma), and decreased level of activity can cause skin lesions/ulcerations or decubitus formation. In addition, malnutrition and immunosuppression delays healing.**
GENERAL PATIENT OUTCOMES:	**Skin integrity maintained/restored.**

INTERVENTIONS	RATIONALE
Independent	
Assess skin daily. Note color, turgor, circulation, and sensation. Describe lesions and observed changes.	Establishes baseline with which changes in status can be compared, and appropriate interventions instituted.
Maintain/instruct in good skin hygiene; for example, wash thoroughly, pat dry carefully, and massage with lotion or appropriate cream.	Maintaining clean, dry skin provides a barrier to infection. Patting skin dry instead of rubbing reduces risk of dermal trauma to dry/fragile skin. Massaging increases circulation to the skin and promotes comfort. Note: Isolation precautions (e.g., gloves, linen, diapers) are required, especially if extensive mucocutaneous herpes lesions are present.

INTERVENTIONS	RATIONALE
Independent	
Reposition frequently. Protect bony prominences with pillows pads, eggcrate mattress, sheepskin protectors.	Reduces stress on pressure points and reduces possibility of ulceration/decubiti.
Maintain clean, dry, wrinkle-free bed.	Skin friction caused by wet or wrinkled sheets leads to breakdown and potentiates infection.
Encourage ambulation/out of bed as tolerated.	Decreases pressure on skin from prolonged bedrest.
Cleanse perianal area. Remove stool with water and mineral oil. Avoid use of toilet paper if vesicles present. Apply protective creams (e.g., zinc oxide, A and D ointment).	Prevents maceration caused by diarrhea and keeps perianal lesions dry. Note: Use of toilet paper may abrade lesions.
Rinse oral mucosal lesions with saline/hydrogen peroxide solutions. Apply lip balm. (Refer to Nursing Diagnosis: Oral Mucous Membranes, alteration in, below.)	Reduces spread of lesions and encrustrations from candidiasis, and promotes comfort.
Use soft toothbrush/gentle brushing.	Rids mouth of microbes without abrading gums.
Cover open pressure ulcers with sterile dressings or protective barrier, as indicated.	May reduce bacterial contamination, promote healing.
Collaborative	
Obtain cultures of open skin lesions.	Identifies infectious pathogens and appropriate treatment needs.
Apply/administer systemic/topical drugs as indicated; for example, acyclovir sodium (Zovirax).	Used in treatment of herpes infectious process. In the event of multidose ointments, care must be taken to avoid cross-contamination.
Cover ulcerated Kaposi's sarcoma lesions with wet-to-wet dressings or antibiotic ointment and telfa, as indicated.	Protects ulcerated areas from contamination and promotes healing.
Provide flotation mattress/bed.	Reduces pressure on skin/tissue.

NURSING DIAGNOSIS:	**Oral Mucous Membranes, alteration in.**
SUPPORTING DATA/CONTRIBUTING FACTORS:	**Presence of Candida, herpes, Kaposi's sarcoma, malnutrition, nausea/vomiting, and side effects of drugs, chemotherapy, contribute to development of oral lesions/ulcerations.**
GENERAL PATIENT OUTCOMES:	**Mucous membranes are intact, pink, and moist; free of inflammation/ulcerations.**

INTERVENTIONS	RATIONALE
Independent	
Note ability to swallow, to handle secretions.	Edema, open lesions, and crusting on oral mucous membranes and throat may cause difficulty with swallowing and increase risk of aspiration.
Provide oral care using soft toothbrush, nonabrasive toothpaste, nonalcohol mouthwash, and lip moisturizer. Use gloves when in direct contact with lesions/secretions.	Reduces risk of further infection, alleviates discomfort, and promotes feeling of well-being. Use of gloves reduces risk to caregiver.
Plan diet to avoid salty, spicy, abrasive, and acidic food or drink. Check for temperature tolerance of foods.	Open lesions will be painful and will be aggravated by salt, spice, acidic foods/beverages. Abrasive foods may open healing lesions. Extreme cold or heat can cause pain to sensitive mucous membranes.
Encourage oral intake of at least 2,500 ml per day.	Maintains hydration, prevents drying of oral cavity.
Collaborative	
Obtain culture specimens as indicated.	Reveals causative organisms and identifies appropriate therapies.
Administer medications, as indicated; for example, nystatin (Mycostatin) solution/troches.	Specific drug choice is dependent on individual situation/infecting organism(s) (e.g., Candida).
Refer for dental consultation, if appropriate.	Gingivitis may require additional therapy to reduce dental losses.

NURSING DIAGNOSIS:	**Activity Intolerance.**
SUPPORTING DATA/CONTRIBUTING FACTORS:	**Malnutrition, weight loss, fever, and CNS involvement can contribute to lethargy, feelings of profound fatigue, and generalized weakness.**
GENERAL PATIENT OUTCOMES:	**During activity, BP and pulse are within patient's normal range; patient is free of dyspnea, syncope, and chest pain.**

INTERVENTIONS	RATIONALE
Independent	
Monitor physiologic response to activity; for example, changes in BP or heart/respiratory rate.	Tolerance may vary greatly, depending on the stage of the disease process, nutrition state, fluid balance, and number/type of opportunistic diseases that the patient has been subject to.
Assist with hygiene, grooming, toileting. Protect patient from injury during activities.	Weakness may make activities of daily living almost impossible for the patient to complete.

INTERVENTIONS	RATIONALE
Independent	
Plan care to allow for rest periods. Plan activities for periods when patient has most energy. Involve patient/significant other(s) in schedule planning.	Planning will allow patient to be active during times when energy level is higher, which may restore a feeling of well-being. Frequent rest periods are needed to restore/conserve energy.
Establish realistic activity goals with patient.	Provides for a sense of control and feelings of accomplishment.
Encourage nutritional intake. (Refer to Nursing Diagnosis: Nutrition, alteration in, less than body requirements, page 308.)	Adequate intake/utilization of nutrients is necessary to meet energy needs for activity.
Collaborative	
Provide supplemental oxygen as indicated.	Presence of anemia/hypoxemia contributes to activity tolerance.

NURSING DIAGNOSIS:	**Thought Processes, alteration in.**
SUPPORTING DATA/CONTRIBUTING FACTORS:	**Hypoxemia, CNS infection, brain malignancies, and/or disseminated systemic opportunistic infection resulting in renal failure, hepatic insufficiency, and severe electrolyte imbalance can produce progressive changes in mental and/or neurologic function.**
GENERAL PATIENT OUTCOMES:	**Alert/oriented. Free of hallucinations.**

INTERVENTIONS	RATIONALE
Independent	
Assess mental/neurologic status: note changes in orientation, level of response to stimuli, ability to solve problems; altered sleep patterns; hallucinations.	Establishes functional neurologic level at time of admission and alerts the nurse to changes in status which may be associated with an opportunistic disease, environmental stressors, psychologic stress, or side effects of drug therapy.
Monitor for signs of CNS infection; for example, headache, nuchal rigidity, vomiting, fever. (Refer to Nursing Diagnosis: Infection, potential for, page 303.)	Central nervous system symptoms associated with disseminated meningitis/encephalitis may range from subtle personality changes to confusion, irritability, drowsiness, stupor, seizures, and dementia.
Maintain a pleasant environment with appropriate auditory and visual stimuli. Reduce provocative/noxious stimuli.	Providing normal environmental stimuli such as radio, television, calendars, and clocks may help in maintaining some sense of reality orientation. If the patient is prone to seizures or increased intracranial pressure, reducing external stimuli may become necessary.

INTERVENTIONS	RATIONALE
Independent	
Reorient as needed. Encourage family/significant other(s) to provide reorientation and current news (e.g., family events).	Frequent reorientation to place and time may be necessary, especially during periods of fever/acute CNS involvement. Familiar contacts are often helpful in maintaining reality orientation, especially if patient is hallucinating.
Maintain safe environment; for example, call bell within patient reach; bed in low position/rails up; seizure precautions; soft restraints if indicated.	Decreases the possibility of patient injury in the presence of seizure activity.
Provide information about care on an ongoing basis. Answer questions simply and honestly. Repeat explanations as needed.	Can reduce anxiety and fear of unknown, enhance patient's understanding and involvement/cooperation in treatment.
Collaborative	
Assist with diagnostic studies (e.g., lumbar puncture, CAT scan), laboratory tests as indicated (e.g., BUN/creatinine, electrolytes, ABGs).	Choice of tests/studies are dependent on clinical manifestations and index of suspicion, inasmuch as changes in mental status may reflect a wide variety of causative factors (e.g., CMV meningitis/encephalitis, drug toxicity, electrolyte imbalances, and altered organ function).
Administer amphotericin B (Fungizone) as indicated.	Antifungal useful in treatment of cryptococcosis meningitis.

NURSING DIAGNOSIS: **Anxiety/Fear.**

SUPPORTING DATA/CONTRIBUTING FACTORS: **The fear and realization of death are ever present, once the diagnosis of AIDS has been made. The patient also may fear transmission of the disease to family/loved ones. Changes in role function and patient's appearance contribute to anxiety and fear.**

GENERAL PATIENT OUTCOMES: **Concerns are being discussed. Patient verbalizes reduced anxiety/fear.**

INTERVENTIONS	RATIONALE
Independent	
Maintain frequent contact with patient. Provide accurate, consistent information regarding prognosis.	Provides assurance that the patient is not alone and fosters trust. Accurate, consistent communication permits patient to make decisions/choices based on realities.
Be alert to signs of denial/depression; for example, withdrawal, angry inappropriate remarks.	Patient may use defense mechanism of denial and express hope that diagnosis is inaccurate. Feelings of

INTERVENTIONS	RATIONALE
Independent	
	guilt and spiritual distress may cause the patient to become withdrawn.
Provide open environment in which patient feels safe to discuss feelings or to refrain from talking.	Needs to feel accepted in present condition without feeling judged.
Permit expressions of anger, fear, despair without confrontation. Give information that feelings are normal and are to be expressed.	Acceptance of feelings allows patient to begin to deal with situation.
Recognize and support stage patient/family is in in the grieving process.	Choice of interventions are dictated by stage of grief, coping behaviors (e.g., anger/withdrawal, denial).
Explain procedures, providing opportunity for questions and honest answers.	Accurate information allows the patient to deal more effectively with the reality of the situation, thereby reducing anxiety and fear of the unknown.
Identify and encourage interaction with support systems. Encourage verbalization/interaction with family/significant other(s).	Reduces feeling of isolation. If direct support systems are not available (e.g., family), outside sources may be needed immediately (e.g., AIDS Task Force).
Provide information and support for significant other(s).	Allows for better interpersonal interaction and reduction of anxiety and fear.
Include significant other(s) as indicated when major decisions are to be made.	Ensures a support system for the patient and allows the significant other the chance to participate in patient's life.
Collaborative	
Refer to psychiatric counseling.	May require further assistance in dealing with diagnosis/prognosis.

NURSING DIAGNOSIS:	**Social Isolation.**
SUPPORTING DATA/CONTRIBUTING FACTORS:	**Major alterations occur in established social/professional/sexual patterns: changes in body image; probable loss of job, finances, home, and insurance; possible loss of acquaintances/friends, and significant other(s). Sometimes physical isolation can contribute to social isolation and potentiate depression.**
GENERAL PATIENT OUTCOMES:	**Expresses increased sense of self-worth and is involved in activities at level of ability/desire.**

INTERVENTIONS	RATIONALE
Independent	
Spend time talking with patient during and between care activities. Be supportive, allowing for verbalization. Treat with dignity and regard for patient's feelings.	Patient may experience physical isolation owing to current medical status and certainly experiences social isolation secondary to diagnosis of AIDS.
Limit/avoid use of mask when possible (e.g., when talking to patient).	Reduces patient's sense of isolation and provides positive social contact, which may enhance patient's self-esteem.
Explain isolation precaution/procedures to patient and family/significant other(s).	Gloves, gowns, mask are not routinely required with a diagnosis of AIDS. Misuse of these barriers enhances feelings of emotional as well as physical isolation. When precautions are necessary, explanations help patient understand reasons for procedures and provides feeling of inclusion in what is happening.
Encourage social activities within tolerated level.	Participation with others can maintain a feeling of belonging.
Encourage active role of contact with significant other(s).	Helps reestablish a feeling of participation in a social relationship. May lessen likelihood of suicide attempts.
Be alert to verbal/nonverbal cues; for example, withdrawal, statements of despair, sense of aloneness. Ask the patient if thoughts of suicide are being entertained.	Patients usually give indicators of despair and suicidal ideation and when confronted are willing to talk about these thoughts, sense of isolation, and hopelessness.

NURSING DIAGNOSIS:	**Powerlessness.**
SUPPORTING DATA/CONTRIBUTING FACTORS:	**The confirmed diagnosis of a terminal disease, with alteration in body image and desired lifestyle, as well as the social ramifications of AIDS, contributes to feelings of loss of control over patient's life. Until and unless the grieving process is completed, the patient will experience a sense of powerlessness. Advancing CNS involvement may contribute to loss of control over all aspects of patient's life.**
GENERAL PATIENT OUTCOMES:	**Verbalizes some feelings of control over situation, expressing feelings of depression/anger/powerlessness.**

INTERVENTIONS	RATIONALE
Independent	
Identify factors that contribute to the patient's feelings of powerlessness; for example, diagnosis of a terminal illness, lack of support systems/isolation, lack of knowledge about present situation.	Patients with AIDS usually are aware of the current literature and prognosis. Fear of AIDS by the general population as well as by the patient's family/significant other(s) is the most profound cause of the patient's isolation. For some patients, this may be the first time that the family has been made aware that the patient has chosen an alternative lifestyle.
Assess degree of feelings of helplessness; for example, verbal/nonverbal expressions indicating lack of control—"It won't make any difference"—flat affect, lack of communication.	Determines the status of the individual patient and allows for appropriate intervention.
Encourage active role in planning activities, establishing realistic/attainable daily goals.	May enhance feelings of control and self-worth.
Encourage patient control and responsibility as much as possible. Show concern for the person. Identify things that the patient can and cannot control.	Many factors associated with the treatments used in this debilitating and ultimately fatal disease process place the patient at the mercy of medical personnel and other unknown people who may be making decisions for and about the patient without regard for the patient's loss of independence.
Provide written and oral explanations of procedures, examinations, and precautions to the patient and significant other(s).	Information can help patient/significant other(s) know what is happening and have a say in decision making.
Maintain strict confidentiality.	Patient's rights are respected.
Collaborative	
Refer to resources; for example, social services, counselors, and AIDS Task Force (local/national).	Establishes support systems, reducing feelings of isolation and powerlessness.

Disseminated Intravascular Coagulation (DIC)

Disseminated intravascular coagulation (DIC) is a unique disorder of coagulation during which hemorrhage and thrombosis occur simultaneously. Fibrin is deposited in the microcirculation, creating multiple thromboses and depleting the blood of essential clotting components. Intravascular clotting leads to circulation problems affecting major organ function and activating the fibrinolytic system in an attempt to lyse the clots. The process of fibrinolysis coupled with the loss of clotting components results in hemorrhage.

PATIENT ASSESSMENT DATA BASE

HISTORY

DIC can occur as a complication of a variety of disorders:

Recent episode of shock; for example, septic, hypovolemic, posttraumatic, or cardiogenic shock.

Acute concurrent infectious process.

Obstetric complications; for example, abruptio placenta, amniotic fluid embolus, retained dead fetus, septic abortion.

Circulatory crises; for example, pulmonary embolus, dissecting aneurysm.

Immunologic problems: transplant/tissue graft rejection, incompatible blood transfusion.

Surgery: cardiothoracic, utilization of extracorporeal circulation.

Trauma: burns, crushing injuries, severe head injury, snake bite, heat stroke.

Congenital conditions: cavernous hemangioma, hyaline membrane disease.

Metabolic/endocrine diseases; for example, renal failure, diabetic ketoacidosis.

Malignant disease; for example, leukemia, solid tumors.

Subjective

Complaints vary and depend on location of hemorrhage(s)/thrombosis. Symptoms may include pain (abdomen, back, muscles, and joints), nausea/vomiting, dyspnea, feelings of impending doom.

PHYSICAL EXAMINATION

Although some patients have no signs except abnormal laboratory values, physical findings are variable, depending on the underlying cause, stage of hemorrhage/thrombus, degree of organ/system involvement.

Inspection

Mentation: altered level of consciousness, coma, convulsions may be noted.

Musculoskeletal: occasionally, facial droop/muscle weakness/hemiparesis may occur, suggestive of cerebral hemorrhage/thrombosis.

Skin: oozing of blood from puncture sites, incisions, body orifices, and mucous membranes, or significant hemorrhage (e.g., epistaxis, hematemesis, melena, and hematuria) often present. Other manifestations may include petechiae, purpura, ecchymosis, hematoma formation. Acral cyanosis/focal gangrene (gray to purplish-black discoloration of fingers, toes, lips, ears) may occur.

Palpation

Peripheral pulses: tachycardia, weak/thready pulses are related to hypovolemia.

Auscultation

Blood pressure: hypotension, decreased pulse pressure, reflecting decreased cardiac output/hypovolemia may be noted.

DIAGNOSTIC STUDIES

CBC may reveal decreased Hct/Hgb, distorted and fragmented red blood cells (schistocytes), and leukocytosis.

Coagulation panel: abnormalities in general tests of coagulation may include the following:

Prothrombin time (PT) and partial thromboplastin time (PTT): prolonged.

Platelets: thrombocytopenia, owing to consumption of platelets.

Fibrinogen: decreased because of excessive utilization/clot formation.

Thrombin time: prolonged time at 1:1 dilution with normal plasma indicates presence of circlating anticoagulants (e.g., fibrin split products).

Fibrin split products (FSP) increase, indicating widespread dissolution of clots.

Antithrombin III: absent.

Factor levels: especially factors V and VIII may be depleted.

Protamine sulfate test: positive result indicative of unstable fibrin (fibrin monomers).

Peripheral blood smear: presence of large platelets, possibly owing to rapid utilization; red cell fragments reflect damage to cells during circulation through areas of fibrin clot formation.

NURSING PRIORITIES

1. Support vital organ functions.
2. Assist with measures to correct/halt abnormal coagulopathy.
3. Prevent/minimize complications.
4. Promote comfort.
5. Provide emotional support to patient/significant other(s).

NURSING DIAGNOSIS:	**Fluid Volume Deficit, potential.**
SUPPORTING DATA/CONTRIBUTING FACTORS:	**Consumption of clotting factors/activation of fibrinolytic system can result in hemorrhage unchecked by normal mechanisms, leading to severe volume depletion. Changes in capillary permeability/osmotic pressure may cause further depletion of circulating fluid volume.**
GENERAL PATIENT OUTCOMES:	**Vital signs within normal range, peripheral pulses palpable and of good quality, urine output greater than 20 to 30 ml per hour.**

INTERVENTIONS	RATIONALE
Independent	
Promote bedrest/limit activity, protect from trauma.	Minor injury/stress may potentiate hemorrhage. (Refer to Nursing Diagnosis: Injury, potential for, continued activation of altered clotting cycle, page 324.)
Assess blood pressure (BP), heart rate, peripheral pulses, capillary refill. Note complaints of dizziness/syncope with movement. Monitor hemodynamic parameters; for example, mean arterial pressure (MAP)/central venous pressure (CVP).	Labile BP/hypotension, tachycardia, weak/thready pulses, delayed capillary refill, low MAP/CVP, suggest hypovolemia.
Evaluate changes in mentation; observe pupils, response to stimuli.	Cerebral anoxia may occur secondary to cerebral or systemic hemorrhage, hypotension, cerebral edema, and hypoxemia. (Refer to Nursing Diagnosis: Tissue Perfusion, page 322.)
Observe arterial and venipuncture sites, surgical incisions, skin, mucous membranes, drains, and tubes for oozing/frank bleeding.	Persistent oozing from multiple sites or increased bloody drainage from tubes, pumps, and drains may indicate developing/increasing coagulopathy.
Hematest secretions/excretions (e.g., sputum, urine, emesis, nasogastric drainage, and stools) for occult blood.	Identify covert bleeding early to initiate therapy/minimize complications.
Assess areas of swelling/distention. Measure circumference of extremities/abdomen as indicated.	Minimal trauma/increased capillary fragility may lead to bleeding into muscles or closed compartments, such as peritoneal space.
Assess ability to move lower extremities. Note presence/absence of joint/muscle pain.	Nerve compression may occur at L2-3 from deep retroperitoneal bleed. Joint/muscle pains may also indicate areas of concealed hemorrhage.
Measure/estimate actual blood loss from drains, tubes.	Assists in determination of fluid volume replacement needs.
Monitor urine output and specific gravity.	Decreased urine output and increased specific gravity may be due to dehydration, hypovolemia, hypotension, or renal microthrombosis.
Monitor total fluid intake. Record subtotals of individual intravenous (IV) components.	Massive fluid resucitation may be required to restore intravascular and extracellular fluid volume at a level that provides optimum BP, cardiac output, and urinary flow. Many fluids may be used; for example, volume expanders, whole blood/blood products, saline solution primers. Subtotals identify continuing needs/excessive replacement of specific components.
Observe for transfusion reactions: hives, chills, fever, facial flush, palpitations, tachycardia, chest pain, dyspnea, headache.	More likely to occur when massive transfusions are required, inasmuch as exposure to multiple donor leukocytes and plasma proteins increases the chance for transfusion reactions.
Note presence/degree of peripheral and dependent edema.	Sudden edema can occur owing to alterations in capillary permeability and osmotic pressure, leading to fluid shifts into tissues. Hypovolemia may be present in spite of apparent edema.

INTERVENTIONS	RATIONALE
Collaborative	
Administer IV fluids/volume expanders (e.g., lactated Ringer's/saline solutions, albumin).	Replacement prevents/corrects hypovolemic shock.
Insert/maintain arterial pressure monitoring lines.	Despite risks of aggravating local bleeding, invasive monitoring may be desired to assess fluid volume and blood pressure and to provide blood specimen aquisition without repeated venipuncture.
Review chest/abdominal x-ray examinations.	Hemothorax, hemoperitoneum may be identified as sources of hemorrhage or result in DIC.
Prepare for/assist with surgical procedures as indicated.	Correction of conditions such as obstetric emergencies and gastric hemorrhage may remove stimulus to coagulation process, terminating DIC.
Administer fresh whole blood, frozen plasma, platelets, and/or specific clotting factors.	Specific components are given according to deficits identified on coagulation panel and existing protocols. Note: Heparin therapy may be initiated prior to blood replacement to prevent consumption of clotting factors/components as they are infused.
Monitor/plot coagulation studies and hematocrit (Hct).	Reveals trends necessary to identify fluid/blood or component replacement needs, to regulate heparin dose, and to evaluate patient's response to therapy. Changes in laboratory values may be evident before bleeding is obvious, and laboratory values may improve before bleeding stops.
Administer IV heparin therapy continuously via infusion pump or intermittently (e.g., minidose protocol).	Heparin helps prevent further thrombus formation, slows coagulation/consumption of clotting factors. It does not lyse clots that have already formed. Heparin should be given IV for an immediate therapeutic effect and for more accurate dose regulation/absorption. Heparin is usually continued until clinical and laboratory evidence suggests that the patient is recovering. Dosage may be reduced/altered to ensure therapeutic effect when heparin clearance is reduced/drug half-life prolonged in presence of renal/liver failure. Note: Fresh forzen plasma may be given prior to/during heparin administration to ensure adequate antithrombin III for interaction with heparin.
Administer vasopressors, monitor effects.	Vasopressors may be used to manage fluid-resistant hypotension.

NURSING DIAGNOSIS:	**Tissue Perfusion, alteration in.**
SUPPORTING DATA/CONTRIBUTING FACTORS:	**Thrombus formation in the microcirculation leads to arterial vasoconstriction and capillary dilation with arteriovenous shunting. Stagnant blood then becomes acidotic as a result of accumulated metabolic pyruvic and**

lactic acids. Tissue damage then can occur as a result of altered oxygen transport/delivery. Systemic perfusion is further impaired by hypovolemia, hypotension, and massive hemorrhage.

GENERAL PATIENT OUTCOMES: **Vital signs and mentation within patient's normal range. Palpable peripheral pulses of good quality. Urine output appropriate for individual situation.**

INTERVENTIONS	RATIONALE
Independent	
Assess neurologic status; for example, changes in level of consciousness, orientation, pupillary reaction, strength/movement of extremities; note complaints of headache or visual impairment.	Changes may be related to hypoxemia, acidosis, and cerebral edema, or may reflect intracranial bleeding or thrombosis, with increased pressure. (Refer to Care Plan: Brain Injury/Increased Intracranial Pressure, page 127.)
Note changes in respiratory rate and depth, or onset of dyspnea, pallor/cyanosis.	Sudden onset of respiratory distress accompanied by rales, dyspnea, cyanosis, and/or hemoptysis may suggest intravascular clotting in the pulmonary system, which can lead to respiratory failure.
Auscultate breath sounds, noting areas of decrease/absence of ventilation, presence of adventitious sounds.	Indicators of developing respiratory complications/failure.
Measure cardiac output (CO), MAP, PCWP.	Hypovolemia, alterations in vascular resistance, or myocardial ischemia can reduce CO and diminish tissue perfusion. Pulmonary hypertension (elevated PCWP) may suggest intrapulmonary vasculature clotting.
Monitor/record cardiac rhythm changes.	Numerous dysrhythmias occur in response to lack of sufficient myocardial perfusion, electrolyte and acid/base disturbance.
Assess/monitor gastrointestinal (GI) function, noting bowel sounds, complaints of abdominal pain, changes in abdominal girth. Observe/guaiac gastric drainage and stools.	Mesenteric ischemia and/or necrosis can result from thrombus formation/hemorrhage. Complications may include obstruction (ileus), GI bleeding with hematemesis and melena, retroperitoneal hemorrhage.
Measure hourly/24-hour urine output, noting decreased output.	Kidneys are the organs most frequently affected by thrombosis, which produces acute tubular necrosis. Renal insufficiency progressing to shutdown may be manifested by oliguria or anuria with or without usual chemical abnormalities of renal failure. However, oliguria also is produced by other factors such as hypovolemia, hypotension, or cardiac failure. (Refer to Care Plan: Acute Renal Failure, page 207.)

INTERVENTIONS	RATIONALE
Independent	
Note equality of pulses, distally and proximally. Observe capillary refill time in fingers/toes.	Multiple/diffuse vascular clot formations may result in loss of adequate circulation to distal extremities.
Examine for petechia, purpura, ecchymosis on skin, buccal membranes, and conjunctiva.	Manifestation of excessive fibrinolytic activity/fibrin deposition in the capillary bed.
Note acral cyanosis/focal gangrene of fingers, toes, lips, ears.	Microvascular thrombosis may result in widespread skin infarctions secondary to thrombotic occlusion of dermal vessels.
Monitor for signs of infection (e.g., fever, purulent secretions, swelling/redness at incision/invasive line insertion sites, positive blood culture).	Sepsis may be a causative factor or potentiate disseminated intravascular coagulation (DIC). (Refer to Care Plan: Sepsis/Septicemia/Septic Shock, page 329.)
Maintain bedrest during bleeding episode.	Orthostatic hypotension often occurs with activity, compromising cerebral perfusion.
Monitor laboratory indices for renal function. Note presence of blood or myoglobin.	Bleeding into urinary system may produce hazy or bright-red urine. Myoglobin is indicative of muscle/tissue destruction. (Refer to Care Plan: Acute Renal Failure, page 207.)
Collaborative	
Administer intravenous (IV) fluids/blood as indicated. (Refer to Nursing Diagnosis: Fluid Volume Deficit, potential, page 320.)	Tissue perfusion is directly related to adequacy of circulating volume.
Review serial electrocardiograms (ECGs). Administer electrolytes/antiarrhythmic drugs as required.	Myocardial ischemia/damage may lead to altered electromechanical function in presence of potassium depletion or decreased myocardial perfusion.

NURSING DIAGNOSIS:	**Injury, potential for, continued activation of altered clotting factors.**
SUPPORTING DATA/CONTRIBUTING FACTORS:	**With consumption of clotting factors and hyperactivity of fibrinolytic system, the patient becomes highly susceptible to trauma/mucosal irritation, which may result in further bleeding and perpetuation of the coagulopathy.**
GENERAL PATIENT OUTCOMES:	**Bleeding is prevented/minimized.**

INTERVENTIONS	RATIONALE
Independent	
Promote bedrest/limit activity.	Reduces risk of trauma/continued bleeding.

INTERVENTIONS	RATIONALE
Independent	
Use extra assistance when moving patient, maintaining proper body alignment and support.	Gentle handling reduces hazard of internal tissue trauma/bleeding.
Provide frequent gentle mouth care and lip lubrication.	Oral mucosa bleeds easily, and membrane ischemia can develop.
Provide liquids and soft foods. Avoid hot/spicy foods and fluids.	Chewing may induce bleeding of the gums and tongue. Heat and spicy foods may be irritating to mucosa.
Give gentle skin care, using mild, nondrying solutions. Use electric razor for shaving. Use paper/silk tape; soft/sheepskin restraints if necessary. Provide gloves as indicated to prevent scratching.	Minimizes skin trauma and localized bleeding.
Teach patient to cough, to sneeze, and to blow nose gently. Avoid Valsalva maneuvers.	Reduces potential for sudden or renewed bleeding by dislodging clot.
Evaluate integrity of orifices containing tubes/devices (e.g., nares, mouth, urethra, anus).	Membranes are fragile and predisposed to ulceration/bleeding.
Use *low* suction to clear respiratory passages if suctioning is required.	Minimizes trauma/bleeding of nasopharynx and trachea.
Limit frequency of cuff BP, and alternate arms if possible.	Recurrent external pressure may cause vascular hemorrhage/hematoma formation.
Use small-gauge needles for necessary venipuncture. Apply pressure to site for at least 10 minutes; then inspect periodically.	Precautions may prevent hemorrhage/reduce hematoma formation.
Apply local pressure, cold compresses, as indicated.	Minimizes blood loss by local vasoconstriction.
Restrict cleansing of incisions and bleeding sites.	Disturbing clots may result in increased bleeding.
Assess for extremity tenderness/swelling.	Thrombosis and/or bleeding into muscle tissue, joint capsules, may occur, necessitating further restriction of activity/exercises.
Collaborative	
Humidify supplemental oxygen/patient environment as indicated.	Drying effects of oxygen/arid climate may potentiate mucous membrane bleeding.
Administer stool softeners. Limit digital manipulation, rectal temperatures, and enemas.	Constipation, straining to produce stool, and rectal irritation can potentiate mucosal bleeding.
Insert/maintain nasogastric tube as indicated. Lavage with cool/room temperature saline per protocol.	Identifies/controls GI bleeding. (Refer to Care Plan: Upper Gastrointestinal/Esophageal Bleeding, page 197.)
Administer antacids, histamine H_2 receptor antagonists, for example, cimetadine (Tagamet), ranitidine (Zantac).	Decreases production and deleterious effect of hydrochloric acid, reducing risk of hemorrhage.
Minimize invasive procedures.	May be necessary to postpone surgery/invasive procedures until hemostasis is adequate, unless indicated to correct underlying cause.

NURSING DIAGNOSIS:	**Gas Exchange, impaired (potential).**
SUPPORTING DATA/CONTRIBUTING FACTORS:	**Fibrin deposition in microcirculation results in red blood cell distruction and creates a hemolytic anemia which reduces oxygen-carrying capacity. Development of acidosis further reduces oxygen release at the cellular level. In addition, ischemic damage of lung parenchyma may occur, resulting in right-to-left shunting and shock lung or adult respiratory distress syndrome (ARDS).**
GENERAL PATIENT OUTCOMES:	**Respiratory rate/depth and arterial blood gases (ABGs) within patient's normal range. Breath sounds clear. Free of cyanosis.**

INTERVENTIONS	RATIONALE
Independent	
Monitor respiratory rate and breathing pattern. Auscultate lungs for adventitious sounds (e.g., crackles/rhonchi).	Tachypnea, dyspnea suggest developing complications such as atelectasis, hypoxia, and acidosis. Crackles may occur with increased congestion related to hydrostatic pressure changes and capillary fragility. Rhonchi/wheezes may be indicative of airway obstruction owing to bronchial edema, presence of secretions.
Observe color/character of tracheal secretions.	Hemoptysis suggests hemorrhage/thrombotic episode in lungs. (Refer to Care Plan: Pulmonary Embolism [Massive], page 95.)
Inspect skin/mucous membranes for cyanosis, pallor.	Hemoglobin desaturation and anemia as well as acidosis contribute to cyanosis by altering oxygen transport/delivery.
Collaborative	
Monitor/graph serial ABGs.	Evaluates therapy needs/effectiveness.
Review serial chest x-ray examinations.	May suggest pulmonary congestion/developing ARDS.
Provide supplemental oxygen via cannula/mask, mechanical ventilator as indicated.	Prevent/correct hypoxemia. Mechanical ventilation may be required in presence of pulmonary complications/respiratory distress. (Refer to Care Plans: Adult Respiratory Distress Syndrome, page 77; Ventilatory Assistance [Mechanical], page 115.)
Administer medications as indicated:	
Bronchodilators (e.g., aminophylline).	Increases intracellular cyclic AMP, resulting in relaxa-

INTERVENTIONS	RATIONALE
Collaborative	
	tion of smooth muscle, dilating bronchial airways and pulmonary blood vessels. This enhances oxygen delivery and gas diffusion.

NURSING DIAGNOSIS: **Comfort, alteration in, pain, acute.**

SUPPORTING DATA/CONTRIBUTING FACTORS: **Bleeding into joints/muscles, hematoma formation, ischemic tissues with areas of acral cyanosis/focal gangrene all contribute to varying degrees of discomfort/pain.**

GENERAL PATIENT OUTCOMES: **Verbalizes increased comfort, demonstrates relaxed posture/facial expression, able to sleep/rest appropriately.**

INTERVENTIONS	RATIONALE
Independent	
Assess verbal/nonverbal cues, noting subtle signs: irritability, restlessness, vital sign changes.	Acutely ill patient may be unable to communicate pain/need for analgesia. Increasing discomfort/new areas of pain suggest complications/continued bleeding.
Provide comfort measures (e.g., gentle skin care, repositioning with pillows/soft bath blankets, use of foot cradle).	Promotes relaxation, decreases pressure on compromised skin/tissue, and provides support for painful joints.
Promote undisturbed rest/sleep periods, limit activity, and assist with self-care needs.	Patients can become easily exhausted because of blood loss, extreme stress of illness, and constant care. This may reduce coping abilities and enhance perception of pain.
Perform active/passive range of motion, as indicated.	Maintains muscle tone and joint mobility but must be performed with caution because of risk of joint hemorrhage.
Provide emotional support to patient/family. Give honest information about measures being used to control bleeding and signs of improvement. (Refer to Care Plan: Psychosocial Aspects of Critical Care, page 379.)	Bleeding is very frightening to patient/family. Fear and anxiety can heighten perception of pain and block effectiveness of patient's usual coping behaviors. Providing information/honest answers can assist patient to manage anxiety/gain some control of situation.
Collaborative	
Administer analgesics in small increments, and monitor effects.	Provides relief of pain. Dosage/frequency may need to be altered for maximal effect without oversedation and hypotension.

INTERVENTIONS	RATIONALE
Collaborative	
Avoid unintentional administration of aspirin-containing products and other platelet-inhibiting medications.	Acetylsalicylic acid inhibits platelet function and may irritate mucosa, potentiating risk of bleeding.
Provide air flotation/foam mattress.	Decreases pressure on skin/bony prominences and may limit development of systemic tissue hypoxia, decubiti.

Sepsis/Septicemia/Septic Shock

Sepsis is a syndrome characterized by clinical signs and symptoms of severe infection which may progress to septicemia and septic shock.

Septicemia implies the presence of a systemic infection of the blood caused by rapidly multiplying microorganisms or their toxins, which can result in profound physiologic changes. The pathogens can be bacteria, fungi, viruses, or rickettsiae. The most common causes of septicemia are gram-negative organisms such as Esherechia coli, Proteus, Klebsiella, Enterobacter, Serratia, and Pseudomonos aeruginosa. If the defense system of the body is not effective in controlling the invading microorganisms, septic shock may result.

Septic shock occurs in approximately one third of patients with septicemia. It is a potentially life-threatening disorder characterized by altered hemodynamics and impaired cellular function, which may progress through stages from a hyperdynamic phase to multiple-system failure.

PATIENT ASSESSMENT DATA BASE

HISTORY

Predisposing factors: chronic health problems such as liver, renal, cardiac disease, diabetes mellitus, alcoholism, malnutrition, and debilitation; malignancy; compromised immunologic system related to drug therapy such as corticosteroids, antimetabolites, radiation; surgical or traumatic wounds; postabortion/postpartal infection; widespread use of antibiotic therapy; soft-tissue infection; prolonged hospitalization.

Invasive manipulation, particularly of the gastrointestinal, genitourinary, or biliary tracts; invasive monitoring devices such as indwelling catheters, central venous and arterial lines, intravenous catheters, endotracheal tubes, tracheostomies; total parenteral nutrition.

Age: infants may be more susceptible owing to immaturity of their defense mechanisms. The elderly, particularly over 65, are at greater risk owing to multiple predisposing factors (e.g., altered organ function and chronic health problems).

Subjective

May complain of malaise, fever, shaking chills, headache, confusion/mental cloudiness.

PHYSICAL EXAMINATION

Hyperdynamic Stage:

Inspection

Mentation: restlessness, apprehension, confusion, disorientation.

Skin: warm, dry, flushed, pink color (vasodilation).

Respirations: tachypnea with decreased respiratory depth.

Urine: output decreased, dark amber color.

Auscultation

Blood pressure: may be in the normal/slightly low normal range, as long as cardiac output remains elevated.

Breath sounds: basilar crackles may indicate onset of cardiac decompensation/developing pulmonary complications.

Palpation

Peripheral pulses: bounding tachycardia often present.

Other

Temperature: usually elevated; occasionally subnormal.

Hypodynamic Stage:

Inspection

Mentation: delirium/coma.

Skin: pale, cold, clammy, mottled (vasoconstriction).

Respirations: tachypnea, dyspnea may occur.

Urine: oliguria, anuria.

Auscultation

Blood pressure: severe hypotension, with narrowing pulse pressure.

Breath sounds: crackles, rhonchi, wheezes may reflect developing failure/respiratory insufficiency.

Heart sounds: dysrhythmias and development of S_3 suggest myocardial dysfunction, effects of acidosis/electrolyte imbalance.

Palpation

Peripheral pulses: weak, thready, easily obliterated; extreme tachycardia.

Other

Temperature: usually subnormal.

DIAGNOSTIC STUDIES

Serum electrolytes: various imbalances may occur owing to acidosis, fluid shifts, and altered renal function.

CBC: Hct may be elevated in hypovolemic states owing to hemoconcentration. Leukopenia (decreased WBCs) occurs early in septicemia, followed by a rebound leukocytosis with increased bands (shift to the left), indicating rapid production of immature WBCs.

Clotting studies:

Platelets: decreased levels (thrombocytopenia) can occur, owing to platelet aggregation.

PT/PTT: may be prolonged, indicating beginning coagulopathy associated with liver ischemia/circulating toxins/shock state.

Serum lactate: elevated in metabolic acidosis, liver dysfunction, shock.

Serum glucose: hyperglycemia occurs, reflecting gluconeogenesis and glycogenolysis in the liver in resposne to cellular starvation caused by the inability of the cells to use glucose, then fat, and finally protein as energy sources.

BUN/creatinine: increased levels are associated with dehydration, renal impairment/failure, and liver dysfunction/failure.

ABGs: respiratory alkalosis and hypoxemia may occur early. In later stages, respiratory and metabolic acidosis occur, caused by failure of compensatory mechanisms.

Urinalysis: presence of WBCs/bacteria suggests infection.

Cultures: wound, sputum, urine, and blood may identify organism(s) causing the sepsis. Sensitivity determines most effective drug choices. Catheter/intravascular line tips may need to be removed and cultured if the portal of entry is unknown.

X-ray examinations: abdominal and lower chest films indicating free air in the abdomen may suggest infection caused by perforated abdominal organ/uterus.

NURSING PRIORITIES

1. Control/eliminate infection.
2. Maintain/restore tissue perfusion and circulatory volume.
3. Minimize/prevent complications.
4. Provide emotional support to the patient/significant other(s).

NURSING DIAGNOSIS:	**Injury, potential for progression of sepsis to septic shock.**
SUPPORTING DATA/CONTRIBUTING FACTORS:	**The risk of sepsis is high in hospitals, especially in critical care areas. Patients may be admitted in septic shock; but frequently they acquire an infection while hospitalized, which overwhelms an already compromised immune system. Failure to recognize/treat infection and/or to exercise proper preventive measures may result in septicemia/septic shock leading to death.**
GENERAL PATIENT OUTCOMES:	**Sepsis is treated. Signs of septicemia/septic shock are absent.**

INTERVENTIONS	RATIONALE
Independent	
Wash hands before/after each care activity.	Reduce risk of cross-contamination.
Wear gloves/gowns when caring for open wounds if soiling possible.	Prevent spread of infection/cross-contamination.
Inspect wounds/site of invasive devices daily. Note signs of local inflammation/infection, changes in color/odor of wound drainage and sputum, cloudy urine.	May provide clue to portal of entry, type of infecting microorganism(s), as well as early identification of secondary infections.
Use sterile technique when changing dressings/suctioning/providing site care (e.g., invasive line, urinary catheter).	Prevents introduction of bacteria, reducing risk of nosocomial infection.
Dispose of soiled dressings/materials in double bag.	Reduces contamination/soilage of area, limits spread of airborne organisms.
Provide isolation/monitor visitors as indicated.	Wound/linen isolation may be all that is required for draining wounds, but reverse isolation/restriction of visitors may be needed to protect the immunosuppressed patient.

INTERVENTIONS	RATIONALE
Independent	
Limit use of invasive devices/procedures when possible.	Reduces number of sites for entry of opportunistic organisms.
Encourage frequent change of position, deep breathing/coughing.	Good pulmonary toilet may prevent pneumonia.
Monitor temperature trends.	Fever (101° to 105° F/38.5° to 40° C) is caused by the effect of endotoxins on the hypothalmus and pyrogen-released endorphins. Hypothermia (less than 96° F/36°C) is usually a grave sign, reflecting advancing shock state/decreased tissue perfusion.
Observe for shaking chills and profuse diaphoresis.	Chills often precede temperature spikes.
Monitor for signs of deterioration of condition/failure to improve during therapy.	May reflect inappropriate/ineffective therapy or overgrowth of resistant/opportunistic organisms.
Collaborative	
Obtain specimens of urine, blood, sputum, wound, invasive lines/tubes for gram stain, culture, and sensitivity, as indicated.	Identification of the portal of entry and the organism causing the septicemia is crucial to effective treatment.
Administer antibiotics as indicated: Broad-spectrum, for example, ampicillin (Omnipen); gram-negative, for example, ticarcillin disodium (Ticar); gram-positive, for example, nafcilin (Nafcil), vancomycin (Vancocin); aminoglycosides, for example, tobramycin (Nebcin), gentamicin (Garamycin); cephalosporins, for example, cefotaxime (Claforan).	Specific antibiotics are determined by culture results, but therapy is usually initiated prior to obtaining culture results, using broad-spectrum antibiotics and based on the most likely infecting organisms. Concomitant use of antimicrobials is often beneficial, but dosage must be balanced against renal function/clearance.
Assist with incision and drainage, wound irrigation, application of warm/moist soaks as indicated.	Facilitates removal of purulent material/necrotic tissue and promotes healing.

NURSING DIAGNOSIS: **Tissue Perfusion, alteration in, decreased.**

SUPPORTING DATA/CONTRIBUTING FACTORS: **The microorganisms that invade the bloodstream stimulate the release of chemical and hormonal substances. Release or activation of these substances initially results in peripheral vasodilation and decreased systemic vascular resistance, creating hypotension. As shock state progresses, tissue perfusion is decreased even more by selective vasoconstriction (reduced organ function) and the systemic effects of acidosis, increased vascular permeability (relative hypovolemia), and vascular occlusion (intimal damage/**

	microemboli). Eventually this leads to myocardial depression, peripheral vascular insufficiency, and tissue ischemia.
GENERAL PATIENT OUTCOMES:	**Blood pressure, cardiac output, heart rhythm/rate within patient's normal range. Usual level of consciousness, urine output greater than 0.5 ml/kg/hour. Skin warm and dry. Active bowel sounds.**

INTERVENTIONS	RATIONALE
Independent	
Monitor trends in blood pressure (BP). Measure/calculate hemodynamic parameters; for example, mean arterial pressure (MAP), cardiac output (CO), systemic vascular resistance (SVR), SVO_2.	Initially decreased arterial blood pressure (MAP) occurs as a result of decreased systemic vascular resistance (SVR), massive peripheral vasodilation, and relative hypovolemia. As shock progresses, CO becomes severely depressed because of major alterations in contractility and preload/afterload, producing profound hypotension. A wide pulse pressure (difference in systolic and diastolic blood pressure) initially exists because of increased CO and decreased SVR. However, in late shock stage, SVR is increased in attempt to reverse hypotension, and a narrow pulse pressure will be seen. Low SVO_2 readings are suggestive of increased oxygen demand and tissue extraction as may occur in hyperdynamic phase. High SVO_2 readings may occur in the hypodynamic phase, reflecting altered cardiorespiratory function/tissue perfusion and reduced cellular utilization of oxygen.
Monitor heart rate, rhythm. Note dysrhythmias.	Tachycardia occurs owing to sympathetic nervous system stimulation secondary to stress response and to compensate for the relative hypovolemia and hypotension. Cardiac dysrhythmias occur later as a result of hypoxia, acid-base/electrolyte imbalance, and/or low flow perfusion state.
Note quality of peripheral pulses.	Initially the pulse is strong/bounding owing to increased CO. Eventually the pulse becomes weak/thready because of sustained hypotension, decreased CO, and peripheral vasoconstriction as the shock state progresses.
Assess respiratory rate, depth, and quality. Note onset of severe dyspnea.	Increased respirations occur in response to direct effects of endotoxins on the respiratory center in the brain, as well as developing hypoxia, stress, and fever. Respirations become shallow as respiratory insufficiency progresses. The result is hypoventilation, which can progress to acute respiratory failure. (Refer to Nursing Diagnosis: Gas Exchange, impaired, page 326.)

INTERVENTIONS	RATIONALE
Independent	
Auscultate breath sounds for presence of crackles, rhonchi, wheezes.	Adventitious sounds such as moist crackles may be noted secondary to pulmonary hypertension, which accelerates the formation of pulmonary edema and development of ARDS. (Refer to Care Plan: Adult Respiratory Distress Syndrome, page 77.) Areas of diminished, absent breath sounds suggest complications (e.g., atelectasis) or respiratory failure.
Note changes in sensorium, such as mental cloudiness, agitation, restlessness, personality changes, delirium, stupor, coma.	Changes reflect alterations in cerebral perfusion, as well as effects of hypoxemia and acidosis.
Assess skin for changes in color, temperature, moisture.	Compensatory mechanism of vasodilitation results in warm, dry, pink skin, which is characteristic of hyperperfusion in hyperdynamic phase of early septic shock. The compensatory mechanism of vasoconstriction, which shunts blood to vital organs, reduces peripheral blood flow and creates cool/cold, clammy, moist, pale/dusky/mottled skin as shock state progresses.
Record hourly urine output and specific gravity.	Decreasing urinary output with increased specific gravity indicates diminished renal perfusion related to fluid shifts and selective vasoconstriction. There may be transient polyuria early in septic shock while CO is elevated. This is followed by oliguria (less than 25 ml hour for an adult) and eventually anuria as the shock state progresses. (Refer to Care Plan: Acute Renal Failure, page 207.)
Auscultate bowel sounds. Monitor gastric pH and hematest for presence of occult blood in stomach contents.	Reduced blood flow to the mesentery (splanchnic vasoconstriction) decreases peristalsis and may lead to paralytic ileus. Stress of illness and use of steroids increase risk of gastric mucosa erosion/bleeding caused by increased acidity, mucosal ischemia, and decreased mucous production.
Note drug effect and monitor for toxicity.	Massive doses of antibiotics are often ordered intravenously which have potentially toxic effects when hepatic/renal perfusion is compromised.
Collaborative	
Administer parenteral fluids. (Refer to Nursing Diagnosis: Fluid Volume Deficit, actual (2), page 335.)	In order to maintain tissue perfusion, large amounts of fluid may be required to support circulating volume.
Administer drugs as indicated:	
Positive inotropic and vasoactive agents; for example, dopamine (Intropin), norepinephrine (Levophed), dobutamine (Dobutrex), neosynephrine (Phenylephrine).	Given to improve myocardial contractile force and to reverse vasodilatation of hyperdynamic phase of septic shock, thereby increasing BP. Dopamine also is used to improve renal and mesenteric perfusion. These agents should be administered concomitantly with parenteral fluids.

INTERVENTIONS	RATIONALE
Independent	
Naloxone (Narcan).	Although use is experimental, Narcan is thought to block endorphin-mediated vasodilatation, thereby increasing BP.
Vasodilators; for example, sodium nitropruside, (Nipride), nitroglycerin (Tridil).	Usually administered in combination with positive inotropic agents to reduce preload and afterload by treating the severe selective systemic vasoconstriction. In addition, coronary perfusion is increased by dilation of coronary arteries, which may improve cardiac function.
Angiotension-converting inhibitors; for example, captopril (Capoten);	Used experimentally to reduce vasoconstriction mediated by angiotension mechanism in severe shock states.
Steroids;	Although controversial, steroids may halt progression to hypodynamic cold shock phase by halting complement activation (kinin/histamine) and its deleterious effects. Other potential advantages include decreased capillary permeability, increased renal perfusion, and inhibition of microemboli formation.
Sodium bicarbonate;	Alterations in perfusion and production of lactate result in metabolic acidosis, requiring base replacement therapy.
Antacids; for example, aluminum hydroxide (Amphojel).	There is increased potential for gastric bleeding owing to stress response. Choice of antacid may be dependent on serum magnesium level.
Indomethacin (Indocin).	Has been used with some success to decrease pulmonary vasoconstriction and to improve pulmonary blood flow. Similar effects may be achieved with use of aspirin.
Monitor ABGs, lactate levels.	Development of respiratory/metabolic acidosis reflects changes in perfusion with loss of compensatory mechanisms (e.g., decreased renal perfusion/hydrogen excretion) and increased production of lactic acid owing to anerobic metabolism secondary to circulatory shunting/stagnation.
Maintain body temperature, using adjunctive aids as necessary (Refer to Nursing Diagnosis: Ineffective Thermoregulation, page 341.)	Temperature elevations increase metabolic/oxygen demand beyond cellular resources, hastening tissue destruction.

NURSING DIAGNOSIS:	**Fluid Volume Deficit, actual (2).**
SUPPORTING DATA/CONTRIBUTING FACTORS:	**Septic shock is associated with massive vasodilatation and increased capillary permeability. Fluid leaks into the interstitial space (third-spacing), resulting in a relative hypovolemia.**

	Note: The potential for a fluid volume excess may exist owing to profound systemic vasoconstriction and myocardial depression, but this is a late, ominous sign in the course of the disease process.
GENERAL PATIENT OUTCOMES:	**Adequate circulatory blood volume maintained as evidenced by vital signs within patient's normal range, palpable peripheral pulses, urine output greater than 0.5 ml per kg per hour, absence of tissue edema.**

INTERVENTIONS	RATIONALE
Independent	
Assess for dry mucous membranes, poor skin turgor, and thirst.	Third-spacing of fluid gives rise to signs of intravascular fluid volume deficit/dehydration.
Observe signs of dependent/peripheral edema in sacrum, scrotum, back, legs.	Fluid losses from the vascular compartment into the interstitial space creates tissue edema.
Monitor BP, heart rate.	Reduction in the circulating fluid volume reduces BP and initiates compensatory mechanisms of tachycardia in order to improve cardiac output and to increase systemic BP.
Palpate peripheral pulses.	Weak, easily obliterated pulses suggest hypovolemia.
Monitor hemodynamic pressures, (e.g., MAP, CVP). Calculate SVR.	Provides information about circulating volume progression of shock state and effects of vasoactive therapy.
Measure/record urine output and specific gravity. Note fluid (intake and output) imbalances and correlate with daily weight.	Urine output of less than 25 ml per hour with a high specific gravity suggests hypovolemia. Continued positive fluid balance with corresponding weight gain may indicate third-spacing and tissue edema formation, suggesting need to alter fluid therapy.
Collaborative	
Administer intravenous (IV) fluids; for example, crystalloids (D5W, N.S.) and colloids (albumin, fresh frozen plasma), as indicated.	Large volumes of fluid usually are required to replace losses from intravascular space caused by peripheral vasodilation, increased insensible losses, reduced oral fluid intake, and possible sequestration of fluid in the peritoneal cavity. Colloids may help mobilize fluids back into the vascular compartment. Note: Solutions containing lactate may be contraindicated because of cumulative effect in presence of rising serum lactate levels.
Monitor laboratory values:	
Hematocrit (Hct)/red blood cell count.	Evaluates changes in hydration/blood viscosity.

INTERVENTIONS	RATIONALE
Collaborative	
Blood urea nitrogen (BUN)/creatinine levels.	Moderate elevations of BUN reflect dehydration, high values of BUN/creatinine may indicate renal dysfunction/failure.

NURSING DIAGNOSIS: **Cardiac Output, alteration in, decreased.**

SUPPORTING DATA/CONTRIBUTING FACTORS: **Initially is increased by sympathetic nervous system stimulation. However, if the sepsis is not controlled, CO falls as a result of decreased circulating volume, reduced venous return, and increased SVR (afterload). In septic shock, decreased CO is associated with myocardial depression caused by hypoxia, complement activation, endorphin/histamine release, and the negative inotropic effect of lysosomal hydralase, a myocardial depressant factor (MDF). In addition, any or all of these factors may result in cardiac dysrhythmias, which further reduce effective cardiac output.**

GENERAL PATIENT OUTCOMES: **Cardiac output within normal limits. Blood pressure and pulse within patient's normal range. Dysrhythmias prevented/controlled.**

INTERVENTIONS	RATIONALE
Independent	
Monitor hemodynamic parameters, including CO and cardiac index (CI).	Although CO measurements initially may be numerically high, CO is inadequate to meet the body's metabolic/oxygen needs. A sustained drop in CO suggests worsening shock state and may reflect myocardial depression.
Record total fluid intake accurately, including flush solutions and cardiac injectate.	Cardiac decompensation may occur in response to small but inappropriate fluid administration when the myocardium is depressed.
Monitor cardiac rhythm continuously; document dysrhythmias.	Dysrhythmias may result from a number of problems; for example, acid-base/electrolyte imbalances, decreased myocardial perfusion/hypoxia. The dysrhyth-

INTERVENTIONS	RATIONALE
Independent	
	mias themselves may alter/further depress myocardial perfusion and CO.
Promote bedrest, assist with activities of daily living.	Decreases myocardial workload/oxygen demand.
Collaborative	
Monitor serum electrolytes.	Potassium imbalances are associated with fluid shifts, acidosis, certain drugs, and may adversely affect cardiac contractility/conduction.
Administer medications as indicated:	
Positive inotropic drugs; for example, digoxin (Lanoxin), dopamine (Intropin), dobutamine (Dobutrex);	Positive inotropic drugs may be given to increase contractile force to overcome the myocardial depression (in conjunction with fluid volume replacement), to increase the cardiac output, to correct hypotension, and thereby to improve systemic perfusion.
Antiarrhythmics; for example, verapamil (Calan), lidocaine.	May be used to treat lethal dysrhythmias while underlying problems are being corrected.
Assist with insertion/maintain intra-arterial balloon pump (IABP). (Refer to Care Plan: Cardiogenic Shock; Nursing Diagnosis Cardiac Output, decreased, page 34.)	May be used to improve CO and hemodynamics while allowing for decreased ventricular work.

NURSING DIAGNOSIS:	**Gas Exchange, impaired (potential).**
SUPPORTING DATA/CONTRIBUTING FACTORS:	**Initially endotoxins produced in sepsis/septicemia affect the respiratory center in the medulla (resulting in hyperventilation/respiratory alkalosis) and increase capillary permeability, leading to pulmonary congestion as fluid shifts to interstitial spaces. Hypoventilation and endotoxin-induced damage to the cells/capillaries interferes with oxygen delivery/utilization in the tissues. Anerobic metabolism causes metabolic acidosis, owing to excess production of lactic acid. Eventually hypoxemia can become intractable to oxygen therapy, and acidosis is both respiratory and metabolic.**
GENERAL PATIENT OUTCOMES:	**Arterial blood gases and respiratory rate within patient's normal range. Absence of dyspnea/cyanosis, breath**

sounds clear, and chest x-ray examinations clear/improving.

INTERVENTIONS	RATIONALE
Independent	
Maintain patent airway.	If ventilations are unassisted, place patient in position of comfort, with head of bed elevated to enhance respiratory effort.
Observe/record changes in rate and depth of respiration, use of accessory muscles/degree of respiratory effort.	Rapid/shallow respirations occur because of hypoxemia, stress, and circulating endotoxins. Hypoventilation and dyspnea reflect ineffective compensatory mechanisms and are indications that ventilatory support is needed.
Auscultate breath sounds. Note crackles, wheezes, areas of decreased/absent ventilation.	Respiratory distress and the presence of adventitious sounds are indicators of pulmonary congestion/ interstitial edema, atelectasis. Note: Respiratory complications, including pneumonia and ARDS, are a prime cause of death. (Refer to Care Plan: Adult Respiratory Distress Syndrome, page 77.)
Note presence of circumoral cyanosis.	Reflects inadequate systemic oxygenation/ hypoxemia.
Monitor alterations in sensorium: agitation, confusion, personality changes, delirium, stupor, coma.	Cerebral function is very sensitive to hypoxemia.
Note cough and purulent sputum production.	Pneumonia is a common nosocomial infection which can occur by aspiration of oropharyngeal organisms or can be spread from other sites.
Facilitate removal of secretions (e.g., turn, cough, deep breathe). Suction with lavage, as indicated.	Frequent pulmonary toilet is necessary to reduce ventilation/perfusion imbalance and to mobilize secretions in order to improve gas exchange.
Monitor SVO_2 if available.	Mixed venous oxygen saturation is an indirect measurement of cardiorespiratory function/tissue perfusion, reflecting tissue utilization of oxygen, and serves as an early indicator of hemodynamic changes/ therapy needs.
Collaborative	
Monitor/graph serial ABGs. Note PaO_2 less than 60 mmHg when patient is receiving supplemental oxygen (suggests ARDS). Note pH below 7.35 and $PaCO_2$ greater than 40 mmHg (respiratory acidosis). Note pH below 7.35 and bicarbonate less than 22 to 24 mEq/liter (metabolic acidosis).	Hypoxemia is related to pulmonary changes (e.g., interstitial edema, atelectasis, and pulmonary shunting). Respiratory acidosis then occurs because of hypoventilation and ventilation-perfusion imbalance. As septic condition worsens, metabolic acidosis arises, owing to build-up of lactic acid from anerobic metabolism.
Administer oxygen as indicated, by nasal cannula, mask, high-flow rebreathing mask, intubation/ mechanical ventilation.	Necessary for correction of hypoxemia with failing respiratory effort/progressing acidosis. High-level oxygen delivery with PEEP via ventilator is usually required to improve tissue oxygenation/saturation of poorly circulating blood. (Refer to Care Plan: Ventilatory Assistance (mechanical), page 115.)

INTERVENTIONS	RATIONALE
Collaborative	
Monitor serial chest x-ray examinations.	Changes reflecting infiltrates/edema formation indicate presence of pulmonary complications.

NURSING DIAGNOSIS:	**Nutrition, alteration in, less than body requirements.**
SUPPORTING DATA/CONTRIBUTING FACTORS:	**Initially a hypermetabolic state exists owing to the stress of infection and excess catecholamine release. Nutritional stores are rapidly depleted as first glucose metabolism, then fat metabolism are impaired. Protein catabolism increases as liver dysfunction progresses, causing increased level of glucose, amino acids, and nitrogeneous waste products. Impaired gastric motility/presence of paralytic ileus may alter effectiveness of enteral feedings. Standard hyperalimentation solutions may potentiate hyperglycemia and azotemia.**
GENERAL PATIENT OUTCOMES:	**Increased nutritional needs will be met, evidenced by positive nitrogen balance, absence of muscle wasting, stabilization of weight.**

Refer to Care Plan: Nutritional Support, page 367.

NURSING DIAGNOSIS:	**Injury, potential for, DIC.**
SUPPORTING DATA/CONTRIBUTING FACTORS:	**Coagulation problems may occur in severe or persistent sepsis related to hematologic changes secondary to accelerated clotting in the microcirculation. These can occur owing to activation of chemical mediators associated with peripheral vascular insufficiency and cell destruction. If massive disseminated intravascular coagulation (DIC) develops, the patient's chances for survival are greatly reduced.**

GENERAL PATIENT OUTCOMES:	Bleeding is prevented/controlled. Complications are prevented.

INTERVENTIONS	RATIONALE
Independent	
Monitor for signs of bleeding: oozing from puncture sites/suture lines, petechiae, ecchymoses, hematuria, epistaxis, hemoptysis, hematemesis.	Associated with coagulapathy/developing DIC. (Refer to Care Plan: Disseminated Intravascular Coagulation, page 319.)

NURSING DIAGNOSIS:	Ineffective Thermoregulation.
SUPPORTING DATA/CONTRIBUTING FACTORS:	In septicemia, circulating endotoxins have a direct effect on the hypothalmus, altering temperature regulation. Dehydration caused by fluid shifts augments the fever response. In addition, the hypermetabolic state results in heat production. As shock progresses, hypothermia may develop as normal responses are overwhelmed/exhausted.
GENERAL PATIENT OUTCOMES:	Temperature within normal range, free of chills.

INTERVENTIONS	RATIONALE
Independent	
Monitor patient temperature, note shaking, chills/profuse diaphoresis.	Temperature usually elevated during hyperdynamic stage; chills often precede temperature spikes.
Monitor environmental temperature. Limit/add bed linens as indicated.	Room temperature/number of blankets should be altered, dependent on stage of shock (e.g., hyperthermia/hypothermia) to maintain near normal temperature.
Provide tepid sponge baths, avoid use of alcohol.	May help reduce fever. Note: Use of ice water/alcohol may cause chills, actually elevating temperature. In addition, alcohol is very drying to skin.
Collaborative	
Administer antipyretics; for example, acetylsalicylic acid (aspirin), acetominophen (Tylenol).	Used to reduce fever by its central action on the hypothalamus, although some sources believe that fever may be beneficial in limiting growth of organism.
Provide cooling blanket.	Used to reduce fever usually greater than 104° to 105° F/39.5° to 40° C when brain damage/seizures can occur.

CHAPTER 12
GENERAL

Chemical Dependency: Alcohol Toxicity/Withdrawal

Patients with alcohol toxicity (markedly elevated blood alcohol level) are often admitted to critical care areas for more obvious medical problems (e.g., multiple trauma or gastric hemorrhage). However, the nurse must be aware that the withdrawal process that follows cessation of alcohol consumption also may become an emergent problem.

PATIENT ASSESSMENT DATA BASE

HISTORY

History of alcohol and/or drug use/abuse. Determine amount of alcohol consumed in last 24 to 48 hours.

Previous hospitalizations for alcoholism and alcohol-related diseases (e.g., cirrhosis, esophageal varices).

History of seizures, with or without anticonvulsant therapy.

Suicide attempts (suicide attempts are 30 percent higher among alcoholics than national average, according to some research).

Present or previous history of recurrent accidents such as falls, automobile, fractures, lacerations, burns.

Precipitating factors of alcohol withdrawal symptoms; for example, lengthy hospitalizations that require more than 48 hours off alcohol (surgery, trauma), and myocardial infarction, which doubles incidence of delerium tremens.

PHYSICAL EXAMINATION

Subjective

Length of time since last drink; for example, currently intoxicated versus early withdrawal with tremors and nausea.

Inspection

Level of consciousness/orientation: confusion, stupor, hyperactivity, distorted thought processes, and slurred/ incoherent speech may be noted.

Eye movements: nystagmus may be present, associated with cranial nerve palsy.

Pupil reaction: constriction may indicate CNS depression.

Affect/mood/behavior: may be fearful, anxious, inappropriate, silly, euphoric, irritable.

Hallucinations: patient may be picking items out of air or responding verbally to unseen person/voices.

Neuromuscular: tremors of face, tongue, and hands are often present; seizures may occur (grand mal most common).

Gait: unsteady walk may be due to thiamine deficiency or cerebellar degeneration.

Skin: scars, ecchymotic areas, spider nevis (impaired portal circulation); fissures at corners of mouth (vitamin deficiency) may be present.

Skeletal: healed or new fractures (signs of recent/frequent trauma).

Edema: generalized tissue edema may be noted, owing to protein deficiencies.

Respirations: patient may be tachypneic in hyperactive state of alcohol withdrawal. Cheyne-Stokes respirations or respiratory depression also may occur.

Temeprature elevation is common, owing to dehydration and sympathetic stimulation accompanied by flushing, diaphoresis.

Abdomen: vomiting, gastric distention may be present; ascites occasionally seen in patients with cirrhosis.

Nutritional state: wasted muscles, dry, dull hair may be noted if malnutrition present.

Palpation

Peripheral pulses may be weak, irregular, rapid.

Abdomen: liver enlargement, abdominal/gastric distention may be noted.

Auscultation

Blood pressure: hypertension is common in early withdrawal stage but may become labile/progress to hypotension.

Breath sounds: presence of diminished/adventitious sounds suggests pulmonary complications; for example, respiratory depression, pneumonia.

Heart sounds: tachycardia common during acute withdrawal. Numerous dysrhythmias may be identified. Other abnormalities depend on underlying heart disease.

Bowel sounds: alterations may occur related to gastric complications, such as gastric hemorrhage or distention.

DIAGNOSTIC STUDIES

Blood alcohol/drug levels: alcohol level may/may not be severely elevated, depending on amount consumed and length of time between consumption and testing. In addition to alcohol, numerous controlled substances may be identified in a poly drug screen (e.g., morphine, Percodan, Quaalude).

CBC may reflect iron-deficiency anemia or acute/chronic gastrointestinal (GI) bleeding. White blood cell count may be decreased, owing to immunosuppression.

Glucose: hyperglycemia/hypoglycemia may be present, related to malnutrition/depletion of liver glycogen stores.

Electrolytes: common disturbances are hypokalemia and hypomagnesemia.

Liver function tests: SGOT, SGPT, and amylase may be elevated, owing to liver or pancreatic damage.

Nutritional tests: albumin may be low, and total protein, decreased. Vitamin deficiencies are usually present, reflecting malnutrition/malabsorption.

Urinalysis: infection may be identified; or ketones may be present owing to breakdown of fatty acids (pseudodiabetic condition).

Chest x-ray examination may reveal right lower lobe pneumonia or chronic lung disorders.

ECG: dysrhythmias, cardiomyopathies, and/or ischemia may be present owing to direct effect of alcohol on the cardiac muscle and/or conduction system.

NURSING PRIORITIES

1. Maintain adequate ventilation.
2. Prevent progression of withdrawal syndrome.
3. Minimize effect of complications.
4. Provide emotional support for patient/significant other(s).

NURSING DIAGNOSIS:	**Breathing Pattern, ineffective (potential).**
SUPPORTING DATA/CONTRIBUTING FACTORS:	**Multiple factors may compromise respiratory function. Central nervous system (CNS) depression can occur as a direct effect of alcohol toxicity; as a result of cumulative effects of anesthesia/narcotic administration and/or of drugs given to control alcohol withdrawal symptoms. In addition, chronic respiratory problems—for example, chronic obstructive pulmonary disease (COPD) and/or development of aspiration pneumonia (associated with loss of consciousness, trauma, vomiting, and gastric hemorrhage)—may further compromise ventilation/oxygenation.**
GENERAL PATIENT OUTCOMES:	**Arterial blood gases (ABGs) are within patient's normal range. Lungs clear. Patient is free of dyspnea/cyanosis.**

INTERVENTIONS	RATIONALE
Independent	
Maintain patent airway. Position on side with head in neutral position. Elevate head of bed. Use airway adjuncts and suction as necessary.	Initial sedative effect of alcohol/drugs potentiates risk of aspiration and relaxation of oropharyngeal musculature.
Monitor/assess rate, depth, and pattern of respirations. Note periods of apnea, Cheyne-Stokes respirations.	Marked respiratory depression can occur, owing to CNS depressant effects from alcohol. This may be compounded by anesthesia, narcotic analgesics, and drugs used to control alcohol withdrawal symptoms. Hyperventilation is common during acute withdrawal phase. Kussmaul respirations are sometimes present, owing to acidotic state associated with vomiting and malnutrition.
Auscultate breath sounds. Note presence of adventitious sounds (e.g., rhonchi, wheezes).	Patient is at risk for atelectasis related to hypoventilation and pneumonia. Right lower lobe pneumonia is

INTERVENTIONS	RATIONALE
Independent	
	common in alcohol-debilitated patients and is often due to aspiration. Chronic lung diseases are also common (e.g., emphysema, chronic bronchitis).
Encourage coughing/deep breathing exercises and frequent position changes.	Enhances lung expansion and mobilization of secretions to reduce risk of atelectasis/pneumonia.
Collaborative	
Administer supplemental oxygen by cannula, mask, mechanical ventilation as indicated.	Hypoxia may occur with CNS depression. Development of severe respiratory depression can require intubation and mechanical ventilation. (Refer to Care Plan: Ventilatory Assistance [Mechanical], page 115.)
Monitor/graph serial ABGs.	Identifies therapy needs and effectiveness.
Review chest x-ray examinations.	Useful in diagnosing/monitoring secondary complications, such as atelectasis/pneumonia.

NURSING DIAGNOSIS:	**Injury, potential for progression of withdrawal.**
SUPPORTING DATA/CONTRIBUTING FACTORS:	**Alcohol withdrawal presents a continuum of symptoms that can range from increased sympathetic activity to hallucinations, seizures, and delerium tremens (DTs). Recognition of early symptoms and prompt intervention are essential for prevention of progression to cardiovascular collapse.**
GENERAL PATIENT OUTCOMES:	**Injury and cardiovascular complications are prevented.**

INTERVENTIONS	RATIONALE
Independent	
Identify stage of alcohol withdrawal symptoms; that is, Stage I is associated with signs/symptoms of hyperactivity (e.g., tremors, sleeplessness, nausea/vomiting, diaphoresis, tachycardia, hypertension). Stage II is manifested by increased hyperactivity plus hallucinations and/or seizure activity. Stage III symptoms include DTs and extreme autonomic hyperactivity with profound confusion, anxiety, insomnia, fever.	Prompt recognition and intervention may halt progression of symptoms and enhance recovery/improve prognosis. In addition, reoccurrence/progression of symptoms indicates need for changes in drug therapy.
Monitor vital signs frequently during acute withdrawal.	Hypertension frequently occurs in acute withdrawal phase. Extreme hyperexcitability accompanied by catecholamine release and increased peripheral vascular

INTERVENTIONS	RATIONALE
Independent	
	resistance raises BP and heart rate. Patients may have underlying cardiovascular disease, which is compounded by alcohol withdrawal and can significantly impair CO, resulting in hypotension and/or symptoms of congestive heart failure.
Auscultate heart sounds. Monitor cardiac rhythm. Document dysrhythmias.	Long-term alcohol abuse may result in cardiomyopathy/congestive heart failure. Tachycardia is common, owing to sympathetic response to increased circulating catecholamines. Dysrhythmias are common, associated with hypoxemia, acid-base/electrolyte disturbances (especially hypokalemia/hypomagnesemia), and sympathetic stimulation.
Evaluate quality of peripheral pulses; assess skin color/moisture.	Vasoconstriction may contribute to reduced peripheral perfusion and pallor. Diaphoresis is common, owing to sympathetic response/fever.
Monitor body temperature.	Elevation may occur, owing to sympathetic stimulation, dehydration, and/or infections.
Monitor intake/output. Note 24-hour fluid balance.	Preexisting dehydration, vomiting, fever, and diaphoresis may result in decreased circulating volume, which can compromise cardiovascular function.
Monitor/document seizure activity. Maintain patent airway. Provide environmental safety (e.g., padded side rails, bed in low position).	Grand mal seizures are most common and may be related to decreased magnesium levels, hypoglycemia, elevated blood alcohol level, or previous history of seizures. A triad of chemical alterations resulting from combined alcohol abuse, drug abuse, and sleep deprivation can precipitate status epilepticus (continual unrelenting seizures), which presents a life-threatening situation.
Be prepared for and assist in cardiopulmonary resuscitation.	Causes of death during acute withdrawal include respiratory depression/arrest, oversedation, excessive psychomotor activity, severe dehydration, and massive infections. Mortality for unrecognized/untreated DTs may be as high as 15 to 25 percent.
Collaborative	
Monitor serum electrolyte levels.	Electrolyte imbalance (e.g., potassium/magnesium) potentiate risk of cardiac dysrhythmias and CNS excitability.
Administer fluids as indicated.	Corrects dehydration and promotes renal clearance of toxins.
Administer medications as indicated,	
Benzodiazepines; for example, chlordiazepoxide (Librium), diazepam (Valium),	Commonly used to control neuronal hyperactivity that occurs as alcohol is detoxified. Intravenous (IV)/oral administration is the route preferred, because intramuscular absorption is unpredictable. Patients initially may require large doses to achieve desired effect, and then the drugs may be tapered and discontinued, usually within 96 hours. Note: These agents must be used

INTERVENTIONS	RATIONALE
Collaborative	
	cautiously in the patient with hepatic disease, because they are metabolized by the liver.
Oxazepam (Serax);	May be drug of choice to decrease withdrawal symptoms in patient with liver disease, because of its shorter half-life.
Phenobarbital (Luminal);	Useful in suppressing withdrawal symptoms as well as an effective anticonvulsant. Use must be monitored to prevent exacerbation of respiratory depression.
Magnesium sulfate.	Reduces tremors and seizure activity by decreasing neuromuscular excitability.

NURSING DIAGNOSIS:	**Sensory-Perceptual Alteration (specify).**
SUPPORTING DATA/CONTRIBUTING FACTORS:	**Acute alcohol withdrawal (sudden cessation of consumption) produces varied/numerous symptoms of mental disturbance, loss of muscular coordination, and behavior problems. Chemical alteration, both endogenous (e.g., electrolyte imbalance, elevated ammonia, elevated blood urea nitrogen) and exogenous (alcohol) can alter sensory reception and/or integration. Sleep deprivation and psychologic stress (anxiety, fear) also may be contributing factors.**
GENERAL PATIENT OUTCOMES:	**Patient is alert and oriented. Auditory/visual hallucinations are absent.**

INTERVENTIONS	RATIONALE
Independent	
Assess level of consciousness; ability to speak, response to stimuli/commands.	Speech may be garbled, confused, or slurred. Response to commands may reveal inability to concentrate, impaired judgment, or muscle coordination deficits.
Observe behavioral responses; for example, hyperactivity, disorientation, confusion, sleeplessness, irritability.	Hyperactivity related to CNS disturbances may escalate rapidly. Sleeplessness is common, owing to loss of sedative effect gained from alcohol usually consumed prior to bedtime. Sleep deprivation may aggravate

INTERVENTIONS	RATIONALE
Independent	
	disorientation/confusion. Progression of symptoms may indicate impending hallucinations (Stage II) or DTs (Stage III).
Check deep tendon reflexes. Assess gait, if possible.	Reflexes may be depressed, absent, or hyperactive. Peripheral neuropathies are common, especially in malnourished patient. Ataxia (gait disturbance) is associated with Werneke's syndrome (thiamine deficiency) and cerebellar degeneration.
Note onset of hallucinations. Document as auditory, visual, tactile.	Auditory hallucinations are reported to be more frightening/threatening to patient. Visual hallucinations occur more at night and often include insects, animals, or faces of friends/enemies. Patients are frequently observed "picking the air." Yelling may occur if patient is calling for help from perceived threat (usually seen in Stage III).
Provide quiet environment. Speak in calm, quiet voice. Regulate lighting as indicated. Turn off radio/television during sleep.	Reduces external stimuli during hyperactive stage. Many patients become more delerious when surroundings cannot be seen, but some respond better to quiet, darkened room.
Provide care by same personnel whenever possible.	Promotes recognition of caregivers and a sense of consistency, which may reduce fear.
Encourage family/significant other(s) to stay with patient whenever possible.	May have a calming effect and may provide a reorienting influence.
Provide frequent reality orientation; for example, to person, place, time, and surrounding environment.	May reduce confusion/misinterpretation of external stimuli.
Minimize bedside discussion concerning patient.	Patient may hear and misinterpret conversation, which can aggravate hallucinations.
Provide environmental safety (e.g., remove articles that can harm patient).	Patient may have distorted sense of reality, be fearful, or be suicidal, requiring protection from self-harm.
Collaborative	
Provide seclusion, restraints, as necessary.	Patients with excessive psychomotor activity, severe hallucinations, violent behavior, and/or suicidal gestures may respond better to seclusion. Restraints are usually ineffective and add to patient's agitation but are sometimes required to prevent self-harm.
Monitor laboratory studies; for example, electrolytes, liver function studies, blood urea nitrogen (BUN), ABGs, glucose, magnesium levels, ammonia.	Changes in organ function may precipitate or potentiate sensory-perceptual deficits. Electrolyte imbalance is common. Liver function often is impaired in the chronic alcoholic patient. Ammonia intoxication can occur if liver is unable to convert ammonia to urea. Ketoacidosis is sometimes present without glycosuria; however, hyperglycemia and hypoglycemia may occur, suggesting pancreatitis or impaired gluconeogenesis in the liver. Hypoxemia and hypercarbia are common manifestations in chronic alcoholic patients (often heavy smokers).

INTERVENTIONS	RATIONALE
Collaborative	
Administer drugs as indicated, for example, thiamine; multivitamins high in vitamin C and vitamin B complex, stress tabs.	Vitamins are depleted because of insufficient intake and malabsorption. Thiamine deficiency is associated with ataxia, loss of eye movement and pupillary response, palpitations, postural hypotension, and exertional dyspnea.

NURSING DIAGNOSIS:	**Nutrition, alteration in, less than body requirements.**
SUPPORTING DATA/CONTRIBUTING FACTORS:	**The chronic alcoholic patient usually has a history of poor dietary intake. Pancreatitis and/or liver disease also may contribute to incomplete utilization of available nutrients. Alcohol exerts an adverse effect on the gastrointestinal (GI) system and can produce a variety of problems, including gastritis, anorexia, malabsorption, nausea, vomiting, and diarrhea.**
GENERAL PATIENT OUTCOMES:	**Adequate nutritional intake as evidenced by appropriate weight gain and positive nitrogen balance. Patient is free of GI complications.**

INTERVENTIONS	RATIONALE
Independent	
Evaluate presence/quality of bowel sounds. Note abdominal distention, tenderness.	Irritation of gastric mucosa is common and may result in epigastric pain, nausea, and hyperactive bowel sounds. More serious effects on GI system may occur secondary to cirrhosis and hepatitis.
Note presence of nausea/vomiting, diarrhea.	Nausea and vomiting are often among first signs of alcohol withdrawal. Fluids and electrolytes are depleted by vomiting and diarrhea and faulty intestinal absorption.
Provide small, frequent feedings/snacks when oral feeding is resumed.	May limit gastric distress, enhance intake.
Record food intake/caloric count.	Determines adequacy of intake and identifies need for supplements or alternate feeding methods.
Weigh daily.	Measures effectiveness of nutritional plan.
Hematest/guaiac gastric contents, stools.	Upper GI bleeding may occur owing to esophagitis, gastritis, ulcers, Mallory-Weiss tear (at esophagogastric junction), or esophageal varices. (Refer to Care

INTERVENTIONS	RATIONALE
Independent	
	Plan: Upper Gastrointestinal/Esophageal Bleeding, page 197.)
Collaborative	
Refer to dietician/nutritional support team.	Coordinates individual nutritional regimen.
Provide diet high in protein with at least one half of calories obtained from carbohydrates.	Stabilizes blood sugar, thereby reducing risk of hypoglycemia.
Maintain nothing-by-mouth (NPO) status if GI bleeding or excessive nausea/vomiting is present.	Decreases effects of gastric/pancreatic stimulation.
Insert/maintain nasogastric tube (Blakemore), if indicated.	Decompresses stomach, reduces gastric acid accumulation, and removes blood, which can produce ammonia in the intestines, thereby potentiating encephalopathy.
Provide nutrition by alternate route if necessary. (Refer to Care Plan: Nutritional Support, page 367.)	Enteral feedings may be needed to supplement oral intake. Hyperalimentation may be preferred or needed if patient is unable to eat or if severe GI/liver complications occur.
Administer medications as indicated; for example, Antacids, antiemetics, antidiarrheals.	Reduce gastric irritation and effects of sympathetic stimulation.

NURSING DIAGNOSIS: **Coping, ineffective, individual/family.**

SUPPORTING DATA/CONTRIBUTING FACTORS: **The alcoholic patient has developed ineffective coping skills to deal with feelings of anxiety, depression, rejection, guilt, and anger. The family also has developed ways of dealing with the alcoholic person that may contribute to the problem. The onset of withdrawal symptoms or DTs may further tax limited coping skills.**

GENERAL PATIENT OUTCOMES: **Verbalizes feelings appropriately. Begins to deal with the reality of the situation. Identifies sources of support/available resources.**

INTERVENTIONS	RATIONALE
Independent	
Assess patient's/family's ability to understand what is happening.	Individuals may be anxious and angry, which can interfere with their participation in care.

INTERVENTIONS	RATIONALE
Independent	
Talk to patient with a calm tone of voice, being non-judgmental.	Minimizes confrontation and helps patient maintain contact with environment.
Provide information regarding therapy and prognosis.	Helps patient/family know what is happening in a situation in which conflicting feelings of anger and fear may be overwhelming.
Encourage patient/significant other(s) to discuss concerns/questions.	Provides opportunity to clarify misconceptions.
Provide opportunities to make choices, and encourage patient to formulate short-term/achievable goals.	Promotes sense of control and individual value/self-worth.
Collaborative	
Refer to hospital psychiatric nurse, social worker, chaplain, and community resources such as Alcoholics Anonymous (AA), AlAnon.	Patient and family/significant other(s) may need additional help/support to develop skills for coping with the situation/necessary lifestyle changes.

Chemical Abuse: Drug Overdose/Poisoning

The focus of this care plan is the acute care of an individual who has ingested, injected, or been exposed to substance(s) which may be toxic/poisonous. Although some overdoses are accidental and may require teaching/learning or assistance with health maintenance, this care plan outlines the psychiatric concerns that may accompany the intentional overdose.

PATIENT ASSESSMENT DATA BASE

HISTORY

Past history of acute/chronic depressive episodes, maladaptive coping mechanisms, suicidal gestures.

Reports of alterations in behavior patterns, changes in problem-solving abilities.

History of chronic pain treated with narcotic analgesics.

Note use of drugs, such as alcohol, methadone, antibuse, illicit drugs.

Simultaneous ingestion of numerous drugs with alcohol.

Ingestion of several drugs containing the same active ingredient (e.g., acetaminophen and cold remedies).

Combination of drugs leading to synergistic effect (e.g., alcohol and major/minor tranquilizers).

Failure to follow medication instructions.

Toxicity resulting from impaired metabolism and excretion.

Subjective

May complain of actual/perceived threat(s) to physical and emotional well-being.

PHYSICAL EXAMINATION

Physical findings vary, depending on causative agent, amount ingested, period of time from ingestion, age, and preexisting condition of patient.

Inspection

Level of consciousness: responses may vary from somnolence (with no voluntary movement) to extreme restlessness, combativeness, and violent behavior (paradoxical hyperexcited state).

Mentation: wide range of response may be noted, including disorientation/complete mental confusion, hallucinations.

Speech: may be unable to speak, have thick slurred speech, or show inability to organize thoughts into words.

Pupils: varying pupil size (constricted/dilated) and reaction, depending on drug ingested. Nystagmus may be present.

Neuromuscular: deep tendon reflexes (DTRs) may vary from hyperresponsiveness to flaccidity. Fine muscle tremors may be noted, or overt seizure activity.

Respirations may be absent, irregular, rapid, and/or shallow.

Urine output may vary, depending on reaction of kidneys to ingested drug and/or fluid balance.

Skin: signs of dehydration may be present (for example, dry mucous membranes), or flushing and diaphoresis may be noted. Pallor and cyanosis may be evident.

Abdomen: nausea, vomiting, and/or gastric bleeding may be present.

Auscultation

Breath sounds may be diminished/absent. Adventious sounds (e.g., crackles/rhonchi) may be present.

Bowel sounds: hypoactive/hyperactive bowel sounds may be present, depending on effects of drug and/or antidote therapies.

Blood pressure: hypotension or hypertension may be present, depending on drug ingested and state of awareness.

Palpation

Peripheral pulses may be weak, thready, if in shock state. Tachycardia, bradycardia, or other irregularities may be noted.

Other

Temperature: hyperpyrexia may be present in sympathomimetic and anticholinergic ingestion. Hypothermia may be present in sedative and hypnotic overdose.

DIAGNOSTIC STUDIES

Toxicology: studies of blood, urine, and gastric contents assist with identification of ingested drug(s).

Urinalysis: alteration in osmolality and pH may be noted.

ABGs: responses vary, depending on patient's previous and present respiratory status and/or drug ingested (e.g., metabolic acidosis is seen in salicylate overdose).

Glucose: hyperglycemia can occur as a response to certain drugs (e.g., salicylates), although hypoglycemia may be the response in children.

Electrolytes may show imbalances; for example, hyperkalemia/hypokalemia and/or hypernatremia/hyponatremia.

BUN and creatinine are elevated in presence of intrinsic renal damage related to effects of nephrotoxic drugs.

Liver enzymes: elevation reflects effects of hepatotoxic drugs.

ECG may reveal ischemia/injury pattern, various dysrhythmias, and/or heart blocks.

Chest x-ray examination may be clear or show infiltrates/varying degrees of congestion (e.g., pulmonary edema).

NURSING PRIORITIES

1. Maintain respiratory/circulatory function.
2. Identify causative agents, prevent further absorption/promote rapid clearance.
3. Prevent further injury to self and/or others.
4. Assess need/initiate referrals for emotional/psychiatric support as indicated.

NURSING DIAGNOSIS:	**Breathing Pattern, ineffective.**
SUPPORTING DATA/CONTRIBUTING FACTORS:	**The majority of overdoses involve drugs that have a depressant effect on the central nervous system (CNS), leading to respiratory insufficiency/failure. Excessive fluid resuscitation to induce rapid diuresis (initial treatment measure) or drug-induced pulmonary**

capillary endothelial damage may result in pulmonary edema/adult respiratory distress syndrome (ARDS). Extreme respiratory distress may occur when caustic agents have been ingested. Aspiration may occur as a result of decreased responsiveness, leading to aspiration pneumonia.

GENERAL PATIENT OUTCOMES: **Spontaneous respirations achieved/maintained. Arterial blood gases (ABGs) are within patient's normal range. Lungs are clear.**

INTERVENTIONS	RATIONALE
Independent	
Maintain patent airway. Position on side with head in neutral position. Insert oral airway, as indicated.	Central nervous system depression can result in loss of motor control off the tongue, which can occlude the oropharynx. Altering patient's position is often all that is needed to open/maintain the airway.
Inspect chest for respiratory rate, depth, and rhythm.	Respirations may be decreased as a result of the effect of depressed CNS function or be rapid/shallow, reflecting hyperexcitability and stimulation of CNS. Alterations in acid-base balance also will affect rate and depth of breathing.
Auscultate lung fields for presence/absence of breath sounds. Note adventitious sounds (e.g., crackles, rhonchi, and wheezes).	Absence of breath sounds in large areas suggests hypoventilation. Small silent spots may indicate atelectasis. Early discovery of changes in breath sounds allows for interventions to minimize pulmonary complications.
Note skin color; observe buccal mucosa, nailbeds, extremities.	Cyanosis is indicative of inadequate oxygenation of blood (desaturated hemoglobin) or may reflect methemoglobinemia from oxidizing agents such as nitroglycerine, chlorates, and sulfonamides. These oxidize hemoglobin to the ferric form and render it incapable of transporting oxygen. A cherry-red skin color indicates carbon monoxide poisoning, which also competes with oxygen for hemoglobin-binding sites.
Change patient's position frequently. Assist with pulmonary toilet; for example, coughing, deep breathing exercises, if patient is not intubated.	Repositioning enhances ventilation and aids in mobilizing secretions to prevent consolidation. Coughing and deep breathing exercises can significantly reduce the tendency to develop atelectasis.
Suction oro-pharyngeal area, as indicated.	Aspiration of secretions/vomitus may occur as a result of diminished gag and swallow reflexes. Severe respiratory distress/depression may require intubation and removal of accumulated secretions by suctioning.

INTERVENTIONS	RATIONALE
Collaborative	
Monitor laboratory studies as indicated; for example, Serial ABGs,	Respiratory acidosis and hypoxia may occur as a result of depressed respiratory effort or may reflect the effects of causative agent (e.g., carbon monoxide). Metabolic acidosis is often present in salicylate poisoning.
Carboxyhemoglobin (COHgb),	Carboxyhemoglobin is produced when carbon monoxide combines with hemoglobin. Levels greater than 15 percent may result in severe complications, including myocardial ischemia/injury.
Methemoglobin (HgbM).	General cyanosis refractory to oxygen administration is seen in overdose of oxidizing agents (e.g., nitrites, nitroglycerine, sulfonamides). HgbM blood levels greater than 50 percent indicate severe toxicity, levels greater than 70 percent are usually fatal.
Administer supplemental oxygen by cannula, mask, or mechanical ventilation as indicated.	Maximizes ventilation and oxygen transport to correct hypoxia caused by hypoventilation, CNS depression, pneumonia, or pulmonary edema. Intubation may be required to protect the airway, even though aspiration of gastric contents may have already occurred.
Administer appropriate antidote; for example, Naloxone (Narcan),	May be administered if the respiratory depressant agent is unknown or if the agent is a narcotic. Narcan is the best narcotic antagonist because of its rapid action, short half-life, and because it can be administered intravenously (IV) or endotracheally.
Methylene blue.	Improves oxygen-carrying capacity of blood by converting methemoglobin to hemoglobin, when methemoglobin levels are greater than 30 percent.
Administer aminophyllin.	Although not an antidote, aminophyllin may be useful in relieving broncospasms, including those secondary to pulmonary microemboli associated with overdose of pentazocine (Talwin)/tripelennamine (Pyribenzamine) known on the street as T's and blues.
Assist with/prepare for hyperbaric oxygen therapy as indicated.	Oxygen under greater pressure than normal atmospheric pressure is used in carbon monoxide poisoning to accelerate the release of carbon monoxide from hemoglobin, thereby improving oxygenation.

NURSING DIAGNOSIS:	**Injury, potential for poisoning.**
SUPPORTING DATA/CONTRIBUTING FACTORS:	**Although overdose has already occurred, poisonous effects of the toxic agent(s) may continue, and without timely intervention, further injury, permanent damage, and/or death may occur.**

GENERAL PATIENT OUTCOMES:	Drug effects are reversed/minimized. Further complications are prevented.

INTERVENTIONS	RATIONALE
Independent	
Ascertain circumstances of overdose (e.g., types and amounts of agents used/available). Request that containers be brought to the hospital if indicated.	Assists with identification of drugs/alerts to possible drug interactions which may occur. The history may be unreliable, and multiple drugs may be involved.
Assess body systems for increasing dysfunction indicative of toxic/adverse effects.	Treatments may need to be altered based on developing changes.
Independent: CNS	
Note deepening coma, loss of pupil reaction/reflexes, changes in blood pressure.	Toxic effects of CNS depressants may be immediately apparent or may develop several hours after treatment is begun.
Note signs of increased CNS stimulation (e.g., hyperactivity, seizures).	Toxic effects of CNS stimulants, hypoxia, and/or withdrawal from certain drugs may result in seizure activity. Sedation may be required to control seizures, especially if frequent or continual.
Monitor body temperature.	Alterations may reflect drug effect on hypothalamus. Hyperpyrexia occurs with salicylate poisoning, sympathomimetic and anticholinergic ingestions. Hypothermia is seen with sedative and hyponotic ingestions.
Independent: Cardiovascular	
Note trends in blood pressure (BP).	Decreased sympathetic tone/vasodilation may occur with some agents, resulting in profound hypotension/cardiovascular collapse (e.g., tricyclic antidepressants). Hypertensive crisis may occur with sympathomimetic overdose.
Monitor cardiac rhythm.	Rhythm disturbances range from tachycardia to severe bradycardia and heart block, especially in presence of tricyclic antidepressant/amphetamine ingestion or hypothermia (associated with barbiturates, sedatives, hypnotics, and tranquilizers).

(Refer to Nursing Diagnosis: Cardiac Output, alteration in, decreased (potential), page 359.)

Independent: Respiratory

Refer to Nursing Diagnosis: Breathing Pattern, ineffective, page 354.)

Independent: Renal

Monitor/calculate hourly and 24-hour output, noting fluid balance.	Changes in urinary output may reflect nephrotoxic effect of agent on the kidney, resulting in acute tubular necrosis (ATN), or reflect prerenal cause (e.g., hypotension with hypoperfusion of kidneys). (Refer to Care Plan: Acute Renal Failure, page 207.)

INTERVENTIONS	RATIONALE
Independent: Gastrointestinal	
Auscultate bowel sounds. Note complaints of abdominal pain, presence of hematemesis/bloody diarrhea.	Severe gastrointestinal (GI) complications can occur; for example, hemorrhagic necrosis, as seen with iron overdose, or massive bowel infarction, as may be seen with tricyclic antidepressant overdose.
Collaborative	
Contact regional poison control center for current treatment/protocol.	These centers have current information regarding detoxification and ways to prevent further absorption and to hasten elimination of toxic substance.
Obtain appropriate specimens for toxicology screening (e.g., blood, urine, gastric contents).	Identifies causative agents and directs therapies/antidotes.
Administer emetics (e.g., ipecac) or assist with gastric lavage, using large amounts saline.	Early removal of drugs from stomach and intestinal tract reduces drug absorption/effect.
Administer absorbents (e.g., activated charcoal) and/or cathartics (magnesium sulfate), as indicated.	Charcoal absorbs/binds with many substances in the GI tract, and a cathartic stimulates gastric motility and evacuation. Note: Charcoal may be contraindicated if an oral antidote is to be given (e.g., N-acetylcysteine [Mucomyst]) and should not be given until effects of ipecac have subsided.
Administer appropriate antidotes as indicated for specific drug and monitor effects per poison control protocol.	Specific antidotes should be obtained from poison control centers. Protocol should be followed and effectiveness monitored by plasma drug levels.
Administer sodium bicarbonate.	Alkalinization of blood to maintain a pH of 7.5 may be useful in correcting some dysrhythmias and conduction disturbances associated with acidic agent overdoses (e.g., tricyclic antidepressants and salicylates). Alkalinization also is used to decrease lipid solubility of salicylates and to decrease uptake by the CNS.
Administer physostigmine salicylate (Antilirium).	Because this is currently the only cholinergic drug known to cross the blood-brain barrier, it is useful in reversing/limiting CNS anticholenergic effects of tricyclic antidepressant (TCA) toxicity. It also possibly reduces the extent of gastric tissue ischemia/injury.
Administer IV fluids in conjunction with	Forced diuresis speeds elimination of agent and reduces its reabsorption in renal tubules. Note: This is contraindicated in presence of renal insufficiency, cardiac disease, and hypokalemia.
Sodium bicarbonate, normal saline, and a diuretic;	Alkaline diuresis is used to promote rapid excretion of acids (e.g., salicylates and barbiturates).
Ascorbic acid, ammonium chloride, and a diuretic.	Acid diuresis may be used to promote rapid excretion of amphetamines and phencyclidine (PCP).
Monitor serum electrolytes and pH as indicated.	Forced diuresis with alteration of pH requires close monitoring to maintain therapeutic range.
Monitor indices of renal/liver function and plasma drug levels.	Evaluates effectiveness of body to clear drug(s). Increasing plasma drug levels, or levels which do not decrease appropriately, may indicate kidney failure/need for dialysis.

INTERVENTIONS	RATIONALE
Collaborative	
Assist with hemoperfusion, exchange transfusion, or hemodialysis/peritoneal dialysis as indicated. (Refer to Care Plan: Renal Dialysis, page 222.)	Drugs that are distributed in plasma proteins and/or have poor systemic clearance (e.g., salicylates) may be cleared by one of these methods. Dialysis may be therapy of choice in presence of massive overdoses and/or cardiac, renal compromise. Hemoperfusion is recommended for sedatives, hypnotics, long-/short-acting barbiturates.

NURSING DIAGNOSIS: **Cardiac Output, alteration in, decreased (potential).**

SUPPORTING DATA/CONTRIBUTING FACTORS: **Drug effect may cause vascular dilatation, resulting in venous pooling and reduced cardiac output. Hypotension, hypoxia, and acidosis affect vital organ perfusion. Dysrhythmias are common and may occur from autonomic and/or direct cardiac effects on conduction and contractility.**

GENERAL PATIENT OUTCOMES: **Vital signs and cardiac output within patient's normal range. Life-threatening dysrhythmias are controlled.**

INTERVENTIONS	RATIONALE
Independent	
Monitor BP and hemodynamic pressures; for example, mean arterial pressure (MAP), central venous pressure (CVP), cardiac output (CO)/index (CI), as indicated.	Provides accurate measurement of fluid status and monitors effects of drugs on cardiovascular system.
Monitor heart rate and rhythm. Record/report dysrhythmias.	Death can occur owing to the life-threatening dysrhythmias, most often seen in overdose of stimulants, cocaine, narcotics, PCP, and tricyclic antidepressants.
Assess mentation, level of consciousness, sensory/motor responses.	Changes may reflect alteration of cerebral perfusion owing to decreasing CO as well as hypoxemia/acid base imbalance or direct effect of drugs.
Note skin color/temperature.	Pallor, central cyanosis, mottling, and cold skin suggest impaired systemic perfusion, possibly owing to decreased CO.
Measure intake and hourly urine outputs and specific gravity.	Decreased urinary output with elevated specific gravity in presence of low blood pressure may indicate hypovolemia/decreased CO. However, continuing oliguria in spite of adequate fluid replacement may suggest acute renal insult/injury.

INTERVENTIONS	RATIONALE
Collaborative	
Monitor blood urea nitrogen (BUN), creatinine, ABGs, and electrolytes.	Blood urea nitrogen and creatinine reflect renal perfusion and ability of the kidneys to excrete waste products/toxins. Hyperemia, acid base, and electrolyte imbalance can produce cardiac dysrhythmias.
Administer IV fluids/plasma expanders/blood as indicated.	Adequate circulating volume is necessary to support CO. Circulating volume may be reduced by side effects of drug; for example, vomiting, diarrhea, diaphoresis, as well as therapies (e.g., forced diuresis).
Administer drugs as indicated:	
Antiarrhythmics, for example, lidocaine hydrochloride (Xylocaine);	Decreases ventricular irritability thereby reducing dysrhythmias. Note: adverse side effects of lidocaine, e.g. hypotension, confusion, may be masked by drug overdose. Pronestyl and Quinidine may be contraindicated in presence of anticholinergic/tricyclic overdose because of myocardial depressive effects and enhanced toxicity.
Isoproterenol (Isuprel);	May be useful temporarily in treating bradycardia/high-degree heart block.
Vasoactive agents, for example, dopamine hydrochloride (Intropin);	May correct hypotension that is refractory to fluid replacement by increasing CO.
Norepinephrine injection (Levophed).	Vasopressor of choice in overdose of phenothiazines or tricyclic antidepressants.
Provide Advanced Cardiac Life Support. Assist with pacemaker insertion as indicated.	Potential for high-degree heart block/full cardiopulmonary arrest is always present in drug overdoses.

NURSING DIAGNOSIS: **Fluid Volume, alteration in, excess (potential).**

SUPPORTING DATA/CONTRIBUTING FACTORS: **Forced diuresis may be employed to enhance elimination of drugs. This can present problems in presence of underlying renal and cardiac disease (especially in geriatric population), which may result in fluid overload.**

GENERAL PATIENT OUTCOMES: **Output approximates intake. Breath sounds clear, dyspnea absent. Vital signs within patient's normal range.**

INTERVENTIONS	RATIONALE
Independent	
Obtain history from previous records, family, significant other, or patient (if able to do so).	History of renal or heart disease is signal for close monitoring of fluid balance/alterations in therapy.
Monitor BP, pulse, and hemodynamic pressures; for example, CVP, PAP, PCWP, if available.	Elevations may indicate hypervolemia/impending cardiac/renal failure.
Record intake and output. Calculate fluid balance.	Positive fluid balance may indicate hypervolemia/fluid retention.
Auscultate lungs, noting presence of adventitious breath sounds (e.g., crackles). Note tachypnea and presence of dyspnea.	Pulmonary congestion suggests hypervolemia.
Auscultate heart sounds.	S_3 may indicate early inability to handle fluid volume/developing congestive heart failure.
Assess for neck vein distention at 45 degrees elevation of head.	Indicator of fluid volume/overload when CVP not available.
Collaborative	
Monitor serum electrolytes.	Decreased sodium may be indicative of dilutional effect of fluid overload.
Administer diuretics as indicated.	Diuretic may be given to reduce total body water or to increase the volume of fluid through the kidney tubules to clear cellular debris, thereby reducing risks of permanent damage (ATN).

NURSING DIAGNOSIS: **Sensory-Perceptual, alteration in (specify).**

SUPPORTING DATA/CONTRIBUTING FACTORS: **Central nervous system depression is a common feature in many overdoses, especially ingestion of sedatives, hypnotics, and narcotics. Confusion, agitation, and disorientation are commonly associated with overdoses of tricyclic antidepressants, PCP, stimulants, and phenothiazines. Agitation and hyperexcitability can interfere with thought processes, resulting in narrowed focus, disruption in ability to concentrate, and distortion of perception.**

GENERAL PATIENT OUTCOMES: **Alert, with confusion/disorientation minimized or absent.**

INTERVENTIONS	RATIONALE
Independent	
Assess mentation/degree of orientation to person, place, and time.	Frequent evaluation is necessary to determine changes in CNS function. For example, inability to maintain orientation may be sign of CNS deterioration/increased drug toxicity.
Provide atmosphere of acceptance, especially when patient has difficulty expressing thoughts and feelings.	Aids in creating a trusting environment and provides opportunity for reflection, which can be helpful in clarifying altered perceptions/disordered thought processes.
Avoid challenging illogical thinking; maintain nondefensive posture. (Refer to Nursing Diagnosis: Violence, potential for, below.)	The patient may not be amenable to logic and may respond defensively to any challenge.
Provide quiet environment, reduce excess stimuli. Approach patient in a calm manner.	The patient may be frightened by distorted perceptions/thought processes, and sudden, unexpected stimuli may precipitate violent response.
Monitor vital signs (e.g., BP, temperature).	Alterations in BP and temperature can affect patient's ability to perceive environment and may alter verbal expression.
Provide seizure precautions; for example, padded siderails, bed in low position, frequent observation.	Central nervous system dysfunction may lead to seizure activity.
Collaborative	
Monitor ABGs, electrolytes, and plasma drug levels.	Hypoxia, acidemia, and electrolyte imbalances as well as direct drug effect can alter sensory perception.
Administer supplemental oxygen, as indicated.	May correct hypoxemia, which alters brain function/perception.
Administer medications as indicated; for example,	
Diazepam (Valium),	Sedative and anticonvulsant, which produces a calming effect on thalamus, hypothalmus, and limbic system. Note: Diazepam may produce synergistic effect in overdoses of sedatives and hypnotics, especially barbituates.
Chlorpromazine (Thorazine),	May be helpful in decreasing agitation/psychosis associated with amphetamine overdose.
Haldoperidol (Haldol),	Manages/reduces psychotomimetic effects of PCP and stimulants. Note: Although Haldol exerts a lesser depressant effect on the respiratory center than Valium, therapeutic levels may be more difficult to achieve because it cannot be given IV.
Diphenhydramine hydrochloride (Benadryl) or benztropine mesylate (Cogentin).	May be effective in treating extrapyramidal effects of phenothiazines.

NURSING DIAGNOSIS: **Violence, potential for.**

SUPPORTING DATA/CONTRIBUTING FACTORS: **Violent behavior is often a side effect of ingested drugs, though individual**

tolerance varies. Decreasing blood levels of certain ingested drugs (withdrawal symptoms) can lead to aggressive/violent behavior. Violent behavior also may reflect anger felt by patient if the overdose was an unsuccessful suicide attempt.

GENERAL PATIENT OUTCOMES: **Violent behavior will be minimized/controlled.**

INTERVENTIONS	RATIONALE
Independent	
Assess frequently for signs of disturbed/violent behavior.	Detection of early signs, including restlessness, irritability, lack of cooperation, and demanding behavior, can aid in prevention of violence.
Observe closely for signs of suicidal intent (e.g., verbalizing intent, attempts at further self-harm).	A drug overdose as an unsuccessful suicide attempt may lead to further suicidal gestures.
Provide quiet, nonthreatening, protective environment. Maintain nonjudgmental, kind approach.	Reducing sensory stimulation can help limit aggressive behavior. Encouraging expression of negative feelings in a nonjudgmental environment can help dissipate feelings of powerlessness, anger, and guilt.
Assess response to visitors; restrict as needed.	Certain visitors may provoke the patient, but others have a calming effect. Goal is to limit and to reduce provocation.
Use physical restraint judiciously, as necessary.	Physical restraint should be used as last resort; however, it may be needed to prevent further injury to patient and/or others.
Collaborative	
Administer drugs as indicated; for example,	
Sedatives and tranquilizers,	May be required in case of uncontrolled violent behavior. Action is to calm patient. Note: Observe for synergistic affect when combined with overdosed drug(s).
Pancuronium bromide (Pavulon).	May be required to suppress life-threatening uncontrollable motor activity seen in PCP overdose. Note: Pancuronium bromide requires mechanical respiratory support.
Refer for psychiatric consultation, if indicated.	Violent behavior may subside as the patient is detoxified. However, exacerbation/reoccurrence of violent behavior may require further therapy/interventions.

NURSING DIAGNOSIS: **Coping, ineffective, individual.**

SUPPORTING DATA/CONTRIBUTING FACTORS: **Patient who is unable to manage internal or environmental stressors prior**

	to overdose event may be further compromised when hospitalized in critical care setting. Suicide attempt may be related to poor problem-solving skills, leading to further inability to deal with stress of current situation. In addition, feelings of anger and guilt about suicide attempt/failure of completion may further compromise coping abilities.
GENERAL PATIENT OUTCOMES:	**Identifies stressors and coping strengths. Initiates steps of problem solving.**

INTERVENTIONS	RATIONALE
Independent	
Assess causative and contributing factors relating to poor coping mechanisms; for example, unwillingness to discuss incident, lack of support system(s), blaming others/difficulty accepting responsibility for own actions.	Identification of causative factors is first step in problem-solving process.
Note expressions of concern/guilt about suicidal attempt. (Refer to Care Plan: Psychosocial Aspects; Nursing Diagnosis: Spiritual Distress, page 386.)	May feel remorseful/guilty because teachings of religious background identify taking own life as wrong.
Demonstrate acceptance by verbal/nonverbal cues.	Patient may be more apt to verbalize when accepting attitude is present in staff providing care.
Offer support by Active Listening, spending time with patient, and encouraging self-expression.	Helps diminish fear and develops a therapeutic environment in which patient can begin to talk about problems leading to decision to overdose.
Validate information by repeating what has been said.	Inaccurate assumptions maybe made unless information is validated.
Assist in identifying problems that can be controlled directly/immediately.	Once problems are identified, solutions may become more visible, thereby restoring some sense of control and hope for further solutions.
Discuss/demonstrate stress-reducing activities (e.g., deep breathing, visualization, progressive relaxation exercises).	Exercise and relaxation techniques help reduce stress and enhance coping abilities.
Support functional coping behaviors (e.g., ability to solve problems, seeking support appropriately from others).	Successful coping mechanisms used in past should be emphasized and built on.
Collaborative	
Refer for psychiatric consultation.	As soon as patient is coherent and recovered from acute overdose, psychiatric consultation should be obtained to identify immediate therapy required and to begin a pertinent treatment program.

NURSING DIAGNOSIS:	**Coping, ineffective family, compromised (potential).**
SUPPORTING DATA/CONTRIBUTING FACTORS:	**Family may be unable to manage stressors associated with overdose event, which sets up a chain of emotions in family/significant other(s), including anger, guilt, fear, and confusion. Inadequate/incorrect information may lead to lack of understanding of overdose event. In addition, when the patient has attempted suicide previously, family may experience feelings of resentment/anger, wishing the patient had succeeded. Accompanying feelings of guilt may compromise the family's ability to deal with the patient's needs.**
GENERAL PATIENT OUTCOMES:	**Family/significant other(s) express feelings, interact positively with patient, providing assistance and support. Family identifies/verbalizes need for support and seeks resources/information.**

INTERVENTIONS	RATIONALE
Independent	
Provide family with necessary information on patient condition.	Accurate/honest information helps initiate coping and supporting process.
Create accepting/supportive environment for family.	Encourages family to express feelings and concerns.
Assess/monitor family interactions, especially during initial visit.	Family may want to be helpful but may be perceived otherwise by patient. It may be necessary to separate patient and family if too unsettling.
Assist with development of effective coping/problem-solving skills through use of repetition and Active Listening.	Family member(s) or significant others are often in shock. Frequent repetition of information and listening to expressions of concern/anger are necessary before the family's level of awareness is raised.
Assess and reinforce family strengths by being available, listening, and noting positive actions/expressions.	May be helpful to gain their confidence so that they are more willing to take risks with self-disclosure related to the situation.
Involve family in care of patient, if appropriate.	Involvement can help build supportive behavior.

INTERVENTIONS	RATIONALE
Collaborative	
Refer to counseling resources as needed; for example, clergy, psychiatric nurse clinician, social services, psychiatrist/psychologist. (Refer to Care Plan: Psychosocial Aspects of Critical Care; Nursing Diagnosis: Coping, ineffective family, compromised, page 391.)	Other resources are often necessary to assist family to deal with what has happened, to learn to solve problems, and to help patient in the most effective manner.

Nutritional Support: Total Parenteral/Enteral Feeding

Specifically designed nutritional therapy is administered by the parenteral or enteral route when the use of standard diets via the oral route is inadequate or not possible. This method is used to prevent/correct protein-calorie malnutrition (defined as a state of impaired function, structural integrity, or development resulting from a discrepancy between the supply of protein, calories, and other essential nutrients and the body's specific metabolic demand for them).

PATIENT ASSESSMENT DATA BASE

HISTORY

Weight: loss of at least 10 percent of body weight within previous six months.

Presence of factors known to alter nutritional requirements/increase energy demands; for example, single or multiorgan failure, sepsis, fever, trauma, extensive burns, use of steroids, use of antitumor agents, immunosuppressants.

Inadequate oral intake owing to medical status or treatment modalities; for example; nothing-by-mouth (NPO) status for 7 to 10 days, long-term use of 5 percent dextrose intravenously; problems with chewing, swallowing, choking, or saliva production. Inadequate oral intake due to educational/social factors; for example, lack of nutrition knowledge/kitchen facilities, reduced/limited financial resources; or illness of psychiatric origin (e.g., anorexia nervosa/bulimia).

Long-term effects of chronic illnesses or treatment may interfere with meeting nutritional requirements; for example, renal dialysis, anorexia/nausea associated with medication use, such as terbutaline sulfate (Brethine); alcohol or other drug use and/or abuse.

Use of medications that cause untoward drug/nutrient interactions; for example, laxatives, anticonvulsives, diuretics, antacids, narcotics, immunosuppressants, chemotherapy.

Protracted protein losses; for example, malabsorption or short gut syndromes with increased diarrhea; renal dialysis, fistulas, protein-losing enteropathies, draining wounds, thermal injuries.

Subjective

May complain of changes in the taste of food, anorexia, nausea/vomiting, diarrhea or constipation, flatulence associated with food intake.

PHYSICAL EXAMINATION

Clinical signs listed below include observations indicative of vitamin/mineral deficiency as well as protein/calorie malnutrition.

Inspection

Actual weight (measured): as compared with usual or preillness weight is less than 90 percent of ideal body weight for height, sex, and age or, equal to or greater than 120 percent of ideal body weight (patient risk is due to tendency to overlook protein and calorie requirements of the obese patient). A distorted actual weight may occur owing to the presence of edema, ascites, organomegaly, tumor bulk, anasarca, amputation.

Mental status: may be lethargic, apathetic, listless, irritable, disoriented, obtunded, comatose.

Hair may be fragile, coarse, lackluster. Alopecia, decreased pigmentation, may be noted.

Eyes may appear sunken, dull, dry, pale conjunctiva. Bitot's spots (triangular shiny gray spots on the conjunctive seen in vitamin A deficiency) or scleral icterus may be noted.

Mouth: mucous membranes may be dry, pale, red, swollen.

Lips may be dry, cracked, red, swollen. Angular stomatitis may be present.

Tongue may be smooth, pale, slick, coated. Color: often magenta, beefy red. Lingual papillae atrophy/swelling may be noted.

Teeth/gums: swollen/bleeding gums, multiple caries may be present. The patient may be edentulous or have dentures that are too large for mouth cavity.

Gag reflex may be decreased/absent (e.g., cerebral vascular accident, head trauma, nerve injury).

Musculoskeletal: skeletal muscle wasting (temporal, intercostal, gastrocnemius, dorsum of hand); thin extremities, flaccid muscles, decreased activity tolerance may be present.

Skin: (any or all of the following may be noted) dry, scaly, tented; flaky paint dermatosis; edema; draining or unhealed wounds, pressure sores; ecchymoses; perifollicular petechiae; subcutaneous fat loss.

Nails may be brittle, thin, flattened, ridged, spoon-shaped.

Respirations: dyspnea, increased sputum production may be noted.

Abdomen: distention/increased girth, ascites may be present.

Stools: may be loose/hard-formed; fatty or clay colored.

Auscultation

Breath sounds: crackles may be noted owing to protein deficiency related fluid shifts.

Bowel sounds may be diminished, hyperactive, or absent.

Palpation

Glands: thyroid, parotid enlargement may be noted.

Pulses: tachycardia, bradycardia may occur.

Abdomen: tender upon palpation.

DIAGNOSTIC STUDIES

Anthropometrics

Weight for height less than 90 percent or equal to or greater than 120 percent ideal body weight per hospital formula.

TRICEP SKINFOLD MEASUREMENT: estimates subcutaneous fat stores; fat reserves less than 10th percentile suggest advanced depletion; levels less than the 30th percentile suggest mild to moderate depletion.

MIDARM MUSCLE CIRCUMFERENCE: measures somatic muscle mass and is used in combination with tricep skin-fold measurement; a decrease of 15 to 20 percentiles from the expected value suggests a significant reduction.

Visceral Proteins

SERUM ALBUMIN: the classic marker measured. Values of 2.7 to 3.4g/dl indicate mild depletion; values of 2.1 to 2.7g/dl, moderate depletion; values of less than 2.1g/dl, severe depletion. Decreased levels are due to poor protein intake, nephrotic syndrome, sepsis, burns, congestive heart failure, cirrhosis, eclampsia, protein-losing enteropathy. Above normal values (greater than 4.5 g/dl) are seen in dehydration.

SERUM TRANSFERRIN: more sensitive to changes in visceral protein stores than albumin; mild depletion = 150 to 200 mg/dl; moderate = 100 to 150 mg/dl; severe = less than 100 mg/dl. Elevated values are seen with iron deficiency, pregnancy, hypoxia, and chronic blood loss. Decreased values are seen with pernicious anemia, chronic infection, liver disease, iron overload, and protein-losing enteropathy. (Note: Value also may be calculated from a formula using Total Iron Binding Capacity (TIBC) value.)

THYROXINE-BINDING PREALBUMIN: reflects rapid changes in hepatic protein synthesis and thus is a more sensitive indicator of visceral protein depletion. Decreased level below 200 mcg/ml is noted with cirrhosis, inflammation, and surgical trauma.

AMINO ACID PROFILE: alterations reflect an imbalance of plasma proteins with depressed levels of branch chain amino acids; amino acid imbalance and altered utilization common with hepatic encephalopathy or sepsis.

Tests of Immune System

TOTAL LYMPHOCYTE COUNT: less than 1500 cells/mm indicates leukopenia and results from decreased generation of T cells, which are very sensitive to malnutrition. Levels are altered by infection and administration of immunosuppressants.

DELAYED CUTANEOUS HYPERSENSITIVITY REACTIONS (DCH): a means of documenting cellular immunity by the observation of the erythematous, indurated skin response to recall antigens (PPD, C.albicans, Trichophyton, SKSD). Failure to react to DCH is called anergy, a negative response that is suggestive of an impaired immune system. Factors other than malnutrition can cause anergy.

Electrolytes/Minerals/Trace Elements

Potassium: deficiency occurs with inadequate intake and with loss of potassium-containing fluids; that is, diarrhea, vomiting, fistula loss, continuous nasogastric suctioning. Potassium also is lost from cells during muscle wasting and is excreted by the kidneys.

Sodium levels are dependent on state of hydration/presence of active loss as may exist in GI suctioning, burns, and so forth.

Phosphorus may be decreased, reflecting inadequate intake, or may be elevated in renal failure.

Magnesium deficiency is common in alcoholics, or in the presence of vomiting and diarrhea; magnesium may be elevated in renal failure.

Calcium levels will be decreased with conditions associated with hypoalbuminemia; for example, renal failure (majority of calcium is bound to albumin). Absorption is decreased by fat malabsorption and low-protein diet.

Zinc deficiency is seen in alcoholic cirrhosis or may be secondary to hypoalbuminemia and GI losses (diarrhea).

Tests Reflecting Protein (Nitrogen) Loss

NITROGEN BALANCE STUDIES: nitrogen excretion (urine, stool, and insensible losses) often exceeds nitrogen (protein) intake in the critically ill, reflecting catabolic response to stress and use of endogenous protein stores for energy production (gluconeogenesis).

BUN may be severely decreased as a result of chronic malnutrition and depletion of skeletal protein stores.

24-HOUR CREATININE EXCRETION: because creatinine is concentrated in muscle mass, there is a good correlation between lean body mass and 24-hour creatinine excretion. Actual values are compared with ideal values (based on height and weight) times 100 percent = Creatinine Height Index (CHI); CHI of 60 to 80 percent = moderate depletion; less than 60 percent = severe depletion.

Tests of Gastrointestinal Function

Tests of malabsorption include Schilling's test, D-xylose test, 72-hour stool fat, GI series.

Chest x-ray examination may be normal or show evidence of pleural effusion; small heart silhouette.

ECG may be normal or demonstrate low voltage, dysrhythmias/patterns reflective of electrolyte imbalances.

NURSING PRIORITIES

1. Minimize/reduce energy losses/needs.
2. Maximize consistent intake of estimated calorie and protein requirements.

3. Restore/maintain body weight; immunocompetence, skin integrity, muscle strength.
4. Minimize/prevent potential complications.
5. Maximize level of nutritional knowledge of patient and/or significant other(s).

NURSING DIAGNOSIS:	**Nutrition, alteration in, less than body requirements.**
SUPPORTING DATA/CONTRIBUTING FACTORS:	**Conditions that interfere with nutrient intake or increase nutrient need/metabolic demand can result in protein/calorie malnutrition. Increased metabolic demand can result in endogenous protein breakdown for use as a caloric source when exogenous nutrient supply is lacking or insufficient. Patient may experience anorexia because of current illness. Medical problems (e.g., cancer and associated treatments, CVA) or surgical procedures involving head and neck region may result in dysphagia/and difficulty swallowing. Depressed mental status/level of consciousness or decreased muscular strength/paralysis may inhibit patient's attempts at self-feeding.**
GENERAL PATIENT OUTCOMES:	**Weight loss stabilized with appropriate weight gains noted. Positive nitrogen balance present.**

INTERVENTIONS	RATIONALE
Independent	
Assess nutritional status during daily nursing care, noting skin, nails, hair. (Refer to Physical Examination, page 367.)	Because nurses spend the most time with critically ill patients, they have the opportunity to observe deviations from normals or patient baseline.
Note admission weight/height; weigh daily.	Establishes baseline. Serial measurements alert one to inappropriate trends in weight loss/gain.
Document oral intake by use of 24-hour recall, food history, calorie counts.	Identify imbalances between estimated nutritional requirements and actual intake.
Assess gag reflex, ability to swallow, motor skills during transitional feedings.	May require retraining by dysphagia expert (e.g., speech therapist) or require long-term tube feeding. Patients with neuromuscular deficits (e.g., post-CVA, brain injury) may require use of special aids developed for feeding.

INTERVENTIONS	RATIONALE
Independent	
Provide optimal environment during attempts at oral intake: remove bedpans, soiled linens. Allow adequate time, provide for socialization/feeding assistance by significant other/nurse. Offer small, frequent feedings, noting patient likes/dislikes and including "home foods" as appropriate.	Oral feedings may be given in conjunction with total parental nutrition (TPN) to meet increased metabolic demands; that is, for burns or during transition from nutritional support. Patients need extra encouragement/assistance to overcome underlying problems such as anorexia, fatigue, muscular weakness.
Schedule activities with adequate rest periods. Promote relaxation techniques.	Conserves energy/reduces calorie needs.
Assure accurate collections of specimens (urine, stool, drainage) for nitrogen balance studies.	Inaccurate collections can alter test results, leading to improper interpretation of patient status.
Assure accurate laboratory results from blood sampling done via multilumen, central venous catheters.	Electrolyte values in particular may be falsely elevated if electrolyte-containing solutions are not turned off prior to blood sampling. Blood flow turbulence around sampling lumen can cause reflux of infusing solutions into the sample.
Be familiar with electrolyte content of parenteral/enteral nutrition solutions.	Metabolic complications of nutritional support often result from a lack of appreciation of the metabolic changes that occur as a result of refeeding (e.g., HHNC, electrolyte imbalances).
Assure that parenteral/enteral nutrition solutions are delivered as prescribed. Use of infusion control device is preferred. Adjust rate to prescribed hourly rate but never "catch up."	Nutrition support prescriptions are based on estimated caloric and protein requirements. A consistent rate of nutrient administration will assure proper utilization with fewer side effects, such as hyperglycemia.
Independent: Enteral	
Assess function and tolerance to enteral feedings: note bowel sounds, complaints of nausea/vomiting, abdominal discomfort, presence of diarrhea/constipation.	Because protein turnover of the GI mucosa occurs approximately every 3 days, the GI tract is at great risk for early dysfunction and atrophy from disease and malnutrition. Intolerance of formula may require change to parenteral administration.
Check gastric residuals. Hold feeding for 1 hour or per protocol for type/rate of feeding used, if residual is greater than 125 ml.	Delayed gastric emptying can be caused by a specific disease process (e.g., paralytic ileus/surgery, shock), by drug therapy (especially narcotics), or the protein/fat content of the individual formula.
Maintain patency of enteral feeding tubes by flushing with warm water or cranberry juice as indicated.	Enteral formulas contain protein that can clog small bore feeding tubes, necessitating removal/replacement of tube.
Independent: Parenteral	
Observe appropriate "hang" time of parenteral solutions per protocol.	Effectiveness of IV vitamins diminishes after 24 hours.
Monitor urine sugar/acetone or finger-stick glucose per protocol.	High glucose content of solutions may lead to pancreatic fatigue, requiring use of supplemental insulin to prevent HHNC. Note: finger-stick determination of glu-

INTERVENTIONS	RATIONALE
Independent	
	cose level is more accurate/may be preferred owing to variations in renal threshold.
Collaborative	
Refer to nutritional team/registered dietitian.	Discussions of patient's nutritional status with physician/dietitian will aid identification of nutrient deficits and need for early parenteral/enteral nutritional intervention.
Calculate basal energy expenditure (BEE) using Harris-Benedict formula based on sex, height, weight, age, and estimated energy/protein requirements.	Combining BEE and physiologic stress, activity, weight gain needs, estimated nitrogen losses, and renal/hepatic functional capacity provides an estimation of calorie and protein needs.
Review results of indirect calorimetry test if available.	State-of-the-art method to measure oxygen consumption reflecting basal or resting metabolic rate to aid in estimating calorie/protein requirements. Note: Rate may be increased by conditions that affect metabolic demand (e.g., fever, sepsis, surgical trauma).
Assist with insertion and confirm proper placement of the central venous catheter tip by chest x-ray examination prior to administration of TPN solutions.	Catheter must lie in superior vena cava. Common complications of insertion include pneumothorax/hemothorax, embolus, or arterial puncture.
Assist with insertion/maintain small-bore feeding tube. Deliver enteral formulas at a continuous hourly rate.	Continuous infusion of enteral formulas is better tolerated than bolus feedings and results in improved absorption.
Assess metabolic response to nutrition support: Monitor laboratory studies; for example, serum glucose, electrolytes, PO_4, BUN/creatinine, liver enzymes, complete blood count (CBC), ABGs.	Untoward effects of refeeding include hypokalemia; hyponatremia and fluid retention; hyperglycemia, hypophosphotemia; increased carbon dioxide production, resulting in respiratory compromise; elevation of liver function tests; renal dysfunction. Note: Although phosphorus deficiency is not a routine occurrence, hypophosphatemia retards the release of oxygen from the hemoglobin molecule at the cellular level, resulting in hemolytic anemia and hemolysis.
Administer intralipid fat emulsions as indicated.	Useful in meeting excessive calorie requirements (e.g., burns) or as a source of essential fatty acids during long-term hyperalimentation. Note: These may be contraindicated in patients with alterations in fat metabolism or in the presence of pancreatitis, liver damage, anemia, coagulation disorders, pulmonary disease.
Administer adjunctive medications, as indicated; for example,	
Insulin,	Alterations in glucose tolerance may require the use of regular insulin.
Diphenoxylate hydrochloride with atropine sulfate (Lomotil), camphorated tincture of opium (paregoric), and metoclopramide hydrochloride (Reglan).	Gastrointestinal side effects of enteral feeding may need to be controlled with antidiarrheal agents (Lomotil/paregoric) or peristaltic stimulants (Reglan) if more conservative measures such as alteration of rate/strength or type of formula are not successful.

INTERVENTIONS	RATIONALE
Collaborative	
Provide calorie-containing beverages, when oral intake is possible (e.g., juices/jello water), dietary supplements (e.g., Sustacal, Ensure), or add Polycose to beverages/water.	Enhances calorie intake when oral intake is limited/restricted.

NURSING DIAGNOSIS: **Infection, potential for.**

SUPPORTING DATA/CONTRIBUTING FACTORS: **Administration of parenteral or enteral nutrition requires the insertion of invasive venous catheters or surgically placed gastrostomy or jejunostomy feeding tubes, thereby disrupting skin integrity and providing route for opportunistic microorganisms to enter the bloodstream. Access devices used for nutritional support are usually in place for extended periods of time, which increases the potential for device-related infection. Finally, improper preparation/handling or contamination of the feeding solution potentiates the risk of bacterial growth/sepsis.**

GENERAL PATIENT OUTCOMES: **Afebrile. Catheter/feeding tube insertion sites clean, free of drainage. No erythema/edema present.**

INTERVENTIONS	RATIONALE
Independent	
Maintain an optimal aseptic environment during bedside insertion of central venous catheters and during changes of TPN bottles and administration tubing.	Catheter-related sepsis may result from entry of pathogenic microorganisms through skin insertion tract or from touch contamination during manipulations of TPN system.
Secure external portion of catheter/administration tubing to outside of dressing with tape. Note intactness of skin suture.	Manipulation of catheter in/out of insertion site can result in tissue trauma (coring) and potentiate entry of skin organisms into catheter tract.
Maintain a sterile occlusive dressing over catheter insertion site. Perform central/peripheral venous catheter dressing care per protocol.	Protects catheter insertion sites from potential sources of contamination. Note: Central venous catheter sites can easily become contaminated from tracheostomy or endotracheal secretions or from wounds of the head, neck, and chest.

INTERVENTIONS	RATIONALE
Independent	
Inspect insertion site of catheter for erythema, induration, drainage, tenderness.	The catheter is a potential irritant to the surrounding skin and subcutaneous skin tract, and extended use may result in insertion site irritation and infection.
Keep manipulations of enteral feeding system to a minimum and wash hands before "breaking system."	Touch contamination by caregiver during enteral formula administration has been shown to cause contamination of formula.
Alternate nares in long-term nasogastric tube feedings.	Reduces risk of trauma/infection of paranasal tissue (especially important in facial trauma/burns).
Provide daily/as necessary site care to abdominally placed feeding tubes.	Gastrointestinal secretions leaking through or around gastrostomy or jejunostomy tube tracts can cause skin breakdown severe enough to require the removal of the feeding tube.
Refrigerate premixed amino acid/dextrose solutions prior to use; observe a 24-hour hang time for amino acid solutions and a 12-hour hang time for intravenous fat emulsions.	Total parental nutrition solutions and fat emulsions have been shown to support the growth of a wide variety of pathogenic organisms once contaminated.
Refrigerate reconstituted enteral formulas prior to use; observe a 4 to 8 hour hang time; discard unused formula after 24 hours.	Enteral formulas easily support bacterial growth and can be contaminated during formula preparation. For example, bacterial growth has been shown to occur within four hours after contamination.
Monitor temperature and urine glucose.	A rise in temperature or loss of glucose tolerance (glycosuria, hyperglycemia) are early indications of possible catheter-related sepsis.
Collaborative	
Aseptically prepare parenteral solutions/enteral formulas for administration.	Total parenteral nutrition solutions should be prepared under a laminar flow hood in the department of pharmacy. Enteral formulas should be mixed in a clean environment in the dietary or pharmacy department, although with the advent of canned/modular formulas this may not be necessary. Note: Additives to TPN solutions as a rule should not be made by staff nurses because of the potential for infection and drug incompatibilities.
Notify physician if signs of infection present. Follow protocol for obtaining appropriate culture specimens (e.g., blood, solutions). Change bottle/tubing as indicated. Administer antibiotics dependent on laboratory results.	Immediate interventions necessary to identify source of infection and appropriate therapy. May require removal of TPN line and culture of catheter tip.

NURSING DIAGNOSIS:	**Fluid Volume, alteration in (fluctuation).**
SUPPORTING DATA/CONTRIBUTING FACTORS:	**Malnourished patients, especially the elderly, often present with severe de-**

hydration. Hypoalbuminemia results in decreased colloidal osmotic pressure that leads to third spacing of fluid (edema). Breakdown of endogenous protein stores releases additional water into circulation. Rapid refeeding may result in a gain of fluid rather than lean body mass, potentiating risk of cardiovascular complications. In addition, high-glucose solutions may result in hyperglycemia, potentiating risk of hyperosmolar nonketotic coma and severe dehydration.

GENERAL PATIENT OUTCOMES: **Mucous membranes moist, urinary output within normal limits, free of edema, excessive weight loss/gain.**

INTERVENTIONS	RATIONALE
Independent	
Assess for clinical signs of dehydration/fluid excess (e.g., thirst, dry skin/mucous membranes, peripheral edema, tachycardia, adventious breath sounds).	Early detection/intervention may prevent occurrence/excessive fluctuation in fluid balance. In severely malnourished patient, left ventricular muscle mass may be diminished, therefore a fluid overload, especially during initial 3 to 5 days of refeeding, may precipitate cardiac decompensation in response to increased cardiac output (CO)/metabolic demand.
Incorporate knowledge of caloric density of enteral formulas into assessment of fluid balance.	Enteric solutions are usually concentrated and may not meet free water needs. With higher calorie formula, additional water is needed to prevent dehydration/hyperosmolar hyperglycemic nonketotic coma (HHNC).
Record intake and output; calculate fluid balance.	Rapid weight gain reflecting fluid retention can predispose the patient to congestive heart failure or pulmonary edema. Excessive urinary losses may reflect developing HHNC. (Refer to Nursing Diagnosis: Nutrition, alteration in, less than body requirements, page 370.)
Record weight change daily.	Gain of greater than 0.5 lbs per day indicates fluid retention and not deposition of lean body mass.
Collaborative	
Monitor serum potassium/phosphorus.	Hypokalemia/phosphatemia can occur owing to intracellular shifts during initial refeeding and may compromise cardiac function if not corrected.

NURSING DIAGNOSIS:	**Injury, potential for, multifactors.**
SUPPORTING DATA/CONTRIBUTING FACTORS:	**Complications that occur owing to nutritional support may be life-threatening. These can include aspiration, air emboli, and septic thrombophlebitis.**
GENERAL PATIENT OUTCOMES:	**Complications associated with nutritional support are prevented/ minimized.**

INTERVENTIONS	RATIONALE
Independent	
Maintain a closed central venous IV system using LuerLok connections/taping of all connections.	Inadvertent disconnection of central IV system can result in lethal air emboli.
Investigate complaints of severe chest pain/coughing. Turn patient to left side in Trendelenburg position if indicated and notify physician.	May indicate presence of air embolus, requiring immediate intervention to displace air into apex of heart away from the pulmonary artery.
Maintain an occlusive dressing on catheter insertion sites for 24 hours after subclavian catheter removed.	Extended catheter use may result in development of catheter skin tract. Once catheter is removed, air embolus is still a potential risk until skin tract has sealed.
Assess catheter for signs of displacement out of central venous position; that is, extended length of catheter on skin surface; leaking of IV solution onto dressing; patient complaints of neck pain, tenderness at catheter site, or swelling of extremity on side of catheter insertion.	Central venous catheter tip may slip out of superior vena cava and position itself into smaller inominate and jugular veins, causing a chemical thrombophlebitis. Incidence of subclavian or superior vena cava thrombosis is increased with extended use of central venous catheters.
Administer appropriate TPN solution via peripheral or central venous route.	Solutions containing high concentrations of dextrose (greater than 10 percent, must be delivered via a central vein, because they will result in chemical phlebitis when delivered through small peripheral veins.
Inspect peripheral TPN catheter site. Change sites at least every 3 days/or per protocol.	Peripheral TPN solutions (although less hyperosmolar) can still irritate small veins and cause phlebitis. Peripheral venous access is often limited in malnourished patients, but site should still be changed if signs of irritation develop.
Monitor patient for potential drug/nutrient interactions.	For example, Digoxin in conjunction with diuretic therapy can cause hypomagnesemia; hypokalemia may result from chronic use of laxatives, mineralocorticosteroids, diuretics, or amphotericin B.
Independent: Enteral	
Assess gastrostomy or jejunostomy tube sites for evidence of malposition.	Indwelling and mushroom catheters are still frequently used for feeding tubes inserted via the abdomen. Migration of the catheter balloon can result in duodenal

INTERVENTIONS	RATIONALE
Independent	
	or jejunal obstruction. Improperly sutured gastrostomy tubes may easily fall out.
Confirm placement of nasoenteral feeding tubes: Determine feeding tube position in stomach by auscultation of injected air prior to intermittent feedings, observe for ability to speak/cough.	Malplacement of nasoenteral feeding tubes may result in aspiration of enteral formula. Patients at particular risk include those who are intubated or obtunded, post-CVA, or following surgery of the head/neck or upper GI system.
Maintain aspiration precautions during enteral feedings: Keep head of bed elevated at 30 to 45 degrees during feeding and at least 1 hour after feeding.	Aspiration of enteral formulas is irritating to the lung parenchyma and may result in infectious pneumonia and respiratory compromise.
Add blue food coloring to enteral formula as indicated.	Helps identify aspiration of enteral formula and/or tracheal esophageal fistula if discovered in sputum/lung secretions. (Note: Avoid use of methylene blue dye, which may cause false-positive guaiac test when assessing for GI bleeding.
Monitor gastric residuals (as previously noted in Nursing Diagnosis: Nutrition, alteration in, less than body requirements, page 370).	Presence of large gastric residuals may potentiate an incompetent esophageal sphincter, leading to vomiting and aspiration.
Note indicators of nasogastric tube intolerance; for example, absence of gag reflex, high risk of aspiration, frequent removal of nasogastric feeding tubes.	May require consideration of surgically placed feeding tubes for maxiofacial trauma, radical neck surgery, patient safety, and consistency of enteral formula delivery.
Collaborative	
Review chest x-ray/kidneys, ureters, bladder (KUB) as indicated.	Central parenteral line placement is routinely confirmed by x-ray. Occasionally gastric positioning of enteral feeding tube also may be assessed by chest x-ray and KUB.
Collaborate with pharmacist in regard to site/time of delivery of drugs whose action might be adversely affected by enteral formula.	For example, vitamin D absorption is decreased by ingestion of mineral oil, which inhibits micelle formation of bile salts, and by neomycin, which inactivates bile salts. Aluminum-containing antacids bind with phosphorus and can cause hypophosphatemia.

NURSING DIAGNOSIS:	**Activity Intolerance.**
SUPPORTING DATA/CONTRIBUTING FACTORS:	**The use of endogenous protein for energy needs results in the loss of skeletal muscle mass. Atrophy of intercostal and extremity muscles presents as exertional dyspnea, early fatigue, and weakness.**
GENERAL PATIENT OUTCOMES:	**Demonstrates measurable increase in physical activity.**

INTERVENTIONS	RATIONALE
Independent	
Provide passive/active range of motion exercises to bedridden patients.	The deposition of lean body mass is dependent on the provision of both isotonic and isometric exercises.
Assist with ambulation at frequent short intervals.	Fatigue is a common sign of malnutrition, and patient will need help with ambulation.
Monitor BP, heart rate/rhythm, respirations.	Physiologic indicators of activity tolerance.
Collaborative	
Obtain physical therapy consultation.	Individualized exercise programs will assist the patient in muscle strengthening.

NURSING DIAGNOSIS: **Knowledge Deficit [Learning Need].**

SUPPORTING DATA/CONTRIBUTING FACTORS: **Although malnutrition usually is not the primary reason for admission, it has great impact on the recovery process. Patients/significant other(s) require information in order to become active participants in resolution of this problem.**

GENERAL PATIENT OUTCOMES: **Verbalizes understanding of condition/disease process and nutritional needs. Demonstrate initial adaptation to treatment.**

INTERVENTIONS	RATIONALE
Independent	
Assess patient's/significant other's knowledge of situation/nutritional state.	Provides baseline for establishing teaching plan.
Provide information regarding:	
Signs/symptoms of malnutrition,	Knowledge of the interaction between malnutrition and critical illness is helpful in understanding need for special therapy.
Reasons for use of parenteral/enteral nutrition support,	May experience anxiety regarding inability to eat and may not comprehend the nutritional value of the prescribed TPN/tube feedings.
Insertion of nutritional support devices,	Patients are often fearful of feeding tubes, comparing their use with prior experiences with endotracheal or nasogastric tubes. Patient cooperation is key to the safe insertion and maintenance of nutritional support access devices.
Importance of transition to oral feedings.	Although patient may have little interest or desire to eat, transition to oral feedings is preferred in view of side effects/complications of nutritional support therapy.

Psychosocial Aspects of Critical Care

The emotional response of the patient in a critical care unit is of extreme importance. Although the stress of this experience is well recognized, the effect on the individual is unpredictable. The mind-body connection is well established; for example, when a physiologic response occurs, a corresponding psychologic response occurs. Also, there are physiologic conditions that have a psychologic component; for example, the emotional instability of Cushing's syndrome/steroid therapy and the irritability of hypoglycemia need to be recognized. It is not necessarily the event but rather the patient's perception of the event that creates problems. Unmet psychologic needs drain energy resources needed for healing.

PATIENT ASSESSMENT DATA BASE

HISTORY

Refer to Assessment Tool, page 13.

PHYSICAL EXAMINATION

Mental status examination measures various aspects of behavior, such as appearance, affect, thought process.

Note physiologic factors that may contribute to psychologic symptoms (anxiety, delirium); for example, endocrine imbalances, medication, therapy.

NURSING PRIORITIES

1. Develop therapeutic nurse/patient relationship.
2. Provide information to patient/significant other(s) to assist in learning about illness/treatment.
3. Support patient/significant other(s) to deal with current situation/begin to plan for the future.

NURSING DIAGNOSIS: **Anxiety.**

SUPPORTING DATA/CONTRIBUTING FACTORS: **The threat of death or permanent changes in health, socioeconomic status, role functioning, and environmental and interaction patterns create a situation in which anxiety is normal for the patient in the intensive care unit. Although personal resources and external (situational) constraints will affect the anxiety level, the patient's perception of the threat to self can be a major determinant of the degree of anxiety experienced. Behavioral manifestations are subject to interpretation by those who observe them; for example, a patient who appears stoic may in fact be very anxious. Although a moderate state of tension can be useful for dealing with stress, severe anxiety can interfere by**

	using energy the patient needs for healing.
GENERAL PATIENT OUTCOMES:	**Verbalizes feelings. Signs of anxiety are decreased/minimized as evidenced by relaxed manner, able to sleep/rest between care/procedures.**

INTERVENTIONS	RATIONALE
Independent	
Assess level of anxiety; observe behavior such as clenched hands, wide eyes, startle response, furrowed brow, clutching/clinging to family/staff, or physical/verbal lashing out.	Individual responses can vary according to culturally learned patterns.
Note palpitations, elevated pulse/respiratory rate.	Changes in vital signs may suggest the degree of anxiety being experienced by the patient or reflect the impact of physiologic factors, such as endocrine imbalances.
Identify patient's/significant other(s) perception(s) of the situation.	Regardless of the reality of the situation, perception affects how they deal with the illness/stress.
Acknowledge reality of the situation as the patient sees it, without challenging the belief.	Patient may need to deny reality until ready to deal with it. It is not helpful to force the patient to face facts.
Evaluate coping/defense mechanisms being used to deal with the perceived/real threat.	May be dealing well with the situation at the moment; for example, denial and regression may be helpful coping mechanisms, but they use energy the patient needs for healing.
Review coping mechanisms used in the past if possible; for example, problem-solving skills, recognizing need/asking for help.	Identify/build on resources the patient/significant other(s) may have available.
Maintain frequent contacts with the patient/significant other(s).	Provides assurance that staff is available for help.
Provide accurate information as appropriate and requested by the patient/significant other(s). Repeat information as necessary.	As opportunities arise and facts are given, individuals will accept what they are ready for.
Be available for listening and talking. Answer questions freely and honestly and in language that is understandable to the patient/significant other(s).	Helps patient/significant other(s) look at realities of the illness and treament, without confronting issues they are not ready to deal with. Complex and/or anxiety-provoking information can be given in manageable amounts over an extended period of time.
Avoid empty reassurances, such as statements of "everything will be all right." Instead, provide specific information; for example, "Your heart rate is regular, your chest pain is being easily controlled, and that is what we want."	These may be interpreted as lack of understanding/honesty and further isolate the patient. Sharing observations used in assessing condition/prognosis provides opportunity for patient/significant other(s) to feel reassured.
Note expressions of concern/anger about treatment/equipment. (Refer to Nursing Diagnosis: Coping, ineffective, individual, page 382.)	Anxiety about self and outcome may be masked by comments/angry outbursts directed at therapy/caregivers.

INTERVENTIONS	RATIONALE
Independent	
Ask the patient/significant other(s) to identify what they can/cannot do about what is happening.	Assists in identifying areas in which control is available, as well as those in which control is not possible.
Provide as much order and predictability as possible in scheduling care/activities, visitors.	Helps patient anticipate and prepare for difficult treatments/movements, as well as look forward to pleasant occurrences.
Provide opportunities for patient to make decisions about care/schedule as much as possible.	Reinforces sense of control over environment, which can help diminish anxiety.
Instruct in ways to use positive self-talk; for example, "I know I am capable of handling this," "I can manage this pain for now."	Internal dialog is often negative. When this is shared out loud, the patient becomes aware and can be directed in the use of positive self-talk, which can help reduce anxiety.
Encourage/instruct in mental imagery/relaxation methods; for example, imagining a pleasant place, use of music/tapes, slow breathing, and meditation.	Will assist in reducing anxiety and maximize coping skills, allowing body to go about its work of healing.
Use touch, Therapeutic Touch, and other adjunctive therapies as indicated.	The use of these skills can assist the patient to feel less anxious. Therapeutic Touch is a method of using the hands to direct human energies to help or to heal.
Acknowledge feelings as they are expressed. If actions are unacceptable, take necessary steps to control/deal with behavior.	Often acknowledging feelings will enable patient to deal more appropriately with situation. May need chemical/physical control for brief periods of time.
Collaborative	
Administer medications as needed; for example, diazepam (Valium), chlordiazepoxide hydrochloride (Librium).	Antianxiety agents may be useful for brief periods of time to assist the patient/significant other(s) to reduce anxiety to manageable levels, allowing for initiation of coping skills.

NURSING DIAGNOSIS:	**Fear.**
SUPPORTING DATA/CONTRIBUTING FACTORS:	**The critical care unit is often viewed as a threatening situation; for example, the patient may see it as a place where people die. The perceived/actual threat of death is often justified. In addition, the patient also may have sensory impairment(s)/drug treatment(s) which intefere with preceptions of environmental stimuli.**
GENERAL PATIENT OUTCOMES:	**Fear is acknowledged/minimized/dealt with.**

INTERVENTIONS	RATIONALE
Independent	
Identify degree and reality of threat to the patient. Discuss situation with patient/significant other(s).	Distorted perceptions of the situation may magnify fear.
Monitor verbal/non-verbal responses and vital signs. Note narrowed focus of attention; for example, patient concentrates on one thing at a time. Validate observations by asking patient "Are you afraid?"	Facial/body expressions, increased pulse/respirations may be indicators of degree of fear. Narrowed focus usually reflects extreme fear/panic.
Encourage patient to identify and to describe fears.	Allows for explanations that may diminish fear.
Acknowledge reality of situation and feelings of fear.	Provides acceptance of the patient's feelings and allows the patient to begin to deal with fear.
Speak in concrete terms that are appropriate to patient/significant other's understanding. Clarify misunderstandings. Repeat explanations as needed.	Avoids misperceptions/interpretations.
Stay with or arrange to have someone stay with the patient. Check on the patient frequently and identify ways in which the patient can get help when needed. (Refer to Nursing Diagnosis: Anxiety, page 379.)	Provides reassurance that someone is available when/if something is needed.

NURSING DIAGNOSIS:	**Coping, ineffective, individual (potential).**
SUPPORTING DATA/CONTRIBUTING FACTORS:	**Being in a critical care setting represents a crisis situation which challenges the patient's previous coping mechanisms/adaptive behaviors. The sick role, pain, or concerns about the diagnosis/outcome can lead to inappropriate use of defense mechanisms (e.g., acting out, depression).**
GENERAL PATIENT OUTCOMES:	**Identifies and uses appropriate coping skills.**

INTERVENTIONS	RATIONALE
Independent	
Note age and developmental stage.	Will influence behavior; for example, some regression is normal during illness/crisis. Age-appropriate behavior is expected; for example, the adolescent may be reluctant to ask for help because independence is a recent critical developmental issue.
Assess ability to understand, noting level of anxiety/functioning and perception of the situation.	Beginning at the patient's level of understanding and function will assist in planning care.

INTERVENTIONS	RATIONALE
Independent	
Observe/record behavior in concrete terms, without being judgmental.	Assists in evaluating current psychologic state and provides clear picture on which to base interventions.
Identify/evaluate coping behaviors being used by the individual.	People usually manage threats by changing the actual stressor, their perception of it or of themselves. Dependent/regressive and angry behaviors may reflect patient's attempts to manage underlying fear. Denial may allow the patient to concentrate on getting well. Regression may help the individual adapt to the dependent situation.
Note limitations without emphasis; for example, "I know you are unable to move/talk."	Acknowledges reality without focusing on problem.
Identify strengths. Provide verbal/nonverbal encouragement.	Helps patient feel more competent to deal effectively with perceived/actual limitations. Caregiver can convey concern/encouragement by facial expressions and/or spending an extra moment talking with the patient.
Give information in clear, concise, specific terms, appropriate to patient's understanding.	Helps patient know what to expect.
Offer explanations of sights/sounds/procedures.	Simple explanations/opportunity to discuss can clarify happenings/perceptions.
Provide for privacy, maintain dignity of patient.	Supports individual's sense of importance.
Schedule activities to allow uninterrupted periods.	Provides patient opportunity to rest and may provide sense of control over some parts of uncontrollable situation.
Ask patient's opinion/choice about music/lighting and other external factors.	Can reduce sensory deprivation/overstimulation as well as enhance patient's sense of control.
Reinforce outside interests as much as possible (e.g., home, family, hobbies).	Redirects patient's attention from problems at hand and provides sense of having a future.

NURSING DIAGNOSIS: **Self-Concept, disturbance in (specify): body image; self-esteem; role performance; personal identity.**

SUPPORTING DATA/CONTRIBUTING FACTORS: **The disruption of an individual's normal lifestyle that occurs with admission to the critical care unit is accompanied by an impact on the components of self-concept. For example, the nature of the illness/trauma and treatments usually requires manipulation of the patient's body, resulting in perceptions of intrusion into personal space and fragmentation**

	into body parts (e.g., "weak heart, failing kidneys"). In addition, actual change in body structure/function (e.g., loss of a part) can negatively affect the individual. The perception of self as a competent person who has a role within a family constellation may be disrupted. For example, the patient experiences concern/fear about the illness itself and its effect on the ability to function in usual lifestyle, to sustain relationship(s), and to work.
GENERAL PATIENT OUTCOMES:	**Indicates (verbally/nonverbally) a sense of self-esteem in current situation/acceptance of body/role changes.**

INTERVENTIONS	RATIONALE
Independent	
Review pathophysiology affecting the patient.	Will determine necessity for intervention and plan of care.
Determine how the patient would like to be addressed, and call by name.	Promotes a sense of dignity and contributes to sense of self.
Listen to what patient says.	Self-valuing/devaluing remarks disclose beliefs about oneself both before and in current situation.
Determine meaning of the loss/change to the patient.	Individuals differ in reaction to a crisis situation. Some may be upset by a small change but take a major trauma with equanimity.
Assess role/status of the patient in the family structure. Ascertain patient's perception of how the current situation is/will affect ability to maintain role.	Illness may necessitate a change in the family system to accommodate tasks usually done by the patient.
Note behavior, especially extremes. Discuss needs openly with patient and develop plan of care together.	Withdrawn/manipulative behavior or anger may be expressions of hopelessness. Passive or aggressive behavior can be indicative of problems of dealing with the situation. (Refer to Nursing Diagnosis: Powerlessness, page 385.)
Assess communication within the family, noting who talks to whom, who makes decisions, and nonverbal interactions between family members (e.g., where members sit/stand in relation to one another). Note expectations patient has of the family and vice versa.	Negative communication patterns can indicate problems such as poor self-esteem, powerlessness, and ineffective coping skills. (Refer to Nursing Diagnosis: Coping, family, potential for growth, page 390; Coping, ineffective, family, compromised, page 391; Coping, ineffective, family, disabled, page 392.)
Provide clear, concise information.	Helps patient/family know what is happening, thereby contributing to feelings of self-esteem.
Encourage individual(s) to make decisions as much as situation allows.	Participation enhances self-esteem.

INTERVENTIONS	RATIONALE
Independent	
Evaluate threat of illness to sexual identity. Note statements that indicate the patient has some concern about how the illness/injury will affect ability to perform in this area; for example, statements of "I don't know if I will be able to do my job," "What if I can't do—?" etc.	Although some illnesses (e.g., myocardial infarction, spinal cord injury) pose a major threat to self-concept/self-esteem and body image, all serious illnesses/injuries affect the patient's sense of self in some way. Sexual identity encompases all feelings, attitudes, and beliefs—not just genital sex, gender, and procreation but also how we see ourselves as male/female, functioning, productive human beings.

NURSING DIAGNOSIS: **Powerlessness.**

SUPPORTING DATA/CONTRIBUTING FACTORS: **A sense of powerlessness on the part of the patient and significant other(s) is produced by the suddenness of the occurrence which brings the patient to a critical care unit; the nature and severity of the illness, insecurity about the outcome; the necessity for multiple procedures and treatments, and the perceived lack of control over what is happening.**

GENERAL PATIENT OUTCOMES: **Patient is involved in some aspects of care and expresses some sense of control over situation and future.**

INTERVENTIONS	RATIONALE
Independent	
Identify locus of control by noting expressions of lack of control/helplessness or, conversely, recognition of one's own responsibility for what can happen.	Provides information about whether control is external or internal. This knowledge of how the patient views control over own destiny will be helpful in developing plan of care that enables patient/significant other(s) to deal with sense of powerlessness.
Note behaviors such as anger, frustration, depression, withdrawal, "giving up."	May be clues to belief that individual does not have power to influence outcome.
Listen for statements of helplessness/hopelessness; expressions of fear.	Indicators useful in assessing degree of powerlessness.
Avoid use of confrontation or logic.	Patient will not accept statements/logic as having potential for making a difference when feeling hopeless/helpless.
Be aware of/deal with manipulative/disruptive behavior by discussing plan of care openly with patient/significant other(s).	Angry/demanding behavior or attempts to influence staff (e.g., play staff against one another) may reflect attempts to gain control when the individual feels powerless.

INTERVENTIONS	RATIONALE
Independent	
Be available to the patient/significant other(s) and show concern for them as an individual.	Creates supportive climate, sends message that caregivers are willing to help.
Use Active-Listening by providing a caring presence and empathic feedback.	Listening to the feelings as well as to the words of the patient's communications can be helpful in moving toward a more hopeful outlook.
Acknowledge reality of feelings.	Provides opportunity for patient to feel understood.
Assist patient/significant other(s) to redefine goals into manageable steps.	Useful in identifying individual's ability to influence situation and to attain goals.
Have patient/significant other(s) identify/list things they can do in the current situation, enlist patient cooperation in concrete ways.	When individual(s) participate in planning for care, they are more apt to feel a sense of control and to follow through with actions.
Involve significant other(s) (someone the patient trusts) in care when possible.	Extends message of caring to the patient and enhances sense of control/reduces feelings of helplessness.
Provide explanations as desired by the individual(s) and keep informed of progress.	Information can help patient/significant other(s) feel more hopeful about situation and more willing to participate in care.

NURSING DIAGNOSIS: **Spiritual Distress (Distress of the Human Spirit).**

SUPPORTING DATA/CONTRIBUTING FACTORS: **Critical illness represents a significant loss for the patient/significant other(s) whether or not it has the potential for a terminal outcome because it is a significant disruption in the patient/family's regular routine. Feelings of guilt, anger, depression may result in serious questioning of previously held beliefs/values.**

GENERAL PATIENT OUTCOMES: **Verbalizes feelings and discusses losses that have occurred or that may occur.**

INTERVENTIONS	RATIONALE
Independent	
Assess perceptions of what is happening, being alert to both verbal/nonverbal cues.	To deal with concerns, it is important to know how the patient/family perceive what is happening, and to remember that they may be afraid to ask openly about concerns.

INTERVENTIONS	RATIONALE
Independent	
Recognize stage of grief patient/significant other(s) may be experiencing.	Knowing stage of grieving is helpful in choosing interventions. For example, behavior such as blaming, anger, withdrawal, and depression may reflect how the individual is currently dealing with events.
Acknowledge reality of feelings. Accept appropriate expressions of feelings/beliefs without judgment. Listen without needing to have answers.	Acceptance of feelings may promote movement toward resolutions. Acceptance of appropriate expression of negative feelings (e.g., anger) conveys the message that caregiver understands it to be an expression of feelings of frustration and helplessness about the situation. Note: Although swearing may be an acceptable expression of feelings, physical violence is not.
Use silence as appropriate.	Silence can convey acceptance and can provide sense of comfort.
Provide open atmosphere in which any question can be asked. Avoid interjecting own attitudes/values.	Fosters communication and gives message that patient/family concerns are important. Negative/judgmental attitudes of caregivers may interfere with care-recovery or may isolate patient/family.
Ask individual(s) what they would like or what they think would be helpful.	Assists them to think through their needs and promotes self-responsibility.
Assist with prayer, readings, and/or meditations.	When patient requests, these can meet a need for spiritual consolation.
Make sure patient knows someone is available at all times.	Provides sense of security.
Use comfort measures/touch as indicated.	Fulfills basic physiologic/psychologic need by providing sense of connection with others.
Collaborative	
Obtain clergy, lawyer, and so forth as patient requires.	Taking care of concrete concerns can help allay distress.

NURSING DIAGNOSIS: **Grieving, anticipatory/dysfunctional.**

SUPPORTING DATA/CONTRIBUTING FACTORS: **The experience of a critical illness forces the patient and/or significant other(s) to face the loss of their normal way of life and to deal with the uncertainty of the outcome with its potential losses. How the experiences will affect their lives/relationships is an unknown factor that engenders fear and anxiety and is influenced by past methods of dealing with loss.**

GENERAL PATIENT OUTCOMES:	Demonstrates (verbally or otherwise) appropriate emotions and begins to identify sense of/ways to deal with loss.

INTERVENTIONS	RATIONALE
Independent	
Identify how patient/significant other(s) are dealing with current happenings.	Nurse needs to know how each individual views what is going on so that interventions are appropriate.
Note verbal/nonverbal communication, and check meaning with the individual.	It can be helpful to clarify observations with the individual. Patient/significant other(s) may express one thing verbally and the opposite nonverbally.
Provide opportunity for patient to discuss meaning the illness/loss has for them.	Information helps the patient clarify the impact of the illness and begin coping with the situation.
Note response of significant other(s) to situation/patient's concerns.	Some responses, such as panic, are nonhelpful and may indicate need for intervention.
Acknowledge appropriate feelings/expressions of grief.	Will help patient/significant other(s) understand normalcy of these feelings and experience release of expressing feelings.
Assist individual(s) to identify strengths/control they have over what is happening.	Promotes development of skills to deal with current situation and to prepare for the future.
Collaborative	
Provide referrals to in-house and appropriate community resources (e.g., clergy, psychiatric counseling, social services).	May be needed to help patient/significant other(s) deal with stress of current situation/uncertainty of outcome.

NURSING DIAGNOSIS:	Thought Processes, alteration in.
SUPPORTING DATA/CONTRIBUTING FACTORS:	Many factors existing in the critical care unit affect the patient's ability to think. Physiologic causes include such factors as chemical imbalance, sleep deprivation, sensory deficits, presence of addictive substances, as well as the disease process itself. In addition, psychologic factors (e.g., anxiety, fear, and sense of powerlessness) can combine with physiologic factors to interfere with thought processes.
GENERAL PATIENT OUTCOMES:	Alterations in thought processes minimized/prevented. Alert/oriented within patient's norm.

INTERVENTIONS	RATIONALE
Independent	
Assess mental status continuously by noting level of consciousness, speech patterns, content of thought, and so forth.	Provides baseline information for planning care.
Determine preillness mental state.	Baseline data aid the caregivers in recognizing changes in behavior/abnormal responses. It also can be of benefit in predicting individual needs.
Provide quiet environment. Approach with a quiet, calm manner.	Patient may be acutely reactive to stimuli because of central nervous system (CNS) stimulation (e.g., withdrawal from addictive substance, or meningitis). Measures to reduce excessive stimulation can improve patient's ability to think more clearly.
Provide ongoing information about treatment and activities that are occurring. Reorient as necessary.	Helps patient evaluate/clarify perceptions and enhances reality orientation.
Use clear, calm communications, avoiding arguments and power struggles.	Provides accurate information without threat. Patient in drug withdrawal may feel threatened, and behavior (withdrawal/aggression) may escalate with confrontation.
Determine if patient is experiencing withdrawal from an addictive substance.	Perceptions may be altered if under the influence of addictive substance(s).
Identify addictive substance, extent of habit, last time taken, and what happens when patient does not take it.	Information necessary to developing treatment plan, providing safe environment, and fostering recovery.
Collaborative	
Monitor laboratory values as indicated; for example, electrolytes, arterial blood gases (ABGs), renal/liver function studies.	Alteration in cerebral circulation, electrolyte balance, hypoxemia, acid-base balance, and metabolic changes are physiologic changes which may affect ability to concentrate/interpret sensory input.
Assist with medical regimen as indicated.	Treatment of the physical factors affecting thought processes may facilitate return to normal, help prevent permanent changes in mentation.

(Refer to Care Plans: Chemical Dependency, Alcohol Toxicity/Withdrawal, page 343; Chemical Abuse: Drug Overdose/Poisoning, page 353.)

NURSING DIAGNOSIS: **Noncompliance (Compliance, alteration in).**

SUPPORTING DATA/CONTRIBUTING FACTORS: **The patient's behavior may reflect an unwillingness to accept care for a variety of personal reasons. For example, the patient may have health beliefs and/or spiritual/cultural values that are in conflict with needs identified by caregivers.**

GENERAL PATIENT OUTCOMES:	**Verbalizes understanding of needs. Makes choice about participation/nonparticipation in treatment plan.**

INTERVENTIONS	RATIONALE
Independent	
Determine reason for behavior/problems which are interfering with treatment.	Many factors may be involved in behavior that is disruptive to the treatment regimen (e.g., fear, pain, anxiety, hypoxemia, chemical imbalance).
Discuss patient's/significant other's view of illness/treatment. Determine cultural/spiritual/health beliefs, as possible.	Provides insight into thoughts/factors related to individual situation.
Review treatment plan with patient/significant other(s). Repeat as necessary.	Provides opportunities to exchange accurate information and to clarify viewpoints/misconceptions.
Be aware of own (caregiver's) response to patient's treatment choices (e.g., refusal of blood or chemotherapy, Living Will).	Negative feelings regarding these choices may be expressed in judgmental behaviors that block or interfere with patient's wishes, comfort, and/or care.
Have same personnel care for patient as much as possible.	Enables relationship to develop in which the patient can begin to trust/participate in care.
Contract with the patient for participation in care.	Patient who agrees to own responsibility is more apt to cooperate.

NURSING DIAGNOSIS:	**Coping, family, potential for growth.**
SUPPORTING DATA/CONTRIBUTING FACTORS:	**The crisis of having a member critically ill presents the family with an opportunity to assess their own values, priorities, goals, and relationships. They may experience a variety of feelings (e.g., self-doubt, guilt, anxiety, and fear), which, when dealt with successfully, can lead to growth.**
GENERAL PATIENT OUTCOMES:	**Expresses desire for help and/or feelings of self-confidence in ability to handle situation. Uses resources/support systems effectively.**

INTERVENTIONS	RATIONALE
Independent	
Orient family to the unit, answering questions, encouraging them to talk. Explain procedures and ask if they want to stay/be involved in care, as possible. Provide quiet place where family can be alone to talk. Let fam-	Familiarity can diminish anxiety, help family deal with situation more effectively. Being able to stay close to the patient and knowing they will be called provides reassurance.

INTERVENTIONS	RATIONALE
Independent	
ily know they will be called if changes occur, and follow through.	
Review individual situation. Listen to family's expressions of concern.	Information about past experiences/ways of dealing with crisis situations will provide clues/affect how current situation is handled. Family needs to know that personnel care about the patient. They also need emotional support and opportunities to vent feelings.
Provide positive information about outcome/prognosis when possible, giving specific facts on a regular basis.	The family needs to feel hopeful.
Help family members be supportive, suggest things they can say or do. Give permission to laugh, joke, touch/hug patient, and to visit as frequently as possible.	Family members may not know what to say to the patient; may say or fear saying things that are detrimental, may be overly protective, or may lack knowledge of how to be supportive.
Note complaints about care; denial; blaming; repetitious questions.	Complaints may suggest that family is seeking reassurance, projecting feelings of anxiety/helplessness, or they may indicate blocking/denial of situation, which may reflect deterioration of coping abilities. (Refer to Nursing Diagnoses: Coping, ineffective family, compromised, below; and Coping, ineffective family, disabled, page 392.)

NURSING DIAGNOSIS:	**Coping, ineffective family, compromised.**
SUPPORTING DATA/CONTRIBUTING FACTORS:	**Family may be so anxious and upset that they are not providing needed support for the patient. The significant other(s) may have to assume the patient's role in the family constellation, which adds additional stress. Family concerns (e.g., finances, child/elderly parent care) also can compromise family coping skills.**
GENERAL PATIENT OUTCOMES:	**Identifies resources within themselves and outside supports that will be helpful in managing current situation.**

INTERVENTIONS	RATIONALE
Independent	
Assess factors that may be contributing to difficulty in dealing with current situation.	Members may express feelings (e.g., guilt and/or anxiety) about actions/situations that happened before the illness/accident occurred. Maturational issues

INTERVENTIONS	RATIONALE
Independent	
	(individual/family) may affect ability to deal with current situation. Resources (financial, emotional, support) can be drained, with additional stresses resulting from a long-standing illness when the person who has been the caregiver is ill and the care of the patient falls on the rest of the family.
Discuss possible underlying reasons for different behaviors that patient is exhibiting. (Refer to Nursing Diagnoses: Coping, ineffective, family, potential for growth, page 390; Coping, ineffective family, disabled, below.)	Helps family/significant other(s) understand and accept/deal with behaviors that may be unusual for the patient.
Collaborative	
Refer to support services as indicated (e.g., psychiatric nurse/psychiatrist, social services, spiritual advisor, community support groups).	May need additional help to resolve problems and to improve coping skills.

NURSING DIAGNOSIS:	**Coping, ineffective family, disabled.**
SUPPORTING DATA/CONTRIBUTING FACTORS:	**Family may have long-standing maladaptive coping skills which are exacerbated by the current situation. Neglecting the patient and/or distorting the situation by denying/exaggerating its seriousness can interfere with the recovery/course of the illness.**
GENERAL PATIENT OUTCOMES:	**Patient/family begin to express more awareness/realistic understanding of the situation.**

INTERVENTIONS	RATIONALE
Independent	
Establish rapport and acknowledge difficulty of the situation for the family.	Promotes situation in which family accepts reality of what is happening and is willing to share problems with staff.
Assess preillness/current behaviors that are interfering with the care/recovery of the patient.	Information about family problems (e.g., divorce/separation, alcoholism, drug abuse, abusive situations) will be helpful in developing an appropriate plan of care.
Collaborative	
Refer for additional help as indicated (e.g., family counseling/therapy, psychotherapy, social services).	Disruption may be so severe that further resources are necessary to deal with/respond to situation.

Pediatric Considerations

PATIENT ASSESSMENT DATA BASE

HISTORY

Note immunization/exposure to measles, rubella, chickenpox, mumps, whooping cough.

Determine child-care situation/exposure to other diseases (e.g., H. influenza, hepatitis, and so forth).

Determine past experience in hospitals; note date and child's reaction.

Nutrition

Note history of recent weight loss and whether it is greater than 5 percent of ideal weight.

Activity

Independent activities: note activities child is able to do independently, such as eating, toileting, washing, dressing. Note how this illness/injury will interfere with child's ability to do normal activities.

Elimination

Bowel habits: note usual frequency, normal character of bowel movements, and any recent changes.

Bladder: note frequency and character of urination and any changes.

Development

Developmental level: note developmental milestones in infant. Observe behavior/learning/verbal skills in relation to age.

Grade/performance in school: note reaction to school; note if continuation of school activities during hospitalization are planned/appropriate.

Family

Family composition: note family members and ages.

Caretaker: note who is primarily responsible for caring for the child.

Problems this family will have owing to this hospitalization: note financial, emotional, transportation, child-care problems, especially if condition is chronic or crippling.

Visitors: note any special visiting privileges or restrictions.

PHYSICAL EXAMINATION

Dependent on specific disease/injury and secondary complications.

Chart of Normal Values

	Vital signs					
	Newborn	Infant	Toddler	Preschooler	School Age	Adolescent
Pulse	70-170	80-160	90-140	80-120	70-110	60-100
Respirations	30-50	26-40	22-34	20-30	18-24	12-20
BP Systolic*	60-90	74-100	80-112	82-110	84-120	94-140
BP Diastolic*	20-60	50-70	50-80	50-78	54-80	62-88

(*Adapted from Hazinski, MF: *Nursing Care of the Critically Ill Child.* CV Mosby, St Louis, 1984.)

Temperature:
  Oral: 97.6°-99.3° F (36.4°-37.4° C)
  R: 97°-100° F (36.2°-37.8° C)
  Ax: 96.6°-98° F (35.9°-36.7° C)

Note: Normal vital signs in the critically ill child suggest loss of compensatory mechanisms. Development of bradycardia/hypotension and lethargy indicate serious deterioration in condition. In addition, small quantitative changes in vital signs may be qualitatively very significant.

DIAGNOSTIC STUDIES

Baseline and specific studies dependent on individual situation/needs.

Laboratory Values Table

Although pediatric laboratory values are often equal to adult values, certain studies may vary according to age, and, therefore, individual laboratories should be consulted to verify abnormal results.

The following are some of the more common laboratory studies with age variations:

ABGs:	pH	PO_2	PCO_2
Infant	7.30	60 to 70 mmHg	26 to 40 mmHg

Acid phosphatase: 2 to 13 yrs: 6.4 to 15.2 IV/ml

Alkaline phosphatase: less than 1 yr: 50 to 260 IU/ml
  2 to 6 yrs: 70 to 160 IU/ml
  7 to 10 yrs: 56 to 258 IU/ml

Ammonia: infant/child: 29 to 80 mcg/dl

BUN: 6 to 23 mg/dl

Creatinine: 6 mos to 2 yrs: 0.2 to 0.7 mg/dl
  2 yrs-12 yrs: 0.3 to 0.8 mg/dl

CBC:	Hgb	Hct	MCV	WBC
6 mos to 1 yr:	11.8	35	77	6,000 to 17,5000
2 to 10 yrs:	12.8	37	80	6,800 to 15,000
11 to 15 yrs:	13.4	39	82	4,800 to 11,000

LDH: 1 mo to 2 yrs: 110 to 244 U/liter
  3 yr-17 yr: 85 to 165 U/liter

Magnesium: child 1.4-1.9 mcq/liter

Osmolality: child 275-296 mOsm/kg serum water

Phosphorus: 1 yr: 4.0-6.8 mg/dl
  5 yr: 3.6-6.5 mg/dl

Sedimentation rate (ESR): infant/child: 3-13 mm/hr

SGOT: 6 mos-1 yr: 16-35 U/liter
  1 yr-5 yrs: 6-30 U/liter

SGPT: infant: < 54 U/liter
  Child: 1-25 U/liter

Cerebrospinal fluid
  Glucose: infant/child: 60 to 80 mg/dl
  Protein, total:
    Child: 10 to 20 mg/dl
    Adolescent: 15 to 30 mg/dl

NURSING PRIORITIES

1. Maintain oxygenation and ventilation.
2. Maintain hemodynamic stability.
3. Promote adequate nutrition.
4. Reduce pain and anxiety.
5. Promote parental coping.

NURSING DIAGNOSIS:	**Airway Clearance/Breathing Patterns, ineffective.**
SUPPORTING DATA/CONTRIBUTING FACTORS:	**Anatomic/physiologic differences in children makes respiratory difficulties more of a problem. Young children have smaller airways, higher airway resistance, and a higher oxygen demand. They cannot increase their tidal volume and instead must increase their respiratory rate. One of the most common causes of cardiac arrest in children is respiratory arrest due to acute airway obstruction and/or respiratory failure. Conditions that most commonly cause respiratory failure differ with age. In the newborn infant the cause may be prematurity with hyaline membrane disease/meconium aspiration. In the child less than two years of age, croup, bronchopneumonia, and inhalation of foreign objects are common causes of obstruction/respiratory failure. After the age of two, respiratory failure may more commonly be caused by epiglottitis (age 2 to 4 years), status asthmaticus, poisoning, near drowning, trauma, and encephalitis. Congenital craniofacial, neck, chest, and airway abnormalities; surgery, trauma, chronic obstructive lung diseases (e.g., cystic fibrosis), and severe allergic reactions can affect the respiratory status of children in all age groups.**
GENERAL PATIENT OUTCOMES:	**Respiratory rate normal for age. Absence of stridor/retractions, cyanosis, adventitious breath sounds.**

INTERVENTIONS	RATIONALE
Independent	
Assess respiratory rate, rhythm, and depth of breathing while child is at rest, when possible. Count respirations for 1 full minute. In verbal child, check how many words can be spoken without needing to breathe.	Children can easily double their respiratory rate without an appreciable difference in the work of breathing. Children also have normal variations in respiratory rhythm which may produce inaccurate results if rates are counted for less than 1 minute. The critically ill child should demonstrate tachypnea. If the respiratory rate begins to slow to "normal" levels, respiratory arrest may be imminent. To identify respiratory difficulties, it is important to note how the child breathes at rest and how this changes when the child is disturbed. The child with severe respiratory difficulty at rest requires immediate intervention. For example, shallow irregular respirations with substernal retractions are a sign of ineffective breathing patterns.
Note tachypnea, nasal flaring, retractions, irritability, and difficulty sucking/swallowing.	Early signs of respiratory distress.
Observe for grunting respirations, jaw tugging, disorientation, lethargy, bradycardia, and slowing respirations.	Signs of significant respiratory distress which may quickly deteriorate into respiratory arrest.
Note sudden choking, ineffective cough, accompanied by labored respirations, stridor, wheezing, retractions, and cyanosis/pallor.	Indicative of respiratory failure secondary to foreign body inhalation, which requires immediate medical intervention to clear the airway.
Assess skin and mucous membrane color.	General indicator of oxygenation. Pallor is associated with hypoxemia and anemia, as well as poor systemic perfusion.
Auscultate all lung fields: front, back, and axillary. Note pitch/duration of breath sounds, presence/absence of stridor or wheezes, and inspiratory/expiratory times.	Breath sounds are easily transmitted through the thin chest wall of the young child. Therefore changes in intensity of breath sounds may be difficult to appreciate. A change in pitch is produced by common problems; for example, fluid accumulation. Decreased and/or adventitious breath sounds may indicate airway obstruction from secretions, edema, or inflammation. Stridor (occasionally heard without a stethoscope) with prolonged inspiratory time indicates an upper airway obstruction. Wheezing with prolonged expiratory time usually indicates a lower airway obstruction.
Position child with head of bed elevated.	Allows for maximum diaphragmatic excursion and chest expansion in infant/small child.
Place roll/pillow under shoulders as indicated.	Promotes extension of neck to prevent airway compression. Note: Hyperextending neck can exacerbate airway obstruction and so should be avoided.
Change patient position at least every 2 hours.	Frequent position changes will help mobilize secretions from different areas of the lungs.
Observe sputum, note changes in color/odor, and note development of fever.	Suggests presence of infectious process.
Suction airway as indicated for no longer than 5 sec-	The child who is not able to cough will need nasopha-

INTERVENTIONS	RATIONALE
Independent	
onds maximum. Maintain appropriate suction pressures; for example, oral/nasopharnygeal suctioning with pressures of 60 to 100 mmHg for infant/100 to 120 mmHg for child; tracheal suctioning with 50 to 95 mmHg for infant/90 to 115 mmHg for child. If sodium chloride tracheal irrigations used, limit to 1 ml for infant/1-5 ml for child.	ryngeal, oropharyngeal, or endotracheal suctioning to assist with removal of secretions. Prolonged suctioning quickly leads to hypoxia, and excessive pressures increase risk of mucosal trauma. Note: Small-caliber endotracheal tubes/tracheostomy tubes require close monitoring, with irrigation and suctioning to prevent plugging by mucus. Avoid suctioning child with croup or epilglottitis, because it may cause laryngospasm and respiratory arrest.
Collaborative	
Monitor laboratory data (e.g., ABGs). Correlate with transcutaneous or pulse oximetry readings.	Increased $PaCO_2$ and decreased PaO_2 may indicate need for artificial airway or support by mechanical ventilation. Transcutaneous blood gas monitoring and pulse oximetry are useful adjuncts to blood gas measurements and should reduce number of blood gas samples needed.
Administer chest physiotherapy and suction as necessary. If patient is able, assist with deep breathing and coughing.	Promotes chest expansion and facilitates removal of tenacious secretions.
Review chest x-ray examinations.	May reflect cause of altered breathing patterns (e.g., airway obstruction or accumulation of secretions).
Administer supplemental oxygen as indicated.	May reduce respiratory rate/effort. Must be used with caution in children with chronic lung problems; for example, cystic fibrosis, BPD. (Refer to Nursing Diagnosis: Gas Exchange, impaired, page 398.)
Assist with insertion of/maintain artificial airway, if indicated.	Airway support may be needed, depending on the site/degree of airway obstruction and may include nasopharygeal, oral, or endotracheal adjuncts. For example, in the infant, a nasopharyngeal endotracheal tube may be ideal because it is easier to stabilize and permits the infant to suck.
Administer medications as indicated:	
Isoetharine hydrochloride (Bronkosol), metaproterenol sulfate (Alupent),	Sympathomimetics which dilate the airways and relieve lower airway obstruction. May be used in asthma.
Racemic epinephrine.	Vasoconstrictor that will relieve soft tissue airway obstruction (e.g., laryngotracheobronchitis or postintubation edema).
Sedation/analgesics, if appropriate. Monitor for effects of respiratory depression.	May be necessary to relieve pain and to assist with deep breathing and coughing. However, these medications also may depress respiratory effort and therefore should be used with caution.
Provide room/tent humidification.	Supplemental moisture can aid mobilization of secretions, reduce irritation of upper airways, especially in upper respiratory infection and croup.

NURSING DIAGNOSIS:	**Gas Exchange, impaired.**
SUPPORTING DATA/CONTRIBUTING FACTORS:	**The elastic tissue in the septae of the alveoli help keep the smaller airways open. Because younger children have decreased muscle tone, there is greater tendency for airway collapse. Collateral pathways of ventilation are not well developed; therefore, airway obstruction is more likely to produce significant abnormalities in gas exchange. In addition, presence of pulmonary edema, near drowning, development of adult type respiratory distress syndrome (ARDS) impede oxygen diffusion. Lastly, anemia (e.g., sickle cell) or blood loss decreases oxygen-carrying capacity of the blood, affecting gas exchange.**
GENERAL PATIENT OUTCOMES:	**Arterial blood gases (ABGs)/respiratory rate and effort are within child's normal range.**

INTERVENTIONS	RATIONALE
Independent	
Assess respiratory rate/effort, especially use of accessory muscles. Note position of comfort for the child.	The child with a partial airway obstruction may be restless and tachypneic, use accessory muscles to breathe. The child in respiratory distress prefers to sit up, although the infant may assume knee/chest or prone position.
Note presence/location of cyanosis (e.g., central versus peripheral).	Cyanosis of mucous membranes, tongue, lips, or nailbeds (central) reflects anatomic or physiologic right-to-left shunts of unoxygenated blood. Peripheral cyanosis may reflect pooling of unsaturated blood related to poor systemic circulation/venous return or cold stress. Note: This may be a normal occurrence in infants.
Auscultate breath sounds.	May be diminished/absent with an airway obstruction/atelectasis/pneumothorax. (Refer to Care Plan: Hemothorax and Pneumothorax, page 88.)
Assess level of consciousness (e.g., anxiety, confusion, agitation, lethargy, stupor).	The child with an increased $PaCO_2$ or decreased PaO_2 will show changes in mentation and level of consciousness. As hypercapnia and/or hypoxemia progresses, the child will become first anxious, agitated, then confused, lethargic, and/or obtunded.

INTERVENTIONS	RATIONALE
Independent	
Monitor heart rate and blood pressure (BP).	Bradycardia and hypotension are late signs of respiratory distress in the child.
Collaborative	
Monitor laboratory data; for example,	
ABGs;	Used to estimate adequacy of alveolar ventilation and to assess degree of hypoxemia, hypercapnia, and acidosis.
A/a gradient (A/a DO_2);	Provides an estimation of intrapulmonary shunting most frequently seen in atelectasis/pneumonia/pulmonary edema.
Hematocrit (Hct)/hemoglobin (Hgb);	Decreased Hct and Hgb reflect decreased oxygen-carrying capacity.
Oxygen saturation (transcutaneous or intra-arterial);	Measures the degree of tissue oxygenation.
End-tidal carbon dioxide values ($PctCO_2$), if available.	Assists in monitoring the degree of hypercapnia in the intubated child.
Review chest x-ray examinations.	May reflect the cause of impaired gas exchange, such as infiltrates or airway obstruction.
Administer supplemental oxygen via cannula, mask, or mechanical ventilator with positive end-expiratory pressure (PEEP) and/or continuous positive airway pressure (CPAP). (Refer to Care Plan: Ventilatory Assistance (Mechanical), page 115.)	Oxygen is the appropriate treatment for hypoxemia. Oxygen is considered a medication, and the effects should be monitored closely. Associated ventilation may be indicated when child is unable to maintain spontaneous ventilation. The addition of PEEP or CPAP reduces airway/alveolar collapse, enhancing gas exchange.
Administer appropriate medications, such as steroids, antibiotics, bronchodilators;	A variety of medications may be used for treatment. However, these three groups of medications are often used together to produce therapeutic effects with smaller doses/fewer side effects.
Sodium bicarbonate 1 mEq/kg.	Use cautiously to correct metabolic acidosis when adequate ventilation is assured.
Assist with insertion of/maintain artificial airway.	May be necessary to maintain airway integrity for optimal oxygen delivery.

NURSING DIAGNOSIS: **Cardiac Output, alteration in, decreased.**

SUPPORTING DATA/CONTRIBUTING FACTORS: **Low cardiac output (CO) is one of the most common cardiovascular problems seen in critically ill pediatric patients and can result from a number of different causes. Hypovolemic shock is the most common cause for decreased**

	CO. Other causes include septicemia, myocardial dysfunction, dysrhythmias, hypothermia, hypoglycemia, hypocalcemia, and congestive heart failure.
GENERAL PATIENT OUTCOMES:	**Vital signs/urine output within normal range for age. Peripheral pulses palpable. Alert mental status.**

INTERVENTIONS	RATIONALE
Independent	
Monitor BP, pulse.	The critically ill child is usually tachycardic, owing to the hypermetabolic state. However, if heart rate exceeds optimal ranges to maximize CO, ventricular filling time and coronary artery perfusion may be so compromised that CO and ventricular function will be decreased. Note: Hypotension is a late sign of decompensation.
Monitor invasive hemodynamic parameters, for example, central venous pressure (CVP), PAP, pulmonary capillary wedge pressure (PCWP), cardiac output (CO), cardiac index (CI).	These parameters help evaluate the degree and cause of decreased CO, guide therapy, and evaluate the child's response to therapy. Cardiac index is the most accurate determinant of systemic blood flow because body surface area is considered. Note: Pressure values are dependent on age (weight and size) and therefore may differ from adult values.
Note decreased core temperature, delayed capillary refill, decreased urinary output, and diminished level of consciousness.	Core temperature is a more reliable indicator of developing shock state because skin temperature may be influenced by environmental factors. The child with vasoconstriction will have cold/mottled extremities and/or pallor. Nailbeds may show a slow capillary refill. Urinary output will decrease as perfusion to the kidneys is decreased. Level of consciousness also may be diminished as perfusion to the brain is decreased.
Weigh daily or more often as indicated and correlate with fluid balance. (Refer to Nursing Diagnosis: Fluid Volume Deficit, actual/potential, page 403.)	A decreased CO is usually a reflection of decreased intravascular volume and/or cardiac dysfunction. Hypovolemia from a variety of causes is common, owing to the fact that the child has a greater percentage of total body water than does an adult.
Monitor electrocardiogram (ECG) continuously as indicated, document dysrhythmias.	Sustained/profound tachycardia, bradycardia, or recurrent dysrhythmias can reduce CO and may lead to cardiac arrest.
Collaborative	
Monitor laboratory data; for example,	
ABGs;	Determines if metabolic acidosis exists (often present with decreased CO, peripheral perfusion).

INTERVENTIONS	RATIONALE
Collaborative	
Electrolytes;	Electrolyte imbalances (e.g., hyperkalemia/hypokalemia) can adversely affect/reduce cardiac conduction/function.
Complete blood count (CBC).	A decreased Hct may reflect hemorrhage loss/decreased circulating volume resulting in decreased arterial oxygen content.
Assist with insertion of/maintain lines for fluid replacement and monitoring.	Insertion of a monitoring line (e.g., Swan-Ganz, CVP, or arterial catheter) assists with determinations of CO and with evaluation of response to therapies (e.g., fluid replacement/drug administration).
Administer fluid therapy as appropriate.	Maintenance of circulating volume is necessary to maximize CO.
Administer medications as indicated; for example, inotropic agents, vasodilators, and/or antiarrhythmic agent (check individual protocol for appropriate dosage): dobutamine (Dobutrex) 2.5 to 10.0 mcg/kg/minute, sodium nitroprusside (Nipride) 0.5 to 8.0 mcg/kg/minute, atropine 0.01 mg/kg, for a minimum dose of 0.1 mg to a maximum of 2 mg, isoproterenol (Isuprel) 0.5 to 0.5 mcg/kg/minute,	If other therapy (e.g., correction of hypovolemia and metabolic acidosis) does not improve CO, drugs may be administered to improve cardiac contractility, to increase heart rate, and/or to reduce afterload. The use of an inotropic agent in combination with a vasodilator may produce a more significant increase in CO than either drug used separately.
Epinephrine 0.01 mg/kg for bolus; 0.05 to 1.0 mcg/kg/minute for drip, lidocaine 1 mg/kg intravenous (IV) for bolus, 20 to 50 mcg/kg/minute for drip.	Antiarrhythmic agents are appropriate for dysrhythmias that interfere with CO. Note: Bolus of epinephrine, atropine, and lidocaine may be given transtracheally if no IV access available.
Assist with insertion/maintenance of pacemaker, as indicated.	May be indicated for support of CO by maintaining adequate heart rate in presence of dysrhythmias such as complete heart block.

NURSING DIAGNOSIS:	**Tissue Perfusion, alteration in, cardiopulmonary, renal, gastrointestinal, peripheral.**
SUPPORTING DATA/CONTRIBUTING FACTORS:	**The same factors that decrease CO also can cause alteration in tissue perfusion. Other factors may include emboli, acidosis, and shock.**
GENERAL PATIENT OUTCOMES:	**Vital signs within normal range for age. Urine output 0.5 to 1.0 ml/kg hour. Peripheral pulses palpable. Alert/responding appropriately. Active bowel sounds present.**

INTERVENTIONS	RATIONALE
Independent	
Assess heart rate, blood pressure; CVP, PAP, PCWP (if available).	Bradycardia/tachycardia and hypotension can decrease blood flow. Left-sided heart failure also will adversely affect blood flow to all organs. An infant who already has cardiovascular compromise may experience heart failure or right-to-left cardiac shunting.
Monitor core temperature and compare with skin temperature.	Although skin temperature may be affected by environmental factors, an early sign of poor systemic perfusion is a rise in core body temperature and a fall in skin temperature.
Provide neutral thermic environment; for example, prevent drafts and unnecessary/prolonged body exposure. Warm IV solutions/blood as indicated.	Environmental factors may potentiate hypothermia. The critically ill infant may not be able to increase oxygen consumption, and therefore cold stress may produce lactic acidosis, hypoxemia, and hypoglycemia.
Assess respirations, noting rate and effort; for example, tachypnea, nasal flaring, retractions, and grunting.	The child with decreased CO and poor tissue perfusion may demonstrate respiratory signs and symptoms related to heart failure.
Record urine output every hour, noting changes in volume and specific gravity.	The kidneys are very sensitive to decreased tissue perfusion, as evidenced by declining/absent urine output. Specific gravity evaluates the child's hydration status as well as renal function.
Assess gastrointestinal function: auscultate bowel sounds, note abdominal girth, nausea/vomiting, feeding intolerance.	Decreased perfusion to the gastrointestinal tract results in decreased gastric motility/functioning. If the child is receiving nasogastric/orogastric feedings, vomiting and/or large residuals may be noted.
Assess for cyanotic or mottled extremities, poor capillary refill, poor or absent pulses, cool/clammy skin.	Poor tissue perfusion/vasoconstriction may be an early sign of decreased CO owing to hypovolemia and/or shock and can result in hypoxia, lactic acidosis.
Collaborative	
Monitor laboratory data: CBC, ABGs, PVO_2 and oxygen saturation.	These data help determine the cause of decreased tissue perfusion (e.g., dehydration, acidosis). They also will help in evaluating organ function (e.g., renal perfusion). Oxygen saturation and PVO_2 help monitor the degree of cellular oxygenation.
Administer medications as indicated:	
Vasopressors,	May be given to increase tissue perfusion/CO.
Vasodilators,	May be used in combination with vasopressors to enhance tissue perfusion.
Antibiotics, steroids, as indicated.	Used for treatment of septic shock. Note: Steroid therapy is controversial. (Refer to Care Plan: Sepsis/Septicemia/Septic Shock, page 329.)
Administer oxygen as necessary.	Correction of hypoxemia/respiratory acidosis enhances oxygen delivery to the tissues.
Assist with dialysis as appropriate. (Refer to Care Plan: Renal Dialysis, page 222.)	The child may develop acute tubular necrosis (ATN) related to decreased perfusion to the kidneys. Perito-

INTERVENTIONS	RATIONALE
Collaborative	
	neal or hemodialysis may be necessary until kidney function is restored.
Insert/maintain nasogastric tube and monitor gastric drainage.	A nasogastric tube should be inserted in the presence of an ileus, to assist with drainage of gastric contents and to prevent vomiting.

NURSING DIAGNOSIS:	**Tissue Perfusion, alteration in, cerebral.**
SUPPORTING DATA/CONTRIBUTING FACTORS:	**Critically ill children may develop cerebral edema for a variety of reasons, such as shock, trauma, mass lesions, or infection. Cerebral edema alters perfusion of brain tissue and may result in permanent damage/death.**
GENERAL PATIENT OUTCOMES:	**Cerebral tissue perfusion is maintained at an adequate level to prevent brain damage/death.**

INTERVENTIONS	RATIONALE
Independent	
Assess changes in level of consciousness/behavior; for example, agitation, lethargy, confusion, coma. Note response to pain.	A change in level of consciousness is often the first sign of increased intracranial pressure. A decreased response to painful stimuli is abnormal in the child.
Note changes in pupil size, equality, and reaction to light.	Compression of the oculomotor nerves causes changes in pupil response to light.
Monitor heart rate, BP, respiratory rate and pattern.	Cushing's reflex (decreased heart rate, increased blood pressure, and alterations in respiratory rate and pattern) is a very late sign of increased intracranial pressure. Hypotension is also a very late sign of increased intracranial pressure.
Assess changes in motor function and reflexes.	The child with increased intracranial pressure may demonstrate decreased motor function along with abnormal posturing and reflexes. As neurologic deterioration progresses, flaccid paralysis will develop. Note: Positive Babinski is normal in infants.
Assess for high-pitched cry, bulging fontanelle, irritability (complaints of headache, nausea, vomiting, or blurred vision).	These signs may be present in infants and children with increased intracranial pressure.
Keep patient positioned with head elevated and in the midline position.	This position promotes venous drainage from the head, limiting edema formation.

INTERVENTIONS	RATIONALE
Collaborative	
Assist with insertion/maintenance of intracranial pressure monitoring device.	This is the most reliable method for determining the presence of increased intracranial pressure and evaluating the response to therapy.
Assist with diagnostic tests such as computerized axial tomography (CAT) scan, magnetic resonance imaging (MRI), electroencephalogram (EEG) and cerebral blood flow studies.	Computerized axial tomography scans/MRI are useful in determining the presence of cerebral edema or infarction. Electroencephalograms are useful in determining the presence of seizure activity. Cerebral blood flow tests/EEGs may be used in the determination of brain death.

(Refer to Care Plan: Brain Injury/Increased Intracranial Pressure, page 127.)

NURSING DIAGNOSIS:	**Fluid Volume Deficit, actual/potential.**
SUPPORTING DATA/CONTRIBUTING FACTORS:	**A child has greater fluid requirements per kilogram of body weight than does an adult because the child has greater insensible water losses. Because the child has larger ratio of body surface area, more fluid is lost to the environment. The child also has a greater percent of total body water than the adult and a larger proportion of this is extracellular. This means that fluid losses such as vomiting, diarrhea, hemorrhage, or increased urinary output from inappropriate antidiuretic hormone (ADH) secretion can quickly produce dehydration/hypovolemia.**
GENERAL PATIENT OUTCOMES:	**Vital signs and urine output are within normal range for age. Mucous membranes are moist.**

INTERVENTIONS	RATIONALE
Independent	
Monitor heart rate, respiratory rate, BP. Note pulse pressure. Measure BP supine and upright in older child.	Signs of hypovolemia include tachycardia, tachypnea, and hypotension. A decreased pulse pressure will be evident before a fall in systolic BP occurs. Orthostatic changes precede hypotension with dehydration.
Monitor hemodynamic pressures, such as CVP, PAP, and PCWP.	Helps evaluate circulating volume as well as cardiac function.

INTERVENTIONS	RATIONALE
Independent	
Assess for dry mucous membranes, decreased urine output, increased urine specific gravity, poor skin turgor, and sunken fontanelle in infants.	Systemic indicators of fluid balance/dehydration.
Measure intake/output, include all sources of fluid losses such as blood drawing, blood loss from chest tubes/other drains, vomiting, diarrhea, or gastric suction.	Small losses can quickly add up to a major fluid deficit. Decreased urine output and increased urine concentration are signs of decreased fluid volume.
Weigh daily, compare with intake/output (fluid balance).	Changes in weight with corresponding positive/negative fluid balance are useful in evaluating continued deficit/rehydration.
Collaborative	
Administer fluids based on the child's calculated needs. Monitor IV rate closely via pump/controlled infusion set.	Fluids are the treatment of choice for hypovolemia/dehydration. Blood loss needs to be considered in terms of the child's total circulating blood volume. For resuscitation, 20 ml/kg of Ringer's lactate is usually administered. The rate of administration should be monitored closely to avoid fluid overload.

NURSING DIAGNOSIS: **Fluid Volume, alteration in, excess.**

SUPPORTING DATA/CONTRIBUTING FACTORS: **Although the child has a larger fluid requirement per unit of body weight, the absolute amount required is small. Too rapid/excessive replacement can result in fluid overload.**

GENERAL PATIENT OUTCOMES: **Intake approximates output, breath sounds clear, free of edema. Alert/responding appropriately.**

INTERVENTIONS	RATIONALE
Independent	
Monitor hemodynamic parameters, such as CVP, PAP, PCWP.	Elevations may reflect fluid excess or cardiac dysfunction.
Assess breath sounds.	Crackles at the end of inspiration indicate fluid accumulation in the lungs.
Assess changes in level of consciousness/behavior (e.g., agitation, lethargy, confusion, coma).	Rapid rehydration may cause cerebral edema as manifested by changes in mentation.
Weigh daily, correlate with intake/output (fluid balance).	Weight gain combined with positive fluid balance suggests fluid excess.

INTERVENTIONS	RATIONALE
Collaborative	
Monitor IV rate closely. Administer fluids via infusion pump.	Fluid overload can happen quickly in the infant/small child because the vascular bed is small.
Administer diuretics as indicated.	Diuretics may be necessary to reduce fluid overload.

NURSING DIAGNOSIS:	**Nutrition, alteration in, less than body requirements.**
SUPPORTING DATA/CONTRIBUTING FACTORS:	**Children have larger obligate energy needs and lower macronutrient stores and are likely to become nutritionally depleted when adequate nutritional support is not provided.**
GENERAL PATIENT OUTCOMES:	**Nutritional support is adequate to provide for weight gain, maintenance of lean body mass and growth, positive nitrogen balance.**

INTERVENTIONS	RATIONALE
Independent	
Inquire about food/fluid intake over last several hours/days prior to admission.	If illness preceded admission, nutritional stores may already be depleted by increased metabolic demands, reduced oral intake, and losses from vomiting/diarrhea.
Measure child's height, weight, and head circumference. Compare with height/weight percentile.	This basic screening should be done to assist with evaluation of nutritional state/need for nutritional consultation.
Weigh daily.	Helps monitor the child's nutritional and fluid status.
Auscultate bowel sounds.	Presence of active bowel sounds in all quadrants suggests readiness for feeding.
Ascertain usual eating patterns, times and favorite foods/beverages. Note use of bottle/type of nipple used by infant. Encourage mother to breastfeed/bring in breast milk for infant if appropriate.	Incorporating familiar foods/usual eating schedule may enhance intake.
Provide small amounts of foods appropriate for age/condition.	Appetite may be decreased and large portions of food are often overwhelming. Toddlers prefer finger foods. Child's/adolescent's intake may need to be encouraged to meet normal growth needs.
Collaborative	
Monitor laboratory studies; for example, Albumin, total protein, glucose, electrolytes.	Evaluates the child's nutritional status and the development of metabolic complications.

INTERVENTIONS	RATIONALE
Collaborative	
Refer to dietician/nutritional support team as indicated.	Aids in establishing nutritional needs and appropriate source.
Administer enteral and/or parenteral nutrition. (Refer to Care Plan: Nutritional Support, page 367.)	The critically ill child is hypermetabolic and often requires support of nutritional reserves. Enteral feeding is preferred because it is more physiologically normal and safer. If enteral feedings are not possible, parenteral nutrition should be initiated.

NURSING DIAGNOSIS: **Comfort, alteration in, pain, acute.**

SUPPORTING DATA/CONTRIBUTING FACTORS: **Children of all ages, including infants, can feel pain. They are exposed to numerous painful procedures in the critical care unit.**

GENERAL PATIENT OUTCOMES: **Pain is minimized/controlled.**

INTERVENTIONS	RATIONALE
Independent	
Assess for increased heart/respiratory rate, BP, and diaphoresis.	These are autonomic responses to pain that can be assessed even in the unconscious child.
Assess for irritability, lethargy, and restlessness.	Additional signs of pain in the infant.
Discuss methods with parents to help minimize/control child's pain. Use comfort measures appropriate for age; for example, pacifier for sucking, tactile stimulation (stroking/cuddling).	Parents are invaluable in helping control child's pain through reassurances and touching/comforting child. This allows parents to be involved in child's care.
Ask child if pain is present and to point to area involved.	Children usually are truthful about presence/perception of pain if adult is caring/listening. However, many preschool/schoolage children may deny pain out of fear of hypodermic injection.
Collaborative	
Administer analgesics as appropriate for situation.	Appropriate at any age to minimize/control pain in the child.

NURSING DIAGNOSIS: **Sleep Pattern Disturbance.**

SUPPORTING DATA/CONTRIBUTING FACTORS: **Children suffer from both sensory overload and sensory deprivation in the intensive care unit (ICU). Many procedures need to be performed**

	around the clock, interrupting the child's sleep.
GENERAL PATIENT OUTCOMES:	**Sleeps/rests between care activities.**

INTERVENTIONS	RATIONALE
Independent	
Plan procedures to allow sleep time, use usual naptime/bedtime in schedule.	Spacing of procedures may allow the child periods of rest.
Provide a sense of day/night for child (e.g., turn out lights, keep noise level down).	A sense of day/night allows the child some sleep time and promotes orientation.
Use familiar objects, bedtime rituals, presleep cues/props (e.g., favorite blanket/toy, rocking chair, pacifier, stories).	Reinforces expected behavior; "now is the time to sleep."

NURSING DIAGNOSIS:	**Anxiety/Fear.**
SUPPORTING DATA/CONTRIBUTING FACTORS:	**The critical care environment is frightening to both child and parents. They are exposed to equipment and procedures that are foreign to them. Child may view hospitalization as punishment for past behavior/thoughts. In addition, fear of bodily injury poses a very real threat in child's mind. Parents often feel frustrated and helpless, especially when prognosis is in question.**
GENERAL PATIENT OUTCOMES:	**Anxiety is minimized as evidenced by behavior of the child; for example, smiling appropriately, interacting with visitors/staff, participating in activities as condition permits.**

INTERVENTIONS	RATIONALE
Independent	
Provide primary nurse.	Better interpretation of responses/needs can be made by having same nurse care for child. Enhances trust in caregiver.
Assess developmental level of the child.	Necessary for identifying appropriate interventions, inasmuch as the fears/anxieties of the child are different during the different developmental stages.

INTERVENTIONS	RATIONALE
Independent	
Provide explanations of procedures and sensations that will be experienced at a level the child understands, include what is expected of child. Use visuals; for example, doll, pictures, or rehearsal, as indicated. Be honest in explanations.	Children deal more effectively with the known—knowing what a procedure involves and what to expect. Younger children often fantasize, which heightens anxiety of the unknown. Dishonesty will destroy the child's trust in the staff.
Provide play activities for the child as appropriate.	Play helps the child work out some of the anger and frustration he/she is experiencing. It also provides diversion.
Minimize separation between parents and child.	Parents provide support and reassurance for their children. Younger children are less tolerant of periods of separation from their parents. Parents are extremely stressed by their child's injury/illness. Their frustrations and anxiety can be alleviated by being allowed to stay with their child.
Maintain "normal" home schedule when possible.	Adherence to usual activity/sleep/eating patterns promotes a sense of normalcy and may be reassuring to the child.
Liberalize visitation policy as indicated, to include siblings/extended family.	Reduces feelings of isolation/separation and reduces anxiety associated with fears of abandonment.
Collaborative	
Administer sedatives as indicated; for example, Diazepam (Valium), lorazepam (Ativan), chloral hydrate (Noctec).	May be helpful in allaying some of the child's anxiety and in helping the child relax.

NURSING DIAGNOSIS:	**Coping, family, potential for growth.**
SUPPORTING DATA/CONTRIBUTING FACTORS:	**The admission of a child to the critical care unit is extremely stressful for parents. For many, it is a crisis situation. With support and guidance, many families can experience growth as they develop coping strategies.**
GENERAL PATIENT OUTCOMES:	**Family members are coping positively with the situation.**

INTERVENTIONS	RATIONALE
Independent	
Assess the stage in the parents' reaction to their child's admission to the ICU; for example, shock, disbelief, denial, guilt, anger, depression.	Parents experience various stages in their reactions. The nurses' strategy for helping parents deal with their feelings depends on the stage they are in.

INTERVENTIONS	RATIONALE
Independent	
Encourage parents to ask questions and ventilate feelings. Be honest in all explanations.	Parents feel a strong need to know what is going on with their child. They need to feel secure in talking about their feelings, good or bad. Honesty is important for them to develop trust in the staff.
Encourage parents to be involved in the child's care as much as possible within their level of comfort.	Parents often feel a loss of control when their child is in the ICU. Allowing them to be involved in their child's care helps them reestablish their role as parents and reduces frustration.
Attempt to find out about siblings and how they are coping with the child's illness/injury.	Siblings are affected by the child's illness. They often feel left out or ignored. They are often fearful about what is happening to the child. By knowing more about the sibling, the nurse can help the parents develop ways to reduce sibling anxiety.
Collaborative	
Identify hospital-based resources for family support (e.g., clergy, social services, nurse counselors).	Provides sources that are readily available for assistance.
Refer family to community support groups, depending on child's diagnosis and prognosis (e.g., Head Injury Support Group, Compassionate Friends).	May need additional help on a long-term/ongoing basis.

NURSING DIAGNOSIS:	**Growth and Development, altered.**
SUPPORTING DATA/CONTRIBUTING FACTORS:	**The age of the child is an important factor in the understanding of the illness/injury that has occurred and why it has happened. Children who do not understand this connection often blame themselves for what has happened. Separation from significant other(s), environmental/stimulation deficiencies, as well as the effects of the dependence and physical disability in the ICU setting, can adversely affect the child and may result in transient developmental regression.**
GENERAL PATIENT OUTCOMES:	**Displays behaviors and self-care skills appropriate for age/development.**

INTERVENTIONS	RATIONALE
Independent	
Note age/developmental level of the child.	Determination of these factors will help with assessment and planning interventions.

INTERVENTIONS	RATIONALE
Independent	
Note effect of illness/injury on child's behaviors; for example, crying, withdrawal, listlessness, anger, regression in self-care/self-control activities appropriate to age.	Although regression/dependence may be a normal expectation, exaggerated behaviors may indicate the presence of problems.
Determine family constellation and type of interactions with the patient.	Identifies support systems available.
Encourage participation in self-care.	Promotes independence and sense of control.
Encourage parents/family to remain with child as much as possible.	Provides sense of consistency/familiarity and avoids effects of separation.
Continue usual home routines as able.	Promotes sense of continuity/security.
Provide opportunity for choices when possible (e.g., beverage to take medicine with, time of bath).	Enhances sense of control.
Set limits as necessary.	Provides for sense of security/safety. Helps child know that adults are going to protect/keep him/her safe.
Provide playtime/diversional activities for age. Allow for release of energy in ways that are acceptable for the situation.	Child may have pent-up energy which needs expression when child is immobilized by illness/injury.
Provide books, activities/games, playthings, and/or schoolwork appropriate for age.	Promotes a sense of normalcy, stimulate thinking/learning.
Recognize need for privacy.	Children develop a sense of modesty and this needs to be respected as much as possible in the setting.
Collaborative	
Refer for counseling; for example, psychiatric nurse, social services, family therapy.	May need additional assistance to prevent future negative effect on growth and development.

Obstetric Considerations

This care plan focuses on the patient who is admitted to the intensive care unit (ICU) for treatment of a life-threatening situation/injury who also happens to be pregnant. The nurse is referred to other care plans appropriate for the primary diagnosis. This care plan provides information related to concerns/considerations that must be taken into account when providing care for this patient and her fetus in order to maintain uterine/placental circulation and maternal/fetal well-being.

PATIENT ASSESSMENT DATA BASE

HISTORY

Last menstrual period (LMP) to determine estimated date of delivery (EDD) and gestational age.

Medications/drugs previously and currently being taken.

Previous complicated pregnancy(s)/delivery(s); for example, gestational diabetes, seizures, pregnancy-induced hypertension, preterm labor, postpartal hemorrhage, cesarean section.

Problems associated with this pregnancy, including exposure to sexually transmitted diseases (STD).

History of present illness/accident.

Existing medical problems (e.g., diabetes mellitus, cardiac, renal).

Subjective (dependent on condition/situation)

May complain of headache, blurred vision, epigastric pain, intense abdominal pain.

May report alteration in frequency/absence of fetal movement.

May verbalize symptoms of spontaneous rupture of membranes (SROM); for example, "gush of water from vagina" or presence of uterine contractions/backache.

PHYSICAL EXAMINATION

Inspection

Venous distention: generalized in pregnancy, reflecting increased plasma volume/cardiac output.

Respirations: usually deeper with increased rate, owing to elevation of diaphragm and reduced lung capacity.

Sterile vaginal examination may reveal bloody show, indicating onset of labor, frank bleeding indicative of hemorrhagic complications such as placental separation, or leakage of fluid suggesting rupture of membranes.

Palpation

Abdomen: rigidity with rebound tenderness suggests intra-abdominal/uterine trauma, although no pain may be present initially following uterine rupture.

Uterus: note presence of uterine contractions. Fundus: height in centimeters is a rough estimate of gestational age after 20 weeks.

Pulses may be reduced in lower extremities, owing to pressure of the uterus on the inferior vena cava and aorta.

Edema: may have pitting edema of lower extremities, dependent edema of sacral area, or facial/periorbital edema. (Digital and periorbital edema are often associated with PIH.)

Auscultation

Breath sounds should be normal/clear but may be diminished in bases, owing to abdominal distention and elevation of diaphragm.

Fetal heart rate (FHR) should be between 120 and 160 per minute.

Bowel sounds: usually decreased, reflecting displacement by the uterus and reduced gastrointestinal motility.

DIAGNOSTIC STUDIES

Hgb/Hct varies, dependent on volume status; pseudoanemia owing to hemodilution may occur normally in pregnancy.

WBC: normally elevated in pregnancy, increases more in labor.

Electrolytes: levels may be slightly lower than normal range, reflecting dilutional effects.

BUN and creatinine are decreased in pregnancy.

Clotting studies: state of hypercoagulability is present. Platelets/fibrinogen/all clotting factors, except II, IV, XI, and XIII, are increased.

Serum blood sugar: patient with diabetes is prone to hypoglycemia in first trimester, hyperglycemia in second and third trimesters.

Liver studies: elevations require evaluation to rule out HELLP syndrome (hemolysis, elevated liver enzymes, low platelets).

Type/crossmatch and Rh factor determination.

Serum/urinary estriol: occasionally done to evaluate placental sufficiency/fetal well-being. Levels drop in presence of pregnancy-induced hypertension (PIH), complicated diabetes.

Kleihauer-Betke test (fetal dex) maternal serum detects transfer of 20 ml or more of fetal blood cells into maternal circulation. Amniocentesis differentiates between maternal/fetal cells and provides an estimate of severity of fetal condition.

Urinalysis: hematuria suggests trauma; elevated WBC may indicate presence of urinary tract infection; presence of albumin is associated with pregnancy-induced hypertension.

Chest x-ray examination usually demonstrates elevation of the diaphragm, heart shifted upward and to the left, and increase in the lung markings owing to an increase in the plasma volume and vascular distention of the pulmonary system.

ECG: axis shifts to the left. Patients are prone to ectopy, and pregnancy lowers the threshold for supraventricular tachycardia.

Echocardiography: demonstrates slightly dilated chambers owing to increased plasma volume.

Doppler: tricuspid regurgitation may be present owing to dilation of the tricuspid anulus.

Fetal ultrasonography determines gestational age, estimates fetal weight and well-being. May also detect intra-abdominal bleeding.

Amniocentesis determines fetal maturity/distress using shake test: L/S ratio; presence of phosphatidylglycerol/phosphatidylinositol (pg/PI), creatinine, bilirubin; Nile blue stain for fetal fat cells and presence of meconium.

Vaginal pool specimen: for gram stain to assess for sepsis; ferning and litmus test (using Nitrazine paper) verify presence of amniotic fluid; shake test, L/S ratio, presence of pg/PI to assess fetal lung maturity.

Culdocentesis: insertion of a needle through the vagina into the peritoneal cavity to determine the presence of bleeding (done in patients with abdominal trauma, suspected of bleeding).

NST (nonstress test): noninvasive test to determine fetal well-being.

CST (oxytocin contraction test) may be done following a nonreactive equivocal NST to determine fetal/placental well-being.

NURSING PRIORITIES

1. Evaluate/stabilize mother's condition.
2. Promote fetal well-being.
3. Correct/prevent complications.
4. Maintain emotional support, assist in the grieving process, if necessary.

NURSING DIAGNOSIS:	**Fluid Volume Deficit, potential/actual.**
SUPPORTING DATA/CONTRIBUTING FACTORS:	**Normal progesterone-induced vasodilation of blood vessels may predispose the patient to increased blood losses before vasoconstriction occurs to stem blood loss. In addition, increased vascularity around the uterus enhances the patient's vulnerability to injury and potentiates the risk of hemorrhage/shock. Pregnancy-induced hypertension (PIH) can cause circulating deficits when fluid shifts from intravascular to interstitial spaces. Lastly, loss of fluid volume can occur from trauma-related injuries or from hemorrhagic complications related to the state of pregnancy; for example, placental separation (abruptio placenta), placenta previa, ectopic pregnancy, hydatidiform mole, abortions, uterine atony, retained placental fragments, or disseminated intravascular coagulation (DIC).**
GENERAL PATIENT OUTCOMES:	**Vital signs and urinary output are within normal limits. Absence of shock syndrome.**

INTERVENTIONS	RATIONALE
Independent	
Note tachycardia, decreased blood pressure, or abnormally low systemic arterial pressure, as well as pallor, decreased capillary refill, and diaphoresis. Monitor hemodynamic pressures; for example, central venous pressure (CVP), pulmonary capillary wedge pressure (PCWP), cardiac output (CO) as available.	Signs/symptoms of hypovolemic shock, but may not be evident until up to 1500 ml of blood is lost because blood volume during pregnancy is usually 30 to 50 percent greater than normal.
Evaluate, record/report amount and nature of vaginal blood loss, if present. Initiate pad count/weigh pads/chux.	Aids in estimation of blood loss. (One gram is equal to approximately 1 ml of blood.)

INTERVENTIONS	RATIONALE
Independent	
Avoid rectal/vaginal examination.	May increase hemorrhage, especially if marginal or total placenta previa is present.
Assess mental status for signs of irritability, mental confusion, agitation. Observe color of mucous membranes.	Cerebral hypoxia associated with hypovolemia may be recognized first by behavior changes, with cyanosis a late manifestation of hypoxia.
Monitor FHR/activity.	Even a transient hypotensive episode can reduce uterine blood flow (which may be decreased by 20 percent before maternal signs of shock are noted) and may be reflected by alterations in FHR and decreased movement.
Monitor intake/output, note urine specific gravity.	Assesses degree of fluid loss. Urinary output less than 0.5 to 1 ml/kg/hr with elevated specific gravity suggests dehydration.
Note history for presence of pregnancy-induced hypertension (PIH) and/or medical condition that may predispose to hypertension (e.g., diabetes, renal/cardiac disease.)	Associated vascular changes/vasoconstriction results in reduced intravascular volume, making client more vulnerable to any blood loss or anesthetic-induced vasodilation.
Investigate complaints of severe abdominal pain/rigidity, reduced fetal activity with/without vaginal bleeding.	Symptoms are suggestive of abruptio placenta. Eighty percent of patients with vaginal bleeding (posttrauma) have placental separation; of these, 20 percent have concealed retroplacental bleeding, resulting in abdominal pain/rigidity.
Note complaint of right upper quadrant (RUQ) pain, in association with nausea/vomiting, epigastric/shoulder pain, abdominal guarding/rebound tenderness.	The enlarged uterus may hide hemorrhage associated with liver/spleen trauma, which should be differentiated from liver involvement owing to PIH (HELLP syndrome). (Refer to Nursing Diagnosis: Fluid Volume, alteration in, excess (potential), page 418.)
Assess for pelvic fracture (e.g., pain on movement).	This is the most common fracture in pregnant patient and is associated with an increased risk of retroperitoneal hemorrhage, related to vascularity of the pelvic region.
Assess for spontaneous bleeding from gums/nose/venipuncture site.	Suggestive of DIC, a potential complication in the prenatal patient who experiences placental separation, eclampsia, sepsis, retention of dead fetus for more than 5 weeks, amniotic fluid emboli, or sepsis.
Position client in left lateral position if possible, or use wedge under right hip. Avoid recumbent/right lateral position.	Left lateral position increases venous return/CO and placental/kidney circulation. Right lateral position interrupts blood flow to heart, and recumbent position aggravates hypotension by compression of inferior vena cava, aorta.
Save expelled tissue/products of conception.	Physician will need to evaluate for possible tissue/membrane retention.
Collaborative	
Monitor laboratory studies; for example,	
Hemoglobin (Hgb)/hematocrit (Hct);	Prenatal plasma levels increase (in greater proportion

INTERVENTIONS	RATIONALE
Collaborative	
	to red blood cell mass,) making assessment by normal parameters difficult. A severe reduction in Hgb/Hct levels may be used as a guideline for blood replacement. Hematocrit levels may be elevated in the client with PIH owing to hemo-concentration resulting from fluid shifts to extravascular space.
Platelets, fibrinogen, and fibrin split products.	Platelet count and fibrinogen level will decrease, but fibrin split products will increase in the presence of coagulopathy (DIC).
Administer fluids as indicated; for example, Ringer's lactate/blood products, fresh frozen plasma and platelets. Start multiple access lines as indicated.	Ringer's lactate (closest to body's electrolyte composition) is usually infused first, followed by whole blood/packed cells/platelets to increase oxygen-carrying capacity/expand volume/replace clotting factors and to maintain/improve renal function.
Avoid use of vasopressors in prenatal client.	Constricts uterine arteries, reduces uterine/placental blood flow, compromising the fetus.
Assist with peritoneal lavage, abdominal ultrasound, as indicated.	Detects possible peritoneal hemorrhage or free fluid in the abdomen.
Prepare for surgical intervention/cesarean delivery.	Dilatation and currettage (D and C) may be indicated for spontaneous/missed/incomplete abortion; cesarean section for partial/complete placenta previa and delivery of fetus, or hysterectomy for ruptured uterus. Surgical treatment of obstetric complications stops hemorrhage/release of thromboplastin, may correct DIC.
Administer heparin if indicated.	Occasionally may be required if surgical correction of underlying cause of coagulopathy is unsuccessful/not possible (e.g., amniotic emboli).

NURSING DIAGNOSIS:	**Gas Exchange, impaired, fetal (potential).**
SUPPORTING DATA/CONTRIBUTING FACTORS:	**Any situation that reduces maternal oxygen levels or maternal circulating volume has similar effects on fetal oxygen levels and placental circulation. With maternal shock, blood is shunted from the fetus as uterine arteries constrict, reducing placental blood flow. Prolonged fetal hypoxia results in anaerobic metabolism/lactic acidosis.**
GENERAL PATIENT OUTCOMES:	**Fetal heart rate, beat-to-beat variability, and movements/activity are**

within normal limits. Non-stress test is reactive.

INTERVENTIONS	RATIONALE
Independent	
Assess FHR for bradycardia (less than 110) lasting longer than 10 minutes or tachycardia (greater than 160).	Tachycardia (normal for a preterm infant) indicates compensatory mechanisms for a hypoxic state in a term infant. Bradycardia indicates severe/prolonged hypoxia.
Monitor for uterine activity, manually/electronically.	Prolonged contractions may decrease blood flow to the fetus and if present may create a periodic pattern associated with cord/head compression, uteroplacental insufficiency.
Use continuous electronic monitoring if fetus is 34 weeks gestation or close to term. Note beat-to-beat variability.	In the event of fetal hypoxia/acidosis, variability (the amount of change from one beat to another) may be reduced from the average 6 to 10 beats per minute, indicating reduced fetal/placental perfusion, compromise.
Check for presence of vaginal discharge, noting color/nature/amount.	May indicate tear/rupture of membrane, resulting in a leaking or gushing of amniotic fluid. Presence of meconium-stained fluid reflects fetal distress/hypoxia and may warn of potential complications for the infant postdelivery.
Note presence of maternal complications that may negatively affect ventilation/placental perfusion (e.g., acute asthma, pulmonary infections, PIH, malnutrition).	A fetus, especially those already partially compromised by prolonged hypoxia/acidosis, may be less able to recover in utero from hypoxia associated with acute hemorrhage/trauma.
Assess extent of maternal blood loss/degree of hypovolemia. (Refer to Nursing Diagnosis: Fluid Volume Deficit, potential, page 413.)	Degree of maternal blood loss/hypovolemia will affect placental circulation/fetal status.
Note changes in maternal mental status or developing cyanosis.	Maternal hypoxemia directly affects fetal status.
Place mother in left lateral position if condition permits, or elevate right hip with wedge. Avoid dorsal recumbent, right lateral position.	Position displaces uterus, preventing compression of inferior vena cava/aorta, which reduces venous return, compromises placental circulation, and causes supine hypotensive syndrome.
Collaborative	
Administer oxygen to the mother.	May increase maternal oxygen levels within the intervillious spaces, providing additional oxygen for fetal uptake even in the case of decreased perfusion.
Monitor maternal serum pH, arterial blood gases (ABGs).	Provides guidelines for assessing therapy needs/effectiveness.
Administer intravenous (IV) fluids/blood products, as indicated.	Maintains adequate CO/placental perfusion. Note: this is especially important if the patient is receiving antihypertensive drugs or an epidural block for pain relief.

INTERVENTIONS	RATIONALE
Collaborative	
Assist with fetal ultrasonography.	Helps estimate gestational age, identify uterine/fetal abnormalities, and determine fetal demise. Gestational age may be criterion for adopting conservative/aggressive management of maternal situation, although life of the mother generally takes precedence over saving life of the fetus.
Assist with NST, using electronic monitor.	A reactive NST (determined by two or more FHR accelerations of at least 15 beats per minute in amplitude and at least 15 seconds duration in a 10-minute period) indicates adequate placental functioning and fetal central nervous system (CNS) integrity.

NURSING DIAGNOSIS: **Cardiac Output, alteration in (decompensation, potential).**

SUPPORTING DATA/CONTRIBUTING FACTORS: **During the second and third trimesters, the plasma volume increases by 30 to 50 percent. Hypertrophy of the cardiac ventricles occurs in response to this increase in the circulating volume, resulting in increased CO, which peaks at 25 to 27 weeks gestation. To compensate for the increased CO, peripheral dilation reduces systemic vascular resistance, lowering the blood pressure. In addition, the resting heart rate is increased by as many as 15 beats per minute near the end of the third trimester. Increases in fluid/stress and/or preexisting cardiac problems can compromsie the system. Increased capillary permeability, hydrostatic pressure, and excess fluid retention potentiates the movement of fluid out of the vascular bed and when combined with a supine recumbent position, reduces venous return/CO.**

GENERAL PATIENT OUTCOMES: **Vital signs/CO within accepted range for gestation. Absence of pathologic edema or pulmonary involvement.**

INTERVENTIONS	RATIONALE
Independent	
Monitor blood pressure (BP) and pulse.	Normally the cardiovascular system compensates for the prenatal increase in circulating volume/CO by increasing pulse rate as many as 15 beats per minute and increasing peripheral dilation. This reduces systemic resistance to CO so that systolic BP readings decrease by 8 mmHg and diastolic pressures usually fall 12 mmHg. Hypertension may suggest fluid overload/cardiac failure.
Measure CO/cardiac index (CI), as indicated.	"Normal" or slightly lower CO/CI actually may indicate severe compromise/reduced perfusion to vital organs, including the uterus and placental circulation, negatively affecting the fetus. Hormonal effects may limit vasoconstrictive response necessary to support decreasing CO.
Auscultate heart sounds, note presence of murmurs.	Systolic murmur may be created by decreased blood viscosity, displacement of the heart/torsion of great vessels caused by abdominal distention.
Monitor intake/output and correlate with daily weight.	Cumulative fluid balances and weight changes are useful in evaluating fluid excess/deficit.
Auscultate lungs for crackles. Note presence of dyspnea, increased respiratory rate/effort.	Pulmonary edema may occur with cardiac failure.
Position patient in left lateral position if possible or place wedge under right hip.	Reducing pressure on the inferior vena cava increases venous return/CO and renal/placental perfusion.
Elevate foot of bed as indicated.	Promotes venous return.
Change position slowly when getting out of bed/chair.	Sudden position changes may result in syncope because blood tends to pool in lower extremities, reducing circulating volume.
Assess for presence of pathologic edema; for example, digits/periorbital, epigastric pain; nausea/vomiting, visual disturbances. (Refer to Nursing Diagnosis: Fluid Volume, excess (potential), below.)	Pathologic edema suggests fluid excess/cardiac compromise.
Collaborative	
Administer IV fluids and plasma expander as indicated.	Corrects fluid volume deficits to improve CO. Note: Use of plasma expanders in presence of edema may compromise cardiac function, owing to fluid overload resulting from mobilization of excess extravascular fluids.

NURSING DIAGNOSIS:	**Fluid Volume, alteration in, excess (potential).**
SUPPORTING DATA/CONTRIBUTING FACTORS:	**During the second trimester, total body water (plasma/red cells) normally**

increases by 1000 ml, owing to estrogen levels stimulating the adrenal gland to secrete aldosterone, which retains sodium and water. By the end of the third trimester, the circulating volume has increased by another 700 ml. This represents a weight gain of approximately 5 pounds, normally without any visible signs of edema. However, rapid or excessive fluid gains can cause edema and may contribute to cardiac decompensation. Although PIH caused by excess fluid retention is not usually seen until the last 10 weeks of the pregnancy, it may develop earlier—especially in the client with predisposing factors such as diabetes, renal disease, hypertension, multiple pregnancies, malnutrition (overweight/underweight), and hydatidiform mole.

GENERAL PATIENT OUTCOMES: Blood pressure within patient's normal prenatal range. Free of signs of pathologic edema/impending convulsive state (eclampsia). Urine negative for albumin; liver enzymes, Hgb/Hct, platelet levels are within normal limits.

INTERVENTIONS	RATIONALE
Independent	
Monitor for increasing BP, pulse.	Elevations may indicate circulatory overload, cardiac involvement. In PIH, significant blood pressure increases may occur (30 mmHg systolic and 15 mmHg diastolic over baseline readings).
Measure invasive hemodynamic pressures, for example, CVP, PAP, PCWP.	Accurately assess circulating volume.
Record intake and output, urine specific gravity.	Output is a sensitive guide to circulating volume/renal function and should approximate intake.
Monitor daily weight.	Conservative management/bedrest in presence of edema may result in up to 4 pounds of fluid loss in first 24 hours.
Monitor for signs/symptoms of pulmonary edema; for example, complaints of dyspnea, increasing restlessness, crackles upon auscultation, cyanosis, or pres-	The most common complication from volume overload is pulmonary edema. Patients with PIH are more susceptible to pulmonary edema, which may be re-

INTERVENTIONS	RATIONALE
Independent	
ence of productive cough.	lated to the decrease in total protein and altered colloid osmotic pressure.
Note location/extent of visible edema and signs of progressive/excessive edema associated with PIH (e.g., epigastric/RUQ pain, visual disturbances, nausea/vomiting, oliguria, elevated liver enzymes/uric acid levels).	Dependent/pedal edema (physiologic edema) commonly occurs owing to decreased venous return from the lower extremities. Digital/periorbital edema suggests fluid overload/developing PIH. Edema of an encapsulated liver manifests as RUQ pain. Cerebral edema may indicate impending eclampsia. Nausea/vomiting may reflect gastrointestinal edema. Oliguria may suggest severe glomeruli spasms.
Test urine for albumin.	Detects vascular involvement associated with glomerular spasms of the kidney, reducing reabsorption of albumin.
Assess reflexes, monitor for eclampsia (convulsive state), onset of labor.	Hyperreflexia (3 to 4+) as well as above signs/symptoms frequently presents just prior to seizure activity.
Initiate seizure precautions (e.g., padded side rails/bite block, supplemental oxygen).	Allows for prompt action in the event of a convulsion. Note: Hypoxia associated with seizure may have serious effect on fetus.
Monitor for signs of abruptio placenta; for example, severe abdominal pain/rigidity with/without vaginal bleeding, reduced fetal activity. (Refer to Nursing Diagnosis: Fluid Volume Deficit, potential, page 413.)	Clients with severe PIH are at risk for abruptio placenta caused by infarcts/necrosis on the maternal portion of the placenta.
Collaborative	
Monitor laboratory studies; for example,	
Hematocrit, total protein, and serum osmolality;	Hematocrit may be used as an indicator of hemoconcentration or dilution but is less reliable because of hematologic changes associated with pregnancy. Generally, levels greater than 41 percent (Caucasian) or greater than 38 percent (black) at sea level are indicative of intravascular fluid shifts to extravascular compartments. Total protein and osmolality can be used in conjunction with the pulmonary capillary wedge pressure (PCWP) to calculate the colloidal osmotic pressure (COP)/wedge gradient. This value may be helpful in determining the risk for developing pulmonary edema.
Blood urea nitrogen (BUN), uric acid, creatinine clearance;	Elevated levels, especially of uric acid, indicate deteriorating renal function.
Liver enzymes.	HELLP (hemolysis, elevated liver enzymes, low platelets) syndrome may be accompanied by liver rupture/maternal death. Treatment involves immediate cesarean delivery of fetus.
Insert indwelling catheter as indicated.	Provides closer evaluation of output, renal function/perfusion.
Administer afterload reducing agents; for example,	May be used in the case of chronic hypertension or

INTERVENTIONS	RATIONALE
Collaborative	
hydralazine hydrochloride (Apresoline),	PIH (e.g., diastolic BP above 110) but must be used with caution because sudden drop in blood with pressure can have deleterious effects on uteroplacental perfusion, potentiating risk of abruptio placenta.
Sodium nitroprusside (Nipride),	Has not been determined safe in pregnancy but may be used short term in hypertensive crisis. Note: Side effects of Nipride mimic progression of eclampsia/abruptio placenta and may potentiate metabolic acidosis, compromising fetal status.
Administer diazepam (Valium).	Useful in prevention/alleviation of seizure activity.
Initiate infusion of magnesium sulfate as indicated.	Magnesium sulfate is a CNS depressant that decreases the amount of acetylcholine released by motor nerve impulses, blocking neuromuscular transmission and reducing the likelihood of eclampsia.
Avoid use of diuretics in patient with PIH unless pulmonary edema creates an emergency situation.	May further contribute to plasma dehydration, thereby reducing circulating blood volume.

NURSING DIAGNOSIS: **Injury, potential for, premature labor.**

SUPPORTING DATA/CONTRIBUTING FACTORS: **Premature labor is defined as labor occurring prior to the 37th week of gestation. Although the actual cause of premature labor has not been determined, many factors have been associated with it, including infection, trauma, dehydration, and severe maternal illness.**

GENERAL PATIENT OUTCOMES: **Preterm labor prevented/identified and pregnancy sustained (if possible) until fetal lungs mature.**

INTERVENTIONS	RATIONALE
Independent	
Note prenatal record for EDD, height of fundus.	Helpful in determining gestational age of fetus.
Assess for uterine activity/contractions periodically. If present, note intensity/duration/frequency. (Refer to Nursing Diagnosis: Comfort, alteration in, pain, page 425.)	Trauma/eclamptic state (convulsions) may precipitate the onset of labor, recognized by contractions (six or more in an hour) or by dilating/effacing of the cervix. Patients may complain of rhythmic cramping, back pain/pelvic pressure, or may be unaware/unable to communicate the presence of their contractions.
Note increased vaginal bleeding accompanied by regular uterine contractions. Save products of	Spontaneous abortion/miscarriage often follows trauma.

INTERVENTIONS	RATIONALE
Independent	
conception/fetus for physician to view. (Refer to Nursing Diagnosis: Coping, ineffective, individual/family (potential), page 427.)	
Maintain bedrest in left lateral position, as indicated.	Promotes relaxation and improves uterine circulation, which may decrease uterine irritability/activity.
Collaborative	
Provide fluids IV/by mouth and administer mild sedation.	Correcting dehydration may enhance uterine perfusion and reduce irritability. Often hydration and mild sedation is all that is required to stop contractions.
Assist with amniocentesis to analyze L/S ratio; presence of pg/PI, and pathogenic organisms. (Administer RhIG to patient postamniocentesis, if patient is RhDu negative).	Lecithin/sphingomyelin ratio of 2.0 indicates fetal lung maturity along with the presence of pg/PI. This information is important if the physician is attempting to stop labor, because stopping labor is not indicated in the presence of a mature fetus or intra-amniotic infection. Mixing of maternal/fetal blood may occur during amniocentesis, causing maternal sensitization in subsequent pregnancies in the Rh negative, Du negative patient.
Administer tocolytics; for example, ritodrine (Yutopar)/terbutaline (Brethine) IV or subcutaneously until contractions cease, then change to oral route.	Beta-mimetics work to relax smooth muscle (the myometrium) and often stop contractions in early premature labor (e.g., the cervix is less than 4 centimeters dilated/50 percent effaced, with membranes intact). Precautions: The use of tocolytics in patients with ruptured membranes is controversial but can be done if the patient is closely monitored for signs of infection.
Monitor for side effects; for example, maternal/fetal tachycardia, tightening of chest, dyspnea, nervousness, decreased diastolic BP, ventricular ectopy.	Development of severe maternal side effects signals need to discontinue tocolytic therapy.
Assess serum potassium/glucose.	Hypokalemia and hyperglycemia may develop with use of tocolytics.
Administer magnesium sulfate, as indicated.	Competes with calcium to relax smooth muscle/inhibit contractions and is used in patients who cannot tolerate the side effects of the beta-mimetics (diabetic patients), patients whose contractions continue with maximum doses of beta-mimetics, or in presence of hemorrhage.
Assess deep tendon reflexes, respiratory rate/serum levels during magnesium sulfate infusion. Note signs of circulatory depression (e.g., hypotension) and CNS effects (e.g., anxiety, drowsiness, lethargy). Have calcium gluconate available.	Therapeutic range of magnesium sulfate is 4 to 7 mg/dl. Toxic levels are manifested by loss of deep tendon reflexes (e.g., patellar, biceps, radial); decreased respiratory rate (less than 12 per minute), indicating need to reduce or discontinue drug/administer antidote.
Administer steroids; for example, betamethasone (Celestone) when gestation is between 28 and 32 weeks. Repeat dose if delivery does not occur within 1 week.	Stimulates the synthesis of fetal surfactant, which promotes fetal lung maturity and thereby reduces risk of respiratory distress syndrome. Note: Concomitant use with tocolytics potentiates risk of maternal pulmonary edema.

INTERVENTIONS	RATIONALE
Collaborative	
Administer antibiotics. (Refer to Nursing Diagnosis: Infection, potential for, below.)	Used if there is evidence of chorioamnionitis and plan for labor induction or cesarean delivery is delayed dependent on fetal age.

NURSING DIAGNOSIS: **Infection, potential for.**

SUPPORTING DATA/CONTRIBUTING FACTORS: **Premature rupture of membranes (PROM) creates risk of ascending maternal infection and fetal sepsis/preterm labor.**

GENERAL PATIENT OUTCOMES: **Mother/fetus free of signs of infection.**

INTERVENTIONS	RATIONALE
Independent	
Assess color/nature/amount of vaginal discharge, test with nitrazine paper. Assess history for possible "gush of water."	Amniotic fluid is alkaline and turns nitrazine paper from yellow to blue. Meconium-stained amniotic fluid suggests fetal distress in response to hypoxia. Large amount of fluid (polyhydramnios) is associated with congential anomalies, diabetes. With prolonged rupture of membranes, ascending infection (endometritis/chorioamnionitis) may result, manifested by foul vaginal discharge.
Provide perineal care to mother as indicated.	Reduces risk of ascending tract infection/chorioamnionitis.
Monitor maternal vital signs.	Increased temperature, pulse, and respiratory rate may be suggestive of infectious process.
Monitor FHR, using continuous electronic monitoring if available.	Fetal sepsis owing to PROM and ascending infection will be manifested by tachycardia: FHR greater than 160 beats/minute.
Collaborative	
Monitor white blood cell (WBC) and differential.	As prenatal patient approaches term, WBC may increase to as high as 20,000, but a patient with sepsis often has leukopenia, which may actually fall within normal limits for the nonpregnant patient. (Note: Increased WBC also can exist in intra-abdominal hemorrhage.)
Collect vaginal pool specimen for gram stain, identification of ferning/nitrazine test.	Gram staining is necessary to identify bacterial growth. If membranes are ruptured, nitrazine paper will turn blue, ferning (arborization) will be microscopically visible on a slide.

INTERVENTIONS	RATIONALE
Collaborative	
Obtain blood cultures as indicated.	Presence of infection or signs/symptoms of sepsis require close monitoring. (Refer to Care Plan: Sepsis/Septicemia/Septic Shock, page 329.)
Administer antibiotic parenterally as indicated.	Treatment of maternal infection (chorioamnionitis) may alleviate likelihood of fetal sepsis developing.
Assist with amniocentesis to determine fetal lung maturity. (Refer to Nursing Diagnosis: Injury, potential for, premature labor, page 421.)	Once membranes have ruptured, establishing fetal maturity is necessary to determine appropriate interventions. Note: If maternal infection develops, the fetus is delivered, regardless of gestational age.

NURSING DIAGNOSIS:	**Tissue Perfusion, alteration in, peripheral (potential for thromboemboli).**
SUPPORTING DATA/CONTRIBUTING FACTORS:	**Chance of thromboembolism is greater in pregnant than in nonpregnant patient owing to natural increase in clotting factors (VII, IX, X, fibrinogen) and a decrease in fibrinolytic activity (clot lysing) as well as increased Hct levels. Immobility/trauma increases likelihood of phlebitis/emboli formation.**
GENERAL PATIENT OUTCOMES:	**Thrombophlebitis and/or pulmonary emboli are prevented.**

INTERVENTIONS	RATIONALE
Independent	
Assess for presence of positive Homan's sign, calf redness/swelling/tenderness.	Pain on passive dorsiflexion of the foot is indicative of deep vein thrombosis, and erythema reflects superficial involvement.
Assess for faintness. Encourage patient to avoid changing position rapidly.	Sudden position changes may result in dizziness as blood pools in lower extremities, reducing circulating volume.
Assist patient with range of motion exercises.	Aids in enhancing venous return. Pregnant patients are prone to venous stasis in the lower extremities owing to pressure of the uterus on the vena cava. This creates the perfect environment for thrombi to form.
Investigate complaints of shortness of breath, severe chest pain.	May reflect presence of pulmonary emboli.

INTERVENTIONS	RATIONALE
Collaborative	
Apply antiembolic hose.	May reduce venous stasis, improve venous return, and reduce risk of thrombophlebitis.
Administer heparin in documented deep vein thrombosis/pulmonary embolus.	Prevents/reduces further clot formation. Heparin can be given safely to obstetric patients because its large molecular size does not cross the placenta, provided it is discontinued 6 to 12 hours prior to delivery. It may be reinstituted 6 hours after vaginal delivery and 12 to 24 hours following cesarean section (these intervals remain controversial).
Avoid use of Coumadin.	Coumadin crosses the placenta and should not be given because of teratogenic effects early in pregnancy and the problem of fetal anticoagulation later in pregnancy.

NURSING DIAGNOSIS:	**Comfort, alteration in, pain, acute.**
SUPPORTING DATA/CONTRIBUTING FACTORS:	**Degree of discomfort/nature of pain and its presence/absence may be helpful in differential diagnosis (e.g., abdominal trauma/abruptio placenta). Signs of labor precipitated by trauma/patient's condition may be accompanied by pain.**
GENERAL PATIENT OUTCOMES:	**Verbalizes relief of pain/discomfort. Signs of labor are detected/treated appropriately.**

INTERVENTIONS	RATIONALE
Independent	
Assess nature/location of pain, obvious injuries. Note nonspecific pain on movement;	Assists in determining differential diagnosis. Helps in determining nature/severity of injuries; for example, nonspecific pain on movement may indicate pelvic fracture (the most common fracture in prenatal patient) and may be responsible for large hemorrhagic losses.
Sharp abdominal/suprapubic pain which then disappears; rapid, shallow breathing; hypotension; reduced/absent fetal heart tones and movement;	Suggests possible uterine rupture, which is preceded by intense pain which then subsides as total rupture occurs.
Persistent/sharp abdominal pain/boardlike abdomen, with visible/concealed (retroplacental) bleeding. May note signs of preterm labor/DIC as sequelae. (Refer to Nursing Diagnosis: Fluid Volume Deficit, potential, page 413.)	Suggests placental separation. If 25 percent of placenta separates, vaginal bleeding and preterm labor often occur. If 50 percent of placenta separates, DIC, uterine tetany, maternal shock, and fetal demise may follow.

INTERVENTIONS	RATIONALE
Independent	
Right upper quadrant pain, nausea/vomiting, abdominal guarding/rigidity, presence/absence of bowel sounds. Distinguish between symptoms related to PIH involvement of organs and trauma injury.	Helps rule out liver/spleen rupture. In pregnancy, stretching of abdominal wall often alters normal responses to intraperitoneal stimuli, making abdominal examination difficult.
Monitor for signs of labor/onset of regular contractions.	Preterm labor often follows injury. (Refer to Nursing Diagnosis: Injury, potential for, premature labor, page 421.)
Collaborative	
Administer medication (e.g., Demerol, Stadol, Nubain) after differential diagnosis is made.	Small, frequent doses of these drugs may alleviate pain without undue sedation/fetal effects.

NURSING DIAGNOSIS: **Anxiety.**

SUPPORTING DATA/CONTRIBUTING FACTORS: **Anxiety/stress, with its stimulation of the adrenal cortex, is accompanied by release of catecholamines, which cause generalized vasoconstriction, possible maternal/fetal tachycardia, hypertension, and reduced placental circulation. Any medical emergency is stress producing, yet the stress level for the pregnant patient/couple may be greater than anticipated because of concern for the well-being of both the mother and her unborn child. Extent of anxiety may be related to the gestation of the fetus and nature/extent of maternal injuries/prognosis for recovery. If the patient is comatose/unable to respond, the husband or supportive other's anxiety may be intensified.**

GENERAL PATIENT OUTCOMES: **Verbalizes fears/concerns for self and fetus. Vital signs (once stabilized) remain within patient normals.**

INTERVENTIONS	RATIONALE
Independent	
Provide primary nurse.	Helps ensure continuity of care, may reduce anxiety, and assist patient to develop trusting relationship and to feel comfortable in identifying/discussing fears.

INTERVENTIONS	RATIONALE
Independent	
Orient to environment/staff/procedures as possible.	Reduces fear associated with the unknown.
Assume unhurried attitude, convey calm in verbal/nonverbal responses.	Facilitates relaxation.
Assess physiologic response to anxiety (e.g., BP, pulse, respirations, FHR).	Prolonged anxiety can result in maternal/fetal tachycardia, elevated BP, pulse, respirations.
Assess stress level associated with the complication/reason for hospitalization. Note perception of illness, clarify misconceptions.	May help identify amount of emotional support necessary (e.g., referral prior to discharge). Misunderstandings may unnecessarily magnify anxiety.
Discuss response to hospitalization/impact on pregnancy.	In the prenatal patient requiring hospitalization, stress levels tend to increase after the first two weeks and remain elevated throughout the remainder of the hospitalization.
Assist patient in relaxation techniques (e.g., breathing, visualization).	Provides opportunity for patient to do something to reduce anxiety and to feel a sense of control.
Provide information as available/requested about extent of injury and treatment. Answer questions directly/honestly. Reinforce positive aspects of maternal/fetal condition.	Anxiety level may be reduced when patient/couple are able to have access to all available information/implications of injury for mother/fetus.
Assess relationship of patient to supportive other/husband/family members, support systems available.	Anxiety will be greater if patient is without necessary family supports and may necessitate resource persons such as social service, clergy.
Provide time alone for couple/family members to verbalize fears/concerns.	Provision for time alone is crucial to promotion of family integration. Each person may be reluctant to honestly share anxieties for fear of upsetting one another.
Collaborative	
Administer mild sedation as indicated.	Anxiety/stress can increase CO and heart rate to the point that the patient can no longer tolerate the increased workload.
Refer to psychiatric nurse clinician/therapist.	May be useful in facilitating expression of concerns and may help couple work through feelings.

NURSING DIAGNOSIS: **Coping, ineffective, individual/family (potential).**

SUPPORTING DATA/CONTRIBUTING FACTORS: **A situational crisis precipitated by the alteration in maternal health can cause severe emotional turmoil for the pregnant patient/couple. Emotional response/ability to cope positively with the traumatic event may depend on effective coping mechanisms developed in dealing with past stressors, availability of support systems/resources, prognosis for both patient**

	and fetus, and events surrounding the injury/event. If the hospitalization is necessitated by trauma/accident, guilt feelings within the patient/couple may be so overwhelming that initially she/they cannot effectively cope with the hospitalization, process information given, or participate in critical decision making. If the prognosis is poor or the outcome fatal for the mother, the fetus, or both, the husband/family/significant other may be overwhelmed with grief and unable to function/make necessary decisions regarding treatment, autopsy requests, and funeral arrangements and may resort to denial for a prolonged period of time rather than begin to move through the stages of grief.
GENERAL PATIENT OUTCOMES:	**Demonstrates initial appropriate grieving/coping with presenting stressors and verbalizes feelings/plans.**

INTERVENTIONS	RATIONALE
Independent	
Evaluate patient/couple's perception/response to events necessitating hospitalization.	Provides information for data base to develop plan of care.
Assess strength/weaknesses of couple's relationship/availability of support systems/religious practices/beliefs.	Strength of marriage/relationship will have impact on short-term and long-term adaptation. In the event of abortion, patient may desire that products of conception be baptized.
Note gestation of current pregnancy.	Prognosis for fetal viability/outcome is better as term approaches.
Evaluate past experiences with conception/childbearing.	Past experiences such as previous child losses, problems with infertility, pregnancy complications may interfere with couple's ability to deal with current stress.
Ascertain previous coping strategies.	Past behaviors may be predictive of ability to cope with current crisis.
Evaluate patient's past/current response to pregnancy/fetus.	Long-term hospitalization may interfere with patient/couple's ability to accomplish the psychologic tasks of pregnancy, placing family at risk for ineffective parenting/attachment to pregnancy/fetus.
Assess coping strategies, initiation of grief process, stage of grieving.	Even with a positive prognosis, patient may experience normal grief for the loss of the uncomplicated pregnancy and continued concerns for fetal well-being.

INTERVENTIONS	RATIONALE
Independent	
Assess for maladaptive behaviors, negative coping. Make appropriate referrals to clergy/counseling.	May indicate a need for more intensive psychologic/spiritual support, especially if life of mother/fetus is threatened.
In the event of fetal/maternal death, offer emotional support/assist in making arrangements for funeral/burial/autopsy.	Stunned/grief-stricken, the husband and/or family may need support/guidance/information about how to proceed.
Collaborative	
Make referrals to appropriate community agencies; for example, social services, parenting classes, Visiting Nurse Association.	May need additional assistance to cope with stressors presented by the unexpected change in events.

NURSING DIAGNOSIS:	**Knowledge Deficit (Learning Need).**
SUPPORTING DATA/CONTRIBUTING FACTORS:	**Lack of understanding/misconceptions related to the nature of injury, pathologic process, prescribed treatment, and prognosis for pregnancy/fetus/patient may cause excess anxiety, concern.**
GENERAL PATIENT OUTCOMES:	**Demonstrates understanding about her condition by verbalizing about physiologic changes/rationale for treatment/potential outcomes for self and the fetus.**

INTERVENTIONS	RATIONALE
Independent	
Assess understanding of hospitalization/protocol of care.	Establishes learning needs.
Correct misconceptions. Provide information about extent of injuries/pathologic process short-term/long-term implications. Explain rationale of care/procedures/tests. Maintain ongoing communication.	Helpful in relieving anxiety associated with the unknown, facilitates cooperation with protocol of care.
Obtain informed consent for necessary treatment.	In the event the patient is unable to sign the consent, the husband/family member may give permission for surgery/emergency treatment.

APPENDIX

FLUID AND ELECTROLYTE IMBALANCES

Assessment Factors and Management

The body's fluid balance depends on the net gain or loss of two components: water and its dominant electrolyte, sodium (Na).

Hypervolemia (Extracellular Fluid Volume Excess)

PATIENT ASSESSMENT DATA BASE

HISTORY

Excess sodium intake/hypertonic fluid replacement.

Excessive, rapid administration of parenteral fluids.

Post surgery (increased release of ADH).

Decreased plasma proteins as may occur with chronic liver disease with ascites, major abdominal surgery, malnutrition/protein depletion.

Chronic kidney disease/acute renal failure.

Congestive heart failure.

Excessive adrenocortical hormone production or hyperaldosteronism.

Subjective

May complain of fatigue, dyspnea, thirst, anorexia, nausea/vomiting, constipation, decreased urinary output.

DIAGNOSTIC STUDIES

Serum sodium may be high, low, or normal.

Urine sodium may be low because of sodium retention.

Total protein: albumin may be decreased.

Serum osmolality: usually unchanged, although hyposmolality may occur.

Serum potassium and BUN: normal or decreased, unless renal damage present.

Urine specific gravity: decreased.

Hct may be normal or decreased, reflecting hemodilution.

Chest x-ray may reveal signs of congestion.

PHYSICAL EXAMINATION

Blood pressure may be elevated.

Pulse may be full/bounding; tachycardia usually present; bradycardia is a late sign of cardiac decompensation.

Heart sounds: extra sounds (S_3) may be noted.

Respirations/breath sounds: tachypneic with/without dyspnea, orthopnea; crackles, productive cough may be present.

Edema: anasarca (generalized), dependent edema; pitting edema, facial edema, periorbital edema.

Neck veins may be distended. CVP increased.

Abdomen: increased girth with fluid wave may be noted.

Weight: acute gain, often in excess of 5 percent of total body weight.

Skin: pale, moist, taut, and cool where edematous.

INTERVENTIONS	RATIONALE
Independent	
Monitor vital signs and hemodynamic parameters; for example, central venous pressure (CVP), pulmonary capillary wedge pressure (PCWP).	Tachycardia and hypertension are common manifestations. Tachypnea usually present with/without dyspnea. Elevations of CVP and PCWP may be noted before dyspnea and adventitious breath sounds occur.
Auscultate lungs and heart sounds. Encourage coughing/deep breathing exercises.	Adventitious sounds (crackles) and extra heart sounds are indicative of fluid excess. Pulmonary edema may develop rapidly. Pulmonary fluid shifts potentiate the risks of respiratory complications.
Assess for presence/location of edema formation.	Edema may be generalized or localized in dependent areas. Elderly patients may develop dependent edema with relatively little excess fluid. Patients in a supine position can have an increase of 4 to 8 liters of fluid before edema is detected.
Note presence of neck vein distention, pitting edema, dyspnea.	Signs of congestive heart failure. Neck vein distention, positive hepatojugular reflex, dyspnea, and pitting edema indicate extracellular fluid excess with cardiac decompensation.
Maintain accurate intake/output. Note decreased urine output, positive fluid balance.	Urine output may be low because of decreased renal perfusion, cardiac insufficiency, and fluid shifts/edema formation.
Weigh as indicated.	Weight gain of 2.2 pounds equals 1 liter of fluid retention.

INTERVENTIONS	RATIONALE
Independent	
Give oral fluids with caution. If fluids are restricted, set up a 24-hour schedule for fluid intake.	Fluid restriction/extracellular shifts can cause drying of mucous membranes, and patient may desire more fluids than is prudent.
Monitor infusion rate of parenteral fluids.	Sudden fluid bolus/prolonged excessive administration potentiates risk of volume overload/cardiac decompensation.
Maintain semi-Fowler's position if dyspnea or ascites is present.	Gravity improves lung expansion by lowering diaphragm and shifting fluid to lower abdominal cavity.
Turn and position frequently. Provide skin care.	Edematous tissue is more prone to breakdown than is normal tissue.
Promote bedrest. Schedule care to provide frequent rest periods.	Limited cardiac reserves result in activity intolerances.
Provide safety precautions as indicated; for example, use of side rails, bed in low position, frequent observation, soft restraints (if required).	Fluid shifts may cause cerebral edema/changes in mentation, especially in the geriatric population.
Collaborative	
Assist with identification/treatment of underlying cause.	Refer to history for listing of predisposing/contributing factors.
Monitor laboratory studies as indicated; for example, electrolytes, blood urea nitrogen (BUN), arterial blood gases (ABGs).	Extracellular fluid shifts, sodium/water restriction, and renal function all affect serum sodium levels. Potassium deficit may occur with diuretic therapy. Blood urea nitrogen may be increased owing to renal dysfunction/failure. Arterial blood gases may reflect metabolic acidosis.
Provide high-protein, low-sodium diet. Restrict fluids as indicated.	Increased serum proteins can enhance colloidal osmotic gradients and promote return of fluid to the vascular space. Restriction of sodium/water decreases extracellular fluid retention.
Administer diuretics; for example, furosemide (Lasix).	Decreases total body water.
Replace potassium losses as indicated.	Potassium deficit may cause lethal cardiac arrhythmias if untreated.
Assist with dialysis/ultrafiltration, if needed.	Provides more rapid reduction of fluid overload, especially in the presence of severe cardiac/renal failure.

Hypovolemia (Extracellular Fluid Volume Deficit)

PATIENT ASSESSMENT DATA BASE

HISTORY

Vomiting, gastric suctioning, diarrhea.

Systemic infections, fever, diaphoresis.

Intestinal obstruction or fistulas.

Decreased fluid intake; for example, preoperative/postoperative NPO status.

Pancreatitis, peritonitis, cirrhosis/ascites.

Wounds or burns, intraoperative fluid loss, hemorrhage.

Kidney disease, diabetic ketoacidosis, HHNC, diabetes insipidus.

Subjective

May complain of thirst, anorexia, nausea/vomiting, constipation (occasionally diarrhea), abdominal cramps. May also report fatigue, tingling of the extremities, vertigo, syncope, generalized weakness.

DIAGNOSTIC STUDIES

Serum sodium may be normal, high, or low.

Urine sodium: usually decreased (less than 10 mEq when losses are from external causes, usually above 20 mEq if the cause is renal or adrenal).

Hct: increased (hemoconcentration) or decreased (hemorrhage).

Serum glucose: normal or elevated.

Serum protein: increased.

BUN and creatinine: increased, with BUN out of proportion to creatinine.

Urine specific gravity: increased.

PHYSICAL EXAMINATION

Blood pressure: postural changes; for example, systolic blood pressure of 10 mmHg lower in sitting or standing than in supine position.

Respirations may be rapid/shallow.

Pulse may be weak/thready. Tachycardia usually present.

Mentation: behavior change, apathy, restlessness, and confusion may be noted.

Neck veins: usually flattened.

Skin may be dry with poor turgor, or pale, moist, clammy (shock). Mucous membranes may be dry; for example, furrows on tongue, decreased tearing and salivation.

Urine: decreased volume and dark/concentrated color. Oliguria (output less than 20 ml per hour or 480 ml in 24 hours) may indicate severe fluid depletion.

Weight: actual weight loss often exceeds 5 percent of total body weight.

Temperature: usually subnormal, although fever may occur.

Abdomen: distention may be present.

INTERVENTIONS	RATIONALE
Independent	
Monitor vital signs/hemodynamic parameters; for example, central venous pressure (CVP), mean arterial pressure (MAP), cardiac output (CO).	Tachycardia is present, as well as varying degrees of hypotension, depending on degree of fluid deficit. Hemodynamic measurements are useful in determining degree of deficit, organ perfusion, and response to therapy.
Observe for signs of shock; for example, pale, cool/	Conditions that contribute to extracellular fluid deficit

INTERVENTIONS	RATIONALE
Independent	
moist skin; changes in mentation; delayed capillary refill.	can result in inadequate organ perfusion to all areas and may cause circulatory collapse.
Monitor urine output. Measure/estimate total fluid losses (e.g., gastric losses, wound drainage, diaphoresis).	A decreased urine output may indicate insufficient renal perfusion/hypovolemia. Fluid replacement needs are based on correction of current deficits and ongoing losses.
Weigh daily and compare with 24-hour fluid balance. Mark/measure edematous areas (e.g., abdomen, limbs).	Changes in weight may not reflect intravascular volume accurately; for example, third spaced fluid accumulation cannot be used by the body for tissue perfusion.
Ascertain patient's beverage preferences and set up a 24-hour schedule for fluid intake. Encourage foods with high fluid content.	Relieves thirst and discomfort of dry mucous membranes and augments parenteral replacement.
Turn frequently, massage skin, and protect bony prominences.	Tissues are more susceptible to breakdown because of vasoconstriction and increased cellular fragility.
Provide skin and mouth care. Bathe every other day with mild soap.	Skin and mucous membranes are dry with decreased elasticity, owing to vasoconstriction and reduced intracellular water.
Provide safety precautions as indicated; for example, use of side rails, bed in low position, frequent observation, soft restraints (if required).	Decreased cerebral perfusion frequently results in changes in mentation/altered thought processes.
Investigate complaints of sudden/sharp chest pain, dyspnea, cyanosis, increased anxiety, restlessness.	Hemoconcentration (sludging) and increased platelet aggregation may result in systemic emboli formation.
Monitor for sudden/marked elevation of blood pressure, restlessness, moist cough, dyspnea, basalar crackles, frothy sputum.	Too rapid a correction of fluid deficit may compromise the cardiopulmonary system, especially if using colloids with general fluid replacement, because increased osmotic pressure potentiates fluid shifts.
Collaborative	
Assist with identification/treatment of underlying cause.	Refer to history for listing of predisposing/contributing factors.
Monitor laboratory studies as indicated (e.g., electrolytes, glucose, pH/$PaCO_2$, coagulation studies).	Depending on the avenue of fluid loss, differing electrolyte imbalances may be present/require correction. Use of glucose solutions in patients with underlying glucose intolerance may result in serum glucose elevation and increased urinary water losses. Alterations in acid-base balance may be further compromised by infusion of lactate solutions.
Administer intravenous (IV) solutions as indicated; for example,	
Isotonic solutions (e.g., normal saline, Lactated Ringer's),	Crystalloids provide prompt circulatory improvement. However, the benefit may be transient because of increased renal clearance. In addition, use of buffered crystalloids (LR) may potentiate the risk of metabolic acidosis.

INTERVENTIONS	RATIONALE
Independent	
Colloids; for example, dextran, plasmanate/albumin, hetastarch (Hespan);	Corrects plasma protein concentration deficits, thereby increasing intravascular osmotic pressure and facilitating return of fluid into vascular compartment.
Whole blood/packed red blood cells.	Indicated when hypovolemia is related to blood loss.
Administer sodium bicarbonate ($NaHCO_3$) if indicated.	May be given to correct severe acidosis while increasing the serum sodium level.

SODIUM

Sodium is the major cation of extracellular fluid (ECF) and is primarily responsible for osmotic pressure in that compartment. Sodium enhances neuromuscular conduction/transmission of impulses and is essential for maintaining acid-base balance.

Hyponatremia (Sodium Deficit)

PATIENT ASSESSMENT DATA BASE

HISTORY

Primary hyponatremia may be due to lack of ingestion of sodium, infusion of sodium-free solutions, salt-wasting renal dysfunction, severe malnutrition. Excessive sodium losses may be through sweating, wounds/trauma (hemorrhage), gastric suctioning, diarrhea, vomiting, adrenal insufficiency (Addison's disease).

Dilutional hyponatremia may be due to excessive water intake/electrolyte-free infusion, water intoxication (IV therapy, tap water enemas), inhalation of fresh water (drowning victim), gastric irrigations with electrolyte-free solutions, SIADH (syndrome of inappropriate antidiuretic hormone), CHF, renal failure/nephrotic syndrome, hepatic cirrhosis, diabetes mellitus (hyperglycemia). Note: A pseudohyponatremia may occur in presence of multiple myeloma, hyperlipidemia, or hypoproteinemia but does not reflect an actual abnormality of water metabolism.

Subjective

May complain of headache, weakness, faintness, muscle cramps, nausea, anorexia, blurred vision.

DIAGNOSTIC STUDIES

Serum sodium: decreased less than 135 mEq/liters, (although symptoms may not appear until levels are 125 or below, as may be noted in SIADH).

Urine sodium: less than 20 mEq/liter unless sodium-wasting nephropathy present.

Serum potassium may be decreased as the kidneys attempt to conserve sodium at the expense of potassium.

Serum chloride//HCO_3: levels are decreased, depending on which ion is lost with the sodium.

Osmolality: commonly low; may be normal (pseudohyponatremia) or high (HHNC).

Urine osmolality: usually less than 100 mOsmol/liter, unless SIADH present, in which case it will exceed serum osmolality.

Urine specific gravity may be decreased less than 1.010, or increased greater than 1.020 (if SIADH present).

Hct is dependent on fluid state; for example, fluid excess versus dehydration.

BUN may be elevated in presence of fluid excess.

PHYSICAL EXAMINATION

Sodium/Water Deficit

Skin: flushed, dry, hot, poor skin turgor; soft/sunken eyeballs.

Mucous membranes: dry, with decreased saliva.

Neuromuscular: muscle twitching may be present.

Respirations: hyperpnea may be noted.

Urine output may be decreased.

Mentation may be lethargic, restless, confused, stuporous.

Sodium Deficit/Water Excess

Blood pressure: hypertension usually present.

Urine output increased.

Skin: generalized edema.

Neuromuscular: general weakness noted.

Severe Sodium Deficit

Blood pressure: hypotension may occur with vasomotor collapse.

Pulse: rapid, thready.

Skin: cold/clammy, fingerprinting on sternum; cyanosis may be noted.

Mentation: coma/convulsions may occur.

INTERVENTIONS	RATIONALE
Independent	
Monitor intake and output. Calculate fluid balance. Weigh daily.	Indicator of fluid balance because either fluid excess or deficit may occur with hyponatremia.
Assess level of consciousness/neuromuscular response.	Sodium deficit may result in decreased mentation to point of coma, as well as generalized muscle weakness/cramps/convulsions.
Maintain quiet environment, provide safety/seizure precautions.	Reduces central nervous system (CNS) stimulation, thereby decreasing risk of injury from neurologic complications (e.g., seizures).
Encourage foods and fluids high in sodium; for example, milk, meat, eggs, carrots, beets, and celery. Use fruit juices and bouillon primarily instead of water.	Unless sodium deficit causes serious symptoms, the patient may benefit from slower replacement by oral method or from removal of salt restriction.
Irrigate nasogastric tube (when used) with normal saline (NS), not water (H_2O).	Isotonic irrigation will minimize loss of gastrointestinal (GI) electrolytes.
Collaborative	
Assist with identification/treatment of underlying cause.	Refer to history for listing of predisposing/contributing factors.

INTERVENTIONS	RATIONALE
Collaborative	
Monitor serum electrolytes/osmolality.	Evaluates therapy needs/effectiveness.
Administer/restrict fluids, depending on fluid volume status.	In presence of hypovolemia, replace volume losses with isotonic saline. In the presence of normal/hypervolemia (SIADH), fluid restriction is indicated.
Administer medications as indicated; for example,	
Furosemide (Lasix),	Effective in reducing fluid excess to correct sodium/water balance.
Sodium chloride,	Small amounts of sodium may need to be replaced for severe symptomatology (e.g., seizures).
Potassium chloride,	Corrects potassium deficit and may enhance action of diuretic.
Demeclocycline (Declomycin).	Useful in treating SIADH in place of severe water restriction, which may not be tolerated by all patients (e.g., chronic obstructive pulmonary disease). Note: This may be contraindicated in patients with liver disease because nephrotoxicity may occur.

Hypernatremia (Sodium Excess)

PATIENT ASSESSMENT DATA BASE

HISTORY

Water loss: polyuria (e.g., diabetes mellitus or insipidus); use of osmotic diuretics, such as Mannitol. Presence of fever; diarrhea; or disease processes that increase extracellular fluid volume (e.g., renal disease, primary aldosteronism, excessive steroids, as in Cushing's disease).

Insufficient water intake/dehydration; administration of tube feedings/high-protein diets with minimal fluid intake; ulcer diets primarily using half and half.

Excessive ingestion of sodium chloride; inhalation of salt water (drowning victim).

Subjective

May complain of thirst unless hypothalamic lesion present.

DIAGNOSTIC STUDIES

Serum sodium: increased greater than 145 mEq/liter. Serum levels greater than 160 mEq/liter may be accompanied by severe neurologic signs.

Serum chloride: increased greater than 106 mEq/liter.

Serum potassium: decreased.

Serum osmolality: greater than 295 mOsmol/liter when dehydrated; lower in presence of extracellular fluid excess.

Hct: may be normal or elevated.

Urine sodium: less than 50 mEq/liter.

Urine chloride: less than 50 mEq/liter.

Urine osmolality: greater than 800 mOsmol/liter.

Urine specific gravity: increased greater than 1.030 if water deficit present, except when hypernatremia is due to polyuria.

PHYSICAL EXAMINATION

Sodium Excess/Water Deficit

Skin: hot, dry, flushed.

Mucous membranes: dry, sticky.

Mentation: irritability; lethargy/coma may occur.

Neuromuscular: rigidity/tremors, generalized weakness.

Blood pressure: postural hypotension may be noted.

Pulse: tachycardia present.

Urine output decreased.

Sodium/Water Excess

Skin: pale, moist, taut, with pitting edema.

Weight gain may be noted.

Mentation: confusion, lethargy may be present.

Blood pressure: elevated.

Respirations may be dyspneic.

Urine output: polyuria may be present.

INTERVENTIONS	RATIONALE
Independent	
Monitor vital signs (e.g., blood pressure).	Either hypertension or hypotension may be present, depending on the fluid status. Presence of postural hypotension may affect activity tolerance.
Monitor intake/output, urine specific gravity. Weigh daily. Assess presence/location of edema.	These parameters are variable, depending on fluid status, and are indicators of therapy needs/effectiveness.
Assess level of consciousness and neuromuscular status (e.g., strength, tone, movement).	In presence of water deficit, rapid rehydration may result in cerebral edema.
Assess mucous membrane/skin turgor, and note color, temperature, moisture.	Water deficit will be manifested by signs of dehydration.
Provide meticulous skin care, massage, lotion, frequent repositioning.	Maintains skin integrity.
Provide frequent oral care. Avoid use of mouthwash/rinse that contains alcohol.	Prevents further drying of mucous membranes.
Maintain seizure precautions.	Sodium excess/cerebral edema increases risk of convulsions.

Collaborative

Assist with identification/treatment of underlying cause.

Refer to history for list of predisposing/contributing factors.

Monitor serum electrolytes and osmolality.

Evaluates therapy needs/effectiveness.

Increase oral/intravenous (IV) fluid intake; for example, 5 percent dextrose in water (in presence of dehydration) or isotonic solutions (0.9 sodium chloride) (if extracellular deficit present).

Replacement of total body water deficit will restore sodium/water balance gradually. Note: Rapid reduction of serum sodium level with corresponding decrease in serum osmolality can cause cerebral edema/convulsions.

Administer diuretics; for example, furosemide (Lasix). Restrict sodium intake in presence of extracellular fluid excess.

Restriction of intake and enhanced renal clearance lowers serum sodium levels.

POTASSIUM

Potassium is the major cation of the intracellular fluid and is responsible for maintaining intracellular osmotic pressure. Potassium also regulates neuromuscular excitability; aids in maintenance of acid-base balance, synthesis of protein, and metabolism of carbohydrates.

Hypokalemia (Potassium Deficit)

PATIENT ASSESSMENT DATA BASE

HISTORY

Renal loss: use of potassium-wasting diuretics, diuresis phase of ATN, healing phase of burns, diabetic acidosis, Cushing's syndrome, nephritis, hypomagnesium, steroid administration.

Gastric loss: vomiting, diarrhea, inflammatory bowel disease, excess use of laxatives, GI suction or fistulas.

Liver disease.

Inadequate intake: starvation, high-sodium diet.

Use of TPN resulting in hypersecretion of insulin.

Severe alkalosis or use of IV glucose/insulin solutions to reverse acidosis (drives potassium into cell, lowering serum level).

Subjective

May complain of muscle pain/cramps, generalized weakness, paresthesia, anorexia, nausea/vomiting.

DIAGNOSTIC STUDIES

Serum potassium: decreased, less than 3.5 mEq/liter.

Serum chloride: often decreased, less than 98 mEq/liter.

Plasma bicarbonate: increased above 29 mEq/liter.

Urine osmolality: decreased.

ECG: low voltage; flat T-wave, appearance of U-wave, depressed S-T segment, peaking of P waves, ventricular dysrhythmias.

PHYSICAL EXAMINATION

Blood pressure: hypotension may be present owing to decreased stroke volume.

Respirations: hypoventilation/decreased respiratory depth owing to muscle weakness; cyanosis may be noted.

Pulses: weak/diminished, may be irregular.

Heart sounds: distant. Dysrhythmias/irregularities noted.

Bowel sounds: decreased.

Abdomen: distention may be present (paralytic ileus).

Mentation: depressed mental state/confusion, apathy, drowsiness, irritability, coma.

Musculoskeletal: hyporeflexia, tetany, paralysis may occur.

Urine: nocturia, polyuria may be present if factors contributing to hypokalemia include CHF or diabetes mellitus.

INTERVENTIONS	RATIONALE
Independent	
Monitor cardiac rhythm. Observe for pulse/electrocardiogram (ECG) changes.	Tachycardia may develop, and potentially life-threatening arrhythmias; for example, PVCs, sinus bradycardia, AV blocks, AV dissociation, and ventricular tachycardia may occur.
Monitor respiratory rate, depth, effort. Encourage cough/deep breathing exercises. Reposition frequently.	Repiratory muscle weakness may proceed to paralysis and eventual respiratory arrest.
Assess level of consciousness and neuromuscular function (e.g., strength, sensation, movement).	Apathy, drowsiness, irritability, tetany, parathesias, and coma may occur.
Auscultate bowel sounds, noting decrease/absence/change.	Paralytic ileus commonly follows gastric losses through vomiting/gastric suction.
Maintain accurate record of urinary, gastric, and wound losses.	Guide for calculating fluid/potassium replacement needs.
Monitor rate of IV potassium administration, using micro/minidrop infusion devices. Check for side effects.	Assures controlled delivery of medication to prevent bolus effect and to reduce associated discomfort (e.g., burning sensation at IV site).
Encourage intake of foods and fluids high in potassium; for example, bananas, orange juice, meat, coffee, colas, tea, leafy vegetables.	Lost potassium may be replaced through the diet if the patient is allowed oral food and fluids.
Dilute oral potassium supplements with 4 oz water/juice and give after meals.	May prevent/reduce gastrointestinal (GI) irritation.
Watch for signs of digitalis intoxication as indicated.	Low potassium enhances effect of digitalis, slowing cardiac conduction. Note: Use of digitalis, diuretics, and a hypokalemia state may produce lethal dysrhythmias.
Observe for signs of metabolic alkalosis, e.g., hypoventilation, tachycardia, dysrhythmias, tetany, changes in mentation, changes in arterial blood gases (ABGs). (Refer to Metabolic Alkalosis, page 454.)	Frequently precedes/follows hypokalemia.

Collaborative

Assist with identification/treatment of underlying cause.	Refer to history for list of predisposing/contributing factors.
Monitor serum potassium and note significant changes.	Levels should be checked frequently during replacement therapy, especially in the presence of insufficient renal function. Sudden excess/elevation may cause cardiac dysrhythmias.
Administer oral and/or IV potassium. Correct acid-base imbalance.	Parenteral replacement should not exceed 40 mEq per 2-hour period. Dietary supplementation also may be used to produce a gradual equilibration if patient is able to take oral food and fluids. Correction of alkalosis will increase serum potassium level and reduce replacement needs. Correction of acidosis will drive potassium back into cells, resulting in decreased serum levels and increased replacement needs.

Hyperkalemia (Potassium Excess)

PATIENT ASSESSMENT DATA BASE

HISTORY

Decreased renal excretion: renal disease/acute failure, hypovolemia. Use of potassium-sparing diuretics or too rapid IV administration of potassium.

Excessive potassium intake: salt substitutes, drugs containing potassium; for example, penicillin.

Release of potassium into serum by destruction of tissue/cells; for example, severe catabolism, burns, crush injuries, myocardial infarction, severe hemolysis, rhabdomyolysis, massive transfusion of banked blood.

Adrenocortical insufficiency (Addison's disease), potassium retained and sodium lost from inadequate amounts of glucocorticoid and mineralocorticoid hormones.

Shifts of potassium out of the cell owing to metabolic acidosis, anoxia.

Insulin deficiency.

Subjective

May complain of nausea, vomiting, diarrhea, generalized weakness, paresthesia.

DIAGNOSTIC STUDIES

Serum potassium: increased greater than 5.5 mEq/liter. Note: Presence of elevated leukocyte or thrombocyte count may cause a pseudohyperkalemia.

Renal function studies may be altered, indicating failure.

ECG changes: T waves elevated and tented, prolonged P-R interval, loss of P waves, widening of QRS complex, and ST segment depression; atrial/ventricular dysrhythmias (e.g., bradycardia, atrial arrest, ventricular fibrillation, cardiac arrest).

PHYSICAL EXAMINATION

Pulse may be irregular.

Musculoskeletal: decreased deep tendon reflexes, progressive flaccid paralysis, twitching, seizures.

Urine volume may be decreased.

Abdomen: hyperactive bowel sounds/increased gastric motility with diarrhea, intestinal colic, nausea, or gastrointestinal (GI) irritability.

INTERVENTIONS	RATIONALE
Independent	
Monitor electrocardiogram (ECG) changes/cardiac rhythm. Be aware that cardiac arrest can occur.	Hyperkalemia depresses myocardial conduction. Bradycardia can progress to cardiac fibrillation/arrest.
Monitor urine output.	In kidney failure, potassium is retained owing to improper excretion. Potassium should not be given if oliguria or anuria is present.
Assess level of consciousness, neuromuscular function (e.g., movement, strength, sensation).	Patient is usually awake and alert, but muscular parathesia, weakness, and flaccid paralysis may occur.
Provide range of motion exercises.	Improves muscular tone and reduces muscle cramps and pain.
Provide frequent rest periods, assist with care activities.	General muscle weakness produces decreased activity tolerance.
Identify/discontinue oral/medicinal sources of potassium (e.g., tomatoes, orange juice, bananas, penicillin).	Facilitates reduction of potassium level and may prevent recurrence of hyperkalemia.
Monitor respiratory rate and depth. Elevate head of bed. Encourage cough/deep breathing exercises.	Patients may hypoventilate and may retain carbon dioxide, leading to respiratory acidosis and respiratory infection. Muscular weakness can affect respiratory muscles and can lead to respiratory complications/respiratory failure.
Collaborative	
Assist with identification/treatment of underlying cause.	Refer to history for list of predisposing/contributing factors.
Administer medications as indicated; for example,	
Intravenous glucose with insulin, sodium bicarbonate;	Short-term emergency measure to move potassium into the cell, thus reducing toxic serum level. Note: Use with caution in presence of CHF or hypernatremia.
Calcium gluconate/chloride;	Temporary measure that antagonizes toxic potassium depressant effects on heart and stimulates cardiac contractility. Note: Calcium is contraindicated in patients on digitalis, because it may result in dysrhythmias.
Sodium chloride,	Enhances renal excretion of potassium.
Diuretics; for example, furosemide (Lasix);	Enhances renal clearance and excretion of potassium.
Hypertonic Kay-exalate, per nasogastric tube/enema, with sorbitol.	Exchange resin, which exchanges potassium for sodium or calcium in the GI tract. Sorbitol enhances evacuation. Note: Use cautiously in patients with CHF, edema, and in elderly patients (contains sodium).

INTERVENTIONS	RATIONALE
Collaborative	
Monitor serum electrolytes, arterial blood gases (ABGs), blood urea nitrogen (BUN)/creatinine as indicated.	Evaluates therapy needs/effectiveness. Note: Hypoventilation may result in respiratory acidosis, thereby increasing serum potassium levels. Unmonitored use of sodium bicarbonate may create excessive alkalosis.
Administer diet low in potassium and protein. Restrict potassium-containing fluids and salt substitutes. Encourage sodium intake unless contraindicated. Increase carbohydrates in diet.	Eliminate exogenous sources of potassium. Sodium intake promotes potassium loss. Sodium deficiency may cause hyperkalemia. Prevents catabolic tissue breakdown with release of cellular potassium.
Provide fresh blood if transfusions required.	Fresh blood has less potassium than banked blood, because breakdown of older red cells releases potassium.
Prepare for/assist with dialysis (peritoneal or hemodialysis).	May be required when more conservative methods fail or are contraindicated (e.g., severe CHF). (Refer to Care Plan: Renal Dialysis, page 222.)

CALCIUM

Calcium is involved in bone formation/reabsorption, neural transmission/muscle contraction, regulation of enzyme systems, and is a coenzyme in blood coagulation.

Hypocalcemia (Calcium Deficit)

PATIENT ASSESSMENT DATA BASE

HISTORY

Excessive gastrointestinal losses: draining gastrointestinal fistula, diarrhea, fat malabsorption, chronic laxative use (particularly phosphate-containing laxatives/enemas).

Massive subcutaneous tissue infections, burns, peritonitis, acute pancreatitis, malignancies.

Extreme stress situations with mobilization and excretion of calcium.

Diuretic and terminal phase of renal failure.

Inadequate dietary intake, lack of milk/vitamin D, excessive protein diet.

Use of anticonvulsants, antibiotics, corticosteroids, excessive citrated blood, calcium-free infusions; rapid infusion of plasmonate.

Primary hypoparathyroidism: hyperphosphatemia, hypomagnesemia.

Malignant neoplasms with bone metastases.

Alkalosis.

Subjective

May report circumoral parathesia, numbness of fingers, muscle cramps, nausea/vomiting, diarrhea, abdominal pain.

DIAGNOSTIC STUDIES

Calcium decreased, less than 4.5 mEq/liter or 8.5 mg/dl.

Urine: Sulkowitch test shows no precipitate.

ECG: prolonged Q-T interval (characteristic). In severe deficiency, T waves may flatten or invert, giving appearance of hypokalemia or myocardial ischemia.

PHYSICAL EXAMINATION

Respirations: labored shallow breathing (bronchospasm may occur).

Musculoskeletal: muscle spasms (carpopedal and laryngo), tetany, tonic/clonic seizures, Trousseau's and Chvostek's signs are positive.

Pulse: weak/decreased, owing to weak cardiac contraction/premature dysrythmias.

Mentation: depression, psychoses may be present.

INTERVENTIONS	RATIONALE
Independent	
Monitor cardiac rhythm/cardiac output.	Calcium deficit weakens cardiac muscle/contractility. Digitalis effect is enhanced by calcium, and patient receiving calcium may develop digitalis intoxication.
Monitor respiratory rate, rhythm, effort. Have tracheostomy equipment available.	Laryngeal stridor may develop and result in respiratory emergency/arrest.
Observe for neuromuscular irritability (e.g., tetany, seizures). Assess for presence of Chvostek's/Trousseau's signs.	Calcium deficit causes repetitive and uncontrolled nerve transmission, leading to spasm of muscle groups.
Provide quiet environment and seizure precautions.	Reduces central nervous system (CNS) stimulation and protects patient from potential injury.
Promote relaxation/stress reduction techniques.	Tetany can be potentiated by hyperventilation and stress. Note: Direct pressure on the nerves also may cause tetany (e.g., tightening blood pressure cuff).
Check for bleeding from any source; for example, GI and genitourinary (GU) tract. Note presence of ecchymosis, petechiae.	Alterations in coagulation can occur as a result of calcium deficiency.
Review use of laxatives/antacids.	Those containing phosphate affect calcium metabolism.
Collaborative	
Assist with identification/treatment of underlying cause.	Refer to history for list of predisposing/contributing factors.
Monitor serum calcium and magnesium.	Evaluates therapy needs/effectiveness.
Administer calcium gluconate/chloride/gluceptate intravenous (IV) or oral preparations; for example, calcium lactate/carbonate.	Provides rapid treatment in acute calcium deficit (especially in presence of tetany/convulsions). Use with caution in digitalized patient because calcium increases cardiac sensitivity to digitalis, thereby increasing risk of toxicity. Oral preparations are useful in correcting subacute deficiencies.

INTERVENTIONS	RATIONALE
Collaborative	
Increase calcium and vitamin D in diet. Restrict phosphorus.	Vitamin D aids in absorption of calcium from intestinal tract.
Administer magnesium sulphate IV/orally if indicated.	Hypomagnesium is a precipitating factor in calcium deficit.

Hypercalcemia (Calcium Excess)

PATIENT ASSESSMENT DATA BASE

HISTORY

Hyperparathyroidism, hyperthyroidism, multiple myeloma/other malignancies, renal disease, skeletal muscle paralysis, parathyroid tumor, sarcoidosis, adrenal insufficiency, tuberculosis.

Excessive administration of vitamins D/A and calcium-containing antacids; prolonged use of thiazides/diuretics, lithium.

Multiple fractures, bone tumors, osteoporosis, osteomalacia, prolonged immobilization, causing release of calcium stores.

Milk-alkali syndrome as a side effect of milk/antacid ulcer therapy.

Hypophosphatasia, hyperproteinemia.

Subjective

May report general malaise, fatigue/weakness, polydipsia, polyuria/nocturia, constipation, anorexia, nausea/vomiting, thirst, epigastric/deep flank or bone pain, headache.

DIAGNOSTIC STUDIES

Serum calcium: increased greater than 5.8 mEq/liter or 10.5 mg/dl.

BUN: increased (calculi can damage kidney).

Serum phosphorus: decreased levels may be noted.

Urine Sulkowitch test shows heavy precipitate.

Urine calcium: increased.

Urine osmolality: decreased.

Urine specific gravity: decreased.

X-ray examinations may reveal evidence of bone cavitation, pathologic fracture, osteoporosis, urinary calculi.

ECG changes: shortened S-T segment and Q-T interval. In severe deficit, QRS may widen and P-R interval lengthen with ventricular prematurities.

PHYSICAL EXAMINATION

Musculoskeletal: hypotonicity/muscular relaxation.

Urine: polyuria, nocturia (occurring because of impaired renal concentrating ability).

Mentation: drowsiness, lethargy, paranoia, personality changes, memory loss, depression, psychosis, lethargy, stupor; coma (with high calcium levels).

INTERVENTIONS	RATIONALE
Independent	
Monitor cardiac rate/rhythm. Be aware that cardiac arrest can occur in hypercalcemic crisis.	Sinus bradycardia, sinus dysrhythmias, wandering pacemaker, and AV block may be noted. Hypercalcemia creates a predisposition to cardiac arrest. Overstimulation of cardiac muscle occurs with resultant dysrhythmias and ineffective cardiac contraction. Note: Digitalis is potentiated by calcium, increasing risk of toxicity.
Assess level of consciousness and neuromuscular status (e.g., muscle movement, strength, tone).	Nerve and muscle activities are depressed. Lethargy and fatigue can progress to convulsions/coma.
Strain urine if flank pain occurs. Provide acid-ash juices, such as cranberry and prune juices.	Large amounts of calcium present in kidney parenchyma may lead to stone formation. Maintaining urine acidity reduces risk of stone formation.
Monitor intake/output, calculate fluid balance.	Efforts to reduce dehydration and to encourage urinary clearance of calcium potentiate the risk of fluid imbalance.
Auscultate bowel sounds.	Hypotonicity leads to constipation when the smooth muscle tone is inadequate to produce peristalsis.
Maintain bulk in diet.	Constipation may be a problem, owing to decreased gastrointestinal tone.
Turn frequently and do range of motion and/or muscle-setting exercises.	Muscle activity may reduce calcium shifting from the bones that occurs during immobilization.
Provide safety measures (e.g., gentle handling when moving/transferring patient).	Reduces risk of pathologic fractures.
Collaborative	
Assist with identification/treatment of underlying cause.	Refer to history for list of predisposing/contributing factors.
Monitor serum electrolytes; for example, potassium and magnesium, in addition to calcium.	Monitors therapy needs/effectiveness. Note: Sodium and potassium losses may occur with diuresis.
Administer isotonic saline and sodium sulfate intravenously (IV)/orally.	Dilutes extracellular calcium concentration, and sodium inhibits tubular reabsorption of calcium, increasing urinary excretion. Note: Salty broth or Gatorade may be given by mouth.
Administer medications as indicated; for example,	
Diuretics; for example, furosemide (Lasix);	Diuresis promotes renal excretion of calcium and reduces risk of fluid excess from isotonic saline infusion.
Sodium bicarbonate,	Induces alkalosis, thereby reducing the ionized calcium fraction.
Phosphate (oral/IV),	Rapid-acting agent that induces calcium excretion and inhibits resorption of bone.
Steroid therapy,	Inhibits intestinal absorption of calcium and reduces inflammation and associated stress response that mobilizes calcium from the bone.
Mithramycin (Mithracin),	Antibiotic that lowers serum calcium by inhibiting bone resorption.

INTERVENTIONS	RATIONALE
Collaborative	
Ethylenediaminetetraacetic acid (EDTA),	Chelating action lowers serum calcium level.
Calcitonin (Calcimar) subcutaneously intramuscularly.	Temporarily reduces serum calcium levels in presence of increased parathyroid hormone.
Prepare for/assist with hemodialysis.	Reduces serum calcium.
Identify/restrict sources of calcium intake, including dairy products, eggs, and spinach.	Foods or drugs containing calcium (e.g., vitamins A and D, alkaline antacids—milk-alkali syndrome) add to calcium load.

MAGNESIUM

Magnesium influences carbohydrate metabolism, secretion of parathyroid hormone, and sodium/potassium transport across the cell membrane; promotes synthesis of protein and nucleic acid; activates ATP and mediates neural transmission within the central nervous system (CNS).

Hypomagnesemia (Magnesium Deficit)

PATIENT ASSESSMENT DATA BASE

HISTORY

Gastrointestinal losses: biliary/intestinal fistula, surgery (bowel resection), impaired GI absorption, prolonged GI suction, malabsorption syndrome, steatorrhea.

Starvation or severe protein malnutrition.

Prolonged intravenous infusion of magnesium-free solutions.

Chronic alcoholism.

Toxemia of pregnancy.

Severe renal disease/diuretic phase of ARF.

Diabetic ketoacidosis, malignancies.

Acute pancreatitis, hypoparathyroidism, SIADH, multiple transfusions with citrated blood.

Primary hyperaldosteronism, hypercalcemia, hyperthyroidism, vitamin D intoxication.

Vigorous and/or prolonged diuresis with mercurial thiazides, gentamicin toxicity.

Subjective

May complain of generalized weakness, vertigo, anorexia, nausea, insomnia.

DIAGNOSTIC STUDIES

Serum magnesium: decreased, less than 1.6 mEq/liter.

Calcium: may be decreased.

ECG: prolonged Q-T interval, broadened T waves.

PHYSICAL EXAMINATION

Musculoskeletal: fasciculations/tremors, neuromuscular irritability/spasticity, spontaneous carpopedal spasms, nystagmus, tetany, convulsions. Chvostek's and Trousseau's signs are positive. Ataxia may be noted.

Pulse: tachycardia present.

ECG: prolonged Q-T interval, broadened T waves, occasional shortened S-T segment.

Blood pressure may be elevated.

Mentation: disorientation, apathy, irritability, depression, may have hallucinations/psychoses.

INTERVENTIONS	RATIONALE
Independent	
Check vital signs frequently. Monitor cardiac rate/rhythm.	Magnesium influences sodium/potassium transport across the cell membrane and affects excitability of cardiac tissue.
Assess level of consciousness, neuromuscular status (e.g., movement, strength, reflexes/tone, sensation, presence of Chvostek's and Trousseau's signs).	Confusion, irritability, and psychosis may occur. However, more common manifestations are muscular (e.g., muscle tremors, spasticity, generalized tetany).
Take seizure/safety precautions (e.g., side rails, bed in low position, frequent observation). Promote bedrest.	Changes in mentation or the development of seizures increases the risk of patient injury.
Provide range of motion exercises as tolerated.	Reduces deleterious effects of muscle weakness/spascity.
Auscultate bowel sounds.	Muscle weakness/spasticity may reduce peristalsis and bowel function.
Observe for signs of magnesium toxicity during intravenous (IV) replacement.	Signs of toxicity include thirst, feeling hot and flushed, diaphoresis, anxiety, drowsiness, increased muscular and nervous system irritability.
Collaborative	
Assist with identification/treatment of underlying cause.	Refer to history for list of predisposing/contributing factors.
Monitor serum magnesium and calcium levels.	Evaluates therapy needs/effectiveness.
Administer magnesium sulfate or magnesium chloride IV.	Intravenous replacement is preferred because absorption of magnesium from intestinal tract varies inversely with calcium absorption.
Administer magnesium sulfate intramuscularly (IM) or magnesium hydroxide orally.	May be given prophylactically or in nonemergent situations.

Hypermagnesemia (Magnesium Excess)

PATIENT ASSESSMENT DATA BASE

HISTORY

Chronic renal disease/failure or untreated diabetic acidosis.

Hyperparathyroidism, aldosterone deficiency, adrenal insufficiency.

Excessive intake/absorption; for example, antacids/laxatives/dialysate.

Aspiration of salt water, hypothermia, shock.

Chronic diarrhea; diseases that interfere with gastric absorption.

Subjective

May complain of generalized weakness, lethargy, nausea/vomiting.

DIAGNOSTIC STUDIES

Serum magnesium: symptomatic at levels greater than 3.0 mEq/liter (increase to 12 to 15 mEq/liter results in death).

ECG: prolonged P-R interval, wide QRS, elevated T waves.

PHYSICAL EXAMINATION

Blood pressure: hypotension.

Respiration: hypoventilation progressing to apnea.

Pulse: slow weak, bradycardia/irregularities (dysrhythmias may be noted).

Mentation: decreased level of consciousness, lethargy progressing to coma.

Musculoskeletal: depressed tendon reflexes progressing to flaccid paralysis.

Skin: vasodilation, flushing, sweating.

INTERVENTIONS	RATIONALE
Independent	
Monitor vital signs. Assess level of consciousness and neuromuscular status; for example, reflexes/tone, movement, strength.	Hypotension is an early sign of toxicity, which may progress to lethargy/coma.
Monitor respiratory rate/depth/rhythm. Encourage coughing/deep breathing exercises. Elevate head of bed as indicated.	Neuromuscular transmissions are blocked by magnesium excess, resulting in muscular weakness manifested by hypoventilation, which may progress to apnea.
Encourage increased fluid intake if appropriate.	Increased diuresis enhances magnesium excretion.
Monitor urinary output.	Renal failure is the primary contributing factor in hypermagnesemia, and if it is present, efforts to increase renal excretion may be contraindicated.
Monitor cardiac rate/rhythm.	Dysrhythmias may develop, progressing to arrest.
Promote bedrest, assist with personal care activities as needed.	Flaccid paralysis, lethargy, and decreased mentation reduce activity tolerance/ability.
Collaborative	
Assist with identification/treatment of underlying cause.	Refer to history for list of predisposing contributing factors.
Monitor serum magnesium levels.	Evaluates therapy needs/effectiveness.
Administer 10 percent calcium gluconate intravenously (IV).	Antagonizes action/reverses symptoms of magnesium toxicity to improve neuromuscular transmission.

INTERVENTIONS	RATIONALE
Collaborative	
Administer IV saline solution/diuretics as indicated.	Expanding extracellular fluid volume and use of diuretics promote renal clearance of magnesium if renal function is normal.
Assist with dialysis as needed.	In the presence of renal disease/failure, dialysis may be needed to lower serum levels.

ACID-BASE IMBALANCES
Assessment Factors and Management

Metabolic Acidosis (Primary Base Bicarbonate Deficit)

Reflects an excess of acid (hydrogen) and a deficit of base (bicarbonate) resulting from acid overproduction, loss of intestinal bicarbonate, inadequate conservation of bicarbonate and excretion of acid, or anaerobic metabolism. Compensatory mechanisms to correct this imbalance include an increase in respirations to blow off excess carbon dioxide, an increase in ammonia formation and acid excretion (hydrogen) by the kidneys, with retention of bicarbonate and sodium.

PATIENT ASSESSMENT DATA BASE

HISTORY

Acidosis from excess accumulation of ketones (acetoacetic acids and other acids) as may occur in diabetes, ketoacidosis, starvation, alcohol intoxication, high-fat diets/lipid administration.

Loss of bicarbonate from the body as may occur in renal acidosis, lactic acidosis from incomplete carbohydrate metabolism, hyperalimentation, vomiting/diarrhea, small bowel/pancreatic fistulas, and ileostomy.

Systemic infections/sepsis, liver failure.

Poisoning; for example, salicylate intoxication (after initial stage), paraldehyde intoxication, and drug therapy (e.g., diamox, NH_4Cl).

Use of IV sodium chloride in presence of preexisting kidney dysfunction.

Use of carbonic anhydrase inhibitors or anion exchange resins; for example, cholestyramine (Questran).

Subjective

Headache, fatigue, drowsiness, decreased mental function, anorexia, nausea/vomiting, diarrhea.

DIAGNOSTIC STUDIES

Arterial pH: decreased, less than 7.35.

HCO_3: decreased, less than 22 mEq/liter.

PCO_2: may be less than 35 to 40 mmHg or normal.

Base excess: decreased, less than −2.

Serum potassium: increased.

Serum chloride: increased.

Serum glucose: may be decreased or increased, dependent on etiology.

Urine pH: decreased, less than 6.0.

ECG: cardiac dysrhythmias (bradycardia) and pattern changes associated with hyperkalemia; for example, tall T wave, prolonged P-R interval, wide QRS.

PHYSICAL EXAMINATION

Blood pressure: hypotension, wide pulse pressure.

Pulse: may be bounding in presence of vasodilation or decreased owing to hypotension. Irregular with cardiac dysrhythmias.

Respirations: may note hyperventilation, dyspnea on exertion, Kussmaul respirations (deep, rapid breathing). If acidosis is due to faulty fat metabolism, the breath will have a "fruity" smell.

Mentation: changes in sensorium include stupor, confusion, lethargy, depression, delirium, coma.

INTERVENTIONS	RATIONALE
Independent	
Monitor vital signs (e.g., blood pressure, hemodynamic parameters—cardiac output).	Arteriolor dilation/decreased cardiac contractility occurs, resulting in systemic shock (e.g., hypotension and tissue hypoxia).
Assess level of consciousness and progressive changes in neuromuscular status (e.g., strength, tone, movement).	Decreased mental function, confusion, seizures, weakness, and flaccid paralysis can occur owing to hypoxia and/or hyperkalemia.
Provide seizure/coma precautions (e.g., bed in low position, side rails, frequent observation).	Protects patient from injury owing to decreased mentation/convulsions.
Monitor electrocardiogram (ECG), noting rate, rhythm, and pattern.	Acidemia may cause serum hyperkalemia, manifested by changes in ECG configuration and presence of tachy or brady dysrhythmias as well as increased ventricular irritability. Life-threatening cardiovascular collapse also may occur owing to arteriolar dilation and decreased cardiac contractility.
Observe for altered respiratory excursion, rate, and depth.	Deep, rapid respirations (Kussmaul) may be noted as a compensatory mechanism to eliminate excess acid. However, as potassium shifts out of cell in an attempt to correct acidosis, respirations may become depressed. Lastly, transient respiratory depression may be the result of overcorrection of metabolic acidosis with sodium bicarbonate.
Assess skin temperature, color, capillary refill.	Evaluates tissue perfusion, effects of hypotension.
Auscultate bowel sounds, measure abdominal girth as indicated.	In the presence of co-existing hyperkalemia, gastrointestinal distress—including distention, diarrhea, and colic—may occur.
Maintain accurate intake/output and daily weight.	Therapy needs are based on underlying cause and fluid balance. For example, polyuria occurring from glycosuria in diabetes can cause circulatory collapse and renal failure owing to hypovolemia.
Test/monitor urine pH.	Kidneys attempt to compensate for acidosis by excreting excess hydrogen in the form of weak acids and ammonia. Maximum urine acidity is pH of 4.0.
Collaborative	
Assist with identification/treatment of underlying cause.	Refer to history for listing of predisposing/contributing factors.

INTERVENTIONS	RATIONALE
Collaborative	
Monitor/graph serial arterial blood gases (ABGs).	Evaluates therapy needs/effectiveness. Blood bicarbonate and pH should slowly increase toward normal levels.
Monitor serum electrolytes; for example, potassium.	As acidosis is corrected, serum potassium deficit may result as potassium shifts back into the cells.
Replace fluids (e.g., D5W/saline solutions), depending on underlying etiology.	Dehydration may be present owing to gastric/urinary losses. Choice of solution varies with cause of acidosis (e.g., diabetic ketoacidosis or gastric suctioning). Note: Lactate-containing solutions may be contraindicated in presence of lactic acidosis.
Administer medications as indicated; for example,	
Sodium bicarbonate or saline intravenously (IV),	Corrects bicarbonate deficit. Used cautiously to correct severe acidosis (pH less than 7.2).
Potassium chloride,	May be required as potassium reenters the cell, causing a serum deficit.
Phosphate,	May be administered to enhance acid excretion in presence of chronic acidosis with hypophosphatemia.
Calcium.	May be given to improve neuromuscular conduction/function and to reduce risk of seizures until other therapy measures are successful.
Modify diet as indicated (e.g., low-protein, high-carbohydrate diet in presence of renal failure, or American Diabetic Association (ADA) diet for diabetic).	Restriction of protein may be necessary to decrease production of acid waste products, and restriction of carbohydrates and use of insulin will correct acid production from metabolism of fats in the diabetic.
Administer exchange resins and/or assist with dialysis as indicated.	May be desired to reduce acidosis by decreasing excess protein and acid waste products (from protein metabolism) if pH is less than 7.1 and bicarbonate therapy is ineffective or CHF develops. (Refer to Care Plan: Renal Dialysis, page 222.)

Metabolic Alkalosis (Primary Base Bicarbonate Excess)

A deficit of hydrogen ions and an excess of bicarbonate occur owing to excessive intake of sodium bicarbonate, gastric/intestinal loss of acid, renal excretion of hydrogen and chloride, or prolonged hypercalcemia. Compensatory mechanisms include slow, shallow respirations to increase carbon dioxide level; and an increase of bicarbonate excretion and hydrogen reabsorption by the kidneys.

PATIENT ASSESSMENT DATA BASE

HISTORY

Prolonged vomiting (stomach contents), gastric lavage, diarrhea (if it has a high chloride content).

Use of potent diuretics with acid loss (hydrogen and potassium).

Excessive use of laxatives, antacids, licorice.

Excessive/overzealous correction of metabolic acidosis with sodium bicarbonate ($NaHCO_3$). Excessive salt use.

Administration of potassium-free IV solutions, citrated blood, transfusion alkalosis.

Primary and secondary hyperaldosteronism.

Adrenocortical hormone disease (e.g., Cushings' syndrome) or corticosteroid therapy.

Prolonged hypercalcemia (nonparathyroid), hypokalemia.

Subjective

May report dizziness, nausea/vomiting, diarrhea.

DIAGNOSTIC STUDIES

Arterial pH: increased, greater than 7.45.

HCO_3: increased, greater than 26 mEq/liter.

PCO_2: slightly increased, greater than 38 mmHg.

Base excess: greater than +2.

Serum chloride: decreased, less than 98 mEq/liter (if alkalosis is hypochloremia), disproportionately to serum sodium decreases.

Serum potassium: decreased.

Serum calcium: usually decreased.

Urine pH: increased, greater than 7.0.

Urine chloride less than 10 mEq/liter suggests chloride-responsive alkalosis, but levels greater than 20 mEq/liter suggest chloride resistance.

ECG may show hypokalemic changes, including peaked P waves, flat T waves, depressed S-T segment, low T wave merging to P wave, and elevated U waves.

PHYSICAL EXAMINATION

Pulse: tachycardia, irregularities/dysrhythmias may be noted.

Respirations: hypoventilation (increases PCO_2 and conserves carbonic acid).

Neuromuscular: hypertonicity of muscles, tetany, tremors, convulsions.

Mentation: confusion, irritability, restlessness, belligerence, coma.

INTERVENTIONS	RATIONALE
Independent	
Monitor vital signs, especially respirations (e.g., rate, rhythm, and depth).	Hypoventilation is a compensatory mechanism to conserve carbonic acid and represents definite risks to the individual (e.g., hypoxemia and respiratory failure).
Assess level of consciousness and neuromuscular status (e.g., strength, tone, movement; presence of Chvostek's/Trousseau's signs).	The central nervous system (CNS) may be hyperirritable, resulting in tingling, numbness, dizziness, restlessness, or apathy and confusion. Hypocalcemia may contribute to tetany (although occurrence is rare).
Monitor electrocardiogram, noting rate, rhythm, pattern.	Atrial/ventricular ectopics and tachyarrhythmias may develop in addition to the effects of co-existing hypokalemia.
Record amount and source of output.	Helpful in identifying source of ion loss; for example,

INTERVENTIONS	RATIONALE
Independent	
	potassium and hydrochloric acid are lost in vomiting and gastrointestinal suctioning.
Reduce/limit gastric suctioning and vomiting. Restrict oral intake/reduce noxious environmental stimuli. Use intermittent/low suction during constant nasogastric suctioning. Irrigate gastric tube with isotonic solutions rather than water.	Limits losses of hydrochloric acid, potassium, and calcium.
Provide seizure/safety precautions as indicated; for example, padded side rails, airway protection, bed in low position, frequent observation.	Changes in mentation/CNS and neuromuscular hyperirritability may result in patient harm, especially if tetany/convulsions occur.
Encourage intake of foods and fluids high in potassium and possibly calcium (dependent on blood level), if oral intake permitted.	Canned grapefruit and apple juices, bananas, cauliflower, dried peaches, figs, and wheat germ are some examples of food useful in replacing potassium losses.
Instruct patient to avoid use of excessive amounts of sodium bicarbonate.	Ulcer patients often take soda and milk of magnesia as well as prescribed alkaline substances.
Collaborative	
Assist with identification/treatment of underlying disorder.	Refer to history for listing of predisposing/contributing factors.
Monitor laboratory studies as indicated; for example, arterial blood gases (ABGs)/pH, serum electrolytes (especially potassium), and blood urea nitrogen (BUN).	Evaluates therapy needs/effectiveness and monitors renal function.
Administer medications, as indicated; for example,	
Sodium chloride orally/intravenously (IV) unless contraindicated,	May be all that is needed to permit kidneys to excrete bicarbonate and to correct alkalosis, but it must be used with caution in patients with CHF or renal insufficiency.
Potassium and chloride (e.g., KCl),	Hypokalemia frequently present. Chloride is needed so kidney can absorb sodium with chloride, enhancing excretion of bicarbonate.
Ammonium chloride or arginine hydrochloride,	Increases amount of circulating hydrogen ions. Monitor administration closely to prevent too rapid a decrease in pH. Note: This may be contraindicated in patients with renal/hepatic failure.
Acetazolamide (Diamox),	A carbonic anhydrase inhibitor that increases renal excretion of bicarbonate.
Spironalactone (Aldactone).	Effective in treating chloride-resistant alkalosis (e.g., Cushing's syndrome).
Avoid/limit use of sedatives or hypnotics.	If respirations are depressed, hypoxia/respiratory failure may result.
Encourage fluids IV/by mouth.	Replace extracellular fluid losses.
Administer supplemental oxygen as indicated.	Respiratory compensation for metabolic alkalosis is hypoventilation, which may cause decreased PaO_2 levels/hypoxia.

INTERVENTIONS	RATIONALE
Collaborative	
Assist with dialysis as needed.	Useful when renal dysfunction prevents clearance of bicarbonate.

Respiratory Acidosis (Primary Carbonic Acid Excess)

Represents an elevation of PCO_2 with resultant excess of carbonic acid (H_2CO_3) owing to primary defects in lung function or changes in normal respiratory pattern. Compensatory mechanisms include an increased respiratory rate; Hb (hemoglobin) buffers carbonic acid, forming bicarbonate ions and deoxygenated hemoglobin; and an increased renal formation of ammonia acid excretions, with reabsorption of bicarbonate.

PATIENT ASSESSMENT DATA BASE

HISTORY

Hypoventilation with retention of carbon dixoide, as in chronic obstructive pulmonary disease, pneumonia, asthma, airway obstructions, smoke inhalation, acute pulmonary edema, hemothorax/pneumothorax, atelectasis, mechanical ventilators, or pickwickian syndrome; excessive carbon dioxide intake (e.g., CVA therapy, rebreathing mask).

Decreased function of respiratory center, such as with head trauma, oversedation, barbiturate poisoning, general anesthesia, and metabolic alkalosis.

Neuromuscular disorders, such as Guillian-Barre Syndrome and myasthensia gravis, botulism, spinal cord injuries, potassium imbalances.

Subjective

May complain of headache, dizziness, visual disturbances, fatigue.

DIAGNOSTIC STUDIES

Arterial pH: decreased, less than 7.35.

HCO_3: normal or increased, greater than 26 mEq/liter.

PCO_2: increased, greater than 45 mmHg.

PO_2: normal or decreased.

Urine pH: decreased, 6.0.

Serum potassium: normal or increased.

Serum calcium: increased.

Serum chloride: decreased.

PHYSICAL EXAMINATION

Mentation: confusion, apprehension, agitation, restlessness, somnolence, coma.

Respiratory effort: increased with dyspnea, nasal flaring/yawning noted.

Respiratory rate: decreased.

Breath sounds: crackles, wheezes, stridor may be present.

Pulse: tachycardia present, irregularities/dysrhythmias may be noted.

Skin: diaphoresis, pallor, and cyanosis may occur in late stage of hypoxia.

Neuromuscular: generalized weakness, tremors, loss of coordination, decreased reflexes.

INTERVENTIONS	RATIONALE
Independent	
Monitor respiratory rate, depth, and effort.	Corresponding hypoxemia leads to respiratory distress/failure.
Auscultate breath sounds.	Identifies area(s) of decreased ventilation/airway obstruction and therapy needs/effectiveness.
Assess for decreased level of consciousness.	Signals severe acidotic state, which requires immediate attention. Sensorium clears slowly because it takes longer for hydrogen ions to clear from cerebrospinal fluid.
Monitor heart rate/electrocardiogram (ECG).	Tachycardia develops in an attempt to increase oxygen delivery to the tissues. Dysrhythmias may occur owing to hypoxia (myocardial ischemia) or electrolyte imbalances.
Note skin color, temperature, moisture.	Diaphoresis, pallor, cool/clammy skin are associated with hypoxemia and may warn of impending respiratory failure.
Encourage turning, coughing, and deep breathing. Place in semi-Fowler's position. Suction as necessary. Provide airway adjunct as indicated.	These measures can improve ventilation and prevent airway obstruction or decreased alveolar diffusion/perfusion.
Collaborative	
Assist with identification/treatment of underlying cause.	Refer to history for listing of predisposing/contributing factors.
Monitor/graph serial arterial blood gases (ABGs).	Evaluates therapy needs/effectiveness.
Administer oxygen as indicated by mask, cannula, or mechanical ventilation. Increase respiratory rate or tidal volume of ventilator.	Prevents/corrects hypoxemia and respiratory failure. Low-flow oxygen is important in obstructive diseases because the respiratory center in the brain is accustomed to increased carbon dioxide levels. When supplemental oxygen is used, it decreases the carbon dioxide (the stimulus for breathing), resulting in carbon dioxide narcosis.
Administer medications as indicated; for example,	
Naloxone hydrochloride (Narcan),	May be useful in arousing patient and stimulating respiratory function in presence of drug sedation.
Sodium bicarbonate ($NaHCO_3$),	Given if pH is less than 7.25 to correct acidosis. Note: Rebound alkalosis may occur.
Potassium chloride (KCl).	Acidosis causes shift of potassium from cells and hydrogen into cells. Correction of acidosis may cause serum hypokalemia as potassium reenters the cell. Either imbalance can impair neuromuscular/respiratory function.
Limit use of hypnotic sedatives or tranquilizers.	In the presence of hypoventilation, respiratory depres-

INTERVENTIONS	RATIONALE
Collaborative	
	sion can occur with the use of sedatives, and carbon dioxide narcosis may develop. Note: Use of pain medication in thoracic surgery may actually improve ventilation and correct acidosis.
Maintain hydration (intravenously/by mouth)/provide humidification.	Assists in thinning/mobilization of secretions.
Provide aggressive chest physiotherapy, including postural drainage and suctioning as indicated.	Aids in clearing secretions, which may improve ventilation, allowing excess carbon dioxide to be eliminated.
Assist with ventilatory aids (IPPB) in conjunction with bronchodilators.	Increase lung expansion and opens airways to improve ventilation, preventing respiratory failure.

Respiratory Alkalosis (Primary Carbonic Acid Deficit)

There is a decrease in PCO_2 with a deficit of carbonic acid (H_2CO_3), owing to a marked increase in the rate of respirations. Compensatory mechanisms include decreased respiratory rate (if the body is able to respond to the drop in PCO_2) to retain carbon dioxide, increased renal excretion of bicarbonate and retention of hydrogen.

PATIENT ASSESSMENT DATA BASE

HISTORY

Hyperventilation caused by nervousness, anxiety, intentional overbreathing, hysteria/extreme emotions; fever; sepsis (usually gram-negative organism), meningitis; severe pain; brain trauma/lesions; multiple pulmonary emboli; or mechanical ventilators.

Restrictive problems, such as asthma, pulmonary fibrosis, pregnancy.

Oxygen lack, such as high-altitude sickness, severe anemia, hypoxemia.

Congestive heart failure, alcoholic intoxication, cirrhosis, thyrotoxicosis.

Paraldehyde or early salicylate intoxication.

Rapid correction of metabolic acidosis (e.g., renal dialysis).

Subjective

May complain of numbness/tingling of face and hands, circumoral paresthesia; muscle cramps; syncope, vertigo; nausea/vomiting.

DIAGNOSTIC STUDIES

Arterial pH: greater than 7.45.

HCO_3: normal or decreased, less than 25 mEq/liter.

PCO_2: decreased, less than 38 mmHg.

Serum potassium: decreased.

Serum chloride: increased.

Serum calcium: decreased.

Urine pH: increased, greater than 7.0.

PHYSICAL EXAMINATION

Neuromuscular: tetany, seizures may be noted.

Mentation: confusion, restlessness, anxiety, obtundation, coma.

Respirations: hyperventilation, dyspnea.

Blood pressure: hypotension present.

Pulse: may be irregular if dysrhythmias present.

INTERVENTIONS	RATIONALE
Independent	
Provide support by calm manner and voice.	May help reassurer and calm the agitated patient, thereby aiding in reduction of respiratory rate.
Demonstrate appropriate breathing patterns and review purpose of ordered treatments (e.g., rebreathing mask/bag).	Decreasing the rate of respirations will restore PCO_2 level.
Assess level of consciousness and neuromuscular status, (e.g., strength, tone, reflexes, and sensation).	Decreased mentation/tetany or convulsions may occur.
Provide safety/seizure precautions, e.g., bed in low position, padded side rails, frequent observation.	Changes in mentation/CNS and neuromuscular hyperirritability may result in patient harm, especially if tetany/convulsions occur.
Collaborative	
Assist with identification/treatment of underlying cause.	Refer to history for listing of predisposing/contributing factors.
Monitor/graph serial arterial blood gases (ABGs).	Identifies therapy needs/effectiveness.
Monitor serum potassium. Replace as indicated.	Hypokalemia may occur as potassium is lost (urine) or shifted into the cell in exchange for hydrogen in an attempt to correct alkalosis.
Provide sedation, as indicated.	May be required to reduce psychogenic cause.
Administer carbon dioxide, or use rebreathing mask as indicated.	Increasing carbon dioxide retention may correct carbonic acid deficit.
Reduce respiratory rate/tidal volume or add additional dead space (tubing) to mechanical ventilator.	These measures will also enhance carbon dioxide retention in the mechanically ventilated patient.

BIBLIOGRAPHY

General

ALSPACH, JG AND WILLIAMS, SM: *ACCN: Core Curriculum For Critical Care Nursing.* WB Saunders, Philadelphia, 1985.
BERK, J, ET AL: *Handbook of Critical Care.* Little, Brown & Co, Boston, 1976.
BRUNNER, LS, AND SUDDARTH, DS: *The Lippincott Manual of Nursing Practice,* ed 4. JB Lippincott, Philadelphia, 1986.
BRUNNER, LS, AND SUDDARTH, DS: *Testbook of Medical-Surgical Nursing.* JB Lippincott, Philadelphia, 1984.
CAMPBELL, C, AND FRISSE, M: *Manual of Medical Therapeutics,* ed 24. Little, Brown & Co, Boston, 1983.
DOENGES, ME, ET AL: *Nursing Care Plans: Nursing Diagnosis in Planning Patient Care.* FA Davis, Philadelphia, 1984.
DOENGES, ME, AND MOORHOUSE, M: *Nurse's Pocket Guide: Nursing Diagnoses with Interventions.* FA Davis, Philadelphia, 1985.
DON, H: *Decision Making in Critical Care.* BC Decker, Philadelphia, 1985.
GAHART, B: *Intravenous Medications: A Handbook for Nurses and Other Allied Health Personnel,* ed 4. CV Mosby, St Louis, 1985.
HUDAK, CM, ET AL: *Critical Care Nursing,* ed 3. JB Lippincott, Philadelphia, 1982.
JOHANSON, BC, DUNGCA, CU, ET AL: *Standards For Critical Care,* ed 2. CV Mosby, St Louis, 1985.
KENNER, CV, ET AL: *Critical Care Nursing: Body-Mind-Spirit,* ed 2. Little, Brown & Co, Boston, 1985.
KIM, MJ, AND MONTZ, DA: *Classification of Nursing Diagnosis: Proceedings of the Third and Fourth National Conferences.* McGraw-Hill, New York, 1982.
KINNEY, M (ED): *AACN's Clinical Reference for Critical Care Nursing.* McGraw-Hill, New York, 1981.
LANGFITT, D: *Critical Care Certification Preparation and Review.* Robert J. Brady, Bowie, MD, 1984.
MATTHEWSON, M: *Pharmacotherapeutics: A Nursing Approach.* FA Davis, Philadelphia, 1986.
MILLAR, S, ET AL: *AACN Procedure Manual for Critical Care,* ed 2. WB Saunders, Philadelphia, 1985.
Nursing86 Drug Handbook. Nursing86 Books, Springhouse Corp, Springhouse, PA, 1986
NURSING REFERENCE LIBRARY: *Assessment.* Nursing84 Books, Springhouse Corp, Springhouse, PA, 1984.
ROGERS, M, ALLO, M, ET AL: *1985 Year Book of Critical Care Medicine.* Year Book Medical Publishers, Chicago, 1985.
SHOEMAKER, WC, THOMPSON, WL, ET AL: *Textbook of Critical Care.* WB Saunders, Philadelphia, 1984.
STROOT, VR, LEE, CA, ET AL: *Fluids and Electrolytes: A Practical Approach,* ed 3. FA Davis, Philadelphia, 1984.
SWEARINGER, P: *Manual of Nursing Therapeutics.* Addison-Wesley, Menlo Park, 1986.
TARTAGLIA, DA: *Nursing diagnosis: Keystone of your careplan,* Nursing85 15(3):34–37, 1985.
THOMAS, C (ED): *Taber's Cyclopedic Medical Dictionary,* ed 15. FA Davis, Philadelphia, 1985.
ULRICH, S: *Nursing Care Planning Guides.* WB Saunders, Philadelphia, 1986.
WILKINS, R, AND LEVINSKY, N: *Medicine: Essentials of Clinical Practice,* ed 3. Little, Brown & Co, Boston, 1983.

Chapter 1: Articles

BARHAM, V, AND SCHNEIDER, W: *Matrix: A unique patient classification system.* J Nurs Admin, December 1968, pp 25–31.
HIGGERSON, N, AND SLYCK, A: *Variable billing for services: New fiscal direction for nursing.* J Nurs Admin, June 1982, pp 20–27.
REINERT, R, AND GRANT, D: *A classification system to meet today's needs.* J Nurs Admin, January 1981, pp 21–25.
LOMBARD, N, AND LIGHT, N: *On-line nursing care plans by nursing diagnosis.* Computers in Healthcare, November 1983, pp 22–23.

Chapter 2: Books

KELLY, MA: *Nursing Diagnosis Source Book.* Appleton-Century-Crofts, Norwalk, CT, 1985.

Chapter 2: Articles

BAER, C (ED): *Nursing diagnosis.* Top Clin Nurs 5(4), January 1984.
GUZZETTA, CE, ET AL: *Nursing diagnosis: Framework, process and problems.* Heart Lung, May 1983.

Chapter 3: Books

BEAL, JM: *Critical Care for Surgical Patients.* Macmillan, New York, 1982.
BERHRENDT, DM, AND AUSTEN, GW: *Patient Care in Cardiac Surgery.* Little, Brown & Co, Boston, 1980.
BRAUNWALD, E: *Heart Disease: A Textbook of Cardiovascular Medicine.* WB Saunders, Philadelphia, 1984.

CARPENITO, LJ: *Nursing Diagnosis: Application to Clinical Practice.* JB Lippincott, Philadelphia, 1983.
CHOW, RK: *Cardiosurgical Nursing Care: Understandings, Concepts, and Principles for Practice.* Springer, New York, 1976.
DUDRICK, SJ, BAUE, AE, ET AL: *Manual of Preoperative and Postoperative Care.* WB Saunders, Philadelphia, 1983.
GIVING CARDIAC CARE. Nursing81 Books, Intermed, Horsham, PA, 1981.
GLENN, WWL, BAUE, AE, ET AL: *Thoracic and Cardiovascular Surgery.* Appleton-Century-Crofts, Norwalk, CT, 1983.
GOULD, KA: *Cardiac critical care nursing.* In YEE, BH, ZORB, SL (EDS): *Cardiac Surgery.* Little, Brown and Co, Boston, 1986, pp 291–318.
HARLAN, BJ, STARR, A, ET AL: *Manual of Cardiac Surgery.* Springer-Verlag, New York, 1980.
HILLIS, LD, FIRTH, BG, ET AL: *Manual of Clinical Problems in Cardiology,* ed 2. Little, Brown & Co, Boston, 1984.
HINCKER, EA, AND MATSANAS, L (EDS): *The Little, Brown Manual of Medical-Surgical Nursing.* Little, Brown & Co, Boston, 1983.
HURST, JW: *The Heart,* ed 6. McGraw-Hill, New York, 1986.
KING, O: *Care of the Cardiac Surgery Patient Surgery Patient.* CV Mosby, St Louis, 1975.
MCCAULEY, K, BREST, A: *McGoon's Cardiac Surgery: An Interprofessional Approach to Patient Care.* FA Davis, Philadelphia, 1985.
Cardiovascular Disorders. Nurse's Clinical Library Series. Nursing84 Books, Springhouse Corp, Springhouse, PA, 1984.
Using Monitors. Nursing Photobook Series. Nursing84 Books, Springhouse Corp, Springhouse, PA, 1984.
Giving Cardiovascular Drugs Safely, Nursing Skillbook Series. Nursing79 Books, Intermed, Horsham, PA, 1979.
REUTHER, MA, AND HANSON, CB: *Cardiovascular Nursing.* Current Clinical Nursing Series. Medical Examination Publishing, 1985.
SCHROEDER, J, AND DAILY, E: *Techniques in Bedside Hemodynamic Monitoring.* CV Mosby, St Louis, 1976.
TURNER, G: *The Cardiovascular Unit: A Guide for Planning and Operation.* John Wiley & Sons, New York, 1978.
UNDERHILL, SL, WOODS, SL, ET AL: *Cardiac Nursing.* JB Lippincott, Philadelphia, 1982.
WENGER, NK, HURST, JW, ET AL: *Cardiology For Nurses.* McGraw-Hill, New York, 1980.
ZSCHOCHE, MJ: *Mosby's Comprehensive Review of Critical Care,* ed 2. CV Mosby, St Louis, 1981.

Chapter 3: Articles

BARHAM, V, AND SCHNEIDER, W: *Matrix: A unique patient classification system.* J Nurs Admin, pp 25–31, December 1980.
Congestive heart failure: Physiology, sign, and symptoms. Nursing83 13(9):44–46, September 1983.
Congestive heart failure—physiology, signs and symptoms. Nursing83 13(9):44–46, September 1983.
HEGGIE, J: *Pulling your patient through congestive heart failure.* RN, pp 31–36, 131–132, September 1980.
HIGGERSON, N, AND SLYCK, A: *Variable billing for services: New fiscal direction for nursing.* J Nurs Admin, pp 20–27, June 1982.
JONES, S, AND BAGG, A: *The drugs you'll use in a code. RN* 48(7):43–46, July 1985.
KLEINHEINZ, T: *The inside story on preload and afterload.* Nursing85, pp 55, May 1985.
LAMB, LS, AND DIGIACOMO, BM: *When your patient is scheduled for mitral valve replacement.* Nursing85 15(1):58–63, January 1985.
LOMBARD, N, AND LIGHT, N: *"On-line nursing care plans by nursing diagnosis.* Computers in Healthcare, pp 22–23, November 1983.
MCCAULEY, K: *Probing the ins and outs of congestive heart failure.* Nursing82, pp 60–65, November 1982.
New concepts in understanding congestive heart failure: How the clinical features arise. AJN, pp 119–142, January 1981.
PUTZIER, DJ, PADRICK, K, ET AL: *Diagnostic reasoning in critical care nursing. Heart Lung* 14(5):430–437, May 1985.
REINERT, R, AND GRANT, D: *A classification system to meet today's needs.* J Nurs Admin, pp 21–25, January 1981.
RN MASTER CARE PLAN: *Helping the patient in shock.* RN 48(7): 26-27, July 1985.
SORENSEN, E: *Why did that ventilator alarm go off?* RN 48(7):38–39, July 1985.
SVENSSON, LG, DECKER, G, ET AL: *A prospective study of hyperamylasemia and pancreatitis after cardiopulmonary bypass.* Ann Thorac Surg 39(5):409–411, 1985.
WHITE, KM: *Completing the hemodynamic picture:* SvO_2*. Heart Lung* 14(3):272–280, March 1985.

Chapter 4: Books

Chest drainage: Clinical assessment and management. Book 3. Argyle, St. Louis.
CLAYTON, BD: *Mosby's Handbook of Pharmacology in Nursing,* ed 3. CV Mosby, St. Louis, 1984.
GUYTON, AC: *Basic Human Physiology: Normal Function and Mechanisms of Disease.* WB Saunders, Philadelphia, 1977.
HINSHAW, H, AND MURRAY, J: *Diseases of the Chest,* ed 4. WB Saunders, Philadelphia, 1980.
HOLLOWAY, NM: *Nursing the Critically Ill Adult.* Addison-Wesley, Menlo Park, 1979.
ISSELBACHER, KJ, ET AL (EDS): *Harrison's Principles of Internal Medicine.* JB Lippincott, Philadelphia, 1982.
MORRISON, ML (ED): *Respiratory Intensive Care Nursing,* ed 2. Little, Brown & Co, Boston, 1979.
SHAPIRO, B, HARRISON, R, TROUT, C: *Clinical Applications of Respiratory Care.* Year Book Medical Publishers, Chicago, 1979.
SHIBEL, EM, AND MOSER, KM (EDS): *Respiratory Emergencies.* CV Mosby, St Louis, 1977.
TILKIAN, SM, CONOVER, MB, ET AL: *Clinical Implications of Laboratory Tests.* CV Mosby, St Louis, 1979.
WADE, JF: *Respiratory Nursing Care: Physiology and Technique.* CV Mosby, St Louis, 1977.

Chapter 4: Articles

BALK, R, AND BONE, RC: *The adult respiratory distress syndrome.* Med Clin North Am 67(3):685–700, 1983.

BOUCHER, BA, AND FOSTER, TS: *The Adult Respiratory Distress Syndrome.* Drug Intell Clin Pharm 18:862–868, November 1984.

CHALIKIAN, J, AND WEAVER, TE: *Mechanical ventilation: Where it's at, where it's going.* AJN, pp 1373–1391, November 1984.

CLINE, B, AND FISHER, M: *ARDS means emergency.* Nursing82, pp 62–67, February 1982.

DAEFFLER, R: *Oral hygiene measures for patients with cancer. I.* Cancer Nurs pp 347–355, October 1980.

DETOLEDO, LW: *Caring for the patient instead of the ventilator.* RN 43:20–23, December 1980.

DIVERTIE, MB: *The adult respiratory distress syndrome.* Mayo Clin Proc 57:371–378, June 1982.

DROPKIN, M: *Compliance in postoperative head and neck patients.* Cancer Nurs, pp 379–384, October 1979.

DUNCAN, C, AND ERICKSON, R: *Pressures associated with chest tube stripping.* Heart Lung 11(2):166–171, March–April, 1982.

GOLDENHEIM, P, AND KAZEMI, H: *Medical intelligence: Current concepts: cardiopulmonary monitoring of critically ill patients.* New Engl J Med, pp 717–720, September 13, 1984.

HAWLEY, HB: *Pulmonary infections in critical care medicine: Challenges and dilemmas. Heart Lung* 15(3): 221–241, May 1986.

KEITH, C: *Wound management following head and neck surgery.* Nurs Clin North Am 14(4):761–778, December 1979.

PETERSON, B: *Application and assessment of O_2 therapy devices.* Nurs Clin North Am, pp 241–258, June 1981.

PETTY, TL, AND FOWLER, AA, III: *Another look at ARDS.* Chest 82:98–104, July 1982.

RAU, JL: *Continuous mechanical ventilation, part I.* Critical Care Update 8(10):10–29, October 1981.

RAU, JL: *Continuous mechanical ventilation, part III.* Critical Care Update 8(11):5–20, November 1981.

Chapter 5: Books

AMERICAN ASSOCIATION OF NEUROSCIENCES NURSES: *Core Curriculum for Neuroscience Nursing,* ed 2. Park Ridge, IL, 1984.

CLOWARD, R: *Acute Cervical Spine Injuries. Clinical Symposa.* CIBA, Summit, NJ, 1980.

Current Concepts in Intensive Care for Neurological Trauma and Diseases. University of Miami School of Medicine Department of Neurological Surgery, 1980.

GOLDBERG, S: *Clinical Neuroanatomy Made Ridiculously Simple,* Medmaster, Miami, 1979.

HOWE, J, DICKASON, E, ET AL: *Handbook of Nursing.* John Wiley & Sons, New York, 1984, pp 770–788.

LARSON, EL, AND VAZQUEZ, M: *Critical Care Nursing.* WB Saunders, Philadelphia, 1983.

MITCHELL, PN, AND PLASTERER, HH: *Neurologic Disorders: AACN's Clinical Reference for Critical Care Nursing.* McGraw-Hill, New York, 1981, pp 637–638.

NIKAS, DL, MITCHELL, PJ, ET AL: *The Critically Ill Neurosurgical Patient.* Churchill-Livingstone, New York, 1982.

Neurologic Disorders. Nursing84 Books, Springhouse Corp, Springhouse, PA, 1984.

Chapter 5: Articles

ANDERSON, M: *My head hurts.* Nursing84 14(9):34–41, 1984.

BRODSLEY, L: *Avoiding a crisis: The assessment.* AJN 82(12):1865–1869, December 1982.

Caring for the patient with elevated intracranial pressure. Nursing82 12(1):48–49, January 1982.

COHN, L: *The hospitalized alcoholic, the hidden diagnosis.* AJN 82(12):1862–1964, December 1982.

COLLINS, A: *Nursing care study: Guillain-Barré syndrome.* Nursing Mirror 156(23):44–47, June 1983.

COOKSLEY, P: *Nursing care study, Guillain-Barré syndrome: Fading away.* Nursing Mirror 152(2):39–43, January 1981.

GRISWOLD, K, GUANCI, MM, ET AL: *An approach to the care of patients with Guillain-Barré syndrome.* Heart Lung 13(1):66–72, January 1984.

HOWARD, M, CORBO-PELAIA, S: *The psychological after effects of halo traction and a review of acute care.* AJN 82(12):1839–1843, December 1982.

JOHNSON, LK: *If your patient has increased intracranial pressure your goal should be: No surprises.* Nursing83 pp 59–63, June 1983.

MAUSS-CLUM, N: *Bringing the unconscious patient back safely: Nursing makes the critical difference.* Nursing82 12(8):34–42, August 1982.

MILLER, RJ: *Guillain-Barré syndrome: Current methods of diagnosis and treatment.* Postgrad Med 77(7):56–64, May 1985.

MILLS, N, AND PLASTERER, HH: *Guillain-Barré syndrome: A framework for nursing care.* Nurs Clin North Am 15(2):257–264, June 1980.

MIRR, MP, JANKOWSKI, K, ET AL: *Nursing management for barbiturate therapy in acute head injuries.* Heart Lung 12(1):52–60, January 1983.

PRYDUN, M: *Guillain-Barré syndrome: Disease process.* Neurosurg Nurs 15(1):27–32, February 1983.

RICHMOND, T: *A critical care challenge: The patient with a cervical spinal cord injury.* Focus on Critical Care 12(2):23–33, April 1985.

ROBINET, K: *Increased intracranial pressure: Management with an intraventricular catheter.* Neurosurg Nurs 17(2):95–103, April 1985.

SAMONDS, RJ: *Guillain-Barré syndrome: Helping the patient in the acute stage.* Nursing80, pp 35–41, August 1980.

STOLARIK, A: *What the comatose patient can tell you.* RN 48(4):26–33, 1985.
SWIFT, N: *Head injury: Essentials of excellent care.* Nursing74 4(9):27–33, September 1974.
YOUNG, MS: *A bedside guide to understanding the signs of intracranial pressure.* Nursing81 11(2):59–62, February 1981.

Chapter 6: Books

DOUGLAS, AP, AND RENNER, IG: *Current Therapy.* WB Saunders, Philadelphia, 1980, pp 388–390.
GIVEN, B, AND SIMMONS, S: *Gastroenterology in Clinical Nursing,* ed 4. CV Mosby, St Louis, 1984.
GUYTON, AC: *Textbook of Medical Physiology,* ed 5. WB Saunders, Philadelphia, 1976.
HAMILTON, H, AND ROSE-MINNIE, B (EDS): *Diseases.* Nurse's Reference Library. Springhouse Corp, Springhouse, PA, 1983.
HOWE, J, DICKASON, E, ET AL: *Handbook of Nursing.* John Wiley & Sons, New York, 1984, pp 1203–1207.
LUCKMAN, J, AND SORENSEN, KC: *Medical-Surgical Nursing—A Pathophysiologic Approach,* ed 2. WB Saunders, Philadelphia, 1980.
MILLER, S: *Methods in Critical Care—The AACN Manual.* WB Saunders, Philadelphia, 1980.
PRICE, SA, AND WILSON, LM: *Pathophysiology: Clinical Concepts of Disease Processes,* ed 2. McGraw-Hill, New York, 1982.
SLEISENGER, MH: *GI Disease.* WB Saunders, Philadelphia, 1983.
WARSHAW, AL, AND RICHTER, JM: *A Practical Guide to Pancreatitis.* Current Problems in Surgery, volume 21, no 12. 1984.

Chapter 6: Articles

AMATO, EJ: *A nursing reference: Gastrointestinal tubes and drains. Part II: Esophageal tubes.* Critical Care Nurse, pp 45–48, January/February 1983.
BONNET F, ROTMAN, N, ET AL: *Changing concepts in the evaluation and treatment of acute severe pancreatitis.* Intensive Care Medicine 11(3):107–109, 1985.
BRIONES, T: *Nursing care plan for the patient with acute gastrointestinal (GI) bleeding.* Critical Care Nurse, pp 22–24, March/April 1984.
BULLAS, JB, AND PJISTER, S: *Upper gastrointestinal hemorrhage.* Critical Care Nurse pp 72–74, May/June 1984.
BUSLEY, HC, AND SEIFFERT, W: *Acute gastrointestinal bleeding.* In HUDAK, CM, ET AL: *Critical Care Nursing,* ed 2. JB Lippincott, Philadelphia, 1982, pp 445–450.
BURKHART, C: *Upper GI hemorrhage: The clinical picture.* AJN, October 1981.
DECKER, S: *The life-threatening consequences of a GI bleed.* RN, October 1985.
DOHERTY, C: *Acute Pancreatitis.* Nursing Mirror 160(25):48–51, June 1985.
DOLAN, P, AND GREENE, HL: *Conquering cirrhosis of the liver.* Nursing76, pp 44–53, November 1976.
DUSEK, JL: *Iced gastric lavage slows bleeding in gastric hemorrhage.* Critical Care Nurse, p 8, July/August 1984.
EIMER KING, D: *How to give your portal hypertension patient a fighting chance.* RN, pp 31–37, July 1983.
FREDETTE, S: *When the liver fails.* AJN 84(1):64–67, January 1984.
GEOKAS, MC: *Acute Pancreatitis.* Ann Intern Med 103:86–100, 1985.
GEVER, L: *Lactulose, a crucial element in treating hepatic encephalopathy.* Nursing82 12(8):76–78, August 1984.
GOLDENBERG, DA: *Management of bleeding esophageal varices.* Critical Care Quarterly, pp. 33–45, September 1982.
MARTIN, DM, AND GALOMBOS, JT: *Fulminant hepatic failure.* Critical Care Quarterly, pp 9–13, September 1982.
MCCONNELL, E: *Curtailing a life-threatening crisis: GI bleeding.* Nursing81 11(70):70–73, April 1981.
MCPHEE, M, *Treatment of acute pancreatitis.* Hosp Pract pp 83–94, June 1985.
PATRAS, A, PAICE, J, ET AL: *Managing GI bleeding, it takes a two-tract mind.* Nursing84 14(7):26–33, July 1984.
PELLEGRINI, CA: *The treatment of acute pancreatitis: A continuing challenge.* N Engl J Med 342(7):436–438, February 14, 1985.
PETLIN, AM, AND CAROLAN, JM: *How to stop a GI bleed.* RN, pp 43–49, April 1981.
RANSON, JH: *Acute pancreatitis: Pathogenesis, outcome and treatment.* Clin Gastroenterol 13(3):843–863, September 1985.
RANSON, JHC: *Risk factors in acute pancreatitis.* Hosp Pract pp 69–73, April 15, 1985.
RICKETSON, CA: *Acute pancreatitis.* Critical Care Update 10(3):40–49, March 1983.
ROBINSON, MK, AND WARDEN, LS: *Hepatorenal syndrome.* Critical Care Nurse, pp 23–26, July-August 1981.
SCHABLICK, K J: *Hepatic failure: Etiologies, manifestations and management.* Critical Care Nurse 5(1):60–86, 1985.
SISKIND, J: Handling hemorrhage wisely. Nursing84 14(8):34–41, January 1984.
STEINBERG, WM: *Acute drug and toxin induced pancreatitis.* Hosp Pract, pp 95–102, May 1985.
TASKES, PP: *Recurrent acute pancreatitis.* Hosp Pract, ppp 85–92, July 1985.
THOMPSON, MA: *Managing the patient with liver dysfunction.* Nursing81, pp 101–107, November 1981.
WHITE, JV, MILAZZO, JV, COMEROTA, AJ: *Management of massive hemorrhage from esophogeal varices.* Critical Care Quarterly, pp 69–80, September, 1985.
WIMPSETT, J: *Trace your patient's liver dysfunction.* Nursing84, 14(8):56–57, August 1984.

Chapter 7: Books

BRUNDAGE, D: *Nursing Management of Renal Problems.* CV Mosby, St Louis, 1980.
DUKE UNIVERSITY HOSPITAL: *Guidelines For Nursing Care: Process and Outcome.* JB Lippincott, Philadelphia, 1983.
HOLLOWAY, NM: *Nursing the Critically Ill Adult.* Addison-Wesley, Menlo Park, 1984.
MILLER, A, AND NORTON, B: *Skills for Professional Nursing Practice.* Appleton-Century-Crofts, Norwalk, CT, 1986.
Personal communication with neprhologists, Department of Internal Medicine, Indiana University Medical Center, Indianapolis.
Personal communication, nursing staff, Renal Intensive Care Unit, Indiana University Medical Center, Indianapolis.
PRICE, SA, AND WILSON, LM: *Pathophysiology: Clinical Concepts of Disease Processes.* McGraw-Hill, New York, 1986.

Chapter 7: Articles

FOSTER, J, *Dialysis: A treatment modality in renal failure.* Critical Care Quarterly 1(2):94–98, September 1978.
FRAHER, J: *Nursing diagnoses and care plans in critical care.* Critical Care Nurse, pp 94–98, November/December 1983.
HAAS, S, AND BERLIN, P: *A participative approach to the care plan problem.* Critical Care Nurse, pp 15–17, July/August 1984.
MARS, DR, AND TRELOAR, D: *Acute tubular necrosis.* Heart Lung 13(2):194–201, March 1984.
PALMER, J, KOOREFIAN, K, ET AL: *Nursing management of continuous arteriovenous hemofiltration for acute renal failure.* Focus on Critical Care 13(5):21–30, October 1986.

Chapter 8: Books

BONAR, JR: *Diabetes—A Clinical Guide,* ed 2. Medical Examination Publishing Co, New York, 1980.
BERKOW, R: *The Merck Manual of Diagnosis and Therapy,* ed 14. Merck, Sharp and Dohme, Rahway, NJ, 1982, pp 1001–1006, 1037–1052.
Managing Diabetes Properly. Nursing Skillbook Series. Springhouse Corp, Springhouse, PA, 1985.
WILLIAMS, R: *Textbook of Endocrinology,* ed 6. WB Saunders, Philadelphia, 1981, pp 117–243.

Chapter 8: Articles

BROWN, SL: *Practical points in the postanesthesia assessment and care of the patient having a thyroidectomy.* Postanesth Nurse 1(3):191–193, August 1986.
BLONDE, L, et al: *Answers to questions on hyperthyroidism.* Hosp Med 20(12):131–1, December 1986.
JOHNSON, D: *Pathophysiology of thyroid storm.* Crit Care Nurse 3(6):80–86, November–December 1983.
LESKE, JS: *Hyperglycemic hyperosmolar nonketotic coma.* Emerg Nurs 10(3):145–150, May/June 1984.
MCADAMS, R, AND BIRMINGHAM, D: *When diabetes races out of control.* RN pp 46–52, May 1986.
MCCARTHY, J: *The Continuum of Diabetic Coma.* AJN, 85(8):878–882, August 1985.
MILLER, V: *Diabetes: Let's stop testing urine.* AJN 86(1):54, January 1986.
ROBERTSON, C: *How to teach patients to monitor blood glucose.* RN 48(12):24–25, December 1985.
ROSENTHAL, N, AND BARRETT, E: *An assessment of insulin action in hyperosmolar hyperglycemic nonketotic diabetic patients.* J Clin Endocrinol Metab 60(3):607–610, 1985.
STOCK-BARKMAN, P: *Confusing concepts—Is it diabetic shock or diabetic coma?* Nursing 83 13(6):33–41, June 1983.
The Patient with Ketoacidosis. RN Master Care Plan. RN, p 53, May 1986.
WINTERS, B: *Nursing implications of hyperosmolar coma.* Heart Lung 12(4):439–446, July 1983.

Chapter 9: Articles

EVERS, J, AND WERPACHOWSKI, D: *Dealing with fractures.* RN 47(11):53-55, 1984.
FARRELL, J: *The trauma patient with multiple fractures.* RN 48(6): 22-25, June 1985.
LARSON, M, LEIGH, J, ET AL: *Detecting compartmental syndrome using continuous pressure monitoring.* Focus on Critical Care 13(5):51–56, October 1986.
SIGMON, H: *Helping your long-term trauma patient travel the road to recovery.* Nursing84 14(1):58–61, January 1984.
STEVENSON, C: *Take no chances with fat embolism.* Nursing85, 15(6):58–63, June 1985.

Chapter 10: Books

ARTZ, CP, MONCRIEF, JA, PRUITT, BA: *Burns: A Team Approach.* WB Saunders, Philadelphia, 1979.
BAXTER, CR: *Crystalloid Resuscitation of Burn Shock.* Little, Brown, & Co, Boston, 1971.
CARPENITO, LJ: *Hnadbook of Nursing Diagnosis.* JB Lippincott, Philadelphia, 1984.
FELLER, I, AND ARCHEMBEAULT, C: *Nursing the Burned Patient.* The Institute for Burn Medicine, Ann Arbor, 1973.
FLETCHER, BJ: *Critical Care Nursing.* JB Lippincott, Philadelphia, 1983.

HOLLOWAY, NM: *Nursing the Critically Ill Adult,* ed 2. Addison-Wesley, Menlo Park, 1984.
LARSON, EL, AND VAZQUEZ, M: *Critical Care Nursing.* WB Saunders, Philadelphia, 1983.
MCCAFFERY, M: *Nursing Management of the Patient in Pain.* JB Lippincott, Philadelphia, 1972.

Chapter 10: Articles

BAXTER, CR, MARVIN, JA, ET AL: *Fluid and electrolyte therapy of burn shock.* Heart Lung 2(5):707, 1973.
FREEMAN, JW: *Nursing care of the patient with a burn injury.* Critical Care Nurse 4(6):52, November/December, 1984.
HURT, R: *More than skin deep, guidelines for caring for the burn patient.* Nursing85, 15(6):52–57, June 1985.
KENNER, C, AND MANNING, S: *Emergency care of the burn patient.* Critical Care Update 7:24, October 1980.
MORATH, MA, MILLER, SF, ET AL: *Interpretation of assessment data in burn patients.* The Bulletin and Clinical Review of Burn Injuries 2(21), 1985.
ROBERTSON, KE, CROSS, PJ, ET AL: Burn care: The crucial first days. AJN 1(30):30–45, January 1985.
ROSEQUIST, CC, AND SHEPP, PH: *Burn care: The nutrition factor.* AJN 1(45):45–47, January 1985.
TOBES, SA, AND BOWDEN, ML: *Teaching coping strategies for pain management.* The Bulletin and Clinical Review of Burn Injuries 2(33), 1985.

Chapter 11: Books

Pneumocystis Pneumoniae. Los Angeles MMWR, 30:250–252, 1981.
ALTMAN, D: *AIDS in the Mind of America.* Anchor Press/Doubleday, New York, 1986.
BEAL, J: *Critical Care of Surgical Patients.* Macmillan, New York, 1982.
BERNALES, V: *City and County of San Francisco, Department of Public Health.* Department of Industrial Relations Labor Commissioner, Case #11-17001-1, September 6, 1985.
CHINN, PL: *Ethical Issues in Nursing.* Aspen Rockville, MD, 1986.
HOLLOWAY, N: *Nursing the Critically Ill Adult,* ed 2. Addison-Wesley, Reading, MA, 1984.
SONNTAG, S: *Illness as a Metaphor.* Farrar, Straus & Giroux, New York, 1978.
South Florida Blood Service, Inc. vs Rasmussen, 467 So. 2nd 798 (Fla. App. 1985).

Chapter 11: Articles

BOND, G, ET AL: *Septicemia from an unexpected source . . . transducer heads.* RN 45:48–49, July 1982.
CENTER FOR DISEASE CONTROL: *Guidelines for surveillance: Acquired immunodeficiency syndrome.* Morbidity and Mortality Weekly Report 34:373–375, 1985.
CENTER FOR DISEASE CONTROL: *Recommendations for preventing transmission of infection with HTTLV-III/LAV in the workplace.* Morbidity and Mortality Weekly Report 34:45, November 5, 1985.
CHAMBERS, J, AND CLICK, *Suspecting and detecting sepsis in the dialysis patient.* Nephrology Nurse, May/June 1982.
CLEARY, T: *Serratio marcescens bacteremias in an Intensive Care Unit.* Infection Control 9(4):107–111, November 1981.
FAUCI, A: *Indicators of cell-mediated immunity in the AIDS and other immunodeficient conditions.* University of Alabama School of Medicine, Birmingham, 1984.
FOX, B, AND STEGALL, B: *Take precautions now—patients receiving total perenteral nutrition (TPN) run the risk of sepsis.* Nursing85, pp 48–49, May 1985.
HALL, KV: *Detecting septic shock before it's too late.* RN, pp 29–32, September 1981.
JAFE, HW, SELIK, RM: *Acquired immune deficiency syndrome in the United States: The first 1,000 cases.* J Infect Dis 148:339–345, 1983.
KIRCHNER, CW: *Two serious complications of neoplasia: Sepsis and disseminated intravascular coagulation.* NCNA, 17(4):595-606, December 1982.
KLEIN, D: *Shock: Physiology, signs and symptoms.* Nursing84, pp 44–45, September 1984.
KLIMEK, J, ET AL: *Enterococcal infections in a large community hospital, with emphasis on bacteremia.* Infection Control, 8(2):58–61, May 1980.
LAMB, LS: *Think you know septic shock? Read this.* Nursing82 12(1):34–43, January 1982.
LARSON, E: *Infection control issues in critical care: An update.* Heart Lung 14(2):149–155, March 1985.
RICE, V: *The critical continuum of septic shock.* Critical Care Nurse, pp 86–109, September/October 1984.
WOLFF, S, AND BUTLER, T: *Gram-negative sepsis.* Topics in Emergency Medicine, pp 36–40, April 1982.

Chapter 11: Personal Communications

Department of Pathology, University of Colorado Health Sciences Center, School of Medicine.
Department of Virology, UCHSC, University Hospital.
Department of Immunology, UCHSC, School of Medicine.

Department of Clinical Laboratories, Information Referral Center, UCHSC, University Hospital.
Department of Respiratory Medicine, Blood Gas Laboratory, UCHSC, University Hospital.

Chapter 12: Books

ALPERS, D, CLOUSE, R, ET AL: *Manual of Nutritional Therapeutics.* Little, Brown & Co, Boston, 1983.
ALTMAN, D: *Aids in the Mind of America.* Anchor Press/Doubleday, Garden City, NY, 1986.
ANWAR, H, FERNANDE, M, ET AL: *Trauma and Pregnancy.* PSG Publishing, Littleton, MA, 1985.
ARIAS, F: *High Risk Pregnancy and Delivery.* CV Mosby St Louis, 1984.
CAMPBELL, C: *Nursing Diagnosis and Interventions in Nursing Practice.* John Wiley & Sons, New York, 1984.
CARPENITO, L: *Nursing Diagnosis: Application to Clinical Practice.* JB Lippincott, Philadelphia, 1983.
CERRA, F: *Pocket Manual of Surgical Nutrition.* CV Mosby, St Louis, 1984.
COHEN-ADDAD, N: *Trauma and Pregnancy.* PSG Publishing, Littleton, MA, 1985.
COUNTEE, R, THOMPSON, J, ET AL: *Trauma and Pregnancy.* PSG Publishing, Littleton, MA, 1985.
DEVITA, VT, HELLMAN, S, AND ROSENBERG, S: *AIDS,* JB Lippincott, Philadelphia, 1985.
GRANT, JB: *Handbook of Total Parenteral Nutrition.* WB Saunders, Philadelphia, 1980.
HAYCOCK, C: *Trauma and Pregnancy.* PSG Publishing, Littleton, MA, 1985.
HAZINSKI, MF: *Nursing Care of the Critically Ill Child.* CV Mosby, St Louis, 1984.
JENSEN, M AND BOBAK, I: *Maternity and Gynecologic Care.* CV Mosby, St Louis, 1985.
LEVIN, D., MORRISS, F, EL AL: *A Practical Guide to Pediatric Intensive Care,* ed 2. CV Mosby, St Louis, 1984.
OLDS, S, ET AL: *Maternal-Newborn Nursing,* ed 2. Addison-Wesley, Menlo Park, 1984.
ROMBEAU, J AND CALDWELL, M (EDS): *Clinical Nutrition, Vol 1. Enteral and Tube Feeding.* WB Saunders, Philadelphia, 1984.
SKILLMAN, J: *Intensive Care.* Little, Brown and Co, Boston, 1975.
SMITH, J: *Pediatric Critical Care.* John Wiley & Sons, New York, 1983.
AMERICAN ASSOCIATION OF CRITICAL CARE NURSES: *Standards for Nursing Care of the Critically Ill.* Reston Publishing, Reston, VA, 1981.
STUART, GW, SUNDEEN, SJ: *Principles and Practice of Psychiatric Nursing,* ed 2. CV Mosby, St Louis, 1983.
WILMORE, D: *The Metabolic Management of the Critically Ill.* Plenum Medical Book Co, New York, 1977.
WILSON, R: *Principles and Techniques of Critical Care,* Upjohn, 1977.
WRIGHT, RA AND HEYMSFIELD, S (EDS): *Nutritional Assessment,* Blackwell Scientific Publications, Boston, 1984.
WYNGAARDEN, J AND SMITH, L: *Textbook of Medicine,* WB Saunders, Philadelphia, 1982.

Chapter 12: Articles

ALLEM, J AND MELLIN, G: *The new epidemic.* AJN, p 1718, November 1982.
AUMANN, G AND BLAKE, G: *Ritodrine hydrochloride in the control of premature labor.* JOGN Nursing, 11:75–79, March/April 1982.
BENNETT, J: *AIDS epidemiology update.* AJN, pp 968–972, September 1985.
BENNETT, J: *HTLV-III AIDS link.* AJN, 85:1086–1089, October 1985.
CARTER, J: *CPR: Breathing life back into a child.* Nursing86 16(10):52–57, October, 1986.
CECCHI, R: *When the system fails.* AJN, pp 45–47, January 1986.
CENTER FOR DISEASE CONTROL: *Reports on AIDS June1981–January 1985.* Morbidity and Mortality Weekly Report, March 1985.
CENTER FOR DISEASE CONTROL: *Guidelines for health care settings.* Morbidity and Mortality Weekly Report, November 1985.
CERRATO, P: *When you think your patient needs TPN.* RN, pp 79–83, May 1985.
CHELSEA PSYCHOTHERAPY ASSOCIATES: *When a friend has AIDS.* Distributed by GMHC.
COUSTAN, D: *The pregnant patient with overt diabetes.* RN, pp 27–33, January/February 1981.
FOX, B, STEGALL, B, ET AL: *Take precautions now (TPN).* Nursing85, pp 48–49, May 1985.
FORLAW, L AND BAYER, L: *Symposia on Nutrition.* Nurs Clin N Am 18(1):3–128, March 1983.
FOSTER, C: *The pregnant trauma patient.* Nursing84 14:58–63, November 1984.
GENT, A AND SANDERSON, P: *Intravenous nutrition.* Nursing Mirror 158(22):19–22, May 1984.
GUINESS, R: *How to use the new small-bore feeding tubes.* Nursing86 16(4):51–56, April 1986.
HAZINSKI, MF: *Nursing care of the critically ill child: The seven point check.* Ped Nurs 2:453, 1985.
HENIG, R: *AIDS, a new disease's deadly odyssey.* New York Times Magazine, February 6, 1986.
HICKEY, M: *What are the needs of families of critically ill patients?* Focus on Critical Care, 12(1):41–43, February 1985.
HOFFMASTER, J: *Detecting and treating pregnancy-induced hypertension.* MCN 8:398–405, November/December 1983.
KENNEDY-CALDWELL, C (ED): *Nutrition support nursing: Core curriculum.* American Society for Parenteral and Enteral Nutrition, 1985.
KLEIBER, C: *Clinical implications of deep and shallow suctioning in neonatal patients.* Focus on Critical Care 13(4):36–39, August 1986.
KOONTZ, W AND CEFALO, R: Dos and don'ts of treating preeclampsia with $MgSO_4$. Contemp Ob/Gyn 25:163–167, October 1983.

LARKIN, M: *Nutrient snatchers.* Health, March 1986.

LUSBY AND SCHIETINGER: *Infection precautions for people with AIDS living in the community.* Distributed by Gay Men's Health Crisis (GMHC).

MAYBERRY, L AND FORTE, A: *Pregnancy-related disseminated intravascular coagulation (DIC).* MCN 10:168–173, May/June 1985.

MUNRO-BLACK, J: *The ABCs of total parenteral nutrition.* Nursing84 14(2):50–56, February 1984.

NEWKIRK, EJ, AND FRY, ME: *Trauma during pregnancy.* Focus on Critical Care, 12(6)31–39, December 1985.

Nursing Grand Rounds: ICU psychosis: helping your patient return to reality. Nursing82, 12(1):58–63, January 1982.

PADBERG, R, RUGGIERO, J, ET AL: *Central venous catheterization for parteral nutrition.* Ann Surgery 193:264–270, 1981.

PEABODY, B: *A mother's perspective.* AJN, pp 45–46, January 1986.

POPKIN, B: *Caring for the AIDS patient—Fearlessly.* Nursing83 pp 50–55, September 1983.

RAMSEY, PW: *Bringing a patient through ICU psychosis.* RN, pp 42–45, September 1986.

THOMAS, D: *The ABCs of pediatric emergencies.* RN, 49(3):34–41, March 1986.

WALL, C: *Making life bearable for your chronic ICU patient.* RN, 48(5):61–68, May 1985.

WEIN AND LOPEZ: *Overview of psychological issues concerning AIDS.* Handout prepared and distributed by Gay Men's Health Crisis (GMHC).

WEINSTEIN, L: *Syndrome of hemolysis elevated liver enzymes, and low platelet count: A severe consequence of hypertension in pregnancy.* Am J Obstet Gynecol pp 159–167, January 1982.

WHITE, M AND RITCHIE, J: *Psychological stressors in antepartum hospitalization: Reports for pregnant women.* Maternal-Child Nursing Journal 13:47–56, Spring 1984.

WILLIS, S: *Hypertension in pregnancy: Pathophysiology.* AJN, pp 792–297, May 1982.

ZOLLI, A AND NEVILLE, W: *Chest Trauma In Pregnancy.* In HAYCOCK, C (ED): *Trauma and Pregnancy.* PSG Publishing Co, Littleton, MA, pp 120–135, 1985.

Appendix: Journals

Clinical Insights: Metabolic acidosis: Physiology, signs and symptoms. Nursing84 14(7):44–45, July 1984.

FOLK-LIGHTY, M: *Fluid imbalances.* Nursing84 14(2):34–41, February 1984.

GAMMON, S: *Respiratory Acidosis.* RN 12(8):68, August 1982.

LANE, G, PEIRCE, A: *When persistence pays off: Resolving the mystery of unexplained electrolyte imbalance.* Nursing82 12(1):44–47, January 1982.

MCADAMS. R, AND MCCLURE, K: *Hypovolemia: When to suspect it.* RN 49(12):34–37, December 1986.

MCADAMS, R, AND MCCLURE, K: *Hypovolemia: How to stop it.* RN 49(12):38–41, December 1986.

RN Master Care Plan: Correcting acid-base imbalance. RN 48(5):39–40, May 1985.

RN Master Care Plan: Preventing electrolyte imbalances. RN 47(11):32–33, November 1984.

INDEX OF NURSING DIAGNOSES

To Samantha, Sarah, and Becca

Contributors

Antonio Abbate, MD, PhD
James C. Roberts, Esquire Professor of Cardiology
VCU Pauley Heart Center
Virginia Commonwealth University
Richmond, Virginia

Dominick J. Angiolillo, MD, PhD
Professor of Medicine
Medical Director, Cardiovascular Research
Director, Interventional Cardiology Fellowship Program
Division of Cardiology
University of Florida College of Medicine—Jacksonville
Jacksonville, Florida

Nandan S. Anavekar, MBBCh, FACC
Associate Professor of Medicine
Department of Cardiovascular Diseases
Department of Radiology
Mayo Clinic
Rochester, Minnesota

Paul W. Armstrong, MD
Distinguished University Professor of Medicine
Founding Director, Canadian VIGOUR Centre
University of Alberta
Edmonton, Alberta, Canada

Kevin R. Bainey, MD, MSc, FRCPC
Assistant Professor of Medicine
Interventional Cardiologist
Director, Interventional Cardiology Fellowship Program
Associate Faculty, Canadian VIGOUR Centre
University of Alberta/Mazankowski Alberta Heart Institute
Edmonton, Alberta, Canada

Jacob F. Bentzon, MD, PhD
Professor
Centro Nacional de Investigaciones Cardiovasculares Carlos III (CNIC)
Madrid, Spain
Associate Professor
Department of Clinical Medicine
Aarhus University
Aarhus, Denmark

Deepak L. Bhatt, MD, MPH, FACC, FAHA, FSCAI, FESC
Executive Director, Interventional Cardiovascular Programs
Heart and Vascular Center, Brigham and Women's Hospital
Senior Investigator, TIMI Study Group
Professor of Medicine, Harvard Medical School
Boston, Massachusetts

Erin A. Bohula, MD, DPhil
TIMI Study Group and Division of Cardiology
Brigham and Women's Hospital
Harvard Medical School
Boston, Massachusetts

Roberto Bolli, MD
Chief, Division of Cardiovascular Medicine
Director, Institute of Molecular Cardiology
Executive Vice Chair, Department of Medicine
University of Louisville
Louisville, Kentucky

Marc P. Bonaca, MD, MPH
Associate Physician
Division of Cardiovascular Medicine
Brigham and Women's Hospital
Instructor, Harvard Medical School
Investigator, TIMI Study Group
Boston, Massachusetts

Jason S. Bradfield, MD, FACC, FHRS
Assistant Professor of Medicine
Director, Specialized Program for Ventricular Tachycardia
UCLA Cardiac Arrhythmia Center
David Geffen School of Medicine at UCLA
Los Angeles, California

Eugene Braunwald, MD, MD(Hon), ScD(Hon), FRCP
Distinguished Hersey Professor of Medicine
Harvard Medical School
Founding Chairman, TIMI Study Group
Brigham and Women's Hospital
Boston, Massachusetts

Una Buckley, MD
Electrophysiology Fellow
UCLA Cardiac Arrhythmia Center
David Geffen School of Medicine at UCLA
Los Angeles, California

Edward T. Carreras, MD
Fellow
Division of Cardiovascular Medicine
Brigham and Women's Hospital
Harvard Medical School
Boston, Massachusetts

Guillaume Cayla, MD, PhD
Professor of Cardiology
Department of Cardiology CHU Nimes
Nimes University Hospital
University of Montpellier
Member of the ACTION Study Group
Nimes, France

Jean Philippe Collet, MD, PhD
Professor of Cardiovascular Medicine
UPMC (PARIS 6)
ACTION Study Group
Institut de Cardiologie
Pitié-Salpêtrière University Hospital
Paris, France

Jeremiah P. Depta, MD, MPHS, FACC
Director of the Advanced Valvular and Structural Heart Disease Program
Sands-Constellation Heart Institute
Rochester General Hospital
Rochester, New York

Marcelo F. Di Carli, MD
Assistant Professor of Radiology and Medicine
Harvard Medical School
Chief, Division of Nuclear Medicine and Molecular Imaging
Director, Noninvasive Cardiovascular Imaging Program
Brigham and Women's Hospital
Boston, Massachusetts

Jacob A. Doll, MD
Division of Cardiology
Duke University Medical Center
Durham, North Carolina

Anique Ducharme, MD, MSc
Professor of Medicine
Université de Montréal
Director, Heart Failure Clinic
Montreal Heart Institute
Montreal, Quebec, Canada

Erling Falk, MD, PhD
Professor
Department of Clinical Medicine
Aarhus University
Department of Cardiology
Aarhus University Hospital
Aarhus, Denmark

James C. Fang, MD
Professor of Medicine
Division of Cardiovascular Diseases
University of Utah
Salt Lake City, Utah

Keith A. A. Fox, MBChB, FRCP, FESC, FACC
Professor of Cardiology
Consultant Cardiologist
University of Edinburgh
Edinburgh, Scotland, United Kingdom

Francesco Franchi, MD
Assistant Professor of Medicine
Division of Cardiology
University of Florida College of Medicine-Jacksonville
Jacksonville, Florida

J. Michael Gaziano, MD, MPH
Chief, Division of Aging, Brigham and Women's Hospital
Scientific Director, Massachusetts Veterans Epidemiology Research and Information Center
Veterans Administration Boston Healthcare System
Professor of Medicine
Harvard Medical School
Boston, Massachusetts

Thomas A. Gaziano, MD, MSc
Assistant Professor
Harvard Medical School
Cardiovascular Medicine Division
Brigham and Women's Hospital
Boston, Massachusetts

Shahab Ghafghazi, MD
Assistant Professor of Medicine
Division of Cardiovascular Medicine and Institute of Molecular Cardiology
Department of Medicine
University of Louisville
Louisville, Kentucky

Christopher B. Granger, MD
Professor of Medicine
Division of Cardiovascular Diseases
Duke University Medical Center
Durham, North Carolina

John D. Grizzard, MD
Associate Professor
Departments of Radiology and Internal Medicine
Charles L. Baird Professor of Non-Invasive Cardiovascular Imaging
VCU Health Systems
Richmond, Virginia

Sharon L. Hale, BS
Assistant Editor
Journal of Cardiovascular Drugs and Therapy
Huntington Medical Research Institutes
Pasadena, California

Timothy D. Henry, MD
Director
Division of Cardiology
Cedars-Sinai Heart Institute
Los Angeles, California

Udo Hoffmann, MD, MPH
Professor of Radiology
Chief, Division of Cardiovascular Imaging
Department of Radiology
Massachusetts General Hospital and Harvard Medical School
Boston, Massachusetts

Allan S. Jaffe, MD
Professor of Medicine and Laboratory Medicine and Pathology
Consultant in Cardiology and Laboratory Medicine and Pathology
Chair, Division of Core Clinical Laboratory Service
Department of Laboratory Medicine and Pathology
Mayo Clinic College of Medicine
Rochester, Minnesota

Stefan James, MD, PhD
Professor of Cardiology
Department of Medical Sciences, Cardiology and Uppsala Clinical Research Center
Uppsala University
Department of Cardiology
Uppsala University Hospital
Uppsala, Sweden

Ik-Kyung Jang, MD, PhD
Professor of Medicine
Harvard Medical School
Cardiology Division
Massachusetts General Hospital
Boston, Massachusetts

Raymond J. Kim, MD
Professor of Medicine and Radiology
Director, Duke Cardiovascular Magnetic Resonance Center
Duke University Medical Center
Durham, North Carolina

Robert A. Kloner, MD, PhD
Vice President for Translation
Director of Cardiovascular Research Institute
Huntington Medical Research Institutes
Pasadena, California
Clinical Professor of Medicine
Division of Cardiovascular Medicine, Department of Medicine
Keck School of Medicine
University of Southern California
Los Angeles, California
Editor-in-Chief
Journal of Cardiovascular Pharmacology and Therapeutics
SAGE Publishing
Thousand Oaks, California

David C. Lange, MD
Fellow
Internal Medicine, Division of Cardiology
Cedars-Sinai Medical Center
Los Angeles, California

Peter Libby, MD
Mallinckrodt Professor of Medicine
Harvard Medical School
Division of Cardiovascular Medicine
Brigham and Women's Hospital
Boston, Massachusetts

Daniel Lindholm, MD, PhD
Uppsala Clinical Research Center, and Department of Medical Sciences, Cardiology
Uppsala University
Department of Cardiology
Uppsala University Hospital
Uppsala, Sweden

Jessica L. Mega, MD, MPH
Associate Professor of Medicine
Harvard Medical School
TIMI Study Group
Brigham and Women's Hospital
Boston, Massachusetts

Todd D. Miller, MD
Professor of Medicine
Department of Cardiovascular Diseases
Mayo Clinic
Rochester, Minnesota

Gilles Montalescot, MD, PhD
Professor of Cardiology
University of Paris VI
Head, Department of Cardiology
Pitie-Salpetriere University Hospital
President of the ACTION Study Group
Institut de Cardiologie
Paris, France

Róisín Morgan, MD
Noninvasive Cardiovascular Imaging
Brigham and Women's Hospital
Boston, Massachusetts

David A. Morrow, MD, MPH
Professor of Medicine, Harvard Medical School
Director, Levine Cardiac Intensive Care Unit
Cardiovascular Division, Brigham and Women's Hospital
Director, TIMI Biomarker Program
Senior Investigator, TIMI Study Group
Boston, Massachusetts

Jack H. Morshedzadeh, MD
Assistant Professor
Division of Cardiovascular Diseases
University of Utah
Salt Lake City, Utah

Christian Mueller, MD
Professor of Cardiology, Internal Medicine, and Intensive Care Medicine
Department of Cardiology and Cardiovascular Research Institute Basel
University Hospital Basel
Basel, Switzerland

Matthias Nahrendorf, MD
Center for Systems Biology
Massachusetts General Hospital
Boston, Massachusetts

L. Kristin Newby, MD
Professor of Medicine
Division of Cardiology
Duke University Medical Center
Durham, North Carolina

Lee Nguyen, MD, MSc
Fellow
Department of Cardiology
Pitié-Salpêtrière University Hospital
University of Paris VI—Pierre & Marie Curie
Paris, France

E. Magnus Ohman, MD
Professor of Medicine
The Kent and Siri Rawson Director, Duke Program for Advanced Coronary Disease
Vice-Chair, Department of Medicine—Development and Innovation
Associate Director, Duke Heart Center
Senior Investigator, Duke Clinical Research Institute
Duke University Medical Center
Durham, North Carolina

Daniel S. Ong, MD
Fellow
Cardiology Division
Massachusetts General Hospital
Harvard Medical School
Boston, Massachusetts

Sunil V. Rao, MD
Associate Professor of Medicine
Duke University Medical Center
Section Chief, Cardiology
Durham VA Medical Center
Durham, North Carolina

Marc S. Sabatine, MD, MPH
Chairman, TIMI Study Group
Physician
Division of Cardiovascular Medicine
Brigham and Women's Hospital
Professor of Medicine
Harvard Medical School
Boston, Massachusetts

Benjamin M. Scirica, MD, MPH
Associate Professor of Medicine
Harvard Medical School
Cardiovascular Division
Senior Investigator, TIMI Study Group
Brigham and Women's Hospital
Boston, Massachusetts

Kalyanam Shivkumar, MD, PhD
Professor of Medicine and Radiology
Director, UCLA Cardiac Arrhythmia Center and EP Programs
Director and Chief, Interventional CV Programs
Director, Adult Cardiac Catheterization Laboratories
Ronald Reagan UCLA Medical Center
UCLA Health System
Los Angeles, California

Johanne Silvain, MD, PhD
Associate Professor of Cardiology
University of Paris VI (UPMC)
Director of the Coronary Care Unit
Pitie-Salpetriere University Hospital (APHP)
Member of the ACTION COEUR Study Group
Institut de Cardiologie
Paris, France

Peter R. Sinnaeve, MD, PhD
Professor of Medicine
Department of Cardiovascular Medicine
University Hospitals Leuven—Campus Gasthuisberg
University of Leuven
Leuven, Belgium

Filip K. Swirski, PhD
Associate Professor
Harvard Medical School
Center for Systems Biology
Massachusetts General Hospital
Boston, Masachusetts

Jean-Claude Tardif, CM, MD, FRCPC, FACC, FAHA, FESC, FCAHS
Director of Research Center
Montreal Heart Institute
Canada Research Chair in Translational and Personalized Medicine
Endowed Research Chair in Atherosclerosis
Professor of Medicine
Université de Montréal
Montreal, Quebec, Canada

Rod S. Taylor, MSc, PhD
Professor of Health Services Research
Director of Exeter Clinical Trials Unit
NIHR Senior Investigator
University of Exeter Medical School
Exeter, United Kingdom

James E. Udelson, MD
Professor of Medicine and Radiology
Tufts University School of Medicine
Chief, Division of Cardiology
The CardioVascular Center
Tufts Medical Center
Boston, Massachusetts

Frans Van de Werf, MD, PhD
Professor of Cardiology
Department of Cardiovascular Sciences
University of Leuven
Leuven, Belgium

Christoph Varenhorst, MD, PhD
Consultant in Clinical and Interventional Cardiology
Department of Medical Sciences, Cardiology and Uppsala Clinical Research Center
Uppsala University
Department of Cardiology
Uppsala University Hospital
Uppsala, Sweden

Amit N. Vora, MD, MPH
Fellow
Division of Cardiovascular Diseases
Duke University Medical Center
Durham, North Carolina

Harvey D. White, MB, ChB, DSc, FRACP, FACC, FESC, FAHA, FHKCC(Hon), FCSANZ, FRSNZ
La'auli (matai), Prince Mahidol Laureate, and John Neutze Scholar
Director of Coronary Care and Green Lane Cardiovascular Research Unit
Green Lane Cardiovascular Service
Auckland City Hospital
Auckland, New Zealand

Ann-Dorthe Olsen Zwisler, MD, PhD
Professor
Cardiologist, Senior Consultant
Head, Danish Knowledge Centre for Rehabilitation and Palliative Care (REHPA)
University Hospital Odense and University of Southern Denmark
Odense, Denmark

Foreword

Early in the twentieth century, coronary artery disease was recognized as a serious condition, but the distinction between its two principal presentations, angina pectoris and acute myocardial infarction, was not clear. By the 1920s, the distinct clinical and pathological manifestations of chronic angina pectoris and acute infarction became clear. In the 1940s, a syndrome intermediate between angina pectoris and acute myocardial infarction, the so-called "intermediate syndrome" (later renamed *unstable angina*), was found to be quite common. By the 1960s, increasing attention was focused on the separation of patients with acute myocardial infarction into those who presented with ST-elevation myocardial infarction (STEMI) and non–ST-elevation myocardial infarction (NSTEMI), then often referred to as "intramural," "non-transmural," or "non–Q wave" MI. All three of these conditions (i.e., unstable angina, STEMI, NSTEMI) were considered to make up the acute coronary syndrome. With the development of more sensitive biochemical markers of myocardial necrosis (i.e., the troponins), the distinction between unstable angina and NSTEMI has become blurred, and an increasing fraction of patients with the former condition actually evolve evidence of myocardial necrosis (i.e., infarction). Thus, it now appears that a large majority of patients with acute coronary syndrome actually have acute myocardial infarction.

Research on this condition has moved forward on many fronts. This text, masterfully edited by David Morrow, an experienced clinician and investigator in this field, captures the major developments, which include the many epidemiological, clinical, pathophysiological, and therapeutic advances in myocardial infarction. Among them are the prehospital assessment and care of patients; the optimal use of cardiac troponins and of a variety of imaging techniques in diagnosis and management of patients with STEMI who cannot receive immediate coronary artery stenting; the optimal timing of revascularization in patients with NSTEMI; the individualization of antiplatelet therapy; the application of mechanical circulatory support for patients with cardiogenic shock; efforts to reverse myocardial infarction–induced ventricular remodeling; and the current status of stem cell therapy in patients after infarction.

The enormous worldwide frequency of acute myocardial infarction and its seriousness places this condition at the very "heart" of cardiology. Indeed, just about every practicing adult cardiologist—whether invasive or noninvasive, whether primarily office- or hospital-based, whether subspecializing in hypertension, heart failure, arrhythmias, prevention, or rehabilitation—encounters patients with myocardial infarction and should stay abreast of the important recent developments in diagnosis and management.

Cardiologists dealing with these patients as well as trainees and clinical investigators will be indebted to Dr. Morrow and his talented authors for providing this important new book. We are proud that it is a companion to *Heart Disease—A Textbook of Cardiovascular Medicine*.

Eugene Braunwald
Boston, Massachusetts
Douglas P. Zipes
Indianapolis, Indiana
Peter Libby
Boston, Massachusetts
Robert O. Bonow
Chicago, Illinois
Douglas L. Mann
St. Louis, Missouri
Gordon F. Tomaselli
Baltimore, Maryland

Preface

From the first description of coronary thrombosis causing acute myocardial infarction in 1910, the classification of myocardial infarction, its epidemiology and natural history, our understanding of its pathobiology, and the landscape of its management have evolved immeasurably. This first edition of *Myocardial Infarction: A Companion to Braunwald's Heart Disease* is aimed at distilling this century of evolution to its most important principles and capturing the contemporary state of the art of clinical care as well as translational and clinical science impacting the management of myocardial infarction. As such, this textbook should be of interest to clinical practitioners, medical trainees, and scientists with an interest in ischemic heart disease and its complications.

All of the contributors who have been involved in the development of this text have labored to produce a book that will serve equally well for comprehensive review and as a readily accessible clinical resource for the busy clinician. We have been impressed by the changing landscape of print and electronic media and have worked to create a forward-looking text that offers both a traditional printed book and an interactive online version that is optimized for tablet and hand-held electronic reading. As such, the authors have molded figures, clinical management algorithms, animations, and videos into engaging, dynamic, and readily accessible educational media for our electronic readers.

The book is framed by the clinical course of care for the patient with myocardial infarction. It is divided into five sections that navigate from the pathobiological underpinnings of atherothrombosis, through the critical initial clinical evaluation and in-hospital management of myocardial infarction, to culminate in the planning of short-term and long-term secondary prevention at the time of hospital discharge. Four of the sections include one or more chapters designated as a "Clinical Practice/Controversy" chapter, which are designed to be management-focused, practical-minded explorations of common, yet challenging, clinical decisions in the care of patients with acute myocardial infarction. In these chapters, internationally recognized leaders in their field have not only reviewed the current evidence and professional guidelines but also offered their own perspective on "best practice" in areas where there is equipoise or controversy.

It has been a tremendous privilege and pleasure to work with the exceptional group of clinical experts, educators, and clinician-scientists who have contributed to this text, and I wish to thank each of them. Foremost, I wish to recognize the sage guidance of Dr. Eugene Braunwald, whose unwavering commitment to excellence is the foundation for *Braunwald's Heart Disease* and each of its companions.

David A. Morrow, MD, MPH
Boston, Massachusetts

Contents

SECTION IV IN-HOSPITAL COMPLICATIONS AND ASSESSMENT

SECTION V DISCHARGE AND BEYOND

Video Contents

Braunwald's Heart Disease Family of Books

BRAUNWALD'S HEART DISEASE COMPANIONS

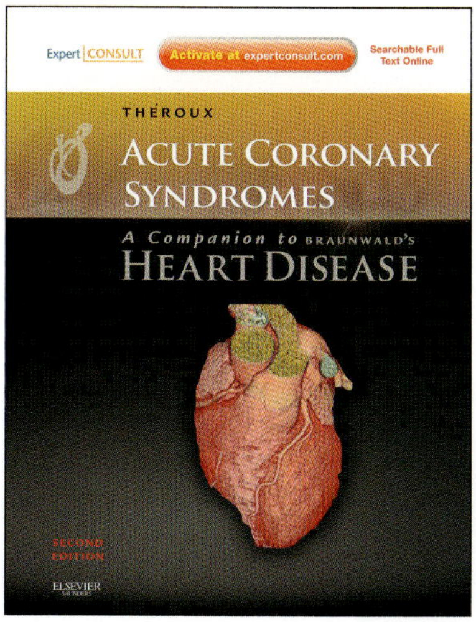

THÉROUX
Acute Coronary Syndromes

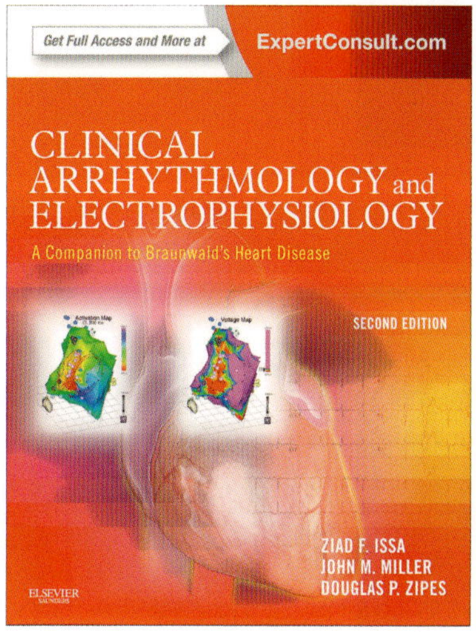

ISSA, MILLER, AND ZIPES
Clinical Arrhythmology and Electrophysiology

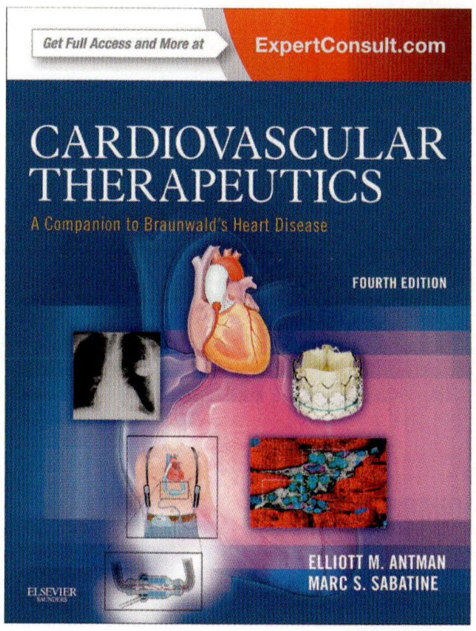

ANTMAN AND SABATINE
Cardiovascular Therapeutics

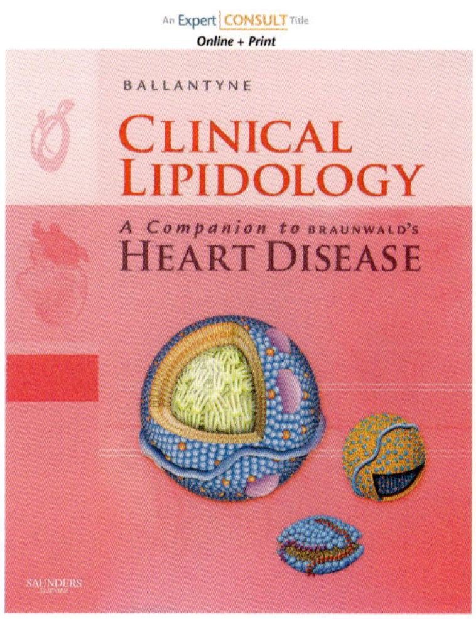

BALLANTYNE
Clinical Lipidology

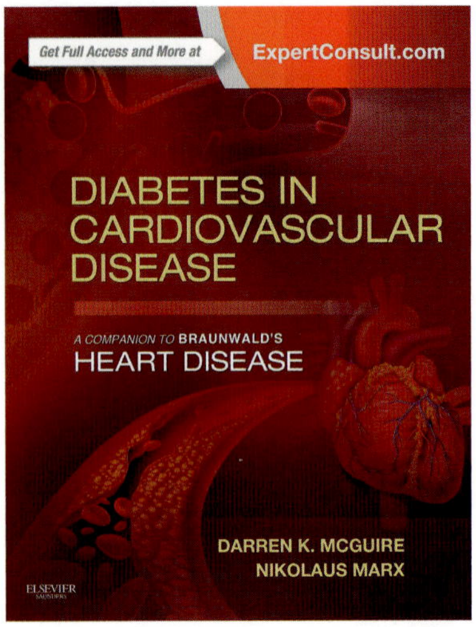

MCGUIRE AND MARX
Diabetes in Cardiovascular Disease

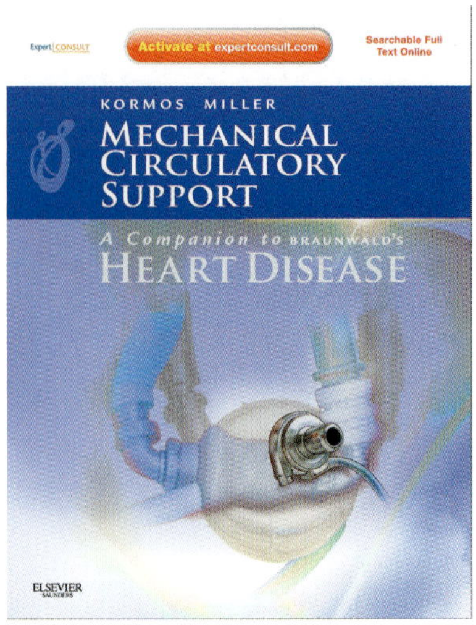

KORMOS AND MILLER
Mechanical Circulatory Support

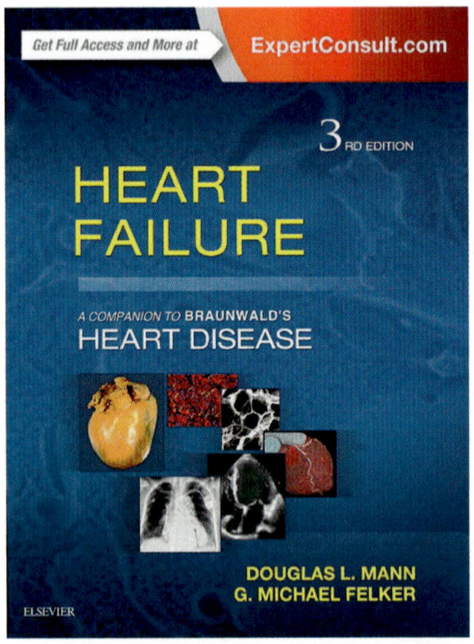

MANN AND FELKER
Heart Failure

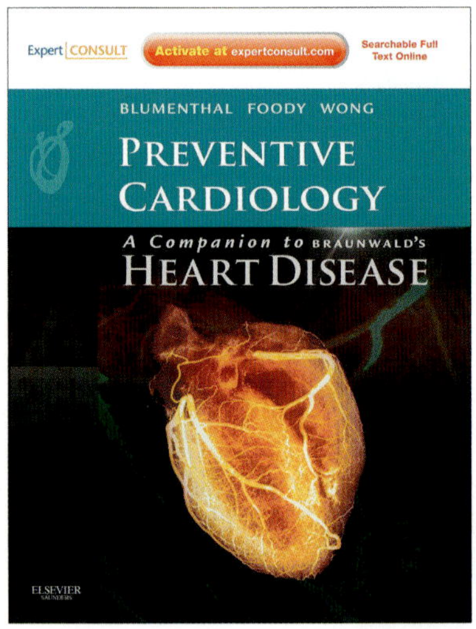

BLUMENTHAL, FOODY, AND WONG
Preventive Cardiology

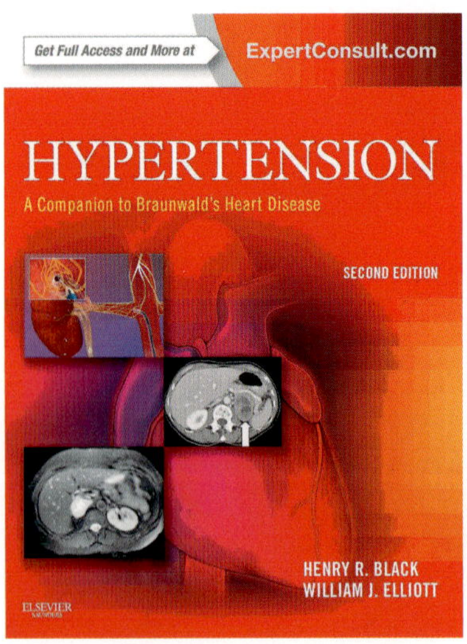

BLACK AND ELLIOTT
Hypertension

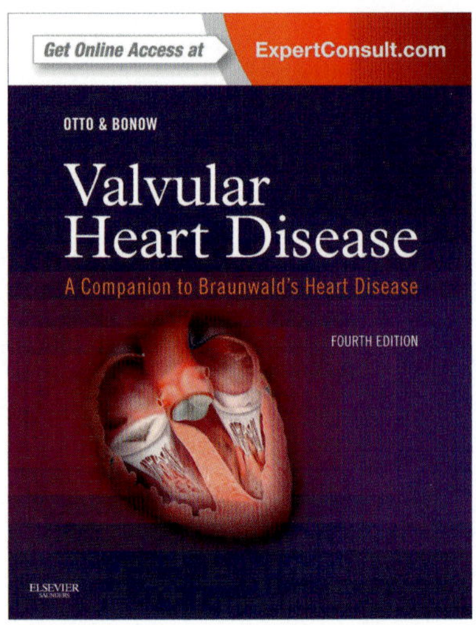

OTTO AND BONOW
Valvular Heart Disease

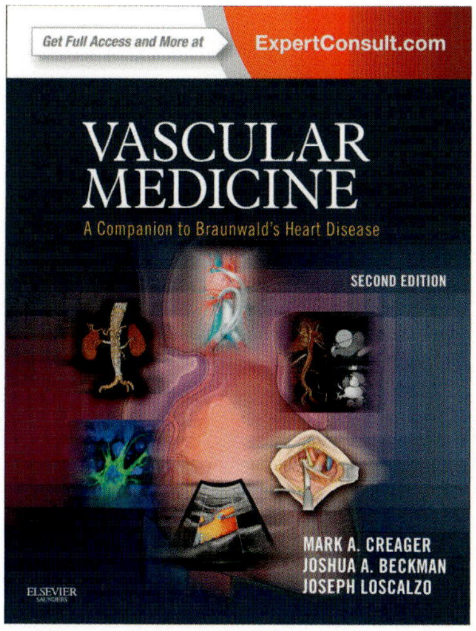

CREAGER, BECKMAN, AND LOSCALZO
Vascular Medicine

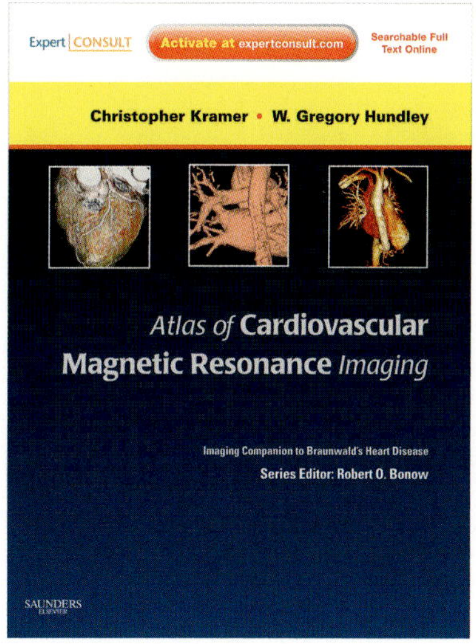

KRAMER AND HUNDLEY
Atlas of Cardiovascular Magnetic Resonance Imaging

BRAUNWALD'S HEART DISEASE REVIEW AND ASSESSMENT

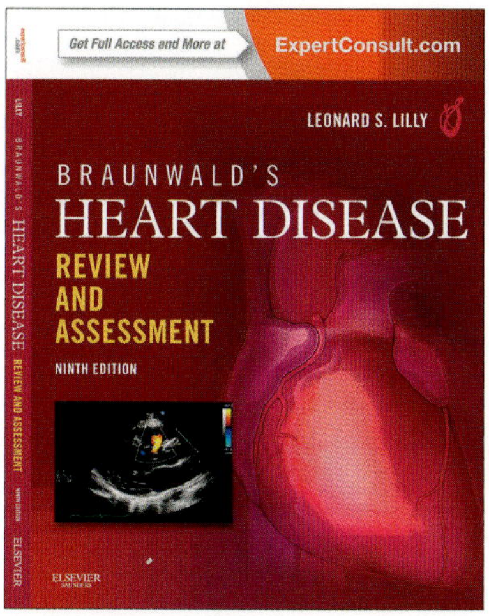

LILLY
Braunwald's Heart Disease Review and Assessment

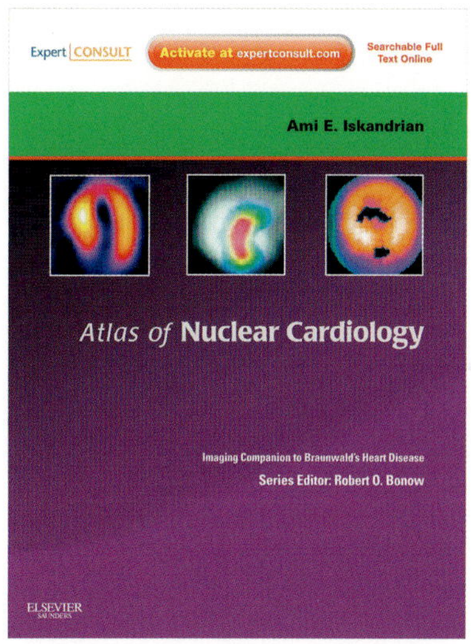

ISKANDRIAN AND GARCIA
Atlas of Nuclear Cardiology

BRAUNWALD'S HEART DISEASE IMAGING COMPANIONS

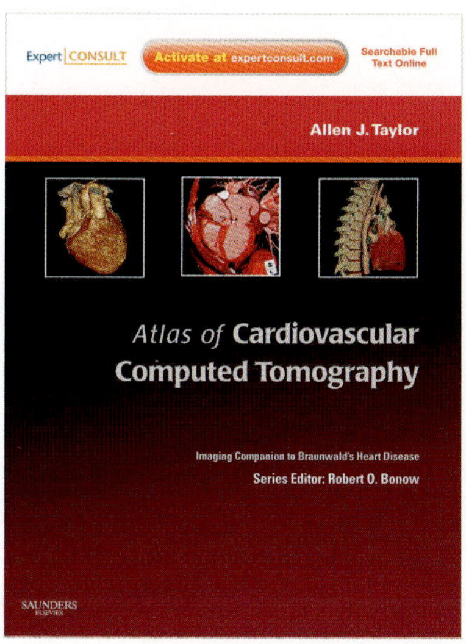

TAYLOR
Atlas of Cardiovascular Computer Tomography

COMING SOON!

BODEN
Chronic Coronary Syndromes

BAKRIS
Hypertension

DE LEMOS
Chronic Coronary Artery Disease

SECTION I

EPIDEMIOLOGY AND PATHOPHYSIOLOGY

1 Classification and Diagnosis of Acute Coronary Syndromes

David A. Morrow and Eugene Braunwald

INTRODUCTION

Until the beginning of 20th century, it was believed that coronary thrombosis was always immediately fatal. In 1910, two Ukrainian physicians described five patients with acute myocardial infarction (MI), in whom three were found to have coronary thrombosis at autopsy. In 1912, James Herrick articulated the first clear description in English of the clinical syndrome of acute MI in his landmark article, "Certain Clinical Features of Sudden Obstruction of the Coronary Arteries." Up to that time, although pathologists had made causal connections between thrombotic coronary occlusion and degenerative changes in the myocardium, a clinical syndrome of MI in surviving patients had not been described. The term acute coronary syndrome (ACS) that emerged more than eight decades later is now used to denote any clinical presentation suggestive of acute myocardial ischemia caused by unstable ischemic heart disease. ACS encompasses both unstable angina (UA) and acute MI, in distinction from chronic stable angina. In addition, some clinicians have adapted use of the term ACS to imply acute coronary atherothrombosis, which is differentiated from ischemia caused by increased myocardial oxygen demand in the presence of stable coronary atherosclerotic lesions.

Over the past century, the classification of ACS, its epidemiology, and our understanding of its pathobiology have evolved considerably.[1–3] The epidemiology and natural history of MI are reviewed in Chapter 2. The pathobiology of ACS is discussed in Chapter 3. Both a historical perspective and a summary of emerging concepts regarding mechanisms of myocardial ischemic injury and healing are provided in Chapter 4. Chapter 7 details the role of cardiac biomarkers of necrosis in the diagnosis of acute MI. In this chapter, we describe the evolution of the clinical classification of ACS, including UA, non–ST-elevation MI (NSTEMI), ST-elevation MI (STEMI), and the additional subclassification of the types of MI as defined in the section on Universal Definition of Myocardial Infarction. This chapter reflects our opinion that in the era of high-sensitivity assays for cardiac troponin (cTn), UA is a disappearing diagnostic entity.[3]

SPECTRUM OF UNSTABLE ISCHEMIC HEART DISEASE

Stable ischemic heart disease (SIHD) is most commonly caused by atheromatous plaque that obstructs or gradually narrows one or more of the epicardial coronary arteries. Although the clinical manifestations of SIHD are variable, stable angina induced by increased effort, as classically described by Heberden in 1772, is typically the predominant symptom. UA is characterized by an accelerated pattern of increasing frequency and tempo of angina or angina at rest in the absence of MI. MI is defined by evidence of myocardial necrosis in a clinical setting consistent with acute myocardial ischemia. Because of the implications for treatment, including reperfusion therapy, MI is classified clinically into those cases in which the clinical presentation includes ST-segment elevation in 2 contiguous leads on the 12-lead electrocardiogram (ECG) and those cases without ST-elevation at presentation, which are designated as NSTEMI. Moreover, because of their indistinguishable clinical and electrocardiographic features (ST-segment depressions and T-wave inversion) and similar management, patients with UA and NSTEMI are commonly grouped together by the term non–ST-elevation ACS (NSTE-ACS) (Figure 1-1; also see the section on Clinical Classification: Electrocardiography).

A nomenclature that incorporates the development of pathological Q waves (Q-wave MI) versus their absence (non–Q-wave MI) on the surface ECG is no longer deemed useful as part of initial management of acute MI; however, the presence of Q waves should be recognized as indicative of late presentation of a large MI. In addition to the categories already described, MI can be classified into various

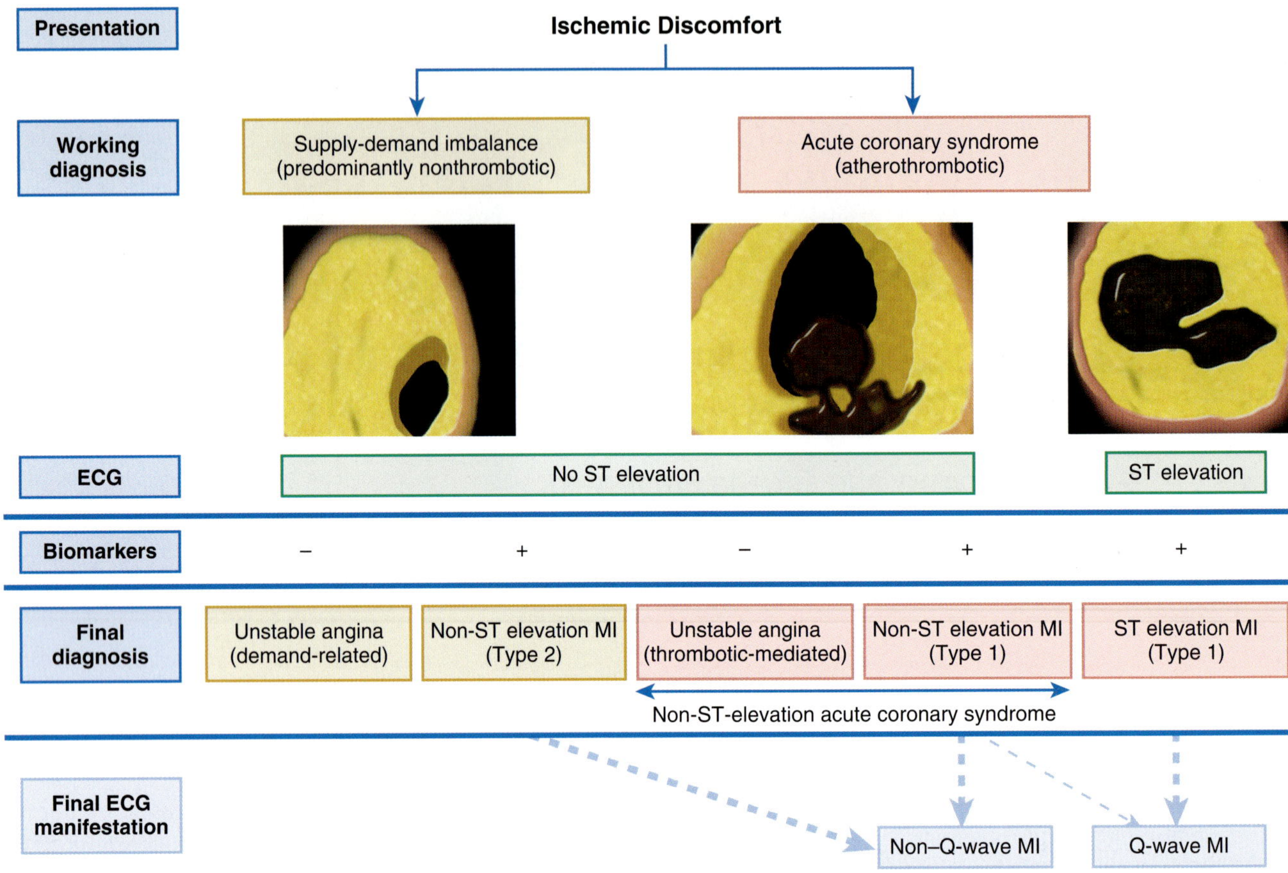

FIGURE 1-1 Myocardial ischemia and infarction. Unstable ischemic syndromes may result from acute changes in either myocardial oxygen demand and/or supply. Predominantly nonthrombotically mediated events (*left side*) typically occur without ST-segment elevation but can result in myocardial infarction (MI) with elevated levels of cardiac biomarkers if the ischemia is sufficiently severe and prolonged (type 2 MI). Myocardial ischemia caused by acute coronary thrombosis (*right side*) may occur with or without ST-segment elevation. The distinction of whether MI has occurred is ultimately determined by the presence or absence of detectable elevation of circulating cardiac troponin. Non–Q-wave MI ultimately develops in most patients with non–ST-elevation MI (NSTEMI); Q-wave MI may develop in a few patients. MI that develops as the result of the atherothrombotic lesion of an acute coronary syndrome is classified as type I MI. *ECG*, Electrocardiography. *(Adapted from Scirica BM, Morrow DA: ST-elevation myocardial infarction: pathology, pathophysiology, and clinical features. In Mann DL, et al, eds:* Braunwald's heart disease: a textbook of cardiovascular medicine, *ed 10, Philadelphia, Saunders, 2015.)*

types, based on pathological, clinical, and prognostic differences, along with different treatment strategies (see the section on Clinical Classification).

Unstable Angina: A Historical Perspective

In the days of Herrick's original clinical description of MI, MI and angina were beginning to be recognized as manifestations of the same underlying disease process.[3] Nevertheless, the conclusions by Russian physicians Obrastzow and Straschesko that "the differential diagnosis of coronary thrombosis from angina pectoris is made by the presence of *status angiosus* with coronary thrombosis and its absence with isolated attacks of *angina pectoris*" reflected the prevailing view at the time that these two diagnoses were quite distinct. This distinction began to blur by 1937, when Sampson and Eliaser and Feil each described several patients with prolonged chest discomfort at rest that differed from stable angina, and appeared sometimes to precede an acute MI.[3] This pattern of symptoms was variously referred to as "pre-infarction angina" or "crescendo angina." In 1948, Wood proposed that this "intermediate coronary syndrome" between stable angina and MI was caused by "a coronary circulation insufficient to meet the full demands at rest yet sufficient to prevent MI." He recognized that, just as for acute MI, coronary thrombosis could be playing a role in this coronary insufficiency. Moreover, he observed that MI or death occurred in 12 of 25 patients with this intermediate coronary syndrome, whereas among 33 patients with the same syndrome whom he treated with oral anticoagulants, only 3 patients died or had an MI. It was nearly 25 years later, in 1971, that Fowler and colleagues introduced the term "unstable angina."

At first, UA was considered to be quite rare, and as late as the 1950s, some experts even questioned its existence. Friedberg, in the leading cardiology textbook at the time, described these patients as "a motley group," which he recommended should be "best classified clinically as angina pectoris (more or less severe or prolonged) or as MI." Despite this debate, in the era predating the development of high-sensitivity assays for cTn, it appeared that UA was common. In 1991, the National Center for Health Statistics reported that UA was responsible for 570,000 hospitalizations annually in the United States, making UA one of the most common reasons for hospital admission.

In 1994, in the first published guidelines on its diagnosis and management, UA was defined as "a clinical syndrome falling between stable angina and MI."[3] Three principal clinical presentations were considered to be typical of UA: (1) angina at rest; (2) new onset of severe exertional angina; and (3) distinct, often sudden, intensification of previously stable angina. Any one of these, in the absence of an acute MI (see the section on Diagnosis of Myocardial Infarction), was the basis for a diagnosis of UA. UA could be further classified

TABLE 1-1 Original Braunwald Classification of Unstable Angina

SEVERITY		A: DEVELOPS IN PRESENCE OF EXTRACARDIAC CONDITION THAT INTENSIFIES MYOCARDIAL ISCHEMIA (SECONDARY UA)	B: DEVELOPS IN THE ABSENCE OF EXTRACARDIAC CONDITION (PRIMARY UA)	C: DEVELOPS WITHIN 2 WKS AFTER ACUTE MYOCARDIAL INFARCTION (POSTINFARCTION UA)
		CLINICAL CIRCUMSTANCES		
I	New onset of severe angina or accelerated angina; no pain at rest	IA	IB	IC
II	Angina at rest within past month but not within preceding 48 hr (angina at rest, subacute)	IIA	IIB	IIC
III	Angina at rest within 48 hr (angina at rest, acute)	IIIA	IIIB Troponin negative IIIB Troponin positive*	IIIC

*Now defined as myocardial infarction if cardiac troponin is more than the 99th percentile upper reference limit.
UA, Unstable angina.
Adapted from Braunwald E: Unstable angina—a classification. Circulation *80:410–414, 1989.*

according to its severity, the clinical circumstances in which it occurred, and the presence or absence of electrocardiographic ST-segment deviations (Table 1-1).

By the beginning of the 21st century, UA was firmly established as one possible manifestation of ACS; however, ambiguity had begun to creep into its definition. As an example, the World Health Organization revision of the definition of MI in 2008 to 2009 characterized UA as "new or worsening symptoms of ischemia (or changing symptom pattern) and ischemic ECG changes…with normal biomarkers," but noted that the "distinction between new angina, worsening angina and unstable angina is notoriously difficult and based on a clinical assessment and a careful and full clinical history."[4] At the same time, the increasing analytical sensitivity of assays for cTn decreased the proportion of patients with ACS with "normal biomarkers" (see the section on Biomarkers of Myocyte Necrosis), resulting instead in the diagnosis of MI.

Diagnosis of Myocardial Infarction

In 1971, the World Health Organization proposed that the diagnosis of MI required the presence of at least two of the following: (1) typical symptoms; (2) a typical ECG pattern involving the development of Q waves; and (3) an initial rise and subsequent fall in serum and/or plasma biomarkers of myocardial necrosis. Patients with similar clinical manifestations of myocardial ischemia as UA, but who exhibited a typical pattern of a rise to abnormally elevated level(s) and subsequent fall in serum biomarkers of necrosis were diagnosed with MI. Subsequently, the emergence of both more sensitive and specific serologic biomarkers of myocardial necrosis and precise imaging techniques prompted a reevaluation of this definition of MI. This effort resulted in an evolution of the definition of MI that placed greater emphasis on the detection of ischemic myocardial necrosis, either with sensitive biomarkers or with cardiac imaging.

In 2000, the First Global MI Task Force, which was a collaborative joint committee of the European Society of Cardiology and the American College of Cardiology, articulated a new definition of MI that was founded on the principle that "any amount of myocardial necrosis caused by ischemia should be labeled as a [myocardial] infarct."[5] In addition, this joint committee confirmed previous guidelines that established the 99th percentile in the distribution of cTn in an apparently healthy population as the upper reference limit (URL) for diagnosis of myocardial injury (see Chapter 7). The task force also recognized that as a consequence of this fundamental premise "an individual who was formerly diagnosed as having severe, stable or unstable angina pectoris might be diagnosed today with a small MI." These principles were refined by the Second Global MI Task Force in 2007, leading to the Universal Definition of Myocardial Infarction, which included a clinical classification of MI that placed emphasis on differentiating the various conditions that might lead to an MI (see the section on Clinical Classification of Myocardial Infarction).[5] Subsequently, the 2012 Third Universal Definition of Myocardial Infarction responded to the development of even more sensitive assays for markers of myocardial necrosis.[6]

The Third Universal Definition of Myocardial Infarction formulated by the European Society of Cardiology, the American College of Cardiology, the American Heart Association, and the World Heart Federation recommends that patients who are suspected on clinical grounds of having ACS should undergo serial sampling for cTn.[6] An MI is defined by a typical rise and/or fall of cTn, with at least one value above the assay's URL, accompanied by at least one other feature of ischemia (e.g., typical symptoms or ECG changes) (Table 1-2).

Biomarkers of Myocyte Necrosis

Contemporary assays for cTn, their related important analytical considerations,[7] and their clinical use in the evaluation of patients with suspected MI are discussed in Chapter 7. This development of progressively more sensitive and precise biomarkers of myocardial necrosis has changed the epidemiology of MI. In the 1980s and 1990s, the myocardial band fraction of creatine kinase (CK-MB) was deemed to be the most sensitive and specific biomarker. Because serial determinations of CK-MB were not part of routine practice at the time in patients with NSTE-ACS, NSTEMI was not adequately excluded in many patients who were given a final diagnosis of UA. Therefore, the high incidence of UA reported in 1991 was likely an overestimate.

TABLE 1-2 Criteria for Acute Myocardial Infarction

The term acute myocardial infarction (MI) should be used when there is evidence of myocardial necrosis in a clinical setting consistent with myocardial ischemia. Under these conditions any one of the following criteria meets the diagnosis for MI:

- Detection of rise and/or fall of cardiac biomarkers (preferably cardiac troponin [cTn]) with at least one value above the 99th percentile upper reference limit (URL) and with at least one of the following:
  - Symptoms of ischemia
  - New significant ST-T changes or new left bundle branch block (LBBB)
  - Development of pathological Q waves in the electrocardiogram (ECG)
  - Imaging evidence of new loss of viable myocardium
  - Identification of an intracoronary thrombus by angiography
- Pathological findings of an acute or a recent MI.

MI in specific settings:

- MI related to sudden cardiac death
  Sudden, unexpected cardiac death, involving cardiac arrest, with symptoms suggestive of myocardial ischemia, or accompanied by presumably new ST elevation, or new LBBB, or evidence of fresh thrombus by coronary angiography and/or at autopsy, but death occurring before blood samples could be obtained, or at a time before the appearance of cardiac biomarkers in the blood.
- MI related to percutaneous coronary intervention (PCI)
  For PCI in patients with normal baseline cTn values (≤99th percentile URL), PCI-related MI is arbitrarily defined by elevations of >5 × 99th percentile URL plus either evidence of ischemia, such as prolonged chest pain or hemodynamic instability, ST changes or new pathological Q waves, angiographic loss of patency of a major coronary artery or a side branch, persistent slow- or no-reflow, or embolization or imaging demonstration of new loss of viable myocardium.
- MI related to stent thrombosis
  PCI-related stent thrombosis is designated MI when detected by coronary angiography or autopsy in the setting of myocardial ischemia and with a rise and/or fall of cardiac biomarkers (preferably cTn) with at least one value above the 99th percentile URL.
- MI related to coronary artery bypass surgery
  For coronary artery bypass surgery (CABG) in patients with normal baseline cTn values (≤99th percentile URL), procedure related MI is arbitrarily defined by elevations of >10 × 99th percentile URL plus either new pathological Q waves or new LBBB, or angiographic documented new graft or native coronary artery occlusion, or imaging evidence of new loss of viable myocardium.

From Thygesen K, Alpert JS, Jaffe AS, et al: Third universal definition of myocardial infarction. J Am Coll Cardiol *60:1581,2012.*

The differentiation between UA and NSTEMI has proven to be of considerable prognostic importance. First demonstrated with CK-MB, and subsequently refined with cTn, patients with unstable ischemic symptoms and biomarker evidence of myocardial necrosis (i.e., NSTEMI) are at significantly higher risk of death or recurrent ischemic events compared with patients presenting with UA, in whom, by definition, biomarkers of necrosis are not elevated (see Chapter 11).

Although, in the 1970s and 1980s, CK-MB was superior to previously available enzymes used as biomarkers of necrosis (total creatine kinase, aspartate aminotransferase, and alanine aminotransferase), it lacked optimal sensitivity and specificity. In 1987, Cummins and colleagues introduced an assay for cardiac-specific troponin I (cTnI), and shortly thereafter, Katus and colleagues developed an analogous assay for cardiac-specific troponin T (cTnT). Troponin I and T are components of the troponin regulatory complex that is bound to actin and modulates the interaction between actin and myosin in myocytes. In contrast to CK-MB, troponin I and T have cardiac isoforms (cTnI and cTnT) that are unique to cardiac myocytes and may be measured by assays that use monoclonal antibodies specific to epitopes of the cardiac form. Because of this greater tissue specificity, cTn allows detection of a faint signal of release from cardiac myocytes against minimal background noise in the circulation, and delivers considerably higher sensitivity and specificity than CK-MB.[5] For example, in the TIMI 3 trial, 25% of the patients classified with UA, based on the absence of abnormally elevated concentrations of CK-MB, had cTnI ≥0.4 ng/ml (the cutpoint of a relatively insensitive assay from the mid-1990s), and therefore, should be reclassified as having had an NSTEMI.[8] Thus, in retrospect, patients with UA made up a smaller percentage of patients with NSTE-ACS than had previously been believed.

Like the earlier classification of ACS patients based on CK-MB, this second wave of reclassification also appeared to be clinically important. Among patients with normal CK-MB, patients with elevated cTn were at higher risk of adverse cardiac events than those without such elevations. In the TIMI 11B trial, we observed a six-fold increase in death or new MI in patients with normal CK-MB who had elevated cTnI compared with patients without such an elevation. The clinical relevance of such reclassification with cTn was reinforced by evidence that patients with ACS who had elevated cTn benefited more from newer therapies than did patients in whom cTn was not detectable. These therapies included an early invasive strategy (see Chapter 16), the addition of platelet glycoprotein IIb/IIIa inhibitors (see Chapter 19), and treatment with a low–molecular-weight heparin rather than unfractionated heparin (see Chapter 18).

Two critical trends in the clinical applications of cTn have since ushered in what we view as a third wave of reclassification of ACS: (1) a move to lower diagnostic cutoffs for cTn; and (2) progressive improvement in the analytical precision of assays for cTn that has further lowered diagnostic and prognostic decision limits.[3,5] At initial approval for clinical use, manufacturer-recommended cutpoints for cTn originated from comparative studies with CK-MB. However, this approach was flawed because the derived cutpoints were based on a comparison with a less sensitive test. For this reason, in 1999, laboratory professional guidelines recommended an additional lower cutpoint based on the distribution of cTn in a healthy reference population. This approach of defining an upper limit of normal at the 97.5th or 99th percentile of a reference population is the method used to establish cutpoints for many clinical laboratory tests. In 2000, cardiology and laboratory professional guidelines endorsed a single cutpoint for diagnosis of MI at the 99th percentile URL for each assay (see Chapter 7).

However, more than 10 years after publication of the first Universal Definition of Myocardial Infarction, many laboratories have continued to report an inconclusive or suggestive range using two cTn cutpoints based on the outdated initial proposal from laboratory guidelines and some package inserts.[9,10] This practice is no longer consistent with present guidelines.[6]

The progressive improvement in analytical precision of assays for cTn during the past 25 years had driven both the limit of detection and the URL downwards. This trend is illustrated by the data from clinical studies that revealed the proportion of patients with NSTE-ACS with a positive cTn result, and hence, a diagnosis of NSTEMI. In 1996, in the TIMI 3 trial, 25% of patients with UA had elevated cTnI (≥0.4 ng/mL). A decade later, in NSTE-ACS patients enrolled into the MERLIN-TIMI 36 trial, which used a widely available current generation sensitive assay for cTnI (URL 0.04 ng/mL), we observed that 65% of patients with NSTE-ACS had a positive

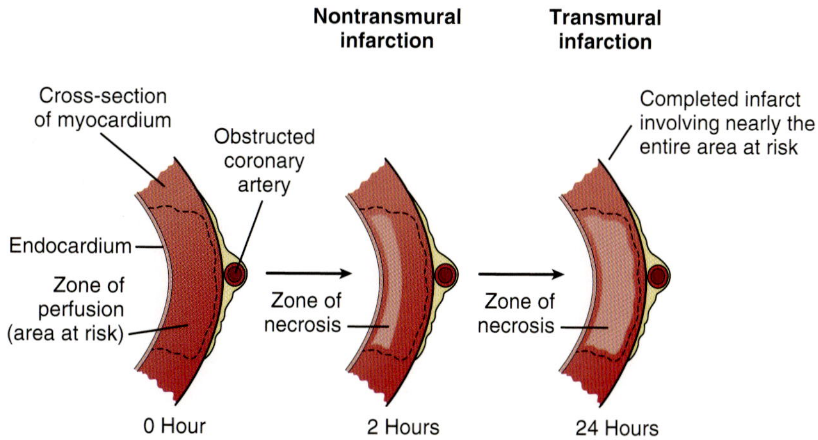

FIGURE 1-2 The progression of myocardial necrosis after coronary artery occlusion. Necrosis begins in a small zone of the myocardium beneath the endocardial surface in the center of the ischemic zone. This entire region of myocardium (*dashed outline*) depends on the occluded vessel for perfusion and is the area at risk. A narrow zone of myocardium immediately beneath the endocardium is spared from necrosis because it can be oxygenated by diffusion from the ventricle. *(Adapted from Schoen FJ, Mitchell, RN: The heart. In Kumar V, et al, eds:* Robbins and Cotran pathologic basis of disease, *ed 8. Philadelphia, Saunders, 2010.)*

cTnI result, approximately 50% of whom would not have been identified with CK-MB.[11] Importantly, the subgroup of patients who had low-level elevations in cTnI that would not have been detected with the previous generation cTn assay turned out to be at similar heightened risk of death or recurrent ischemic events. Using the earlier assay, these patients did not have detectable elevations of cTn and would therefore have been considered to have UA, but were later classified as NSTEMI and were found to have a commensurately increased risk.[11]

With yet another decade of evolution, high-sensitivity assays with improved analytical precision have progressively lowered the URL and enabled detection limits as low as 0.0002 ng/ml (0.2 ng/L) with consequent detection of cTn above the URL in 82% to 99% of patients with putative UA; again, data demonstrate a graded rise in the rate of adverse outcomes.[12,13] Such clinical studies have established that most patients with clinical manifestations of myocardial ischemia, with pain at rest, but without elevated cTnI by a previous generation assay, have detectable dynamic concentrations of circulating cTnI measured by a high-sensitivity assay, and therefore, would be reclassified from UA to NSTEMI. Clinically, there is a need to distinguish acute increases in cTn that occur in MI from chronic, relatively stable, low-level concentrations that can exist in patients with SIHD or other structural heart disease, but which are not necessarily indicative of ACS (see Chapter 7, Table 7-2).[14]

CLASSICATION OF MYOCARDIAL INFARCTION

Pathological Description

The pathological diagnosis of MI requires evidence of myocardial cell death. Characteristic findings of myocyte necrosis include coagulation necrosis and contraction band necrosis, usually with patchy areas of myocytolysis at the periphery of the infarction (see Figure 4-2). During the acute phase of MI, most of the myocyte loss occurs via coagulation necrosis, with ensuing inflammation, phagocytosis of necrotic myocytes, and repair eventuating into scar formation (see Chapter 4).

MI can be classified pathologically on gross examination as transmural, in which myocardial necrosis involves the full thickness (or nearly full thickness) of the ventricular wall, and subendocardial (nontransmural) infarcts, in which the necrosis involves the subendocardium, the intramural myocardium, or both, without extending all the way through the ventricular wall to the epicardium (Figure 1-2). Transmural infarction is more likely when coronary thrombosis is completely occlusive and is localized to the distribution of a single coronary artery. Subendocardial infarctions may result from severely narrowed, but still patent, coronary arteries, or when significant collateral circulation to the infarcted region exists. Patchy subendocardial infarction may arise from reperfusion of an originally occlusive thrombus with restoration of blood flow before the wavefront of necrosis has extended from the subendocardium across the full thickness of the ventricular wall (see Chapter 24).

Clinical Classification

Electrocardiography

Abnormalities of the surface ECG during myocardial ischemia or infarction may include the PR segment, the QRS complex, the ST-segment, or the T-wave. The earliest manifestation of myocardial ischemia is typically hyperacute T-wave amplitude followed by ST-segment changes. The loss of electromotive forces caused by myocardial necrosis leads to R-wave loss in the ECG territory of the MI. The development of Q-waves is a result of delayed conduction through an ischemic area or conduction around an area of infarction, leading to recording potentials from the opposite ventricular wall. Criteria for Q-waves consistent with previous MI are shown at the bottom of Table 1-3. Transient Q-waves may be observed during an episode of acute ischemia or (rarely) during acute MI with successful reperfusion.

The term Q-wave infarction was often used synonymously with transmural infarction, whereas non–Q-wave infarctions were believed to be indicative of subendocardial infarctions. However, studies that used cardiac magnetic resonance imaging (see Chapter 33) indicate that the development of Q-waves on the ECG is influenced more by the size of the infarction than the extent of transmural involvement (see Figure 1-1). Moreover, the classification of MI on the basis of Q-waves has been supplanted by a focus on the presence or absence of initial ST-segment elevation

TABLE 1-3 Electrocardiographic Manifestations of Myocardial Infarction

ECG Manifestations of Acute Myocardial Ischemia (in Absence of LVH and LBBB)
ST Elevation
New ST elevation at the J point in two contiguous leads with the cutpoints: ≥0.1 mV in all leads other than leads V_2 to V_3 In leads V_2 to V_3 ≥0.2 mV in men ≥40 years, and ≥0.25 mV in men <40 years, or ≥ 0.15 mV in women
ST Depression and T-Wave Changes
New horizontal or down-sloping ST depression ≥0.05 mV in two contiguous leads and/or T inversion ≥0.1 mV in two contiguous leads with prominent R wave or R/S ratio >1
ECG Changes Associated with Previous Myocardial Infarction (Q Waves)
• Any Q wave in leads V_2 to V_3 ≥0.02 sec or QS complex in leads V_2 and V_3 • Q wave ≥0.03 sec and ≥ 0.1 mV deep or QS complex in leads I, II, aVL, aVF, or V_4 to V_6 in any two leads of a contiguous lead grouping (I, aVL, V_1–V_6, II, III, aVF)* • R wave ≥ 0.04 sec in leads V_1 toV_2 and R/S ≥1 with a concordant positive T wave in the absence of a conduction defect

*The same criteria are used for supplemental leads V_7 to V_9, and for the Cabrera frontal plane lead grouping.
ECG, Electrocardiography; *LBBB*, left bundle branch block; *LVH*, left ventricular hypertrophy.
From Thygesen K, Alpert JS, Jaffe AS, et al: Third universal definition of myocardial infarction. J Am Coll Cardiol *60:1581,2012.*

TABLE 1-4 Universal Definition Classification of Myocardial Infarction

Type 1: Spontaneous Myocardial Infarction
Spontaneous myocardial infarction related to ischemia caused a primary coronary event, such as plaque rupture, erosion, fissuring, or dissection.
Type 2: Secondary Myocardial Infarction
Myocardial infarction secondary to ischemia caused by increased oxygen demand or decreased supply (e.g., coronary endothelial dysfunction, coronary artery spasm, coronary embolism, tachy-/brady-arrhythmias, anemia, respiratory failure, hypotension, and hypertension with or without LVH).
Type 3: Myocardial Infarction Related to Sudden Cardiac Death
Sudden unexpected cardiac death with symptoms suggestive of myocardial ischemia, accompanied by presumably new ST elevation, or new LBBB, or evidence of fresh thrombus in a coronary artery by angiography or at autopsy, but death occurs before blood samples could be obtained, or at a time before the appearance of cardiac biomarkers in the blood
Type 4a: Myocardial Infarction Related to PCI
Type 4b: Myocardial Infarction Related to Stent Thrombosis
Type 5: Myocardial Infarction Related to CABG

CABG, Coronary artery bypass graft; *LBBB*, left bundle branch block; *LVH*, left ventricular hypertrophy; *PCI*, percutaneous coronary intervention.
From Thygesen K, Alpert JS, Jaffe AS, et al: Third universal definition of myocardial infarction. J Am Coll Cardiol *60:1581,2012.*

(see the section on Spectrum of Ischemic Heart Disease). Nonetheless, the development of Q-waves during the subsequent evolution of an MI adds to other clinical data suggesting a larger infarction.

Deviation of the ST-segment is the most consistent ECG finding during severe myocardial ischemia, and it is the result of the development of a voltage gradient between the normal and ischemic zones of the myocardium. The voltage gradient leads to a flow of current between regions of myocardium, resulting in the injury current recorded on the surface ECG. When acute ischemia is transmural, which is usually associated with complete coronary occlusion, the overall ST vector is most often shifted in the direction of the epicardial layers, producing ST-segment elevation. In contrast, when ischemia is confined to the subendocardium, the ST vector usually shifts toward the ventricular cavity, which results in ST-segment depression in the overlying leads. Clinical studies have established the benefit of immediate reperfusion therapy in patients with ST-segment elevation (see Chapter 13). Because of this fundamental tie to therapeutic strategy for patients with acute MI, current nomenclature focuses on classifying patients at the time of presentation as STEMI or NSTEMI (see Figure 1-1). Criteria for diagnostic ST-segment elevation are shown in Table 1-3. Lesser degrees of ST-segment deviation should also be recognized by the clinician and integrated into the overall clinical assessment of the patient with suspected MI (see Chapter 6).

Universal Definition of Myocardial Infarction Classification of Myocardial Infarction Type

In addition to establishing criteria for the diagnosis of MI, the Universal Definition of Myocardial Infarction classifies definite MI into various types, based on proposed pathological, clinical, and prognostic differences (Table 1-4).[6] Importantly, these classifications are intended to be useful for determining therapeutic strategy, which is expected to differ, for example, between spontaneous MI and MI secondary to an increase in myocardial oxygen demand or coronary vasospasm (Figure 1-3; also see Chapter 13).

Spontaneous Myocardial Infarction (Type 1)

Type 1 MI is an event related to atherothrombosis, including plaque rupture, ulceration, fissuring, erosion, or dissection, with resulting coronary thrombus in one or more of the coronary arteries (see Chapter 3). The Universal Definition of Myocardial Infarction also classifies distal platelet microemboli as type 1 MI. Type 1 MI is the classic paradigm of ACS with an atherothrombotic cause for which early reperfusion therapy for STEMI and antithrombotic therapies and invasive evaluation for NSTEMI and STEMI are of proven benefit. Patients with type 1 MI may have underlying severe epicardial coronary artery disease (CAD) but nonobstructive or minimal CAD may be found at angiography in 5% to 20% of patients, particularly among women (see the section on Myocardial Infarction with Nonobstructive Coronary Arteries).

Myocardial Infarction Secondary to an Ischemic Imbalance (Type 2)

Type 2 MI is defined as an MI that occurs as a result of an imbalance between myocardial oxygen supply and demand, which is contributed to by a condition other than CAD (see Figure 1-3). Type 2 MI may occur in the setting of stable underlying coronary atherosclerosis that results in supply–demand mismatch only in the context of increased myocardial oxygen demand or reduced oxygen delivery. Examples include MI in the presence of uncontrolled hypertension, markedly increased heart rate caused by arrhythmia, or severe anemia. Other contributors may include respiratory failure, bradycardia, and hypotension. Type 2 MI also encompasses reduced myocardial blood oxygen supply that results from coronary vasospasm, endothelial dysfunction, or coronary

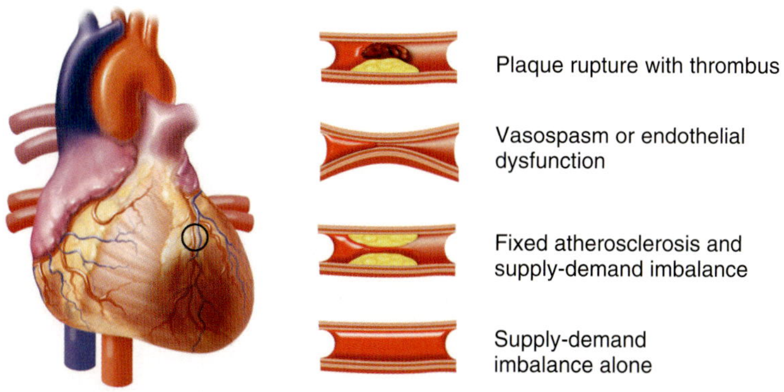

FIGURE 1-3 Differentiation between myocardial infarction (MI) types 1 and 2 according to the condition of the coronary arteries. Myocardial ischemia and infarction can result from various coronary disease processes, including erosion or rupture of vulnerable atherosclerotic plaque leading to acute thrombus formation and subsequent ischemia (type 1 MI, *top*), or predominantly nonthrombotic supply–demand mismatch from any of the following (type 2 MI): coronary vasospasm; increased myocardial demand in the setting of a fixed coronary lesion; or supply–demand imbalance in the absence of critical epicardial disease, such as in patients with microvascular disease or endothelial dysfunction. *(From Thygesen K, Alpert JS, Jaffe AS, et al: Third universal definition of myocardial infarction.* J Am Coll Cardiol *60:1581, 2012.)*

embolism, as well as ischemia that occurs in patients with extreme increases in myocardial oxygen demand in the absence of recognized coronary abnormalities (also see the section on Myocardial Infarction in Nonobstructive Coronary Arteries). Nonischemic etiologies of myocardial injury caused by direct myocardial toxicity of circulating substances in the setting of acute illness or stress-induced cardiomyopathy (Takotsubo myopathy) are both *not* classified as type 2 MI, but they may be very difficult to distinguish from myocardial ischemia because of increased myocardial demand (see Table 7-2).

Estimates of the proportion of MIs that are type 2 vary widely from 3.5% to 72%, depending on the setting and approaches to diagnostic categorization. Among patients with established ischemic heart disease and recent ACS, less than 5% of recurrent infarctions appear to be type 2.[15] In hospitalized patients with elevated cTn, the proportion of type 2 MIs increases from 10% to 30%, and among all-comers to the emergency department who have cTn evaluated, the proportion has been reported to be as high as approximately 70%.[16] Although approaches that incorporate specific criteria for heart rate, blood pressure, hemoglobin, and oxygenation have been proposed,[17] there is no established gold standard for type 2 MI. Efforts to establish rigid criteria are likely to be unsuccessful because the severity of increased myocardial oxygen demand necessary to cause ischemic injury will vary substantially based on the severity of any underlying coronary abnormalities. For example, a heart rate of 110 beats/min may cause ischemia in a patient with severe left main coronary disease, but others may tolerate a heart rate of 150 beats/min without any ischemia. Presence of a clearly identifiable cause (e.g., infection, or acute change in heart rate or blood pressure) or situational signs or symptoms may all be used as evidence for a type 2 cause. Diagnostic coronary imaging may not be appropriate in many cases, such as patients with severe noncardiac illness, but it is often helpful when performed.

Few studies have examined the near- and long-term prognosis in patients with type 2 MI. Among patients with established ischemic heart disease and a previous ACS, cardiovascular mortality associated with type 2 MI appears similar to that for recurrent type 1 MI (Figure 1-4).[15] Moreover, among unselected patients hospitalized with MI, patients with type 2 MI appear to have worse long-term survival than patients with type 1 MI (Figure 1-5).[17]

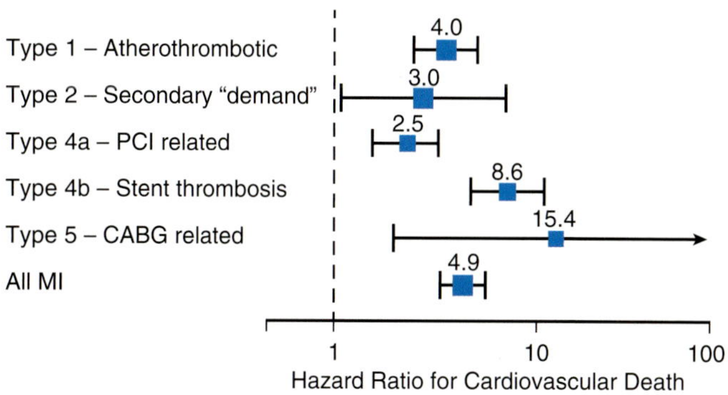

FIGURE 1-4 Prognosis associated with myocardial infarction (MI) classified by the Universal MI Classification System. Data are from 1218 new or recurrent MIs occurring in a clinical trial of patients with acute coronary syndrome. Adjusted hazard ratio for cardiovascular (CV) death at 180 days during study follow-up by the universal definition of MI subtypes (type 1: spontaneous atherothrombotic; type 2: demand related; type 3: sudden unexpected cardiac death; type 4a: percutaneous coronary intervention [PCI] related; type 4b: stent thrombosis; and type 5: coronary artery bypass grafting [CABG] related). Referent for type 5 MI was the cohort of patients who underwent CABG but did not have an MI during follow-up. Analyses were adjusted for known risk indicators of age, sex, diabetes, hypertension, dyslipidemia, renal function, previous heart failure, previous MI, randomization group, severity of coronary artery disease at the index angiogram, and presenting syndrome (unstable angina, non–ST-elevation MI, or ST-elevation MI). *(From Bonaca MP, Wiviott SD, Braunwald E, et al: American College of Cardiology/American Heart Association/European Society of Cardiology/World Heart Federation universal definition of myocardial infarction classification system and the risk of cardiovascular death: observations from the TRITON-TIMI 38 trial [Trial to Assess Improvement in Therapeutic Outcomes by Optimizing Platelet Inhibition With Prasugrel-Thrombolysis in Myocardial Infarction 38].* Circulation *125:577–583, 2012.)*

This observation may be explained by the generally older age and greater number of comorbid medical conditions in the population with type 2 MI, as well as the common presence of an acute noncardiac illness that contributes to the onset of ischemia. In general, management of type 2 MI should be directed at the underlying contributors to a supply–demand mismatch. Because of the poor prognosis of patients with type 2 MI, long-term cardiovascular risk stratification is often appropriate once a primary noncardiac illness is treated.

Cardiac Death Caused by Myocardial Infarction (Type 3)

In some instances, patients with symptoms suggestive of myocardial ischemia accompanied by presumed new ischemic ECG changes or new left bundle branch block (LBBB) may experience sudden death before blood samples for biomarkers can be obtained or before circulating cardiac

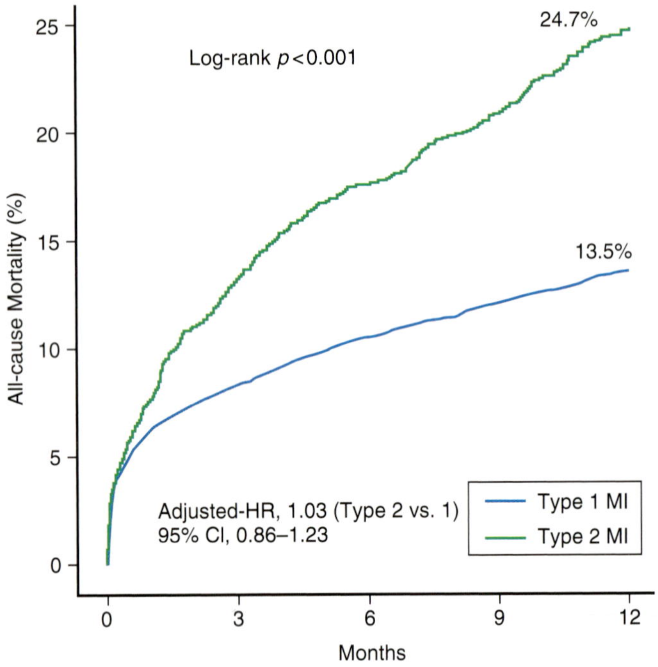

FIGURE 1-5 Survival among patients with type 1 and type 2 myocardial infarction. Data are from 20138 patients hospitalized in 2011 in Sweden with an acute myocardial infarction (MI) stratified into MI type 1 (88.5%) and type 2 (7.1%). All-cause mortality through 1 year after hospital admission is shown. The adjusted risk of type 1 and type 2 MI were very similar after accounting for the greater comorbid conditions of patients with type 2 MI. Nevertheless, the risk of death after a type 2 MI was no less than that after a type 1 MI. *CI*, Confidence interval; *HR*, hazard ratio. *(From Baron T, et al: Type 2 myocardial infarction in clinical practice.* Heart *101:101-106, 2015.)*

biomarkers become elevated. In such cases of a presentation with clinical features of myocardial ischemia, or presumed new ischemic ECG changes, patients should be classified as having had a fatal MI, even in the absence of diagnostic cardiac biomarkers.

Myocardial Infarction Associated with Revascularization Procedures (Types 4 and 5)

Periprocedural myocardial injury or infarction may occur during mechanical revascularization, either by percutaneous coronary intervention (PCI) (type 4) or coronary artery bypass graft (CABG) (type 5). MIs related to PCI are further classified as periprocedural MI (type 4a) and stent thrombosis (type 4b). PCI and CABG-related MIs are arbitrarily defined by specific thresholds above the URL (see Table 1-2) in conjunction with either evidence of ischemia, demonstrated loss of myocardium, or overt clinical complications. Elevated cTn values that do not meet these thresholds may be evident after revascularization procedures or may occur in the absence of clear evidence of ischemia. The Universal MI Committee has concluded that it is likely that limitation of such an injury is optimal; however, in the absence of overt procedural complications, a specific threshold for an asymptomatic rise in circulating cTn or CK-MB that is associated with worse clinical outcomes has not been conclusively defined.[6]

The clinical significance of periprocedural myocardial injury is controversial and has led to the development of multiple alternative definitions for types 4 and 5 MI by various stakeholders.[18] It is our interpretation of the available evidence that there is an increasing gradient of risk associated with increasing concentrations of CK-MB or cTn after coronary revascularization procedures; however, the associated mortality risk, for type 4a MI in particular, although measurable, is less than that for spontaneous (type 1) MI (see Figure 1-4). In part, the controversy stems from seemingly conflicting data from observational studies in which some have shown no association with adverse outcomes in patients with biomarker elevation post-PCI (see Chapter 23). However, it is likely that the risk associated with periprocedural injury may vary across settings (e.g., elective PCI compared with primary PCI in STEMI). Moreover, discrimination of new periprocedural injury from elevated concentrations of cTn or CK-MB preprocedure, if they are caused by a presenting MI or chronic structural heart disease, is complicated and pivotal to accurately estimating the risk associated with type 4 and type 5 MI.

Definitions that incorporate criteria for dynamic increases, which are clearly separate from myocardial injury preceding the procedure, and that use higher biomarker thresholds for diagnosis of MI, appear to improve specificity and have an association with cardiovascular mortality.[19,20] Despite the controversy, the consensus view across committees participating in the development of professional guidelines and/or definitions is that when associated with clinical evidence of ischemia (e.g., persistent ST-changes, symptoms, or angiographic loss of flow in a major vessel or branch), elevation of cTn or CK-MB establishes the diagnosis of periprocedural MI; however, the criteria for biomarker elevation differ between these recommended definitions.[6,21,22]

The treatment of periprocedural MI depends on the underlying cause. For example, with acute stent thrombosis, immediate re-dilation of the occlusion with or without stenting is highly effective in reducing the size of the infarction. Dissection and side branch occlusion can be treated with dilation and stenting of the occlusive lesions. In most cases, a periprocedural myocardial injury is silent and not detected during the procedure, but recognized afterwards. Specific therapeutic guidelines for such patients have not been developed.

Classification by Myocardial Infarction Size

In addition to classification by MI type, the Universal Definition Classification System also has proposed categories of MI size based on the peak concentration of the cardiac biomarker (cTn preferred).[6] Data using both scintigraphy and cardiac magnetic resonance (CMR) suggest that peak cTn values correlate well with infarct size determined from imaging approaches. As for CK-MB, the correlation between cTn and MI size by CMR is less strong in NSTEMI than in STEMI. However, correlation ranges are good (0.8–0.93) and are better than the correlations reported for CK-MB. Clinicians should recognize that because of the improved sensitivity of cTn (compared with CK-MB) elevations relative to the URL differ between cTn and CK-MB in terms of the size of the infarct reflected (i.e., a twofold elevation of cTn reflects a substantially smaller amount of necrosis than a twofold elevation of CK-MB). The relative relationship between the two biomarkers will differ between each assay. As an approximation, in one comparative study of cTn and CK-MB based on prognosis rather than imaging of infarct size, a 3-fold elevation of CK-MB was equivalent in frequency and 1-year mortality risk to a 60-fold elevation of cTn.[20] As discussed in Chapter 7 and Chapter 11, the risk associated with elevation of cTn is, nonetheless, evident at even one- to two-fold elevations above the URL in patients with a clinical syndrome consistent with myocardial ischemia (Figure 1-6).

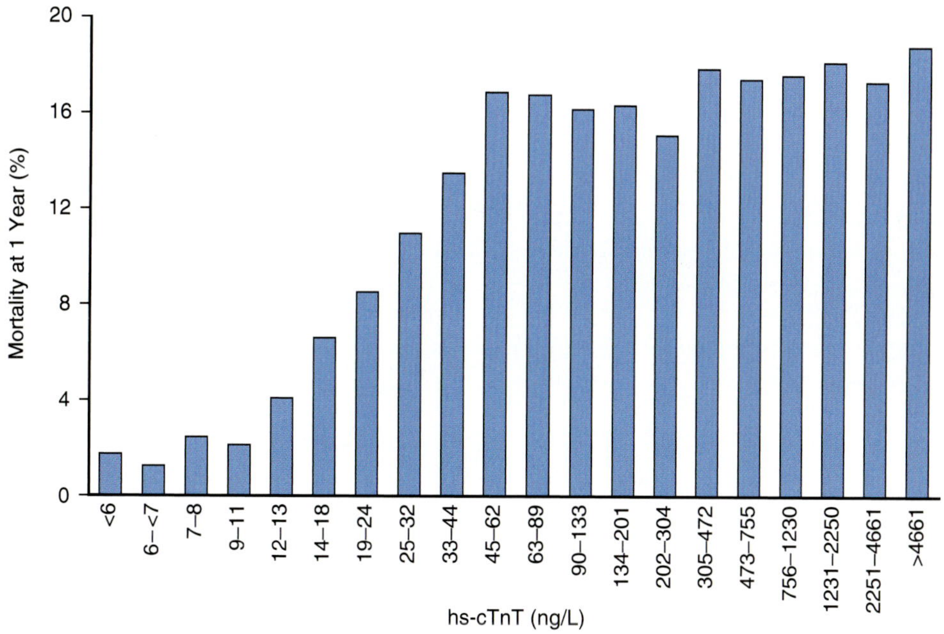

FIGURE 1-6 Crude all-cause mortality at 1 year, stratified according to the level of maximal high-sensitivity cardiac troponin T (hs-cTnT), among 48,594 patients with suspected acute coronary syndrome followed in the SWEDEHEART registry. The risk began increasing at 12 to 13 ng/L of hsTnT (99th percentile upper reference limit = 14 ng/L). *(From Melki D, et al: Implications of introducing high-sensitivity cardiac troponin T into clinical practice data from the SWEDEHEART Registry.* J Am Coll Cardiol *65:1655–1664, 2015.)*

Myocardial Infarction in the Setting of Nonobstructive Coronary Arteries

Up to 20% (average approximately 6%) of participants in registries of patients with a clinical diagnosis of MI are found to have no evidence of obstructive epicardial coronary atherosclerosis at coronary angiography.[23] Such patients with suspected MI with nonobstructive coronary arteries (MINOCA) are very difficult to discriminate from patients with nonischemic mechanisms of acute myocardial injury. In a meta-analysis of 28 studies, patients with MINOCA were more likely to be younger and female, and less likely to have dyslipidemia than patients with critical coronary atherosclerosis. Other coronary abnormalities are moderately prevalent in this population. Among 402 patients with MINOCA, 28% had inducible coronary vasospasm. CMR among 1801 patients with suspected MINOCA revealed delayed hyperenhancement consistent with MI in 24% and features of myocarditis in 33%, illustrating the challenging clinical overlap between patients with probable type 2 MI and those with other causes of myocardial injury.[23] For this reason, CMR imaging is emerging as a valuable tool when it becomes clinically important to perform additional diagnostic evaluation in patients with suspected MINOCA (see Chapter 6 and Chapter 33). In general, the prognosis of patients with MINOCA is more favorable than that of patients with obstructive coronary disease, but less so in comparison to individuals without cardiac disease or patients with chest pain without MI.[23] Because of the heterogeneous contributors to MINOCA, there are as yet no well-defined algorithms for treatment.

SUMMARY

The terminology and epidemiology that describes unstable ischemic heart disease continues to evolve. Current nomenclature has shifted in focus toward alignment with discrete lines of clinical management. The term ACS captures the spectrum of unstable angina, NSTEMI, and STEMI. Although present guidelines remain silent on this issue, we favor reserving the term ACS for unstable ischemic syndromes of atherothrombotic causes to differentiate patients with acute thrombosis from the increasingly recognized, large group of patients with nonthrombotic, mostly demand-related ischemia and infarction (see Figure 1-1).

Initial classification of the patient with suspected ACS should be made on the basis of the ECG to identify patients with STEMI who are candidates for immediate reperfusion therapy. Among patients with NSTE-ACS, the advent of more sensitive assays for cTn has shifted the epidemiology, such that the proportion of patients with NSTE-ACS who have demonstrable myocardial injury, and thus are classified as NSTEMI rather than UA, has steadily increased. In our view, when high-sensitivity assays for cTn are applied, it is an extremely small proportion of patients with unstable ischemic symptoms who do not manifest at least small amounts of myocardial injury, and for this reason, UA has all but disappeared. Because the distinction between UA and NSTEMI has become highly dependent on the particular assay used for detecting cTn, the term UA has increasing ambiguity and means different things to different people. With this shift, the epidemiology of ACS has come full circle back to before the 1930s when two principal manifestations of symptomatic ischemic heart disease were recognized: SIHD and acute MI.

Because of an accompanying increase in the heterogeneity of patients with MI, it has become even more important to classify every MI. Equally important, MI must be distinguished from myocardial injury caused by primarily nonischemic causes, in which setting we advocate being descriptive for the purposes of clinical clarity (e.g., "myocardial injury caused by decompensated heart failure" or "myocardial injury caused by myocarditis"). The classification of MI based on the setting and suspected underlying pathology as captured by the Universal Definition of Myocardial Infarction classification system is an important step toward defining rational pathways for treatment of the varied group of patients with MI encountered in clinical practice. A diagnosis of "acute MI" is no longer sufficient; instead, for example, a diagnosis of a "type 2 NSTEMI in the setting of uncontrolled hypertension" is substantially more useful to formulating a treatment plan and communicating with colleagues.

Classic References

Heberden W: *Commentaries on the history and cure of diseases*, London: Printed for T. Payne, Mews-Gate; 1802.

Herrick JB: *A short history of cardiology*, Springfield, MA: Charles C. Thomas; 1942.

Herrick J: Certain clinical features of sudden obstruction of the coronary arteries, *Transactions of the American Association of Physicians* 27:100–116, 1912.

Levine SA: *Coronary thrombosis: its various clinical features*, Baltimore, 1929, The Williams & Wilkins Company.

Obrastzow WP, Straschesko ND: Zur Kenntnis der Thrombose der Koronararterien des Herzens, *Z Klin Med* 71:116–132, 1910.

References

1. Nabel EG, Braunwald E: A tale of coronary artery disease and myocardial infarction, *N Engl J Med* 366:54–63, 2012.
2. Falk E, Nakano M, Bentzon JF, et al.: Update on acute coronary syndromes: the pathologists' view, *Eur Heart J* 34:719–728, 2013.
3. Braunwald E, Morrow DA: Unstable angina: is it time for a requiem? *Circulation* 127:2452–2457, 2013.
4. Mendis S, Thygesen K, Kuulasmaa K, et al.: World Health Organization definition of myocardial infarction: 2008-09 revision, *International J Epidemiology* 40:139–146, 2011.
5. Morrow DA: Clinical application of sensitive troponin assays, *N Engl J Med* 361:913–915, 2009.
6. Thygesen K, Alpert JS, Jaffe AS, et al.: Third universal definition of myocardial infarction, *Eur Heart J* 33:2551–2567, 2012.
7. Christenson RH, Bunk DM, Schimmel H, et al.: Point: put simply, standardization of cardiac troponin I is complicated, *Clin Chem* 58:165–168, 2012.
8. Antman EM, Tanasijevic MJ, Thompson B, et al.: Cardiac-specific troponin I levels to predict the risk of mortality in patients with acute coronary syndromes, *N Engl J Med* 335:1342–1349, 1996.
9. Collinson PO, van Dieijen-Visser MP, Pulkki K, et al.: Evidence-based laboratory medicine: how well do laboratories follow recommendations and guidelines? The Cardiac Marker Guideline Uptake in Europe (CARMAGUE) study, *Clin Chem* 58:305–306, 2012.
10. McKeeman GC, Auld PW: A national survey of troponin testing and recommendations for improved practice, *Ann Clin Biochem* 52(Pt 5):527–542, 2015.
11. Bonaca M, Scirica B, Sabatine M, et al.: Prospective evaluation of the prognostic implications of improved assay performance with a sensitive assay for cardiac troponin I, *J Am Coll Cardiol* 55:2118–2124, 2010.
12. Wilson SR, Sabatine MS, Braunwald E, et al.: Detection of myocardial injury in patients with unstable angina using a novel nanoparticle cardiac troponin I assay: observations from the PROTECT-TIMI 30 Trial, *Am Heart J* 158:386–391, 2009.
13. Bonaca MP, O'Malley RG, Murphy SA, et al.: Prognostic performance of a high-sensitivity assay for cardiac troponin I after non-ST elevation acute coronary syndrome: Analysis from MERLIN-TIMI 36, *European Heart Journal Acute Cardiovasc Care* 4:431–440, 2015.
14. Omland T, de Lemos JA, Sabatine MS, et al.: A sensitive cardiac troponin T assay in stable coronary artery disease, *N Engl J Med* 361:2538–2547, 2009.
15. Morrow DA, Wiviott SD, White HD, et al.: Effect of the novel thienopyridine prasugrel compared with clopidogrel on spontaneous and procedural myocardial infarction in the Trial to Assess Improvement in Therapeutic Outcomes by Optimizing Platelet Inhibition with Prasugrel-Thrombolysis in Myocardial Infarction 38: an application of the classification system from the universal definition of myocardial infarction, *Circulation* 119:2758–2764, 2009.
16. Sandoval Y, Smith SW, Thordsen SE, et al.: Supply/demand type 2 myocardial infarction: should we be paying more attention? *J Am Coll Cardiol* 63:2079–2087, 2014.
17. Saaby L, Poulsen TS, Hosbond S, et al.: Classification of myocardial infarction: frequency and features of type 2 myocardial infarction, *Am J Med* 126:789–797, 2013.
18. White H: Avatar of the universal definition of periprocedural myocardial infarction, *J Am Coll Cardiol* 62:1571–1574, 2013.
19. Bonaca MP, Wiviott SD, Braunwald E, et al.: American College of Cardiology/American Heart Association/European Society of Cardiology/World Heart Federation universal definition of myocardial infarction classification system and the risk of cardiovascular death: observations from the TRITON-TIMI 38 trial (Trial to Assess Improvement in Therapeutic Outcomes by Optimizing Platelet Inhibition With Prasugrel-Thrombolysis in Myocardial Infarction 38), *Circulation* 125:577–583, 2012.
20. Tricoci P, Leonardi S, White J, et al.: Cardiac troponin after percutaneous coronary intervention and 1-year mortality in non-ST-segment elevation acute coronary syndrome using systematic evaluation of biomarker trends, *J Am Coll Cardiol* 62:242–251, 2013.
21. Moussa ID, Klein LW, Shah B, et al.: Consideration of a new definition of clinically relevant myocardial infarction after coronary revascularization: an expert consensus document from the Society for Cardiovascular Angiography and Interventions (SCAI), *J Am Coll Cardiol* 62:1563–1570, 2013.
22. Kappetein AP, Head SJ, Genereux P, et al.: Updated standardized endpoint definitions for transcatheter aortic valve implantation: the Valve Academic Research Consortium-2 consensus document, *J Thorac Cardiovasc Surg* 145:6–23, 2013.
23. Pasupathy S, Air T, Dreyer RP, et al.: Systematic review of patients presenting with suspected myocardial infarction and nonobstructive coronary arteries, *Circulation* 131:861–870, 2015.

2 Global Evolving Epidemiology, Natural History, and Treatment Trends of Myocardial Infarction

Thomas A. Gaziano and J. Michael Gaziano

INTRODUCTION

Cardiovascular disease (CVD) was the single most important cause of death worldwide in 2013, when it was responsible for 17 million deaths and the loss of 329 million disability-adjusted life-years (DALYs).[1] Of all causes of CVD, *ischemic heart disease* (IHD) remains the major contributor, accounting for half of all CVD-associated morbidity and mortality. IHD as measured by the Global Burden of Disease project is driven predominantly by acute myocardial infarction (MI) and, to a lesser extent, angina. Over the past two decades, while age-standardized IHD mortality in most world regions has decreased,[2,3] the global burden of IHD has increased by 29 million DALYs (representing a 29% increase), owing in large part to overall population growth and to the aging of the population.

This chapter presents a review of the global burden of IHD, with an emphasis on low- and middle-income countries (LMICs). Also considered are the trends in management of acute MI. Concluding the chapter is a discussion of challenges that IHD poses to the global community and solutions that may help to reduce IHD morbidity and mortality.

Data Sources

Data for mortality and DALYs come from the Global Burden of Diseases, Injuries, and Risk Factors Study 2010 (GBD), which obtained and analyzed mortality data for 187 countries from 1980 to 2010,[2,4,5] and the World Health Organization (WHO) Mortality Data Base.[6] Although the GBD study made extensive efforts to standardize mortality data, these estimates should be interpreted cautiously, because the methodology of coding deaths varies globally, potentially leading to significant misclassification.[7] The World Bank has divided the world into seven regions: one region consisting of high-income countries (HICs) and six geographic regions consisting of low- and middle-income countries (LMICs). The information on demographic and social indices presented here is from the World Bank's World Development Indicators (WDIs), and data on gross national income (GNI) per capita were derived using the Atlas method in 2011 U.S. dollars (USD).

MORTALITY AND MORBIDITY DUE TO MYOCARDIAL INFARCTION

Age-adjusted IHD death rates in HICs are declining; however, the current high burden of IHD is primarily the consequence of deaths among 85% of the world's population living in LMICs (Figure 2-1). Globally, between 1990 and 2010, the age-adjusted death rate decreased by 21% from 131/100,000 to 106/100,000, but the number of IHD-associated deaths is increasing. In this same period, the number of deaths increased by 35%. Approximately a third of the increase in DALYs attributable to IHD is due to aging of the world population, and another 22% is due to population growth.[3] Globally, the incidence of acute MI declined over the period 1990 to 2010, dropping from 222.7/100,000 to 195.3/100,000 for males and from 136.3/100,000 to 115.0/100,000 for females (Figure 2-2). The greatest declines occurred in HICs, with only modest declines in LMICs, whereas increases in acute MI incidence were observed in Eastern Europe (Figure 2-3). Despite a meaningful decline in age-adjusted IHD deaths, the DALYs lost due to IHDs have decreased only marginally, by 0.6%, from 1895/100,000 to 1884/100,000.[5]

The reduction in MI mortality appears to be a result of a reduction in both the age-adjusted MI incidence and the case-fatality rate. In a study of the four communities in the Atherosclerosis Risk in Communities (ARIC) Study in the United States, rates in both in-hospital and out-of-hospital mortality declined.[8] Over the period 1987 to 2008, the age-adjusted MI incidence decreased in black and white men and in women, but at different rates. Adjusted for biomarkers, the rates of decline were 4.3%, 3.8%, 2.9%, and 1.5% among white men, white women, black women, and black men, respectively. Age-adjusted in-hospital deaths declined annually by an average of 7.2% for men and 6.9% for women, with most of the reductions coming in the later years (1997 to 2008) compared with the earlier time period (1987 to 1996). Out-of-hospital mortality also declined by 4.9% and 3.7% per year for men and women, respectively. The Kaiser Permanente Northern California health care system reported a 24% decline in MI incidence from 1999 to 2008.[9] This reduction was almost entirely driven by reductions in ST-elevation MIs (STEMIs) from 133 per 100,000 person-years

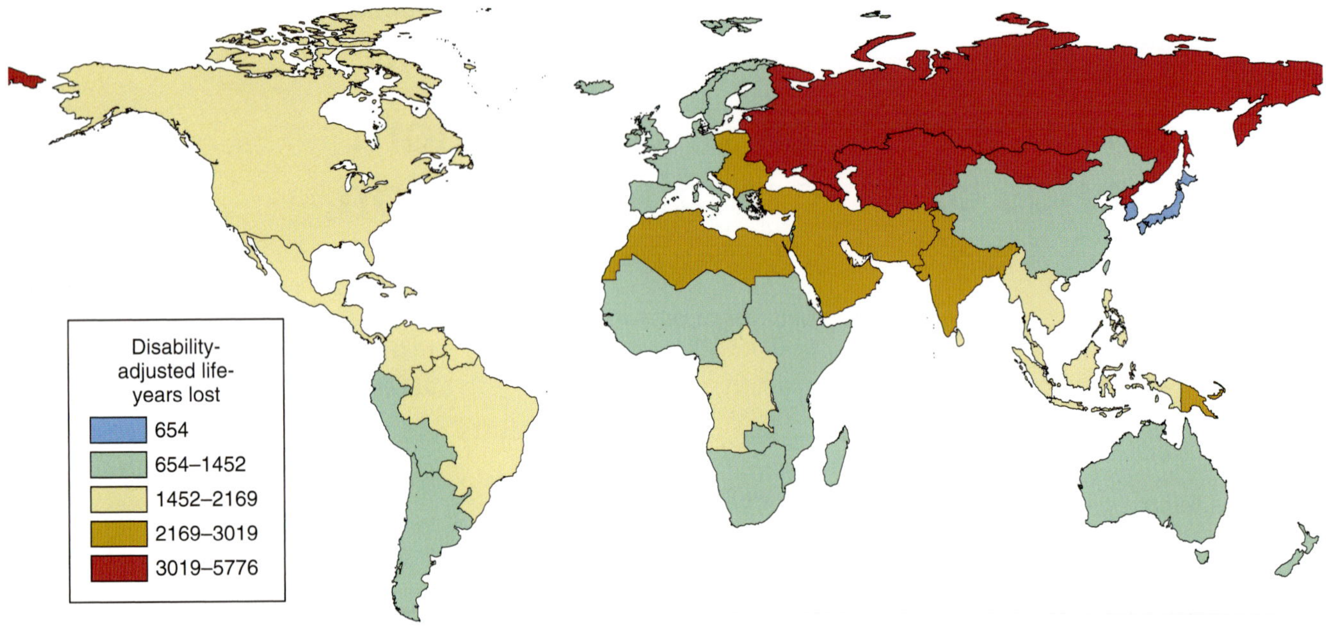

FIGURE 2-1 **Disability-adjusted life-years (DALYs) lost owing to ischemic heart disease (IHD) in 2010, in 21 Global Burden of Disease study regions.** *(From Moran AE, Forouzanfar MH, Roth GA, et al: The global burden of ischemic heart disease in 1990 and 2010: The Global Burden of Disease 2010 study.* Circulation *129: 1493-1501, 2014.)*

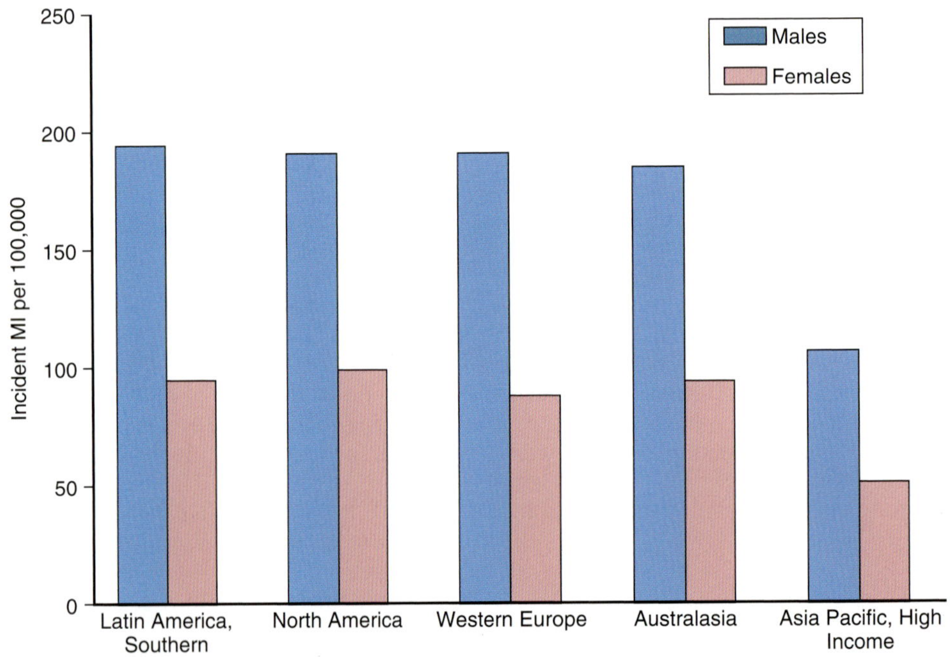

FIGURE 2-2 **Global regional variance in acute myocardial infarction (MI) incidence per 100,000 population.** *(From Moran AE, Forouzanfar MH, Roth, GA, et al: The global burden of ischemic heart disease in 1990 and 2010: The Global Burden of Disease 2010 study.* Circulation *129[14]:1493–1501, 2014.)*

in 1999 to 50 per 100,000 person-years in 2008 (Figure 2-4). Thirty-day mortality also declined, with an odds ratio of 0.76 on comparing 2008 rates to 1999 rates. Over a similar time period in the Worcestor, Massachusetts area, STEMI incidence declined by nearly 50%, with no significant change in that of non ST-elevation MI (NSTEMI).[10] In England, the reduction in MI mortality appears to be split between reductions in MI incidence and in case-fatality rate.[11] From 2000 to 2010, MI case-fatality rates dropped by approximately 3.6% and 4.2% annually, respectively, for men and women, and MI incidence declined by 4.8% and 4.5%, respectively, for men and women. Similarly, over a 25-year period (1984 to 2008) in a large Danish study of more than 234,000 patients with first-time MI, MI incidence declined by 48% and 37% for men and women, respectively, and 30-day mortality declined by greater than 50% in both men and women in the same time period[12] (Figure 2-5).

In addition to the decline in incidence and case-fatality rates over recent decades, the morbidity associated with MI also has changed. For example, patients with MI in Olmsted County, Minnesota, presented with lower severity of heart failure despite more comorbid conditions.[13] Furthermore, the incidence of heart failure (HF) developing both early (within 7 days of MI) and late (8 days up to 5 years later) declined dramatically by 5.7% and 5.8%, respectively, in absolute terms over the time frame 1990 to 1996, compared with 2004 to 2010

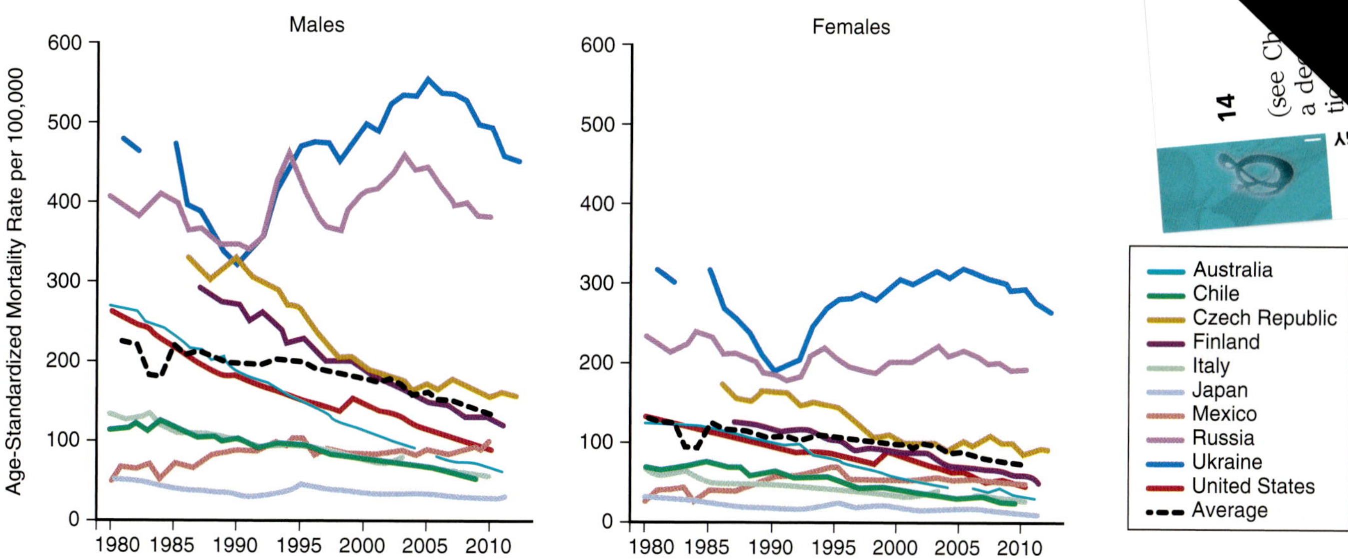

FIGURE 2-3 Age-standardized mortality rate per 100,000 population for ischemic heart disease among males and females in 10 selected representative countries, 1980 to 2012. *(From Ali MK, et al:* Health Aff (Millwood) *34:1444-1455, 2105. Copyright Project HOPE—The People to People Health Foundation, Inc.)*

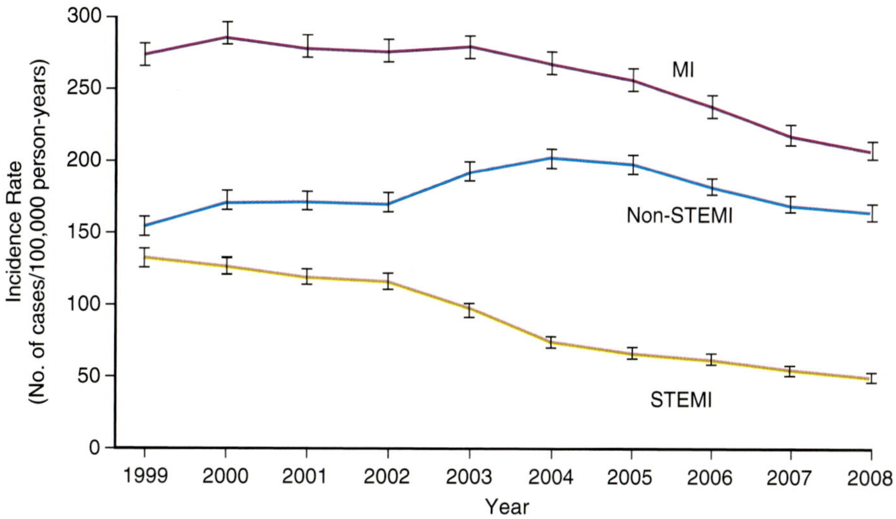

FIGURE 2-4 Age- and sex-adjusted incidence rates of acute myocardial infarction, 1999 to 2008. *I bars* represent 95% confidence intervals. *MI,* Myocardial infarction; *Non-STEMI,* non–ST-elevation myocardial infarction; *STEMI,* ST-elevation myocardial infarction. *(From Yeh RW, Sidney S, Chandra M, et al: Population trends in the incidence and outcomes of acute myocardial infarction.* N Engl J Med *362[23]:2155-2165, 2010.)*

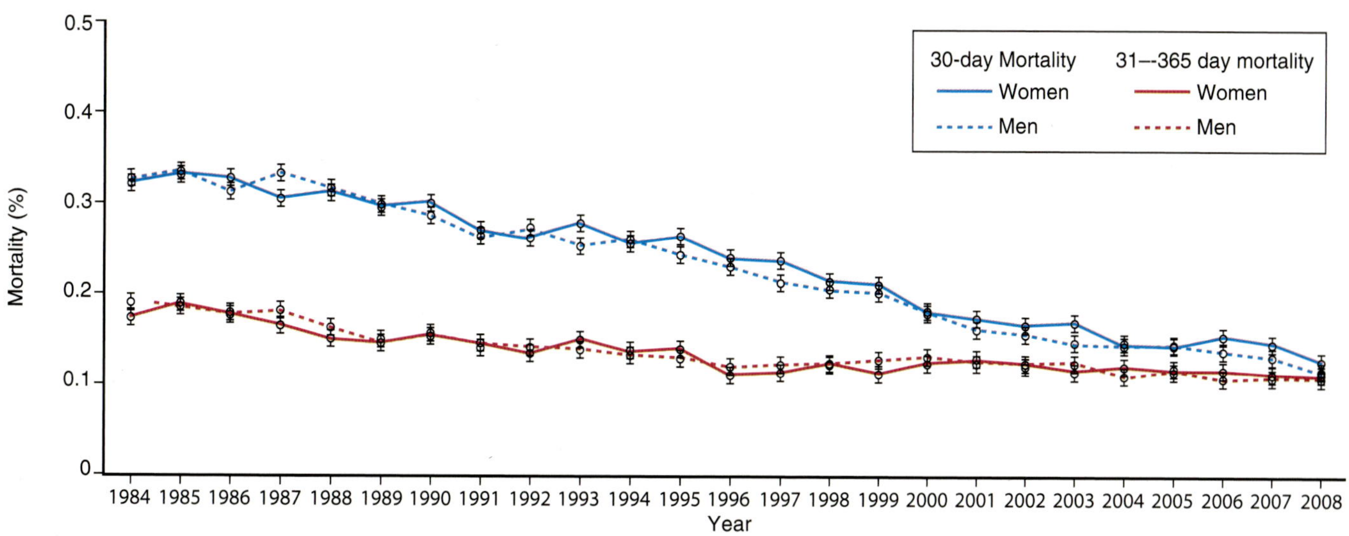

FIGURE 2-5 Standardized 30-day and 31- to 365-day mortality after first-time hospitalization for myocardial infarction among Danish men and women between 1984 and 2008. *(From Schmidt M, Jacobsen JB, Lash TL, et al: 25 year trends in first time hospitalisation for acute myocardial infarction, subsequent short and long term mortality, and the prognostic impact of sex and comorbidity: A Danish nationwide cohort study.* BMJ *344:e356, 2012.)*

apter 25). The entire decline was accounted for by creased frequency of HF associated with reduced ejec- on fraction, because no decline was observed in the risk of HF with preserved ejection fraction after MI. An analogous decline in HF during the index admission for MI also was seen in Worcester, Massachusetts, after 1991.[14]

VARIATION IN THE GLOBAL BURDEN OF ISCHEMIC HEART DISEASE

Although global trends show a larger IHD burden in LMICs in comparison with HICs, significant variation in IHD burden is evident across the six LMIC regions, and among countries within a given region or World Bank income category. Described next are those regional variations in acute MI incidence and burden.

High-Income Countries

For the GBD 2010 Study, HICs were divided into five regions: Asia Pacific, High Income; Europe, Western; Australasia; North America, High Income; and Latin America, Southern. Among males in 2010, the regions from highest to lowest in terms of MI incidence per 100,000 were Latin America, Southern (194.47), North America (191.28), Western Europe (191.04), Australasia (185.21), and Asia Pacific, High Income (106.84). Among females the MI incidence rates were lower with the rate per 100,000 females in each region: Latin America, Southern (95.15), North America (98.91), Western Europe (88.24), Australasia (93.61), and Asia Pacific, High Income (50.77). In all regions the male-to-female ratio was approximately 2:1 (Figure 2-6). All of these regions had declines of approximately 22% (Asia Pacific) to 40% (Europe, Western) from 1990 rates. The age-standardized loss in DALYs attributed to IHD decreased, with Japan, South Korea, and France reporting the lowest DALYs lost among high-income countries.[15]

Low- and Middle-Income Countries

East Asia and the Pacific

In 1990, IHD was the fourth major cause of death in the East Asia and Pacific (EAP) region, but by 2010, it was the leading cause. The MI incidence varied among the EAP subregions in

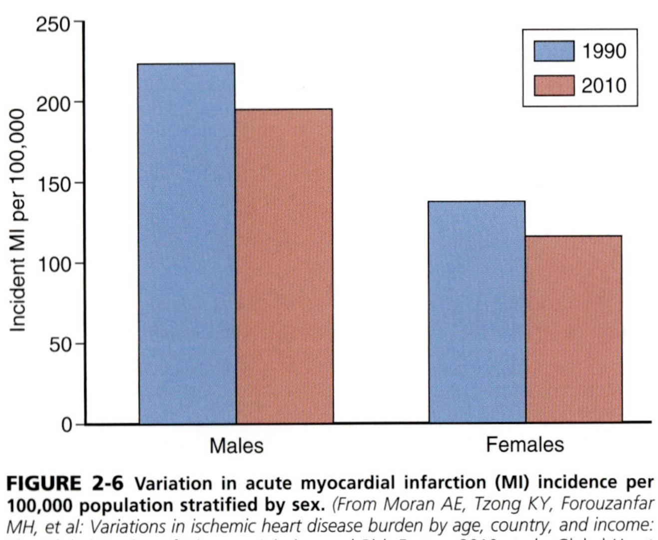

FIGURE 2-6 Variation in acute myocardial infarction (MI) incidence per 100,000 population stratified by sex. *(From Moran AE, Tzong KY, Forouzanfar MH, et al: Variations in ischemic heart disease burden by age, country, and income: The Global Burden of Diseases, Injuries, and Risk Factors 2010 study.* Global Heart *9[1]:91-99, 2014.)*

2010, ranging from highest at 212/100,000 males in Oceania, to 167/100,000 males in Southeast Asia, and lowest at 133/100,000 males in East Asia. The rates mildly declined by approximately 10% in Oceania and Southeast Asia and remained similar to those reported in 1990 in East Asia. For women, as in the HICs, overall incidence was lower than in men. Rates of MI/100,000 females were 130, 101, and 78 for Oceania, Southeast Asia, and East Asia, respectively. Southeast Asian women had a 20% decline, and East Asian women saw only mild declines in their incidence rates. Oceanian women saw a mild increase compared with 1990.[15] Furthermore, CVD accounts for the largest proportion of DALYs lost in the region, with 26 million lost in Southeast Asia and 67 million lost in East Asia.[2]

Central and Eastern Europe and Central Asia

The highest CVD mortality rate occurs in this region and was 866/100,000 in Eastern Europe and 604/100,000 in Central Europe.[15a] As seen in other regions, the number of CVD-related deaths varies across countries. In Ukraine, Bulgaria, Belarus, and Russia, CVD rates have reached an alarming 800/100,000 for men.[16] Also as in other regions, the largest component of CVD mortality is acute MI. MI incidence is highest in the world, at 410/100,000 males in Eastern Europe, followed by 341/100,000 males in Central Asia and 265/100,000 males in Central Europe. Rates for males increased by 16% in Eastern Europe, mildly increased in Central Asia, and declined by 30% in Central Europe. The incidence rates per 100,000 females were 199, 189, and 138 for Eastern Europe, Central Asia, and Central Europe, respectively. Like the males, females in Central Europe demonstrated a large 25% decline in incidence, with 10% increase in Eastern Europe and a minimal decline of 3% in Central Asia.

Latin America and the Caribbean

The Latin America and Caribbean (LAM) region has a high CVD burden[17]; in 2010, CVD was responsible for 29% of all deaths, and IHD was the leading cause of DALYs lost, representing a 36% increase over 1990 rates.[18] Rates of MI incidence in 2010 were similar per 100,000 males in Central America (198), Tropical Latin America (205), and Caribbean Latin America (210) and considerably lower in the Andean subregion (149). Declines in incidence in this region ranged from nearly 20% in Tropical Latin America to only approximately 7.5% in Central America. For women, the Caribbean rate was highest at 140/100,000, compared with 124/100,000, 119/100,000, and 102/100,000, respectively, for Central America, Tropical Latin America, and the Andean subregion. Declines were similar to those for males across the region compared with 1990 data.

North Africa and the Middle East

In 2010, IHD accounted for 93 deaths per 100,000 population, representing a 15% increase in IHD mortality rates. In addition to increased mortality, CVD and IHD were responsible for 17.2 million and 6.8 million DALYs lost, respectively. Individual country data show that 12 of the 19 countries in North Africa and the Middle East are ranked in the top 50 countries worldwide for age-adjusted IHD mortality rates. Overall, the region had an MI incidence rate of 257/100,000 males and 153/100,000 females in 2010. These rates represented 20% and 15% decreases, respectively, for males and females since 1990.

South Asia

CVD accounts for 20% of all deaths in the South Asian Region (SAR), of which IHD is responsible for more than 50%.

In 2010, IHD was responsible for 1.8 million deaths, or 10.6% of all fatalities. In addition to mortality, CVD also was responsible for 60.5 million of DALYs lost in 2010. India, with a population of 1.2 billion, is the largest country within this region and has an extremely high burden of IHD. In 1990, 1.18 million people died from IHD; this increased to 2.03 million in 2010, and it is estimated that CVD represents 25% of deaths in India. South Asia has the third highest MI incidence of all regions, with 245/100,000 in males and 155/100,000 in females. Women have seen an approximately 8% decline, whereas the rate for men declined by little over 3% compared with 1990 rates.

Sub-Saharan Africa

Of all the subregions in sub-Saharan Africa, Southern Africa has the highest number of CVD deaths, currently at 13%; in Western Africa, CVD accounts for 7.5% of all deaths. Overall, across sub-Saharan Africa, the mortality rates are lower than global averages, with the exception of Southern Africa, where the rates have increased from 129/100,000 to 136/100,000. Sub-Saharan Africa is divided into Central, East, Southern, and West subregions. For men, the MI incidence rates per 100,000 are 223, 172, 174, and 181, respectively. For women, the rates are 165, 139, 118, and 147, respectively. For both men and women in West and Central Africa, there was either no change or mild increases in MI incidence compared with 1990 rates. Men and women in East and Southern sub-Saharan Africa saw drops in MI incidence of approximately 10% from 1990 rates. As part of the WHO's Global Action Plan for Prevention and Control of Noncommunicable Diseases 2013-2020, it is estimated that a combination of cost-effective health interventions, with an implementation cost of $1 per capita in low-income countries (LICs) and up to $3 per capita in HICs, could help to reduce the burden of CVD and diabetes in Africa .[19]

ECONOMIC BURDEN OF ISCHEMIC HEART DISEASE

The economic burden of IHD is significant and can be measured in at least three ways: first, by financial costs incurred in the health care system and described in "cost-of-illness" studies; second, by microeconomic studies that assess the household impact of health events such as MIs; and, third, by macroeconomic analyses that assess worker productivity or loss of economic growth from individual patients or their caregivers being partially or completely out of work as a consequence of illness. The literature on the first and second measures in LMICs is sparse, and no published microeconomic studies have focused exclusively on IHD. Many LMICs lack extensive insurance plans, and government-funded plans may be inadequate, requiring people to pay out of pocket for health services in the acute setting, for medications, and for outpatient follow-up care.[20]

Relatively more information is available on the economic burden from a macroeconomic perspective.[21] The LIMCs are earlier in the epidemiologic transition, so IHD occurs at younger age than in HICs. Accordingly, although data are limited, the macroeconomic burden for each IHD event is likely to be higher. In China, annual direct costs of CVD are estimated at more than $40 billion, which translates into 4% of their GNI. In South Africa, 25% of the health care expenditure is devoted to CVD. Relatively few cost-of-illness studies have been done in other regions of the world, but information on the costs associated with risk factors for IHD is available. Globally, health care costs related to hypertension were estimated at $370 billion in 2001, a staggering figure that was estimated to increase to $1 trillion in direct costs and up to $4 trillion for indirect costs by 2011, or nearly a doubling over a decade.[22] Although the cost of managing risk factors is immense, the cost of long-term management of IHD is equally high. Heart failure, the most common sequela of IHD, is estimated to cost $108 billion annually.[23-25]

INTERVENTIONS

Success in reducing CVD mortality rates depends on improved primary and secondary prevention strategies (see Chapter 34). Approximately 25% to 50% of the reduction in CVD-associated mortality is related to treatments, and the remainder is due to changes in risk factors.[26] Improvements in acute care reduce case fatality but also increase the chronic IHD population in need of secondary prevention. Considered next are individual-level interventions for management of MI globally and their cost-effectiveness (Table 2-1).

Acute Management

Several factors contribute to the optimal management of MI, starting with the quality of prehospital care available to those experiencing cardiac symptoms (see Chapter 5). Although the literature on this topic for LMICs is sparse, a survey of emergency medicine leaders in 13 LMICs in Africa, Asia, and Latin America showed that the availability of emergency medical transport (e.g., ambulances) is limited and the rates of use are low, particularly in rural areas, largely attributable to deficiencies in funding and administrative leadership.[27] Additional studies are required to elucidate those factors contributing to low availability and to identify barriers to use of formal emergency medical transport systems in LMICs. Recognizing the high proportion of persons with MI dying before reaching a hospital, a modeling study from China estimated that even optimal use of standard hospital-based treatments would have a limited impact on IHD-associated mortality.

The medical management of MI has been well established through clinical trials and involves the use of aspirin, beta blockers, statins, angiotensin receptor blockers (ARBs) or angiotensin-converting enzyme (ACE) inhibitors, other antiplatelet agents, fibrinolytics, and anticoagulants (see Chapter 13). The availability of and adherence to clinical guidelines vary significantly in different world regions. A retrospective analysis of studies involving 50,310 patients with STEMI from 63 countries showed that the rate of use of aspirin and beta blockers ranges from 75% to 95% in middle-income countries.[28] These findings are consistent with data from the Gulf RACE (8176 adults, 6 countries), ACCESS (11,731 adults, 19 countries), and ZESCA (127 adults, 4 countries) studies, which showed that 68% to 96% of patients received aspirin, beta blockers, an ACE inhibitor, and a statin.[29-31] Several countries have increased the use of evidence-based medications, as seen in the expanded GRACE2 registry in 31,982 adults in 25 countries[32] and in the study of 1025 patients with acute coronary syndromes (ACS) managed at a tertiary care hospital in Lebanon,[33] which may be due to quality improvement measures, as seen in the BRIDGE-ACS study of 1150 patients in Brazil.[34] Despite the availability and

TABLE 2-1 Cost-Effectiveness of Interventions at the Individual Level

INTERVENTION	SOURCE FOR ESTIMATE: COUNTRY OR WORLD BANK REGIONS STUDIED	LOW-INCOME COUNTRIES (GNI PER CAPITA*: ≤$1045)		MIDDLE-INCOME COUNTRIES (GNI PER CAPITA*: $1045 TO $12,746)	
		Very Cost-Effective Up to 1× GNI/QALY	Cost-Effective Up to 3× GNI/ QALY (up to $3135)	Very Cost-Effective Up to 1× GNI/QALY	Cost-Effective Up to 3× GNI/ QALY (up to $38,238)
Aspirin + beta blocker	All non–high-income regions	$11 to $22			
Aspirin + beta blocker + SK	All non–high-income regions	$634 to $734			
Aspirin + beta blocker + tPA	All non–high-income regions				$15,860 to $18,893
Aspirin + beta blocker + statin + ACE inhibitor	All non–high-income regions	$300 to $400			
†Aspirin + beta blocker + statin + ACE inhibitor	China		$ 3100	$ 3100	
†Clopidogrel	China				$17,600
†Primary PCI	China				$9000 to $23,000
Coronary artery bypass graft surgery	South Asia, sub-Saharan Africa, and East Asia and the Pacific				$24,040 to $33,846 (ICER compared with four medications: aspirin, beta blocker, statin, and ACE inhibitor)
Nicotine replacement therapy	All non high-income regions	$55 to $761			
Community pharmacist–based smoking cessation program	Thailand	*Men*: $500 with 0.18/LY gained *Women*: $614 with 0.24/LY gained			
Nicotine-based gum	Seychelles	$599			
Bupropion-based	Seychelles	$227			
ICD	United States				$17,000
CRT in heart failure	Brazil				I$15,723
CRT	Argentina	I$34 (ICER compared with medical therapy)			

*GNI per capita, as defined by the World Bank: low-income countries: $1045 or lower; middle-income countries: $1045 to $12,746; high-income countries: $12,746 or higher.
†ICER compared with current treatment.
ACE, Angiotensin-converting enzyme; *CRT,* cardiac resynchronization therapy; *GNI,* gross national income; *ICER,* incremental cost-effectiveness ratio; *ICD,* implantable cardioverter-defibrillator; *I$,* international dollar; *IHD,* ischemic heart disease; *LY,* life year; PCI, percutaneous coronary intervention; *QALY,* quality-adjusted life-year; *SK,* streptokinase; *tPA,* tissue plasminogen activator..

proven use of these drugs, certain patient groups are less likely to receive appropriate therapy, as seen among persons of lower socioeconomic status in the CREATE Prospective Registry Study compared with those in the ACCESS study,[31] and among women in a study of 6 countries in the Middle East,[35] resulting in higher mortality. The effect that income may have on differential use of different accurate treatments and time to use, such as for fibrinolytics and secondary treatments, is manifest in the relationship between gross national income (GNI) and overall mortality[28] (Figure 2-7).

Cost-Effectiveness of Acute Management Strategies

The cost-effectiveness of four incremental strategies for the treatment of MI has been evaluated: (1) aspirin; (2) aspirin and atenolol; (3) aspirin, atenolol, and streptokinase; and (4) aspirin, atenolol, and tissue plasminogen activator (tPA). The incremental cost per quality-adjusted life-year (QALY) gained for the combination of aspirin plus a beta blocker (strategy 2) was less than $25 for all 6 LMIC regions; the cost per QALY gained for streptokinase ranged from $630 to $730, and the incremental cost-effectiveness ratio (ICER) for tPA was approximately $16,000/QALY gained, when compared with streptokinase (see Chapter 15). Furthermore,

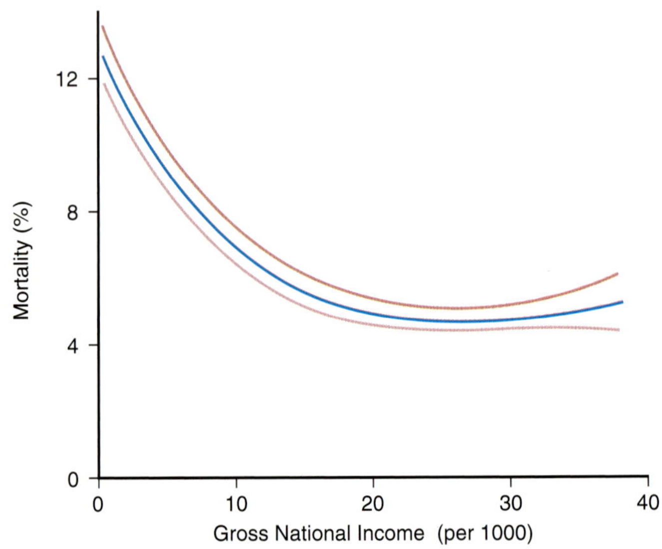

FIGURE 2-7 Relationship between gross national income (GNI) and 30-day mortality rate as a continuous function of GNI. *Blue* and *red lines* represent 30-day mortality and 95% confidence interval, respectively. *(From Orlandini A, Díaz R, Wojdyla D, et al: Outcomes of patients in clinical trials with ST-segment elevation myocardial infarction among countries with different gross national incomes.* Eur Heart J*27[5]:527-533, 2006.)*

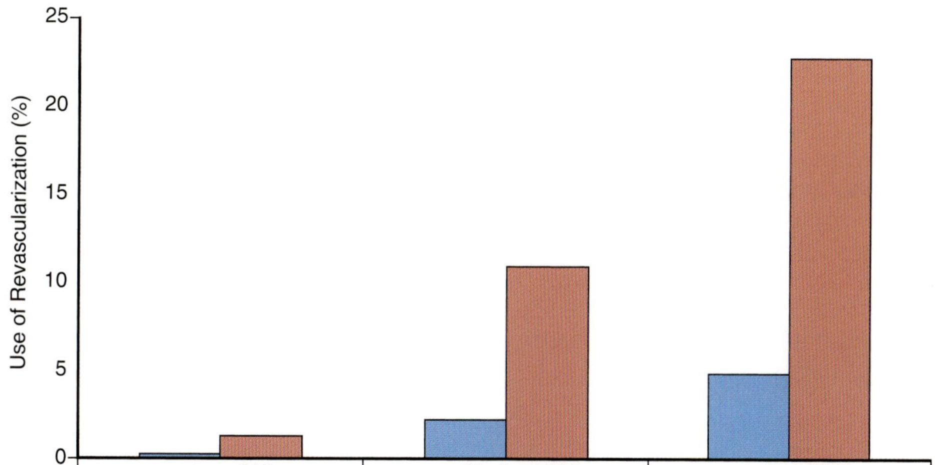

	Low GNI	Medium GNI	High GNI
CABG	0.2	2.2	4.8
PCI	1.3	10.9	22.7

FIGURE 2-8 Coronary artery bypass graft (CABG) surgery and percutaneous coronary intervention (PCI) rates among patients with ST-elevation myocardial infarction (STEMI) by gross national income (GNI). *(From Orlandini A, Díaz R, Wojdyla D, et al: Outcomes of patients in clinical trials with ST-segment elevation myocardial infarction among countries with different gross national incomes.* Eur Heart J *27[5]: 527-533, 2006.)*

recent Markov modeling of optimal medical management of in-hospital ACS showed that optimal use of aspirin, beta blocker, ACE inhibitor, and a statin had an ICER of less than $3100.[36]

In addition to the foregoing medication regimens, management of MI may require reperfusion therapy with either a fibrinolytic or percutaneous coronary intervention (PCI), the use of which varies by LMIC region (see Chapter 15). In LMICs, fibrinolytics are more commonly used than PCI, although the time to initiation of fibrinolytic therapy is longer than in their higher-GNI counterparts (4.3 hours versus 2.8 hours).[28] The rates of PCI and coronary artery bypass grafting (CABG) are higher in high-income than in low-income patients (Figure 2-8). In a study of 13,591 patients enrolled in the National Cardiovascular Disease Registry Ministry of Health hospitals in Malaysia, the use of streptokinase was more common for minorities (Chinese and Indians) than among local Malaysians, who were more likely to get PCI.[37] In India, the overall use of PCI was low, and even lower for persons of low socioeconomic status, reflecting inequity in care even within a country.[38] In the Thai Registry, the Kerala ACS Registry (based in India), and the Gulf RACE study, approximately 40% to 80% of patients with STEMI received fibrinolytic therapy.[30,39,40] Remarkably, in the ACCESS study of 11,731 adult subjects from 19 countries in Africa, Latin America, and the Middle East, approximately 40% of patients with confirmed MI did not receive PCI or fibrinolytic therapy, resulting in a higher mortality rate.[31] In Europe, PCI is emerging as the primary choice in most countries (see Chapter 17).[41,42]

Overall, fibrinolysis with streptokinase remains a cost-effective strategy in LMICs.[26] From the foregoing studies and the GRACE registry,[32] it is evident that the use of fibrinolytics and PCI varies significantly. In the appropriate MI setting, PCI has been reported to be as cost-effective as medical management[36]; however, additional studies are required to further evaluate this finding. In some LMIC regions, the use and quality of PCI care are improving despite several barriers,[43] whereas in other countries, such as India, treatment continues to rely on fibrinolytics until PCI-based infrastructure, access to services, and quality of cardiac care improve.[44] Inhabitants of several LMICs may reside in areas without timely access to a PCI facility; simulation analysis of a hypothetical nonurban population in Canada showed that building a new PCI facility is associated with a cost of $7478/QALY gained in comparison with ambulance transport.[44a] Future studies in LMICs are required to estimate costs associated with building new facilities.

In comparison with reports on use of fibrinolytics and PCI, data on the number of cardiac surgeries performed and their outcomes are sparse. Although CABG is a cost-effective intervention in HICs, its incremental cost-effectiveness ratio relative to a combination of four medications—aspirin, beta blocker, statin, and ACE inhibitor—may be attractive to middle-income countries ($24,040 to $72,345/QALY gained), but it may be available only to a smaller proportion of the population.[26,45]

Independent of the intervention used, in several instances, patients may require management in a coronary care unit (CCU), where they can be monitored closely. When appropriately triaged, cardiac intensive care is cost-effective despite increased staffing and facilities but may not be as widely available in all LMIC regions.

Secondary Prevention of Myocardial Infarction

Primary prevention strategies for CVD include population-based and individual-level interventions. Population-based interventions often are directed toward cessation of tobacco use, reduction in dietary salt and trans fatty acid consumption, and increased physical activity. Individual-level interventions for primary prevention include management of cholesterol, hypertension, obesity, and diabetes, as well as targeted smoking cessation programs.

Strategies for secondary prevention can take advantage of some of these population-based efforts but generally are more focused on individual-level interventions. In addition, revision of regional or national government health policies to improve chronic care services are important. Individual-level interventions typically are aided by increasing access and adherence to essential CVD medications, increasing availability of cardiac resynchronization/defibrillation therapy (see Chapter 28), and increasing access to and the use of cardiac rehabilitation (see Chapter 34). Discussed next are a few key population- and individual-level interventions.

Access to Essential Medications for Secondary Prevention of Cardiovascular Disease

In addition to management of risk factors, several evidence-based medication regimens are effective in the secondary prevention of CVD. Such regimens include aspirin, beta blockers, ACE inhibitors/ARBs, cholesterol-reducing agents (for example, statins), and more recently, multidrug combination pills. Several studies have shown that the use of medications for secondary prevention varies significantly across LMIC regions, despite their inclusion in the WHO Model List of Essential Medications. The WHO-PREMISE Study in 10 LMICs showed that among patients with IHD, only 81.2% were prescribed aspirin, 48.1% a beta blocker, 39.8% an ACE inhibitor, and 29.8% a statin.[46] A survey of nine European countries (the EUROASPIRE III study) showed that among patients with IHD, only 71% and 78% were on a statin and an ACE inhibitor/ARB, respectively.[47] The most recent PURE prospective study (153,996 adults in 3 HICs and 14 LMICs) showed that only 25.8% were receiving an antiplatelet medication, 20.4% a beta blocker, 20.0% an ACE inhibitor/ARB, and 16.7% a statin.[48] The range across income groups is quite significant, however, with HICs having more than three to four times the proportion of patients on appropriate therapy compared with LICs (Figure 2-9). The results are even more concerning in India, where a survey of 53 villages found that 14% of patients were on aspirin, 41% on a blood pressure–lowering medication, and 5% on a cholesterol-lowering medication.[49] Supporting this finding was an observational study of statin use in India, which showed that although the use of statins had increased over the period 2006 to 2010, only 8% of patients with CHD were on a statin.[50]

Several factors are responsible for the low rate medication use, including inadequate availability and access to affordable medications, limited number of health care providers, and complicated regimens of medications. In many LMICs, the cost of a month's supply of generic secondary prevention medications ranges from 1.5 to 18.4 days' wages for government workers, and the availability of cardiovascular medications ranges from 25% in the public sector to 60% in the private sector.[51,52] Availability of generic medications was influenced by the Trade-Related Aspects of Intellectual Property Rights (TRIPS) Agreement in 1995, which obliged World Trade Organization (WTO) members to protect pharmaceutical patents for 20 years from when they are filed.[53] The subsequent Doha Declaration in 2003 granted nations compulsory licenses to domestically manufacture essential medications without permission of the patent holder,[54] a trend that appeared to have increased until 2006.[55] Canada is the only country that has issued a compulsory license to export generic medications to poorer nations,[55] which has helped to increase their availability. More recent studies have shown that over the period 2001 to 2011, generic medications in the private sector of 19 LMIC (in Latin America, Middle East, and South Africa) represented approximately 70% to 80% of the market share, which is larger than in most European countries.[56]

A majority of patients with CVD should receive several medications, and to increase the availability of these medications in LMICs, the concept of the polypill, with fixed dose combinations of different cardiac medications, was developed as a possible mechanism to increase adherence and availability.[57-59] Analysis of studies shows that improved access to pharmaceuticals, improved use of insurance policies, and aligning incentives for physicians, consumers, and drug vendors may increase the uptake of generic medications.[60] Additionally, higher availability of trained professionals may help with improving patients' access to medications.

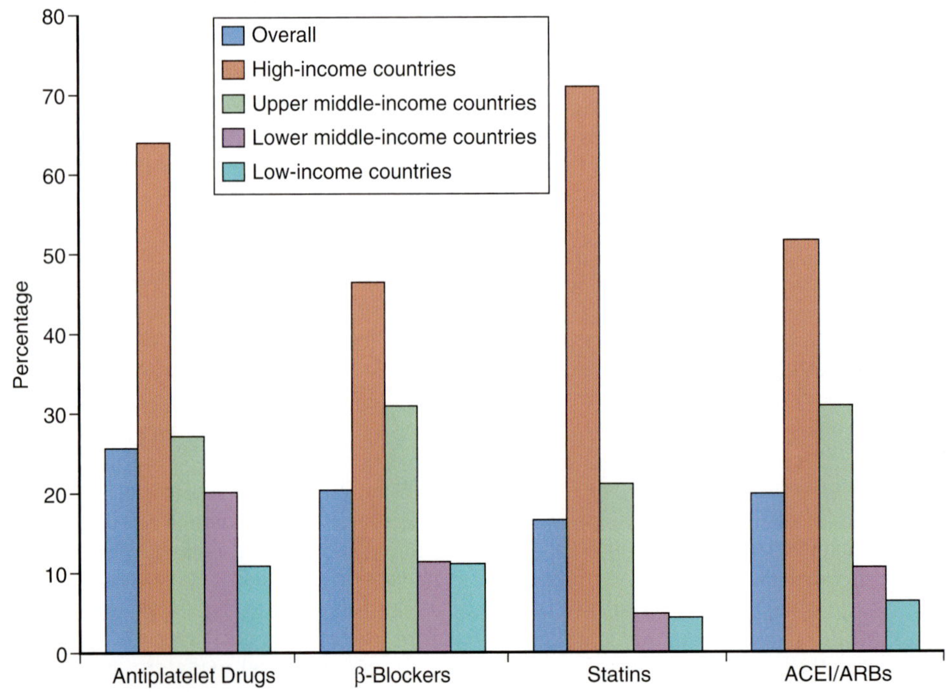

FIGURE 2-9 Use of secondary medications by income. *ACEIs,* Angiotensin-converting enzyme inhibitors; *ARBs,* Angiotensin receptor blockers. *(From Yusuf S, Islam S, Chow CK, et al: Use of secondary prevention drugs for cardiovascular disease in the community in high-income, middle-income, and low-income countries (the PURE Study): A prospective epidemiological survey.* Lancet *378[9798]:1231-1243, 2011.)*

Medications are cost-effective in the treatment of MI and in the secondary prevention of IHD. The combination of aspirin, ACE inhibitor, beta blocker, and a statin is cost-effective in LMIC and is associated with $300 to $400/QALY gained, even in the absence of a polypill.[61,62]

Medication Adherence

Medication adherence refers to whether or not patients take medications in the required frequency and for the required duration; patients who have medications available for at least 80% of the time are considered to be adherent.[63] Approximately 60% of people (in different world regions) who are prescribed medications show adequate adherence.[64,65] The PURE study observed the lowest medication use in LICs, possibly owing to poor availability of and adherence to medications.[49] Adequate medication adherence is associated with a 10.1% to 17.8% reduction in cost between high- and low-adherence groups[66] and is associated with lower mortality rates, as was seen in the REACH International Registry.[67]

Data regarding interventions to improve medication adherence are limited. Recent research suggests that reduced out-of-pocket expenses, better case management, patient education with behavioral support, mobile phone messaging, support by broader guidelines, and regulatory and communication-based policies may improve medication adherence.[68-71] The MI FREEE trial in the United States has shown that elimination of copayments for drugs after an MI results in higher medication adherence, increasing from 35.9% to 49%.[72] Furthermore, insurance plans that targeted high-risk patients, offered wellness programs, and made these benefits available for medications ordered by mail were associated with a 4% to 5% higher medication adherence.[50] Although these studies are promising, future research will reveal if these models can be successfully replicated in LMICs.

The so-called polypill is one possible intervention to improve medication adherence. A randomized controlled trial with 2004 participants in India and Europe showed that use of a polypill (containing aspirin, statin, and two blood pressure–lowering agents) versus usual care was associated with improved medication adherence (86% versus 65%), with concurrent reduction in systolic blood pressure (by 2.6 mm Hg) and low-density lipoprotein (LDL) cholesterol (by 4.2 mg/dL).[73] Several other secondary prevention trials are under way, including the Indian Polycap-K Trial (in men and women in India), Kanyini Guidelines Adherence with Polypill (in indigenous and nonindigenous peoples in Australia), and the Trial in Secondary Prevention (in Spain and Latin American countries).[58,74] These and other studies will provide information on the effectiveness of polypills in the secondary prevention of CVD and may raise the suggestion that polypills be included in the WHO Model List of Essential Medications.[75]

Smoking Cessation

Although the use of tobacco products represents a major risk factor for CVD, a significant proportion of the global population continues to smoke.[76-78] Worldwide, approximately 1.1 billion people smoke, of whom 82% reside in LMICs. To address the significant morbidity and mortality associated with smoking, the WHO Assembly adopted the WHO Framework Convention on Tobacco Control (FCTC) in 2003, making this the first global tobacco treaty to regulate smoking. Several countries have implemented FCTC measures to curb the use and effects of smoking.

The price of tobacco products is a major determinant in smoking uptake and cessation.[77] The International Agency for Research on Cancer (IARC) has shown that a 50% increase in inflation-adjusted tobacco price reduces consumption by 20% in LMICs.[77] In LMICs, low specific excise tax is the main reason that cigarettes are approximately 70% cheaper.[77] Tobacco taxation represents the most cost-effective antismoking intervention[79]; however, strong political opposition in many countries remains a major barrier to wider implementation of higher tobacco taxes.[80]

In addition to increased taxation, regulating advertisements and smoking in public spaces also can limit the use of tobacco products. Advertising bans can result in a significant decline in smoking,[81] and legislation-based smoking bans can result in reduced hospital admissions for cardiac events.[82] Furthermore, effective public health efforts have shown a 15% to 30% long-term cumulative decline in smoking rates, with a 6% reduction in the demand for tobacco.

Although population level interventions can be effective, several individual-level interventions including nicotine replacement therapy (NRT), non–nicotine-based products, and behavioral modification also have been implemented (see Chapter 34). Systematic reviews of studies in HICs and LMICs show that NRT can increase the rate of cessation by 50% to 70% and is effective in sustained smoking abstinence.[83] In addition to NRT, bupropion and nortriptyline, which are non–nicotine-based medications, were shown to have efficacy similar to that of NRT[84]; however, these medications are not on the WHO Model List of Essential Medications (the current list includes nicotine), and additional studies are required to determine the availability of these medications to large populations in LMICs.

Cost-Effective Interventions

Information on cost-effectiveness is essential for countries to be able to set priorities given scarce resources. Overall, several cost-effective interventions are available for acute and chronic management of ACS and for the long-term management of IHD risk factors (see Table 2-1). The WHO Commission on Macroeconomics and Health has recommended choosing interventions that cost less than three times the GNI per capita of the concerned country. Most data on cost-effectiveness come from studies based in HICs; however, studies directed at estimating cost-effectiveness at the regional and countrywide levels in LMICs are emerging.[62,85-87] Comparative effectiveness and cost-effectiveness information should guide the implementation of the components of MI care, to maximize accessibility and to achieve equitable distribution.

Of all tobacco cessation interventions discussed, taxation represents the most cost-effective intervention to reduce smoking[62,79] (Table 2-2), although NRTs also are cost-effective depending on their price and availability. Jha and colleagues analyzed the cost-effectiveness of tobacco control using a cohort of smokers alive in 2000. The cost-effectiveness value associated with this reduction is $3 to $42/QALY saved for tax increases (not including tax revenue), $55 to $761/QALY for NRT, and $54 to $674 for nonprice measures. Data on cost-effective interventions in LMIC are limited; however, a

TABLE 2-2 Cost-Effectiveness of Interventions to Reduce Tobacco Use at the Population or Health Systems Level

		LOW-INCOME COUNTRIES (GNI PER CAPITA*: ≤$1045)		MIDDLE-INCOME COUNTRIES (GNI PER CAPITA*: $1045 TO $12,746)	
INTERVENTION	COUNTRY OR WORLD BANK REGIONS	Up to 1× GNI/QALY	Up to 3× GNI/QALY (up to $3135)	Up to 1× GNI/QALY	Up to 3× GNI/QALY (up to $ 38,238)
Tax increase on tobacco	All non–high-income regions	$3 to $42			
Nonprice measure	All non–high-income regions	$54 to $674			
Tobacco tax strategy	South Africa	$ 31			
Tobacco indoor air strategy	South Africa	$410			

*GNI per capita, as defined by the World Bank: low-income countries: $1045 or lower; middle-income countries: $1045 to $12,746; high-income countries: $12,746 or higher.
GNI, Gross national income; *QALY,* quality-adjusted life-year.

few country-specific studies have been reported. In South Africa, the tobacco tax and indoor air policies are highly cost-effective, with an ICER of $31 (USD) per DALY averted (in 2000) for the tobacco tax strategy and $410 per DALY averted for the indoor air strategy.[62,88] In Seychelles, a cohort study showed that the incremental cost per life-year saved was $599 USD for nicotine-based gum and $227 USD for bupropion.

These studies show that the effectiveness of a strategy may vary across different world regions, and that additional studies are required to identify cost-effective interventions in other regions.

SUMMARY AND FUTURE DIRECTIONS

Despite progress in age-adjusted rates, IHD, including MI as the principal component, remains one of the most common causes of death and disability around the globe. Regional variation presents different problems and challenges. Although rates are falling in HICs, the numbers of MIs continue to rise owing to the aging of the population. Acute MI in LMICs strikes at a younger age and has a much greater impact on economic development. Available treatments and primary and secondary preventive measures also vary widely.

To cope with the multiple challenges, availability of good data, from all over the world, is essential. Although access to data on rates of MI and other noncommunicable diseases (NCDs) as well as risk factors is generally improving, accurate data are lacking in some geographic areas. As outlined in this chapter, various economic and other factors have been identified as important drivers of change, including that leading to informed decision-making regarding country-specific allocation of resources in combating this global epidemic. In addition, specific interventions, at both individual-patient and population-based levels, are now recognized as potential strong contributors to improved management of MI in different parts of the world.

References

1. GBD 2013 Mortality and Causes of Death Collaborators, Naghavi M, Wang H, et al.: Global, regional, and national age-sex specific all-cause and cause-specific mortality for 240 causes of death, 1990-2013: A systematic analysis for the Global Burden of Disease STUDY 2013, *Lancet* 385(9963):117–171, 2015.
2. Lozano R, Naghavi M, Foreman K, et al.: Global and regional mortality from 235 causes of death for 20 age groups in 1990 and 2010: A systematic analysis for the Global Burden of Disease Study 2010, *Lancet* 380(9859):2095–2128, 2012.
3. Moran AE, Forouzanfar MH, Roth GA, et al.: The global burden of ischemic heart disease in 1990 and 2010: the Global Burden of Disease 2010 study, *Circulation* 129(14):1493–1501, 2014.
4. GBD 2013 DALYs and HALE Collaborators, Murray CJ, Barber RM, et al.: Global, regional, and national disability-adjusted life years (DALYs) for 306 diseases and injuries and healthy life expectancy (HALE) for 188 countries, 1990-2013: Quantifying the epidemiological transition, *Lancet* 386(10009):2145–2191, 2015.
5. Murray CJ, Vos T, Lozano R, et al.: Disability-adjusted life years (DALYs) for 291 diseases and injuries in 21 regions, 1990-2010: A systematic analysis for the Global Burden of Disease Study 2010, *Lancet* 380(9859):2197–2223, 2012.
6. Ali MK, Jaacks LM, Kowalski AJ, et al.: Noncommunicable diseases: Three decades of global data show a mixture of increases and decreases in mortality rates, *Health Aff Aff (Millwood)* 34(9):1444–1455, 2015.
7. Pagidipati NJ, Gaziano TA: Estimating deaths from cardiovascular disease: a review of global methodologies of mortality measurement, *Circulation* 127(6):749–756, 2013.
8. Rosamond WD, Chambless LE, Heiss G, et al.: Twenty-two year trends in incidence of myocardial infarction, CHD mortality, and case-fatality in four US communities, 1987 to 2008, *Circulation* 125(15):1848–1857, 2012.
9. Yeh RW, Sidney S, Chandra M, et al.: Population trends in the incidence and outcomes of acute myocardial infarction, *N Engl J Med* 362(23):2155–2165, 2010.
10. McManus DD, Gore J, Yarzebski J, et al.: Recent trends in the incidence, treatment, and outcomes of patients with ST and non-ST-segment acute myocardial infarction, *Am J Med* 124(1): 40–47, 2011.
11. Smolina K, Wright FL, Rayner M, Goldacre MJ: Determinants of the decline in mortality from acute myocardial infarction in England between 2002 and 2010: linked national database study, *BMJ* 344:d8059, 2012.
12. Schmidt M, Jacobsen JB, Lash TL, et al.: 25 year trends in first time hospitalisation for acute myocardial infarction, subsequent short and long term mortality, and the prognostic impact of sex and comorbidity: A Danish nationwide cohort study, *BMJ* 344:e356, 2012.
13. Gerber Y, Weston SA, Berardi C, et al.: Contemporary trends in heart failure with reduced and preserved ejection fraction after myocardial infarction: A community study, *Am J Epidemiol* 178(8):1272–1280, 2013.
14. McManus DD, Chinali M, Saczynski JS, et al.: 30-year trends in heart failure in patients hospitalized with acute myocardial infarction, *Am J Cardiol* 107(3):353–359, 2011.
15. Moran AE, Tzong KY, Forouzanfar MH, et al.: Variations in ischemic heart disease burden by age, country, and income: the global burden of diseases, injuries, and risk factors 2010 study, *Global Heart* 9(1):91–99, 2014.

15a. Institute for Health Metrics and Evaluation (IHME): GBD compare, 2015, IHME, University of Washington. http://vizhub.healthdata.org/gbd-compare.

16. Mirzaei M, Truswell A, Taylor R, Leeder SR: Coronary heart disease epidemics: Not all the same, *Heart* 95(9):740–746, 2009.
17. Glassman A, Gaziano TA, Buendia CPB, de Aguiar FCG: Confronting the chronic disease burden in Latin America and the Caribbean, *Health Affairs* 29(12):2142–2148, 2010.
18. Institute for Health Metrics and Evaluation: Global Burden of Disease (GBD) database. http://www.healthdata.org/data-tools.
19. Mendis S, Chestnov O: Costs, benefits, and effectiveness of interventions for the prevention, treatment, and control of cardiovascular diseases and diabetes in Africa, *Prog Cardiovasc Dis* 56(3):314–321, 2013.
20. Kruk ME, Goldmann E, Galea S: Borrowing and selling to pay for health care in low-and middle-income countries, *Health Aff (Millwood)* 28(4):1056–1066, 2009.
21. Gaziano TA, Bitton A, Anand S, et al.: Growing epidemic of coronary heart disease in low- and middle-income countries, *Curr Prob Cardiol* 35(2):72–115, 2010.
22. Gaziano TA, Bitton A, Anand S, et al.: The global cost of nonoptimal blood pressure, *J Hypertens* 27(7):1472–1477, 2009.
23. Cook C, Cole G, Asaria P, et al.: The annual global economic burden of heart failure, *Int J Cardiol* 171(3):368–376, 2014.
24. Miller G, Randolph S, Forkner E, et al.: Long-term cost-effectiveness of disease management in systolic heart failure, *Med Decis Making* 29(3):325–333, 2009.
25. Safraj S, Ajay VS, Prabhakaran D: Heart failure: Meeting the challenges of surveillance and knowledge translation in resource-poor settings, *Curr Cardiol Rev* 9(2):99–101, 2013.
26. Ford ES, Capewell S: Proportion of the decline in cardiovascular mortality disease due to prevention versus treatment: public health versus clinical care, *Annul Rev Public Health* 32(1):5–22, 2011.
27. Nielsen K, Mock C, Joshipura M, et al.: Assessment of the status of prehospital care in 13 low-and middle-income countries, *Prehosp Emerg Care* 16(3):381–389, 2012.
28. Orlandini A, Diaz R, Wojdyla D, et al.: Outcomes of patients in clinical trials with ST-segment elevation myocardial infarction among countries with different gross national incomes, *Eur Heart J* 27(5):527–533, 2006.
29. Shimony A, Grandi SM, Pilote L, et al.: Utilization of evidence-based therapy for acute coronary syndrome in high-income and low/middle-income countries, *Am J Cardiol* 113(5):793–797, 2014.
30. Zubaid M, Rashed WA, Almahmeed W, et al.: Management and outcomes of Middle Eastern patients admitted with acute coronary syndromes in the Gulf Registry of Acute Coronary Events (Gulf RACE), *Acta Cardiol* 64(4):439–446, 2009.
31. ACCESS Investigators: Management of acute coronary syndromes in developing countries: Acute coronary events—a multinational survey of current management strategies, *Am Heart J* 162(5):852–859.e22, 2011.
32. Goodman SG, Huang W, Yan AT, et al.: The expanded Global Registry of Acute Coronary Events: Baseline characteristics, management practices, and hospital outcomes of patients with acute coronary syndromes, *Am Heart J* 158(2):193–201.e5, 2009.
33. Abdallah M, Karrowni W, Shamseddeen W, et al.: Acute coronary syndromes: Clinical characteristics, management, and outcomes at the American University of Beirut Medical Center, 2002-2005, *Clin Cardiol* 33(1):E6–E13, 2010.

34. Berwanger O, Guimaraes HP, Laranjeira LN, et al.: Effect of a multifaceted intervention on use of evidence-based therapies in patients with acute coronary syndromes in Brazil: The BRIDGE-ACS randomized trial, *JAMA* 307(19):2041–2049, 2012.
35. El-Menyar A, Zubaid M, Rashed W, et al.: Comparison of men and women with acute coronary syndrome in six Middle Eastern countries, *Am J Cardiol* 104(8):1018–1022, 2009.
36. Wang M, Moran AE, Liu J, et al.: Cost-effectiveness of optimal use of acute myocardial infarction treatments and impact on coronary heart disease mortality in China, *Circ Cardiovasc Qual Outcomes* 7(1):78–85, 2014.
37. Lu HT, Nordin RB: Ethnic differences in the occurrence of acute coronary syndrome: Results of the Malaysian National Cardiovascular Disease (NCVD) Database Registry (March 2006-February 2010), *BMC Cardiovasc Disord* 13(1):97, 2013.
38. Xavier D, Pais P, Devereaux PJ, et al.: Treatment and outcomes of acute coronary syndromes in India (CREATE): A prospective analysis of registry data, *Lancet* 371(9622):1435–1442, 2008.
39. Mohanan PP, Mathew R, Harikrishnan S, et al.: Presentation, management, and outcomes of 25 748 acute coronary syndrome admissions in Kerala, India: Results from the Kerala ACS Registry, *Eur Heart J* 34(2):121–129, 2013.
40. Srimahachota S, Boonyaratavej S, Kanjanavanit R, et al.: Thai Registry in Acute Coronary Syndrome (TRACS)—an extension of Thai Acute Coronary Syndrome registry (TACS) group: Lower in-hospital but still high mortality at one-year, *J Med Assoc Thai* 95(4):508, 2012.
41. Kristensen SD, Laut KG, Fajadet J, et al.: Reperfusion therapy for ST elevation acute myocardial infarction 2010/2011: Current status in 37 ESC countries, *Eur Heart J* 35(29):1957–1970, 2014.
42. Schiele F, Hochadel M, Tubaro M, et al.: Reperfusion strategy in Europe: Temporal trends in performance measures for reperfusion therapy in ST-elevation myocardial infarction, *Eur Heart J* 31(21):2614–2624, 2010.
43. Ranasinghe I, Rong Y, Du X, et al.: System barriers to the evidence-based care of acute coronary syndrome patients in China: Qualitative analysis, *Circ Cardiovasc Qual Outcomes* 7(2):209–226, 2014.
44. Dalal J, Sahoo PK, Singh RK, et al.: Role of thrombolysis in reperfusion therapy for management of AMI: Indian scenario, *Indian Heart J* 65(5):566–585, 2013.
44a. Potter B, Weinstein MC, Gaziano TA: Unpublished work, 2014.
45. Gaziano TA: Cardiovascular disease in the developing world and its cost-effective management, *Circulation* 112(23):3547–3553, 2005.
46. Mendis S, Abegunde D, Yusuf S, et al.: WHO study on Prevention of REcurrences of Myocardial Infarction and StrokE (WHO-PREMISE), *Bull World Health Organ* 83(11):820–829, 2005.
48. Kotseva K, Wood D, De Backer G, et al.: EUROASPIRE III: A survey on the lifestyle, risk factors and use of cardioprotective drug therapies in coronary patients from 22 European countries., *Eur J Cardiovasc Prev Rehabil* 16(2):121–137, 2009.
48. Yusuf S, Islam S, Chow CK, et al.: Use of secondary prevention drugs for cardiovascular disease in the community in high-income, middle-income, and low-income countries (the PURE Study): A prospective epidemiological survey, *Lancet* 378(9798):1231–1243, 2011.
49. Joshi R, Chow CK, Raju PK, et al.: Fatal and nonfatal cardiovascular disease and the use of therapies for secondary prevention in a rural region of India, *Circulation* 119(14):1950–1955, 2009.
50. Choudhry NK, Dugani S, Shrank WH, et al.: Despite increased use and sales of statins in India, per capita prescription rates remain far below high-income countries, *Health Aff (Millwood)* 33(2):273–282, 2014.
51. Cameron A, Roubos I, Ewen M, et al.: Differences in the availability of medicines for chronic and acute conditions in the public and private sectors of developing countries, *Bull World Health Organ* 89(6):412–421, 2011.
52. van Mourik MS, Cameron A, Ewen M, Laing RO: Availability, price and affordability of cardiovascular medicines: A comparison across 36 countries using WHO/HAI data, *BMC Cardiovasc Disord* 10:25, 2010.
53. Smith RD, Lee K, Drager N: Trade and health: An agenda for action, *Lancet* 373(9665):768–773, 2009.
54. Lybecker KM, Fowler E: Compulsory licensing in Canada and Thailand: Comparing regimes to ensure legitimate use of the WTO rules, *J Law Med Ethics* 37(2):222–239, 2009.
55. Beall R, Kuhn R: Trends in compulsory licensing of pharmaceuticals since the Doha Declaration: a database analysis, *PLoS Med* 9(1):129, 2012.
56. Kaplan WA, Wirtz VJ, Stephens P: The market dynamics of generic medicines in the private sector of 19 low and middle income countries between 2001 and 2011: A descriptive time series analysis, *PloS One* 8(9):e74399, 2013.
57. Bautista LE, Vera-Cala LM, Ferrante D, et al.: A 'polypill' aimed at preventing cardiovascular disease could prove highly cost-effective for use in Latin America, *Health Aff (Millwood)* 32(1):155–164, 2013.
58. Lonn E, Bosch J, Teo KK, et al.: The polypill in the prevention of cardiovascular diseases: Key concepts, current status, challenges, and future directions, *Circulation* 122(20):2078–2088, 2010.
59. Yusuf S, Pais P, Afzal R, et al.: Effects of a polypill (Polycap) on risk factors in middle-aged individuals without cardiovascular disease (TIPS): A phase II, double-blind, randomised trial, *Lancet* 373(9672):1341–1351, 2009.
60. Kaplan WA, Ritz LS, Vitello M, Wirtz VJ: Policies to promote use of generic medicines in low and middle income countries: a review of published literature, 2000-2010, *Health Policy* 106(3): 211–224, 2012.
61. Gaziano TA, Opie LH, Weinstein MC: Cardiovascular disease prevention with a multidrug regimen in the developing world: A cost-effectiveness analysis, *Lancet* 368(9536):679–686, 2006.
62. Gaziano TA, Pagidipati N: Scaling up chronic disease prevention interventions in lower- and middle-income countries, *Annu Rev Public Health* 34:317–335, 2013.
63. Ho PM, Bryson CL, Rumsfeld JS: Medication adherence: Its importance in cardiovascular outcomes, *Circulation* 119(23):3028–3035, 2009.
64. Bowry AD, Shrank WH, Lee JL, et al.: A systematic review of adherence to cardiovascular medications in resource-limited settings, *J Gen Intern Med* 26(12):1479–1491, 2011.
65. Chowdhury R, Khan H, Heydon E, et al.: Adherence to cardiovascular therapy: A meta-analysis of prevalence and clinical consequences, *Eur Heart J* 34(38):2940–2948, 2013.
66. Bitton A, Choudhry NK, Matlin OS, et al.: The impact of medication adherence on coronary artery disease costs and outcomes: A systematic review, *Am J Med* 126(4):e27–357.e7, 2013.
67. Kumbhani DJ, Fonarow GC, Cannon CP, et al.: Predictors of adherence to performance measures in patients with acute myocardial infarction, *Am J Med* 126(1):e9–74.e1, 2013.
68. De Jongh T, Gurol-Urganci I, Vodopivec-Jamsek V, et al.: Mobile phone messaging for facilitating self-management of long-term illnesses, *Cochrane Database Syst Rev*(12):CD007459, 2012.
69. Laba TL, Bleasel J, Brien JA, et al.: Strategies to improve adherence to medications for cardiovascular diseases in socioeconomically disadvantaged populations: A systematic review, *Int J Cardiol* 167(6):2430–2440, 2013.
70. Tajouri TH, Driver SL, Holmes Jr DR: 'Take as directed'—strategies to improve adherence to cardiac medication, *Nat Rev Cardiol* 11(5):304–307, 2014.
71. Viswanathan M, Golin CE, Jones CD, et al.: Interventions to improve adherence to self-administered medications for chronic diseases in the United States: A systematic review, *Ann Intern Med* 157(11):785–795, 2012.
72. Choudhry NK, Avorn J, Glynn RJ, et al.: Full coverage for preventive medications after myocardial infarction, *N Engl J Med* 365(22):2088–2097, 2011.
73. Thom S, Poulter N, Field J, et al.: Effects of a fixed-dose combination strategy on adherence and risk factors in patients with or at high risk of CVD: The UMPIRE randomized clinical trial, *JAMA* 310(9):918–929, 2013.
74. Sanz G, Fuster V: Fixed-dose combination therapy and secondary cardiovascular prevention: Rationale, selection of drugs and target population, *Nat Clin Pract Cardiovasc Med* 6(2):101–110, 2009.
75. Huffman MD, Yusuf S: Polypills: Essential medicines for cardiovascular disease secondary prevention? *J Am Coll Cardiol* 63(14):1368–1370, 2014.
76. Giovino GA, Mirza SA, Samet JM, et al.: Tobacco use in 3 billion individuals from 16 countries: An analysis of nationally representative cross-sectional household surveys, *Lancet* 380(9842): 668–679, 2012.
77. Jha P, Peto R: Global effects of smoking, of quitting, and of taxing tobacco, *N Engl J Med* 370(1):60–68, 2014.
78. Ng M, Freeman MK, Fleming TD, et al.: Smoking prevalence and cigarette consumption in 187 countries, 1980-2012, *JAMA* 311(2):183–192, 2014.
79. Ruger JP, Lazar CM: Economic evaluation of pharmaco- and behavioral therapies for smoking cessation: a critical and systematic review of empirical research, *Annu Rev Public Health* 33:279–305, 2012.
80. Jamison D, Breman J, Measham J, et al.: *Disease control priorities in developing countries*, ed 2 New York, Oxford University Press and The World Bank, 2006.
81. Higashi MH, Truong KD, Barendregt JJ, et al.: Cost effectiveness of tobacco control policies in Vietnam, *Appl Health Econ Health Policy* 9(3):183–196, 2011.
82. Callinan JE, Clarke A, Doherty K, Kelleher C: Legislative smoking bans for reducing secondhand smoke exposure, smoking prevalence and tobacco consumption, *Cochrane Database Syst Rev*(4): CD005992, 2010.
83. Moore D, Aveyard P, Connock M, et al.: Effectiveness and safety of nicotine replacement therapy assisted reduction to stop smoking: Systematic review and meta-analysis, *BMJ* 338:b1024, 2009.
84. Hughes JR, Stead LF, Hartmann-Boyce J, et al.: Antidepressants for smoking cessation, *Cochrane Database Syst Rev*(1):CD000031, 2014.
85. Huffman MD, Baldridge A, Bloomfield GS, et al.: Global cardiovascular research output, citations, and collaborations: A time-trend, bibliometric analysis (1999-2008), *PLoS One* 8(12):e83440, 2013.
86. Myers L, Mendis S: Cardiovascular disease research output in WHO priority areas between 2002 and 2011, *J Epidemiol Global Health* 4(1):23–28, 2014.
87. Suhrcke M, Boluarte TA, Niessen L: A systematic review of economic evaluations of interventions to tackle cardiovascular disease in low-and middle-income countries, *BMC Public Health* 12(1):2, 2012.
88. Bitton A, Gaziano TA: *The cost-effectiveness of selective tobacco control policies in South Africa*, Society of General Internal Medicine 34th Annual Meeting: Building 21st Century Medicine Through Education, Research, Policy and Practice, Phoenix, Ariz, 2011, pp 353–354.

3 New and Emerging Insights into the Pathobiology of Acute Myocardial Infarction

Erling Falk and Jacob F. Bentzon

INTRODUCTION

Atherosclerosis is a lipoprotein-driven chronic inflammatory disease of arteries that leads to the accumulation of fibrotic, necrotic, and calcified tissue in the arterial intima, which is described as an atherosclerotic lesion or plaque. These plaques cause clinical disease by luminal narrowing or sudden precipitation of arterial thrombi that obstruct blood flow to the heart (coronary heart disease [CHD]), brain (ischemic stroke), or legs (peripheral artery disease [PAD]). The most common of these manifestations is CHD, such as stable angina pectoris and the acute coronary syndromes (ACS), including acute myocardial infarction (MI) (see Chapter 2).

Figure 3-1 shows a case example of ACS in a previously healthy 58-year-old man who suddenly developed chest pain and soon thereafter a lethal arrhythmia. The autopsy revealed an acute thrombus precipitated by an atherosclerotic lesion that had otherwise developed quietly, probably for many decades preceding the event. Each such fatal case is a missed opportunity. If the protagonist had known that the disease would lead to fatal complications, there would have been ways of retarding its development by lifestyle adjustments and preventive drug therapy (see Chapter 34). The key mechanisms underlying the development of atherosclerosis are currently known, and most clinical events should, in principle, be preventable if this knowledge is translated into effective preventive measures.

This chapter offers an introduction to the causes and central disease mechanisms of atherosclerosis, and describes what we know and have yet to learn about why some plaques suddenly precipitate life-threatening thrombosis. Furthermore, we discuss the terms plaque burden, activity, and vulnerability, which are commonly used to characterize the state and expected fate of individual lesions or patients. The pathobiology of myocardial injury, healing, and remodeling are discussed in Chapter 4 and Chapter 36.

MULTIFACTORIAL CAUSES

An increased blood concentration of apolipoprotein B (apo B)–containing lipoproteins, of which low-density lipoproteins (LDLs) is usually the most prevalent form, is necessary for atherosclerosis to develop, but many other factors can facilitate the development of atherosclerosis and MI (see Chapter 2).[1–5] None of these other risk factors alone are sufficient to cause atherosclerosis, but because most individuals in modern societies have LDL levels that are permissive for development of atherosclerosis, the presence of other risk factors explains much of the occurrence of the disease. The central disease mechanisms discussed in the following sections are assumed to be the same, irrespective of the set of causal factors in a particular patient, but the presence of individual risk factors influences the course of the disease and the mode of presentation. For example, cigarette smoking predisposes to thrombotic complications and increases the risk more for MI than for stable angina,[6] hypertension is an exceptionally powerful risk factor for stroke,[7] and smoking and diabetes account for most of the risk of developing lower extremity PAD.[8]

MECHANISMS OF PLAQUE FORMATION

The mechanisms leading to atherosclerotic plaque development are complex, involving lipoprotein retention, inflammatory cell recruitment, foam cell formation, apoptosis and necrosis, smooth muscle cell (SMC) proliferation and matrix synthesis, calcification, angiogenesis, arterial remodeling, fibrous cap rupture, thrombosis, and more (Animation 3-1).[9] Some of these are necessary steps in lesion progression (e.g., lipoprotein retention and vascular inflammation) and represent already exploited or potential targets for medical therapies. Other processes may be innocent bystanders (e.g., plaque calcification); although these are useful as a characteristic feature to identify atherosclerosis by imaging, they do not appear to be centrally involved in the genesis of

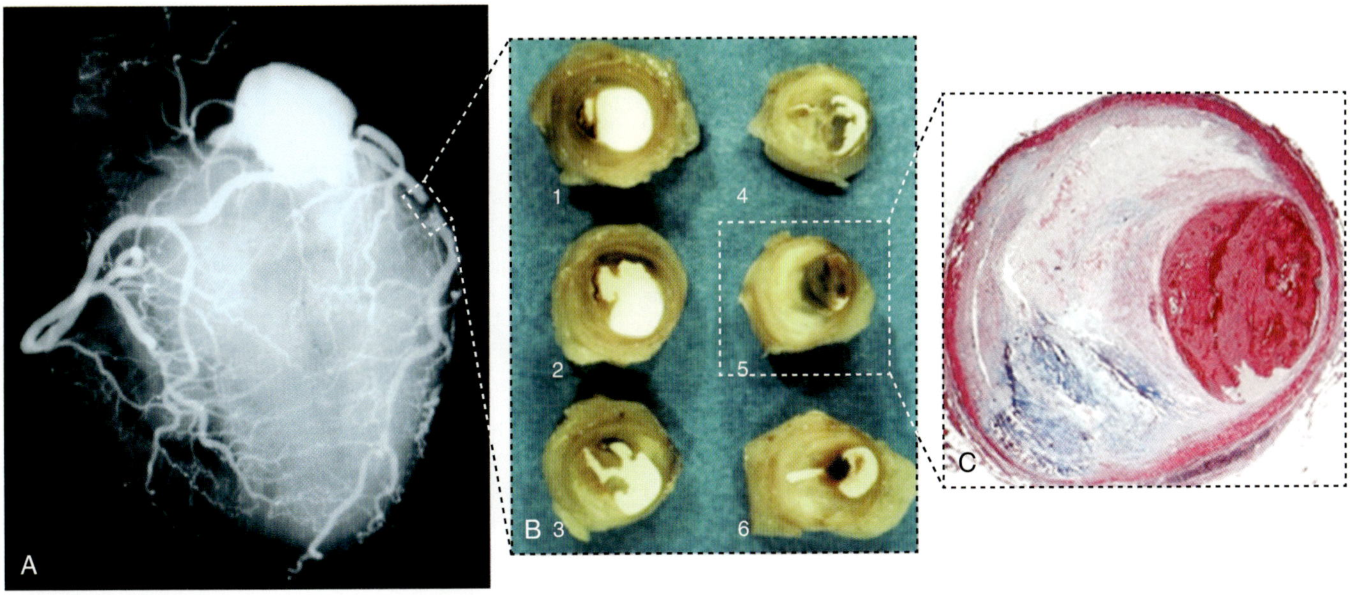

FIGURE 3-1 A fatal case of atherothrombosis. (**A**) A postmortem coronary angiogram shows a filling defect in the proximal left anterior descending artery. (**B**) Consecutive cross sections of the affected region of the left anterior descending artery reveal massive atherosclerotic plaques with macroscopically visible rupturing and a near-occluding thrombus. (**C**) The thrombus and the underlying plaque in a histological section. Elastin-trichrome stain.

lesions or their clinical complications. The combination of fat deposition and necrosis that lead to soft necrotic cores (*atheré*: gruel or porridge [Greek]) and that of calcification and fibrosis that lead to hard tissue components (*scleros*: hard [Greek]), distinguish atherosclerosis from other arteriosclerotic diseases, such as media sclerosis and arteriolosclerosis, and gave the disease its name.

It is important to realize that major parts of our understanding of the initiation and progression of atherosclerosis are deduced from studies in animal models. Experiments are necessary to demonstrate causal mechanisms, and although some experiments can be performed in humans or substituted by Mendelian randomization studies of randomly segregating gene variants,[10] most are referred to exploration in animal models. Animals do not spontaneously develop atherosclerosis, but the disease can be induced in most species by increasing the level of LDL or other apo B–containing lipoproteins by feeding atherogenic diets or by genetic modification. Mouse models in particular have been essential because of the efficiency by which gene function can be probed in the living organism through genetic modification. Today our understanding of atherosclerotic lesion development in the mouse clearly surpasses similar insight into any other organism.

Knowledge of the disease in animal models is an important steppingstone for insight into human atherosclerosis, because the overall architecture of the disease processes is likely to be the same. However, it would be bold to assume that the molecular mechanisms are identical, and perhaps even more unlikely to think that the rate-limiting processes, and thus, the best targets for drug treatment, are conserved. Furthermore, because current models only feature some aspects of atherosclerosis, our mechanistic knowledge has important blind spots. There is in-depth knowledge of how LDL causes atherosclerotic lesion formation, but considerably less is known about the paths by which such lesions cause clinical disease through thrombosis or luminal narrowing, simply because this progression does not occur reproducibly in animals. Moreover, mechanistic insight into the effects of other causal factors, such as hypertension and diabetes, remains rudimentary.

Lesion Classification

Atherosclerosis is a progressive disease that begins early in life, but the speed of progression is highly dependent on vascular localization and varies markedly among different individuals. Even under the most facilitating conditions, it usually takes several decades to develop symptomatic lesions. The abdominal aorta, coronary arteries, ilio-femoral arteries, and carotid bifurcations are typically the most heavily affected.

By examining the same vascular sites in decedents of different age groups, pathologists have inferred a sequence of lesion development and have suggested criteria to classify lesions into types based on morphological criteria. Two classification schemes are commonly used. The American Heart Association (AHA) classification (types I to VIII) is based on a detailed microscopic analysis of human atherosclerosis at different stages of development and lends itself particularly well to studies that focus on the initiation and progression of lesions.[11] A modified version, which is more direct in describing the link between lesion morphology and clinical complications, was later introduced by Virmani and colleagues (Figure 3-2).[12] A single patient with advanced disease will harbor many of these different lesion types across the vascular bed, reflecting the variability in the time of initiation, speed, and course of lesion development at different sites of the vasculature.

Lipoprotein Retention

LDL causes atherosclerosis by accumulating in the arterial intima. This accumulation does not occur uniformly throughout the vasculature, but is initially restricted to predilection sites near branch points and along inner curvatures. In these regions, the flow of blood exerts low or oscillatory shear stress on the endothelium, and these are further characterized by changes in endothelial turnover

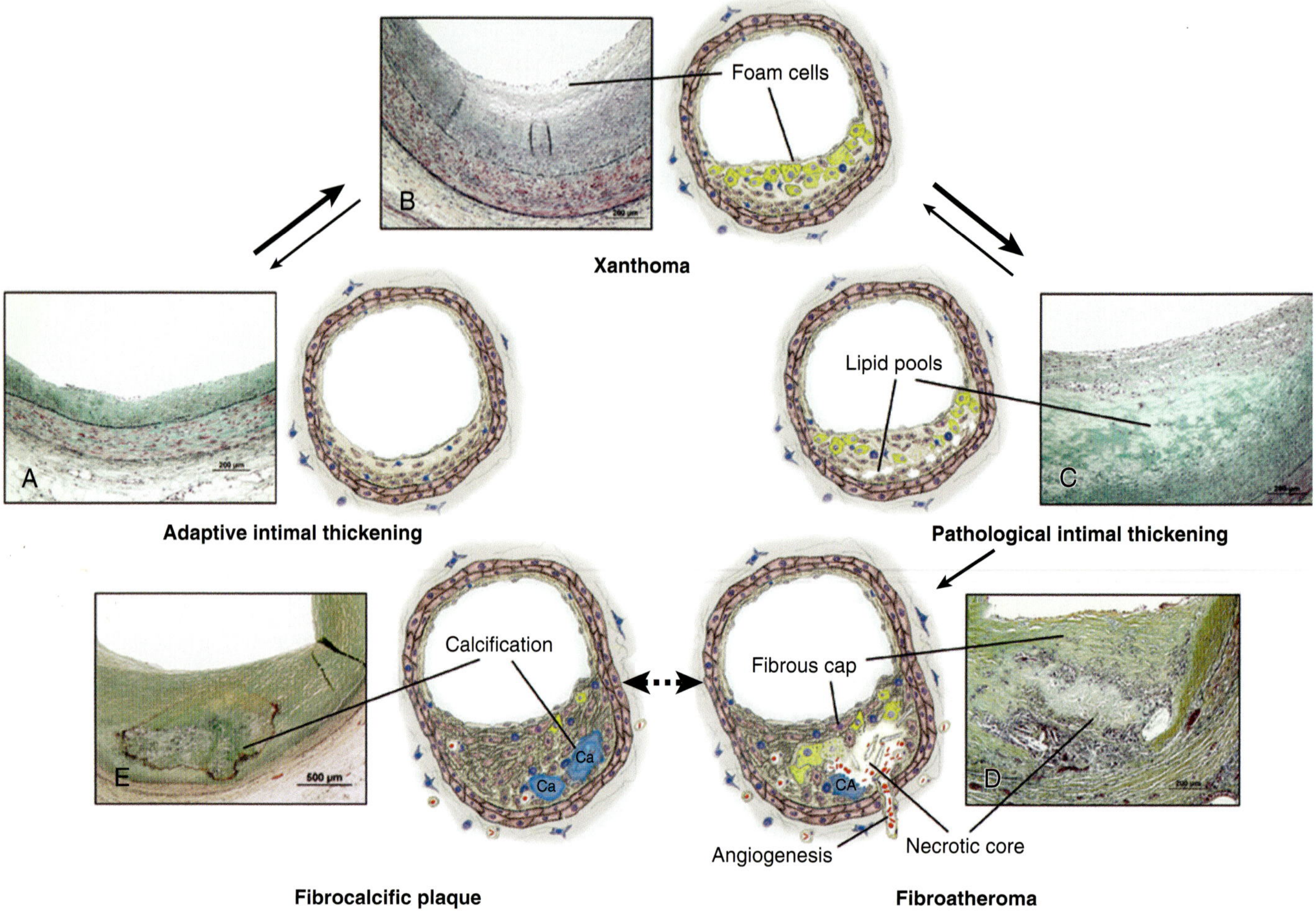

FIGURE 3-2 Lesion types of atherosclerosis and a proposed sequence of their development. (**A**) Adaptive intimal thickening characterized by smooth muscle cell accumulation within the intima. (**B**) Intimal xanthoma corresponding to the accumulation of foam cell macrophages within the intima. (**C**) Pathologic intimal thickening denotes the accumulation of extracellular lipid pools in the absence of apparent necrosis. (**D**) Fibroatheroma indicating the presence of a necrotic core. The necrotic core and surrounding tissue may eventually be calcified, which forms the fibrocalcific plaque shown in (**E**). Because some of the advanced lesion types (fibroatheromas and fibrocalcific plaques) evolve simultaneously in life, their interrelationships are difficult to resolve in autopsy studies. Movat pentachrome stain. *Ca*, Calcium. *(From Bentzon J, et al: Mechanisms of plaque formation and rupture.* Circ Res *114:1852, 2014.)*

and gene expression, presence of subendothelial dendritic cells, and in humans, by the development of adaptive intimal thickening in the first months of life (see Figure 3-2A). Intimal thickenings may grow to be as thick as the underlying media, consisting of a subendothelial proteoglycan-rich layer and a deeper musculo-elastic layer with SMCs and elastic fibers. It is tempting to speculate that these specialized areas of the vasculature serve physiological roles in vascular homeostasis or host defense in the normal body,[13] but in the presence of supraphysiological levels of circulating LDL, they become the hotbed for atherogenesis. They are affected early during atherogenesis, and the rate of progression is higher here than at other arterial sites. With time, the disease spreads to the adjacent intima, and in older adult patients dying from MI, the epicardial coronary arteries are often "diffusively" affected by confluent plaques.

The ability of adaptive intimal thickenings to bind and retain insudating LDL particles from the blood may at least partly explain the propensity of these sites for the development of atherosclerosis. Studies in mice have revealed that local binding of LDL particles to proteoglycans is an important step in disease initiation, and extracellular lipid droplets in the proteoglycan-rich layer of adaptive intimal thickenings is the first microscopic sign of lesion development in children and young adults.[14] As the disease evolves, the endothelium becomes more leaky, and the expression of bridging molecules (e.g., lipoprotein lipase) and proteoglycans with longer side chains promote the ability of the lesion to sequester LDL from the blood.[14] This construct predicts that a higher LDL level is needed to induce the disease than to maintain and progress it once lesions have formed, and interestingly, is consistent with the strong relationship between LDL levels in young adulthood and the risk of developing CHD later in life.[15]

Inflammation

LDL retained in the arterial intima is subject to oxidation and other types of modification, and thereby, acquires molecular epitopes (danger-associated molecular patterns) that are identical to or mimic epitopes on microbes and cell debris. These molecular epitopes are recognized by membrane-bound and cytoplasmic pattern recognition receptors and natural antibodies of the innate immune system.[16] Adaptive immunity also reacts to modified LDL and mounts a multifaceted immune response.[17] The endless supply of LDL from the blood and the formation of modified LDL in the intima provide a persistent proinflammatory stimulus that leads to chronic nonresolving inflammation in the vascular wall. Initially, endothelial cells and SMCs are induced to express adhesion molecules, chemoattractants, and growth factors that interact with receptors on monocytes and stimulate their homing, migration, and differentiation into macrophages and dendritic cells.[18]

Foam Cells

In the intima, the recruited cells take up modified LDL through scavenger receptors and possibly by other mechanisms as well.[19] This process clears modified LDL from the extracellular space, but leads to foam cell formation, with massive accumulation of cholesterol and cholesteryl ester droplets in the cytoplasm. Local SMCs also accumulate intracellular fat droplets, possibly by similar mechanisms.[20,21]

Foam cell formation may itself be accompanied by proinflammatory activation, mediated by intracellular cholesterol crystals activating the NLRP3 inflammasome,[22] but recruited macrophages may also be activated in a proinflammatory M1 direction by the binding of modified LDL to toll-like receptors. The activated cells in turn secrete proinflammatory cytokines (e.g., interleukin [IL] 1-β and tumor necrosis factor-α [TNF-α]), reactive oxygen species and enzymes that promote further retention and modification of LDL (e.g., myeloperoxidase), and many other mediators that have been shown to play a role in atherosclerosis (e.g., plasminogen activators, cathepsins, and matrix-metalloproteinases).[18] Other macrophages in the intima are polarized in an anti-inflammatory M2 direction and secrete proteins and small molecules (e.g., transforming growth factor-β and proresolving lipids) that favor resolution of inflammation.[18,23]

T-helper 1 cells reacting toward modified LDL and other autoantigens related to the atherosclerotic process appear in the human intima coincident with the first foam cells, and they secrete proinflammatory cytokines (e.g., interferon-γ) that accentuate vascular inflammation in mouse models.[16] However, other immune cell types, such as regulatory T cells and possibly B cells, may ameliorate it. In human, but not murine, lesions, cytotoxic T cells are abundant, albeit of unknown functional consequence to plaque development.[24]

The description of the inflammatory response to modified LDL has become increasingly more complex with the recognition of multiple macrophage polarization phenotypes and T-cell subtypes, some with proinflammatory and some with anti-inflammatory activities. Importantly, as well as soothing to anyone trying to keep pace with the field, drastic LDL lowering has the potential to quickly resolve the inflammation. In atherosclerotic mice and rabbits that are reversed to normal LDL levels, plaque macrophages quickly reduce in number.[25,26]

Fatty Streaks

Accumulating macrophage foam cells, which are easily recognized using a microscope, are telltales of lipoprotein-driven inflammation that occurs in the vascular wall. Foam cells initially accrue in the luminal, proteoglycan-rich layer of the intima, and when several layers have formed, they are visible to the unaided eye on the intimal surface as yellow-colored xanthomas or fatty streaks (see Figure 3-2B). Xanthomas are harmless, and they are fully reversible. They are present in some infants in the first 6 months of life, probably reflecting the risk factors of the mother, but their number declines in subsequent years. At adolescence, they reappear in atherosclerosis-prone regions of the coronary arteries and the aorta in most people.

Necrosis

Many xanthomas do not progress further, but some, especially among those developing in adaptive intimal thickenings, develop necrotic foci with accumulation of acellular, lipid-rich material. Such lesions are collectively known as progressive atherosclerotic lesions and are further subdivided into pathological intimal thickening and fibroatheromas depending on the extent of necrosis. In pathological intimal thickening, only smaller lipid pools are present in the musculo-elastic layer beneath the layers of foam cells without gross disruption of the normal structure of the intima (see Figure 3-2C). Such changes are commonly seen at 20 to 30 years of age in atherosclerosis-prone regions of the coronary arteries. In some lesions, the isolated lipid pools grow into confluent necrotic cores (also known as lipid cores), and large areas of the original intima are destroyed, probably by invading macrophages. Morphologically, this process can be characterized as being in an early or late stage of necrosis, with the former showing some presence of the original intimal matrix with macrophage infiltration, whereas in the latter, only a matrix-devoid, acellular gruel of lipids (cholesteryl esters, free cholesterol, phospholipids, and triglycerides) and cell debris are seen.[9] When one or more necrotic cores are present, the lesion is a fibroatheroma (see Figure 3-2D).

Death of SMCs and infiltrating macrophages are believed to be the main mechanism responsible for lipid pools and necrotic cores.[27,28] Apoptotic SMCs and macrophages become detectable co-incident with the occurrence of acellular regions in human lesions, and cell death, both apoptotic and other forms, can be seen at the margin of the necrotic core. Many factors able to induce apoptosis in vitro are present in plaques (e.g., endoplasmic reticulum stress and oxidized lipids from modified LDL), and it is reasonable to assume that several of these cooperate to cause apoptosis in vivo.[28,29] The presence of free apoptotic remnants in the tissue (i.e., not associated with phagocytic cells) indicates that impaired removal of apoptotic remnants (efferocytosis) contribute to the growth of the necrotic core.[30] Instead of being phagocytosed by neighboring cells, remnants are left to undergo secondary necrosis, and the lipid-rich and proinflammatory cargo is consequently deposited in tissue.

The chemical composition of the necrotic core indicates that other sources of lipid may be important co-contributors, including direct accumulation of cholesteryl esters from insudating LDL and free cholesterol–rich erythrocyte membranes that are derived from intraplaque hemorrhages.[31]

Necrosis of lesions is a critical part of lesion development, because it predisposes to clinical events. In its absence, the development of atherosclerosis would be a much less dangerous disease. Why necrosis occurs in some, but not other lesions, is not well understood, and apparently, the causal factors are at least partly dissociated from those that cause the initial xanthoma. For example, men and women develop similar amounts of coronary xanthomas early in life, but adult men have more lesions with lipid pools and necrotic cores than women of similar age.[9]

Plaque Angiogenesis and Intraplaque Hemorrhage

The center of many atherosclerotic lesions become hypoxic, and cells respond by expressing hypoxia-inducible factor-1α (HIF-1α) and vascular endothelial growth factor, thereby providing a stimulus for the recruitment of neovessels into the base of progressive atherosclerotic lesions.[32,33] The new vessels originate mainly from the adventitial vasa vasorum, and they are fragile and leaky, without supporting mural cells, giving rise to local extravasation of plasma proteins and erythrocytes, as well as providing an entry path for immune cells.[34] Intraplaque bleeding from neovessels is common in fibroatheromas and may expand the necrotic core and promote inflammation.[31] Another common source of plaque hemorrhage is extravasation of blood through a ruptured fibrous cap.

Lysis of red blood cells leads to spilling of free hemoglobin and heme moieties into tissues. Both components are oxidative and proinflammatory, and efficient defense systems have evolved to neutralize them.[35] Free hemoglobulin is bound by haptoglobin, and the complex is internalized through CD163 in macrophages, whereas heme is bound by hemopexin and scavenged through the LDL receptor–related protein 1 (LRP1) in a variety of cell types.[36] Inside cells, toxic heme is degraded by heme oxygenase-1, which leads to release of bilirubin and deposition of iron in the form of ferritin.

Histology shows that defense systems are in place to counteract the effects of intraplaque hemorrhage. Macrophages at sites of hemorrhage are polarized to a hemoglobin-scavenging type characterized by expression of CD163 and heme oxygenase-1.[37,38] These cells lack typical markers of proinflammatory M1 macrophages (TNF-α and inducible nitric oxide synthase) and express the mannose receptor typical of M2-like macrophage differentiation, suggesting that they may dampen the proinflammatory effects of the hemorrhage. Lesions, especially fibroatheromas, also often contain abundant cellular ferritin.

The finding of associations between haptoglobin variants and cardiovascular disease supports the importance of an efficient defense against free hemoglobin in the atherosclerotic plaque. The human haptoglobin gene has a common polymorphism, which consists of an intragenic duplication of two exons. In addition to Hp1.1, which resembles haptoglobin in other mammals, it gives rise to larger multimeric haptoglobin variants, Hp2.1 and Hp2.2, which differ in their ability to neutralize hemoglobin, especially when hemoglobin is glycosylated.[39] Several studies, although not all, have indicated that the cardiovascular risk in general, and the inflammatory response to intraplaque hemorrhage in particular, is accentuated in patients with diabetes who express the Hp2.2 variant.[39,40]

Fibrosis

The connective tissue of lesions is initially that of the normal arterial intima or adaptive intimal thickening, but gradually this loose fibrocellular tissue is replaced and expanded by collagen-rich fibrous tissue, which often grows to become the quantitatively dominant component of plaques. Pieces of tissue that lie between a necrotic core and the surface of the plaque are called fibrous caps (see Figure 3-2).

The collagen, elastin, and proteoglycans of the fibrous matrix are mainly produced by SMCs, and the secretory function of lesional SMCs is reflected by their ultrastructural phenotype, characterized by an abundant rough endoplasmic reticulum and Golgi complex, and only sparse myofilaments. This phenotype has been termed synthetic in contrast to the contractile phenotype of medial SMCs. Few synthetic SMCs are present in the normal intima, but they increase substantially in number during lesion development, probably both by local proliferation and by migration of medial SMCs that subsequently undergo phenotypic modulation to the synthetic phenotype.[41] Notably, the number of SMCs in plaques at all stages may be grossly underestimated because many synthetic SMCs do not contain detectable levels of the contractile proteins routinely used to recognize SMCs in tissue sections (e.g., smooth muscle alpha-actin [SMαA]).[42,43]

Classical studies of X chromosome inactivation patterns found plaque SMCs to be arranged in large clonal populations, but these studies could not decide whether the precursor of these clones were patches of vessel wall with a single embryological cell origin, from which multiple SMCs migrated into lesions, or whether the atherosclerosis involved massive clonal expansion of a few SMCs. However, genetic tagging studies in the mouse indicate the last explanation is correct; SMCs undergo massive expansion during atherosclerotic lesion development.[21] Marked cell proliferation may explain why plaque SMCs have shortened telomeres and express multiple other markers of senescence,[44] and why the fibrous tissue eventually loses most of the SMCs that produce it, leaving behind large areas of hypocellular fibrosis.

Many plaques at autopsy consist exclusively of fibrous and sometimes calcified tissue without extracellular lipid pools or a necrotic core. The genesis of these fibrocalcific plaques is not fully understood (see Figure 3-2E). Some pathologists believe that the development of a necrotic core is the prerequisite of fibrosis, and sequential sectioning often reveals that a necrotic core is present in the upstream or downstream vicinity of the section with fibrocalcific plaque. Where this is not the case, an originally formed core may have calcified or disappeared because of local quiescence of the atherosclerotic process or through silent plaque rupture with extrusion of the core (see the section on Mechanisms of Plaque Rupture).

Calcification

Calcification is a characteristic feature of progressive atherosclerotic lesions and increases steadily with age. Microscopic hydroxyapatite granules are initially seen, especially in the basal parts of lesions within lipid pools and at the rim of developing necrotic cores.[45] Matrix vesicles, apoptotic cell bodies, and cell debris from dying SMCs and macrophages in these areas appear to act as nidi for the initial calcium precipitation in a process resembling dystrophic calcification of other soft tissues undergoing injury. The dense calcifications that develop later mostly have an underlying acellular fibrous matrix without any signs of a necrotic core, inflammation, or angiogenesis.

Active cell-mediated processes akin to bone formation have been suggested to be involved in plaque calcification,

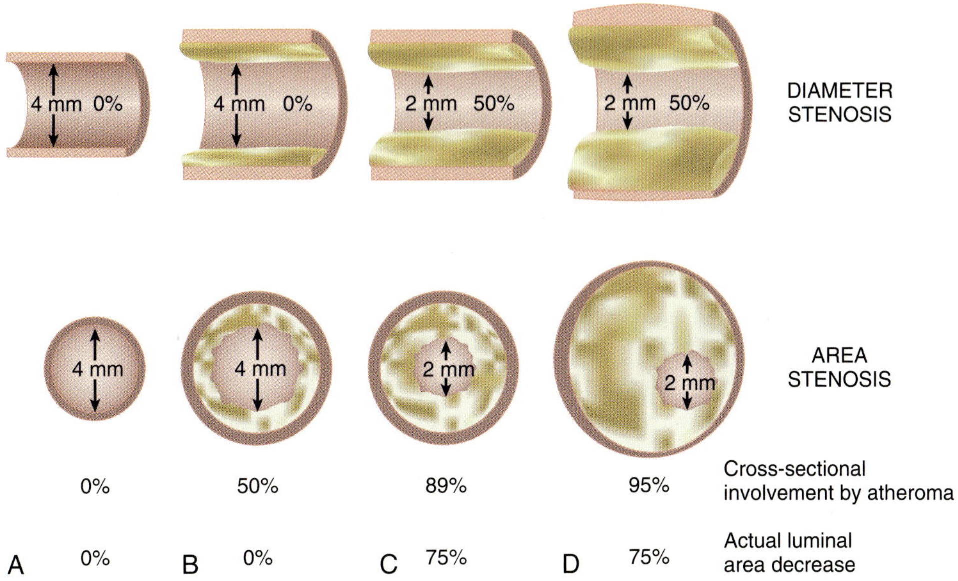

FIGURE 3-3 Angiographic and cross-sectional evaluations of the arterial lumen. *Top row*, Angiographic views. The examples (**A** to **D**) illustrate how angiography cannot be used to determine the presence or size of atherosclerotic plaques because of arterial remodeling. *Bottom row*, Cross-sectional views. The same segments seen under the microscope illustrating how the lumen stenosis cannot be determined because of arterial remodeling. A less than 50% angiographic stenosis may look severely obstructed. *(Redrawn from Fishbein MC, Siegel RJ: How big are coronary atherosclerotic plaques that rupture?* Circulation *94:2662, 1996.)*

but the structure of the initial calcification granulae is different from that of bone.[46] However, cell-mediated processes may be involved in the subsequent conversion of the microgranulae to larger lumps and plates of calcium deposits, and osseous metaplasia are occasionally seen in lesions that are heavily calcified, sometimes including bone marrow.[45] Interestingly, some studies suggest that statins promote coronary artery calcification.[47]

Arterial Remodeling

During atherosclerotic lesion formation, the local vessel segment may either expand and thereby preserve or even increase the lumen (expansive remodeling) or shrink to diminish it (constrictive remodeling). Expansive remodeling is the general rule and explains why so few, even large, plaques cause severe stenosis. It may partly be a homeostatic response of the nondiseased vessel wall at sites of eccentric plaque formation to maintain normal shear stress. However, increasing evidence suggests that it is predominantly a pathophysiologic process in which proteolytic enzymes secreted by plaque macrophages cause the underlying media to thin and yield. This hypothesis is supported by the observation that plaque growth is frequently followed by a paradoxical increase in lumen area, and the fact that the direction and extent of remodeling is associated with the composition of the local plaque. Expansive remodeling is more often seen with fibroatheromas, and the extent of enlargement is positively correlated to plaque inflammation, medial atrophy, and the size of the necrotic core.[9] The mechanisms underlying constrictive remodeling are not well understood, but it mostly occurs with fibrocalcific plaques and may be related to scar-like contraction of SMCs during plaque healing (see the section on Healed Plaques and Incorporated Thrombi). Interestingly, expansive remodeling may be reduced in patients with diabetes.[48] The association between remodeling and atherosclerosis is a two-way process. As plaques develop and the arterial wall remodels as a result, local flow patterns change, and in turn, may influence the progression of the disease and ultimately the fate of lesions.[49]

Because of remodeling, angiography is not useful for diagnosing the presence of atherosclerotic plaque or measuring changes in atherosclerotic plaque size with medical intervention (see Chapter 10). Similarly, single histological sections examined at autopsy cannot be used to make inferences about stenosis severity. As depicted in Figure 3-3, the use of the term stenosis or histological stenosis in the pathology literature has little to do with the obstruction to blood flow.

CLINICAL MANIFESTATIONS OF ATHEROSCLEROSIS

Most people in industrialized societies die with progressive atherosclerotic lesions, but only a minority die because of them. The mechanisms discussed so far in this chapter are often without clinical consequences and the developed lesions asymptomatic throughout life; however, some lesions end up being obstructive to blood flow, and a few elicit life-threatening thrombotic complications.

Severe stenosis, which may present as stable angina, is often caused by a fibroatheroma or a fibrous plaque. The plaque may be substantially calcified, and the local vessel segment is often negatively remodeled, but the relationship between plaque morphology, arterial remodeling, and stenosis formation is not consistent. The obstruction is rarely fatal, except in cases in which scarring of the myocardium may predispose to lethal arrhythmia. MI and other types of ACS are predominantly caused by a luminal thrombus imposed on an atherosclerotic plaque.[31] Other rare causes of MI are emboli, artery dissection, tunnel coronary arteries, vasculitis, cocaine abuse, or trauma.[50]

Plaque rupture is the most frequent mechanism precipitating thrombosis (see Animation 3-1). In plaque rupture, a structural defect (i.e., a gap) in the fibrous cap of a fibroatheroma exposes the highly thrombogenic core to the blood (Figures 3-4 and 3-5). Necrotic core material is

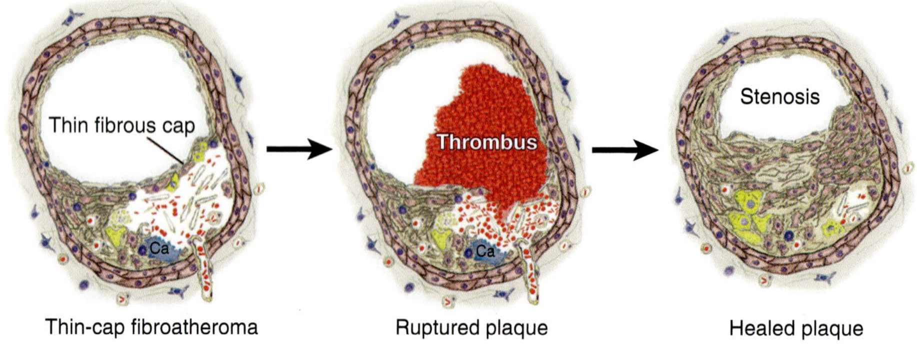

FIGURE 3-4 Plaque rupture. Rupture of a thin-cap fibroatheroma with nonfatal thrombus and subsequent healing with fibrous tissue formation and constrictive remodeling. *(From Bentzon J, et al: Mechanisms of plaque formation and rupture.* Circ Res *114:1852, 2014.)*

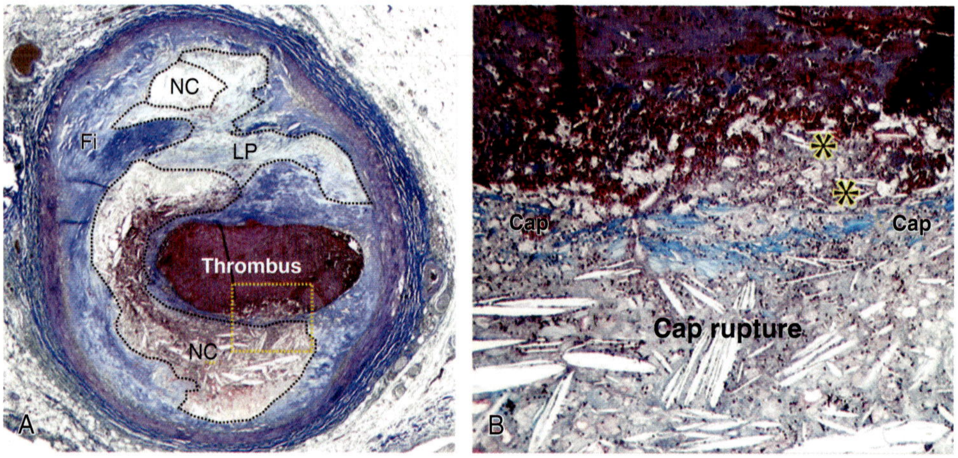

FIGURE 3-5 Thrombosis caused by plaque rupture. (**A**) The culprit plaque is a fibroatheroma consisting of large amounts of hypocellular fibrous tissue (Fi), areas dominated by extracellular lipid pools (LP), and fully developed necrotic cores (NC). The lumen is occluded by thrombus. (**B**) Larger magnification of the inset in (**A**). The thin fibrous cap covering the large NC has ruptured, and the core material, including cholesterol crystals (*asterisk*), has been propelled into the lumen where it can be found at the base of the thrombus. Elastin-trichrome stain (collagen: *blue*). *(From Bentzon J, et al: Mechanisms of plaque formation and rupture.* Circ Res *114:1852, 2014.)*

sometimes found expelled from the plaque and embedded in the thrombus, indicating that the rupture and thrombosis coincided, which supports the cause-and-effect relationship. Plaque rupture is a well-defined term, whereas other terms, such as plaque disruption and fissuring, are used ambiguously in the literature.[31]

In rare cases, nodular calcifications (calcified nodules) are found protruding into the lumen through a ruptured "fibrous cap." Although controversial, such protruding calcified nodules have been suggested as a separate precipitating mechanism of thrombosis.[12,31] When no plaque rupture can be identified despite a thorough microscopic search throughout the thrombosed vascular segment, the term plaque erosion is used (Figure 3-6). This term was chosen because the endothelium is typically missing beneath the thrombus, but whether it vanished before or after thrombosis is unknown. Both pathological intimal thickening and fibroatheromas may be complicated by plaque erosion.

A compilation of autopsy data totaling 1847 cases from around the world showed that most fatal coronary thrombi are associated with plaque rupture regardless of the clinical presentation (MI: 79%; sudden coronary death: 65%), age (older than 60 years: 77%; younger than 60 years: 64%; unknown: 73%), sex (men: 76%; women: 55%), and continent (Europe: 72%; United States: 68%;

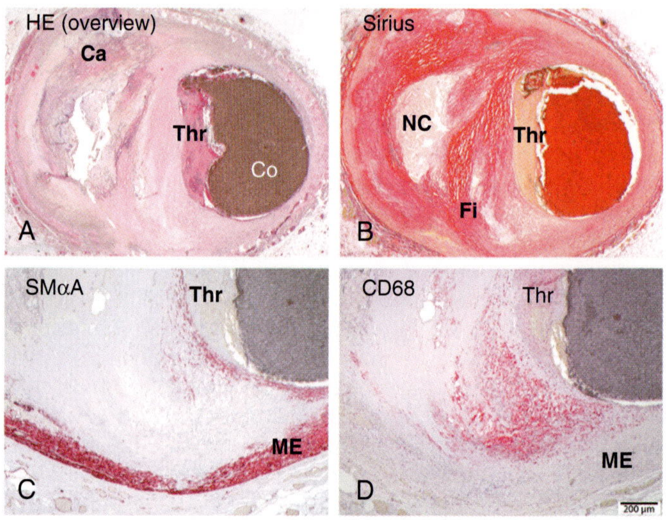

FIGURE 3-6 Thrombosis not caused by plaque rupture: plaque erosion. (**A** and **B**) The culprit plaque is a fibroatheroma consisting of fibrous tissue (Fi), calcification (Ca), and a small necrotic core (NC) recognized by its complete lack of supporting collagen on Sirius-stained sections (collagen: *red*). Mural thrombosis (Thr) has formed over an intact thick fibrous cap. Contrast (Co) in the residual lumen. (**C**) Staining for the contractile protein SMαA (smooth muscle cells, *red*) reveals their preferential location near the endothelium. (**D**) Staining for the CD68 receptor (macrophages; *red*) reveals ongoing inflammation in the shoulder region of the lesion. *HE*, Hematoxylin and eosin; *ME*, media.

Asia 81%).[31] The age and sex difference is interesting, and rupture has been found to be a particularly infrequent mechanism behind the few fatal thrombi occurring in premenopausal women. This difference in pathology might reflect the protective effect of female gender on atherosclerosis development and the fact that erosion occurs on earlier types of lesions, including pathological intimal thickening, more commonly than does plaque rupture for which fibroatheromas are the only substrate. Whether this point can be extended to other low-risk populations is unknown. Some studies have reported that diabetes, smoking, and the level of hyperlipidemia are associated with the mechanism of thrombosis in MI, but no consistent relationships, except for gender and menopause, have been demonstrated.[31]

Autopsy data may not be representative of MI cases in general, because autopsies are only performed in the dead and mostly in cases in which death was unexpected. With the development of intravascular optical coherence tomography catheters, which have the ability to visualize the luminal parts of coronary lesions at high resolution, it is now possible to detect plaque rupture in the living (see Chapter 10). Such studies have shown that plaque rupture is also the main cause of thrombosis in survivors, with the highest proportion found among those presenting with ST-elevation MI.[51]

Mechanisms of Plaque Rupture

Plaque rupture occurs where the cap is thinnest and most infiltrated by macrophages and macrophage foam cells; in eccentric plaques, the weakest spot is often the cap margin or "shoulder region." Only extremely thin fibrous caps are at risk of rupturing. As assessed by microscopic examination, the average thickness of ruptured caps in the coronary arteries is only 23 μm (the diameter of only one foam cell), and 95% of ruptured fibrous caps are less than 65 μm. Based on these observations, Virmani and colleagues introduced the term thin-cap fibroatheromas (TCFAs) for coronary fibroatheromas with a fibrous cap thickness of less than 65 μm.[12] By introducing this category, most lesions that are not TCFAs can be classified as unlikely candidates for producing plaque rupture in the near future.

Thin-Cap Fibroatheroma

Conceptually, the development of TCFAs and their subsequent rupture might best be understood as an expansion of the necrotic core until it reaches the surface, and like early necrotic core formation, the degradation of the fibrous cap is characterized by cell death and macrophage infiltration. Ruptured caps contain fewer SMCs and less collagen than intact caps, and SMCs are usually absent at the actual site of rupture. At the same time, proteolytic enzymes, such as plasminogen activators, cathepsins, and matrix metalloproteinases, secreted from infiltrating macrophages destroy the collagen-rich cap matrix.[25,28] Although the macrophage density in ruptured caps is usually high, whole-plaque macrophage density rarely exceeds a few percent because ruptured caps are tiny, and thus, it is a misconception that ruptured plaques are always highly inflamed. Whether degradation of the fibrous cap takes decades to evolve or is much more dynamic is not known. However, the fact that fibroatheromas are commonly seen at 30 years of age, a time at which MI is exceedingly rare, seems to indicate that it is a slow, smoldering process.

Rupture of a thin cap and subsequent thrombosis may occur spontaneously, but in some cases a temporary increase in emotional or physical stress provides the final triggering of the event. Recognized triggers include physical and sexual activity, anger, anxiety, work stress, earthquakes, war and terror attacks, temperature changes, infections, and cocaine use. Also simple daily activities or the circadian rhythm of biological pathways may determine the onset of MI, which is most frequent in the morning. The triggering pathways may include activation of the sympathetic nervous system with increased heart rate and blood pressure leading to plaque rupture, or increased coagulability and platelet reactivity leading to an accentuated thrombotic response on already ruptured plaques.[9,52] It is important to note that although triggers temporarily increase the relative risk of MI in susceptible individuals, the impact on absolute risk is extremely small because the exposure is transient and uncommon.[52] Furthermore, it is likely that many coronary events that are not precipitated by a trigger would have occurred in the absence of triggers within a few weeks.[9]

Mechanisms of Plaque Erosion

The mechanism(s) leading to thrombus without rupture is one of the most important unresolved questions within atherosclerosis research. The surface endothelium under the thrombus is usually missing, but no distinct morphological features of the underlying plaque have been identified, and why endothelium is lost and thrombosis precipitated remains elusive. Eroded plaques in cases of sudden death are often scarcely calcified, are rarely associated with expansive remodeling, and are less inflamed than ruptured plaques. In addition, the part of the lesion in close proximity to the thrombus is often rich in SMCs, versican, hyaluronan, and type III collagen.[12,53] However, others have reported focused inflammation immediately beneath the superimposed thrombus in fatal MI.[31] The age of the thrombus and the possibility of thrombosis-induced inflammation could potentially explain some of these differences, but it is also possible that erosion does not represent a single, but several different, mechanisms that lead to thrombosis.

Vasospasm has been suggested as the cause of the endothelial damage, and erosions are typically seen with lesions that show a well-developed media with contractile SMCs, which differs from other lesion types, including ruptured lesions where the underlying media is thin and disorganized. Furthermore, the high hyaluronan content may render endothelial cells susceptible to apoptosis, and together with recruited neutrophils and neutrophil extracellular trap formation, may drive endothelial desquamation.[54]

Morphology identical to that of plaque erosion can often be found in sections up- or downstream of plaque rupture with a fatal superimposed thrombus,[12] and it is possible that some of the mechanisms leading to thrombus with plaque erosion can help stabilize and accentuate thrombus formation after rupture. Autopsy studies indicate that only a minority of ruptures lead to clinical symptoms, whereas the others heal silently with only mural thrombus.[55] Hypothetically, loss of the antithrombotic properties of the plaque surface, which in its extreme may present as plaque erosion, could be a determining factor between these outcomes, together with circulating thrombogenic factors.

Plaque Thrombogenicity and Thrombosis

There are three major determinants of coronary thrombosis—the local thrombogenic substrate (plaque), local flow disturbances (stenosis), and the systemic thrombotic propensity (blood)—which is known as the Virchow triad.[56]

The necrotic core exposed to the blood by plaque rupture appears to be highly thrombogenic, which is most likely caused by a high content of tissue factor and prothrombotic apoptotic microparticles.[57] Rapid flow and high shear forces promote arterial (vs. venous) thrombosis via shear-induced platelet activation, and the importance of platelets, coagulation, and fibrinolysis is documented by the protective effects of antiplatelet agents and anticoagulants in patients at risk of coronary thrombosis.[58] In case of plaque rupture and erosion, circulating tissue factor and prothrombotic microparticles may influence the ensuing thrombotic response.[57] Cigarette smoking predisposes individuals to CHD at least partly through increasing systemic thrombotic propensity.[4]

Plaque material is sometimes found interspersed in the thrombus, indicating that severe thrombosis occurred immediately after plaque rupture. However, the layering of most coronary thrombi and the presence of thromboemboli in the myocardium distal to evolving thrombi indicate that usually the thrombotic response is dynamic. Waves of thrombosis and thrombolysis, often with concomitant vasospasm, occur on the time scale of days before producing the fatal occlusion (Figure 3-7). The initial flow obstruction is usually caused by platelet aggregation, but subsequently, fibrin may stabilize the platelet-rich thrombus. Smaller mural thrombi may heal silently. Nonocclusive or transiently occlusive thrombi are common in MI without ST-segment elevation, and more stable and occlusive thrombi prevail in ST-elevation MI. A critical thrombotic component is also common in culprit lesions responsible for out-of-hospital cardiac arrest and sudden coronary death (see Chapter 13 and Chapter 28).[31]

Healed Plaques and Incorporated Thrombi

A nonuniform or layered pattern of dense type I (older) and loosely arranged type III (younger) collagen, which is judged to indicate a healed plaque rupture, can be identified in many coronary plaques, particularly in those that cause chronic high-grade stenoses.[9] Other plaques may have a multilayered appearance consistent with a history of incorporation and organization of thrombus on eroded plaques.

These observations are indicative, and it is possible that similar morphology can result from a burst of plaque growth without rupture and thrombosis. Notably, multilayered plaques ("buried fibrous caps") are also seen in mouse models in which rupture and thrombosis are exceedingly rare. However, by accepting this caveat, the combined findings indicate that silent plaque ruptures and erosions are important for plaque growth and development of chronic stenosis (see Figure 3-4). This notion may explain why chronic coronary stenosis often develops in a phasic rather than linear manner, forming at sites that were only insignificantly narrowed in an antecedent angiography.[59]

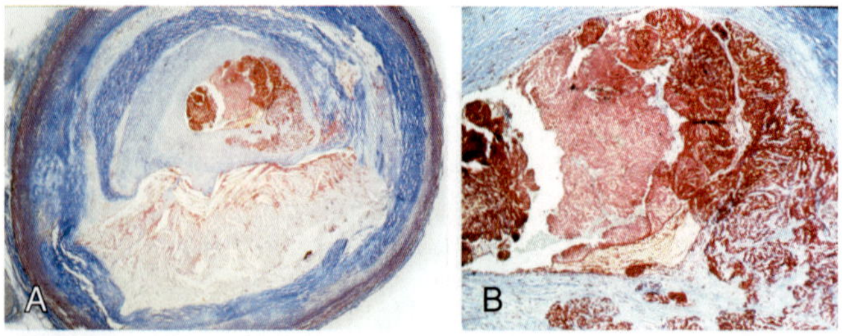

FIGURE 3-7 Coronary thrombosis. (**A**) The thrombotic response to plaque rupture is often dynamic, revealed by a layered structure of the thrombus and distal thromboembolism. (**B**) The layered thrombus at higher magnification. Local vasomotion may contribute to the dynamic flow obstruction caused by an atherothrombotic culprit lesion. Trichrome stain (thrombus: *red*, collagen: *blue*, necrotic core: *colorless*).

Plaque Regression

Lowering of LDL in patients with CHD reduces the risk of recurrent events, but changes in plaque size are slow and modest in magnitude.[60] Instead, the beneficial effects are explained by changes in plaque morphology. Analyses of carotid endarterectomy specimens, imaging and animal experiments have shown that efficient LDL lowering leads to resolution of inflammation, loss of neovessels, and reductions in extracellular lipids and the necrotic core, whereas the amount of calcification both in animals and humans may increase.[25,47] It is comprehensible that these changes lower the risk of plaque rupture. Whether the risk of thrombosis by erosion is also reduced has yet to be established.

PLAQUE BURDEN

In research and clinical practice, there is a need to characterize atherosclerosis or individual plaques for a few important and measurable characteristics that convey the status of the disease process and the risk of progression. Such variables can be used as endpoints for clinical trials and as risk prediction tools to guide decisions about therapies. Some of the terms used in this area are plaque burden, activity, and vulnerability.

Plaque burden is a measure of the extent of atherosclerosis in the body or in a particular vascular bed irrespective of the cellular composition and activity of plaques, and it is an important estimator of the risk for MI.[55,61] It can be measured directly as plaque volume, exemplified by coronary intravascular ultrasound (see Chapter 10) or three-dimensional ultrasound of the carotids, or by some proxy that is correlated with the extent of atherosclerosis, such as the measurement of coronary calcium score by computed tomography (see Chapter 9) or the ankle–brachial pressure index. Because atherosclerosis is a multifocal disease that affects the entire vasculature, having a high plaque burden in one vascular territory (e.g., the carotids or lower limbs) is a marker for advanced disease in other territories, especially in the coronary arteries, because of their high susceptibility to atherosclerosis.[62,63]

PLAQUE ACTIVITY

The activity of the disease or individual plaques is an important, but poorly defined concept. It is important because the ability to faithfully measure disease activity (e.g., by noninvasive imaging [see Chapter 10] or a circulating biomarker [see Chapter 8]) would be an important tool for the discovery of new causative factors and for demonstrating efficacy of new therapies in small "proof-of-concept" clinical trials. Furthermore, not having to rely on clinical endpoints to measure effect would pave the way for research and possibly preventive treatment at earlier stages of the disease, where we appear to know more about the pathophysiological processes and where the disease may potentially be more modifiable.

Atherosclerotic disease activity does not have a simple, defined meaning.[64] It is often taken to mean inflammation, measured for instance, as the density of macrophages in plaques. This conceptualization is reasonable because of the central role of vascular inflammation in plaque development. However, there is a vast difference in clinical importance between the inflammation of an early atherosclerotic lesion and the focused inflammation of a fibrous cap that may lead to rupture and thrombosis. Several other processes in atherosclerotic plaques could be included under the heading of plaque activity, including plaque necrosis, which constitutes the perhaps most detrimental activity of the disease. Neovascularization (angiogenesis), leaky endothelium, and plaque hemorrhage often accompany inflammation and constitute other potential biomarkers of disease activity.[65]

PLAQUE VULNERABILITY

Much effort has been put into recognizing the pathological features of vulnerable plaques (or synonymously thrombosis-prone or high-risk plaques) to predict which plaques are at risk of precipitating thrombosis and to understand the mechanisms leading to their formation (i.e., those plaques at high short-term risk of thrombosis).[31]

Notably, causing thrombosis is not the same as causing MI. Many ruptures and erosions are asymptomatic in the short term, although they may sometimes lead to gradual coronary narrowing (see Figure 3-4).[55] The vulnerable patient is a term used to describe patients at high short-term risk of an acute clinical event. This high risk depends on plaque burden, plaque vulnerability, systemic thrombotic propensity, and the myocardial susceptibility to ischemia and arrhythmia.

In the next sections, we briefly discuss the features of plaques assumed to be at a high risk of rupture. The other types of vulnerable plaques predisposing to thrombosis with erosion or possibly calcified nodule remain poorly understood. For the clinician, it is important to know that the mere presence of intravascular ultrasound (IVUS)–detected calcified nodules in the intima are not associated with an increased future risk of thrombi.[66]

RUPTURE-PRONE PLAQUES

Table 3-1 outlines features for which statistically significant differences have been reported between ruptured and nonruptured fibroatheromas. The prototypical ruptured plaque is a TCFA with a large necrotic core and macrophage infiltration in the cap (Figure 3-8). Because only a few TCFAs typically exist simultaneously,[67] the risk of rupture is limited to a small group of lesions at any point in time. Consistent with their importance for precipitating fatal coronary plaque ruptures, TCFAs tend to cluster in the proximal segments of the major coronary arteries, where also most plaque ruptures and thrombi are seen.[31]

Necrotic Core

If no necrotic core is present, there is no overlying fibrous cap to rupture. Consistently, not having necrotic cores among nonculprit lesions in the proximal coronary arteries indicates a favorable prognosis after MI.[68] However, a larger necrotic core also confers greater risk than a small one.[9] The importance of necrotic core size for plaque stability is comprehensible, because the total lack of supporting collagen in the lipid-rich core confers greater tensile stress to the overlying fibrous cap. A large necrotic core may also increase the thrombogenecity of the plaque material, and hence, the risk of a clinical event in case of plaque rupture.[57]

Plaque Size and Severity of Stenosis

Retrospective angiographic studies and the prospective PROSPECT (Providing Regional Observations to Study Predictors of Events in the Coronary Tree) study have shown that plaques with severe stenosis carry a higher per-plaque risk for producing clinical events than plaques that cause no or nonsevere stenosis.[69] However, such lesions are few, and overall, most ACS are precipitated by plaques without significant stenosis on an antecedent angiography weeks or months before.[69] This epidemiology is consistent with the distribution of TCFAs, as shown by a combined

TABLE 3-1 Features of Ruptured Plaques*

Thrombus
Large necrotic core (>30% of plaque)
Fibrous cap covering the necrotic core
Thin (thickness usually <65 μm)
High macrophage density
Few smooth muscle cells
Expansive remodeling preserving the lumen
Neovascularization from the vasa vasorum
Plaque hemorrhage
Adventitial/perivascular inflammation
"Spotty" calcification

*The same features, except rupture of the cap and luminal thrombus, are assumed to characterize vulnerable plaques of the rupture-prone type.

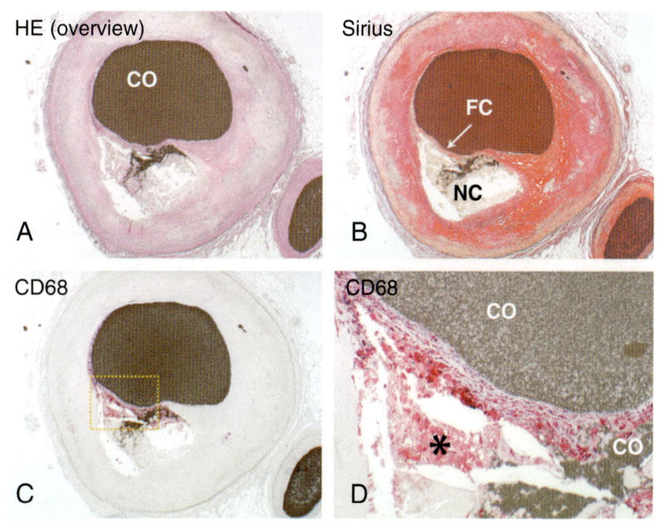

FIGURE 3-8 Thin-cap fibroatheroma with inflammation in the cap. (**A** and **B**) The plaque is composed predominantly of fibrous tissue and a necrotic core (NC) with an extremely thin fibrous cap (FC). (**C**) Staining for CD68 (macrophages: *red*) visualizes abundant macrophages in the fibrous cap, but other parts of the plaque are not inflamed. (**D**) Larger magnification of inset in (**C**). The cap contains very few smooth muscle cells (not shown). Dead macrophages without nuclei are seen within the necrotic core (*asterisk*). Penetration of the contrast medium (CO) injected postmortem from the lumen into the NC reveals that in this particular case an FC rupture is present in an adjacent segment. *HE*, Hematoxylin and eosin. *(From Bentzon J, et al: Mechanisms of plaque formation and rupture.* Circ Res *114:1852, 2014.)*

angiography and optical coherence tomographic imaging study of nonculprit lesions (see Chapter 10).[70] Lesions that caused severe stenosis were twice as likely to be TCFAs than lesions with only nonsevere stenosis, but the total number of TCFAs with nonsevere stenosis was three times higher than those with severe stenosis. The mild preexistent stenosis of most TCFAs and ruptured plaques is explained by expansive remodeling, because such lesions are, on average, large.

The long-held notion that mild to moderate obstructive coronary lesions are responsible for the majority of MIs has been challenged by studies that described significant narrowing in the days preceding MI.[59,71] However, significant narrowing shortly before MI may be a result of (rather than a precursor) for rupture.[9,71] Plaque rupture is followed not only by dynamic luminal thrombosis (with or without vasospasm), but also high-pressure hemorrhage into the plaque through the ruptured surface, giving rise to rapid plaque expansion that is unresponsive to thrombolysis and aspiration thrombectomy, and as discussed previously, the temporal relationship between plaque rupture and MI is often protracted.

Other Associated Features

Other features that are associated with ruptured lesions include neovascularization, plaque hemorrhage, a "spotty" pattern of calcifications, and adventitial inflammation.[31] These features are not independently associated with ruptured plaques but correlate with necrotic core size and expansive remodeling. However, a special importance of these features lies in the fact that they are credible targets for noninvasive imaging, in contrast to fibrous cap thickness, which is far below the resolution limit of noninvasive techniques (see Chapter 10).

Predictive Value of Vulnerable Plaque Features

The absence of TCFAs in a patient indicates a low imminent risk for plaque rupture and thrombosis, but what risk is conferred by their presence? In the PROSPECT study, only a minority of virtual histology (VH)-TCFAs identified by VH-IVUS led to coronary events (mostly progressive angina) at a median follow-up of 3.4 years.[69] Another serial VH-IVUS study found that VH-TCFAs arise and disappear more dynamically than what was previously believed.[72] Both these studies weaken the rationale for a targeted therapeutic approach to rupture-prone plaques.[55] However, it is important to note that the performance and resolution of VH-IVUS does not permit the identification of TCFAs as pathologists define them,[73] and the use of more precise methods in future studies may lead to different results. The other vulnerable plaque features are not sufficiently specific for predicting the fate of individual lesions, but it is possible, although not yet established,[55] that a high prevalence of vulnerable plaque features, such as large necrotic cores, among lesions in an individual may indicate a higher risk than would be predicted by measurements of plaque burden alone.

PERSPECTIVES FOR PREVENTION

Pathology teaches us that atherosclerosis is a life-long progressing disease, and living a long life is the single most important risk factor for dying or developing symptoms from atherosclerosis. The longer individuals live, the more likely it is they will experience the consequences of a life's burden of risk factor exposure. A longer lifespan, because of improvements in socioeconomic conditions and health care, is the central cause of the global epidemic of cardiovascular disease.[74] The age-adjusted mortality from CHD has declined substantially in recent decades, but because the decline is partly explained by improved survival after MI, and more people are becoming at risk of CHD because of an aging population, it is still only a half victory (see Chapter 2).[75–77] The sustained search for new insights into the pathobiology of atherothrombosis may define new avenues for diagnosis, risk stratification, and therapy.

Classic References

Falk E, Shah PK, Fuster V: Coronary plaque disruption, *Circulation* 92:657, 1995.

Stary HC, et al.: A definition of advanced types of atherosclerotic lesions and a histological classification of atherosclerosis. A report from the Committee on Vascular Lesions of the Council on Arteriosclerosis, American Heart Association, *Circulation* 92:1355, 1995.

Virmani R, et al.: Lessons from sudden coronary death: a comprehensive morphological classification scheme for atherosclerotic lesions, *Arterioscler Thromb Vasc Biol* 20:1262, 2000.

References

1. Martin SS, Blumenthal RS, Miller M: LDL cholesterol: the lower the better, *Med Clin North Am* 96:13, 2012.
2. Nordestgaard BG, et al.: Familial hypercholesterolaemia is underdiagnosed and undertreated in the general population: guidance for clinicians to prevent coronary heart disease: consensus statement of the European Atherosclerosis Society, *Eur Heart J* 34:3478, 2013.
3. Lim SS, et al.: A comparative risk assessment of burden of disease and injury attributable to 67 risk factors and risk factor clusters in 21 regions, 1990-2010: a systematic analysis for the Global Burden of Disease Study 2010, *Lancet* 380:2224, 2012.
4. Willey J, Gonzalez-Castellon M: Cholesterol level and stroke: a complex relationship, *JAMA Intern Med* 173:1765, 2013.
5. Mazzone T: Intensive glucose lowering and cardiovascular disease prevention in diabetes: reconciling the recent clinical trial data, *Circulation* 122:2201, 2010.
6. Barua RS, Ambrose JA: Mechanisms of coronary thrombosis in cigarette smoke exposure, *Arterioscler Thromb Vasc Biol* 33:1460, 2013.
7. Go AS, et al.: Heart disease and stroke statistics–2014 update: a report from the American Heart Association, *Circulation* 129:e28, 2014.
8. Fowkes FGR, et al.: Comparison of global estimates of prevalence and risk factors for peripheral artery disease in 2000 and 2010: a systematic review and analysis, *Lancet* 382:1329, 2013.
9. Bentzon JF, et al.: Mechanisms of plaque formation and rupture, *Circ Res* 114:1852, 2014.
10. Jansen H, Samani NJ, Schunkert H: Mendelian randomization studies in coronary artery disease, *Eur Heart J* 35:1917, 2014.
11. Stary HC: Natural history and histological classification of atherosclerotic lesions: an update, *Arterioscler Thromb Vasc Biol* 20:1177, 2000.
12. Virmani R, et al.: Lessons from sudden coronary death: a comprehensive morphological classification scheme for atherosclerotic lesions, *Arterioscler Thromb Vasc Biol* 20:1262, 2000.
13. Randolph GJ: Mechanisms that regulate macrophage burden in atherosclerosis, *Circ Res* 114:1757, 2014.
14. Fogelstrand P, Boren J: Retention of atherogenic lipoproteins in the artery wall and its role in atherogenesis, *Nutr Metab Cardiovasc Dis* 22:1, 2012.
15. Hartiala O, et al.: Adolescence risk factors are predictive of coronary artery calcification at middle age: the cardiovascular risk in young Finns study, *J Am Coll Cardiol* 60:1364, 2012.
16. Lichtman AH, et al.: Adaptive immunity in atherogenesis: new insights and therapeutic approaches, *J Clin Invest* 123:27, 2013.
17. Libby P, Lichtman AH, Hansson GK: Immune effector mechanisms implicated in atherosclerosis: from mice to humans, *Immunity* 38:1092, 2013.
18. Libby P, et al.: Inflammation and its resolution as determinants of acute coronary syndromes, *Circ Res* 114:1867, 2014.
19. Steinberg D: The LDL modification hypothesis of atherogenesis: an update, *J Lipid Res* 50(Suppl): S376, 2009.
20. Allahverdian S, et al.: Contribution of intimal smooth muscle cells to cholesterol accumulation and macrophage-like cells in human atherosclerosis, *Circulation* 129:1551, 2014.
21. Feil S, et al.: Transdifferentiation of vascular smooth muscle cells to macrophage-like cells during atherogenesis, *Circ Res* 115:662, 2014.
22. Sheedy FJ, et al.: CD36 coordinates NLRP3 inflammasome activation by facilitating intracellular nucleation of soluble ligands into particulate ligands in sterile inflammation, *Nat Immunol* 14:812, 2013.
23. Stöger JL, et al.: Distribution of macrophage polarization markers in human atherosclerosis, *Atherosclerosis* 225:461, 2012.
24. van Dijk RA, et al.: A change in inflammatory footprint precedes plaque instability: a systematic evaluation of cellular aspects of the adaptive immune response in human atherosclerosis, *J Am Heart Assoc* 4:e001403, 2015.
25. Libby P: Mechanisms of acute coronary syndromes and their implications for therapy, *N Engl J Med* 368:2004, 2013.
26. Peled M, Fisher EA: Dynamic aspects of macrophage polarization during atherosclerosis progression and regression, *Front Immunol* 5:579, 2014.
27. Clarke MC, Bennett MR: Cause or consequence: what does macrophage apoptosis do in atherosclerosis? *Arterioscler Thromb Vasc Biol* 29:153, 2009.
28. Moore KJ, Tabas I: Macrophages in the pathogenesis of atherosclerosis, *Cell* 145:341, 2011.
29. Seimon TA, et al.: Atherogenic lipids and lipoproteins trigger CD36-TLR2-dependent apoptosis in macrophages undergoing endoplasmic reticulum stress, *Cell Metab* 12:467, 2010.
30. Tabas I: Macrophage death and defective inflammation resolution in atherosclerosis, *Nat Rev Immunol* 10:36, 2010.
31. Falk E, et al.: Update on acute coronary syndromes: the pathologists' view, *Eur Heart J* 34: 719, 2013.
32. Marsch E, Sluimer JC, Daemen MJ: Hypoxia in atherosclerosis and inflammation, *Curr Opin Lipidol* 24:393, 2013.

33. Moreno PR, Purushothaman M, Purushothaman KR: Plaque neovascularization: defense mechanisms, betrayal, or a war in progress, *Ann N Y Acad Sci* 1254:7, 2012.
34. Sluimer JC, et al.: Thin-walled microvessels in human coronary atherosclerotic plaques show incomplete endothelial junctions relevance of compromised structural integrity for intraplaque microvascular leakage, *J Am Coll Cardiol* 53:1517, 2009.
35. Jeney V, Balla G, Balla J: Red blood cell, hemoglobin and heme in the progression of atherosclerosis, *Front Physiol* 5:379, 2014.
36. Nielsen MJ, Møller HJ, Moestrup SK: Hemoglobin and heme scavenger receptors, *Antioxid Redox Signal* 12:261, 2010.
37. Boyle JJ, et al.: Coronary intraplaque hemorrhage evokes a novel atheroprotective macrophage phenotype, *Am J Pathol* 174:1097, 2009.
38. Finn AV, et al.: Hemoglobin directs macrophage differentiation and prevents foam cell formation in human atherosclerotic plaques, *J Am Coll Cardiol* 59:166, 2012.
39. Cahill LE, et al.: Haptoglobin genotype is a consistent marker of coronary heart disease risk among individuals with elevated glycosylated hemoglobin, *J Am Coll Cardiol* 61:728, 2013.
40. Purushothaman M, et al.: Genotype-dependent impairment of hemoglobin clearance increases oxidative and inflammatory response in human diabetic atherosclerosis, *Arterioscler Thromb Vasc Biol* 32:2769, 2012.
41. Campbell JH, Campbell GR: Smooth muscle phenotypic modulation—a personal experience, *Arterioscler Thromb Vasc Biol* 32:1784, 2012.
42. Bentzon JF, et al.: Smooth muscle cells in atherosclerosis originate from the local vessel wall and not circulating progenitor cells in apoE knockout mice, *Arterioscler Thromb Vasc Biol* 26:2696, 2006.
43. Gomez D, et al.: Detection of histone modifications at specific gene loci in single cells in histological sections, *Nat Meth* 10:171, 2013.
44. Bennett MR: Life and death in the atherosclerotic plaque, *Curr Opin Lipidol* 21:422, 2010.
45. Otsuka F, et al.: Has our understanding of calcification in human coronary atherosclerosis progressed? *Arterioscler Thromb Vasc Biol* 34:724, 2014.
46. Bertazzo S: Nano-analytical electron microscopy reveals fundamental insights into human cardiovascular tissue calcification, *Nat Mater* 12:576, 2013.
47. Puri R, et al.: Impact of statins on serial coronary calcification during atheroma progression and regression, *J Am Coll Cardiol* 65:1273, 2015.
48. Puri R, et al.: The distinctive nature of atherosclerotic vascular disease in diabetes: pathophysiological and morphological insights, *Curr Diab Rep* 12:280, 2012.
49. Stone PH, et al.: Prediction of progression of coronary artery disease and clinical outcomes using vascular profiling of endothelial shear stress and arterial plaque characteristics: the PREDICTION study, *Circulation* 126:172, 2012.
50. Bastante T, et al.: Nonatherosclerotic causes of acute coronary syndrome: recognition and management, *Curr Cardiol Rep* 16:543, 2014.
51. Jia H, et al.: In vivo diagnosis of plaque erosion and calcified nodule in patients with acute coronary syndrome by intravascular optical coherence tomography, *J Am Coll Cardiol* 62:1748, 2013.
52. Mittleman MA, Mostofsky E: Physical, psychological and chemical triggers of acute cardiovascular events: preventive strategies, *Circulation* 124:346, 2011.
53. Kramer MC, et al.: Relationship of thrombus healing to underlying plaque morphology in sudden coronary death, *J Am Coll Cardiol* 55:122, 2010.
54. Quillard T, et al.: TLR2 and neutrophils potentiate endothelial stress, apoptosis and detachment: implications for superficial erosion, *Eur Heart J* 36:1394, 2015.
55. Arbab-Zadeh A, Fuster V: The myth of the "vulnerable plaque": transitioning from a focus on individual lesions to atherosclerotic disease burden for coronary artery disease risk assessment, *J Am Coll Cardiol* 65:846, 2015.
56. Badimon L, Vilahur G: Thrombosis formation on atherosclerotic lesions and plaque rupture, *J Intern Med* 276:618, 2014.
57. Rautou PE, et al.: Microparticles, vascular function, and atherothrombosis, *Circ Res* 109:593, 2011.
58. Weitz JI: Insights into the role of thrombin in the pathogenesis of recurrent ischaemia after acute coronary syndrome, *Thromb Haemost* 112:924, 2014.
59. Puri R, et al.: High-risk coronary atheroma - the interplay between ischemia, plaque burden and disease progression, *J Am Coll Cardiol* 63:1134, 2014.
60. Nicholls SJ, et al.: Effect of two intensive statin regimens on progression of coronary disease, *N Engl J Med* 365:2078, 2011.
61. Baber U, et al.: Prevalence, impact, and predictive value of detecting subclinical coronary and carotid atherosclerosis in asymptomatic adults: the BioImage study, *J Am Coll Cardiol* 65:1065, 2015.
62. Hussein AA, et al.: Peripheral arterial disease and progression of coronary atherosclerosis, *J Am Coll Cardiol* 57:1220, 2011.
63. Sillesen H, et al.: Carotid plaque burden as a measure of subclinical atherosclerosis: comparison with other tests for subclinical arterial disease in the High Risk Plaque BioImage study, *JACC Cardiovasc Imaging* 5:681, 2012.
64. Fryburg DA, Vassileva MT: Atherosclerosis drug development in jeopardy: the need for predictive biomarkers of treatment response, *Sci Transl Med* 3:72cm6, 2011.
65. Sluimer JC, Daemen MJ: Novel concepts in atherogenesis: angiogenesis and hypoxia in atherosclerosis, *J Pathol* 218:7, 2009.
66. Xu Y, et al.: Prevalence, distribution, predictors, and outcomes of patients with calcified nodules in native coronary arteries: a 3-vessel intravascular ultrasound analysis from Providing Regional Observations to Study Predictors of Events in the Coronary Tree (PROSPECT), *Circulation* 126:537, 2012.
67. Cheruvu PK, et al.: Frequency and distribution of thin-cap fibroatheroma and ruptured plaques in human coronary arteries: a pathologic study, *J Am Coll Cardiol* 50:940, 2007.
68. Dohi T, et al.: Non-fibroatheroma lesion phenotype and long-term clinical outcomes, *JACC Cardiovasc Imaging* 6:908, 2013.
69. Stone GW, et al.: A prospective natural-history study of coronary atherosclerosis, *N Engl J Med* 364:226, 2011.
70. Tian J, et al.: Prevalence and characteristics of TCFA and degree of coronary artery stenosis: an OCT, IVUS, and angiographic study, *J Am Coll Cardiol* 64:672, 2014.
71. Niccoli G, et al.: Are the culprit lesions severely stenotic? *JACC Cardiovasc Imaging* 6:1108, 2013.
72. Kubo T, et al.: The dynamic nature of coronary artery lesion morphology assessed by serial virtual histology intravascular ultrasound tissue characterization, *J Am Coll Cardiol* 55:1590, 2010.
73. Falk E, Wilensky RL: Prediction of coronary events by intravascular imaging, *JACC Cardiovasc Imaging* 5:S38, 2012.
74. Murray CJ, Lopez AD: Measuring the global burden of disease, *N Engl J Med* 369:448, 2013.
75. Fuster V, Mearns BM: The CVD paradox: mortality vs prevalence, *Nat Rev Cardiol* 6:669, 2009.
76. Nabel EG, Braunwald E: A tale of coronary artery disease and myocardial infarction, *N Engl J Med* 366:54, 2012.
77. Heidenreich PA, et al.: Forecasting the future of cardiovascular disease in the United States: a policy statement from the American Heart Association, *Circulation* 123:933, 2011.

4 Mechanisms of Myocardial Ischemic Injury, Healing, and Remodeling

Matthias Nahrendorf, Filip K. Swirski, and Peter Libby

EVOLUTION OF CONCEPTS REGARDING MECHANISMS OF MYOCARDIAL INFARCTION

Historical Perspective

The scientific study of the mechanisms of myocardial infarction (MI) occurred surprisingly recently. Heberden published his strikingly contemporary description of angina pectoris in 1772. The very first article in the predecessor of the *New England Journal of Medicine*, published in 1812, described a North American case of angina pectoris that came to autopsy. The author, John Warren, concluded that because the coronary arteries were enlarged, they were "not essentially connected with angina pectoris; and, therefore… not the cause of the disease." In contrast, British observers previously proposed an association between "ossification" of the coronary arteries and angina pectoris based on anecdotal autopsy observations.

Although physicians from the time of Morgangni and Corvisart and the great nineteenth century German pathologists described cardiac aneurysms or "fatty degeneration," the link among angina pectoris, coronary artery disease, and MI came together only at the beginning of the 20th century. The Russian physicians Obrastzow and Straschesko articulated the connection between coronary thrombosis and prolonged angina pectoris. In 1912, James Herrick described the survival of individuals with coronary thrombosis, a situation that was previously considered invariably fatal. Samuel A. Levine, a cardiologist at Boston's Peter Bent Brigham Hospital (currently Brigham and Women's Hospital), in his 1929 monograph on "Coronary Thrombosis" reviewed the connection between coronary artery disease and MI. Levine published a report of two cases of coronary thrombosis, including one diagnosed antemortem in 1918 that clearly connected this pathological finding with MI (Figure 4-1). The advent of electrocardiography in the early part of the 20th century also helped clarify the entity of MI by providing a noninvasive method of detection of myocardial injury, ischemia, and infarct. Herrick's 1942 monograph on the history of cardiology highlighted the confusion that previously prevailed with regard to the acute coronary syndromes (ACS) and their pathogenesis. He stated, "It was long before it was realized that the Ariadne thread that guided one through the maze of angina pectoris, infarct, rupture, certain forms of pericarditis, and of acute and chronic heart failure was disease of the coronary artery."

As late as the 1970s, controversy still brewed regarding the causality of coronary thrombosis in MI.[1] The ascendancy of selective coronary arteriography heightened interest in coronary vasospasm as a pathogenic process that led to myocardial ischemia. The introduction of calcium channel blockers as pharmacologic tools to treat vasospasm spurred this interest. The advent of fibrinolytic agents and their success in restoring coronary flow in some patients with ST-elevation MI (STEMI) brought thrombosis to the forefront as a pathological mechanism for MI.

In evaluating the current state of knowledge put forth in this chapter, readers should reflect that this history illustrates the degree to which pathophysiological constructs depend on the tools of the time, and how concepts evolve as new methodologies emerge. Today's tools likely similarly constrain our vision, and the synthesis we provide here will doubtless require revision as we learn more.

The Concept of Mutability of Myocardial Infarction: Oxygen Supply and Demand Balance, Reperfusion, and Remodeling

As late as the 1970s, most regarded MI as an "all or none" event. Individuals transitioned from apparent good health or stable angina to acute MI suddenly, as if struck by lightning. Treatment focused on symptom relief and did not encompass efforts to modify the infarction, then considered completed at presentation. In the late 1950s to 1960s, rigorous physiologic investigations delineated the factors that determine the myocardial requirements for oxygen. This area of inquiry provided a scientific basis for conceiving of myocardial ischemia as an imbalance between oxygen supply and demand.[2] Some of the determinants of oxygen requirements seemed modifiable. The frequency, force of contraction (inotropic state), and afterload contributed to myocardial oxygen demand. This recognition led to the exploration of carotid sinus stimulation and intervention that reduced blood pressure and heart rate as a treatment for angina pectoris.[3] Implantation of a carotid sinus nerve stimulator could provide relief from angina pectoris.

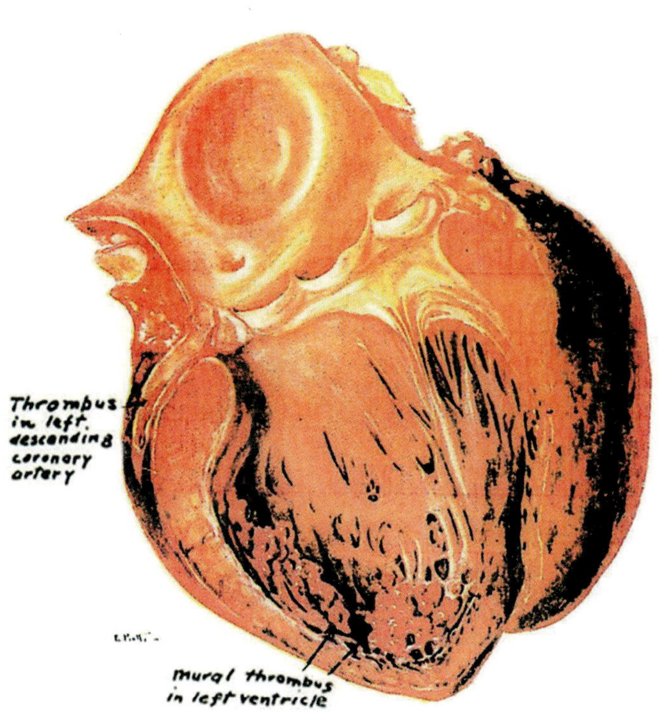

FIGURE 4-1 Coronary thrombus associated with myocardial infarction. The frontispiece of Samuel A. Levine's 1929 monograph on "Coronary Thrombosis" shows a thrombus in the left anterior descending coronary artery with apical thinning and a large mural thrombus in the left ventricle. *(From Levine SA:* Coronary thrombosis: its various clinical features, *Baltimore, The Williams & Wilkins Company, 1929.)*

These early efforts represented pioneering developments in device therapy.

The introduction of β-adrenergic blocking agents in the 1960s provided a pharmacologic tool for manipulating myocardial oxygen requirements (see Chapter 13).[4] Blocking β-adrenergic stimuli could both lower heart rate and reduce the force of contraction of the left ventricle, which are two key determinants of myocardial oxygen requirements. Experimental studies in dogs with coronary artery ligation affirmed the concept that interventions that decreased myocardial oxygen requirements could limit myocardial injury following coronary artery ligation as determined by electrocardiographic, histologic, and biochemical criteria (see also Chapter 24).[5] If performed with sufficient haste, coronary artery reperfusion could mitigate the consequences of coronary artery ligation in dogs.[6]

These observations affirmed the principle of mutability of the consequences of a given coronary occlusion. Further physiologic studies on experimental MI conducted in rats disclosed a previously unrecognized aspect of the myocardial response to coronary artery ligation: expansive geometric remodeling (see Chapter 36). Following ligation of the left anterior descending coronary artery, the left ventricular cavity of rat hearts showed regional expansion.[7] This consequence of coronary artery ligation also proved mutable. Pioneering observations showed that interruption of the renin-angiotensin system, as affected by administration of angiotensin-converting enzyme inhibitors, could reduce the expansive remodeling in the left ventricles of rats following coronary artery ligation.[8] Clinical pilot observations affirmed the translatability of these results. Ultimately, large-scale clinical trials confirmed improvement in long-term outcomes in patients treated with interventions that interrupted the renin-angiotensin-aldosterone axis.

These brief summaries of bodies of work conducted in the 1970s and 1980s reveal how recent concepts regarding the mutability of MI emerged. The experimental findings, which were rapidly reduced to practice, ushered in the era of reperfusion achieved first by biologically derived fibrinolytic agents (e.g., streptokinase), thrombolytic agents derived through recombinant DNA technology (e.g., tissue plasminogen activator), and were followed by fibrinolytic agents (see Chapter 15). Percutaneous intervention to achieve reperfusion and "salvage" infarcting myocardium came in successive waves—percutaneous balloon angioplasty, bare metal stents, drug-eluting stents, and currently, bioabsorbable stents (see Chapter 17). This entire revolution in our fundamental understanding of the relationship between coronary artery occlusion and MI, the recognition of its mutability, and the translation to clinical practice occurred in a compressed time scale, only over the last three or four decades. Built on a burgeoning scientific foundation, the treatment of MI has transformed from mere symptomatic relief to pharmacologic and mechanical interventions that modify the disease and its downstream consequences, including arrhythmias and the development of heart failure (see Chapter 13).

New Insights into the Mechanisms of Coronary Thrombosis

Understanding of the mechanisms of coronary thrombosis that most often lead to MI has evolved hand-in-hand with the evolution of our concepts with regard to MI. Chapter 3 reviews in detail the current state of the pathophysiology of coronary artery thrombosis, as do authoritative reviews.[9,10]

PATHOLOGICAL FINDINGS DURING THE EVOLUTION AND HEALING OF MYOCARDIAL INFARCTION

The traditional concept of the cellular sequence of events in myocardial infarction focused primarily on myocyte injury, death, and "replacement fibrosis," which are the formation of granulation tissue, provisional scar, and ultimately, a fully healed scar. Morphologic appearance characterized various stages of myocyte injury (Figure 4-2 and Table 4-1). During the first 12 hours, myocyte necrosis occurs, accompanied by edema manifested microscopically by an increased spacing between sarcomere bundles. After 12 to 24 hours, neutrophils accumulate, myocytes die, and contraction bands appear. In the ensuing days, myocyte death continues, and mononuclear phagocytes begin to engulf the remains of dying cells, particularly near the border zone of the infarct. After the first week, granulation tissue begins to form, characterized by neoangiogenesis and extracellular matrix accumulation. After several weeks, a well-organized collagenous extracellular matrix replaces the functioning myocardium in the center of the infarct.

In the current era, many patients with ACS undergo reperfusion, altering this classical sequence of events that characterizes infarct healing. Reperfusion can salvage myocardial tissue in a manner that depends on the time of reestablishing blood flow following the onset of ischemia (see Chapter 13). Reperfused regions of infarcts can show accentuation of hemorrhage. Reperfusion can also hasten the death of irreversibly injured myocytes and accentuate

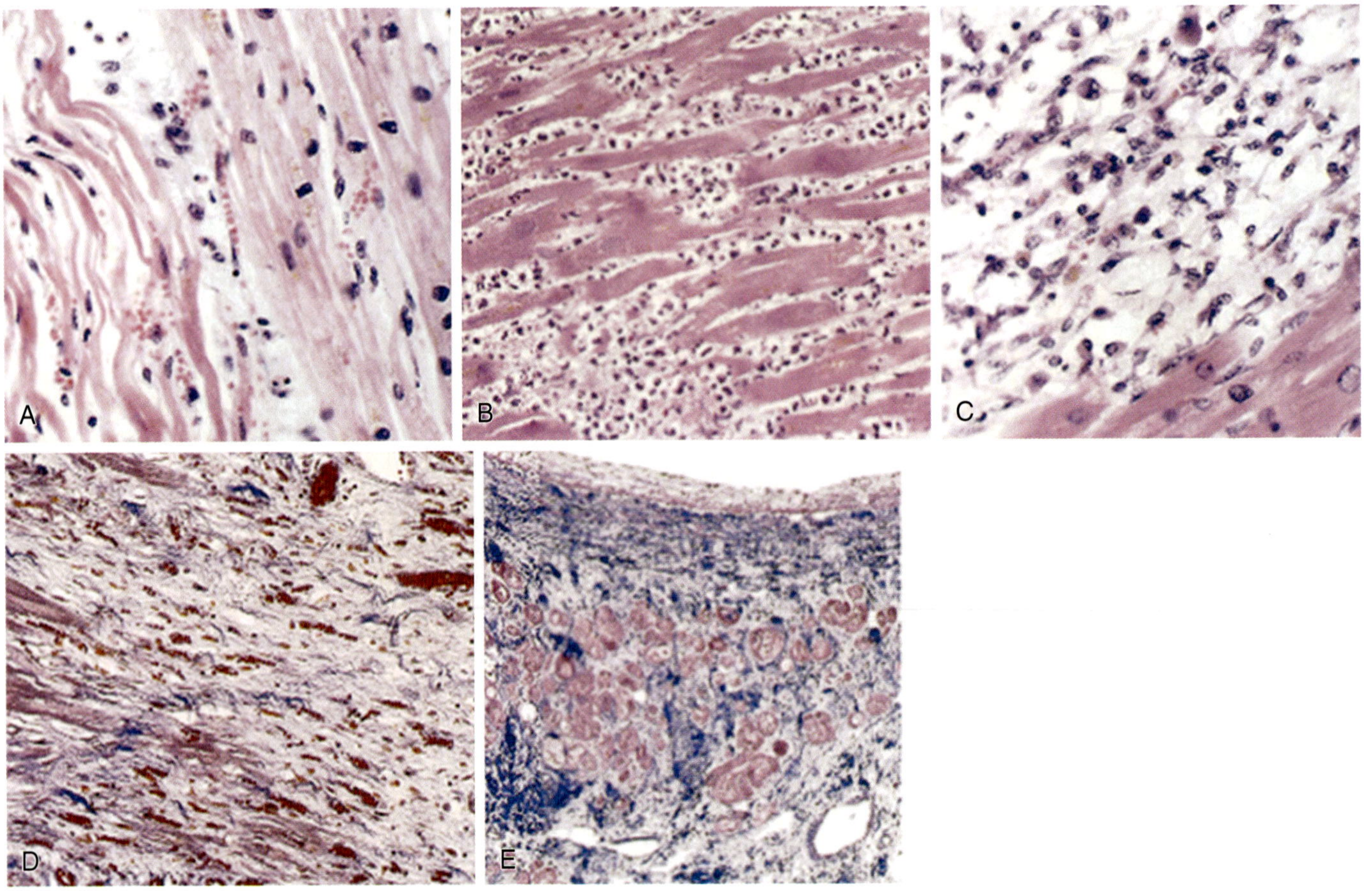

FIGURE 4-2 The sequence of pathological findings during myocardial infarction. (**A**) Section of myocardium 1 day postinfarction shows myocyte necrosis along with "wavy fibers" (*left*, elongated and narrow) compared with adjacent normal fibers (*right*). Widened spaces between the dying fibers contain edema fluid and neutrophils, the "first responders" during ischemic injury. (**B**) Plentiful polymorphonuclear leukocytes populate infarcting myocardium after 3 to 4 days. (**C**) Nearly complete destruction of myocardial architecture characterizes the most severely affected portions of the myocardium 7 to 10 days after presentation. (**D**) Granulation tissue contains collagen (*blue*) and neo-vessels. (**E**) A healed myocardial infarction shows regions of replacement of myocytes by a collagenous scar. Only a few cardiac muscle fibers persist in this section. *(Adapted from Schoen FJ, Mitchell RN: The heart. In Kumar V, AK Abbas, JC Aster, eds.* Pathologic basis of disease, *ed 9, Philadelphia, Saunders, 2015.)*

TABLE 4-1 Functions of Monocyte Subtypes

MONOCYTE SUBTYPE	PROTEOLYSIS	PHAGOCYTOSIS	INFLAMMATION	FIBROSIS	ANGIOGENESIS
$Ly6C^{high}$ $CD14^{++}$ $CD16^{-}$	High	High	High	Less	Less
$Ly6C^{low}$ $CD14^{+}$ $CD16^{+}$	Less	Less	Less	More	More

contraction band formation. Even when intervention reestablishes epicardial flow, microvascular dysfunction can cause distal microvascular occlusion, yielding the "no reflow" phenomenon (see Chapter 24).

THE CURRENT ERA: THE ROLE OF INFLAMMATION IN THE EVOLUTION AND HEALING OF MYOCARDIAL INFARCTION

The remarkable revolutions in understanding and treating MI, as recounted previously, emerged from application of classical physiologic and pharmacologic concepts and investigations. These advances, which were predicated primarily on approaches to realign a mismatch between oxygen supply and demand, accorded little weight to the response of the myocardial tissue itself. The cardiovascular community expended strenuous efforts to comprehend and modify either coronary artery perfusion or the oxygen requirements of the heart muscle. This undertaking focused on aspects of myocardial intermediary metabolism, and the regulation of the force and frequency of cardiac contraction, but largely relegated the myocardium itself to the role of bystander. Moreover, although the cardiac myocyte received detailed attention from physiologic and biochemical investigators, the other cellular constituents of the heart, with the possible exception of the endothelial cells, received relatively little attention from clinical investigators.

The last decade witnessed the dawning of an increased interest in the response of myocardial tissue to ischemic injury viewed through the lens of inflammation. The balance of this chapter reviews some of these more recent observations and concepts. Perhaps the study and clinical translation of the principles elucidated in this work will provide a platform for future advances in mitigating MI, as classical physiologic and pathological studies allowed in previous years.

Inflammatory Response to Myocardial Infarction

The first forays implicating inflammation in MI depended on careful clinical observations and classical pathological investigation. Samuel Levine in his 1929 monograph on "Coronary Thrombosis" stated, "In the great majority of acute cases of coronary thrombosis, there quickly develops a fever and leukocytosis." He deduced "...that infarcted tissue...probably liberates toxic products that produce leukocytosis and fever," whereas he remarked that "the leukocyte count is apt to run hand in hand with the fever." He further noted "...a distinct increase in the polymorphonuclear ratio, which rises to 80% and sometimes even to 90%...." His careful clinical observations led him to conclude "the presence of a leukocytosis is one of the most constant findings in coronary thrombosis."

Following Levine's astute clinical observations, pathologists at the Boston City Hospital formally studied the sequence of inflammatory cell appearance in the infarcting myocardium based on histopathological study of human hearts postmortem.[11] They established the well-defined sequence of microscopic changes in the previously described infarct region. In the first hours to days following presentation, polymorphonuclear leukocytes accumulated in the infarcting myocardium. After several more days, mononuclear phagocytes predominated. In the second and subsequent weeks following presentation, fibroblasts and "connective tissue" appeared (Figure 4-3A). These findings, together with the clinical observations that documented peripheral leukocytosis in patients who experienced MI, called attention to the potential role of inflammatory cells in MI.

Early studies also supported the involvement of inflammation in acute MI by monitoring biomarkers of the acute phase response. In particular, C-reactive protein elevation, recognized in the mid-20th century, indicated that an inflammatory state ensued following MI.[12] Only recently have investigations suggested that inflammation may not merely follow MI as a consequence, but that inflammatory processes may modulate the tissue response to ischemic injury as discussed in the following.

In the 1980s and 1990s, many studies of ischemia–reperfusion injury focused on the recruitment of leukocytes as a potential therapeutic target, including inhibition of leukocyte adhesion molecules.[13] Yet, these studies focused little on the effector functions of various classes of leukocytes in different phases of myocardial ischemic injury, nor did they address the origins of leukocytes that accumulate in the infarcting myocardium.

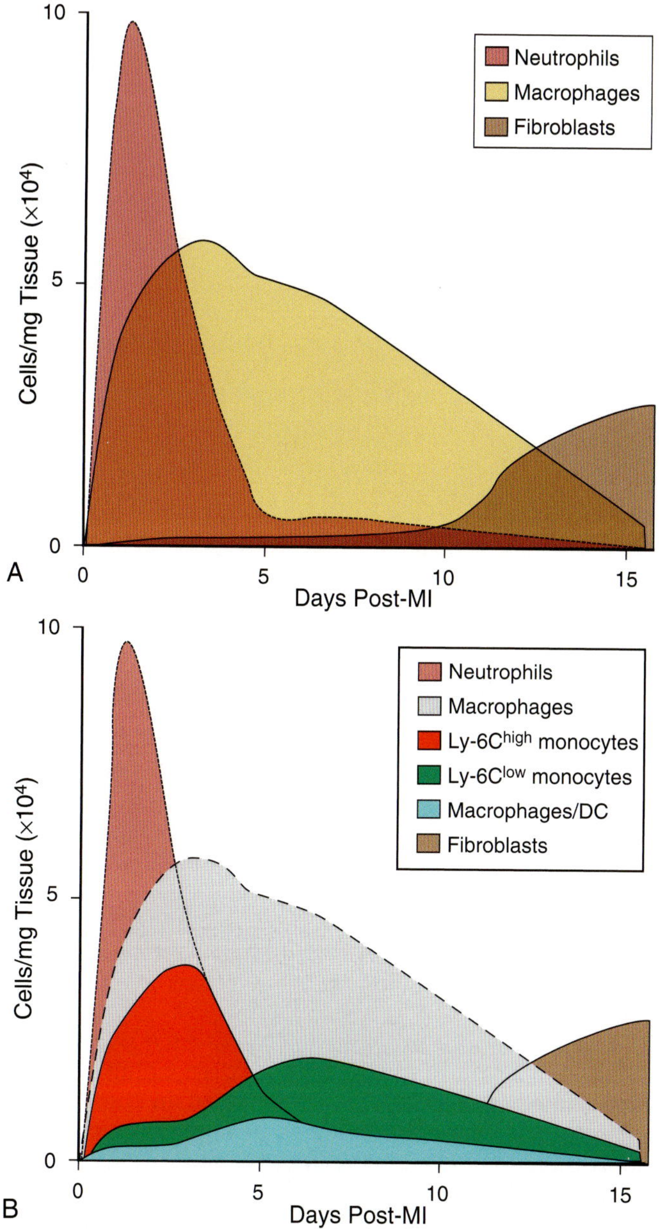

FIGURE 4-3 The temporal sequencing of cell populations following myocardial infarction. (**A**) Classical sequencing of a first wave of polymorphonuclear leukocytes, followed by mononuclear phagocytes, and ultimately, fibroblasts and connective tissues, that emerged from observations by pathologists. (**B**) Resolution of the mononuclear phagocytes population into two peaks, an initial proinflammatory population followed by the predominance of a less inflammatory subset of mononuclear phagocytes that exhibit reparative functions. *DC*, Dendritic cell; *MI*, myocardial infarction. *(Adapted from Nahrendorf M, et al: The healing myocardium sequentially mobilizes two monocyte subsets with divergent and complementary functions.* J Exp Med *204:3037–3047, 2007.)*

Inflammatory Cells and Infarct Healing

Experimental studies have deepened our understanding of the participation of inflammatory mechanisms in myocardial ischemic injury. Traditionally, such inquiries focused on the acute inflammatory response mediated by polymorphonuclear leukocytes. More recent studies have called attention to the participation of mononuclear phagocytes that participate not only acutely, but also in the more chronic phases of healing of myocardial injury. This work has shown that the normal myocardium possesses a resident population of these mononuclear cells, indicating a role in ongoing immune surveillance or other unknown functions.[14]

Role of Specific Leukocyte Classes

Inflammation biologists have increasingly recognized the functional diversity of various leukocyte classes.[15,16] In particular, monocytes, which are key responders to tissue injury that participate in repair processes, exist in various states that express varied palettes of mediators and functions. The polarization of leukocyte function into subsets often shows clearer demarcation in mice than in humans. In mice, a particularly proinflammatory subset of monocytes expresses high levels of a surface marker denoted as Ly-6C. Human cells with a high concentration of a cell surface marker known as CD14, with low levels of CD16,

TABLE 4-2 Evolution of Morphologic Changes in Myocardial Infarction

TIME	GROSS FEATURES	LIGHT MICROSCOPE	ELECTRON MICROSCOPE
Reversible Injury			
0–0.5/ hr	None	None	Relaxation of myofibrils; glycogen loss; mitochondrial swelling
Irreversible Injury			
0.5–4/hr	None	Usually none; variable waviness of fibers at border	Sarcolemmal disruption; mitochondrial amorphous densities
4–12/hr	Dark mottling (occasional)	Early coagulation necrosis; edema; hemorrhage	
12–24/hr	Dark mottling	Ongoing coagulation necrosis; pyknosis of nuclei; myocyte hypereosinophilia; marginal contraction band necrosis; same neutrophilic infiltrate	
1–3 days	Mottling with yellow-tan infarct center	Coagulation necrosis, with loss of nuclei and striations; more substantial neutrophil accumulation	
3–7 days	Hyperemic border; central yellow-tan softening	Disintegration of dead myofibers, with dying neutrophils; phagocytosis of dead cells by macrophages in infarct border zone	
7–10 days	Maximally yellow-tan and soft, with depressed red-tan margins	Robust phagocytosis of dead cells; granulation tissue at margins	
10–14 days	Red-gray depressed infarct borders	Well-established granulation tissue with new blood vessels and collagen deposition	
2–8/wk	Gray-white scar, progressive from border toward core of infarct	Increased collagen deposition, with decreased cellularity	
>2/mo	Scarring complete	Dense collagenous scar	

Adapted from Schoen FJ, Mitchell RN: The heart. In Kumar V, AK Abbas, JC Aster, eds: Pathologic basis of disease, *ed 9, Philadelphia, Saunders, 2015.*

resemble the Ly-6C^{high} monocyte subset in mice.[17] Human monocytes that have low surface amounts of CD14 and higher concentrations of CD16 may resemble the Ly-6C^{low} population of monocytes in mice. Table 4-2 shows the characteristics of the proinflammatory subsets of monocytes and macrophages.

Initial studies of experimental MI in mice showed that following ligation of the left anterior descending coronary artery, leukocytes promptly accumulated in the evolving infarct.[18] As observed in humans, polymorphonuclear leukocytes predominated in the first hours following coronary artery ligation. Subsequently, a population of proinflammatory monocytes appears in the evolving infarct. In later days (days 5 to 7), the mononuclear phagocytes in the infarcting zone display markers of alternatively activated or less intensely inflammatory cells (see Figure 4-3B). As discernable from Table 4-2, the proinflammatory subset of monocytes exhibits characteristics that could prove salutary in an early phase of myocardial ischemic injury. In particular, the proinflammatory monocytes have high phagocytic and proteolytic activity. These functional features could promote the clearance of dead cardiocytes and their detritus. Proteolytic cleavage of proteins released by dying cells and of the surrounding extracellular matrix could pave the way for subsequent healing and fibrosis. An overly aggressive proteolytic response could hasten thinning of the infarcting left ventricular wall and foster friability that could, in the extreme, promote expansive left ventricular remodeling, predispose to aneurysm formation, and potentiate the formation of pseudoaneurysms, ventricular septal defects, or ventricular rupture (see also Chapter 36).

Following the advent of the proinflammatory monocytes, a less inflammatory or alternatively activated subset of monocytes and/or macrophages predominates, characterized by low surface expression of Ly-6C. These Ly-6C^{low} mononuclear phagocytes in the evolving infarct can further "clear" dead myocytes. Genetic manipulations that interfere with this process, known as efferocytosis, can impair healing and function of the infarcted myocardium in mice.[19] This subset of mononuclear phagocytes exhibits functions that could contribute to myocardial healing by formation of granulation tissue and the extracellular matrix. In particular, this less inflammatory subset of mononuclear phagocytes has relatively less proteolytic potential, but it produces transforming growth factor-β (TGF-β), which is a strong stimulus to extracellular matrix gene expression and an inhibitor of inflammation. These Ly-6C^{low} cells also secrete angiogenic molecules such as vascular endothelial growth factor, which is a mediator implicated in neoangiogenesis, a characteristic of granulation tissue (see Table 4-2). Figure 4-4 depicts postulated functions of proinflammatory monocytes in the early phase of myocardial ischemic injury (see Figure 4-4A) and the less inflammatory mononuclear phagocytes in the latter phase (see Figure 4-4B). In mice, extreme hypercholesterolemia impairs healing of MI, which is likely related to a striking Ly-6C^{high} monocytosis.[20,21] Adaptive immunity may also modulate the function of mononuclear phagocytes in MI. Regulatory T cells, a subset that elaborates TGF-β, interleukin (IL)-10, and IL-13, can slant the macrophage population in experimental MI in mice toward an "M2" palette of functions that may foster healing and improve survival.[22]

Monocyte Origins in Myocardial Infarction

Because of the rapid appearance of monocytes in the infarcting myocardium, further studies sought to delineate the origin of these cells. These investigations disclosed the existence in mice of a preformed pool of proinflammatory monocytes in the subcapsular region of the red pulp of the spleen.[23] Following coronary artery ligation, intravital

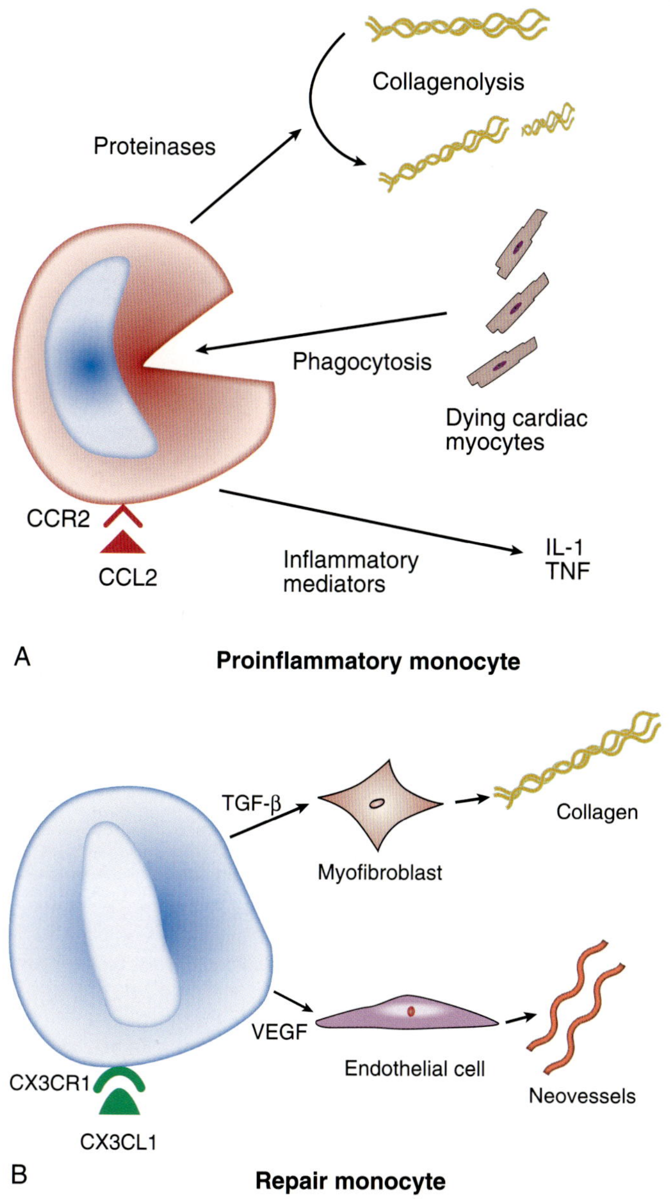

FIGURE 4-4 Subtypes of mononuclear phagocytes exhibit distinct functional palettes in the infarcting myocardium. (**A**) A proinflammatory monocyte (marked by high levels of Ly-6c in mice and high levels of CD14 with low levels of CD16 in humans). These cells possess high phagocytic capacity that permits them to clear the debris of dead and dying cells, acting as a "demolition" crew following acute ischemic myocardial injury. These cells also produce hydrolytic enzymes at high concentrations that permit them to degrade macromolecules released by dead or dying cells and also to remodel the extracellular matrix to prepare the way for production of a provisional extracellular matrix, and ultimately, scar formation. (**B**) A less inflammatory monocyte characterized in particular by high concentrations of transforming growth factor (TGF-β), which is a potent stimulus to extracellular matrix synthesis needed for repair and scar formation. These less inflammatory cells also elaborate angiogenic mediators, such vascular endothelial growth factor (VEGF), that promote the formation of new microvessels. Fibrosis and microvascularization characterize granulation tissue, long recognized as part of the healing response of injured tissues. The appropriate balance between the proinflammatory and reparative subset of mononuclear phagocytes can influence both the structure and function of the myocardium following coronary occlusion and critically modulate the healing process. *IL*, Interleukin; *TNF*, tumor necrosis factor.

microscopic and cell-tracking studies showed the traversal of these proinflammatory monocytes from the spleen to the infarcting myocardium. Thus, the spleen warehouses a set of monocytes poised to respond to tissue injury on an emergency basis. Subsequent studies indicated that in the mouse spleen, extramedullary hematopoiesis can furnish and replenish this pool of proinflammatory monocytes that provide "early responders" to acutely injured tissues such as the infarcting myocardium.[24]

Further investigation identified specific hematopoietic factors that regulate this extramedullary hematopoiesis. Retention of hematopoietic progenitors in the spleen rely on the interaction of VLA-4 with vascular cell adhesion molecule-1 (VCAM-1), which is expressed by $CD169^+$ splenic macrophages. Ablation of these cells, or silencing of VCAM-1 using in vivo RNAi, leads to a loss of progenitor cells from the spleen.[25] In addition, post-MI splenic myelopoiesis depends on IL-1β. A recently recognized subpopulation of B lymphocytes, known as innate response activator B cells, elaborate the hematopoietic growth factors, such as granulocyte-monocyte colony stimulating factor, that engender extramedullary hematopoiesis in the context of atherosclerosis, and possibly in MI as well.[26] Cytokines unleashed during tissue injury (e.g., IL-1β) increase bone marrow hematopoietic stem cell proliferation after coronary artery ligation in mice by direct actions on hematopoietic cells and by modulating the microenvironment in the bone marrow niche.[27] Myeloid precursor cells that bear the chemokine receptor CCR2 appear to be pivotal to the development of macrophages in mouse MI that participate in tissue healing and influence the development of heart failure post-MI.[28]

Efforts to unravel further layers of the control of emergency leukopoiesis following coronary artery ligation in mice focused on the recruitment of precursors of the myeloid cells from niches in the bone marrow. These investigations revealed a hitherto unsuspected connection between activation of the sympathetic nervous system following coronary artery occlusion and mobilization of these progenitors of myeloid cells from the bone marrow.[29] The results implicated β_3 adrenergic activation of bone marrow niche cells as a stimulus that activates these precursors of leukocytes found in the myocardium during ischemic injury and the bone marrow. These studies elucidated a novel neuro-splenic-myocardial axis that operates during MI in mice (Figure 4-5).

"Cardiosplenic" Axis in Humans

Do these observations in mice relate to MI in humans? Although indirect, preliminary observations support the translatability of these concepts derived from mouse experiments to humans who are responding to stress and sustain an MI. The spleens of patients who have an MI contain more cells bearing markers of myeloid precursors (C-kit positive) that also manifest markers of mitosis (Ki67).[29] These observations indicate increased extramedullary hematopoiesis in the spleen of humans who have experienced MI. Humans hospitalized for acute MI who received treatment with β-adrenergic blocking agents before their event (in a nonrandomized allocation) had lower total leukocyte and monocyte counts in peripheral blood in a post hoc analysis. This observation, although subject to several types of confounding factors, supports a link between β-adrenergic signaling and leukocyte biology in humans.[29]

Studies of psychological stress produced experimentally both in mice and in medical residents subjected to emotional stress because of rotations in intensive care units showed increased peripheral leukocyte counts, and in the case of mice, leukopoiesis.[30] Finally, recent human observations supported the operation of a "cardiosplenic" axis in humans who experienced an acute MI.[31] Using fluorodeoxyglucose-18 (^{18}F-FDG) uptake as a marker of inflammatory

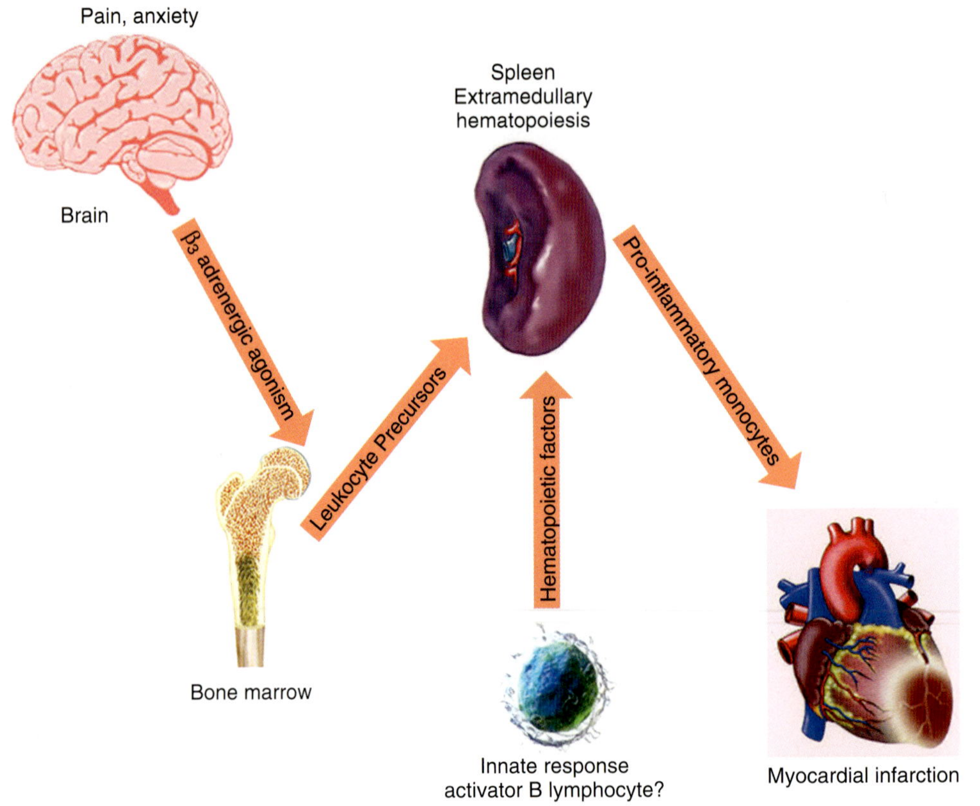

FIGURE 4-5 Activation of extra cardiac organs following myocardial infarction: a cardio-spleno-neuro-medullary network. Coronary ligation elicits a hyperadrenergic state caused by activation of the sympathetic nervous system in response to pain and hemodynamic alterations. β_3-adrenergic signaling can mobilize myeloid precursor cells from a bone marrow niche to the spleen where they can multiply in response to hematopoietic growth factors, some of which arise from innate response activator B cells. The spleen, in an angiotensin II–dependent manner in mice, can rapidly mobilize proinflammatory monocytes from a preformed pool to migrate to injured tissues (e.g., the infarcting myocardium) and engage in a first phase of tissue remodeling that may help to restore homeostasis. The myeloid precursor cells mobilized from bone marrow provide the precursors of mature leukocytes in the spleen where they undergo expansion by extramedullary hematopoiesis. Hematopoietic growth factors that promote the expansion of leukocyte populations may derive in part from innate response activator B cells.

activation, patients (n = 22) with an ACS and an equal number of sex-matched control subjects without ACS, but who had atherosclerotic disease, underwent positron emission tomography scanning to assess ^{18}F-FDG uptake. The spleens of ACS patients displayed a statistically significant increase in the ^{18}F-FDG signal compared with the control subjects (P = .03). These results corroborated the concept of altered splenic metabolic activity in patients with ACS. These investigators further retrospectively studied a cohort of approximately 500 patients who underwent ^{18}F-FDG imaging for various clinical indications. The investigators dichotomized this cohort into those who had splenic uptake of ^{18}F-FDG above or below the median. The analysis showed a striking and statistically significant increase in cardiovascular events in individuals who exhibited ^{18}F-FDG uptake above the median (P = .002). In this cohort, which was followed up for cardiovascular events, the ^{18}F-FDG uptake in various arteries correlated well with splenic uptake of ^{18}F-FDG. These findings supported the relationship between metabolic activity in the spleen and in arteries. These results, taken together, indicated an altered metabolism associated with macrophage activation, or perhaps even monocyte production, in the spleens of patients with ACS. They further corroborated the potential clinical implications of metabolic activity in the spleen of ACS patients. Further analyses indicated that messenger RNAs that encode a number of inflammation-related genes in the peripheral leukocytes of patients with ACS were correlated significantly with the uptake of ^{18}F-FDG in the spleen. The patients with above-median splenic ^{18}F-FDG uptake had significantly more cardiovascular events during follow-up in a post hoc analysis.

This ensemble of results supports the notion that MI elicits a systemic inflammatory response and can alter functions of remote organs (e.g., the spleen) that participate in the regulation of inflammation and immunity. The interruption of renin-angiotensin signaling by administration of angiotensin-converting enzyme inhibitors limits the recruitment of proinflammatory monocytes from the spleen to the infarcting myocardium in mice.[32] Thus, the observations that support the operation of a cardiosplenic axis in humans provides novel insight into the mechanisms by which existing therapies might modify MI. Similarly, some of the benefits observed in survivors of MI because of the administration of β-adrenergic blocking agents might result from modulation of leukopoiesis and the flux of inflammatory cells, as indicated by the animal experiments.

Areas of Ongoing Investigation

This blossoming of new knowledge regarding the roles of leukocytes in the healing of MI and previously unsuspected links between the central nervous system, the bone marrow, the spleen, and the ischemic myocardium represents a panel of new potential therapeutic targets for modifying outcomes after MI beyond restoration of blood flow or interventions to reduce the oxygen requirements of the myocardium. Initial forays into modifying the functions of leukocytes using nanoparticles that target receptors involved in recruiting proinflammatory subsets of leukocytes (the chemokine receptor CCR2) provide experimental validation of the concept that targeting leukocyte functions following MI might mitigate ischemic injury.[33]

The sequence of an initial recruitment of proinflammatory leukocytes and the subsequent appearance of less inflammatory leukocytes raises the question of the origin of the alternatively activated or less inflammatory subset of mononuclear phagocytes in the latter phases of response to acute ischemic injury to the myocardium. Do the less inflammatory cells arise because of a second wave of recruitment, caused perhaps by engagement of the chemokine receptors that help distinguish this less inflammatory subset from their proinflammatory counterparts? For example, the fractalkine receptor CX3CR1 exists at high levels on the less inflammatory monocytes, whereas the chemokine receptor CCR2 that responds to MCP-1/CCL2 predominates in the proinflammatory monocyte subset.[14,34,35] Alternatively, the proinflammatory cells could give rise to the less inflammatory subset by changing their functional palette. Recent experiments in mice support the possibility that proinflammatory monocytes serve as a precursor of the less inflammatory cells. In particular, a specific transcription factor, a member of the nuclear hormone receptor family known as nuclear receptor subfamily 4-group a-member 1 (Nr4a1), regulates a transition from proinflammatory monocytes to the reparative population. The Ly-6C^{low} macrophage population depends in part on activation of Nr4a1 (also known as Nur77).[36] Some Ly-6C^{high} monocytes that infiltrate the infarcting myocardium early will mature into cardiac macrophages. They can also give rise to the Ly-6C^{low} cells that then can multiply within the myocardium and expand the population of these mononuclear phagocytes that exert reparative functions. Animals deficient in Nr4a1 show an impaired transition of proinflammatory to reparative mononuclear phagocyte populations. They further show functional impairment as illustrated by accentuated declines in ejection fraction, increases in both systolic and diastolic dimensions, larger scars, and decreased collagen concentration. These results not only provide insight into the mechanisms by which the less inflammatory mononuclear phagocytes accumulate in the infarcting myocardium, but they also illustrate the functional importance of the sequence of monocyte subset populations in determining aspects of cardiac structure and function associated with outcomes in humans.

SUMMARY

In contrast to the venerable recognition of angina pectoris, the elucidation of the relationship between acute MI and coronary artery disease came about only a century ago. The initial fatalistic view that MI immediately produced irreversible injury gave way to an era of a more nuanced understanding of the pathophysiology of MI that has transformed clinical care by use of pharmacologic and mechanical interventions, most of which target improvements in the balance of oxygen supply and demand.

We have now entered a new area of understanding of the biological responses of the myocardium itself, and particularly the inflammatory cells, which are predominantly myeloid cells that populate the evolving infarct and likely critically influence the extent of tissue injury and the quantity and quality of myocardial healing. Harnessing these novel insights in the development of new therapies may help improve further outcomes in patients who have survived MIs.[37] In particular, because of advances in revascularization strategies and management of arrhythmias, more patients survive MIs. Yet, chronic impairment of ventricular function promotes the development of heart failure caused by ischemic cardiomyopathy. Perhaps manipulation of the inflammatory response during acute MI could help forestall the development of left ventricular dysfunction that fuels the growing epidemic of heart failure confronted by contemporary cardiology.

ACKNOWLEDGEMENTS

The authors thank F. J. Schoen, PhD, MD, and R. N. Mitchell, MD, PhD, for permission to adapt Figure 12-14 and Table 12-5 from Chapter 12 of *Pathologic Basis of Disease* (9e).

Classic References

Braunwald E: Thirteenth Bowditch lecture. The determinants of myocardial oxygen consumption, *Physiologist* 12:65–93, 1969.

Fye WB: *Classic papers on coronary thrombosis and myocardial infarction*. Birmingham, AL: The Classics of Cardiology Library; 1991.

Heberden W: *Commentaries on the history and cure of diseases*. London: Printed for T. Payne, Mews-Gate; 1802.

Herrick J: Certain clinical features of sudden obstruction of the coronary arteries, *Transactions of the American Association of Physicians* 27:100–116, 1912.

Herrick JB: *A Short History of Cardiology*, Springfield, MA., 1942, Charles C. Thomas.

Leibowitz J: *The history of coronary heart disease*, Berkeley, CA, 1970, University of California Press.

Levine SA: *Coronary thrombosis: its various clinical features*, Baltimore, 1929, The Williams & Wilkins Company.

Obrastzow WP, Straschesko ND: Zur Kenntnis der Thrombose der Koronararterien des Herzens, *Z Klin Med* 71:116–132, 1910.

Warren J: Remarks on angina pectoris, *New England Journal of Medicine and Surgery* 1:1–11, 1812.

References

1. Roberts W: Editorial: coronary thrombosis and fatal myocardial ischemia, *Circulation* 49:1–3, 1974.
2. Braunwald E: 50th anniversary historical article. Myocardial oxygen consumption: the quest for its determinants and some clinical fallout, *J Am Coll Cardiol* 34:1365–1368, 1999.
3. Braunwald E, et al.: Relief of angina pectoris by electrical stimulation of the carotid-sinus nerves, *N Engl J Med* 277:1278–1283, 1967.
4. Black J: Nobel lecture in physiology or medicine–1988. Drugs from emasculated hormones: the principle of syntopic antagonism, *In Vitro Cell Dev Biol* 25:311–320, 1989.
5. Braunwald E, Maroko PR, Libby P: Reduction of infarct size following coronary occlusion, *Circ Res* 35(Suppl 3):192–201, 1974.
6. Maroko P, et al.: Coronary artery reperfusion: I. Early effects on local myocardial function and the extent of myocardial necrosis, *J Clin Invest* 51:2710–2717, 1972.
7. Pfeffer MA, Pfeffer JM: Ventricular enlargement and reduced survival after myocardial infarction, *Circulation* 75:IV93–97, 1987.
8. Pfeffer JM, Pfeffer MA, Braunwald E: Influence of chronic captopril therapy on the infarcted left ventricle of the rat, *Circ Res* 57:84–95, 1985.
9. Falk E, et al.: Update on acute coronary syndromes: the pathologists' view, *Eur Heart J* 34:719–728, 2013.
10. Libby P: Mechanisms of acute coronary syndromes and their implications for therapy, *N Engl J Med* 368:2004–2013, 2013.
11. Mallory GK, White PD, Salcedo-Salgar J: The speed of healing of mycardial infarction: a study of the patholigic anatomy in seventy-two cases, *Am Heart J* 18:647–671, 1939.
12. Kroop IG, Shackman NH: The C-reactive protein determination as an index of myocardial necrosis in coronary artery disease, *Am J Med* 22:90–98, 1957.
13. Simpson PJ, et al.: Reduction of experimental canine myocardial reperfusion injury by a monoclonal antibody (anti-Mo1, anti-CD11b) that inhibits leukocyte adhesion, *J Clin Invest* 81: 624–629, 1988.
14. Swirski FK, Nahrendorf M: Leukocyte behavior in atherosclerosis, myocardial infarction, and heart failure, *Science* 339:161–166, 2013.
15. Weber C, Zernecke A, Libby P: The multifaceted contributions of leukocyte subsets to atherosclerosis: lessons from mouse models, *Nat Rev Immunol* 8:802–815, 2008.
16. Libby P, et al.: Diversity of denizens of the atherosclerotic plaque: not all monocytes are created equal, *Circulation* 117:3168–3170, 2008.
17. Libby P, Nahrendorf M, Swirski FK: Monocyte heterogeneity in cardiovascular disease, *Semin Immunopathol* 35:553–562, 2013.
18. Nahrendorf M, et al.: The healing myocardium sequentially mobilizes two monocyte subsets with divergent and complementary functions, *J Exp Med* 204:3037–3047, 2007.
19. Wan E, et al.: Enhanced efferocytosis of apoptotic cardiomyocytes through myeloid-epithelial-reproductive tyrosine kinase links acute inflammation resolution to cardiac repair after infarction, *Circ Res* 113:1004–1012, 2013.
20. Swirski FK, et al.: Ly-6Chi monocytes dominate hypercholesterolemia-associated monocytosis and give rise to macrophages in atheromata, *J Clin Invest* 117:195–205, 2007.
21. Panizzi P, et al.: Impaired infarct healing in atherosclerotic mice with Ly-6Chi monocytosis, *J Am Coll Cardiol* 55:1629–1638, 2010.
22. Weirather J, et al.: Foxp3+ CD4+ T cells improve healing after myocardial infarction by modulating monocyte/macrophage differentiation, *Circ Res* 115:55–67, 2014.
23. Swirski FK, et al.: Identification of splenic reservoir monocytes and their deployment to inflammatory sites, *Science* 325:612–616, 2009.
24. Leuschner F, et al.: Rapid monocyte kinetics in acute myocardial infarction are sustained by extramedullary monocytopoiesis, *J Exp Med* 209:123–137, 2012.
25. Dutta P, et al.: Macrophages retain hematopoietic stem cells in the spleen via VCAM-1, *J Exp Med* 212:497–512, 2015.

26. Hilgendorf I, et al.: Innate response activator B cells aggravate atherosclerosis by stimulating TH1 adaptive immunity, *Circulation* 129:1677–1687, 2014.
27. Sager HB, et al.: Targeting interleukin-1β reduces leukocyte production after acute myocardial infarction, *Circulation* 132:1880–1890, 2015.
28. Dutta P, et al.: Myocardial infarction activates CCR2(+) hematopoietic stem and progenitor cells, *Cell Stem Cell* 16:477–487, 2015.
29. Dutta P, et al.: Myocardial infarction accelerates atherosclerosis, *Nature* 487:325–329, 2012.
30. Heidt T, et al.: Chronic variable stress activates hematopoietic stem cells, *Nat Med* 20:754–758, 2014.
31. Emami H, et al.: Splenic metabolic activity predicts risk of future cardiovascular events: demonstration of a cardiosplenic axis in humans, *JACC Cardiovasc Imaging* 8:121–130, 2015.
32. Leuschner F, et al.: Angiotensin-converting enzyme inhibition prevents the release of monocytes from their splenic reservoir in mice with myocardial infarction, *Circ Res* 107:1364–1373, 2010.
33. Leuschner F, et al.: Silencing of chemokine (C-C motif) receptor 2 in myocarditis, *Eur Heart J* 36:1478–1488, 2015.
34. Gordon S: Macrophage heterogeneity and tissue lipids, *J Clin Invest* 117:89–93, 2007.
35. Jia T, et al.: Additive roles for MCP-1 and MCP-3 in CCR2-mediated recruitment of inflammatory monocytes during Listeria monocytogenes infection, *J Immunol* 180:6846–6853, 2008.
36. Hilgendorf I, et al.: Ly-6Chigh monocytes depend on Nr4a1 to balance both inflammatory and reparative phases in the infarcted myocardium, *Circ Res* 114:1611–1622, 2014.
37. Leuschner F, et al.: Therapeutic siRNA silencing in inflammatory monocytes in mice, *Nat Biotechnol* 29:1005–1010, 2011.

SECTION II

Initial Evaluation and Risk Stratification

5 Prehospital Assessment and Systems of Care

Timothy D. Henry and David C. Lange

CASE VIGNETTE

A 56-year-old riverboat captain experienced sudden onset of shortness of breath and diaphoresis at 1:30 AM while on his boat near Red Wing, Minnesota (Figure 5-e1). Emergency Medical Services (EMS) were activated from the boat, and at 2:26 AM, the first responders from the Red Wing Fire Department arrived on scene. At 2:38 AM, a 12-lead electrocardiogram (ECG) (Figure 5-e2) was obtained showing a large inferior-posterior ST-elevation consistent with ST-elevation myocardial infarction (STEMI). By 3:09 AM, a helicopter arrived to transport the patient to the Minneapolis Heart Institute Regional STEMI Center 55 miles away, in Minneapolis, Minnesota. The patient was loaded in the helicopter at 3:20 AM; treated with aspirin 325 mg, clopidogrel 600 mg, and a weight-based intravenous bolus of unfractionated heparin; and arrived at the STEMI center at 3:38 AM. He underwent emergent cardiac catheterization, which revealed a 100% thrombotic occlusion of the mid-right coronary artery (Figures 5-e3A and 5-e3B) and had a successful primary percutaneous coronary intervention (PPCI). Post-PPCI, his left ventricular ejection fraction was 65% with mild hypokinesis of the inferior wall. The prehospital ECG-to-device time was 101 minutes, and the door-to-device time was 41 minutes. He was discharged from the hospital the following day and was asymptomatic at 1-year follow-up.

In summary, a 56-year-old with acute onset of shortness of breath in the middle of the night, in the middle of the Minneapolis River, 55 miles from the nearest PPCI center, was able to receive guideline-directed medical therapy and PPCI in a timely fashion with an excellent outcome, as a result of a regionalized STEMI system with prespecified standardized protocols and transfer agreements in place.

INTRODUCTION

Nearly 500,000 Americans experience an acute STEMI each year in the United States (see Chapter 2). A decade ago, many of these patients did not receive appropriate treatment for this life-threatening condition. Approximately 30% of STEMI patients did not receive any form of reperfusion therapy (PPCI or fibrinolysis). Of those who underwent PPCI, only 40% were treated within the recommended time frame (medical contact-to-device time ≤90 minutes). For patients who received fibrinolytics, less than 50% met the recommended door-to-needle time of ≤30 minutes.[1,2] Care for STEMI patients has evolved dramatically over the past 30 years (see Chapter 13). The 1990s was a period of rapid evolution in STEMI care, from fibrinolytics to coronary angiography with balloon angioplasty, and subsequently, coronary stenting. However, it was not until the past decade that the systems for delivery of care became a focus of attention.

Regional STEMI systems of care have drastically changed the approach to health care delivery for acute coronary syndromes (ACS), providing access to PPCI for an increasing proportion of the population. This evolution has resulted in dramatic improvements in time to treatment (Figure 5-1) and cardiovascular outcomes (Figure 5-2).[1,3–7] Chapter 13 provides an overview of the principles of care for acute MI, including the critical relationship between time to treatment and outcomes in STEMI (see Figure 13-3). Selection among the approaches to reperfusion therapy is addressed in Chapter 14. Treatment with fibrinolytic therapy is discussed in Chapter 15, and PPCI is discussed in Chapter 17. In this chapter, we describe the design and implementation of complex regional systems of care and examine the individual components of any successful STEMI system of care that include: (1) rapid and thorough prehospital evaluation and triage, typically performed by EMS; (2) referring hospitals and clinics ("referral centers"); and (3) regional, tertiary care receiving centers capable of PPCI, preferably with surgical backup ("receiving centers") (Figure 5-3).

Although these critical elements of triage, transportation, referral centers, and receiving centers are integral components of a STEMI system, no two STEMI systems are alike. Diversity in geography, politics, and sociodemographics across the United States and throughout the world result in a wide variety of STEMI systems, which are all directed toward the same goal—to increase access to timely reperfusion with PPCI for STEMI by reducing delays inherent in systems of care (see also Chapter 13 and Figure 14-1). In the United States, current American College of Cardiology Foundation (ACCF)/American Heart Association (AHA) guidelines (see Figure 13-5) recommend EMS transportation of STEMI patients directly to a receiving center hospital for PPCI, with an ideal first medical contact to PPCI device (FMC-to-balloon) time goal of less than 90 minutes (class I, level of evidence B).[8] Furthermore, for patients presenting to a non–PPCI-capable hospital, immediate transfer to a receiving center hospital for PPCI is the recommend reperfusion strategy with a goal FMC-to-device time of less than 120 minutes (class I, level of evidence B).[8]

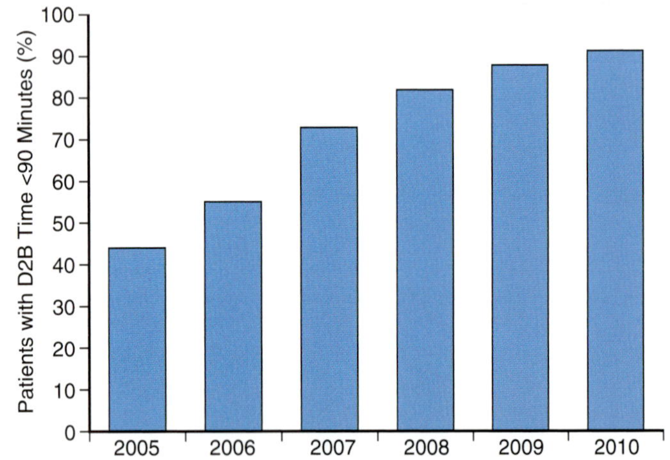

FIGURE 5-1 **Trends in door-to-balloon (D2B) time among U.S. hospitals (2005 to 2010) showing marked improvement in the percentage of patients with D2B time of less than 90 minutes.** *(From Krumholz H, et al: Improvements in door-to-balloon time in the United States, 2005 to 2010.* Circulation *124:1038–1045, 2011.)*

PREHOSPITAL EVALUATION

Evolution of Emergency Medical Services

The first U.S. Civilian ambulance service was formed in 1865 in Cincinnati, Ohio. It was comprised of local hospital interns who drove a horse-drawn carriage (Figure 5-e4). The first "rescue squad," designed to deliver basic first aid to civilians was formed in the late 1920s in Roanoke, Virginia. However, there were few advances in emergency care services until the late 1960s. In 1966, the National Academy of Sciences published a statement that many deaths in the United States were preventable and could be reduced through community education, safety standards, and prehospital coordination. This recognition, along with advances in the field of cardiopulmonary resuscitation (CPR) and management of out-of-hospital cardiac arrest (OHCA), served as the impetus for the first statewide EMS system in Maryland, thanks in large part to the efforts of R. Adams Cowley. In 1968, St. Vincent's Hospital in New York City built the nation's first mobile coronary care unit, staffed initially with physicians and later by paramedics. This unit was the first to evaluate and triage patients with cardiac complaints and included a portable, battery-powered cardiac monitor and defibrillator, as well as supplies for intravenous access, mobile oxygen, and medications. From here, the modern day EMS system was born. Today, EMS providers in the United States

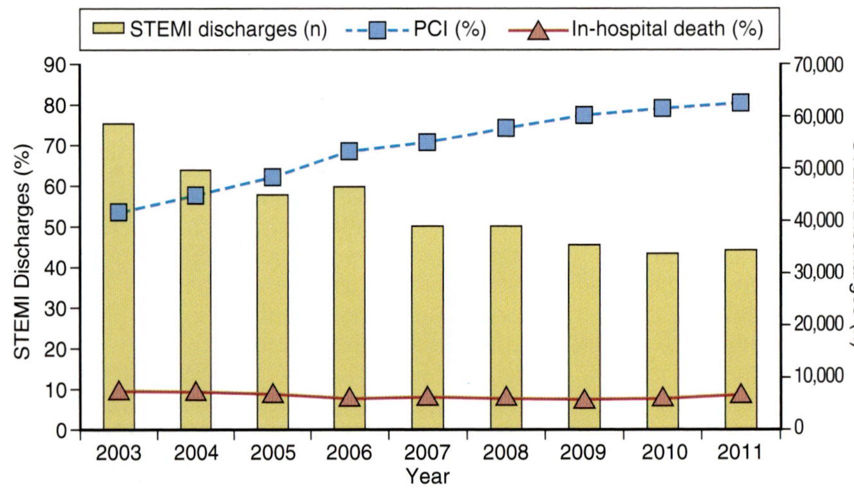

	2003	2004	2005	2006	2007	2008	2009	2010	2011
STEMI discharges (n)	58,644	49,515	44,840	46,238	39,014	38,910	35,292	33,619	34,182
PCI (%)	53.57	57.13	61.69	68.32	70.23	74.03	77.12	78.84	79.99
In-hospital death (%)	9.49	9.22	8.77	7.76	8.06	7.61	7.17	7.74	8.25

FIGURE 5-2 **Trends in U.S. ST-elevation myocardial infarction (STEMI) care from 2003 to 2011. Use of primary PCI increased to 80% with decreasing mortality.** *PCI, percutaneous coronary intervention. (From Shah RU, et al: Increasing percutaneous coronary interventions for ST-segment elevation myocardial infarction in the United States.* J Am Coll Cardiol Intv *8:139–146, 2015.)*

care for an estimated 22 million patients per year. The incorporation of various vehicles, including ambulance vans, helicopters, and airplanes, has allowed for rapid mobilization and transportation of patients over great distances in short periods of time.

With the development of formal EMS systems throughout the country, the framework was in place to build complex regional systems of care for a variety of medical conditions. The first systems of care were designed for trauma patients and acute cardiovascular emergencies, such as STEMI and stroke. The integration of EMS and the incorporation of the prehospital phase for ACS evaluation and diagnosis are integral components of any regionalized STEMI system of care. EMS providers and other first responders have four primary responsibilities: (1) prehospital evaluation, (2) treatment, (3) triage, and (4) transfer (Figure 5-4).

Prehospital Systems

The prehospital evaluation should consist of a focused history and physical examination, including a complete assessment of vital signs and a prehospital 12-lead electrocardiogram (PHECG). Earlier STEMI diagnosis based on the PHECG facilitates in-hospital STEMI treatment.[9–11] Hospitals with the shortest door-to-balloon (D2B) times are those that have incorporated prehospital STEMI diagnosis with pre-activation of the cardiac catheterization laboratory (CCL). This strategy requires a multidisciplinary team approach in which either the emergency physician or specially trained EMS providers activate the CCL without cardiology consultation.[12]

However, the rapid transport of STEMI patients to the nearest PPCI-capable facility may be limited by several factors.[15] First, only a minority (≤5%) of EMS transported patients with chest pain actually have STEMI. Second, an inadequate number (~50%) of EMS systems have PHECG capabilities.[15,16] Third, in some regions a mandate still exists for transport of patients with suspected STEMI to the nearest facility, even if that facility does not provide PPCI. Fourth, evolution toward a more integrated process of prehospital care is complicated by the fact that there are 329 different EMS regions in the United States, with more than 993 hospital-based EMS systems.[15] Remarkably, hospital-based EMS systems represent only 6.5% of all EMS providers, with the remainder comprised of private, third party systems (48.6%) and fire station–based systems (44.9%).

Integrated Emergency Medical Systems

Although the transport time to a specialized PPCI center may appear long, the benefits outweigh the drawbacks when an integrated EMS system incorporates pre-notification, termed "parallel processing." Some have proposed doubling the allotted transport time for suspected STEMI patients, to allow transportation of these patients directly to a "center of excellence," where the target D2B time is ≤60 minutes. Process efficiency can be achieved only through an integrated system for STEMI care that incorporates the PHECG for earlier diagnosis, expedited triage, and readily available, rehearsed transport systems. A more uniform evolution toward integrated STEMI care has been impeded by a lack of funding, diverging incentives, a lack of coordinated objectives, and at times, competing strategies. For example, in many regions, particularly those without state-regulated certificate of need requirements, there has been a proliferation of new catheterization laboratories for the provision of PPCI without regard for PPCI volume or surgical backup.[17] Conversely, other regions have developed integrated EMS systems that focus on prehospital diagnosis, triage, and transfer to an established center of excellence proficient in both primary and elective PCI.[18–20] Although expansion of PPCI-capable centers can improve access to care, more efficient use of existing PPCI centers through prehospital–EMS integration has been proven to be a more cost-effective strategy. Only recently have sophisticated modeling techniques been used to compare the relative efficacy and/or cost of these competing strategies for the care of STEMI patients.[21] Importantly, a strategy focused on EMS integration, prehospital diagnosis, triage, and transportation with more effective use of existing PPCI facilities was found to be more effective

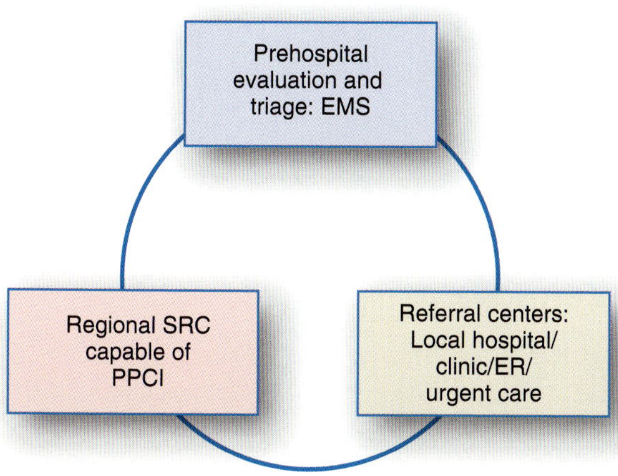

FIGURE 5-3 Components of a successful system-of-care for ST-elevation myocardial infarction (STEMI). *EMS*, Emergency medical services; *ER*, emergency room; *PPCI*, primary percutaneous coronary intervention; *SRC*, STEMI-receiving center.

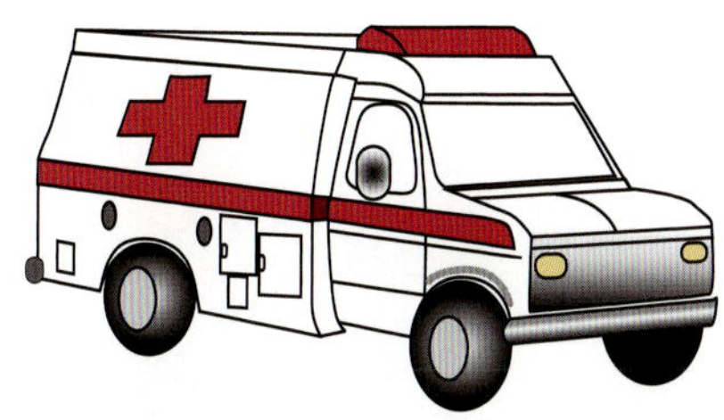

Evaluate	• Focused history and exam, including vital signs • Prehospital 12-lead ECG
Treat	• Per standardized protocols: aspirin, $P2Y_{12}$ receptor antagonist
Triage	• PPCI-capable center for all STEMIs
Transfer	• From field to closest PPCI-capable center • From "referral center" to "receiving center"

FIGURE 5-4 The four major responsibilities of EMS providers in a regional ST-elevation myocardial infarction (STEMI) receiving center (SRC) network. *ECG*, Electrocardiogram; *EMS*, emergency medical services; *PPCI*, primary percutaneous coronary intervention.

and less costly than a strategy of creating new PPCI facilities[21] (Figure 5-e5).

The coordination of strategies, as well as the integration of essential prehospital and in-hospital resources for ACS care on the state level has been the focus of the AHA Mission: Lifeline initiative, which was created as a response to missed opportunities for prompt, appropriate STEMI treatment.[15] The Mission: Lifeline goal is to improve outcomes for STEMI patients by building integrated care networks through community outreach, training, and education of civilians and EMS personnel. The AHA Mission: Lifeline also provides a blueprint for hospitals and administrators to implement systems of care. At present, approximately 65% of U.S. citizens have access to a Mission: Lifeline system of care, the number of which has increased greatly over the past decade (Figure 5-5).[2]

Although the AHA's Mission: Lifeline has been instrumental in the proliferation of STEMI systems of care throughout the country, the ACC's Door-to-Balloon Alliance sought to improve D2B times in PPCI hospitals. The D2B Alliance was launched in 2006, in partnership with the Institute for Healthcare Improvement. This Alliance provided hospitals with evidence-based strategies and supporting tools needed to reduce D2B times through a focus on process improvement, parallel processing, and interdisciplinary collaboration. The keys to reducing D2B times are (1) the emergency department (ED) physician (or EMS PHECG) activates the CCL, (2) one call activates the entire team, (3) the CCL team is ready within 30 minutes of receiving the activation call, (4) prompt data feedback, and (5) a team-based approach with commitment from all levels. When launched, the initial goal was to achieve D2B times of ≤90 minutes for 75% of STEMI patients presenting to a PPCI facility. In the decade since its inception, the D2B Alliance has facilitated dramatic improvements in D2B times across the country (see Figure 5-1).[1,22,23] Through the efforts of these organizations, as well as the individual efforts of countless nurses, doctors, administrators, and EMS providers, the STEMI receiving network system of care model has blossomed both domestically and abroad.

SYSTEMS OF CARE IN PRACTICE

ST-Elevation Myocardial Infarction Systems of Care: The European Experience

The rapid restoration of normal coronary blood flow, via pharmacological and/or mechanical recanalization of an occluded coronary artery, limits the extent of myocardial necrosis and reduces the mortality of patients who present with STEMI (see Figure 13-3). PPCI has demonstrated more frequent, complete, and durable coronary reperfusion in both randomized controlled clinical trials and observational studies (see Chapter 14 and Chapter 17). For these reasons, PPCI is the preferred revascularization modality as long as an experienced operator can provide it in a timely manner (Figure 5-6; also see Figure 13-5).[8,24] On the basis of these principles, the first randomized controlled trials, which compared long-distance transport to PPCI centers with primary fibrinolysis performed at local hospitals, were performed in Europe in the early 2000s.[25] Overall, these studies, which are discussed in Chapter 14, demonstrated that transferring patients with STEMI to a tertiary angioplasty facility could be both safe and effective. In context, transfer-related delays were generally more than 1 hour and FMC-to-device times were more than 2 hours (Figures 5-e6A and 5-e6B and 5-e7A and 5-e7B). Transfer-related delays that prolong the time for initiation of

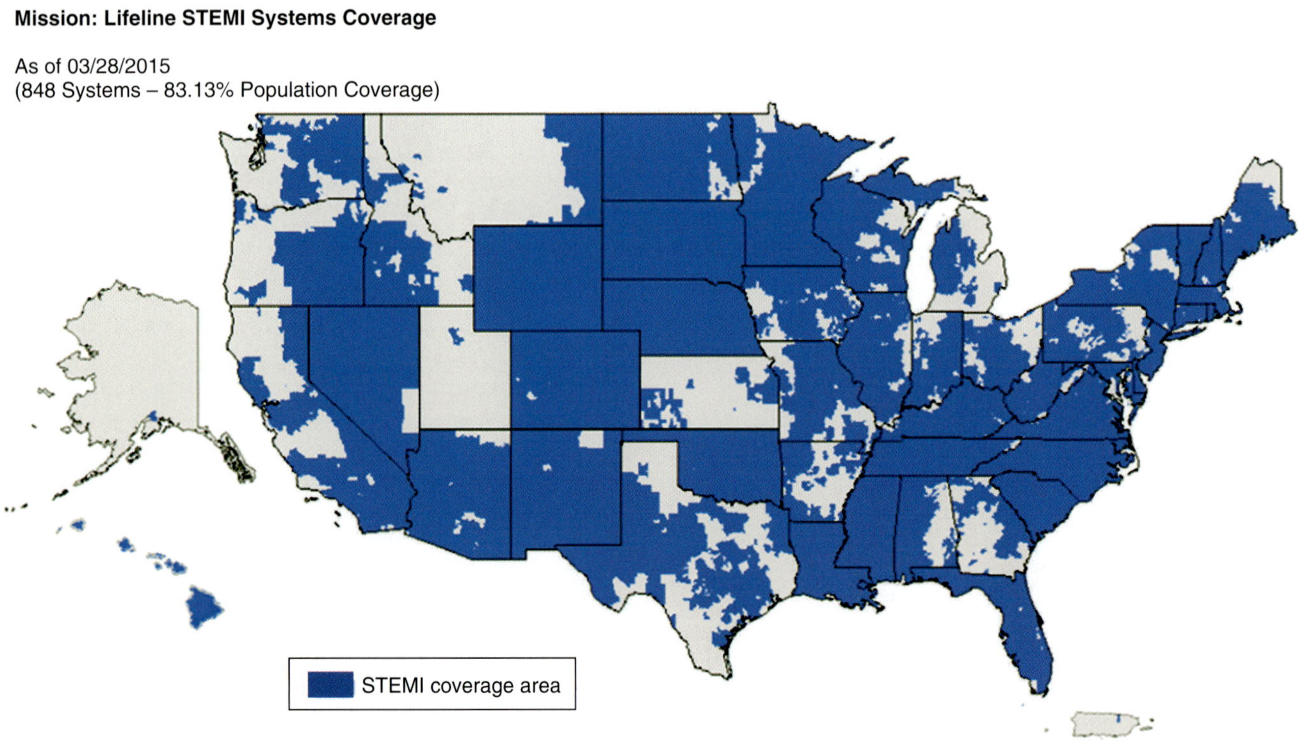

FIGURE 5-5 Mission: Lifeline coverage map. All system data, including coverage area, are self-reported data. Note: Cardiac Resuscitation Coverage Areas listed are also indicative of an ST-elevation myocardial infarction (STEMI) system in place. Mission: Lifeline does not recognize Cardiac Resuscitation Systems that are not also associated with an active STEMI System. *(Source: American Heart Association. Centers for Disease Control and Prevention, National Center for Health Statistics: Compressed mortality file 1999-2006. CDC Wonder Online Database. ICD10 121-122, 2015.)*

reperfusion by more than 90 minutes appear to favor fibrinolytic therapy (see Chapter 14 and Figure 14-9).[26–28]

Contemporary STEMI systems of care in Europe include the VIENNA STEMI network and the SAMU system in Paris.[29] The former is based on a rotational call between the only two high-volume PPCI centers available. In the latter, physicians routinely staff the ambulances and initiate prehospital care. A pharmaco-invasive strategy that uses prehospital fibrinolytic therapy is commonly used in these two systems, particularly for patients presenting early after STEMI (<3 hours).[26–29] These and other international STEMI systems of care are summarized in Table 14-e1.

Despite the results of these trials, many were pessimistic that such a system would work within the construct of U.S. health care because of geographic, political, and financial barriers. In addition, the only U.S. STEMI transfer trial (air-PAMI) reported a total median D2B of 155 minutes with equivocal results, although the trial was small and underpowered.[25]

ST-Elevation Myocardial Infarction Systems of Care: The United States

In the early 2000s, there was mounting evidence that STEMI care within the United States was inadequate. In 2004, the ACC/AHA guidelines for the care of STEMI patients made a class I, level of evidence B recommendation that "the delay from patient contact with the healthcare system (typically, arrival at the Emergency Department (ED) or contact with EMS) to initiation of fibrinolytic therapy should be less than 30 minutes" (Figure 5-6; also see Figure 13-5). Alternatively, if PPCI was chosen, "the delay from patient contact with the health care system (typically, arrival at the ED or contact with EMS) to balloon inflation should be less than 90 minutes." This marked the first time such a recommendation regarding the timing of reperfusion appeared in the ACC/AHA guidelines.[8] Despite this strong recommendation, data from the National Registry of Myocardial Infarction revealed that D2B times in the United States were too slow, in particular for patients who were transferred for PPCI. With a median D2B time of 180 minutes, only 15% of transfer patients achieved a D2B time of less than 120 minutes, and only 4% of patients had a D2B time that met the recommended standard of less than 90 minutes. In 2006, the Institute of Medicine (IOM) published a report titled "Hospital Based-Emergency Care: At the Breaking Point." In this report, the IOM concluded that overcrowding of emergency rooms, as well as "fragmented" care and inaccessibility of specialists were the largest barriers to improving emergency medical care. The IOM called for drastic changes in coordination of care, policy, funding, and research practices.

Fortunately, despite the many obstacles, there were firm believers in the potential of STEMI systems that were willing to invest incredible time, energy, and resources into building functional STEMI systems within the United States. In 2003, the Minneapolis Heart Institute (MHI) at Abbott Northwestern Hospital began to build one of the first regional STEMI systems in the United States. The system was modeled after successful regional trauma systems and was built on the premise that accelerated diagnosis, streamlined processes, and standardized care protocols were the keys to implementing and maintaining a successful STEMI system within the United States. The MHI system functioned as a "wheel-and-spoke" model, with MHI at the center of the system. Referral hospitals and clinics within a 60-mile

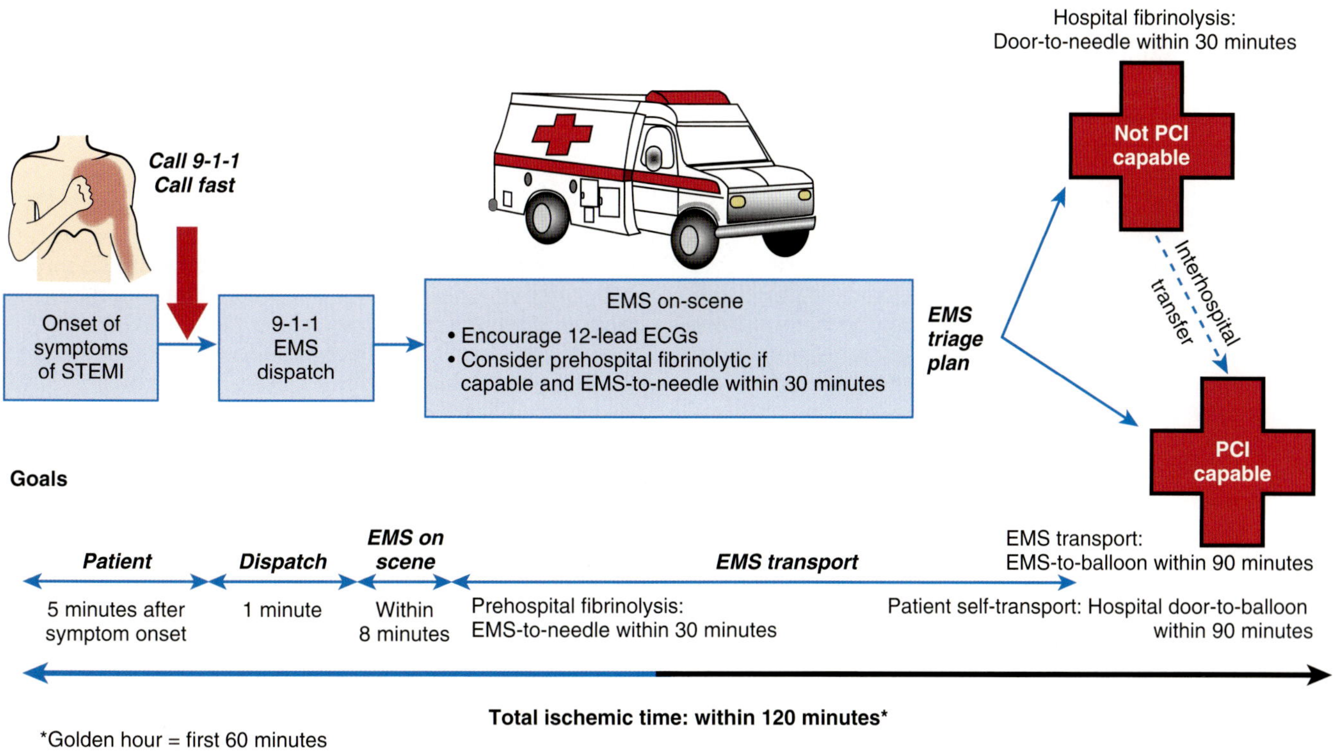

FIGURE 5-6 Goals for early reperfusion therapy. Patients are encouraged to call 911 no later than 5 minutes after the onset of symptoms. Emergency medical services (EMS) is encouraged to perform a prehospital 12-lead electrocardiogram (ECG), and in some instances, administer prehospital fibrinolytics. Patients should be preferentially transported to a percutaneous coronary intervention (PCI)-capable hospital when possible, often bypassing a non-PCI hospital, with an EMS-to-balloon time of less than 90 minutes. If transported to a non-PCI hospital, that facility may administer fibrinolytics with a door-to-needle time of less than 30 minutes or transfer to a PCI-capable hospital. The goal is a total ischemic time of less than 120 minutes. *STEMI*, ST-elevation myocardial infarction. *(From Vavalle JP, Granger CB: The need for regional integrated care for ST-segment myocardial infarction.* Circulation *124:851–856, 2011.)*

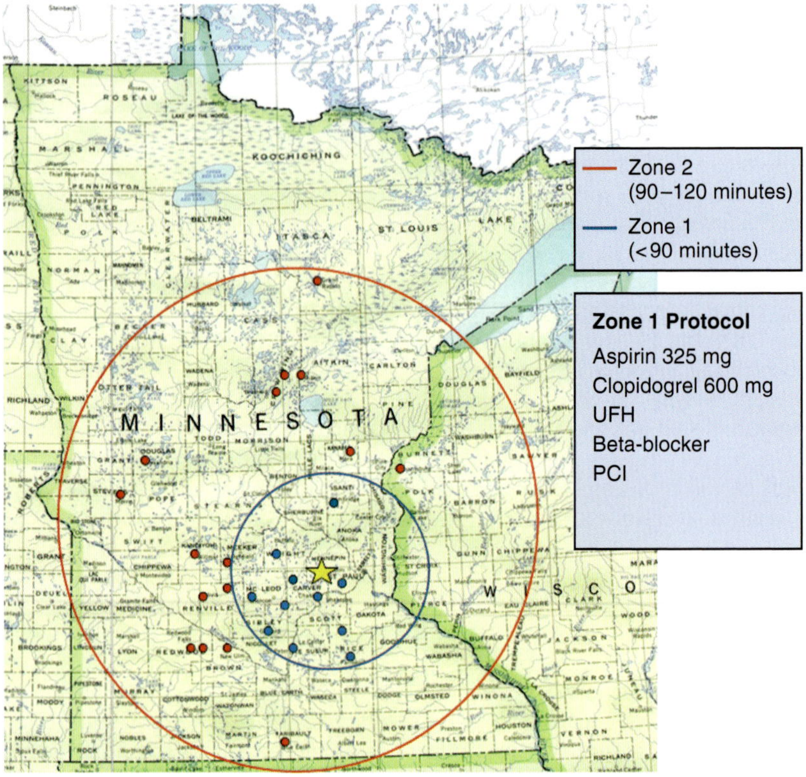

FIGURE 5-7 Map of Minnesota with the primary percutaneous coronary intervention (PPCI) center in Minneapolis (*star*), Zone 1 hospitals (<60 miles from PPCI hospital) (*blue circle*), and Zone 2 hospitals (60 to 210 miles from PCI hospital) (*red circle*). The pharmacological protocols for the PPCI center and Zone 1 hospitals are shown. See text for discussion of the Zone 2 protocol. *UFH*, Unfractionated heparin. *(From Minneapolis Heart Institute, Minneapolis, Minnesota.)*

radius of MHI were considered Zone 1, with a standardized protocol that included evidence-based adjunctive medications (aspirin, clopidogrel, weight-based intravenous bolus of unfractionated heparin, and intravenous β-blockers) and a prespecified transfer plan from each site. The regional STEMI-system grew quickly and expanded to Zone 2, which included referral hospitals within a 60- to 210-mile radius, using a similar standardized protocol with the addition of one-half dose of intravenous tenecteplase and immediate transfer to MHI for pharmaco-invasive PCI (Figure 5-7; see Chapter 14).[18,27,30] In addition to the standardized protocol, the MHI group placed high priority on gathering data for quality assurance purposes and feedback. Through the next several years, the MHI group was able to demonstrate marked improvements in a variety of outcomes, including death, re-infarction, stroke, and length of hospital stay.

Within the next 5 years, regional systems of care for STEMI patients were developed throughout the United States (Figure 5-8).[31] These systems were built individually and tailored to the unique political, geographical, and socioeconomic landscapes of the various regions. Some were built in a wheel-and-spoke fashion similar to MHI, whereas others were built more as a "web" network, with multiple different tertiary centers serving as hubs for PPCI in the area (Figures 5-e8A and 5-e8B; also see Table 14-e1). Despite their differences in structure, organization, and providers, these systems demonstrated a combined rate of D2B time of ≤90 minutes in 86% of STEMI patients (see Figure 5-8).[31] In addition, each region individually surpassed the ACC's D2B Alliance benchmark of more than 75% of STEMI cases achieving D2B of ≤90 minutes.[31] Thus, these systems were able to demonstrate that, through a variety of models, regional STEMI Receiving Center Networks were able to provide diverse communities with timely access to quality STEMI care (see Figures 5-8A and 5-8B).

Importantly, these systems were not formed solely from preselected, high-performing centers. For example, in Los Angeles County (LAC), less than 50% of STEMI patients had a D2B time of ≤90 minutes before the implementation of the LAC STEMI receiving network. Within 1 month of implementing the STEMI network, more than 90% of the STEMI patients had a D2B time of ≤90 minutes (see Figure 5-e8B).[31] To effectively triage patients to the appropriate hospital (STEMI Receiving Center vs. closest available hospital), LAC became one of the first STEMI systems to integrate PHECGs into the EMS care plan, with the computer read determining the destination of patient triage.

In North Carolina, collaborators built the first statewide STEMI system, which included both PPCI and fibrinolytic-based strategies (Figure 5-e9).[19] Through this integrated approach, the RACE providers were able to demonstrate significant improvements in reperfusion rates and time-to-treatment metrics. Outcome data trended toward improvement as well, but these measures did not reach statistical significance.

Professional Society Guidelines

The successes in Minnesota, North Carolina, and California were replicated across the United States and contributed to a change in the ACCF/AHA Guidelines for STEMI patients. Current guidelines give a class I, level of evidence B recommendation that "all communities should create and maintain a regional system of STEMI care."[8] The same level of recommendation is given for performance of a 12-lead ECG by EMS personnel.[8] The AHA Mission: Lifeline and the ACC D2B Alliance played

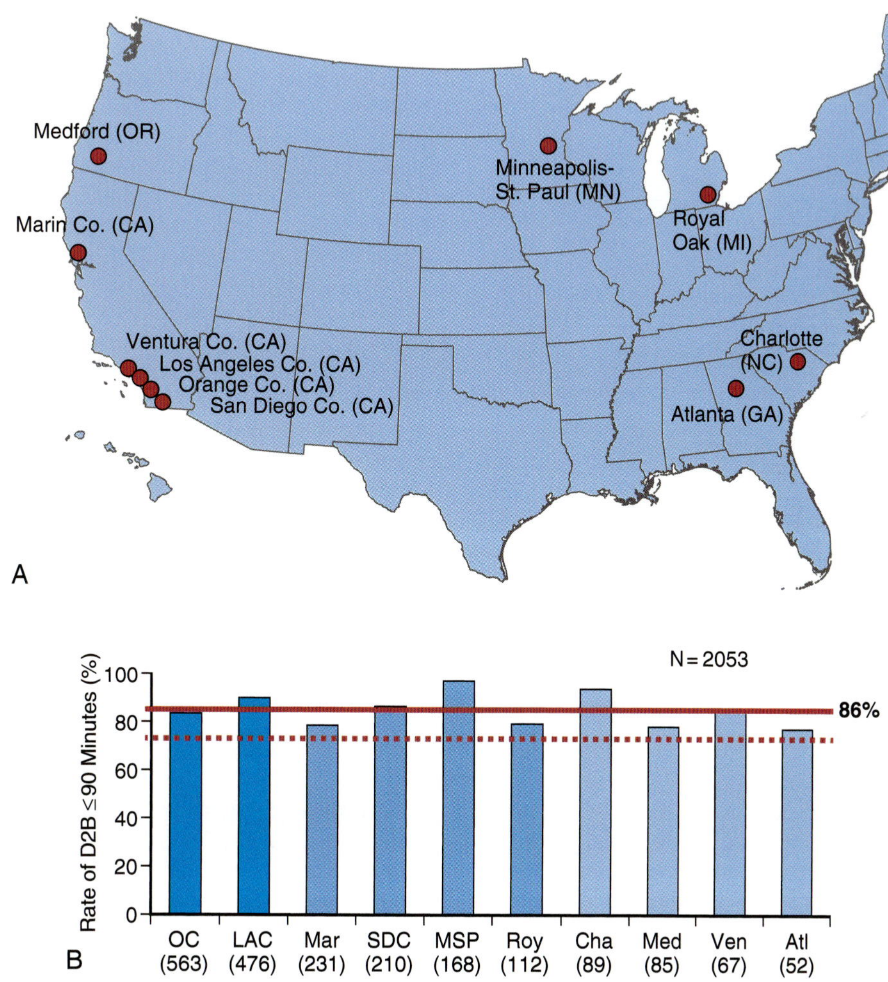

FIGURE 5-8 (**A**) U.S. ST-elevation myocardial infarction (STEMI) Receiving Networks in 2009. (**B**) Rate of door-to-balloon (D2B) time ≤90 minutes in U.S. STEMI-Receiving Networks in 2009 on the basis of total number of patients in each region who had a prehospital electrocardiogram (+) for STEMI and underwent primary percutaneous coronary intervention through August 31, 2007. Regional databases with more than 400, 400 to 100, and less than 100 primary percutaneous coronary intervention patients are denoted in *dark blue, blue,* and *light blue*, respectively. The *dashed red line* represents D2B Alliance benchmark rate of 75%. The *solid red line* denotes 86% rate of D2B ≤90 minutes for all 10 regions combined (n = 2053). *(From Rokos IC, et al: Integration of pre-hospital electrocardiograms and ST-elevation myocardial infarction receiving (SRC) networks: impact on door-to-balloon times across 10 independent regions.* J Am Coll Cardiol Cardiovasc Intv *2:339–346, 2009.)*

crucial roles in the growth and expansion of STEMI systems of care. The successes of regional STEMI systems has stimulated the application of new systems of care for other cardiovascular emergencies, including OHCA, aortic dissection, and stroke.[32]

UNITED STATES CARDIOVASCULAR SYSTEMS OF CARE: THE CURRENT LANDSCAPE

The Mission: Lifeline program has established criteria for EMS, referral centers, and receiving centers.[2] The PPCI center must have a CCL with staffing available to perform PPCI 24 hours a day, 7 days a week, 365 days a year. These centers should be able to perform PPCI in a timely fashion and should meet the ACC's D2B Alliance criteria of having a D2B time of ≤90 minutes in at least 75% of nontransfer STEMI patients. These centers must be capable of providing supportive care on-site for STEMI and its complications; however, surgical backup is not required at all sites. For PPCI centers without on-site surgical backup, these centers should have a standing agreement in place with a tertiary care center that has 24-hour surgical support available. PPCI center administrators must demonstrate adequate support and oversight of the PPCI center performance, including, but not limited to, having a multidisciplinary team that performs ongoing quality assurance review. The PPCI center should have a robust and ongoing program in support of continuing medical education. The PPCI centers should meet current ACC/AHA program requirements, including performing (as an institution) at least 36 PPCIs and a total of at least 400 PCIs per year. The PPCI STEMI program should be clearly described in the institution's manual of operations, and the PPCI center must have mechanisms in place for monitoring and improving the performance of the program (Table 5-1).[2]

In addition to these institutional requirements, the interventional cardiologists of the PPCI center should meet the current ACC/AHA guidelines for competency in PPCI, which include at least 11 PPCIs annually and a total of at least 75 PCIs per year. Furthermore, these physicians and staff should have a formal call schedule that clearly delineates who is responsible for on-hours and after-hours care of STEMI (see Table 5-1).[2]

The Ideal System of Care Network

There are certain key features that are common among successful systems of care.[33] The success of any system of care is predicated upon the performance and the

TABLE 5-1 Requirements of an SRC PPCI Center: Institutional and Physician

Institutional
PCI available 24/7/365
PCI performed as soon as possible (DTB Alliance goal, 75%; DTB <90 min)
Able to provide supportive care on-site for STEMI and complications
• Agreement with tertiary care center for any PPCI center that does not have surgical backup on-site
Commitment by hospital administration in support of SRC program participation
• Mechanisms for monitoring program performance
• Multidisciplinary team for quality assurance review
CME program
ACC/AHA program requirements: 36 PPCI and 400 total PCI per year
PPCI program described in a manual of operations
Physician
Interventionalists should meet ACC/AHA guidelines for competency: 11 PPCIs per year and 75 total PCIs per year
Formal on-call schedule

ACC/AHA, American College of Cardiology/American Heart Association; *CME*, continuing medical education; *DTB*, Door-to-Balloon; *PPCI*, primary percutaneous coronary intervention; *SRC*, STEMI Receiving Center; *STEMI*, ST-elevation myocardial infarction.
From American Heart Association: Mission: Lifeline, *2015. http://www.heart.org/HEARTORG/HealthcareResearch/MissionLifelineHomePage/LearnAboutMissionLifeline/STEMI-Systems-of-Care_UCM_439065_SubHomePage.jsp.*

commitment of its individual members. This committed membership includes the general public, EMS personnel, physicians, and allied health professionals at both the referral centers and receiving centers. In the ideal system of care, the patients and community members would recognize the signs and symptoms of a cardiac emergency and appropriately respond by activating EMS (via 911) immediately. Automated external defibrillators should be available in public places and should be intuitive enough to be used by both lay people and medical professionals. If appropriate, the public would recognize the need for and would initiate CPR. These objectives can only be achieved through community outreach and education.

The ideal EMS agency would have standardized "point-of-entry" protocols that clearly delineate which patients should be transported to the nearest referral hospital and which patients should be transported to the nearest receiving hospital. This decision-making would be based, in part, on the acquisition, interpretation, and transmission of a PHECG. Successful implementation of such protocols is dependent not just on the acquisition of the PHECG, but the accurate interpretation followed by appropriate activation of the CCL. This goal can be accomplished by a computer algorithm with or without EMS overread or by transmission to the receiving center. These protocols are ideally created through the joint efforts of EMS personnel, emergency physicians, cardiologists, hospital administrators, and staff. They should be supported by the payers and administrators within the system. For patients who self-present to a referral center, EMS activation via 911 should occur to facilitate rapid transport of these patients to a receiving facility that can provide definitive therapy (see Figure13-5). In systems where PPCI is not available at all or in a timely fashion, the use of fibrinolytics as reperfusion therapy should be included as an alternative in the protocol (see Figure 14-12).

In an ideal system of care, the referring hospitals should also have standardized point-of-entry protocols that clearly delineate which patients should be transferred to a referral center based on patient-specific risk criteria, indications and contraindications to alternative therapies, and the proximity to the nearest receiving center. Furthermore, these centers should have integrated plans for the return of patients to their local community hospitals and care centers for pre- and postdischarge follow-up care. The referral centers should have mechanisms that promote efficient transfer of data (medical records, study results, and so on) to the receiving centers for purposes of continuity of care and to avoid redundancies in the system. Referral and receiving centers should have standardized protocols in place to ensure the efficient delivery of evidenced-based therapies for all patients, while minimizing variability in the delivery of care.

The ideal receiving center must have the facilities, expertise, equipment, and training to administer definitive therapy for each acute cardiovascular condition. These centers should meet minimal performance guidelines and should be involved in ongoing assessment and quality improvement efforts. These receiving centers should also have mechanisms to promote efficient transfer of data (medical records, study results, and so on) back to the referral centers to promote continuity of care and avoid redundancies in the system. They should also follow standardized protocols to minimize variability in the delivery of evidence-based care and should clearly and consistently promote bidirectional feedback between the various members of the system.

In addition to these individual components, the ideal system of care should have common features that are applicable to all members and components of the system itself. First, all members of the system must share a sense of teamwork and singular common purpose—to provide the highest quality care in the timeliest fashion possible. To do this, system members must share a mutual respect for each individual player and must understand that for the system to succeed, each member plays a critical role. Every member of the team is crucial, and improvements to the system require input and leadership at every level. The need for education, training, and retraining cannot be underestimated because of the large number of people involved and ongoing changes in both personnel and new data.

Standardized protocols and order sets designed by use of guideline-based therapies ensure that the highest percentage of eligible patients receive the highest quality care. However, the same system needs to allow flexibility to address the individual needs of patients and physicians. Systems must be activated in a timely and uniform fashion; a single phone call or page should alert all pertinent members of the system to provide any pertinent updates on the patient's condition and status. All parties within the system would ideally be involved in ongoing data collection and research for quality assurance and improvement purposes. Feedback is a key component; this could include the transporting paramedics observing an angiogram, the interventional cardiologist calling the ED physician immediately following the procedure, and communication the following day among the system coordinators, EMS, and ED managers. The primary cardiologist should communicate with the primary care physician as well. Monthly, quarterly, and yearly quality reports provide ongoing and system-wide quality improvement. Financial and moral support from hospital administration is essential, and if missing, can create a major stumbling block. Perhaps the most important link in the chain is a passionate leader at every level.[33]

Systems of Care: Successes and Advantages

The advantages to a "systems of care" approach include increased access to tertiary care for patients with complex, high-risk conditions (Table 5-2).[32] This access decreases the number of "eligible but untreated" patients in a wide geographic region. Standardized protocols within systems of care improve time to treatment, including FMC-to-device time, while also providing clear communication and expectations for patients based on their point-of-entry. Furthermore, systems of care have consistently shown improvements in important outcomes, including all-cause mortality, cardiovascular mortality, re-infarction, stroke, and length of hospitalization.[34] STEMI systems are now being implemented throughout the world with consistently positive results.[29,35,36]

Systems of Care: Current Challenges, Gaps, and Barriers

Terkelsen and colleagues introduced the idea of "system delays," which focuses on the time from FMC to the initiation of reperfusion therapy (see Figure 14-1).[37] They performed a retrospective analysis of 6209 patients with STEMI or bundle branch block MI who were admitted for PCI between 2002 and 2008 using public medical databases from Western Denmark; they found that systems delays were independently associated with a 10% increase in long-term mortality for every 60-minute time interval of delay (Figure 5-9).[37] The authors argued that outcomes based on symptom onset to reperfusion were subject to selection bias, information bias, recall bias, and confounding, whereas the total system delay provided a modifiable target that might improve clinical outcomes.[37]

Systems Delays

A major challenge for STEMI systems is the total D2B time for patients who are transferred from a referral hospital. "Door-in-door-out" (DIDO) time at the referral hospitals appears to be the major system delay and is a well-identified target for improvement. Wang and colleagues studied more than 14,000 patients between 2007 and 2010 using the "Action Get with the Guidelines" registry and found that the median DIDO time was 68 minutes (interquartile range, 43 to 120 minutes). Only 11% of patients had DIDO times of less than 30 minutes (Figure 5-10A).[38] Furthermore, longer DIDO times were associated with increased mortality (see Figure 5-10B).[38] Similarly, Herrin and colleagues reviewed 2009 Centers for Medicare and Medicaid data and found that the median DIDO time was 66 minutes, and only 9.7% of patients had DIDO times of less than 30 minutes.[39]

System delays are heterogeneous in terms of their duration and association with outcomes. Miedema and colleagues described the frequency, magnitude, and clinical impact of specific delays in 2034 STEMI patients transferred for PPCI (Figure 5-11).[30] The most frequent delays occurred at the referral hospital and were related to awaiting transport and ED delay. The longest delays were related to nondiagnostic initial ECGs and diagnostic dilemmas, but the delays that had clinical impact were related to cardiac arrest and cardiogenic shock. Frequently, the cardiac arrest and/or shock was the cause of the delay rather than a result of the delay (Table 5-3).[30]

TABLE 5-2 Advantages and Successes of ST-Elevation Myocardial Infarction Systems of Care

Improve access to tertiary care facilities
Decrease the number of "eligible, but untreated" patients
Shorter time-to-treatment through standardized protocols
Improved patient outcomes, including all-cause mortality, cardiovascular mortality, reinfarction, stroke, and length of hospitalization

From American Heart Association: Mission: Lifeline, *2015. http://www.heart.org/HEARTORG/HealthcareResearch/MissionLifelineHomePage/LearnAboutMissionLifeline/STEMI-Systems-of-Care_UCM_439065_SubHomePage.jsp.*

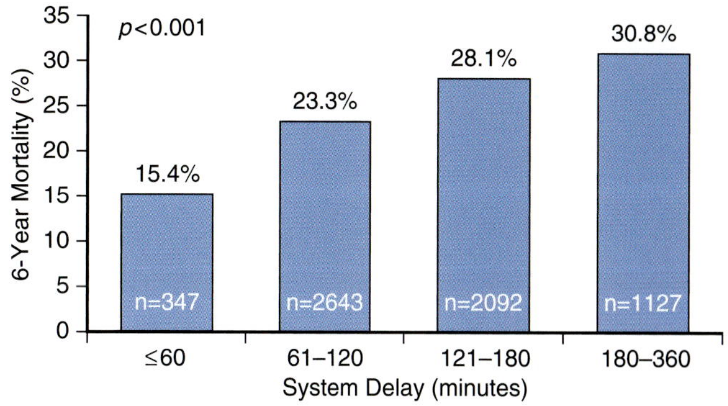

FIGURE 5-9 Mortality based on duration of system delay in ST-elevation myocardial infarction. (From Terkelsen CJ, Sorensen JT, Maeng M, et al: System delay and mortality among patients with STEMI treated with primary percutaneous coronary intervention, *JAMA* 304:763–771, 2010.)

Resources for Staffing, Research, and Quality Improvement

In addition to delays, there are challenges with the ability of PPCI centers to accept all patients because of limitations of CCL staffing and facility availability. Maintaining adequate staffing requires a great deal of manpower, in addition to large financial overhead to operate these systems of care. Reimbursement is a common challenge, because many different hospitals and providers may take care of a single patient during their stay within a system of care.

Participation in research and quality improvement measures takes time, effort, and financial backing. Perhaps this accounts for the current gaps in knowledge regarding cost-effectiveness and certain outcome measures. Incomplete data collection and inadequate exchange of information are ongoing issues for many systems of care. Underreporting of outcomes and "scrubbing" data do little to enhance our understanding of patient outcomes.[40] Multiple isolated medical record systems, both electronic and handwritten, are often forced to interact with one another within a given system of care.

Public Policy and Consideration of Need

Public policy and oversight is another arena that provides unique challenges to each system of care. Regional transportation systems need to be developed in many areas of the country, and ongoing clarification on what constitutes an acceptable "receiving" center and "referring" center is needed. Public education and community outreach is necessary to teach patients and community members to recognize the signs and symptoms of a cardiac emergency and appropriately respond by activating EMS (via 911) immediately.

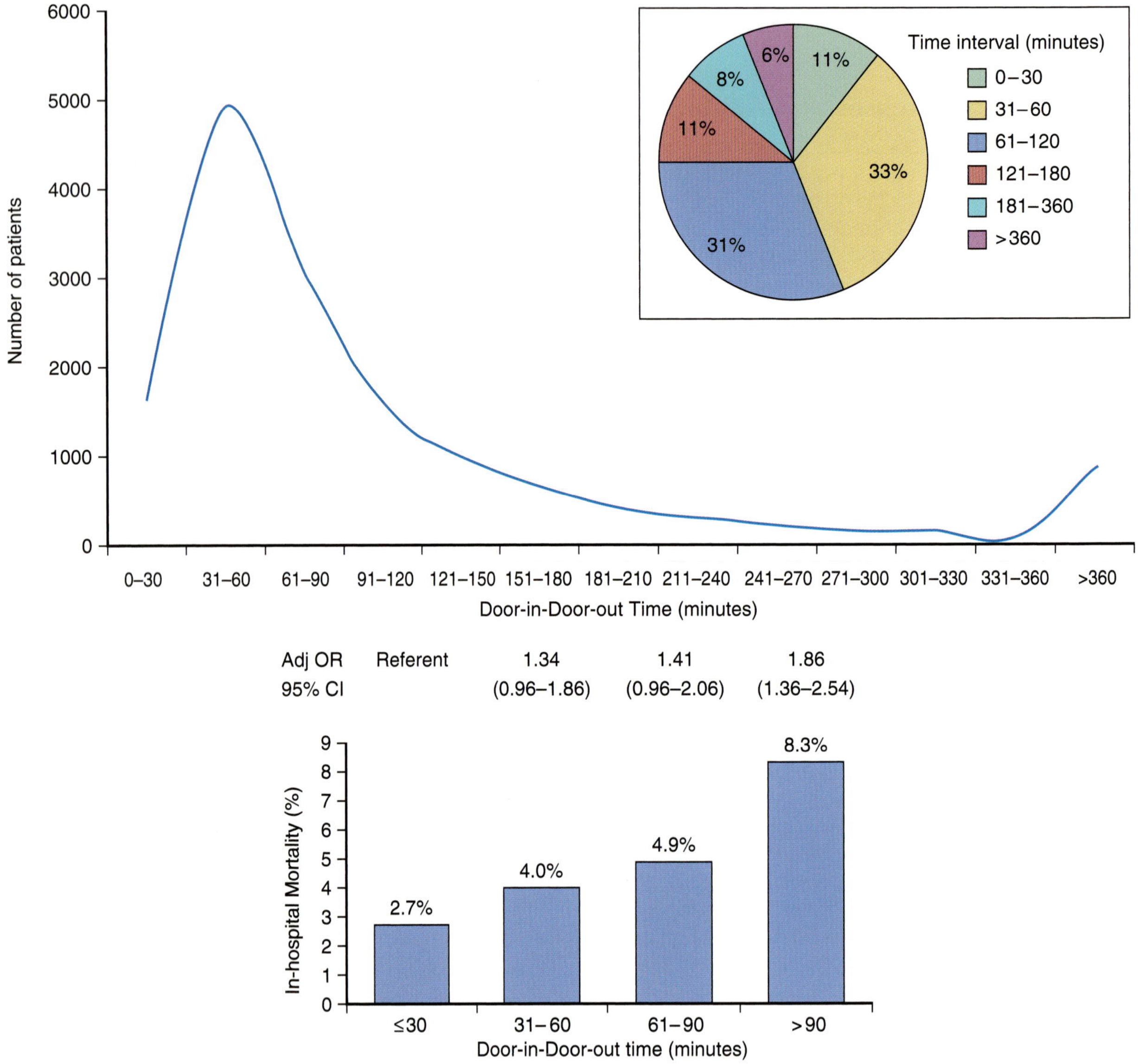

FIGURE 5-10 (**A**) Door-in-door-out times from Action Get with the Guidelines registry data. (**B**) Mortality associated with Door-in-door-out times. *CI*, Confidence interval; *OR*, odds ratio. (From Wang TY, Nallamothu BK, Krumholz HM, et al: Association of door-in door-out time with reperfusion delays and outcomes among patients transferred for primary percutaneous coronary intervention, *JAMA* 305:2540–2547, 2011.)

Accurate mapping and denotation of receiving centers and referral centers is necessary to identify regions in need of more robust systems of care. This would also allow for new partnerships and would facilitate linking these hospitals into a more cohesive system of care.[41] Furthermore, delineation of daytime PPCI centers and 24-hour PPCI centers is critical to reduce confusion and facilitate patient triage in a timely fashion.

Other Issues: In-Hospital ST-Elevation Myocardial Infarction and False Activations

STEMIs that occur in-hospital are a recently identified problem and are associated with longer time-to-treatment than STEMI patients who drive to the hospital (76 minutes vs. 66 minutes) (Figure 5-e10) and markedly worse clinical outcomes. These outcomes can be improved with standardized "in-house" STEMI protocols.[42,43] Finally, false or inappropriate activations have become a very challenging issue, with rates of inappropriate activations from 10% to as high as 40%, depending on definitions and regions.[44–47] Reasons for false activations vary and include abnormal repolarization, nondiagnostic ECG, pericarditis, left bundle branch block, left ventricular hypertrophy, and previous MI, among others. Clinical predictors and outcomes for this emerging population have not been well characterized, and solutions for minimizing the false-positive rates without increasing the rates of missed STEMIs are complex at best. Refining these systems to improve the specificity of our STEMI selection process without sacrificing the sensitivity is one of the greatest challenges that STEMI systems face.

FUTURE DIRECTIONS AND STRATEGIES FOR IMPROVEMENT

The advent of complex regional STEMI systems is a major achievement that has helped to improve the quality of cardiovascular care. Looking forward, ideally, the entire U.S. population will have locally designed regional systems not only to provide timely access to PPCI for all STEMI patients, but also to care for all acute cardiovascular emergencies.[32] This

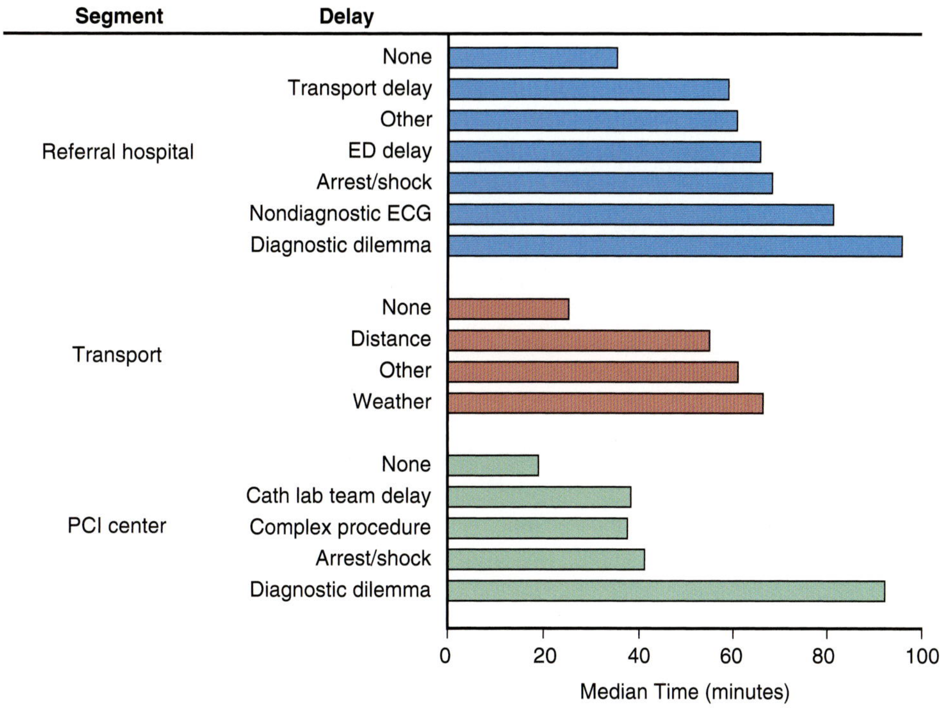

FIGURE 5-11 Median times for individual delays at each of the three treatment segments. *ED*, Emergency department; *ECG*, electrocardiogram; *PCI*, percutaneous coronary intervention. *(From Miedema MD, et al: Causes of delay and associated mortality in patients transferred with ST-elevation myocardial infarction.* Circulation *124:1636–1644, 2011.)*

TABLE 5-3 Frequency, Magnitude, and Mortality Associations of Specific Delays at the Referral Hospital. Referring Hospital (Door-in to Door-out Delays) and PPCI Center (DTB Delays)

CHARACTERISTIC	PATIENTS N (%)	MAGNITUDE (MIN) MEDIAN (25TH–75TH PERCENTILE)	IN-HOSPITAL MORTALITY (%)	1-YEAR MORTALITY (%)
Referring Hospital				
No delay (<45 min)	730 (36.0)	35 (28–41)	4.0	8.1
Awaiting transport	535 (26.4)	59 (51–72)	3.9	7.3
ED delay	289 (14.3)	65.5 (56–83.5)	3.8	6.9
Nondiagnostic ECG	184 (9.1)	81 (64–110.5)	0	3.3
Diagnostic dilemma	177 (8.7)	95.5 (72–127)	7.3	12.4
Cardiac arrest/shock	111 (5.5)	68 (56–86)	30.6	38.7
Other	2 (0.1)	06.5 (58–63)		
Total	2028			
PCI Center				
No delay (<30 min)	1696 (84.3)	19 (15–23)	3.5	7.3
Catheterization laboratory team delay	143 (7.1)	38 (34–50)	5.6	9.1
Complex procedure	117 (5.8)	38 (34–45)	8.6	14.5
Cardiac arrest/shock	43 (2.1)	41 (35–46)	44.2	55.8
Diagnostic dilemma	14 (0.7)	92.5 (59–131)	7.1	7.1
Total	2013			

DTB, Door-to-balloon; *ECG*, electrocardiogram; *ED*, emergency department; *PPCI*, primary percutaneous coronary intervention.
From Miedema MD, et al: *Causes of delay and associated mortality in patients transferred with ST-elevation myocardial infarction.* Circulation *124:1636–1644, 2011.*

lofty goal is not only possible, but within our grasp in the next decade. We envision these same systems providing similar care, including standardized protocols and transfer plans, for all acute cardiovascular emergencies, including OHCA, aortic dissection, pulmonary embolism, stroke, abdominal aortic aneurysms, and non–ST-elevation ACS. With an added emphasis on data collection and monitoring, we are optimistic that we will identify new targets for improvement in care and clinical outcomes. In addition, this expansion would enable the growth of large registry databases, such as the ACTION-Get With the Guidelines and Cath-PCI registries. Advances in technology and migration toward electronic medical record systems should allow for further integration of medical information, more comprehensive data, and more transparent communication among providers, patients, and families. Further streamlining of processes, including giving all EMS providers access to PHECG systems, might allow for further reduction in FMC-to-device times. Finally, there are obvious areas for improvement that we can begin to target, particularly with regard to in-hospital STEMIs and false activations.

To quote Albert Einstein, "We cannot solve our problems with the same thinking we used when we created them." With novel approaches and further refinements to our current systems of care, we no doubt can solve the many challenges that we face today and look forward to the next set of challenges that might follow.

References

1. Krumholz H, et al.: Improvements in door-to-balloon time in the United States, 2005 to 2010, *Circulation* 124:1038–1045, 2011.
2. American Heart Association: STEMI Systems of Care, *Mission: Lifeline*, 2015. http://www.heart.org/HEARTORG/HealthcareResearch/MissionLifelineHomePage/LearnAboutMissionLifeline/STEMI-Systems-of-Care_UCM_439065_SubHomePage.jsp.
3. Menees DS, et al.: Door-to-balloon time and mortality among patients undergoing primary PCI, *N Engl J Med* 369:901–909, 2013.
4. Bates ER, Jacobs AK: Time to treatment in patients with STEMI, *N Engl J Med* 369:889–892, 2013.
5. Nallamothu BK, et al.: Relation between door-to-balloon times and mortality after percutaneous coronary intervention over time: a retrospective study, *Lancet* 385:1114–1122, 2015.
6. Masoudi FA, et al.: Cardiovascular care facts: a report from the National Cardiovascular Data Registry, *J Am Coll Cardiol* 2013(62):1931–1947, 2011.
7. Shah RU, et al.: Increasing percutaneous coronary interventions for ST-segment elevation myocardial infarction in the United States, *J Am Coll Cardiol Intv* 8:139–146, 2015.
8. O'Gara PT, et al.: 2013 ACCF/AHA guideline for the management of ST-elevation myocardial infarction: a report from the American College of Cardiology Foundation/American Heart Association Task Force on Practice Guidelines, *J Am Coll Cardiol* 61:e78–140, 2013.
9. Daudelin DH, et al.: Improving use of prehospital 12-lead ECG for early identification and treatment of acute coronary syndrome and ST-elevation myocardial infarction, *Circ Cardiovasc Qual Outcomes* 3:316–323, 2010.
10. Diercks DB, et al.: Utilization and impact of pre-hospital electrocardiograms for patients with acute ST-segment elevation myocardial infarction: data from the NCDR (National Cardiovascular Data Registry) ACTION (Acute Coronary Treatment and Intervention Outcomes Network) Registry, *J Am Coll Cardiol* 53:161–166, 2009.
11. Pitta SR, et al.: Using prehospital electrocardiograms to improve door-to-balloon time for transferred patients with ST-elevation myocardial infarction: a case of extreme performance, *Circ Cardiovasc Qual Outcomes* 3:93–97, 2010.
12. Bradley EH, et al.: National efforts to improve door-to-balloon time: results from the Door-to-Balloon Alliance, *J Am Coll Cardiol* 54:2423–2429, 2009.
13. Pedersen SH, et al.: Field triage reduces treatment delay and improves long-term clinical outcome in patients with acute ST-segment elevation myocardial infarction treated with primary percutaneous coronary intervention, *J Am Coll Cardiol* 54:2296–2302, 2009.
14. Le May MR, et al.: A citywide protocol for primary PCI in ST-segment elevation myocardial infarction, *N Engl J Med* 358:231–240, 2008.
15. Jollis JG, et al.: Systems of care for ST-segment elevation myocardial infarction: a report from the American Heart Association's Mission: Lifeline, *Circ Cardiovasc Qual Outcomes* 5:423–428, 2012.
16. Henry TD, Gibson CM, Pinto DS: Moving toward improved care for the patient with ST-elevation myocardial infarction: a mandate for systems of care, *Circ Cardiovasc Qual Outcomes* 3:441–443, 2010.
17. Langabeer JR, et al.: Growth in percutaneous coronary intervention capacity relative to population and disease prevalence, *JAHA* 2:e000370, 2013.
18. Henry TD, et al.: A regional system to provide timely access to percutaneous coronary intervention for ST-elevation myocardial infarction, *Circulation* 116:721–728, 2007.
19. Jollis JG, et al.: Expansion of a regional ST-segment-elevation myocardial infarction system to an entire state, *Circulation* 126:189–195, 2012.
20. Aguirre FV, et al.: Rural interhospital transfer of ST-elevation myocardial infarction patients for percutaneous coronary revascularization: the Stat Heart Program, *Circulation* 117:1145–1152, 2008.
21. Concannon TW, et al.: Comparative effectiveness of ST-segment elevation myocardial infarction regionalization strategies, *Circ Cardiovasc Qual Outcomes* 3:1–8, 2010.
22. American College of Cardiology: *Door-to-Balloon Alliance*. http://cvquality.acc.org/Initiatives/D2B.aspx, 2015.
23. Hildebrandt DA, Larson DM, Henry TD: The critical imperative: pre-hospital management of the ST-elevation myocardial infarction patient, *Interventional Cardiology Clinics* 1:599–608, 2012.
24. Vavalle JP, Granger CB: The need for regional integrated care for ST-segment myocardial infarction, *Circulation* 124:851–856, 2011.
25. De Luca G, Biondi-Zoccai G, Marino P: Transferring patients with ST-segment elevation myocardial infarction for mechanical reperfusion: a meta-regression analysis of randomized trials, *Ann Emerg Med* 52:665–676, 2008.
26. Pinto DS, et al.: for the National Registry of Myocardial Infarction Investigators. Benefit of transferring ST-segment-elevation myocardial infarction patients for percutaneous coronary intervention compared with administration of onsite fibrinolytic declines as delays increase, *Circulation* 124:2512–2521, 2011.
27. Larson DM, et al.: Safety and efficacy of a pharmaco-invasive reperfusion strategy in rural ST-elevation myocardial infarction patients with expected delays due to long distance transfers, *Eur Heart J* 33:1232–1240, 2012.
28. Madan M, et al.: Relationship between time to invasive assessment and clinical outcomes of patients undergoing an early invasive strategy after fibrinolysis for ST-segment elevation myocardial infarction: a patient-level analysis of the randomized early routine invasive trials, *J Am Coll Cardiol Intv* 8:166–174, 2015.
29. Huber K, et al.: Enhancing the efficacy of delivery reperfusion therapy: a European and North American experience with STEMI networks, *Am Heart J* 165:123–132, 2013.
30. Miedema MD, et al.: Causes of delay and associated mortality in patients transferred with ST-elevation myocardial infarction, *Circulation* 124:1636–1644, 2011.
31. Rokos IC, et al.: Integration of pre-hospital electrocardiograms and ST-elevation myocardial infarction receiving (SRC) networks: impact on door-to-balloon times across 10 independent regions, *J Am Coll Cardiol Intv* 2:339–346, 2009.
32. Graham KJ, et al.: Has the time come for a national cardiovascular emergency care system? *Circulation* 125:2035–2044, 2012.
33. Henry TD: From concept to reality: a decade of progress in regional ST-segment elevation myocardial infarction systems, *Circulation* 126:166–168, 2012.
34. Henry TD, Jacobs AK, Granger CB: Regional systems of care for ST-elevation myocardial infarction: do they save lives? *Am Heart J* 166:389–391, 2013.
35. Solla DJ, et al.: Integrated regional networks for ST-segment elevation myocardial infarction care in developing countries: the experience of Salvador, Bahia, Brazil, *Circ Cardiovasc Qual Outcomes* 6:9–17, 2013.
36. Benedek IS, Gyongyosi M, Benedek T: A prospective regional registry of ST elevation myocardial infarction in Central Romania: impact of the Stent for Life Initiative recommendations on patient outcomes, *Am Heart J* 166:457–465, 2013.
37. Terkelsen CJ, Sorensen JT, Maeng M, et al.: System delay and mortality among patients with STEMI treated with primary percutaneous coronary intervention, *JAMA* 304:763–771, 2010.
38. Wang TY, et al.: Association of door-in door-out time with reperfusion delays and outcomes among patients transferred for primary percutaneous coronary intervention, *JAMA* 305:2540–2547, 2011.
39. Herrin J, et al.: National performance on door-in door-out time among patients transferred for primary percutaneous coronary intervention, *Arch Intern Med* 171:1879–1886, 2011.
40. Campbell AR, et al.: ST-elevation myocardial infarction: which patients do quality assurance programs include? *Circ Cardiovasc Qual Outcomes* 2:648–655, 2009.
41. Rokos IC, et al.: Mission: Lifeline STEMI networks geospatial information systems (GIS) maps, *Crit Path Cardiol* 12:43–44, 2013.
42. Kaul P, et al.: Association of inpatient vs. outpatient onset of ST-elevation myocardial infarction with treatment and clinical outcomes, *JAMA* 312:1999–2007, 2014.
43. Garberich RF, et al.: ST-elevation myocardial infarction diagnosed after hospital admission, *Circulation* 129:1225–1232, 2014.
44. Garvey JL, et al.: Rates of cardiac catheterization cancelation for ST-segment elevation myocardial infarction after activation by emergency medical services or emergency physicians: results from the North Carolina Catheterization Laboratory Activation Registry, *Circulation* 125:308–313, 2012.
45. Rokos IC, et al.: Appropriate cardiac cath lab activation: optimizing electrocardiogram interpretation and clinical decision-making for acute ST-elevation myocardial infarction, *Am Heart J* 160:995–1003, 2010. 1003.e1–8.
46. Larsen DM, et al.: False positive cardiac catheterization laboratory activation among patients with suspected ST-segment elevation myocardial infarction, *JAMA* 298:2754–2760, 2007.
47. McCabe JM, et al.: Prevalence and factors associated with false-positive ST-segment elevation myocardial infarction diagnoses at primary percutaneous coronary intervention–capable centers: a report from the Activate-SF registry, *Arch Intern Med* 172:864–871, 2012.

6

Clinical Practice/Controversy

Clinical Approach to Suspected Acute Myocardial Infarction

David A. Morrow

INTRODUCTION

Chest symptoms suspicious for acute myocardial infarction (MI) are among the most common reasons for emergency evaluation, accounting for six to seven million emergency department (ED) visits each year in the United States. The initial assessment of nontraumatic chest discomfort is challenging because of the broad range of possible causes (Figure 6-1). The primary aim of the ED assessment is to rapidly identify the minority of patients whose symptoms are the manifestation of a life-threatening condition that should not be missed and to initiate appropriate therapy. More than 60% of patients who present with chest symptoms suspicious for MI are hospitalized for further testing, and the remainder undergo additional investigation in the ED. However, in most series of unselected populations, only 5% to 15% are ultimately determined to have an acute coronary syndrome (ACS), and less than 10% are found to have other life-threatening cardiopulmonary conditions. Therefore, an efficient but effective evaluation of this population of patients that avoids the excessive use of testing and minimizes empiric treatment is important.

Pathways for the triage and management of patients with ST-segment elevation on the presenting electrocardiogram (ECG) are described in Chapter 5. In contrast, strategies for evaluating low-risk patients with a low probability of MI are discussed in Chapter 12. The present chapter provides a general framework for the clinical approach to the assessment of patients with an intermediate or high probability of MI. Risk factors for MI are discussed in Chapter 2. The optimal use of cardiac troponin (cTn) is detailed in Chapter 7, and other biomarkers are considered in Chapter 8. Diagnostic imaging in the ED is described in Chapter 9. Chapter 11 provides an in-depth discussion of tools for risk stratification of the patient with established MI.

GOALS OF THE INITIAL ASSESSMENT OF SUSPECTED MYOCARDIAL INFARCTION

The fundamental goals of the initial assessment of the patient with chest symptoms suspicious for myocardial ischemia are (1) to assess the probability that the symptoms are caused by underlying myocardial ischemia (diagnosis), and (2) to determine the probability of major cardiovascular complications if the cause of the patient's presentation is myocardial ischemia (risk stratification).[1–3] These two concurrent probabilistic assessments rely on the clinical history, the physical examination, ECG, and initial cardiac biomarkers, and are intertwined because each of these elements provides information that influences both the diagnostic and prognostic probabilities (see the section on Clinical Approach to the Patient). Together, these two probabilistic assessments guide subsequent diagnostic testing, including the use of invasive coronary angiography, triage, and the initiation of empiric medical therapies while the diagnosis is established (Figure 6-2).

CAUSES OF CHEST DISCOMFORT

The characteristics of symptoms caused by myocardial ischemia are discussed in this section. The major alternative causes of chest discomfort are summarized in Table 6-1 and described briefly in this section. In general, the initial diagnostic assessment of patients with acute chest discomfort centers around three categories: (1) myocardial ischemia; (2) other cardiopulmonary causes (pericardial disease, aortic emergencies, and pulmonary conditions); and (3) noncardiopulmonary chest pain. High-risk conditions, other than acute MI, to be considered in the differential diagnosis include acute aortic syndrome, pulmonary embolism, tension pneumothorax, and pericarditis with tamponade.

Myocardial Ischemia

Onset of myocardial ischemia is precipitated by an imbalance between myocardial oxygen requirements and myocardial oxygen supply, which results in insufficient delivery of oxygen to meet the heart's metabolic demands. Chest discomfort caused by myocardial ischemia is termed *angina pectoris,* often referred to simply as angina. The causes and classification of myocardial ischemia into stable angina, unstable angina, non–ST-elevation MI (NSTEMI), and ST-elevation MI (STEMI) are addressed in Chapter 1. The pathobiology of unstable ischemic heart disease is discussed Chapter 3 and Chapter 4.

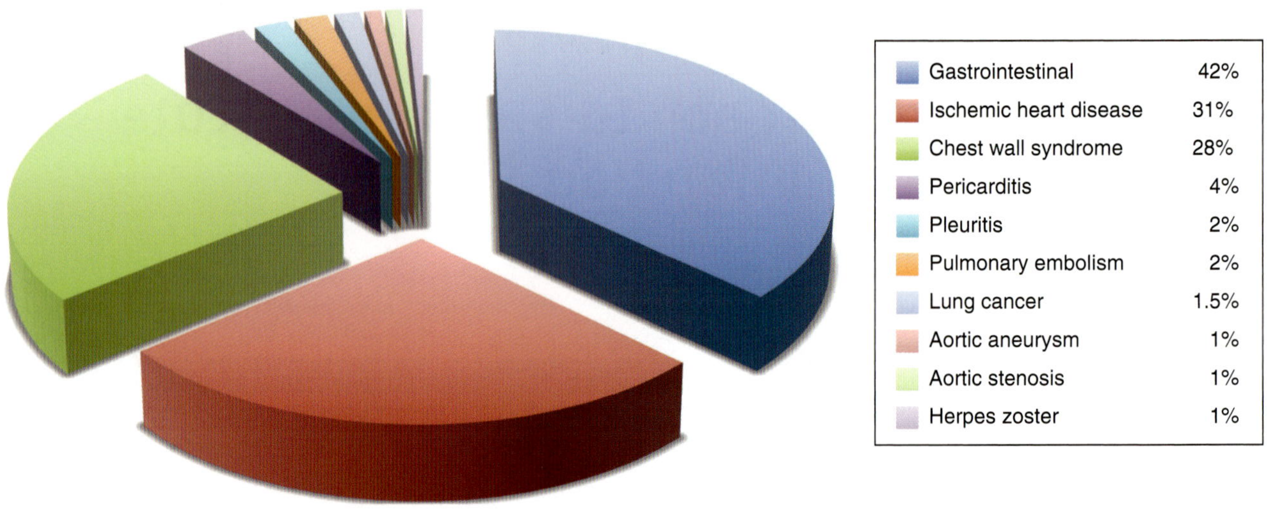

FIGURE 6-1 Distribution of final discharge diagnoses in patients with nontraumatic acute chest pain. *(Data from Fruergaard P, et al: The diagnoses of patients admitted with acute chest pain but without myocardial infarction.* Eur Heart J *17:1028,1996.)*

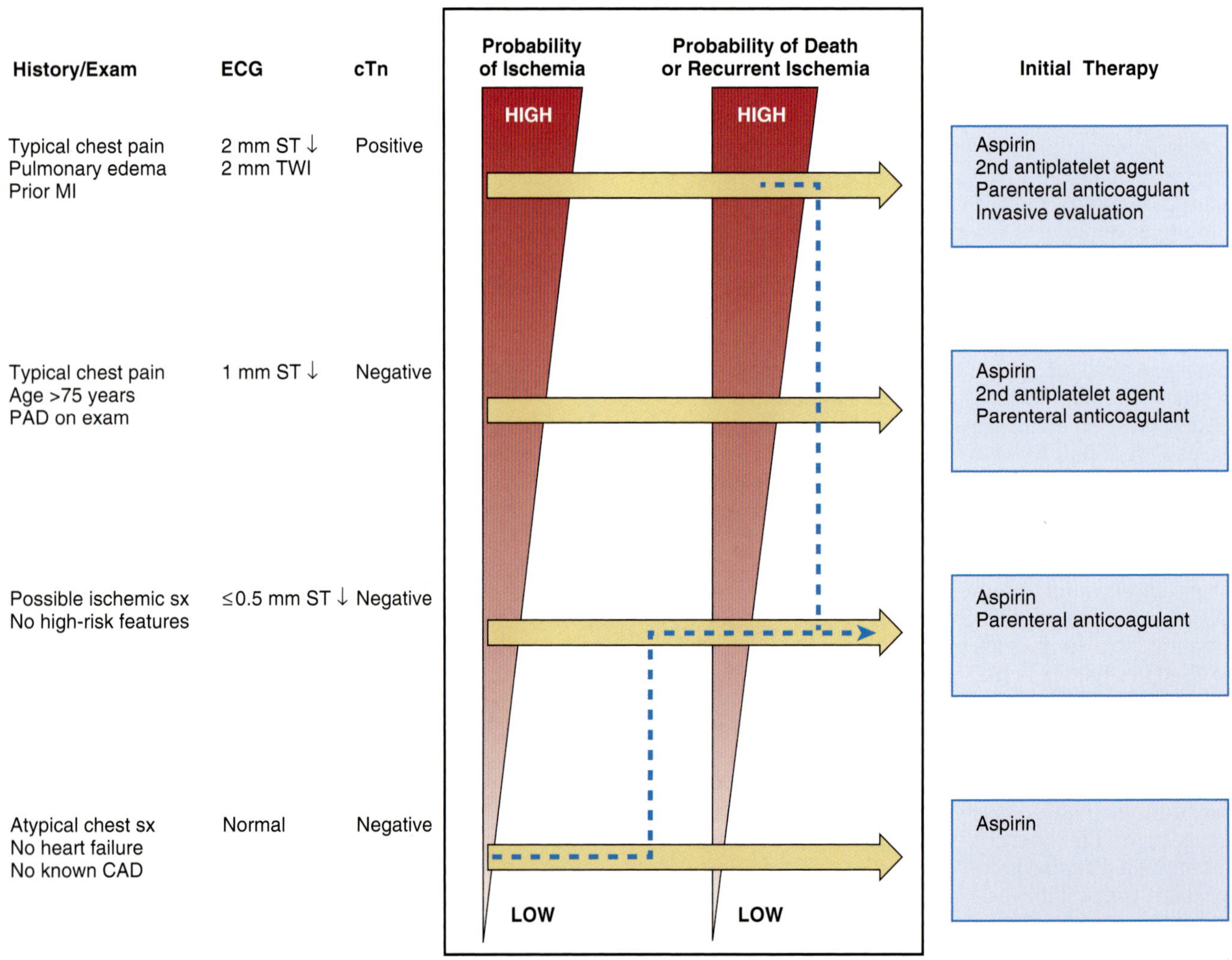

FIGURE 6-2 Integrated assessment of the patient with possible myocardial infarction (MI). The history of symptoms (sx), examination, electrocardiogram (ECG), and biomarkers are used to assess both the probability that the presenting symptoms are a manifestation of myocardial ischemia and the risk of death or recurrent ischemic events. Examples of high-, intermediate-, and low-risk features are provided (see text for additional details). These two probabilities drive decision-making regarding therapy. The *solid thick arrows* illustrate decisions regarding therapy in patients in whom the probability of ischemia and risk are concordant. The *dotted blue line* illustrates the possible therapeutic approach in patients with a lower clinical probability of MI (see *bottom origin of the dotted line*) who nonetheless fall into a high-risk group (see *upper origin of the dotted line*) based on other clinical features. Similarly, a patient with a good clinical story for ischemia, but otherwise low-risk features might also be treated without invasive coronary evaluation. *CAD*, Coronary artery disease; *PAD*, peripheral artery disease; *TWI*, T-wave inversion.

TABLE 6-1 Typical Clinical Features of Major Causes of Acute Chest Discomfort

SYSTEM	CONDITION	ONSET/DURATION	QUALITY	LOCATION	ASSOCIATED FEATURES
Cardiopulmonary					
Cardiac	Myocardial ischemia	Stable angina: Precipitated by exertion, cold, or stress; 2–10 min; Unstable angina: Increasing pattern or at rest; MI: Usually >30 min	Pressure, tightness, squeezing, heaviness, burning	Retrosternal, often radiation to neck, jaw, shoulders, or arms; sometimes epigastric	S_4 gallop or mitral regurgitation murmur (rarely) during pain; S_3 or rales if severe ischemia or complication of MI
	Pericarditis	Variable; Hours to days; may be episodic	Pleuritic, sharp	Retrosternal or toward cardiac apex; may radiate to left shoulder	May be relieved by sitting up and leaning forward; Pericardial friction rub
Vascular	Acute aortic syndrome	Sudden onset of unrelenting pain	Tearing or ripping; knifelike	Anterior chest, often radiating to back, between shoulder blades	Associated with hypertension and/or underlying connective tissue disorder; murmur of aortic insufficiency, loss of peripheral pulses
	Pulmonary embolism (PE)	Sudden onset	Pleuritic; may be heaviness with massive PE	Often lateral, on the side of the embolism	Dyspnea, tachypnea, tachycardia, and hypotension
	Pulmonary hypertension	Variable; often exertional	Pressure	Substernal	Dyspnea, signs of increased venous pressure
Pulmonary	Pneumonia or pleuritis	Variable	Pleuritic	Unilateral, often localized	Dyspnea, cough, fever, rales, occasional rub
	Spontaneous pneumothorax	Sudden onset	Pleuritic	Lateral to side of pneumothorax	Dyspnea, decreased breath sounds on side of pneumothorax
Noncardiopulmonary					
Gastrointestinal	Esophageal reflux	10–60 min	Burning	Substernal, epigastric	Worsened by postprandial recumbency; Relieved by antacids
	Esophageal spasm	2–30 min	Pressure, tightness, burning	Retrosternal	Can closely mimic angina
	Peptic ulcer	Prolonged; 60–90 min after meals	Burning	Epigastric, substernal	Relieved with food or antacids
	Gallbladder disease	Prolonged (h); generally steady and subsides spontaneously	Aching or colicky	Epigastric, right upper quadrant; sometimes to the back and lower chest or scapula	May follow meal
Neuromuscular	Costochondritis	Variable	Aching	Sternal	Sometimes swollen, tender, warm over joint; May be reproduced by localized pressure on examination
	Cervical disk disease	Variable; may be sudden	Aching; may include numbness	Arms and shoulder	May be exacerbated by movement of neck
	Trauma or strain	Usually constant	Aching	Localized to area of strain	Reproduced by movement or palpation
	Herpes zoster	Usually prolonged	Sharp or burning	Dermatomal distribution	Vesicular rash in area of discomfort
Psychological	Emotional and psychiatric conditions	Variable; may be fleeting or prolonged	Variable; often tightness and dyspnea with feeling of panic or doom	Variable; may be retrosternal	Situational factors may precipitate symptoms; history of panic attacks depression

From Morrow DA: Chest discomfort. In Kasper DL, et al, eds: Harrison's principles of internal medicine, *ed 19, New York, McGraw Hill, 2015.*

Characteristics of Myocardial Ischemia

Myocardial ischemia can usually be identified from the patient's history and from the ECG. Possible ischemic symptoms include various combinations of chest, upper extremity, mandibular, or epigastric discomfort, or an ischemic equivalent, such as dyspnea or fatigue (see the section on Clinical Approach: History). When myocardial ischemia is sufficiently severe and prolonged in duration (e.g., as short as 20 to 30 minutes), irreversible cellular injury occurs, resulting in MI. Often, the discomfort is diffuse—not localized, nor positional, nor affected by movement of the region—and it may be accompanied by diaphoresis, nausea, or syncope. Because of their prevalence among other common conditions, these symptoms may be incorrectly attributed to

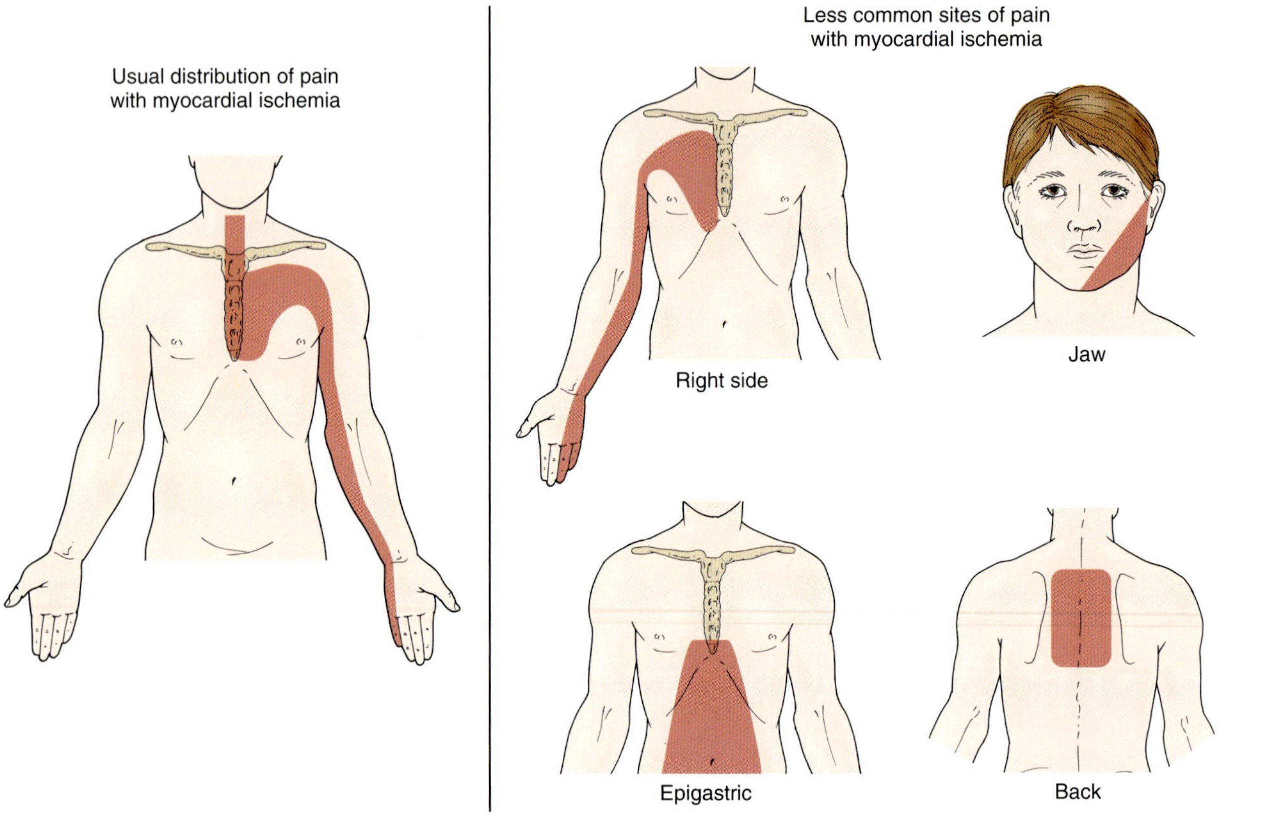

FIGURE 6-3 Pain patterns with myocardial ischemia. The usual distribution is referral to all or part of the sternal region, the left side of the chest, and the neck and down the ulnar side of the left forearm and hand. With severe ischemic pain, the right chest and right arm are often involved as well; however, isolated involvement of these areas is rare. Other sites sometimes involved, either alone or together with other sites, are the jaw, epigastrium, and back. *(From Braunwald E: The history. In Braunwald E, et al, eds:* Heart disease, *ed 6, Philadelphia, Saunders, 2001, p. 33.)*

gastrointestinal, neurological, pulmonary, or musculoskeletal disorders (see Table 6-1). In addition, MI may occur with atypical symptoms or may be asymptomatic. Such atypical presentations are more common in women, older adults, patients with diabetes, or postoperative and critically ill patients.

The clinical characteristics of angina pectoris are highly similar whether the ischemic discomfort is a manifestation of stable ischemic heart disease, unstable angina, or MI, with exceptions being differences in the pattern and duration of symptoms associated with these syndromes. Heberden initially described angina as a sense of "strangling and anxiety." Chest discomfort characteristic of myocardial ischemia is usually described as aching, heavy, squeezing, crushing, or constricting. However, in a substantial minority of patients, the quality of discomfort is very vague and may be described as a mild tightness, or merely an uncomfortable feeling that sometimes is experienced as numbness or a burning sensation. The site of the discomfort is usually retrosternal, but radiation is common, and usually occurs down the ulnar surface of the left arm; the right arm, both arms, neck, jaw, or shoulders may also be involved (Figure 6-3). These and other characteristics of ischemic chest discomfort pertinent to discrimination from other causes of chest pain are discussed later in this chapter (see the section on Approach to the Patient).

Stable angina usually begins gradually and reaches its maximum intensity over a period of minutes before dissipating within several minutes with rest or with nitroglycerin. The discomfort typically occurs predictably at a characteristic level of exertion or psychological stress. By definition,

TABLE 6-2 Three Principal Presentations of Unstable Ischemic Heart Disease

CLASS	PRESENTATION
Rest angina	Angina occurring at rest and prolonged, usually >20 min
New-onset angina	New-onset angina of at least CCS class III Severity
Increasing (crescendo) angina	Angina that has become distinctly more frequent, longer in duration, or lower in threshold (increased by 1 or more CCS class to at least CCS class III severity)

CCS, Canadian Cardiovascular Society.
From Anderson JL, Adams CD, Antman EM, et al: ACC/AHA 2007 guidelines for the management of patients with unstable angina/non-ST-elevation myocardial infarction. J Am Coll Cardiol *50:e1–e157, 2007.*

unstable angina manifests by self-limited symptoms that may be exertional, but that occur at increased frequency with progressively lower intensity of physical activity or at rest (Table 6-2).[4] Chest discomfort associated with MI is typically more severe, is prolonged (usually ≥30 minutes), and is not relieved by rest.

Triggers of Myocardial Ischemia

Myocardial ischemia may be triggered by acute coronary atherothrombosis (see Chapter 3), increased myocardial oxygen demand, such as during intense psychological stress, or fever, or by decreased oxygen delivery due to anemia, hypoxia, or hypotension (see Chapter 1). Other contributors to stable and unstable ischemic heart disease, such as endothelial dysfunction, microvascular disease, and vasospasm, may also exist alone or in combination with coronary atherosclerosis and may be the dominant cause of myocardial ischemia in some patients. Nonatherosclerotic processes, including congenital abnormalities of the coronary vessels, myocardial bridging, coronary arteritis, and radiation-induced coronary disease, can also lead to coronary obstruction.[5] In addition, conditions associated with extreme myocardial oxygen demand and impaired endocardial blood flow, such as in patients with aortic valve disease, hypertrophic cardiomyopathy, or idiopathic dilated cardiomyopathy, can precipitate myocardial ischemia in patients with or without underlying obstructive atherosclerosis. In the course of their history and physical examination, clinicians should consider each of these potential contributors to the onset of myocardial ischemia.

Nonischemic Causes of Chest Discomfort

Cardiopulmonary Causes

Pericardial and Myocardial Diseases

Inflammation of the pericardium can cause acute chest discomfort. The pain of pericarditis is believed to arise primarily from associated pleural inflammation, and is consequently more common in infectious compared with noninfectious causes of pericarditis, because the former more often involve the pleura. The pain of pericarditis is usually a pleuritic discomfort that is exacerbated by breathing, coughing, or changes in position, and is often referred to the shoulder and neck.

Acute inflammatory and other nonischemic myocardial diseases can also produce chest symptoms (see Table 6-1). Takotsubo stress–related cardiomyopathy can cause the abrupt onset of chest pain and shortness of breath, and may mimic acute MI because of associated ECG abnormalities, including ST-segment elevation and elevated biomarkers of myocardial injury.

Acute Aortic Syndromes

Acute aortic syndromes, including aortic penetrating ulcer, intramural hematoma, and frank dissection, are less common but important causes of chest pain (see Table 6-1). Acute aortic syndromes typically present with thoracic pain that is often severe, sudden in onset, sometimes described as tearing in quality, and can occur in the midline of the anterior chest. Dissections that begin in the ascending aorta and extend to the descending aorta tend to cause pain in the front of the chest that extends toward the back, between the shoulder blades. Aortic aneurysms without dissection are most often asymptomatic, but these can cause chest pain by compressing adjacent structures. This pain tends to be steady, deep, and occasionally severe. Aortitis, in the absence of dissection, is a rare cause of chest discomfort.

Pulmonary Embolism

Pulmonary and pulmonary vascular conditions that cause chest discomfort usually do so in conjunction with dyspnea. The symptoms are usually pleuritic in nature and may be lateral, in the case of smaller pulmonary emboli, or may be severe and substernal, in the case of massive pulmonary embolism. Massive or submassive pulmonary embolism may also cause syncope, hypotension, and signs of right heart failure.

Other Pulmonary Causes

Primary spontaneous pneumothorax is a rare cause of chest discomfort. The symptoms are usually sudden in onset and dyspnea may be mild. Most pulmonary diseases, including pneumonia and malignancy, that can involve the pleura may cause pleurisy, a knifelike pain that is worsened by inspiration or coughing. Chronic pulmonary hypertension can cause chest pain that may be very similar to angina in its characteristics. Reactive airways diseases can also cause chest tightness, with associated breathlessness.

Noncardiopulmonary Causes

Gastrointestinal Conditions

Gastrointestinal disorders are the most common cause of nontraumatic chest discomfort (see Figure 6-1 and Table 6-1). In some cases, the symptoms can be quite difficult to discern from myocardial ischemia. Esophageal disorders, in particular, may cause an intense squeezing discomfort that is similar to angina in the character and location. Like angina, esophageal discomfort may be relieved by nitroglycerin or calcium channel blockers. Gastroesophageal reflux and disorders of esophageal motility are common disorders that should be considered in the differential diagnosis of chest pain. Hepatobiliary disorders may also mimic myocardial ischemic pain (see Table 6-1).

Musculoskeletal

Chest discomfort can be produced by any musculoskeletal disorder involving the chest wall, or nerves of the chest wall, neck, or upper limbs. Costochondritis, cervical radiculitis, shoulder tendinitis or bursitis may all mimic angina. Pain in a dermatomal distribution should prompt consideration of herpes zoster.

Panic Disorder

As many as 10% of patients who present to EDs with acute chest discomfort have a panic disorder or related condition. The symptoms may include tightness or aching that is associated with a sense of anxiety and difficulty breathing.

CLINICAL APPROACH TO THE PATIENT

History

Assessment of the patient with chest symptoms suspicious for MI relies heavily on the clinical history and physical examination to direct the diagnostic evaluation. The quality, location, radiation, onset, pattern, and duration of the pain, as well as any provoking or alleviating factors provide information that shapes both the probability that the symptoms are ischemic and yields information about prognosis (see Figure 6-1).

Quality of the Pain

The quality of chest discomfort is not sufficiently accurate to establish a diagnosis. However, the characteristics of the pain are pivotal in formulating an initial clinical impression of the probability of MI (Figure 6-4). Although pressure or tightness is a typical presentation of myocardial ischemic pain, some patients with ischemic chest symptoms deny any "pain," but rather complain of shortness of breath or a vague

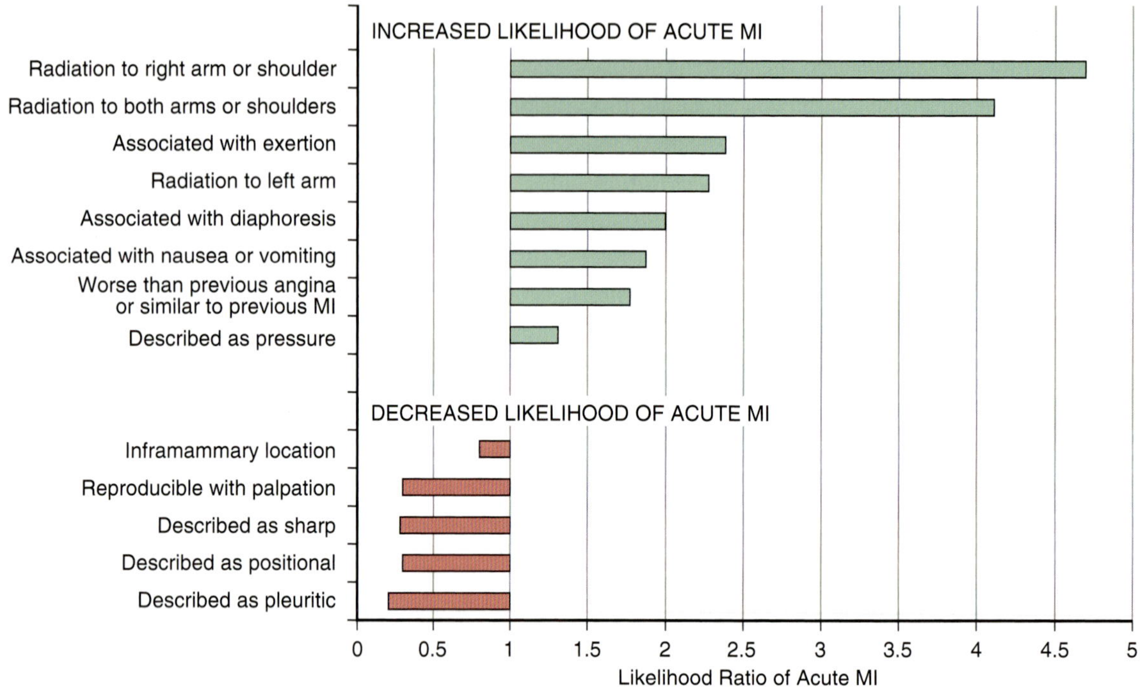

FIGURE 6-4 Association of chest pain characteristics with the probability of acute myocardial infarction (MI). *(Data from Swap CJ, Nagurney JT: Value and limitations of chest pain history in the evaluation of patients with suspected acute coronary syndromes, JAMA 294:2623–2639, 2005.)*

sense of anxiety. The similarity of the symptoms to previous ischemic presentations may be useful, but greater severity of pain does not improve diagnostic accuracy. It is unusual for angina to be sharp, as in knifelike, stabbing, or pleuritic; however, patients sometimes use the word "sharp" to convey the severity of discomfort. Pleuritic discomfort is suggestive of a condition involving the pleura, including pericarditis, pulmonary embolism, or pulmonary parenchymal diseases (see also the section on Causes of Chest Discomfort), and is the quality with the strongest negative predictive value for ischemia (Figure 6-4). "Tearing" or "ripping" pain should prompt consideration of acute aortic dissection. However, acute aortic emergencies also present commonly with severe, knifelike pain. A burning quality raises the possibility of a gastrointestinal cause, but may also occur with MI.

Location of the Discomfort

Myocardial ischemic discomfort is typically substernal in location with radiation to the neck, jaw, shoulder, or arms (Figure 6-3). Nevertheless, some patients present with aching only in sites of radiated pain. Pain that is highly localized, such as being able to be demarcated by the tip of one finger, is highly unusual for myocardial ischemia. Pain that occurs solely above the mandible or below the epigastrium is rarely angina. The typical distribution of symptoms of discomfort according to cause is illustrated in Figure 6-5. Severe pain radiating to the back, particularly between the shoulder blades, should prompt consideration of an acute aortic syndrome. Radiation to the trapezius ridge is a characteristic site of radiation of pericardial pain and is uncommon with myocardial ischemia.

Pattern

Symptoms caused by myocardial ischemia usually develop over minutes, and are exacerbated by activity and relieved by rest. Pain that peaks in intensity at its onset is more characteristic of aortic dissection, pulmonary embolism, or spontaneous pneumothorax. Pain that lasts only a few seconds is rarely caused by myocardial ischemia. In the absence of developing clinical consequences, (e.g., elevation of cardiac biomarkers, heart failure, or hypotension), discomfort that is constant in pattern and steady in intensity over many hours to days is not likely to be the cause of myocardial ischemia. The onset of MI has a circadian pattern, with the peak incidence ranging between midnight and 6 AM. Most patients with MI have an antecedent history of exertional chest symptoms, and more than 80% have a history of coronary artery disease. However, MI may be the first symptomatic presentation of coronary atherosclerosis for some patients.

Provoking and Alleviating Factors

Patients with pain caused by myocardial ischemia often report a history of exacerbation by exertion and relief or improvement with rest. Positional changes in the pain are infrequent with angina. Changes in the discomfort with movement of the upper extremities and neck suggest a musculoskeletal cause. The pain of pericarditis is often increased when the patient is supine and relieved when the patient sits upright and leans forward. Gastroesophageal reflux may be exacerbated by alcohol, some foods, or by a reclined position. Although postprandial angina has been described, worsening symptoms provoked by eating usually suggests a gastrointestinal cause (see Table 6-1). Pain related to peptic ulcer disease typically emerges 1 to 2 hours after a meal and is usually relieved promptly by acid-reducing therapies.

Relief of chest discomfort within minutes after administration of nitroglycerin is suggestive, but not sufficiently sensitive nor specific to make a definitive diagnosis of myocardial ischemia. Complete relief after a longer delay (e.g., >10 minutes) after nitroglycerin points away from myocardial ischemia. Esophageal discomfort can also be relieved by nitroglycerin.

Associated Symptoms

Diaphoresis, dyspnea, nausea, fatigue, faintness, and belching can all accompany chest pain caused by myocardial

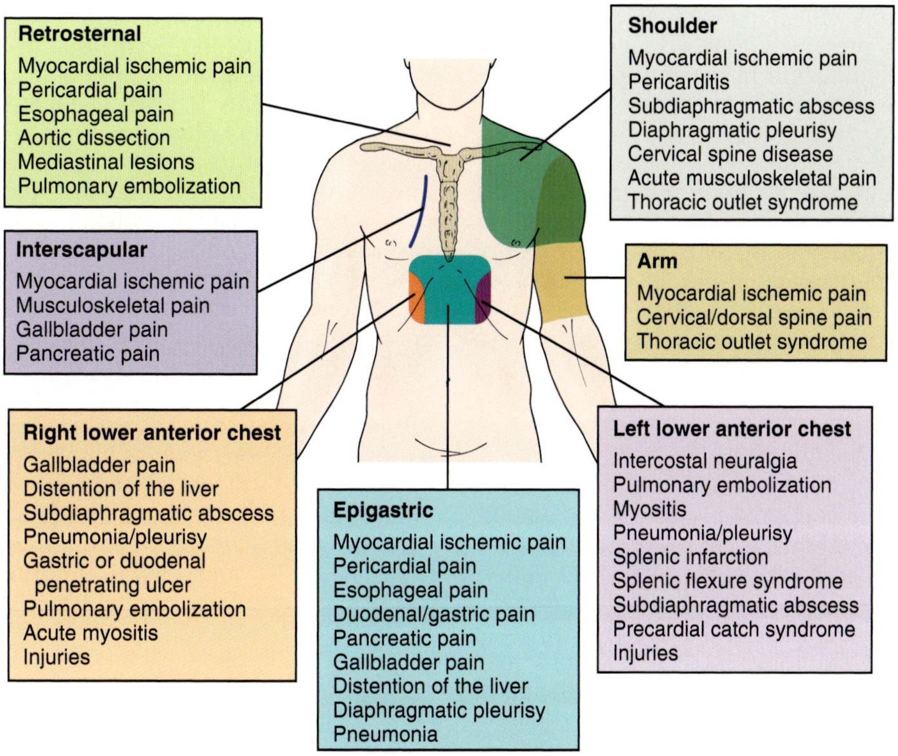

FIGURE 6-5 Differential diagnosis of chest pain according to the location of the discomfort. Serious intrathoracic or subdiaphragmatic diseases are usually associated with pains that begin in the left anterior chest, left shoulder or upper arm, interscapular region, or epigastrium. *(From Braunwald E: The history. In Zipes DP, et al, eds:* Heart disease, *ed 7, Philadelphia, Saunders, 2005, p. 68.)*

ischemia, or may exist alone as ischemic equivalents, particularly in women and older adults. Dyspnea is not specific for myocardial ischemia, but the presence of dyspnea as a symptom is important because it points to a cardiopulmonary cause, and when it accompanies myocardial ischemia, is an indicator of a higher risk of fatal complications (see Chapter 11). Sudden onset of significant respiratory distress should prompt consideration of pulmonary embolism and spontaneous pneumothorax. Presentation with syncope or presyncope should raise consideration of hemodynamically significant pulmonary embolism or aortic dissection, as well as ischemic arrhythmias. Although nausea and vomiting suggest a gastrointestinal disorder, these symptoms may occur with an MI (more commonly inferior MI), and are presumably related to vagal reflexes or stimulation of ventricular receptors as part of the Bezold-Jarisch reflex.

Medical History and Review of Systems

The patient should be assessed for risk factors for coronary atherosclerosis and conditions that may predispose the patient to specific other processes that may cause chest discomfort. For example, a history of connective tissue diseases (e.g., Marfan disease) should heighten the clinician's suspicion for an acute aortic syndrome or spontaneous pneumothorax. Review of the medical history should also include surveying for conditions that might contribute to myocardial supply–demand mismatch. Emotional stressors can also be a trigger for MI.

Physical Examination

The physical examination of patients with chest discomfort can provide indirect evidence for myocardial ischemia by identifying contributors to supply–demand, such as uncontrolled hypertension, or consequences of ischemia, such as heart failure. In addition, the examination may help to identify specific alternative causes (e.g., pneumothorax or pneumonia) and provide an overall assessment of the clinical stability of the patient. However, because the physical examination may be normal in patients with unstable ischemic heart disease, an unremarkable physical examination does not reliably exclude MI as a cause of chest discomfort.

General

Patients with acute MI often appear anxious, uncomfortable, or diaphoretic. In patients with early complications of MI, cyanosis or pallor may also be evident. Patients who are massaging or clutching their chests may describe their pain with a clenched fist held against the sternum (the Levine sign, named after Dr. Samuel A. Levine). Tachycardia and hypotension in the setting of an MI are indicative of important hemodynamic consequences of the MI and should prompt consideration of emerging cardiogenic shock (see Chapter 25) because of impaired left ventricular function or mechanical complications (see Chapter 26). The presence of low-grade fever should not dissuade consideration of MI as a diagnosis, because fevers may occur with acute infarction.

Cardiopulmonary

The jugular venous pulse is often normal in patients with acute MI. Palpation of the chest may reveal a dyskinetic ventricle in patients with large infarctions or previous MI. Cardiac auscultation may reveal a third or, more commonly, a fourth heart sound, reflecting myocardial systolic or diastolic dysfunction. Murmurs of mitral regurgitation or a harsh murmur of a ventricular septal defect may indicate mechanical complications of MI (see Chapter 26). Murmurs may reveal underlying cardiac disorders that contribute to ischemia (e.g., aortic stenosis or hypertrophic cardiomyopathy).

Pericardial friction rubs reflect pericardial inflammation that may occur in late presentations of MI. Findings of pulmonary edema on examination in patients with MI are a harbinger of very poor prognosis (see Chapter 11).

Vascular

Pulse deficits may reflect underlying chronic atherosclerosis, which increases the likelihood of coronary artery disease. However, findings of acute limb ischemia, including loss of the pulse and pallor, particularly in the upper extremities, should prompt consideration and immediate evaluation for aortic dissection. The presence of peripheral artery disease is also an indicator of a higher risk of poor cardiovascular outcomes in the short and long term.

Other Elements of the Examination

The remaining elements of the examination, including the abdominal examination and musculoskeletal evaluation, may reveal evidence for alternative causes of chest discomfort, and thus, are critical components of the evaluation, together with the cardiopulmonary and vascular examinations. Localized swelling, redness, or marked tenderness of the costochondral and chondrosternal articulations may occur in patients with costochondritis. Pain on palpation of these joints is a useful clinical sign; however, deep palpation may elicit pain in the absence of costochondritis, and chest wall tenderness does not exclude myocardial ischemia.

Electrocardiography

The ECG is pivotal for identifying patients with ongoing ischemia and is valuable for risk stratification. Professional society guidelines recommend that the first ECG be obtained within 10 minutes of first medical contact (see Chapter 5), with the primary goal of identifying patients with ST-segment elevation diagnostic of STEMI. ST-segment depression and symmetric T-wave inversions at least 0.2 mV in depth are useful for detecting myocardial ischemia in the absence of STEMI and are also indicative of higher risk of death or recurrent ischemia (see Chapter 11). Serial acquisition of ECGs (e.g., every 15 to 30 minutes) is recommended in the emergency evaluation of suspected MI. In addition, an ECG with right-sided lead placement should be considered in patients with a clinical suspicion of ischemia, as well as a nondiagnostic standard 12-lead ECG. Despite the value of ECG, its sensitivity for ischemia is as low as 20% in some studies.[5]

The J-point is used to determine the magnitude of the ST-segment deviation. For diagnosis of STEMI, ST-segment elevation should be present in at least two anatomically related leads. Criteria for diagnostic ST-elevation are listed in Table 1-3. Occasionally, ST-segment shifts caused by myocardial ischemia may meet the criteria in only one lead, with elevation less than the required ST-deviation in a contiguous lead. The clinician should recognize that lesser degrees of ST-deviation or T-wave inversion do not exclude acute myocardial ischemia or evolving MI. ST-segment deviation can be dynamic in the setting of myocardial ischemia. This variability is the rationale for serial recordings of the ECG in patients with a high clinical suspicion of MI and an initially nondiagnostic ECG. Continuous computer-assisted 12-lead ECG recording and ST-segment monitoring may also be useful. An ECG should also be repeated for patients with recurrence of symptoms after an asymptomatic interval. The evolution of ST-T waveforms and development of Q waves, when present, assist the clinician in estimating the time from the onset of the event, identifying the infarct-related artery, and gauging the amount of myocardium at risk. Each of these elements is also useful for assessing prognosis (see Chapter 11).[1] More profound ST-segment deviation or T-wave inversion involving multiple leads and vascular territories is associated with a worse prognosis. The ECG may also detect the onset of arrhythmias, or intraventricular and atrioventricular conduction delays, which are discussed in Chapter 26 and Chapter 28.

Abnormalities of the ST segment and T wave may occur in a variety of conditions other than MI, including pulmonary embolism, ventricular hypertrophy, acute and chronic pericarditis, myocarditis, electrolyte imbalance, and metabolic disorders. ST-deviation may also be present in patients with chronic conditions such as left ventricular hypertrophy, left bundle branch block, Brugada syndrome, stress cardiomyopathy, and early repolarization patterns. Hyperventilation occurring in patients with panic disorder can also lead to nonspecific ST- and T-wave abnormalities. Q waves may occur because of myocardial fibrosis and cardiomyopathy in the absence of coronary artery disease.

Cardiac Biomarkers

Laboratory testing in patients with chest symptoms suspicious for MI focuses on the detection of myocardial injury (see Chapter 1). In some cases, biomarkers that reflect the underlying contributors (e.g., inflammation) or consequences of ischemia (e.g., increased wall stress and end-diastolic pressures) may be useful (see Chapter 8). The optimal use of cardiac troponin (cTn) is discussed in a detailed manner in Chapter 7. In brief, with most current generation assays for cTn, assessment at hospital arrival and 3 to 6 hours after presentation is sufficient to detect or exclude MI. Creatine kinase-MB does not add to cTn for the diagnostic assessment of these patients. For patients with recurrent symptoms that are suspicious for ischemia, later serial measurements (e.g., q6-8h from 6 to 24 hours) should be obtained in most cases. Moreover, in patients for whom the pretest probability of acute myocardial ischemia is particularly high, additional evaluation is warranted even if the initial cardiac biomarkers are normal. It is not necessary or advisable to measure cTn in patients without suspicion for ACS, unless it is being used for the specific purpose of risk stratification, such as in pulmonary embolism or heart failure.

Rapid rule-out protocols using 1- or 2-hour testing of cTn are an emerging application of high-sensitivity assays for cTn and are described in Chapter 7. Although such testing schemes are likely to be useful for the safe discharge of patients with a negative predictive value, more investigation is needed before these approaches can be endorsed for routine use in the United States.[6] Moreover, such rapid rule-out strategies must incorporate clinical characteristics of the patient and the presentation (Figure 6-6). These integrated tools for diagnostic assessment are described in Chapter 12.

Because of the higher negative predictive value of high-sensitivity assays for cTn, there is a tradeoff for detecting myocardial injury in a larger proportion of patients with non-ACS cardiopulmonary conditions than with the previous generations of assays. Because of this evolution in the analytical sensitivity, other aspects of the clinical evaluation are critical for the physician to formulate a probability that the symptoms represent ACS. In addition, the evaluation of

HEART Score		
History	Highly suspicious Moderately suspicious Slightly suspicious	2 1 0
ECG	Significant ST-depression Nonspecific abnormality Normal	2 1 0
Age	≥ 65 years >45 – <65 years ≤45 years	2 1 0
Risk factors	≥ 3 risk factors 1–2 risk factors None	2 1 0
Troponin (serial)	≥3 x 99th percentile 1–<3 x 99th percentile ≤ 99th percentile	2 1 0
	TOTAL	
	Low risk: 0 to 3 **Not low risk:** ≥ 4	

North American Chest Pain Rule	
High-risk criteria	**Y/N**
Typical symptoms of ischemia	
ECG: acute ischemic changes	
Age ≥ 50 years	
Known coronary artery disease	
Troponin (serial) > 99th percentile	
Low risk: All no **Not low risk:** Any yes	

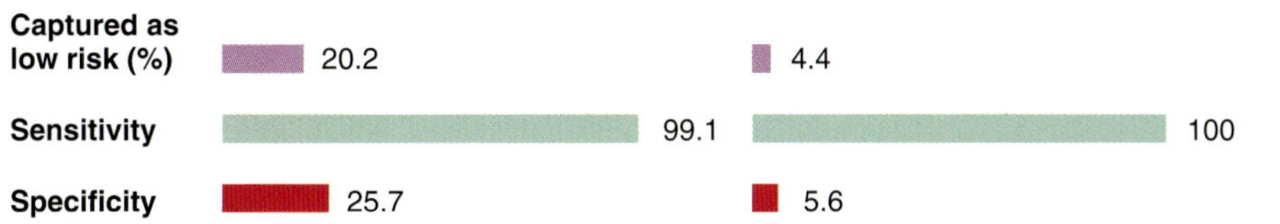

FIGURE 6-6 **Decision aids used in conjunction with serial measurement of cardiac troponin for evaluation of acute chest pain.** *ECG*, Electrocardiography. *(Data from Mahler et al: Identifying patients for early discharge: performance of decision rules among patients with acute chest pain,* Int J Cardiol *168:795–802, 2013.)*

serial values of cTn for evidence of a dynamic (rising and/or falling) pattern is important in discriminating acute causes of myocardial injury from chronic elevation caused by underlying structural heart disease, end-stage renal disease, or interfering antibodies (see Chapter 7).[6] The finding of an elevated concentration of cTn is virtually always associated with a poorer prognosis; however, when it is the result of a chronic condition causing myocardial injury, the time course of that risk is over the long term and may warrant disease-modifying preventive therapies rather than acute invasive evaluations and interventions.[5]

Chest Radiography

The chest radiograph is often unremarkable in patients with acute MI. When present, pulmonary edema is a poor prognostic indicator. The chest radiograph is useful for excluding other potential causes of chest symptoms. Specific findings include pulmonary parenchymal processes, widening of the mediastinum in some patients with aortic dissection, Hampton hump or Westermark sign in patients with pulmonary embolism, or pericardial calcification in chronic pericarditis.

Formulating a Clinical Probability of Myocardial Infarction

Ultimately, the clinician must formulate a clinical impression of the probability that a patient's symptoms represent an acute MI. In patients with ST-segment elevation that meet diagnostic criteria (see Table 1-3), the probability of MI is extremely high, although up to 5% of such patients will end up having an MI excluded (see Chapter 1). Among patients without ST-segment elevation, establishing an initial diagnosis is more challenging. The clinician relies on the history, physical examination, and ECG with interpretation of cardiac biomarkers in that clinical context. Appropriate interpretation of cTn, which is a marker of myocardial injury that is not specific to ischemia, requires a "pretest" assessment of the likelihood that the patient's symptoms represent myocardial ischemia. Clinical experience and sound judgment continue to play a critical role in the evaluation of patients with suspected MI.

Because of the inherent challenges and high clinical stakes, multiple clinical algorithms have been developed to aid in decision-making during the assessment and triage of patients with chest pain suspicious for myocardial ischemia (see Figure 6-6). Such decision aids are most commonly used to identify patients with low clinical probability of ACS who are candidates either for early provocative testing for ischemia or discharge from the ED (see Chapter 12). The common elements to these tools are (1) symptoms typical for myocardial ischemia, (2) known atherosclerosis or risk factors for atherosclerosis, including older age, (3) ischemic ECG abnormalities, and (4) elevated cTn. Reflecting their lack of specificity, the overall diagnostic performance of such decision aids is poor (area under the receiver-operating curve 0.55 to 0.65). However, the negative predictive performance of some such instruments is very high (>99%).[7] Nevertheless, no such decision aid (or single clinical factor) is sufficiently sensitive and well validated to use as a sole tool for clinical decisions.

Clinicians should differentiate between the diagnostic algorithms discussed previously in this chapter and in

Chapter 12 and the clinical risk scores (e.g., the TIMI and GRACE risk scores discussed in Chapter 11) derived for assessment of prognosis in patients with an established diagnosis of ACS. These latter risk scores were not developed for the purpose of diagnostic assessment.

In conjunction with formulation of the previously described diagnostic and prognostic estimates, the clinician must also make decisions regarding additional testing, noninvasive and invasive, and initial empiric therapy. Because delay of treatment in patients with ACS is associated with adverse outcomes, timely initiation of therapy is a priority. As such, treatment, such as aspirin and an anticoagulant, is often initiated in patients with suspected MI while diagnostic testing continues. Figure 6-1 illustrates the interplay of the assessment of likelihood of MI and risk status with respect to therapeutic decision-making. For example, a patient with a low probability of an acute MI, but with a high-risk profile should the patient have unstable ischemic heart disease, may be treated similarly to a patient with a moderate probability of acute MI who is at moderate risk of complications. Patients with a moderate or greater suspicion for acute MI or who are at high risk, and in whom MI has not been excluded, warrant initiation of treatment (see Figure 6-1 and Chapter 13).

DECISIONS REGARDING ADDITIONAL TESTING

Invasive Coronary Evaluation

Patients with ST-segment elevation and a clinical presentation consistent with ischemia should undergo emergent cardiac catheterization when available in a timely fashion in an experienced STEMI center (see Chapter 5 and Chapter 14). Decision-making regarding invasive coronary angiography in patients without diagnostic ST-segment elevation is discussed in Chapter 16. In general, patients with refractory symptoms or high-risk features should undergo coronary angiography for treatment if a diagnosis of MI has been established or for completion of the diagnostic assessment when an alternative cause has not been identified. In patients at lower risk or in whom patient preferences or appropriateness for coronary angiography do not favor invasive evaluation, additional noninvasive assessment may be useful to establish the diagnosis and for risk assessment.

Provocative Testing for Ischemia

Exercise ECG with or without imaging is commonly used for completion of risk stratification in patients who have undergone an initial evaluation that has not revealed a specific cause of chest discomfort and has identified them as having a low, or in some cases intermediate, probability of MI (see also Chapter 12). Early exercise testing is safe in patients without high-risk findings after 8 to 12 hours of observation and can assist in refining their prognostic assessment. For example, in low-risk patients who underwent exercise testing in the first 48 hours after presentation, those without evidence for ischemia had a 2% rate of cardiac events through 6 months compared with 15% in patients with either clear evidence for ischemia or an equivocal result. Patients who are unable to exercise may undergo pharmacological stress testing with either nuclear perfusion imaging or echocardiography (see Chapter 9). Notably, some experts have deemed the routine use of stress testing for low-risk patients as unsupported by direct clinical evidence and a potentially unnecessary source of cost.[8]

Professional society guidelines identify ongoing chest pain as a contraindication to stress testing. In selected patients with persistent pain and nondiagnostic ECG and biomarker data, myocardial perfusion images can be taken at rest. The absence of any perfusion abnormality substantially reduces the likelihood of coronary artery disease. In some centers, early myocardial perfusion imaging is performed as a part of a routine strategy for evaluating patients at low or intermediate probability of ACS in parallel with other testing (see Chapter 9). In this strategy, normal perfusion images can identify patients for expedited discharge and outpatient exercise stress testing, if indicated.

Other Noninvasive Studies

The selective use of noninvasive cardiac imaging, to provide additional diagnostic and prognostic information in patients with suspected MI is described in Chapter 9. In addition, the individual modalities of echocardiography, computed tomographic angiography, and cardiac magnetic resonance imaging (CMR) are discussed in Chapter 9, Chapter 31, and Chapter 33. These techniques can provide information regarding myocardial function, myocardial perfusion, scar formation, and mechanical complications of MI that are valuable for refining the diagnostic and prognostic assessment. Typically, echocardiography is the most widely and rapidly available cardiac imaging modality for the initial assessment. Computed tomographic angiography of the chest can be useful for the "triple rule out," with simultaneous assessment for coronary artery obstruction, pulmonary embolism, and aortic dissection. CMR provides the most comprehensive cardiac imaging and myocardial characterization, which can be particularly useful in evaluating patients with increases in cTn that are deemed due to causes other than myocardial ischemia.

CRITICAL PATHWAYS

Because of the challenges inherent in reliably identifying the small proportion of patients with acute MI, while not exposing the large number of low-risk patients to unnecessary testing and extended in-hospital evaluations, many medical centers have adopted critical pathways to expedite the evaluation of patients with nontraumatic chest pain, sometimes in dedicated Chest Pain Units. At the same time as offering efficient pathways for assessment of the low-risk patient (see Chapter 12), medical providers must also follow strategies to rapidly identify patients with acute MI and initiate evidence-based therapies (see Chapter 5 and Chapter 13).

SUMMARY

The clinical approach to patients with suspected MI relies on formulation of an assessment of the likelihood of myocardial ischemia based on the patient's history, examination, and ECG. Ischemic symptoms include various combinations of chest, upper extremity, or mandibular discomfort, and may be accompanied by or manifested solely as atypical symptoms such as dyspnea, abdominal malaise, diaphoresis, nausea, presyncope, or fatigue. The discomfort associated with acute MI usually lasts more than 20 minutes. Ischemic symptoms may easily be confused for those from neurological, pulmonary, or musculoskeletal disorders. Concurrent assessment of the probability of ischemia and the risk of early cardiovascular complications if the symptoms are due to MI are the foundation of prudent decision-making.

References

1. Morrow DA: Cardiovascular risk prediction in patients with stable and unstable coronary heart disease, *Circulation* 121:2681–2691, 2010.
2. Amsterdam EA, Wenger NK, Brindis RG, et al.: 2014 AHA/ACC guideline for the management of patients with non-st-elevation acute coronary syndromes: a report of the American College of Cardiology/American Heart Association Task Force on Practice Guidelines, *J Am Coll Cardiol* 64:e139–228, 2014.
3. O'Gara PT, Kushner FG, Ascheim DD, et al.: 2013 ACCF/AHA guideline for the management of ST-elevation myocardial infarction: a report of the American College of Cardiology Foundation/American Heart Association Task Force on Practice Guidelines, *J Am Coll Cardiol* 61: e78–140, 2013.
4. Braunwald E, Morrow DA: Unstable angina: is it time for a requiem? *Circulation* 127: 2452–2457, 2013.
5. Thygesen K, Alpert JS, Jaffe AS, et al.: Third universal definition of myocardial infarction, *Eur Heart J* 33:2551–2567, 2012.
6. Morrow DA, Bonaca MP: Real-world application of "delta" troponin: diagnostic and prognostic implications, *J Am Coll Cardiol* 62:1239–1241, 2013.
7. Mahler SA, Riley RF, Hiestand BC, et al.: The HEART Pathway randomized trial: identifying emergency department patients with acute chest pain for early discharge, *Circulation Cardiovascular Quality and Outcomes* 8:195–203, 2015.
8. Amsterdam EA, Kirk JD, Bluemke DA, et al.: Testing of low-risk patients presenting to the emergency department with chest pain: a scientific statement from the American Heart Association, *Circulation* 122:1756–1776, 2010.

7 Optimal Use of Cardiac Troponin in Patients with Chest Discomfort

Allan S. Jaffe

INTRODUCTION

Cardiac troponin (cTn) is the biomarker of choice for the evaluation of patients with symptoms suggestive of acute myocardial ischemia. Increases in cTn are necessary for the diagnosis of acute myocardial infarction (MI).[1] Some even have opined that with the advent of high-sensitivity assays that the diagnosis of acute unstable coronary disease will eventually require an increasing pattern of cTn values, assuming timing permits such an evaluation.[2] The present chapter attempts to provide clinicians with the data and skills necessary to understand and use cTn values optimally in patients with possible unstable ischemic heart disease. The selection of appropriate patients in whom to measure cTn and the interpretation of cTn results in the context of other features of the clinical presentation are discussed in Chapter 6. The use of cTn in conjunction with other cardiovascular biomarkers is addressed in Chapter 8.

BASIC CONSIDERATIONS ABOUT CARDIAC TROPONIN FOR CLINICIANS

All cTn assays are different, and values from one assay cannot be extrapolated to another. Even assays that seem to identify a similar number of patients in a given clinical situation are calibrated differently; they often use different antibodies, and thus the values will not be the same between assays[3] (Tables 7-1 and 7-2). There have been attempts to standardize assays, but they are unlikely to be successful in the near term.[4] Thus, clinicians need to learn to use the assay(s) that are employed locally. Physicians should know a variety of characteristics as described in the following. Different assays have different issues in regard to specificity, interferences, and sensitivity.

Specificity and Interferences

There may be a small number of patients in whom cTnT has some skeletal muscle interference because the proteins that occur in response to skeletal muscle and injury may be re-expressed, and therefore, cause false positives.[5] The frequency of this phenomenon is unclear, and only a handful of cases have been reported. However, a systematic and scientifically robust evaluation of this issue has not been accomplished. cTnI assays do not have this problem, but these assays are more prone to interference from heterophilic antibodies (see the following) and also from antibodies that can block binding and lead to reduced values. For some assays, this phenomenon is estimated to occur in as high as 0.5% of all positives.[6] All assays can be affected by fibrin interference, which on rare occasions, can cause high values that are not repeatable and do not fit with the clinical picture.

Interfering Proteins

The most common analytical source of spurious cTn elevations, which are more common with cTnI assays, are related to cross-reacting antibodies, the heterophilic antibodies, which are antibodies to the protein from which the assay is developed. These phenomena normally cause high values that do not change over time. They can be easily unmasked in the laboratory, where additional blocking antibodies can be added and/or with dilution studies. When there is such interference, the sample will not dilute at all until such time as the interfering substance is totally gone, and then the value will become undetectable.[7] There also are rare cases of macrotroponemias, which are troponin–immunoglobulin complexes that can cause analytical false positive results.[8] These have rarely been a problem with conventional assays, but could become more common with high-sensitivity assays for troponin I (hsTnI).[9]

Impact of Blood Sampling

With the increased sensitivity of modern cTn assays, quality control of sampling is important. For example, hemolysis will decrease cTnT levels and may increase levels of cTnI with some assays.[7] Thus, avoiding blood draws from indwelling catheters (the most common cause of hemolysis) is advised as much as possible. It is not unreasonable to ask good laboratories to quality assure values that appear peculiar to a given clinical setting or circumstance, or violate what is known about the kinetics of cTn.

TABLE 7-1 **Metrics for Cardiac Troponin Assays Cleared by the Food and Drug Administration**

COMPANY/ PLATFORM/ ASSAY	99TH PERCENTILE (ng/L)	DOES 10% CV FALL ABOVE OR BELOW 99TH PERCENTILE
Abbott AxSYM ADV	0.04 μg/L	>
Abbott ARCHITECT	0.028 μg/L	>
Abbott i-STAT	0.08 μg/L	>
Alere Triage	<0.05 μg/L	>
Beckman Access AccuTnI	0.04 μg/L	>
bioMérieux Vidas Ultra	0.01 μg/L	>
Mitsubishi Pathfast	0.029 μg/L	<
Ortho Vitros ECi ES	0.034 μg/L	=
Radiometer AQT90 cTnI	0.023 μg/L	>
Radiometer AQT90 cTnT	0.017 μg/L	>
Response RAMP	<0.01 μg/L	>
Roche Elecsys TnT Gen 4	<0.01 μg/L	>
Roche Elecsys TnI	0.16 μg/L	>
Siemens Centaur Ultra	0.04 μg/L	<
Siemens Dimension RxL	0.07 μg/L	>
Siemens Immulite 2500	0.2 μg/L	>
Siemens Stratus CS	0.07 μg/L	<
Siemens Vista	0.045 μg/L	<
Tosoh AIA	<0.06 μg/L	>

CV, Coefficient of variation.

TABLE 7-2 **High-Sensitivity Cardiac Troponin Assays Not Approved by the Food and Drug Administration**

COMPANY/ PLATFORM/ASSAY	99TH PERCENTILE (ng/L)	DOES THE 10% CV FALL ABOVE OR BELOW 99TH PERCENTILE
hsTnI		
Abbott ARCHITECT*	16	<
Beckman Access	8.6	=
Nanosphere MTP	2.8	<
Singulex Erenna	10.1	<
Siemens Vista	9	<
hsTnT†		
Roche Elecsys*	14	<

CV, Coefficient of variation; *hsTn*, high-sensitivity cardiac troponin.
*Available for use worldwide, but not cleared by the U.S. Food and Drug Administration for use in the United States.
†Some would question the classification of this assay as high sensitivity; see text.

Sensitivity

It is critical to understand the different levels of sensitivity of cTn assays. The best available approach to classification of the sensitivity of cTn assays is based on the number of normal individuals detected with a given assay.[10] In this framework, assays that detect values in more than 50% of apparently normal individuals are termed high-sensitivity assays (Figure 7-1). This classification framework also indicates that assays with less imprecision, that have a level of a 10% coefficient of variation (CV) ≤99th percentile should be preferred; these are called "clinically acceptable." Assays with a CV between 10% and 20% are called usable, and assays with a CV at the 99th percentile of more than 20% are not acceptable.[3] Assays that deliver a CV of less than 20% at the values of interest have been shown not to increase the frequency of false-positive results.[3] Nevertheless, even greater precision of the assay improves the ability to recognize a changing pattern.

Although this framework for classification is the most commonly used, it is not perfect. There is an apparent discordance between the proportion of normal individuals with detectable levels of cTn and those with disease who have detectable concentrations. In comparative studies, the hsTnT assay that detects cTn in a relatively low proportion of normal individuals compared with other hsTn assays (see Figure 7-1). However, the hsTnT assay appears to detect more elevations in patients with cardiac disease than a cTnI assay that delivers detectable values in a far greater number of normal individuals.[11] This observation suggests that clinical sensitivity and the proportion of normal individuals detected with the cTn assay are not the same. Alternative reasons for this apparent discordance include the possibility of false-positive cTnT values (e.g., due to skeletal muscle damage or false-negative cTnI values, which are caused by the previously mentioned anti-cTnI antibodies). Despite these caveats, in general, the proportion of normal individuals with detectable cTn can be used to decide the relative sensitivity of a particular assay (see Figure 7-1). From that perspective, the hsTnT assay appears more similar to standard "sensitive" assays now in contemporary practice than to other assays classified as high sensitivity.

The 99th Percentile Reference Limit

It is important to know the 99th percentile of a normal reference population for your local assay (see Table 7-1). This upper reference limit (URL) value, rather than the 97.5 percentile, which was the typical convention with most laboratory tests, was recommended when cTn was first codified in the Universal Definition of MI. This higher URL was selected to minimize the frequency of elevations that were not associated with cardiovascular pathology.[12] In many hospital systems, cut points at concentrations higher than the 99th percentile have been arbitrarily assigned or are based on outdated benchmarks and reported as definite MI. However, use of such a higher cut point will reduce the clinical sensitivity for identifying patients with MI. For this reason, clinical providers should be familiar with the 99th percentile decision limit for the assay used locally. In addition, in knowing the 99th percentile URL for your assay, the clinician must also understand the importance of identifying a rising or falling pattern of cTn values (see the section on Definition of a Changing Pattern of Cardiac Troponin Values).

Advanced Considerations

For assays that are not high-sensitivity assays, the 99th percentile tends to work well in practice as the diagnostic cut point for MI. However, some experts have questioned whether the 99th percentile URL is ideal or if the value should be lowered to the 97.5% value in the high-sensitivity assays currently available in Europe, and which are expected to come to the United States. This issue is a complicated one and in part depends on how the 99th percentile is defined.[6]

The details of methods for determining the 99th percentile in the normal population are beyond the scope of this chapter, but it should be understood that the more rigorously a clinician screens for occult cardiovascular disease by history, physical examination, measurement of other biomarkers

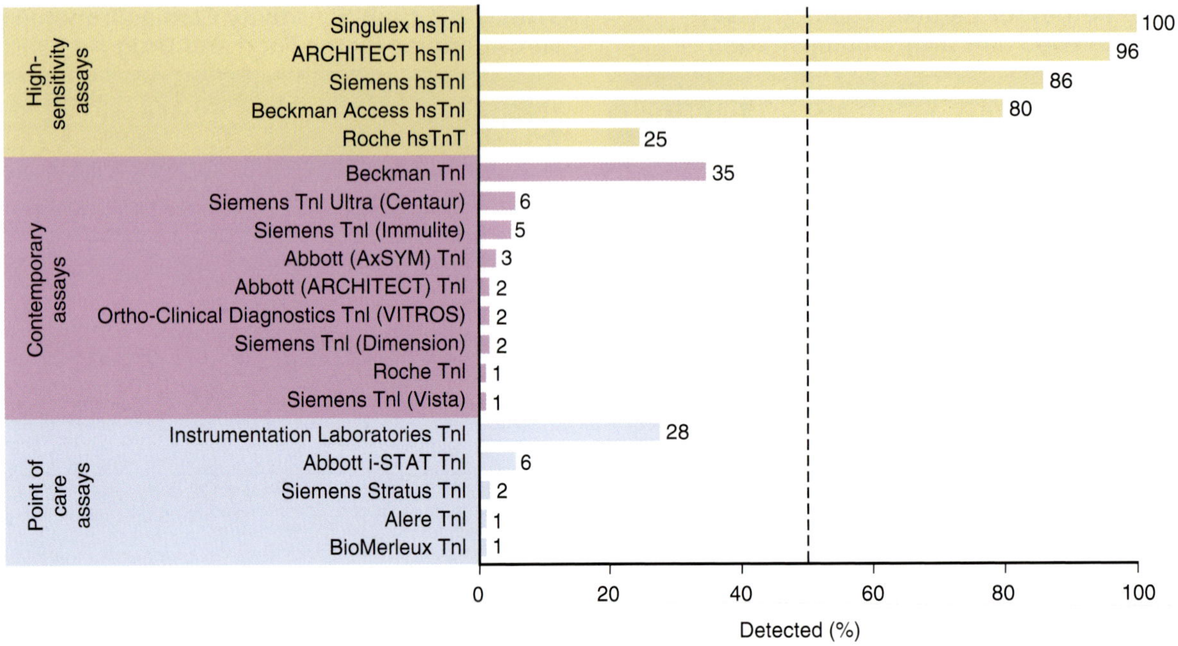

FIGURE 7-1 Frequency of normal individuals with detectable values for cardiac troponin (cTn). Samples were provided by Apple and colleagues and run by the diagnostic companies. Some would question the classification of high-sensitivity (hsTnT) as a "high-sensitivity" assay because less than 50% of normal individuals had a detectable value. *(Adapted from Apple FS, Ler R, Murakami MM: Determination of 19 cardiac troponin I and T assay 99th percentile values from a common presumably healthy population.* Clin Chem *58:1574-1581, 2012.)*

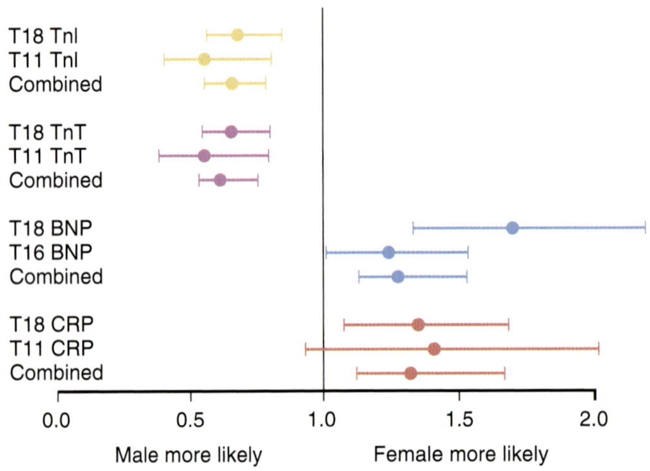

FIGURE 7-2 Relative probability of elevations of various biomarkers by gender from the TIMI trials. Numbers (11, 16, and 18) designate the specific TIMI trial numbers. High-sensitivity troponin (Tn) assays were not used. *BNP*, Brain natriuretic peptide; *CRP*, C-reactive protein. *(Adapted from Wiviott SD, Cannon CP, Morrow DA, et al: Differential expression of cardiac biomarkers by gender in patients with unstable angina/non–ST-elevation myocardial infarction.* Circulation *109:583, 2004, Fig. 2.)*

(e.g., natriuretic peptides), assessment of renal function, and cardiovascular imaging, the more apt a clinician will be able to identify a truly normal population, absent any underlying cardiovascular abnormalities. With more rigorous screening, the value for the 99th percentile of the population distribution becomes lower and lower.[7,13] Thus, with high-sensitivity assays, because few manufacturers have used such rigorous approaches to screening, some confidence boundaries around the estimated 99th percentile URL will likely be necessary. As such, the reported 99th percentile values in package inserts for hsTn assays may be higher than those observed in a more intensively screened population.

For patients with unstable ischemic heart disease, the values of hsTn are likely to be high, so this issue is unlikely to influence the diagnosis of MI significantly.[14] For more chronic disease states, it may well be that a value lower than the 99th percentile URL would be optimal for clinical decision-making. However, regardless of how these issues related to determination of the URL are viewed, the key to interpretation of hsTn is to use not only the 99th percentile value but also determine whether a changing pattern is present along with the clinical circumstances of the patient's presentation (see the sections on Definition of a Changing Pattern of Cardiac Troponin Values and Importance of Clinical Context).

Sex-Specific Cutoffs

Sex-specific cutoff values will be needed with hsTn assays. It has been known for some time that the frequency of elevations of cTn with conventional assays in patients with acute coronary syndrome (ACS) are much greater in men than in women (Figure 7-2).[15] With hsTn assays, it is now clear that women have lower 99th percentile URL values. The clinical relevance can be debated for the diagnosis of MI.[15,16] Nevertheless, because of differences in the pathogenesis of atherosclerotic coronary artery disease between the sexes, it is likely that sex-specific cut points for cTn will be important across all clinical settings, especially in emerging clinical applications in chronic heart disease.[15]

Definition of a Changing Pattern of Cardiac Troponin Values

The concentration of cTn is now measurable in most of the population with high-sensitivity assays (by definition), and chronic elevations of cTn are apparent in many patients with underlying structural heart disease. Therefore, the ability to define and identify changing concentrations of cTn (a delta) is important to discriminating acute myocardial injury, including MI, from chronic disease or normal.[17] The optimal definition of a changing value continues to be debated and is a focus of ongoing investigation. However, at present, some best available practical approaches can be outlined for clinical practice.

With conventional cTn assays, a delta criterion of at least three SDs of the variation around the value has been advocated to be sure that any two values are analytically different from each other. It is from this concept that the criterion of a 20% relative change was developed. This criterion works well with conventional assays when values are elevated. However, a 20% relative change is likely too small as a delta criterion when the values are near the 99th percentile URL (see the following). For high-sensitivity assays, I recommend using a criterion of a 50% relative change when near the 99th percentile URL, which is a lower relative change criterion if the baseline value is elevated. An absolute value that is similar in magnitude to a 50% change also appears to work well near the 99th percentile, but may be superior especially when baseline values are elevated (Figure 7-3).[17]

The clinician must recognize that with imprecise assays, noise in the results may exceed these change criteria. This limitation highlights why it is important to have good precision at the 99th percentile URL. Moreover, some patients with acute MI will have a changing pattern that is smaller in magnitude.[17] Additional important caveats to interpreting changes in cTn are described in the next section.

Challenges in Defining a Change Criterion

With conventional assays for cTn, when values are not elevated, imprecision is much greater and the 20% relative change criterion will be too small and must be individualized for each assay. Nevertheless, assays that do not have an imprecision at less than 10% at the 99th percentile URL can still be used and do not cause false-positive elevations.[1]

With high-sensitivity assays, determination of the optimal criteria for a changing value has become much more complicated. With the ability to measure values in normal individuals, biologic variation has an impact on this evaluation. When biologic variation is taken into account, it is clear that the reference change value (RCV), which is the value where one can be sure that the values are different, increases from 50% to 85%. For some assays, to increase complexity, imprecision depends not only on the reagents but on the piece of equipment used to make the measurement.[18] Although a criterion of a 50% relative change or an absolute value that is similar appears to work fairly well around the upper range of normal, when cTn values are substantially elevated, which usually means patients have presented late after the onset of acute MI, a delta may not be found at all if the concentrations are around the peak values or on the downslope of the curve. In addition, once cTn values are elevated, the relative (percent) rise is not nearly as robust because values may not be able to increase further. Therefore, in those circumstances, I recommend use of an absolute criteria or a lower percentage (e.g., 20%). In my opinion, it is likely that a change criterion based on the absolute concentration will

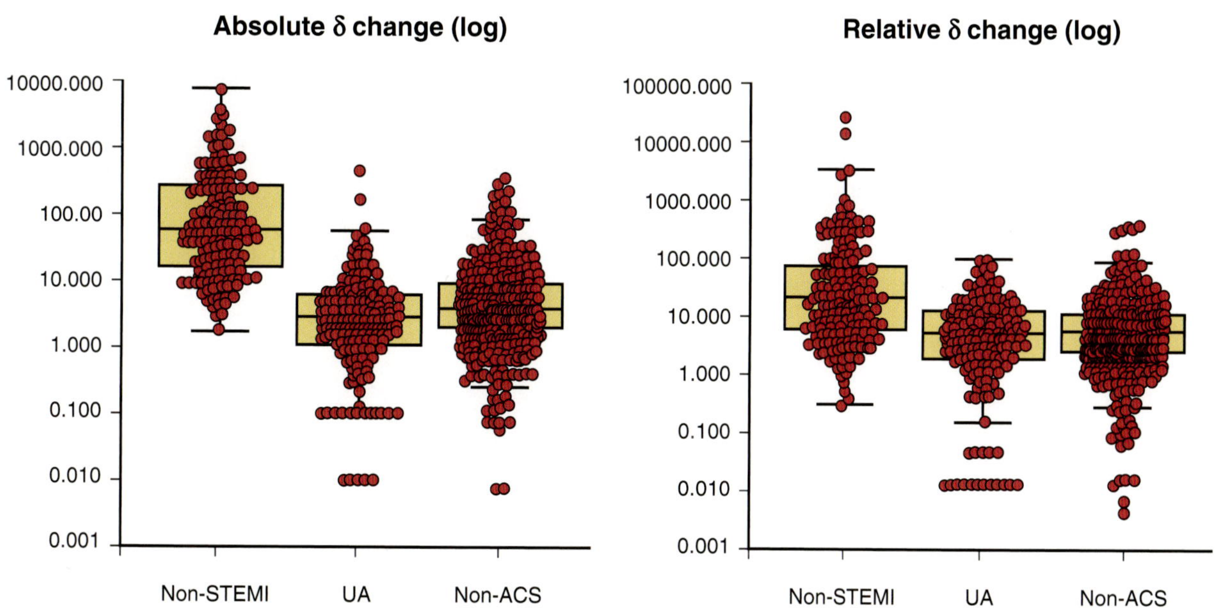

FIGURE 7-3 Distribution of the relative and absolute changes in high-sensitivity cardiac troponin T concentration among patients presenting with suspected acute coronary syndrome (ACS). The advantage of absolute values was driven mostly by those who presented late after symptoms and had elevated baseline high-sensitivity cardiac troponin T values. *Non-STEMI*, Non–ST-elevation myocardial infarction; *UA*, unstable angina. *(Adapted from Mueller M, Biener M, Vafaie M, et al: Absolute and relative kinetic changes of high-sensitivity cardiac troponin T in acute coronary syndrome and in patients with increased troponin in the absence of acute coronary syndrome.* Clin Chem *58:209–218, 2012.)*

turn out to be optimal for diagnosis when baseline cTn values are elevated.

As indicated previously, there will be a group of patients in whom some clinical judgment will be necessary. At present, many of the approaches advocated for defining changing values have been predicated on data collected by convenience registries, which are less rigorous than ideal.[17] In addition, some of the criteria are based on a flawed approach of using validated changes over 6 hours and extrapolating those changes over shorter periods of time. cTn release is blood flow–dependent, and the assumption that cTn release is consistent assumes that blood flow does not change over time. That assumption is not proven and likely incorrect. In addition, some of the delta criteria are based on such small values that even the best assays may not be capable of providing sufficiently accurate values.[17] Thus, caution is suggested with the use of these approaches, especially in patients who present early after the onset of symptoms. Nonetheless, with hsTn assays, the preceding suggestions are likely to be valid even in more rigorous studies. However, it is likely that the optimal criteria will be assay-dependent. Finally, the use of any criteria less than the RCV will result in a tension between sensitivity and specificity.[7] Using delta criteria less than the RCV will include some patients who do not have acute ischemic heart disease, but who may have other acute diseases that can cause elevations or more chronic disease with myocyte injury (see the section on Situations That May Be Confused with Myocardial Infarction). Decisions about how to manage these issues in practice should be made conjointly by emergency department (ED) physicians, cardiologists, and laboratorians.

Sampling and Reporting

To provide a consistent approach to measurement of cTn, a set sampling interval is recommended. The optimal sampling interval between the first 1 and 3 hours differs from one that might be advocated for the period between 3 and 24 hours after presentation with suspected MI.[3] I favor a strategy of 0, 3, and 6 hours, an approach that is recommended in current professional guidelines. Moreover, it is very helpful to have laboratory reports indicate whether a changing pattern of cTn values is present.[1] In addition, to avoid difficulties associated with large numbers of zeroes, as assay sensitivity improves, whole numbers, (generally, in units of nanograms per liter or picograms per milliliter) should be used rather than complex decimal type values for hsTn assays.[3]

THE IMPORTANCE OF CLINICAL CONTEXT

Elevations in cTn, although indicative of myocyte injury, are not solely caused by ischemic heart disease. There are a huge number of patients with increased values that reflect other cardiac pathophysiological disturbances (Table 7-3; see also Chapter 6).[19] For example, left ventricular hypertrophy (LVH) increases the amount of troponin per gram of myocardium, and therefore, is associated with higher values.[20] Metabolic perturbations, such as those that occur with renal failure, often in association with LVH, are also associated with elevations in cTn that are not necessarily caused by ischemic heart disease.[20] Similarly, in acute circumstances such as sepsis, the elaboration of a variety of cytokines and tumor necrosis factor can cause elevations. In addition, drug toxicities, such as carbon monoxide poisoning and cardiotoxic chemotherapy (e.g., adriamycin and herceptin) cause elevations that are likely caused by injury to myocytes. Therefore, proper interpretation requires that the cause of any given increase of cTn be considered within the clinical context in which it occurs.

Chronic elevations, such as those seen in renal failure, do not change substantially, but those that are associated with sepsis, for example, may manifest a rising and/or falling pattern. However, in general, with the exception of an unusual renal failure patient and rare analytical artifacts, marked elevations are usually caused by ischemic heart disease and/or myocarditis.[21] With high-sensitivity assays, the frequency of elevated values will increase markedly, allowing for better triage and decision-making. For example, this application may turn out to be useful in patients who have atrial fibrillation[22] and those at risk for the development of heart failure,[23] but only if clinicians interpret the information in the appropriate clinical context and do not assume all elevations are caused by ischemic heart disease.

A Bayesian Approach to the Chest Pain Patient

The optimal way to use troponin is to evaluate patients before obtaining samples for cTn to identify those at high risk compared with those at intermediate and low risk (see also Chapter 6).[24] The reasons for this are Bayesian. For example, if the most specific characteristic in one ED study that was optimal with a hazard ratio of 2.5 (radiation of chest pain to the left arm) is used and applies it to a group of patients with an overall population risk that is low (e.g., 10% to 15%), then the post-test probability of acute MI is raised to only 27%.[25] Similar statements can be made in regard to negative predictors such as pleuritic chest pain, which has a low hazard ratio of 0.20; however, when applied in a

TABLE 7-3 Acute Causes of Elevated Troponin Levels

ACUTE MYOCARDIAL INFARCTION	NONISCHEMIC ACUTE MYOCARDIAL INJURY
Type 1 MI	Congestive heart failure
Type 2 MI	Infection
Hypertension	Myocarditis
Tachyarrhythmia	Endocarditis
Severe anemia	Inflammation
Decreased supply (±ACS)	Pericarditis
Spasm	Malignancy and cancer therapy
Embolism	Trauma
Drugs	Electrical injury including ablation
Cocaine	Infiltrative diseases
Methamphetamines	Stress cardiomyopathy
Procedure-related	Pulmonary embolism
PCI	Sepsis
CABG	Renal failure
TAVR	Stroke, including subarachnoid bleed
	Acute respiratory failure

ACS, Acute coronary syndrome; *CABG*, coronary bypass grafting; *MI*, myocardial infarction; *TAVR*, transcatheter aortic valve replacement.
Adapted from De Lemos JA: Increasingly sensitive assays for cardiac troponins. A review. JAMA *309:2262–2269, 2013.*

high-risk patient, this factor would not lower the likelihood of an event enough to be comfortable excluding acute MI. Therefore, more complete risk stratification is needed at presentation (see Chapter 6 and Chapter 11).

Once the pretest probability of the disease is developed, the evaluation of the troponin measurements can begin. Regardless of the specific risk stratification scheme, an important issue to keep in mind is that all patients are not the same, and the patient mix at any given institution will vary.[26] Thus, it is up to the local physicians to think through and modify the available proposals so they are optimized for use in their given facilities.[27]

Rapid Rule-Out Protocols Using Troponin in Low-Risk Patients

It is the feeling among ED physicians that they are obligated to rarely miss anyone with MI. If ED physicians are polled, they believe that they should have an event rate at 30 days that is less than 1%.[28] Therefore, ED staff measure troponin in large numbers of individuals to make sure no one is missed because of an atypical presentation. Consequently, a large number of low-risk patients are evaluated; this explains in part why the frequency of MI in unselected chest pain patients is almost invariably in single digits and sometimes even in the low single digits.[29] For this reason, a variety of approaches have been developed to facilitate the ruling out of low-risk patients (Table 7-4, and see Chapter 12). Unfortunately, the data supporting these schema are not always ideally accurate.

Standard Troponin Assays

With standard troponin assays, the guidelines suggest that samples up to 6 hours be used to rule out acute MI as the standard of care.[1] However, in low-risk patients, data suggest that 2- or 3-hour samples, if totally unremarkable, can be used reasonably to exclude MI.[30,31] There are a variety of caveats if such a strategy is embraced. These caveats include the fact that most patients do not come to the hospital early. Thus, many studies that support rapid rule-out protocols have been based on datasets that contained mostly patients who went to the ED many hours after the onset of symptoms.

There is general agreement that once a patient is 6 hours after the onset of symptoms, a normal cTn excludes acute MI. Most patients with MI will have elevated troponin by that time.[27] However, it should be appreciated that if recurrent symptoms are present, the timing of sampling must start de novo.[17] However, particularly with less sensitive assays, the finding of a normal cTn result at that time cannot exclude the possibility of unstable angina. Several studies have supported a clinical strategy of using serial testing of cTn through 6 hours to make a discharge decision. With such a strategy, and adequate clinical scrutiny for the possibility of a late rule out/rule in and/or unstable angina, the frequency of adverse events is low.

However, limitations of such studies should be recognized. The data reported are often simply the metrics used to accomplish the rule out without comparison to a gold standard approach that uses longer sampling times.[30,31] Most patients enrolled in such studies have been very low risk (e.g., TIMI risk scores of 0 or 1). In addition, information about how these patients were evaluated during follow-up after discharge is not presented or appreciated as an element of the strategy. For example, in the study by Than et al,[30] short-term follow-up evaluations occurred in almost all patients. Seventy-five percent had additional investigations, 81% had stress tests, 18% had changes in their therapeutic regimen, and 2% had angiographic procedures. Thus, early rule-out strategies using conventional assays can be very effective, but they rely on clinical judgment to identify patients with unstable angina and include good follow-up. However, the most important elements of ideal follow-up are currently unclear and unsure whether exercise stress testing or computerized coronary angiography is necessary (see Chapter 12).

TABLE 7-4 Strategies to Rule Out Myocardial Infarction

APPROACH	CAVEATS
Standard Assays	
No value >99th% URL in patients >6 h of symptoms	Cannot rule out unstable angina
No changing pattern of cTn results after 6 h	Could be late (>24 h) of symptom onset
Normal cTn values that are 2 h apart	Only for low-risk patients. Good short-term follow-up essential. Care required for early presenters.
hsTn Assays	
No value >99th% URL in patients >6 h of symptoms	Unstable angina unlikely
Very low or undetectable value at presentation	Care required for early presenters. Key value will vary by assay. Only works for low-risk patients. Caution in those who present atypically (e.g., women with possible SCAD)
Lack of an elevated hsTn value >1–3 h	Care required for early presenters. Caution advised if rising pattern but values not yet >99th% URL.
No changing pattern of elevated cTn results after 6 h	Could be late (>24 h) of symptom onset

hsTn, High-sensitivity cardiac troponin; *URL*, upper reference limit.

High-Sensitivity Assays for Troponin

The application of rule-out strategies is more effective with high-sensitivity assays. Not only do these assays more sensitively detect cardiac injury, and therefore, are more apt to detect a rising and/or falling pattern, but their values also tend to increase (albeit not out of the normal range) when comorbidities related to cardiovascular disease are present.[20] Accordingly, low or undetectable values with hsTn assays, assuming the timing of the analysis is correct, not only reflect the absence of an increasing pattern of hsTn, but also make it less likely that comorbidities associated with the development of atherosclerotic disease (e.g., diabetes, hypertension, hyperlipidemia) are present.[20] Therefore, some have advocated the use of low values using an hsTn assay, even on an initial sample, to exclude acute MI.[32–34]

This proposal for clinical application of cTn for rapid rule out has been mostly promulgated with the moderately sensitive hsTnT assay (see Figure 7-1 and the section on Sensitivity).[10] For that particular assay, an undetectable value (<5 ng/L) is believed to exclude acute MI. An example of a 1-hour algorithm is shown in Figure 7-4; the numbers are specific to the hsTnT assay only. The limitations of these studies should be considered. First, the frequency of an undetectable hsTnT has been as high as 61% in one study from Scandinavia,[34] but a prospective study has suggested that the frequency of undetectable troponin is substantially lower when a more structured prospective evaluation is performed.[35] Second, it is likely that most of these patients in such studies arrived at the ED reasonably late after the onset of symptoms.[33–35] Moreover, the subgroup of patients who present within the first hour of symptoms have not been well reported in many of these evaluations.

In addition to these considerations related to individual studies and patient characteristics, analytical issues are also important to evaluating rapid diagnostic strategies using cTn. Unfortunately, different assays have different frequencies of detection. Several of the newer high-sensitivity assays detect values in almost everyone. In that circumstance, an undetectable value as a rule-out criterion cannot be used. Thus, each assay will need to develop and define the low-level value that might be associated with a facile rule-out protocol. In addition, several studies have examined 1-, 2-, and 3-hour rule out strategies.[38] Again, the principles are the same; if the patient is more than 6 hours from presentation, an undetectable value offers an extremely high negative predictive value. If the patient assessment is earlier than that, then two values that are below the URL with high-sensitivity assays seem to rule out acute MI.[36-38] At present, additional markers to facilitate the rule-out process have been advocated, and many have been proposed. Copeptin appears to have some utility as a rule-out marker, but at times it can be falsely negative (see Chapter 8).[39,40]

Caveats for Clinical Application of Rapid Rule-Out Strategies

Physicians should exercise caution in applying a 1- or 2-hour rule-out algorithm in the early presenting patient. These approaches all are predicated on accurate timing of the troponin measurements. However, patients who present when the timing of the onset of symptoms is ambiguous can be problematic. If there is ambiguity, then the time of onset should be considered the initial time of presentation in the ED. Similarly, for patients who have recurrent chest pain, the clock should restart after each episode.[27] If hsTn values are rising, even within the normal range, additional values may be necessary. Again, clinicians should consider the frequency of low- versus high-risk presentations that occur in any given locale to individualize this approach, if it is to be used it in clinical practice. As well, specific metrics will need to be developed for individual assays. Nonetheless, it is likely that this approach using high-sensitivity assays will emerge as a viable strategy for the early discharge of many patients.

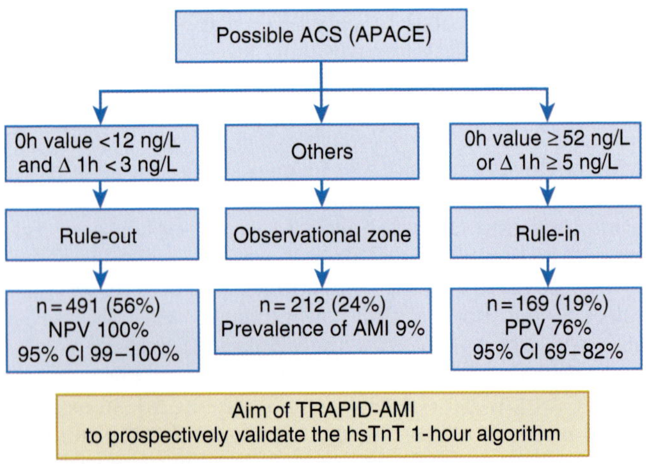

FIGURE 7-4 Proposed 1-hour algorithm using zero hour (h) and 1-h measurements for the evaluation of patients with possible acute coronary syndrome (ACS) using high-sensitivity cardiac troponin T (hsTnT). See text. *AMI,* Acute myocardial infarction; *APACE,* advantageous predictors of acute coronary syndrome evaluation; *CI,* confidence interval; NPV, negative predictive value; *PPV,* positive predictive value. *(Adapted from Reichlin T, Schindler C, Drexler B, et al: One-hour rule-out and rule-in of acute myocardial infarction using high-sensitivity cardiac troponin T.* Arch Intern Med *172:1211–1218, 2012.)*

High-Risk Patients

In high-risk patients, the focus of testing has more to do with confirming the diagnosis of acute MI and facilitating how rapidly diagnosis can occur (Table 7-5). In general, high-risk patients are not good candidates for the early rapid exclusion of acute MI. Such patients are underrepresented in the clinical studies performed to date.[17]

Contemporary Assays

For ruling-in with contemporary assays, patients who present near the 6-hour mark should have an easily detectable rise and/or fall in cTn with sensitive or insensitive assays.[41] Usually, the rising pattern of cTn is readily apparent. A delta criterion of more than 20% is reasonable if the initial cTn value is elevated.[1] However, a higher threshold should be used with conventional assays near the 99th percentile URL when there is greater imprecision of the assay.[1] In hospitals using insensitive assays, the clinician should consider whether some of these patients who do not rule in could have unstable angina. It may be reasonable to reassess cTn beyond 6 hours in patients for whom there is a high index of suspicion of acute MI; there may be an occasional patient who has a total occlusion with poor blood flow without effective washout of the cardiac marker, resulting in late increases in cTn. Such testing beyond 6 hours should be reserved for a relatively small subset of patients.

High-Sensitivity Assays

With high-sensitivity assays, for patients presenting during the first 6 hours of symptom onset, the sensitivity of cTn for MI is high because unstable ischemic heart disease usually results in marked changes in values.[41] Thus, most, but not all patients, will rule in within 3 hours. If the timing is

TABLE 7-5 Strategies to Rule In Myocardial Infarction

APPROACH	CAVEATS
Standard Assays	
cTn >99th% URL with a rising and/or falling pattern	May take up to 6 h or at times more. Rise and/or fall may be missing if late presenter. At times later samples may be necessary. Generally an invasive strategy to treatment is pursued.
hsTn Assays*	
hsTn >99th% URL with a rising and/or falling pattern of ≥50% from a value >99th%	Absolute values should work as well and may be better, but will need to be assay-specific.
hsTn >99th% URL with a rising and/or falling pattern of ≥20% from a value >99th% URL	Absolute values are likely better, but will need to be assay-specific.
Unchanging hsTn elevations	Could be caused by MI if they are late presenters.

hsTn, High-sensitivity cardiac troponin; *MI,* myocardial infarction; *URL,* upper reference limit.

*With hsTn assays, patients with higher values should undergo invasive treatment. Those with lower values must be individualized (see text).

appropriate, the absence of a rising pattern of hsTn probably excludes unstable angina as well.[2] An example of such an algorithm is shown in Figure 7-4.

Considerations regarding the change criteria are otherwise similar to those detailed in the previous section for low-risk patients. Limitations of studies to be considered include limited examination of subsets based on timing of presentation, inappropriate gold standards for the diagnosis of acute MI, and incomplete acquisition of serial samples. Use of an insensitive gold standard will select patients with larger MIs and potentially make hsTn assays appear better than they really are when the full spectrum of detectable MIs are considered.[17] These effects have led to an exaggeration of how early patients rule in.[17]

The distinction among patients who have pulmonary embolism, sepsis, and/or a variety of other acute diseases that can cause cTn elevations is a clinical one (see Chapter 6). However, because ischemic heart disease generally results in much higher values than most of those entities (see the section on Situations That May Be Confused with Myocardial Infarction), high values and marked changes should be considered acute ischemic heart disease with a higher probability that changes are in a middle range, where a more disciplined evaluation of possibilities other than MI is recommended. Additional considerations regarding cTn change, or delta, criteria were discussed in the section on Challenges in Defining Change Criteria. Particularly in high-risk patients, the physician should be astute about whether the values being used to define a change were measured near peak values, and thus may not appear to manifest a changing pattern. In addition in patients presenting late after the onset of symptoms, the cTn concentrations could be on the downslope of the time–concentration curve, and it could be difficult to see a changing pattern. In this situation, it is difficult to know whether an acute event was missed or whether a given patient had a chronically elevated cTn, which is particularly common with high-sensitivity assays and can be related to structural heart disease alone or structural heart disease with some degree of coronary instability.[17] In this situation, some of these individuals may still warrant the designation of having unstable angina.

Once patients have ruled in for MI, it is difficult, if not impossible, to use cTn values to detect injury related to interventions such as percutaneous coronary intervention (PCI) unless the values are shown to be stable before the procedure.[43] At that time, a 20% change would be considered significant. If the baseline value is normal, a fivefold increment is suggested by the guidelines.[1] It is controversial as to whether there is any prognostic significance for post-PCI elevations.[43]

Patients with Intermediate Risk

The considerations already described regarding testing of cTn apply equally; however, there may be even more ambiguity of clinical decision-making for the intermediate-risk patient. Additional scrutiny may be necessary among patients who have an elevated cTn that does not change. Additional information is needed to make a more definitive diagnosis in these circumstances.

Special Subsets with Possible Myocardial Infarction

Women

Women present less typically and have lower levels of cTn (see the section on Sex-Specific Cutoffs).[15,27] From the available data, it does not appear as if separate change

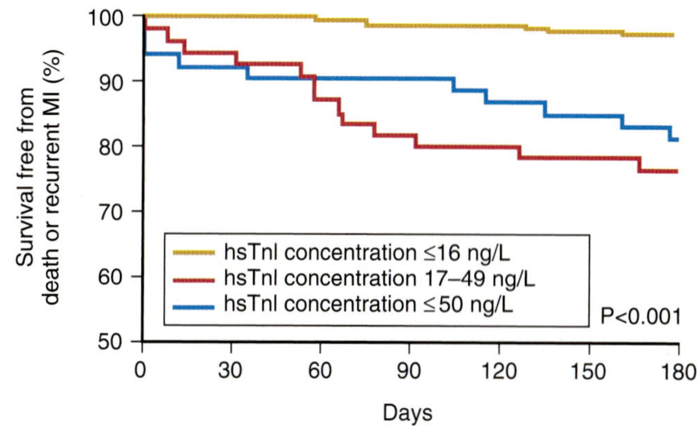

FIGURE 7-5 Influence of the cutoff value used to diagnose acute myocardial infarction. Values for women between the gender-specific and the overall cutoff values were associated with the same number of events as values above the overall cutoff value, supporting the importance of using sex-specific cutoff values with high-sensitivity troponin I (hsTnI) assays. Ideally, a cutoff of 26 ng/L should have been used. *(Adapted from Shah ASV, Griffiths M, Lee KK, et al: High sensitivity cardiac troponin and the under-diagnosis of myocardial infarction in women: prospective cohort study.* Br Med J *350:g7873, 2015.)*

values are necessary for women, but the 99th percentile cutoff values in women will be lower with high-sensitivity assays. Using the proper cutoff value is key to detecting disease in women (Figure 7-5).[16] There may be many more women with events who initially have lower values. Therefore, there needs to be particular concern about women in terms of perhaps not fitting ideally into the early rule-out algorithms.

Renal Failure

Patients with renal failure provide another illustrative subgroup. It has been shown with contemporary assays that even when patients have chronic cTn elevations that the diagnosis of MI is easily made based on a rising and/or falling pattern.[1] Consideration of whether there is a changing pattern is particularly important in this group, who are very likely to have ubiquitous elevations of hsTn using high-sensitivity assays.[44]

Older Patients

Similar approaches should be taken for older adults, who will also have substantial elevations in hsTn at baseline, which is likely caused by comorbidities.[13] Raising the cutoff value will simply disadvantage those who have aged well and who do not have elevated values. Thus, in older individuals, it is the change from baseline that is important. However, clinicians should understand that older patients frequently will have elevated values, and that fact should be taken into account during their evaluation.

TYPE 1 VERSUS TYPE 2 ACUTE MYOCARDIAL INFARCTION AND CARDIAC INJURY

Elevations in cTn can come from a variety of causes (Table 7-3),[1] reflecting chronic heart disease related to underlying coronary disease, left ventricular hypertrophy, and increased wall stretch, such as might occur with left ventricular dilation. Thus, not all elevations are caused by unstable ischemic heart disease. In addition, it is now recognized that there are different types of MIs (see Chapter 1). In 2007, the distinction was made in the Universal Definition to

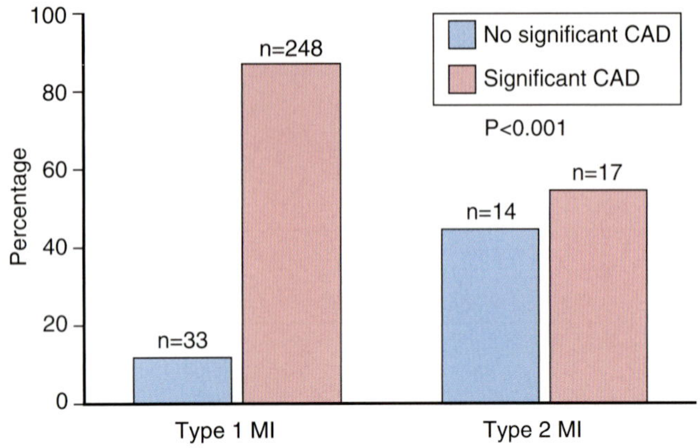

FIGURE 7-6 Frequency of coronary artery disease in patients with type 1 (n = 386) compared with type 2 (n = 144) myocardial infarction (MI) from 533 patients with acute MI and 4449 patients included in the evaluation. Patients with type 2 MI often do not have significant coronary artery disease (CAD). *(From Saaby L, Poulsen TS, Hosbond S, et al: Classification of myocardial infarction: frequency and features of type 2 myocardial infarction.* Am J Med *126:789–797, 2013.)*

distinguish between so-called type 1 MI, which is caused by an acute plaque rupture event, from MI caused by a variety of other causes, which include coronary endothelial dysfunction, vasospasm, supply–demand imbalance, and spontaneous coronary dissection (see also Chapter 1).[1] These distinctions have become increasingly important because research has begun to be developed concerning the characteristics of these two entities.

With conventional sensitive assays, the data previously developed suggest that patients who present with an acute ischemic presentation and elevated cTn are better served with an invasive interventional strategy.[27] These data do not mean that all individuals with elevated cTn or even all individuals who may have a rising pattern of cTn must have coronary angiography, because it is clear that a pattern of increasing acute elevations can be seen in patients with sepsis, pulmonary embolism, and myocarditis. However, because of the appropriate clinical findings, a rising and/or falling pattern of cTn in a high-risk patient with an elevated value or in a patient who presents late after the onset of symptoms should lead, assuming there are no contraindications, to an invasive strategy (see Chapter 16). Notably, a percentage of patients (in some studies as high as 28%) may not have a culprit lesion.[27,45] Many of these patients likely have a variety of other mechanisms for acute MI (see Chapter 1), including type 2 MI.

The frequency of type 2 acute MIs likely will increase with high-sensitivity assays. Type 2 MIs elaborate less cTn than type 1 acute MIs, so their relative abundance will increase.[46] A large percentage of these patients may not have coronary artery disease that requires intervention (Figure 7-6). Rather, treatment is aimed at an underlying problem, whether it is supply–demand imbalance caused by hypertension or tachycardia, or endothelial dysfunction, coronary spasm, or even coronary dissection.[46,47]

For the present time, my suggested approach is to define a value at your own institution that correlates with the concentrations identified previously with less high-sensitivity assays and use that value as a cutoff value for those who need urgent angiography. Patients with ischemic heart disease who have values above that level should receive aggressive care and probably urgent invasive evaluation. Those with values below that level should be individualized; some may need cardiac catheterization, some may not. However, among patients with a high suspicion for type 1 MI, any elevation of cTn above the 99th percentile URL should lead to an invasive evaluation (see Chapter 6 and Chapter 16).

Unfortunately, there are no Current Procedure Terminology codes to distinguish type 2 acute MIs and no good code for cardiac injury. Coding these events as acute MIs often leads to the concept that hospitals are not providing adequate MI care, because many of these patients may not always receive conventional MI therapy.

SITUATIONS THAT MAY BE CONFUSED WITH MYOCARDIAL INFARCTION

See also Chapter 6.

Pulmonary Embolism

Patients with pulmonary embolism (PE) can have symptoms, ECG changes, and elevations of cTn. Individuals with PE who have elevated cTn are a high-risk group.[49] It is clear that these patients benefit from more aggressive treatment such as thrombolysis, but they also have more bleeding, so the net clinical benefit is still unclear.[50] In general, the elevations are modest and short lived (they are often gone by 72 hours).

Aortic Dissection

Aortic dissection is another potential mimicker of acute MI. If proximal, it can involve the coronary arteries (usually the right coronary artery) and cause marked cTn elevations. However, even in the absence of coronary involvement, elevations of cTn can occur and are likely related to the usually present acute or chronic severe hypertension.[51] It is an adverse prognostic sign.

Carbon Monoxide Poisoning

Patients with carbon monoxide poisoning can present with elevations of cTn acutely.[52]

Acute Heart Failure

Patients with acute heart failure and elevated cTn are a common source of confusion. Many such patients have elevations of cTn on admission with a rising and/or falling pattern, and the frequency with which this occurs will increase significantly with hsTn assays. Despite the fact that a common cause for heart failure is coronary artery disease, most of these patients do not have acute MI.[53] Elevations of cTn are most often not different between those who have heart failure caused by ischemic heart disease and those who have it because of dilated cardiomyopathy[53]; some may be the result of acute ventricular dilation.[53] Thus, consideration of acute MI in this group depends on the clinical characteristics of the presentation and other measures and cannot be predicated on cTn alone.

Critical Illness

In addition, for critically ill patients who simply have a cardiac injury, it is likely multifactorial, such as patients with sepsis or acute respiratory failure. The prognosis is clearly adverse, likely because the paradigms used to treat these entities are not sensitive to the need to find a balance between best therapy of the underlying disease and best therapy of the underlying disease that accommodates the fact that there is concomitant cardiovascular disease. In the long run, we will no doubt eventually begin to define specific therapies for each of these groups.[48] Currently, the best one can do is to individualize by scrutinizing each of these patients; this is something cardiologists should be able to do and recommend with a fair degree of accuracy.

Management

An invasive approach to evaluation is not appropriate for individuals who do not have an ischemic cause for their troponin elevations, but who instead have sepsis or PE, myocarditis, or underlying structural cardiac abnormalities. The cTn elevations are likely multifactorial.[42] However, for such patients with a nonischemic cause of elevated cTn, their risk for adverse outcomes is high in the short and long term. Nevertheless, they rarely require urgent coronary intervention. This supposition does not mean that they should never have invasive coronary evaluation, but as a general rule, treatment of these patients should be oriented toward the underlying disease and not the coronary anatomy. In general, such patients with nonischemic causes of elevation of cTn should not be diagnosed with type 2 MI, but instead as patients with cardiac injury. Clinical individualization is essential.[42]

SUMMARY

If used properly, cTn values will markedly facilitate the diagnosis and management of almost all patients. Learning the basics about how to use it properly will markedly improve the practice of clinicians. Ignoring the lessons of troponin is likely to be associated with confusion for clinicians and adverse effects in patients. High-sensitivity assays markedly improve the use of cTn for a variety of entities, most of which are more chronic rather than acute. Because there are more elevations, hsTn requires greater sophistication in its use for the evaluation of patients with chest pain, and clinicians who are not accustomed to using a rising and/or falling pattern of values to aid in diagnosis may find hsTn problematic. However, there are compensatory benefits, such as the ability to rule out patients at an early point in time and the ability to subset patients with chronic disease in a more intelligent manner. Obviously, there are many issues yet to be totally studied and definitive guidelines to be articulated. Physicians need to be wary of the one-size-fits-all approach promulgated by some investigators. However, it is likely that the previously articulated principles for all Tn assays will, in the long run, guide the clinical use of this important biomarker.

References

1. Thygesen K, Alpert JS, Jaffe AS, Simoons ML, et al.: Writing Group on behalf of the Joint ESC/ACCF/AHA/WHF Task Force for the Universal Definition of Myocardial Infarction Third Universal Definition of Myocardial Infarction, *J Am Coll Cardiol* 61:1581–1598, 2012.
2. Braunwald E, Morrow DA: Unstable angina: is it time for a requiem? *Circulation* 127:2452–2457, 2013.
3. Apple FS, Jaffe AS, Collinson P, Mockel M, et al.: International Federation of Clinical Chemistry (IFCC) Task Force on Clinical Applications of Cardiac Bio-Markers. IFCC educational materials on selected analytical and clinical applciations of high sensitivity cardiac troponin assays, *Clin Biochem* 48:201–203, 2015.
4. Apple FS: Counterpoint: standardization of cardiac troponin I assays will not occur in my lifetime, *Clin Chem* 58:169–171, 2012.
5. Jaffe AS, Vasile VC, Milone M, et al.: Diseased skeletal muscle: a noncardiac source of increased circulating concentrations of cardiac troponin T, *J Am Coll Cardiol* 58:1819–1824, 2011.
6. Ungerer JP, Marquart L, O'Rourke PK, et al.: Concordance, variance, and outliers in 4 contemporary cardiac troponin assays: implications for harmonization, *Clin Chem* 58:274–283, 2012.
7. Korley FK, Jaffe AS: Preparing the United States for high sensitivity cardiac troponin assays, *J Am Coll Cardiol* 61:1753–1758, 2013.
8. Legendre-Bazydlo LA, Haverstick DM, Kennedy JLW, et al.: Persistent increase of cardiac troponin I in plasma without evidence of cardiac injury, *Clin Chem* 56:702–705, 2010.
9. Savukoski T, Engström E, Engblom J, et al.: Troponin-specific autoantibody interference in different cardiac troponin I assay configurations, *Clin Chem* 58:1040–1048, 2012.
10. Apple FS, Ler R, Murakami MM: Determination of 19 cardiac troponin I and T assay 99th percentile values from a common presumably healthy population, *Clin Chem* 58:1574–1581, 2012.
11. Aldous SJ, Florkowski CM, Crozier IG, et al.: Comparison of high sensitivity and contemporary troponin assays for the early detection of acute myocardial infarction in the emergency department, *Annals Clin Biochem* 48:241–248, 2011.
12. Jaffe AS: The 10 commandments of troponin, with special reference to high sensitivity assays, *Heart* 97:940–946, 2011.
13. McKie PM, Heublein DM, Scott CG, et al.: Defining high-sensitivity cardiac troponin concentrations in the community, *Clin Chem* 13(59):1099–1107, 2013.
14. Korley FK, Schulman SP, Sokoll LJ, et al.: Troponin elevations only detected with a high-sensitivity assay: clinical correlations and prognostic significance, *Acad Emerg Med* 21:727–735, 2014.
15. Jaffe AS, Apple FS: High-sensitivity cardiac troponin assays: isn't it time for equality? *Clin Chem* 60:7–9, 2014.
16. Shah ASV, Griffiths M, Lee KK, et al.: High sensitivity cardiac troponin and the under-diagnosis of myocardial infarction in women: prospective cohort study, *Br Med J* 350:g7873, 2015.
17. Jaffe AS, Moeckel M, Giannitsis E, et al.: In search for the holy grail: suggestions for studies to define delta changes to diagnose or exclude acute myocardial infarction: a position paper from the study group on biomarkers of the Acute Cardiovascular Care Association, *Eur Heart J: Acute Card Care* 4:313–316, 2014.
18. Frankenstein L, Wu AHB, Hallermayer K, et al.: Biological variation and reference change value of high-sensitivity troponin T in healthy individuals during short and intermediate follow-up periods, *Clin Chem* 57:1068–1071, 2011.
19. de Lemos JA: Increasingly sensitive assays for cardiac troponins: a review, *JAMA* 309:2262–2269, 2013.
20. de Lemos JA, Drazner MH, Omland T, et al.: Association of troponin T detected with a highly sensitive assay and cardiac structure and mortality risk in the general population, *JAMA* 304:2503–2512, 2010.
21. Twernbold R, Jaffe AS, Reichlin T, et al.: High-sensitivity tropnin T measurements: what do we gain and what are the challenges? *Eur Heart J* 33:579–586, 2012.
22. Hijazi Z, Oldgre J, Siegbahn A, et al.: Biomarkers in atrial fibrillation: a clinical review, *Eur Heart J* 34:1475–1480, 2013.
23. McKie PM, AbouEzzeddine OF, Scott CG, et al.: High-sensitivity troponin I and amino-terminal pro–b-type natriuretic peptide predict heart failure and mortality in the general population, *Clin Chem* 60:1225–1233, 2014.
24. Diamond GA, Kaul S: How would the Reverend Bayes interpret high-sensitivity troponin? *Circulation* 121:1172–1175, 2010.
25. Sara JDS, Holmes Jr DR, Jaffe AS: Fundamental concepts of effective troponin use: important principles for internists, *Am J Med* 128:111–119, 2014.
26. Poku JK, Bellamkonda-Athmaram VR, Fernanda Bellolio M, et al.: Failure of prospective validation and derivation of a refined clinical decision rule for chest radiography in emergency department patients with chest pain and possible acute coronary syndrome, *Acad Emerg Med* 19:E1004–E1010, 2012.
27. Amsterdam EA, Wenger NK, Brindis RG, et al.: 2014 AHA/ACC guideline for the management of patients with non–St-elevation acute coronary syndromes: a report of the American College of Cardiology/American Heart Association Task Force on Practice Guidelines, *Circulation* 130:e344–e426, 2014.
28. Than M, Herbert M, Flaws D, Cullen L, et al.: What is an acceptable risk of major adverse cardiac event in chest pain patients soon after discharge from the emergency department? *Int J Cardio* 166:752–754, 2013.
29. Jaffe AS, Apple FS: High-sensitivity cardiac troponin: hype, help, and reality, *Clin Chem* 56:342–344, 2010.
30. Than M, Cullen L, Aldous S, et al.: A 2-hour accelerated diagnostic protocol to assess patients with chest pain symptoms using contemporary troponins as the only biomarker: the ADAPT Trial, *J Am Coll Cardiol* 59:2091–2098, 2012.
31. Goodacre S, Bradburn M, Cross E, et al.: RATPAC Research Team. The Randomised Assessment of Treatment using Panel Assay of Cardiac Markers) trial: a randomised controlled trial of point-of-care cardiac markers in the emergency department, *Heart* 97:190–196, 2011.
32. Body R, Carley S, McDowell G, et al.: Rapid exclusion of acute myocardial infarction in patients with undetectable troponin using a high-sensitivity assay, *J Am Coll Cardiol* 58:1332–1339, 2011.
33. Rubini Giménez M, Hoeller R, Reichlin T, et al.: Rapid rule out of acute myocardial infarction using undetectable levels of high-sensitivity cardiac troponin, *Int J Cardiol* 168:3896–3901, 2013.
34. Bandstein N, Ljung R, Johansson M, Holzmann MJ: Undetectable high-sensitivity cardiac troponin T level in the emergency department and risk of myocardial infarction, *J Am Coll Cardiol* 63:2569–2578, 2014.
35. Body R, Burrows G, Carley S, et al.: High sensitivity cardiac troponin T levels below the limit of detection to exclude acute myocardial infarction: a prospective evaluation, *Clin Chem* 61:983–989, 2015.
36. Reichlin T, Schindler C, Drexler B, et al.: One-hour rule-out and rule-in of acute myocardial infarction using high-sensitivity cardiac troponin T, *Arch Intern Med* 172:1211–1218, 2012.
37. Reichlin T, Cullen L, Parsonage WA, et al.: Two-hour algorithm for triage toward rule–out and rule-in of acute myocardial infarction using high-sensitivity cardiac troponin T, *Am J Med* 128:369–379, 2015.
38. Hamm CW, Bassand JP, Agewall S, et al.: ESC Committee for Practice Guildeines. ESC Guidelines for the management of cute coronary syndromes in patients presenting without persistent ST-segment elevation: The Task Force for the management of acute coronary syndromes (ACS) in patients presenting without persistent ST-segment elevation of the European Society of Cardiology (ESC), *Eur Heart J* 32:2999–3054, 2011.
39. Maisel A, Mueller C, Neath S-X, et al.: Copeptin helps in the early detection of patients with acute myocardial infarction: primary results of the CHOPIN trial (Copeptin Helps in the Early Detection of PAtients with Acute Myocardial Infarction), *J Am Coll Cardiol* 62:150–160, 2013.
40. Mockel M, Searle J, Hamm CW, et al.: Early discharge using single cardiac troponin and copeptin testing in patients with suspected acute coronary syndrome (ACS): a randomized, controlled clinical process study, *Eur Heart J* 36:369–376, 2015.
41. Mueller M, Biener M, Vafaie M, et al.: Absolute and relative kinetic changes of high-sensitivity cardiac troponin T in acute coronary syndrome and in patients with increased troponin in the absence of acute coronary syndrome, *Clin Chem* 58:209–218, 2012.
42. Alpert JS, Thygesen KA, White HD, Jaffe AS: Diagnostic and therapeutic implications of type 2 myocardial infarction: review and commentary, *Am J Med* 127:105–108, 2014.
43. Jaffe A, Apple FS, Lindahl B, et al.: Why all the struggle about CK-MB and PCI? *Eur Heart J* 33:1046–1048, 2012.
44. Jacobs LH, van de Kerkhof J, Mingels AM, et al.: Haemodialysis patients longitudinally assessed by highly sensitive cardiac troponin T and commercial cardiac troponin T and cardiac troponin I assays, *Ann Clin Biochem* 46:283–290, 2009.

45. Ong P, Athanasiadis A, Hill S, et al.: Coronary artery spasm as a frequent cause of acute coronary syndrome: The CASPAR (Coronary Artery Spasm in Patients with Acute Coronary Syndrome) study, *J Am Coll Cardiol* 52:523–527, 2008.
46. Saaby L, Poulsen TS, Hosbond S, et al.: Classification of myocardial infarction: frequency and features of type 2 myocardial infarction, *Am J Med* 126:789–797, 2013.
47. Saaby L, Poulsen TS, Diederichsen ACP, et al.: Mortality rate in type 2 myocardial infarction: observations from an unselected hospital cohort, *Am J Med* 127:295–302, 2014.
48. Landesberg G, Jaffe AS, Gilon D, et al.: Troponin elevation in severe sepsis and septic shock: the role of left ventricular diastolic dysfunction and right ventricular dilatation, *Crit Care Med* 42:790–800, 2014.
49. Lankeit M, Jiménez D, Kostrubiec M, et al.: Predictive value of the high-sensitivity troponin T assay and the simplified pulmonary embolism severity index in hemodynamically stable patients with acute pulmonary embolism: a prospective validation study, *Circulation* 124:2716–2724, 2011.
50. Meyer G, Vicaut E, Danays T, et al.: Fibrinolysis for patients with intermediate-risk pulmonary embolism, *N Engl J Med* 370:1402–1411, 2014.
51. Rapezzi C, Longhi S, Graziosi M, et al.: Risk factors for diagnostic delay in acute aortic dissection, *Am J Cardiol* 102:1399–1406, 2008.
52. Teksam O, Gumus P, Bayrakci B, et al.: Acute cardiac effects of carbon monoxide poisoning in children, *Ann Emerg Med* 17:192–196, 2010.
53. Januzzi Jr JL, Filippatos G, Nieminen M, Gheorghiade M: Troponin elevations in patients wtih heart failure: on behalf of the third universal definition of myocardial infarction Global Task Force: Heart Failure Section, *Eur Heart J* 33:2265–2271, 2012.

8 Other Biomarkers and the Evaluation of Patients with Suspected Myocardial Ischemia

Christian Mueller

INTRODUCTION

Cardiac troponin (cTn) is the preferred biomarker for the evaluation of patients with suspected acute myocardial infarction (MI) (see Chapter 7).[1–4] In addition, it makes sense that other biomarkers that reflect the varied causes and consequences of MI, such as inflammation, activation of coagulation, endothelial dysfunction, and hemodynamic stress, might contribute information that is complementary to the detection of myocyte injury with cTn. Hence, other biomarkers believed to reflect these underlying pathobiological processes have been studied extensively with respect to their ability to add to cTn for diagnosis or risk stratification. In particular, additional cardiovascular biomarkers have been proposed to help address the most important limitation of conventional cTn assays: a deficit in sensitivity within the first hours after onset of acute MI.[1–10]

Despite the compelling a priori rationale and translational science behind them, few biomarkers have yet proven valuable in routine clinical practice when added to use of a contemporary assay for cTn. As such, the current clinical role of alternative biomarkers is less than what was anticipated 10 years ago. This chapter discusses the rationale for investigating cardiovascular biomarkers other than cTn and the available evidence regarding their diagnostic and prognostic applications, with more depth given to the few biomarkers that are in present clinical use for these indications in some regions of the world.

RATIONAL SEARCH FOR CARDIOVASCULAR BIOMARKERS

Although cTn is the prototypical cardiovascular biomarker because of its value for diagnosis and clinical decision-making, cTn and other biomarkers of necrosis are detectable only once myocardial injury has occurred, and they give no insight into the pathobiological causes of the myocardial injury. Because the increase of cTn concentrations in peripheral blood are inherently delayed by the time required for destruction of the myocyte cytoskeleton, strategies using conventional assays for cTn require serial sampling and prolonged monitoring for 6 to 12 hours in a significant number of patients (see Chapter 7). However, the clinical introduction of sensitive and high-sensitivity assays for cTn has substantially reduced and modified this aspect of unmet clinical need.[1–10] Also, because cTn is an integral part of the definition of MI,[3,4] in the absence of any other "gold standard," diagnostic studies inherently favor cTn and render it virtually impossible for any alternative biomarker to replace cTn.[4,5]

Therefore, a more likely role for alternative biomarkers is to complement rather than replace cTn in clinical practice.[4,5] Theoretically, some time delay between the onset of MI (coronary plaque rupture with distal embolization and/or coronary occlusion) and the appearance of cTn as a structural protein in the peripheral circulation should still remain.[4,5] In addition, because detection of circulating cTn using currently available assays signals cardiomyocyte injury regardless of the underlying cause, multiple nonischemic conditions can challenge the interpretation of increases in cTn, particularly mild increases.[1–5] Therefore, alternative biomarkers that reflect other pathophysiological signals (e.g., plaque rupture and/or plaque erosion) (see Chapter 3), other signals that are consistently present at the onset of acute MI (e.g., endogenous stress), biomarkers that reflect myocardial ischemia without necrosis (for the detection of unstable angina), or biomarkers that are associated with a specific pathobiology present in only a subset of MI patients have the potential to help differentiate among the various subtypes of MI (particularly type I vs. type II; see Chapter 1) and allow more personalized and targeted patient management (Figure 8-1).[1–5]

DIAGNOSTIC APPLICATIONS

The search for biomarkers of myocardial necrosis that are more sensitive or rise earlier than cTn has proven predominantly unsuccessful. In this author's opinion, only one alternative biomarker, copeptin, has matured enough to currently justify possible routine clinical use for the early diagnosis of acute MI; therefore, it is discussed in greater detail.[5–13]

Biomarkers Indicative of Ischemia

Copeptin

Copeptin is a blood biomarker that has entered the clinical arena because of the development of an analytically reliable method to measure a signal that is released stochiometrically with the biologically active vasopressin.[5–10]

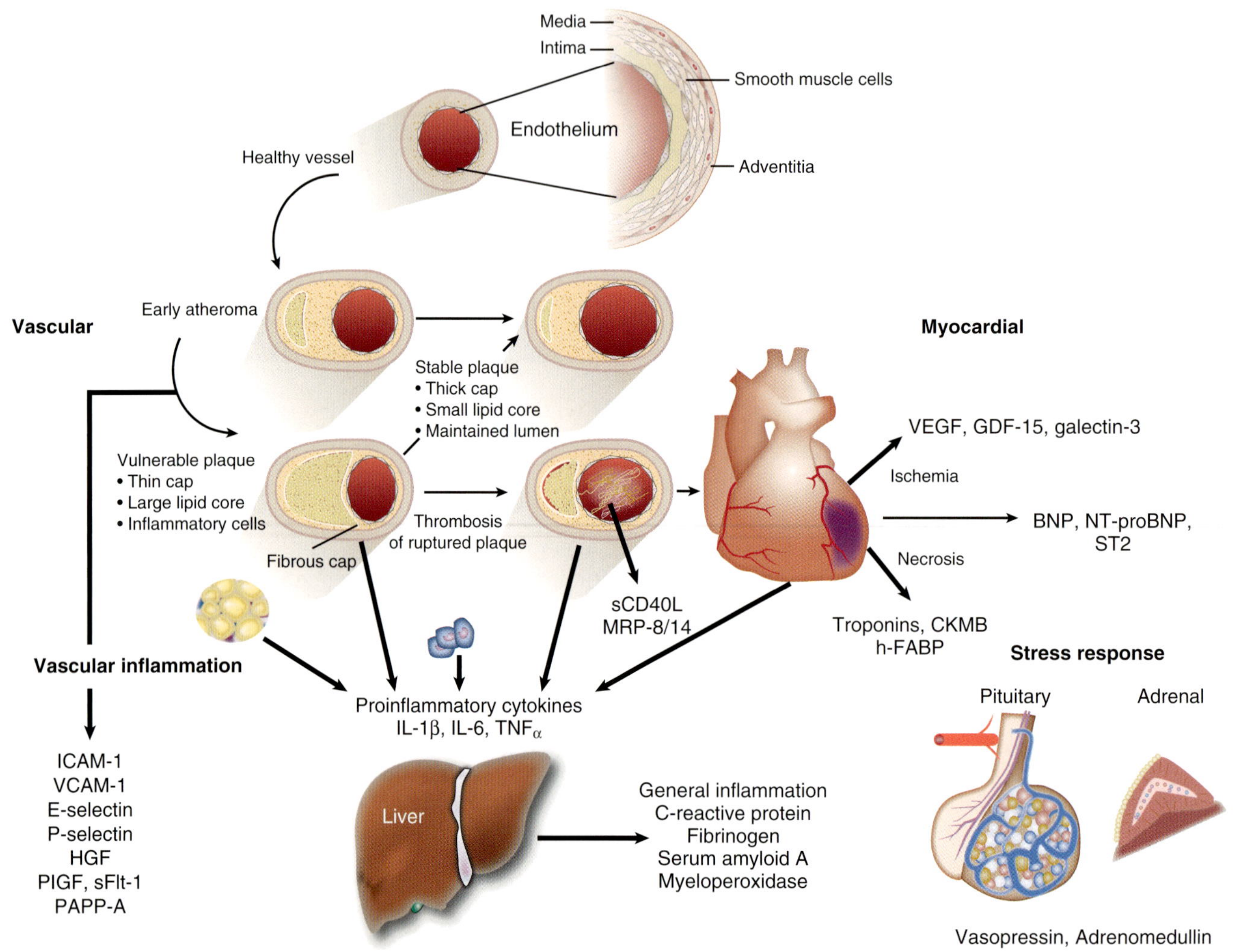

FIGURE 8-1 The pathobiology of acute myocardial infarction and critical points where vascular and systemic inflammation, thrombosis, myocardial injury, myocyte stress, and hemodynamic perturbation may lead to elaboration of candidate biomarkers. *BNP*, Brain natriuretic peptide; *CKMB*, creatine kinase-myocardial band; *GDF-15*, growth-differentiation factor-15; *h-FABP*, heart-type fatty acid-binding protein; *HGF*, hepatocyte growth factor; *ICAM-1*, intercellular adhesion molecule-1; *IL*, interleukin; *MRP*, myeloid-related protein; *NT-proBNP*, N-terminal BNP; *PAPP-A*, pregnancy-associated plasma protein-A; *PlGF*, placental growth factor; *sFlt*, soluble fms-like tyrosine kinase; *TNF*, tumor necrosis factor; *VCAM-1*, vascular cell adhesion molecule-1; *VEGF*, vascular endothelial growth factor.

Arginine vasopressin (AVP) plays an important role in fluid balance by mediating antidiuretic effects (thus, its previous name "antidiuretic hormone") and vascular tone by causing strong arteriolar vasoconstriction. It is secreted as a prohormone from the pituitary gland and then cleaved from its precursor (Figure 8-e1). The remaining part of the prohormone is called copeptin, and from an analytical viewpoint, it offers a distinct advantage, because it is much more stable than AVP.

The current concept is that endogenous stress is the main trigger of AVP and/or copeptin release. Because endogenous stress is already present at the onset of acute MI, copeptin has the theoretical advantage over necrosis biomarkers because it is able to identify acute ischemia and MI early after symptom onset, even when cTn (measured by a conventional assay) is still normal (Figure 8-2).[5–10] Because the time course of endogenous stress and detectable cardiomyocyte damage seems to be reciprocal, copeptin seems to be an ideal marker to compensate for the deficit in sensitivity with conventional cTn assays in patients who present early after the onset of MI. When used in conjunction with conventional fourth-generation cTnT, the added value of copeptin for diagnostic accuracy at the time of initial presentation is substantial (Table 8-1 and Figure 8-3A).[5–10] These findings in a pilot study were subsequently confirmed by several large diagnostic studies, an open-label randomized management trial, and a meta-analysis that summarized findings from 14 studies in more than 9000 patients.[5–10] However, the sensitivity of the cTn assay used in combination with copeptin is an important determinant of the magnitude of any incremental clinical value of copeptin.[5–10] When used with conventional cTn assays, copeptin significantly increases diagnostic accuracy; however, when tested in conjunction with high-sensitivity cTn, the gain in accuracy is much smaller (see Figure 8-3B).

Levels of copeptin are also strongly associated with the risk of death. An elevation in copeptin carried a similar associated risk of all-cause mortality with that associated with an elevation in cTn (odds ratio 5.6 vs. odds ratio 6.8, respectively).[9] In addition, copeptin seems to modify the risk of death associated with levels of cTn (Figure 8-4).

The potential application in which copeptin seems to have the greatest appeal to clinicians is its use within a

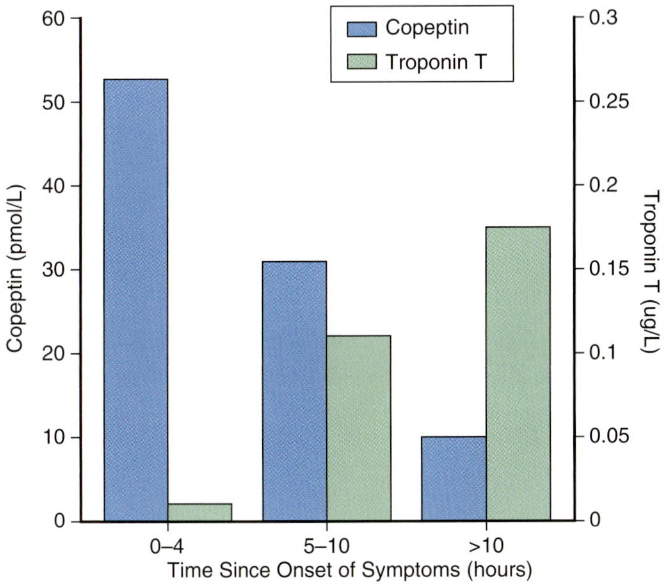

FIGURE 8-2 **Levels of copeptin and cardiac troponin in patients with acute myocardial infarction according to the time since chest pain onset.** *(From Reichlin T, et al: Incremental value of copeptin for rapid rule out of acute myocardial infarction.* J Am Coll Cardiol *54:60–68, 2009.)*

TABLE 8-1 Biomarkers in the Diagnosis of Acute Myocardial Infarction*

CHARACTERISTICS	AUC (95% CI)	AUC (95% CI) IN COMBINATION WITH HS-cTnT
hs-cTnT and hs-cTnI	0.96 (0.94–0.98)	
c-TnT	0.90 (0.86–0.94)	
Copeptin	0.75 (0.69–0.81)	0.96 (0.94–0.98)
Copeptin + c-TnT	0.97 (0.95–0.98)	
h-FABP	0.59 (0.48–0.70)	0.88 (0.86–0.90)
sFlt-1	0.70 (0.64–0.76)	0.96 (0.95–0.98)
PlGF	0.60 (0.54–0.66)	0.96 (0.95–0.98)
MPO	0.63 (0.59–0.68)	0.95 (0.92–0.97)
MRP8/14	0.65 (0.60–0.69)	0.95 (0.92–0.97)
PAPP-A	0.62 (0.57–0.67)	0.95 (0.93–0.97)
CRP	0.59 (0.54–0.64)	0.95 (0.93–0.97)

AUC, Area under the curve; *CI*, confidence interval; *cTn*, cardiac troponin; *CRP*, C-reactive protein; *h-FABP*, heart-type fatty acid-binding protein; *hs*, high sensitivity; *MPO*, myeloperoxidase; *MRP*, myeloid-related protein; *PAPP-A*, pregnancy-associated plasma protein-A; *PlGF*, placental growth factor; *sFlt*, soluble fms-like tyrosine kinase.
*For levels of biomarkers obtained at presentation to the emergency department.
Adapted from Rubini Gimenez M, Twerenbold R, Mueller C: Beyond cardiac troponin: recent advances in the development of alternative biomarkers for cardiovascular disease. Expert Rev Mol Diagn *15:547–556, 2015.*

dual-marker strategy for early rule-out of acute MI. Patients with acute chest pain presenting to the emergency department (ED) with negative initial values of cTn (below the 99th percentile) and also low levels of copeptin (e.g., <10 pmol/L) have a low probability of a final diagnosis of MI. Therefore, this combination of negative biomarker results yields a commensurately high negative predictive value (98% to 99% if using high-sensitivity cTn assays) for acute MI and may be considered to facilitate rapid discharge from the ED without the need for serial cTn testing. An open-label multicenter randomized controlled study that evaluated the safety and efficacy of this approach compared with standard of care (second cTn measurement after 3 to 6 hours) supported the safety of this strategy.[8] Among 920 patients with suspected acute coronary syndrome (ACS), the rates of major adverse cardiovascular events by 30 days were 5.17% (95% confidence intervals, 3.30% to 7.65%) in the standard group and 5.19% (95% confidence intervals, 3.32% to 7.69%) in the copeptin group. The rate of adverse events in those with low copeptin who were discharged was 0.6%. However, clinicians should be aware that because of the rapid decline in copeptin after resolution of ischemia, false negative results are possible when patients present late (e.g., >6 hours) after symptoms.

Other Putative Biomarkers of Ischemia

Other biomarkers of ischemia, such as ischemia-modified albumin or unbound free-fatty acids, that have been studied for diagnostic application in patients with suspected MI have not sustained consistent evidence for incremental value and are therefore not recommended for clinical use. See the section Forward Outlook for a discussion of ongoing investigation of microRNA as a candidate biomarker family.

Biomarkers of Necrosis

General Considerations

At present, biomarkers of necrosis other than cTn appear to have no additive diagnostic role for acute MI. When cTn is not available, the next best alternative is creatine kinase-MB (CK-MB) (measured by mass assay). Because CK-MB constitutes 1% to 3% of the CK in skeletal muscle and is present in minor quantities in the intestine, diaphragm, uterus and prostate, the specificity of CK-MB is impaired in the setting of major injury to these organs, especially skeletal muscle. Although of historical significance, because of their low specificities for cardiac injury, lactate dehydrogenase, aspartate aminotransferase, and total CK should not be used for the diagnosis of MI. Myoglobin shares this limitation because of its high concentration in skeletal muscle. Because of its small molecular size and rapid rise in the setting of myocardial necrosis, myoglobin has a historical interest as an early marker of MI; however, this application of myoglobin has now been shown not to add diagnostically to sensitive and high-sensitivity assays for cTn.

Heart-Type Fatty Acid-Binding Protein

Heart-type fatty acid-binding protein (h-FABP), a small soluble cytosolic protein involved in the transportation of long-chain fatty acids into the cardiomyocyte, is released rapidly into the circulation in the setting of cardiomyocyte injury.[5] Because of its solubility and small size (15 kDa), h-FABP can be released more rapidly than structurally-bound molecules like cTn.[5,11–14] Thus, h-FABP is regarded as an early sensitive marker of MI.[5] Most of the promising data regarding the potential clinical value of h-FABP were obtained before the clinical introduction of sensitive and high-sensitivity cTn assays. When studied in conjunction with sensitive and high-sensitivity cTn, the available data are heterogeneous as to whether h-FABP provides added diagnostic value in patients presenting with suspected MI, including in the challenging subgroup of patients who present early.[5,11–14] h-FABP is available for clinical use in some countries and is used routinely in some centers.

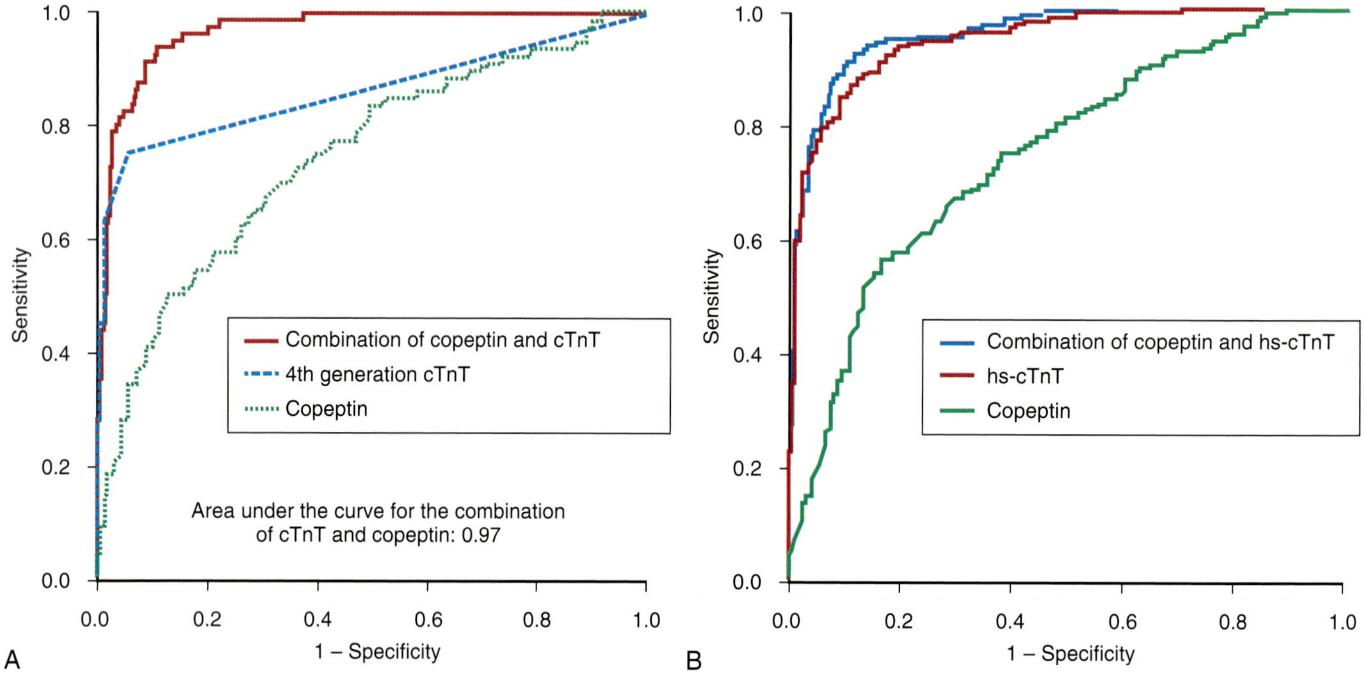

FIGURE 8-3 Copeptin substantially increases diagnostic accuracy as quantified by the area under the receiver-operating characteristics curve when used with conventional cardiac troponin (cTn) assays, such as the (**A**) fourth-generation cTnT assay, but only marginally when used with (**B**) high-sensitivity (hs) cTn. *(Adapted from Reichlin T, et al: Incremental value of copeptin for rapid rule out of acute myocardial infarction.* J Am Coll Cardiol *54:60–68, 2009.)*

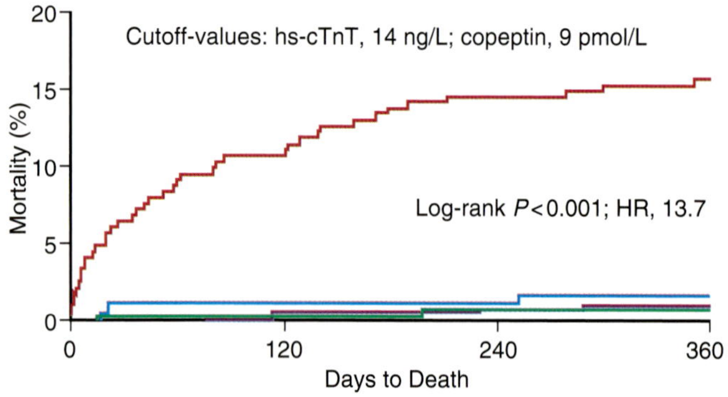

FIGURE 8-4 Mortality in patients presenting with suspected acute myocardial infarction to the emergency department stratified according to levels of high-sensitivity cardiac troponin T (hs-cTnT) and copeptin. Patients with elevation in both markers are at high-risk (*red*), whereas patients with elevations of only hs-cTnT (*blue*), only copeptin (*green*), or with normal levels for both markers (*purple*) are at low risk of death. *HR*, Hazard ratio. *(Courtesy of C. Mueller, unpublished data.)*

Biomarkers of Plaque Instability

Inflammation plays a key role in atherosclerotic plaque formation (see Chapter 3) and contributes to plaque destabilization and plaque disruption that precedes cardiomyocyte damage by minutes to potentially hours or days. For this reason, biomarkers of plaque instability are logical candidates to provide added value in the early diagnosis of acute MI (see Figure 8-1).[5,15–19] Among the biomarkers believed to be associated with plaque instability, assays have been developed for at least six candidates that allowed their evaluation in clinical studies: C-reactive protein (CRP), myeloperoxidase (MPO), myeloid-related protein 8/14 (MRP-8/14), pregnancy-associated plasma protein-A (PAPP-A), and the angiogenetic factors vascular endothelial growth factor receptor 1, also called fms-like tyrosine kinase (Flt-1), and placental growth factor (PlGF).[5,15–19] Despite the strong underlying pathophysiological rationale, methodologically robust diagnostic studies have not been able to show consistently compelling diagnostic clinical utility for CRP, MPO, MRP-8/14, PAPP-A, or the angiogenic markers (see Table 8-1).[5,15–26] In particular, their lack of specificity for coronary arterial inflammation, or even cardiovascular inflammatory processes, has been a major limitation, resulting in extremely poor positive predictive value and a limited overall impact on diagnostic accuracy. Pertinent examples of relevant studies are discussed in more detail in the sections that follow.

Myeloperoxidase

MPO is a hemoprotein that is produced by polymorphonuclear neutrophils and macrophages in response to inflammatory stimuli, and that catalyzes the conversion of chloride and hydrogen peroxide to hypochlorite.[27] MPO is involved in the oxidation of lipids within low-density lipoprotein particles, and it is believed to promote the formation of foam cells in atherosclerotic plaques. Inflammatory cells producing MPO are found more frequently and in higher concentrations in the culprit lesions of patients with ACS than in patients with stable disease. Together with metalloproteinases, MPO contributes to the degradation of the collagen layer of atheroma and the risk of erosion or rupture.[28]

MPO concentration is increased in patients with coronary heart disease, with a gradient of increasing concentration among patients with stable coronary artery disease, those with unstable angina, and patients with acute MI. Elevated levels of MPO are associated with a future risk of developing coronary heart disease and a higher risk of major cardiovascular events in patients who present with ACS. In a cohort of 604 patients who presented with suspected ACS, increasing concentrations of MPO were associated with a higher risk of major cardiovascular events and a greater likelihood of a final diagnosis of unstable angina or MI.[28] On the basis of these findings, high-throughput assays for MPO for clinical use were introduced. However, in practice, MPO had limited clinical use because of its lack of clinical specificity. MPO concentrations are elevated whenever there is activation of neutrophils and macrophages, such as those that can occur in infectious, inflammatory, or infiltrative disease processes.

Angiogenic Factors

Angiogenic factors not only are important in the development and progression of atherosclerosis, but they also seem to be involved in the pathogenesis of MI.[5,15–19] Flt-1 is expressed on endothelial cells and macrophages, and binds not only to the vascular endothelial growth factor but also to PlGF, a platelet-derived protein. PlGF appears to promote the inflammatory process of atherosclerosis, which includes the recruitment of circulating macrophages and atherosclerotic intimal thickening. In patients with acute MI, PlGF is increased, regardless of cTn concentrations, implying that it is a biomarker of the atherothrombotic substrate, such as plaque instability, plaque disruption, or impending thrombosis (Figure 8-e2).[5,15–19] Soluble Flt-1 (sFlt-1), a type of Flt-1 without the transmembrane and intracellular tyrosine kinase domain, is a potential endogenous opponent of PlGF. sFlt-1 is believed to be able to capture PlGF and thereby reduce the amount available to bind to the receptor located on macrophages and endothelial cells.[5,15–19]

Because both sFlt-1 and PlGF have also demonstrated changes in their blood concentrations during ongoing MI, they have a strong rationale as diagnostic tools. A multicenter study that enrolled patients who presented with symptoms suggestive of MI compared sFlt-1 and PlGF concentrations with the results of a fourth-generation cTnT assay and a high-sensitivity cTnT assay. For the diagnosis of MI, the combination of cTnT and sFlt-1 improved the performance of cTnT alone and led to a negative predictive value of 98.3% at time of presentation, but the combination of sFlt-1 and PlGF did not add diagnostic information when used together with high-sensitivity cTnT (area under the curve of 0.96 in both cases) (see Table 8-1).[19] Because sensitive and high-sensitivity cTn assays have become the clinical standard in most countries, sFlt-1 and PlGF do not seem to have clinical relevance in the diagnosis of MI, despite a strong and independent association with long-term mortality. However, their association with plaque instability and coronary artery disease may render them helpful in the distinction of type I MI (plaque rupture) from type II MI (conditions with increased oxygen demand).[5,19] This hypothesis is the subject of ongoing investigation.

PROGNOSTIC APPLICATIONS

Although most candidate cardiovascular biomarkers studied over the past two decades have failed to improve diagnostic accuracy compared with cTn, a broad range of blood markers have been recognized to identify patients with coronary heart disease, including acute MI, who have a heightened risk for death and recurrent major cardiovascular events. As shown in Table 8-2, several of these biomarkers can improve prognostic discrimination beyond the detection of myocardial injury alone. Nevertheless, these biomarkers (other than lipids and cTn) do not presently have a prominent role in the clinical care of patients once the diagnosis of MI is established. The best available evidence has supported that the most important management decisions (e.g., decisions regarding early invasive evaluation) can be based on cTn as the sole biomarker.[20] Despite their prognostic associations, biomarkers other than cTn have no clear-cut clinical implications that affect patient management in the setting of acute MI. Consequently, at present, none of these biomarkers are recommended for routine measurement in patients with suspected or established MI. However, measurement of natriuretic peptides is reasonable in patients for whom the clinician wishes additional information for risk stratification.

Biomarkers of Hemodynamic Stress

Natriuretic Peptides

Natriuretic peptides (NPs) have consistently predicted death and the development of heart failure independently of other clinical and imaging data, including left ventricular ejection fraction.[21,22] NPs are quantitative markers of hemodynamic cardiac stress and therefore are quantitative markers of heart failure (clinical or subclinical). For three NPs (brain NP [BNP], N-terminal proBNP [NT-proBNP], and midregional-pro-atrial natriuretic peptide [MR-proANP]), mature assays with well-validated cutoff values are available clinically. All three have high and comparable diagnostic accuracy for acute heart failure. NPs are released from the left and right ventricles, as well as the atria, in response to pressure or volume overload (Figure 8-5). Their levels seem to integrate the presence and extent of left ventricular systolic dysfunction, left ventricular diastolic dysfunction, valvular dysfunction, and right ventricular dysfunction.

In patients with both non–ST-elevation myocardial infarction (NSTEMI) and ST-elevation myocardial infarction (STEMI), elevated concentrations of BNP or NT-proBNP identify patients with up to a fivefold higher risk of death and new and/or recurrent heart failure. Data from more than 10 clinical studies consistently revealed that BNP and NT-proBNP are among the most robust predictors of death and heart failure after MI. In a contemporary analysis of more than 41,000 patients from the US National Cardiovascular Data Registry, patients with NSTEMI and STEMI who had a BNP concentration in the highest quartile had a risk of death in-hospital that exceeded 10% compared with those with a BNP in the lowest quartile who had in-hospital mortality rates of 1.3% and 1.9% after presenting with NSTEMI or STEMI, respectively (Figure 8-6).[29]

Despite the consistent evidence supporting the use of BNP and NT-proBNP to identify patients at risk for death and heart failure after MI, more sparse data are available to guide clinicians with respect to the therapeutic implications of these findings. An aggressive approach to coronary revascularization following ACS may be of benefit for patients with BNP or NT-proBNP elevation.[30] However, two retrospective studies that evaluated the use of BNP and NT-proBNP to select patients for an invasive management strategy have shown seemingly conflicting results. In a substudy of the TACTICS-TIMI 18 trial, in which BNP levels were strongly associated with the risk for death after presenting with ACS, BNP did not identify a subgroup who derived particular benefit from the early invasive management strategy. In contrast, in a FRISC II substudy, patients who presented with ACS and elevated plasma levels of NT-proBNP and interleukin-6 (IL-6) had a survival benefit when they were assigned to an early invasive strategy instead of to an early conservative strategy (Figure 8-7). Although such findings from a single study are supportive of the concept that high-risk patients with elevated NPs have the most to gain from invasive evaluation and revascularization, the data are insufficient to warrant routine application of NPs in this manner.

TABLE 8-2 Comparison of Selected Cardiovascular Biomarkers

CHARACTERISTICS	PROGNOSTIC IMPACT	DIAGNOSTIC IMPACT	THERAPEUTIC IMPACT
Markers of Necrosis			
Creatine phosphokinase-MB	+++	+++	++
Myoglobin	+	+	+
Cardiac troponin	++++	++++	++++
Markers of Myocardial Dysfunction or Stress			
Atrial natriuretic peptide	++	++*	?
B-type natriuretic peptides	++++	++++*	+++
Copeptin	++	+++	?
Proadrenomedullin	++	+	?
Markers of Inflammation			
Adiponectin	++	?	?
C-reactive protein	+++	?	++
Growth differentiation factor-15	+++	?	+
Interleukin-6	+++	?	?
Soluble ST2	++	?	?
Tumor necrosis factor-α	++	?	?
Markers of Ischemia			
Choline	+	?	?
Heart-type fatty acid-binding protein	++	++	?
Ischemia modified albumin	+	+	?
Markers of Plaque Destabilization/Rupture			
Lipoprotein associated phospholipase A2	++	?	?
Matrix metalloproteinase-9	++	?	?
Myeloperoxidase	++	++	?
Placental growth factor	++	?	?
Pregnancy-associated plasma protein A	+++	+	?
Secretory phospholipase A2	+	?	?
Soluble intercellular adhesion molecule 1	+++	?	?
Markers of Platelet Activation			
Soluble CD40 ligand	++/?	?	?
Soluble P-selectin	++	?	?

+, Some evidence by small studies; ++, intermediate evidence from several studies or one large study or trial; +++, good evidence from several large studies or trials; ++++, excellent evidence; ?, conflicting results or no results available or not applicable.
*For stratification of patients with heart failure.
From Hochholzer W, Morrow DA, Giugliano RP: Novel biomarkers in cardiovascular disease: update 2010. Am Heart J *160:583–94, 2010.*

Therefore, in the absence of definitive treatment implications, clinical use of BNP and NT-proBNP in patients with MI is presently limited to risk stratification, for which it is a reasonable option to enhance prognostic assessment along with cTn and other clinical risk indicators.

Novel Biomarkers of Hemodynamic Stress

Clinical outcomes in patients with MI are dominated by the degree of impairment of left ventricular function (see Chapter 11 and Chapter 13). Therefore, noninvasive tools that reflect the severity of myocardial stress related to ischemia or infarction could plausibly contribute information to guide prognostication and possibly therapy. In addition to the NPs, several other candidate biomarkers of hemodynamic stress have emerged as potent predictors of adverse outcomes, particularly death and heart failure. Such stress markers have been identified either by the finding that they are induced by hemodynamic stress or that they correlate with hemodynamic parameters in vivo. These candidate markers reflect a broad range of pathobiological sequelae of increased stress on cardiac myocytes (Figure 8-8). ST2 and adrenomedullin are two such interesting markers that are available for cardiovascular applications in some countries.

ST2

ST2, also known as IL-1 receptor-like-1, is a mechanically regulated protein that is a member of the IL-1 receptor family. The soluble form of ST2 has a signal sequence that enables its secretion from a variety of cell types, including cardiac myocytes subjected to mechanical strain. A larger membrane-anchored form is denoted ST2L. The ligand for ST2 appears to be IL-33, which is also induced and released by stretched myocytes. Binding of IL-33 to ST2L, in response to cardiac disease or injury, has elicited a cardioprotective effect in experimental models. Soluble ST2 appears to act as a decoy receptor, binding to circulating IL-33 and thereby dampening its actions by making it unavailable to ST2L for cardioprotective signaling. ST2 is markedly upregulated as early as 1 hour

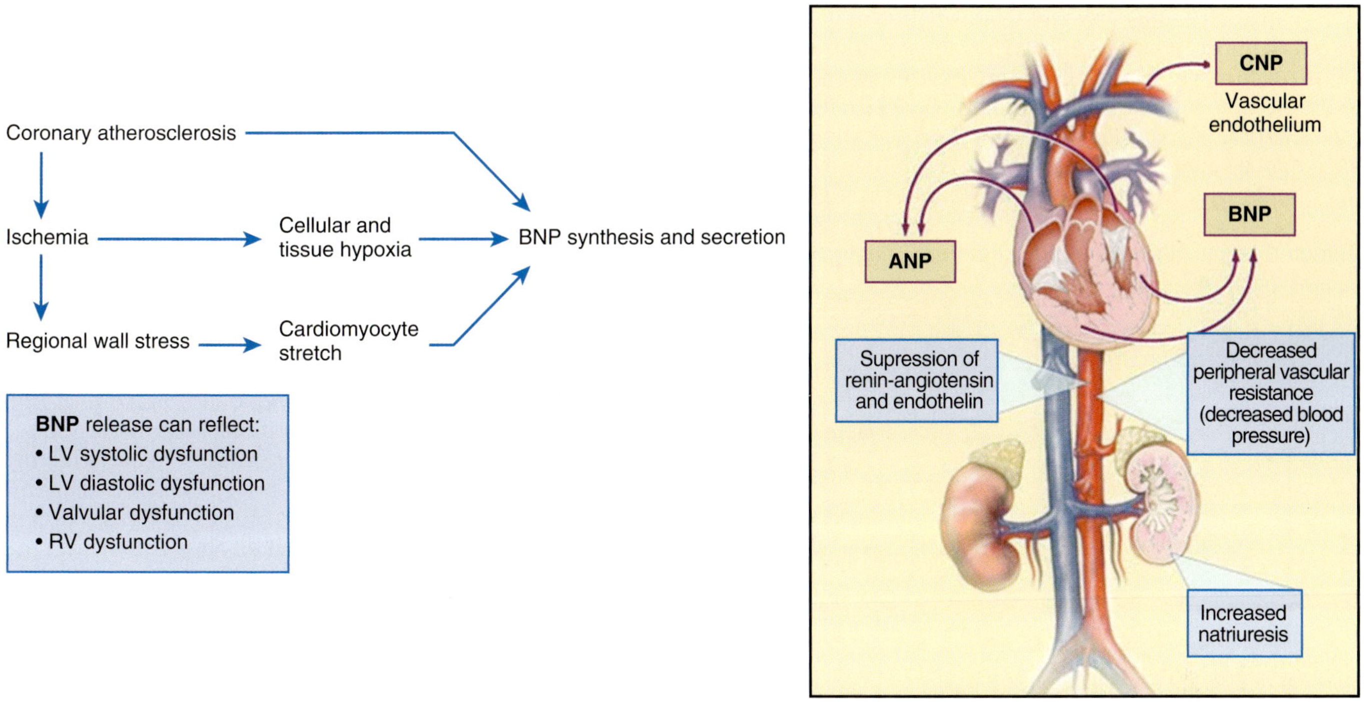

FIGURE 8-5 Proposed mechanisms of natriuretic peptide release in coronary ischemic disease. Blood concentrations of natriuretic peptides quantify cardiac hemodynamic stress by summarizing the extent of left ventricular (LV) systolic dysfunction, LV diastolic dysfunction, valvular dysfunction, and right ventricular (RV) dysfunction. *ANP*, Atrial natriuretic peptide; *BNP*, brain natriuretic peptide; *CNP*, C-type natriuretic peptide. *(Adapted from Abdullah SM, de Lemos JA: Natriuretic peptides in acute and chronic coronary artery disease. In Morrow DA, editor:* Cardiovascular biomarkers: pathophysiology and disease management. *Humana Press, Totowa, NJ, 2006.)*

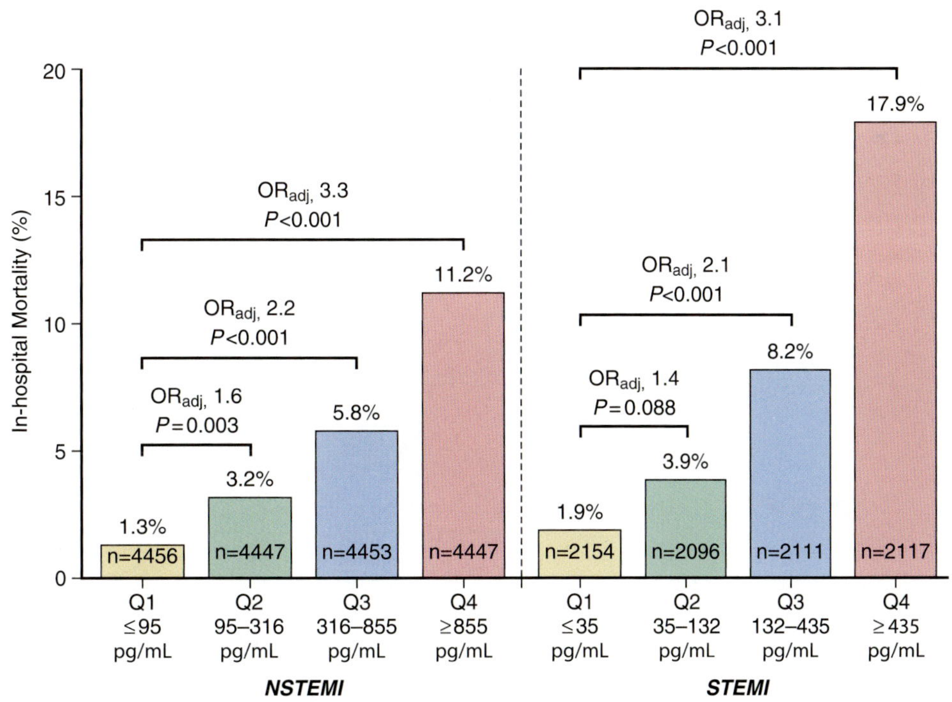

FIGURE 8-6 In-hospital mortality according to the quartile (Q) of brain natriuretic peptide in 41,683 patients with non–ST-elevation myocardial infarction (NSTEMI) and 27,860 patients with STEMI at 309 U.S. hospitals from the ACTION Registry–GWTG between July 2008 and September 2009. The odds ratios (OR) are adjusted for age, serum creatinine, systolic blood pressure, cardiac troponin, heart failure, shock, ST-deviation, heart rate, and a history of peripheral artery disease. *(From Scirica BM, et al: Association between natriuretic peptides and mortality among patients admitted with myocardial infarction: a report from the ACTION Registry(R)-GWTG™.* Clin Chem *59:1205–1214, 2013.)*

following mechanical strain in patients with acute MI, and has been associated with adverse remodeling in this population. In patients with MI, a high ST2 level at presentation identifies patients with a more than threefold higher risk of cardiovascular death or heart failure as early as 30 days and through 1 year after onset.[31] Although ST2 concentrations are higher in patients with greater myocardial injury, ST2 is only weakly correlated with peak cTn as an indicator of infarct size; this suggests that ST2 is not purely a marker of hemodynamic stress, but may also reflect inflammation, fibrosis, and adverse myocardial remodeling, likely through pathways distinct from those detected by established biomarkers.

Because ST2 may integrate information regarding the extent of injury, the inflammatory response, and mechanical stress on cardiac myocytes, ST2 has the theoretical potential to be useful to guide therapies aimed at adverse remodeling (see Chapter 36), or the ST2 and/or IL-33 signaling pathway itself may be a target for intervention. A small study (n = 100) in patients with STEMI demonstrated that increases of ST2 concentration were associated with adverse remodeling detected by cardiac magnetic resonance imaging over 12 to 24 weeks. Moreover, the study suggested that the aldosterone antagonist eplerenone could reduce medium-term adverse remodeling in high-risk patients with elevated ST2. At present, professional society guidelines make no specific recommendation for the use of ST2 in patients with acute MI.

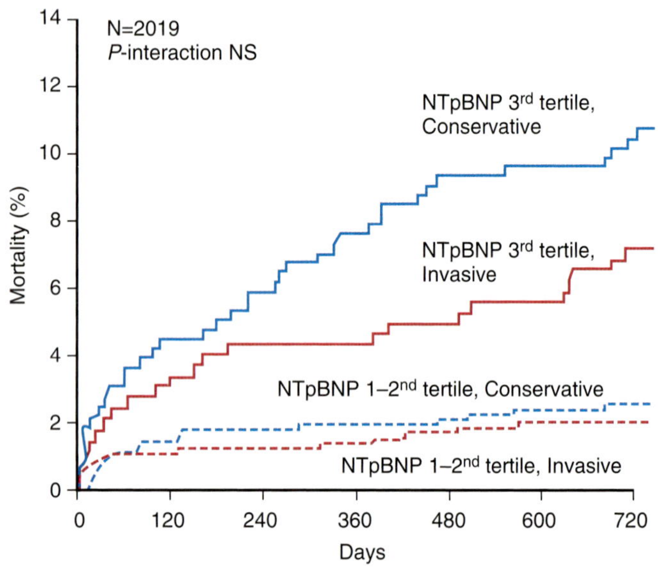

FIGURE 8-7 Mortality at 2 years in a nested biomarker analysis among patients randomized to an early invasive strategy versus conservative strategy for management of non–ST-elevation acute coronary syndromes. Data are stratified by baseline concentration of N-terminal brain natriuretic peptide (NTpBNP). *(Adapted from Jernberg T, et al: N-terminal pro-brain natriuretic peptide in relation to inflammation, myocardial necrosis, and the effect of an invasive strategy in unstable coronary artery disease.* J Am Coll Cardiol *42:1909–1916, 2003.)*

Mid-Region Pro-Adrenomedullin

The peptide adrenomedullin is a potent vasodilator that also influences cardiac contractility, diuresis, and natriuresis. Its precursor, pre-proadrenomedullin, is synthesized and present in the heart, adrenal medulla, lungs, and kidneys. The production of adrenomedullin is stimulated by both cardiac pressure and volume overload. Because of its greater stability than adrenomedullin, the midregional fragment of pro-adrenomedullin (MR-proADM) is more reliably measured. In patients with acute MI, MR-proADM is independently associated with the risk of cardiovascular death or heart failure; MR-proADM performs as well as established cardiac biomarkers (e.g., NPs), improving discrimination and reclassification of risk for these events.[32] Importantly, like ST2, MR-proADM shows a more modest association with the risk of recurrent ischemic events (Figure 8-9).

Although a potential therapeutic interaction with MR-proADM and an angiotensin-converting enzyme inhibitor has been reported in patients with stable ischemic heart disease,[33] the notion that MR-proADM may be useful for guiding therapies for adverse remodeling in patients with MI is a hypothesis that requires prospective evaluation.

Inflammatory Biomarkers and Prognosis

Motivated by multiple lines of evidence that implicate inflammatory processes as central contributors to acute atherothrombosis, mediators of the inflammatory response, including acute phase proteins, cytokines, and cellular

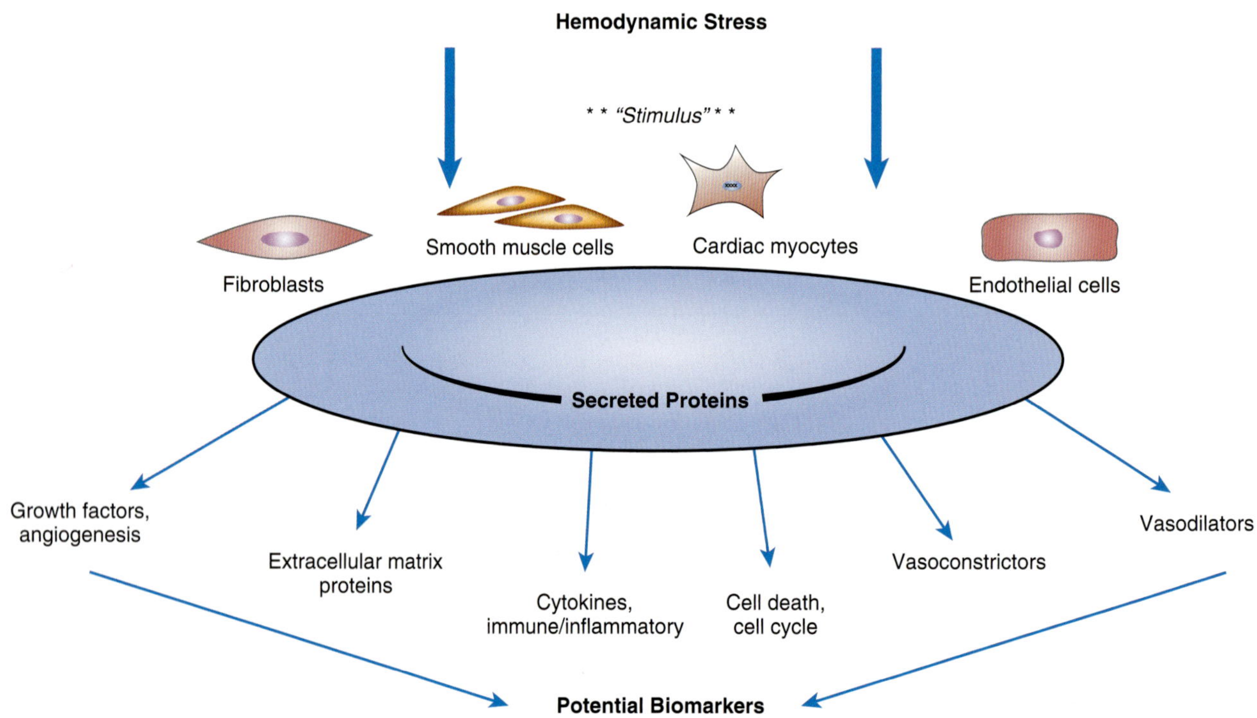

FIGURE 8-8 Hemodynamic stress is a stimulus for the production of secreted proteins from multiple functional classes; when detected in plasma and/or serum, they are potential biomarkers of hemodynamic stress.

adhesion molecules have been evaluated as risk indicators in patients with MI. As the prototypical acute phase reactant, CRP was the focus of initial investigation in this area. More than 12 clinical studies demonstrated the predictive capacity of high-sensitivity CRP (hs-CRP) levels with respect to cardiovascular outcome either during the initial hospitalization or long-term follow-up after ACS. Several, but not all, studies indicated that the relationship between hs-CRP and outcome is strongest with respect to mortality and heart failure, with a weaker relationship to recurrent MI.[30] Although such findings are conceptually important and support the relevance of inflammation to prognosis in patients with ACS, the lack of specificity of hs-CRP has been an important limitation to clinical application in this patient population.

Although hs-CRP was the first and is arguably the best studied of the inflammatory markers in the setting of MI, other biomarkers that putatively participate more directly in the inflammatory pathobiology of the natural history of ACS have been investigated. MPO was discussed earlier in this chapter. Growth-differentiation factor-15 (GDF-15), as an example of an emerging candidate biomarker in this category, is discussed in the following.

Growth-Differentiation Factor-15

GDF-15 is a member of the transforming growth factor-β superfamily and was originally identified in activated macrophages. GDF-15 is involved in regulating inflammatory and apoptotic pathways needed for development, differentiation, and tissue repair in a variety of organs. GDF-15 is up-regulated in a range of malignancies and in many tissues following injury, ischemia, and other forms of stress. Cardiomyocytes express and secrete GDF-15 in the setting of ischemia and reperfusion. GDF-15 is also associated with reduced endothelium-dependent vasodilatation, increased plaque burden and left ventricular mass, reduced left ventricular ejection fraction, and clinical manifestations of coronary artery disease and heart failure.

Multiple studies have provided consistent evidence for a relationship between GDF-15 and adverse outcomes in patients with MI. As an example, circulating blood concentration of GDF-15 was a strong independent marker of 1-year mortality in an analysis of 2081 patients with NSTE-ACS. Approximately two-thirds of patients in the study presented with GDF-15 levels above the upper limit of normal in healthy controls (1200 ng/L); one-third presented with levels of more than 1800 ng/L. Increasing tertiles of GDF-15 were associated with an increasing cumulative risk of death at 1 year, ranging from 1.5% to 14.1%. Furthermore, this prognostic relationship was incremental to that attained by cTn, NT-proBNP, CRP, and clinical factors. Compared with the other biomarkers, GDF-15 demonstrated the highest c-statistic of 0.76 for 1-year mortality (c-statistic for NT-proBNP, 0.74; CRP, 0.63). These findings were confirmed in another cohort of 1142 patients with MI and a cohort of 479 unselected patients with acute chest pain (30% with acute MI). GDF-15 also significantly improves the discriminatory capacity of the GRACE risk score (see Chapter 11).

With respect to treatment, a subgroup analysis of the FRISC-II trial that randomized patients with NSTE-ACS to an invasive or conservative strategy demonstrated the potential impact of GDF-15 on clinical decision-making. Patients with an elevated cTn, but with a GDF-15 of less than 1200 ng/L were at a low risk and did not have a detectable benefit from invasive management. In contrast, in patients with higher GDF-15 levels, the occurrence of death or nonfatal MI was reduced by an invasive strategy (Figure 8-10). Thus, GDF-15 has the potential to become a clinically useful novel biomarker because it provides not only independent prognostic information, but may also affect therapeutic decision-making. However, this observation warrants confirmation in additional studies.

Prognostic Markers and Clinical Decision-Making

Because of the strong independent prognostic relationships held by several candidate biomarkers, why is it that their prognostic value is insufficient to result in widespread clinical adoption in acute MI? In the author's opinion, seven reasons are relevant. First, in clinical practice,

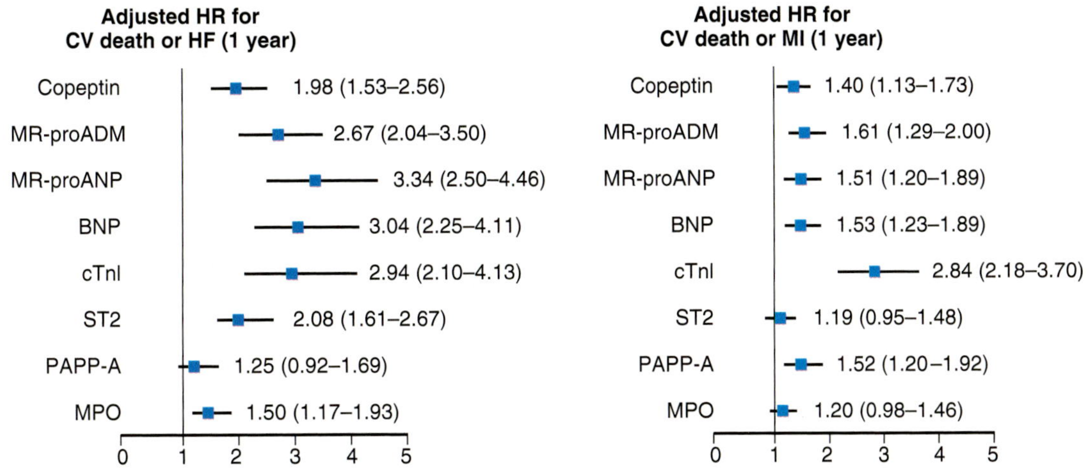

FIGURE 8-9 Concurrent assessment of multiple candidate biomarkers in 4432 patients with non–ST-elevation acute coronary syndrome randomized to ranolazine or placebo in the MERLIN-TIMI 36 trial and followed for 1 year. Adjusted risk of 1-year adverse cardiovascular outcomes associated with elevation of individual biomarkers of necrosis, inflammation, and hemodynamic stress. Clinical model includes age older than 65 years, coronary artery disease (CAD), CAD risk factors, ≥2 episodes of pain at rest, chronic aspirin use, ST depression, history of heart failure, and creatinine clearance less than 60. Each biomarker added to clinical model individually. *BNP*, brain natriuretic peptide; *cTnI*, cardiac troponin I; *CV*, cardiovascular; *HR*, hazard ratio; *MI*, myocardial infarction; *MPO*, myeloperoxidase; *MR-proADM*, midregional fragment of pro-adrenomedullin; *MR-proANP*, midregional-pro-atrial natriuretic peptide; *PAPP-A*, pregnancy-associated plasma protein-A. *(From O'Malley RG, et al: Prognostic performance of multiple biomarkers in patients with non-ST-segment elevation acute coronary syndrome: analysis from the MERLIN-TIMI 36 trial [Metabolic Efficiency With Ranolazine for Less Ischemia in Non-ST-Elevation Acute Coronary Syndromes-Thrombolysis In Myocardial Infarction 36].* J Am Coll Cardiol *63:1644–1653, 2014.)*

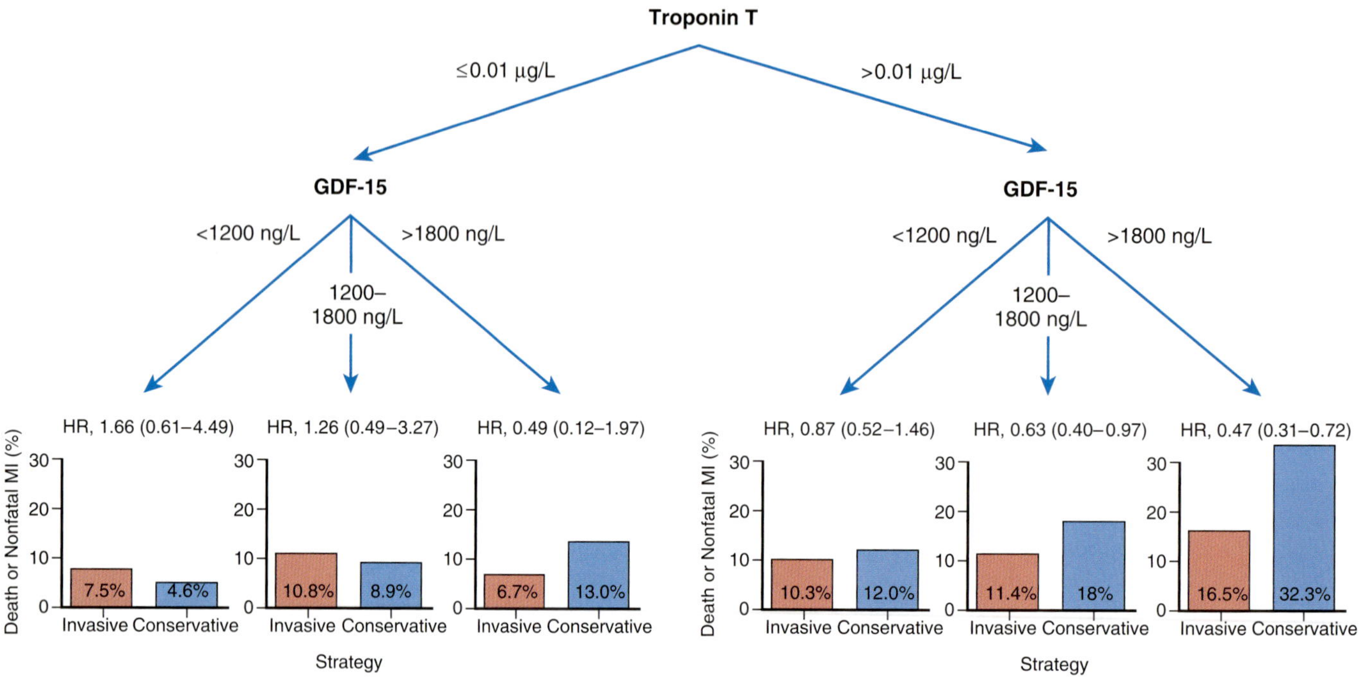

FIGURE 8-10 Levels of growth differentiation factor-15 (GDF-15) and impact of therapy strategy. Incidence of death and nonfatal myocardial infarction (MI) during 2-year follow-up according to troponin and GDF-15 levels and therapy strategy. Comparison between conservative and invasive therapy strategy by Cox regression analysis. *HR*, Hazard ratio. *(From Hochholzer W, et al: Novel biomarkers in cardiovascular disease: update 2010.* Am Heart J *160:583–594, 2010.)*

clinicians are mandated to make a diagnosis, but they are not mandated to make an accurate risk estimate regarding death or other adverse events. Second, clinical risk stratification tools, such as the GRACE score and TIMI Risk Scores (see Chapter 11), are easily and widely available as inexpensive, excellently validated approaches to risk stratification. Third, current guidelines recommend imaging to characterize left ventricular function in all patients with acute MI.[2] This liberal recommendation for imaging renders it difficult for NPs or other "hemodynamic stress" markers to provide intuitive incremental value. Fourth, the lack of consistent interaction with benefit from a specific treatment according to phenotyping by the alternative biomarker is critical. Fifth, widespread use of angiotensin-converting enzyme inhibitors and angiotensin receptor blockers for the treatment of arterial hypertension reduces the proportion of patients that might benefit from an upgrade in treatment with these drugs because of elevated levels of biomarkers of myocardial stress. Sixth, at least in Europe, additional testing with those biomarkers that are clinically available is costly compared with other blood tests. Seventh, insufficient medical education regarding the clinical use of biomarkers has resulted in a relevant gap in existing knowledge and their implementation into clinical practice.

FORWARD OUTLOOK

The biomarkers that this chapter introduced and other interesting candidate biomarkers are still looking for their appropriate clinical indications in patients with acute MI. For several of these biomarkers, precise and rapid assays are already clinically available or about to be implemented in modern laboratory platforms.[16–18,23–26] These biomarkers include galactin-3, fibroblast growth factor-23 (FGF-23), GDF-15, MR-proADM, PAPP-A, and ST2.[16–18,23–26] In addition to the issues raised in the preceding section, open questions related to these biomarkers include the exact pathophysiology of their release into blood, including the quantification of the predominant contributor organs. None of these biomarkers are cardiac specific. All of them identify MI patients with increased risk of death and/or heart failure. Future studies need to identify which changes in patient management can be justified upon the information provided by these biomarkers.

A first glimpse into the future was provided by an analysis in 3627 patients with stable coronary artery disease randomly assigned to trandolapril or placebo within the PEACE trial, which revealed that FGF-23 might help identify patients who derive greater clinical benefit from angiotensin-converting enzyme inhibitor therapy.[5,23] FGF-23 is an endocrine regulator of mineral metabolism, and markedly elevated levels are associated with cardiovascular events in patients with chronic kidney disease. Among patients in the top quartile of FGF-23 levels, trandolapril significantly reduced cardiovascular death or incident heart failure (hazard ratio, 0.45), whereas there was no clinical benefit in the remaining patients (hazard ratio, 1.07; P for interaction = .0039).[5,23] This interaction was independent of and additive to stratification based on renal function. In addition to identifying FGF-23 as an emerging biomarker of interest, this study illustrated the potential role for cardiovascular biomarkers in targeting a specific pharmacotherapy.

MicroRNA

MicroRNAs, which are a unique class of endogenous noncoding RNAs, are highly conserved across species, repress gene translation upon binding to messenger RNA (which therefore influence many biological processes in the heart), and are increasingly investigated as diagnostic and/or therapeutic tools.[34–37] In contrast to most biomarkers described in this chapter, pre-analytical and analytical considerations

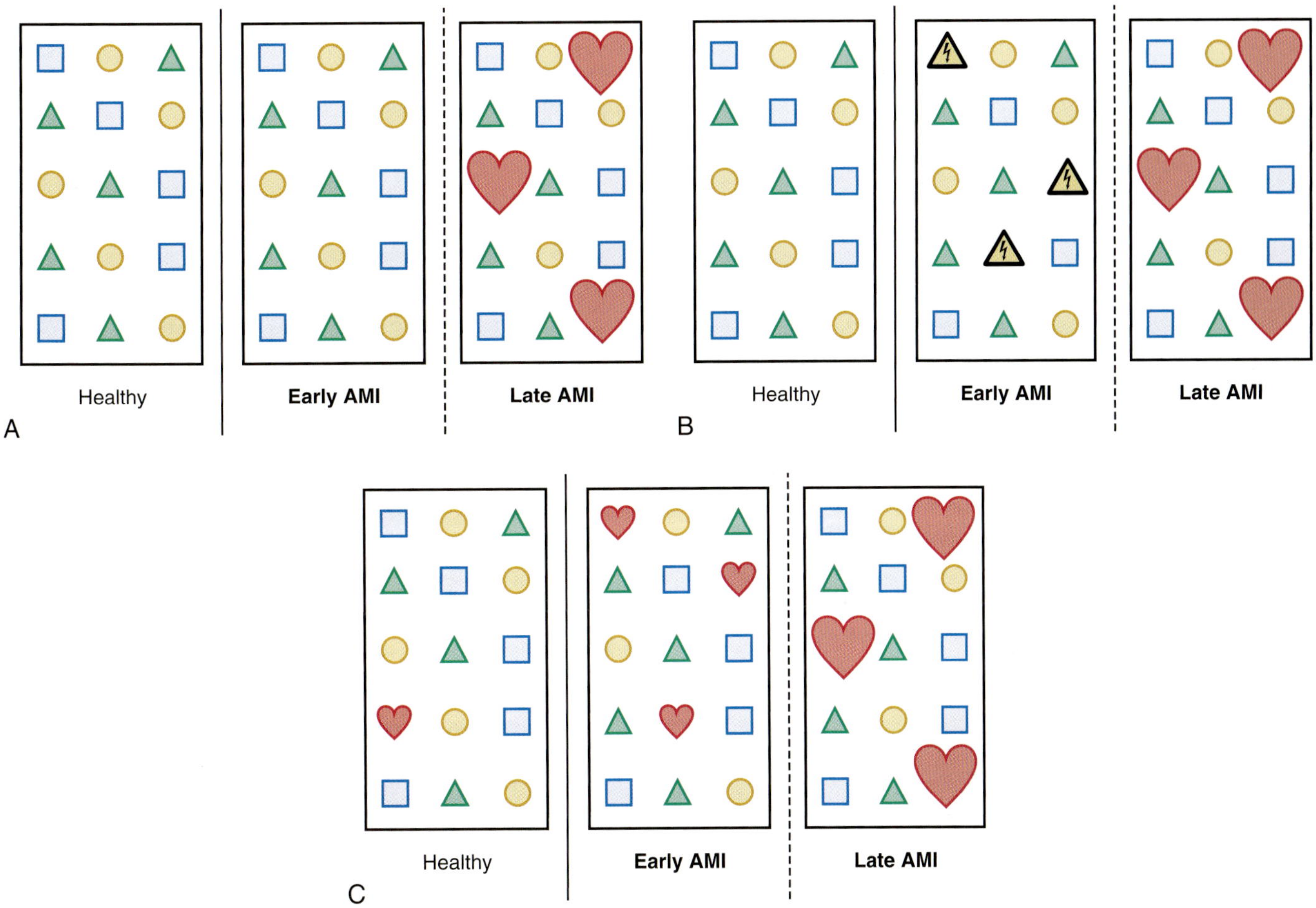

FIGURE 8-11 **Scheme of proteins detected in blood in healthy individuals, patients with acute myocardial infarction (AMI) soon (e.g., 2 hours) after chest pain onset, and patients with AMI late (e.g., 6 hours) after chest pain onset.** (**A**) Using conventional cardiac troponin (cTn) assays, myocardial injury (*red hearts*) is detected only later after presentation with AMI. (**B**) Using the "team or dual-marker approach" combining copeptin as a marker of endogenous stress with cTn, cardiac stress (*yellow triangles*) is detected in patients early after onset of AMI. (**C**) Using high-sensitivity cTn, myocardial injury is now detected in early AMI and is measurable in apparently healthy patients. *(Courtesy of Tobias Reichlin, MD.)*

are less established for microRNA and may, at least in part, account for some of the differences observed in the early pilot studies. Although the complex biological functions of microRNAs are incompletely understood, microRNAs seem to present in a tissue- and cell-specific manner.[34–37]

MicroRNAs, whose release is believed to be not only a consequence of cell death and plasma membrane disruption but also of an active release as a response to myocardial ischemia,[34–37] have emerged as biomarkers of possible clinical value in the early diagnosis of acute MI and/or unstable angina. Prospective diagnostic studies have shown that currently known microRNAs seem unable to compete with cTn in the early diagnosis of acute MI,[36,37] but may be helpful in the detection of unstable angina.[35] Using a three-phase approach comprising (1) profiling of microRNAs in patients with unstable angina and control groups, (2) replication of significant microRNAs in an independent patient cohort, and (3) validation of a multi-microRNAs panel in a third cohort, a panel of three microRNAs with diagnostic value emerged. Of 25 microRNAs selected for replication, 8 microRNAs remained significantly associated with unstable angina. In a validation phase, a microRNA panel including miR-132, miR-150, and miR-186 showed the highest discriminatory power (area under the curve, 0.91). Further comparative studies are needed to explore the diagnostic and prognostic value of microRNAs.

SUMMARY

In conclusion, the sensitivity deficit of conventional cTn assays (Figure 8-11A) has sparked the interest in alternative biomarkers. Copeptin, if used in combination with cTn, helps to overcome the sensitivity deficit in early presenters (see Figure 8-11B), and therefore, provides an alternative rapid rule-out approach. Further studies are necessary to define the role of copeptin and all other alternative biomarkers when used in conjunction with high-sensitivity cTn assays (see Figure 8-11C). Sensitive and high-sensitivity cTn assays have become the standard of care in most countries worldwide and have reduced, as well as modified, the possible clinical use of alternative biomarkers. Current unmet needs, and therefore, areas of ongoing research include whether such novel biomarkers have a role in directing the management of patients presenting with mild elevations of high-sensitivity cTn or in the differentiation of type I and type II acute MI.

References

1. Morrow DA, de Lemos JA: Benchmarks for the assessment of novel cardiovascular biomarkers, *Circulation* 115:949–952, 2007.
2. Roffi M, Patrono C, Collet J-P, et al: 2015 ESC guidelines for the management of acute coronary syndromes in patients presenting without persistent ST-segment elevation, *Eur Heart J* 37:267–315, 2016.
3. Thygesen K, et al.: Third universal definition of myocardial infarction, *Eur Heart J* 33:2551–2267, 2012.
4. Thygesen K, et al.: How to use high-sensitivity cardiac troponins in acute cardiac care, *Eur Heart J* 33:2252–2257, 2012.

5. Rubini Gimenez M, Twerenbold R, Mueller C: Beyond cardiac troponin: recent advances in the development of alternative biomarkers for cardiovascular disease, *Expert Rev Mol Diagn* 15:547–556, 2015.
6. Reichlin T, et al.: Incremental value of copeptin for rapid rule out of acute myocardial infarction, *J Am Coll Cardiol* 54:60–68, 2009.
7. Balmelli C, et al.: Comparison of the performances of cardiac troponins, including sensitive assays, and copeptin in the diagnosis of acute myocardial infarction and long-term prognosis between women and men, *Am Heart J* 166:30–37, 2013.
8. Mockel M, et al.: Early discharge using single cardiac troponin and copeptin testing in patients with suspected acute coronary syndrome (ACS): a randomized, controlled clinical process study, *Eur Heart J* 36:369–376, 2015.
9. Lipinski MJ, et al.: A systematic review and collaborative meta-analysis to determine the incremental value of copeptin for rapid rule-out of acute myocardial infarction, *Am J Cardiol* 113:1581–1591, 2014.
10. Maisel A, et al.: Copeptin helps in the early detection of patients with acute myocardial infarction: primary results of the CHOPIN trial (Copeptin Helps in the early detection Of Patients with acute myocardial INfarction), *J Am Coll Cardiol* 62:150–160, 2013.
11. Bruins Slot MH, et al.: Heart-type fatty acid-binding protein in the early diagnosis of acute myocardial infarction: a systematic review and meta-analysis, *Heart* 96:1957–1963, 2010.
12. Reiter M, et al.: Heart-type fatty acid-binding protein in the early diagnosis of acute myocardial infarction, *Heart* 99:708–714, 2013.
13. Schoenenberger AW, et al.: Incremental value of heart-type fatty acid-binding protein in suspected acute myocardial infarction early after symptom onset, *Eur Heart J Acute Cardiovasc Care*, 2015 Feb 13. pii: 2048872615571256. [Epub ahead of print].
14. Kagawa Y, et al.: Comparison of heart-type fatty acid binding protein and sensitive troponin for the diagnosis of early acute myocardial infarction, *Int J Cardiol* 166:347–351, 2013.
15. Schaub N, et al.: Markers of plaque instability in the early diagnosis and risk stratification of acute myocardial infarction, *Clin Chem* 58:246–256, 2012.
16. Bonaca MP, et al.: Prospective evaluation of pregnancy-associated plasma protein-a and outcomes in patients with acute coronary syndromes, *J Am Coll Cardiol* 60:332–338, 2012.
17. von Haehling S, et al.: Value of serum pregnancy-associated plasma protein A for predicting cardiovascular events among patients presenting with cardiac chest pain, *Canadian Medical Association Journal* 185:E295–E303, 2013.
18. O'Malley RG, et al.: Prognostic performance of multiple biomarkers in patients with non-ST-segment elevation acute coronary syndrome: analysis from the MERLIN-TIMI 36 trial (Metabolic Efficiency With Ranolazine for Less Ischemia in Non-ST-Elevation Acute Coronary Syndromes-Thrombolysis In Myocardial Infarction 36), *J Am Coll Cardiol* 63:1644–1653, 2014.
19. Hochholzer W, et al.: Impact of soluble FMS-like tyrosine kinase-1 and placental growth factor serum levels for risk stratification and early diagnosis in patients with suspected acute myocardial infarction, *Eur Heart J* 32:326–335, 2011.
20. Morrow DA, et al.: Ability of minor elevations of 3770 troponins I and T to predict benefit from an early invasive strategy in patients with unstable angina and 3771 non-ST elevation myocardial infarction: results from a randomized trial, *JAMA* 286:2405–2412, 2001.
21. Maisel A, et al.: State of the art: using natriuretic peptide levels in clinical practice, *Eur J Heart Fail* 10:824–839, 2008.
22. de Lemos JA, et al.: The prognostic value of B-type natriuretic peptide in patients with acute coronary syndromes, *N Engl J Med* 345:1014–1021, 2001.
23. Udell JA, et al.: Fibroblast growth factor-23, cardiovascular prognosis, and benefit of angiotensin-converting enzyme inhibition in stable ischemic heart disease, *J Am Coll Cardiol* 63:2421–2428, 2014.
24. Schaub N, Reichlin T, Meune C, et al.: Markers of plaque instability in the early diagnosis and risk stratification of acute myocardial infarction, *Clin Chem 58*(1):246–256, 2012.
25. Sanchez-Mas J, et al.: Galectin-3 expression in cardiac remodeling after myocardial infarction, *Int J Cardiol* 172:e98–e101, 2014.
26. Lassus J, et al.: Incremental value of biomarkers to clinical variables for mortality prediction in acutely decompensated heart failure: the Multinational Observational Cohort on Acute Heart Failure (MOCA) study, *Int J Cardiol* 168:2186–2194, 2013.
27. Chen K, Keaney Jr JF: Evolving concepts of oxidative stress and reactive oxygen species in cardiovascular disease, *Curr Atheroscler Rep* 14:476–483, 2012.
28. Schindhelm RK, et al.: Myeloperoxidase: a useful biomarker for cardiovascular disease risk stratification? *Clin Chem* 55:1462–1470, 2009.
29. Scirica BM, et al.: National Cardiovascular Data Registry. Association between natriuretic peptides and mortality among patients admitted with myocardial infarction: a report from the ACTION Registry(R)-GWTG™, *Clin Chem* 59:1205–1214, 2013.
30. NACB Writing Group, Wu AH, et al.: NACB Committee, Cannon CP, Storrow AB. National Academy of Clinical Biochemistry laboratory medicine practice guidelines: use of cardiac troponin and B-type natriuretic peptide or N-terminal proB-type natriuretic peptide for etiologies other than acute coronary syndromes and heart failure, *Clin Chem* 53:2086–2096, 2007.
31. Kohli P, et al.: Role of ST2 in non-ST-elevation acute coronary syndrome in the MERLIN-TIMI 36 trial, *Clin Chem* 58:257–266, 2012.
32. O'Malley RG, et al.: Prognostic performance of multiple biomarkers in patients with non-ST-segment elevation acute coronary syndrome: analysis from the MERLIN-TIMI 36 trial (Metabolic Efficiency With Ranolazine for Less Ischemia in Non-ST-Elevation Acute Coronary Syndromes-Thrombolysis In Myocardial Infarction 36), *J Am Coll Cardiol* 63:1644–1653, 2014.
33. Sabatine MS, et al.: Evaluation of multiple biomarkers of cardiovascular stress for risk prediction and guiding medical therapy in patients with stable coronary disease, *Circulation* 125:233–240, 2012.
34. Notari M, Pulecio J, Raya Á: Update on the pathogenic implications and clinical potential of microRNAs in cardiac disease, *Biomed Res Int* 2015:105620, 2015.
35. Zeller T, et al.: Assessment of microRNAs in patients with unstable angina pectoris, *Eur Heart J* 35:2106–2114, 2014.
36. Devaux Y, et al.: Diagnostic and prognostic value of circulating microRNAs in patients with acute chest pain, *J Intern Med* 277:260–271, 2015.
37. D'Alessandra Y, et al.: Circulating microRNAs are new and sensitive biomarkers of myocardial infarction, *Eur Heart J* 31:2765–2773, 2010.

9 Cardiac Imaging for Patients with Acute Chest Pain in the Emergency Department

Udo Hoffmann and James E. Udelson

INTRODUCTION

Previous chapters have detailed the important roles of clinical presentation (see Chapter 6), cardiovascular risk factors, electrocardiography (ECG), and biomarkers (see Chapter 7 and Chapter 8) in the initial assessment of patients who present with acute chest pain to the emergency department (ED). However, even all of this information does not allow accurate exclusion or diagnosis of acute myocardial infarction (MI) in a substantial proportion of patients. This chapter reviews the clinical utility, strengths, and weaknesses of the major imaging modalities that have been studied in this setting.

The use of imaging techniques in the evaluation of patients with chest pain in the ED has increased steadily. Between 1999 and 2008, the use of advanced medical imaging in the ED increased more than fourfold beyond standard x-ray testing.[1] Because less than 10% of patients with an inconclusive initial ED evaluation are subsequently diagnosed with MI, the primary goal is to safely and efficiently identify those without MI. In the United States, the standard of safety for patients and ED physicians has been defined as a risk of an adverse event of less than 1% within 30 days after discharge.[2] However, imaging should be held to a higher standard than this and not only provide diagnostic information, but also prognostic information that may help tailor medical therapy even in those without acute MI.

Available tests include functional testing at rest and stress, anatomic coronary assessment by computed tomographic angiography (CTA), and myocardial perfusion and viability by cardiac magnetic resonance imaging (CMR). Currently, the role of CTA and anatomic assessment is restricted to de novo acute chest pain presentations, whereas stress test–based assessment of myocardial ischemia is favorable in those who have had previous events. It is further important to emphasize that it is a small proportion of patients who present with chest pain that have a final diagnosis of acute coronary syndrome (ACS), and that most patients who undergo imaging are classified as having unstable angina (85%) with few non–ST-elevation MIs (NSTEMIs) (15%), although this epidemiology is shifting (see Chapter 1 and Chapter 6).[3]

Rationale for Functional and Anatomic Assessment

Functional Imaging

In the so-called "ischemic cascade," the earliest manifestation of ischemia is a perfusion abnormality. As supply–demand mismatch worsens, left ventricular diastolic abnormalities develop, and then later, systolic wall motion abnormalities. Ischemic changes on the ECG, increases in troponin, and onset of angina are late events. The ability to use imaging to detect regional differences in myocardial blood flow (with perfusion imaging) and regional variation in systolic function allows for identification of myocardial ischemia in patients before, or even in the absence of, ECG changes.

Anatomic Assessment of Coronary Artery Disease

Overall, most ACS occur as a result of rupture of an atherosclerotic plaque (see Chapter 3).[4] However, most patients in whom plaque rupture occurs in a large, previously nonobstructive vessel will present with STEMI and will be referred immediately to the catheterization laboratory. In contrast, candidates for imaging will more likely present with an acute exacerbation of an already existing luminal narrowing. A minority of patients referred for imaging will eventually develop troponin elevation and be diagnosed with an MI.

FUNCTIONAL IMAGING

Gathered over 40 years, data that have assessed functional imaging for the evaluation of patients with chest symptoms presenting to the ED are predominantly observational in nature. However, some randomized comparative effectiveness trials have been performed.

Rest Radionuclide Myocardial Perfusion Imaging

Early reports of rest radionuclide myocardial perfusion imaging (MPI) to assess patients with chest pain in the ED using thallium-201 planar imaging in patients with unstable angina and suspected MI date back to the 1970s. Because the redistribution of thallium-201 requires imaging to be completed relatively quickly after injection, this tracer is challenging for imaging ED patients. Subsequently, technetium-99 (Tc99m)–based agents with only minimal redistribution, such as sestamibi and tetrofosmin, have enabled rest perfusion imaging in the ED setting.

Rest-Only Myocardial Perfusion Imaging in Suspected Acute Coronary Syndromes

During the 1990s, a series of studies that used Tc99m-sestamibi at rest established that hypoperfused myocardium before thrombolysis in patients with STEMI represented the area-at-risk of infarct. Subsequently, Tc99m-sestamibi imaging was established as a marker of infarct size in clinical trials of therapeutic agents for patients with MI.[5] Tc99m-sestamibi imaging at rest demonstrated a high negative predictive value in patients who presented to the ED with suspicion for ACS to exclude MI, as well as had a higher sensitivity than the ECG recorded during symptoms for predicting the presence of a coronary stenosis on subsequent angiography. In addition, a normal perfusion study identified patients at low risk for subsequent cardiovascular events.[6] Examples of normal and abnormal studies are shown for applications of rest-only MPI in Figures 9-1 and 9-2. Examples of stress MPI are shown in Figures 9-e1 and 9-e2.

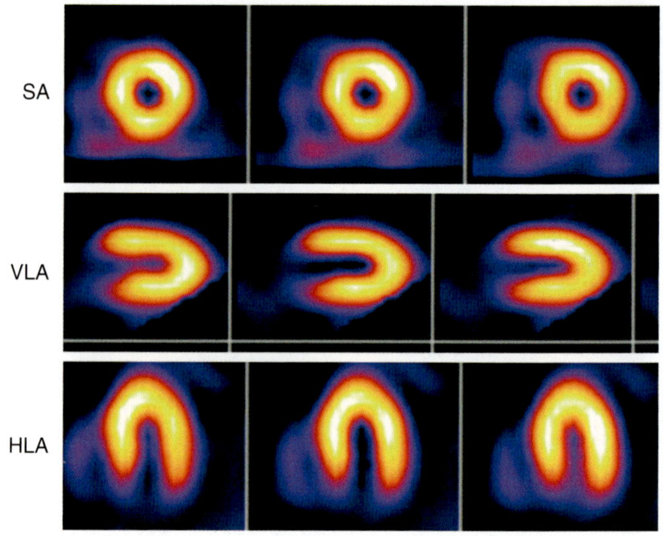

FIGURE 9-1 A normal resting myocardial perfusion imaging study shows homogeneous tracer distribution in all myocardial territories, as seen in the short-axis (SA), vertical long-axis (VLA), and horizontal long-axis (HLA) tomographic views. Based on a large observational literature database, the likelihood of unstable angina or acute myocardial infarction in such a patient is very low.

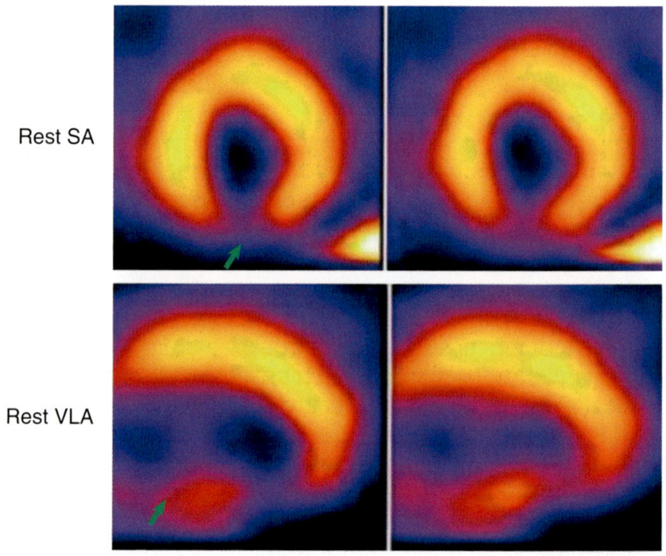

FIGURE 9-2 Abnormal rest myocardial perfusion imaging study, showing an inferior wall perfusion defect at rest (*green arrows*), in the short-axis (SA) and vertical long-axis (VLA) views. This finding would be consistent with reduced resting perfusion and ischemia or new infarct in the inferior wall. It could also represent a remote infarct, so that this testing strategy is most useful in those without a history of myocardial infarction.

Subsequently, in a larger study[7] in which approximately 1200 ED patients with ECGs that were nondiagnostic for ischemia or infarction and possible or probable unstable angina had perfusion scans performed; the sensitivity of MPI for MI was 100% (95% confidence interval [CI], 64% to 100%), and the negative predictive value for MI or revascularization over 1 year of follow-up was 97% (95% CI, 95% to 98%). Including revascularization, the total event rate at 12-month follow-up was 0.9% in patients with a normal resting scan and 42% in those with abnormal findings. These data added weight to the concept that a normal perfusion study when performed immediately in the ED identified a low-risk group that were potentially eligible for early discharge.

Randomized Trials of Myocardial Perfusion Imaging in the Emergency Department

To critically assess the application of single-photon emission computed tomography (SPECT) MPI in the ED, several randomized effectiveness trials were conducted to study the effect on clinical decision-making when using the test versus when not using the test in a more real-life setting, where clinicians were not directed in their decisions by protocol (Table 9-1).

The ERASE Chest Pain (Emergency Room Assessment of Sestamibi for the Evaluation of Chest Pain) multicenter trial enrolled approximately 2500 patients in an effectiveness trial to test whether providing results of rest MPI to ED clinicians for patients with low-to-intermediate likelihood of ACS would improve clinical decision-making, which was defined as the appropriateness of an admitting decision.[8] An appropriate admission was defined as admission of a patient who was ultimately found to have a final diagnosis of ACS (blindly adjudicated), whereas an unnecessary admission was defined as the admission of a patient who was ultimately found to have a final diagnosis of "not ACS." Among patients randomized to the imaging strategy who ultimately were found to not have ACS, unnecessary admissions were significantly reduced (relative risk, 0.84; 95% CI, 0.77 to 0.92), whereas there was no change in appropriate admission for those with ACS. The results of this large, multicenter randomized effectiveness trial provided strong evidence that incorporating rest MPI in this setting could improve triage decisions.

TABLE 9-1 Randomized Controlled Trials Incorporating Rest and/or Stress Myocardial Perfusion Imaging into Clinical Decision-Making for Emergency Department Chest Pain Patients

AUTHOR/ REFERENCE	NO. OF PTS	INTERVENTION	CONTROL	TIMING OF INTERVENTION	EFFECTIVENESS?*	ENDPOINT(S)	RESULTS
Stowers (2000)	46	Rest MPI	SOC	After ED	No, clinical decisions driven by protocol	In-hospital costs and length of stay	Rest MPI-guided strategy had lower median in-hospital costs and shorter median LOS
Udelson (2002)	2475	Rest MPI	SOC	In ED	Yes	% Unnecessary admissions	Group randomized to rest MPI had fewer unnecessary admissions (in those without ACS)
Lim (2013)	1508	Stress/rest MPI	SOC	After 6 h of negative serial biomarkers/ ECGs	Yes	Admission rate	Stress MPI group had lower admission rate

ACS, Acute coronary syndrome; *ECGs*, electrocardiograms; *ED*, emergency department; *LOS*, length of stay; *MPI*, myocardial perfusion imaging; *SOC*, standard of care.
*"Effectiveness" refers to whether the clinical decisions that followed knowledge of the randomized test results were protocol-driven. In the trial by Stowers and colleagues, the steps of care after the initial imaging results (or control group without imaging) were directed by the research study protocol. In the trials by Udelson and colleagues and Lim and colleagues, the test results were given to clinicians who then incorporated the results into their own decision-making, not directed by protocol. This latter, more real-life scenario is consistent with an effectiveness trial.

Appropriate Use Criteria, Guidelines, and Clinical Role

Appropriate use criteria for the use of radionuclide imaging from the American College of Cardiology Foundation (ACCF), the American Society of Nuclear Cardiology (ASNC), the American College of Radiology (ACR), the American Heart Association (AHA), and the Society of Nuclear Medicine (SNR), among others, rate the use of rest-only MPI as appropriate in the setting of acute chest pain suspicious for ACS, provided that the initial ECG is nondiagnostic or normal, the initial troponin is negative, and pain is ongoing or recent.[9]

Resting Echocardiography

A major strength of resting two-dimensional (2-D) echocardiography in the evaluation of acute chest pain is its widespread availability and portability; however, a skilled operator is needed to acquire images, and experience is required for expert interpretation of images. Similarly to MPI, evaluation of suspected ACS by resting 2-D echocardiography is based on the concept that a perfusion abnormality will result in abnormal regional wall motion and myocardial thickening. Because regional wall motion abnormalities may resolve relatively soon after resolution of angina, 2-D echocardiography should be performed as early as possible, optimally in patients with ongoing symptoms, to provide high sensitivity (up to 90%). Although the exact time frame during which regional wall motion abnormalities will resolve after the offset of myocardial ischemia is unknown, studies suggest that the high sensitivity can be maintained within a window of 4 hours of arriving to the ED, and will drop to 64% sensitivity after resolution of chest pain.[10]

Echocardiography in Acute Coronary Syndrome

ED providers often use ultrasound in their initial evaluation, including for those patients with chest pain. The focused cardiac ultrasound examination is intended to rapidly identify pericardial effusion, assess global systolic function, discover significant left or right ventricular enlargement, and assess intravascular volume through identification of the diameter and degree of collapse of the inferior vena cava. The American Society of Echocardiography (ASE) consensus statement reports that the examination is not intended to replace a comprehensive echocardiogram, and most providers who perform the test will not be vigorously trained in the acquisition and interpretation of ultrasound imaging to identify regional wall motion abnormalities.[11] As of yet, there are no strong data to support the use of handheld ultrasound in the initial evaluation of suspected MI, without concomitant high suspicion of dissection or pericardial effusion.

Echocardiographic Imaging with Contrast

Echocardiographic contrast consists of gas microbubbles that are encapsulated and create a nonlinear vibration from contact with the ultrasound wave emitted from the transducer.[12] The use of contrast echocardiography for opacification of the left ventricular cavity is safe in the setting of ACS. In the left ventricle, this opacification provides a contrast to the surrounding myocardium and allows for improved identification of the endocardial border, enhancing the assessment of regional wall motion abnormalities especially when imaging is technically difficult.

Beyond the use of contrast for left ventricular cavity opacification, it has also been investigated for evaluation of myocardial perfusion. The gas microbubbles of echocardiographic contrast also enter the myocardial circulation. The bubbles are fragile, and if a strong ultrasound pulse is generated, they will burst. Careful imaging of the myocardium in the cycles after the ultrasound pulse will demonstrate a new contrast agent entering the myocardial microvasculature. This influx can be visualized and analyzed based on the time to reperfuse, and correlates with myocardial blood flow to various segments.[13]

Although not approved by the Food and Drug Administration (FDA) for the indication of assessing myocardial perfusion, myocardial contrast echocardiography has been extensively studied, and the data suggest that its use is safe and may provide useful and simultaneous data regarding myocardial perfusion and wall motion.[14] The perfusion and wall motion data derived from contrast perfusion echocardiography in the setting of ACS correlate with radionuclide MPI. Specifically, both wall motion and perfusion with echocardiographic contrast show a more than 80% agreement with SPECT imaging of perfusion. When results of the two imaging modalities are discordant, contrast echocardiography is typically abnormal and SPECT is normal, probably because of the destruction of bubbles closest to the ultrasound transducer often causing the appearance of a perfusion defect in the anterior wall and apex.

Appropriate Use Criteria, Guidelines, and Clinical Role

The 2011 appropriate use criteria for echocardiography rate the evaluation of acute chest pain with suspected MI and nondiagnostic ECG when a resting echocardiogram can be performed during pain as appropriate.[15] In the absence of pain, but with other features of an ischemic equivalent or positive biomarkers, the use of echocardiography is similarly appropriate.

Stress Testing with or without Imaging in the Emergency Department

Stress Radionuclide Myocardial Perfusion Imaging

In patients unable to exercise, or those with an uninterpretable ECG, the addition of an imaging modality to stress is warranted. One study for the evaluation of chest pain in the ED reported a protocol that used a multistep process, including history and physical, 2-hour biomarker levels, serial ECGs, and stress MPI for select patients based on risk category. The sensitivity and specificity for the diagnosis of ACS at 30 days for those patients who underwent stress testing was 99% and 87%, respectively.[16]

In a randomized trial that incorporated stress MPI into the evaluation pathway,[17] following a negative observation period involving serial ECG monitoring and serial biomarkers, 1508 patients were allocated to the use of stress MPI in the ED or to complete a standard clinical evaluation. Overall, fewer patients who had stress imaging performed were admitted (18.5% vs. 10.2%). However, event rates were low in both groups, and most patients were able to exercise and had an interpretable ECG. The predictive value of exercise ECG was similar to stress MPI, so although it is effective, the additional costs of imaging should be considered in such a situation under clinical conditions.

Stress Echocardiography

A study of 377 patients with a normal or nondiagnostic ECG and negative serial biomarker levels at 6 hours examined the ability of early dobutamine stress echocardiography in the ED to predict outcomes.[18] Testing was not possible in 23 of 404 patients because of poor acoustic windows, a proportion similar to the general population. With dobutamine stress testing, 39 patients tested were unable to complete the protocol because of intolerable side effects, such as arrhythmia, severe hypertension, or hypotension. The overall event rate, including death, MI, rehospitalization, or revascularization, was 31% in patients with a positive stress echocardiogram and 4% in patients with a negative study. The negative predictive value was 96%, slightly lower than that reported in studies of radionuclide imaging.

Dobutamine stress echocardiography may be a cost-effective strategy compared with exercise treadmill testing alone.[10] Nucifora and colleagues[19] reported on 190 patients with chest pain, serial negative biomarkers, and nondiagnostic ECG results who were randomized to undergo either dobutamine stress echocardiography or exercise ECG testing. There was a higher event rate in patients who were discharged after negative exercise ECG testing compared with dobutamine stress echocardiography (11% vs. 0%; P = .004). Costs were lower in the dobutamine echocardiography group at both 1- and 2-month follow-up compared with exercise ECG testing (\$1026 ± \$253 vs. \$1329 ± \$1288; P = .03 at 1 month and \$1029 ± \$253 vs. \$1684 ± \$2149; P = .005 at 2 months). Lower costs in the dobutamine stress echocardiography group were believed to be caused by shorter length of stay and less need for follow-up testing for indeterminate results, which are more likely with exercise ECG testing alone.

Appropriate Use Criteria, Guidelines, and Clinical Role

The 2011 ACC/AHA guidelines present a class I recommendation, that in patients with suspected ACS, if the follow-up 12-lead ECG and cardiac biomarkers measurements are normal, a stress test (exercise or pharmacological) to provoke ischemia should be performed in the ED, in a chest pain unit, or on an outpatient basis in a timely fashion as an alternative to inpatient admission. Also, patients with possible ACS and negative cardiac biomarkers who are unable to exercise or who have an abnormal resting ECG should undergo a pharmacological stress test with imaging.[3] The 2009 appropriate use criteria for cardiac radionuclide imaging rate the use of stress MPI in the setting of possible ACS with a (1) normal or nondiagnostic ECG; (2) either low or high clinical risk based on Thrombolysis In Myocardial Infarction (TIMI) score; and (3) either negative, borderline, equivocal, or minimally elevated troponin all as appropriate.[20] The 2008 appropriate use criteria for stress echocardiography rate the use of stress echocardiography as appropriate for the indication of acute chest pain in the setting of an intermediate pretest probability of coronary artery disease (CAD) and an ECG without dynamic ST changes when serial cardiac enzymes are negative.[21]

Figure 9-3 illustrates points in the triage algorithm when rest and stress functional imaging could be used. Although the efficacy and effectiveness, especially of rest perfusion imaging, has been demonstrated, these techniques are not widely deployed. Rather, the more common strategy has been to assess serial biomarkers in the ED or in an Observation Unit, followed by stress testing (see Chapter 12).

CARDIAC COMPUTED TOMOGRAPHY ANGIOGRAPHY

In most patients who are ultimately diagnosed with ACS, acute chest pain develops because of myocardial ischemia after the erosion or rupture of a coronary atherosclerotic plaque (see Figure 3-5). Moreover, a significant coronary stenosis can be detected by invasive coronary angiography in most patients with ACS (>80%), whereas ACS is rare in the absence of coronary atherosclerosis.[3] To assess for obstructive CAD and reach a confident diagnosis, clinicians have typically relied on the patient's history and presentation, followed by noninvasive stress testing, and in some cases, invasive coronary angiography. For the first time, the advent of high-quality cardiac computed tomography angiography (CCTA) has provided clinicians with the ability to visualize the coronary arteries without the risks of invasive angiography. During the preceding decades of care for patients with acute chest pain, such insight into coronary anatomy has been considered the holy grail of cardiac imaging. However, now that CCTA is available, the benefits of this technology have been vigorously disputed. Because of the low efficiency of functional testing as a gatekeeper,[22] proponents have argued that CTA allows more precision and individually tailored care, because, on one hand, CCTA is be able to

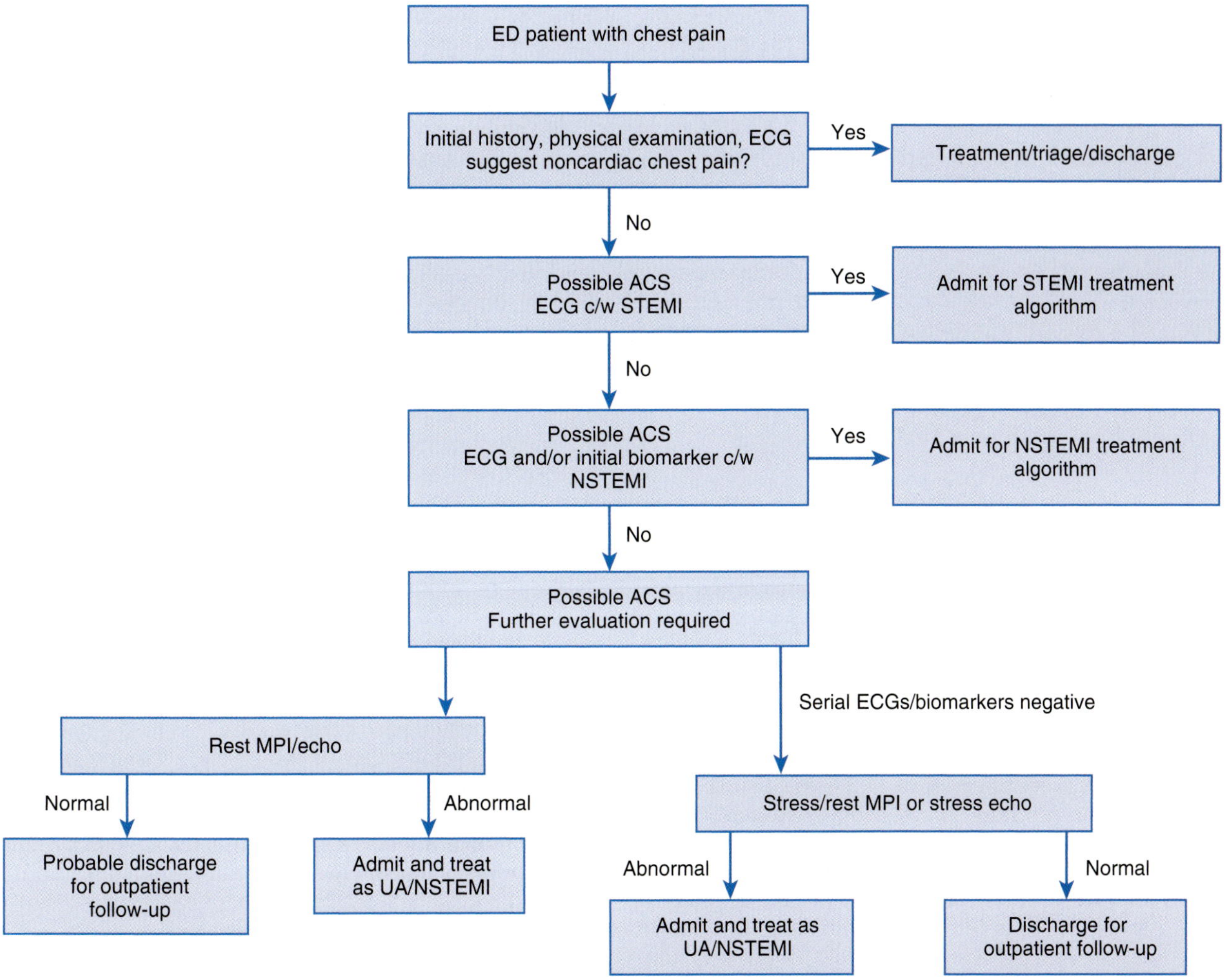

FIGURE 9-3 Flow diagram illustrating points in triage algorithm where rest and stress functional imaging could be used. In a patient presenting to the emergency department (ED) with a chest pain syndrome, if the initial history, physical, and electrocardiogram (ECG) suggest a clear noncardiac or nonischemic source of pain, then treatment and triage can be planned accordingly, facilitating rapid discharge from the ED. If ST-elevation is present in the ECG, then an ST-elevation myocardial infarction (STEMI) treatment algorithm can begin immediately. Similarly, if the initial ECG and/or initial biomarkers are diagnostic of unstable angina (UA) or non–ST-elevation MI (NSTEMI), the patient can be admitted and treated, consistent with the extant guidelines. However, if there is not a clearly diagnostic initial ECG or biomarker for NSTEMI, then the patient can be considered as having "possible" acute coronary syndrome (ACS), and further evaluation is needed. Rest myocardial perfusion imaging (MPI) can be used in this situation before using serial biomarkers, before there is no stress testing involved. If the rest study is normal, substantial data suggest that the likelihood of UA/NSTEMI is very low, and the patient could be considered for rapid discharge with outpatient follow-up for further assessment. An abnormal resting perfusion study suggests that the symptoms are likely related to a myocardial perfusion abnormality and a UA/NSTEMI syndrome. Such a patient can be admitted and treated. A caveat involves the possibility that the abnormality may also represent an old MI. However, in the absence of history of MI, treatment should presume an acute abnormality. Some centers prefer a strategy of obtaining serial biomarker studies to rule in or out ACS. If positive, such patients are considered to have an NSTEMI and treated accordingly. If serial ECGs and biomarkers are negative, NSTEMI is ruled out, although there remains a possibility of "troponin-negative UA." Many such patients can be discharged for outpatient stress testing, or tested while in an observation status. If a stress/rest MPI study or a stress echocardiogram is normal, it makes both ACS and significant underlying coronary artery disease (CAD) unlikely. If abnormal, the results suggest that the presenting episode may have been ACS, and the patient can be treated as such. There is also the possibility although that the presenting symptoms were noncardiac in origin, that the stress test reflects underlying CAD not related to the presenting symptoms. In such a case, clinical judgment needs to be involved to assess the relation between the test result and symptoms.

exclude the most common reason for ACS in many patients. On the other hand, CCTA can identify patients potentially needing urgent revascularization, whereas the patients without significant obstructive disease could avoid a test that, for them, provides risk but no possibility of benefit. Greater efficiency might well also lead to lower total costs of care. Skeptics counter that CTA is too sensitive and will detect many patients with bystander CAD, and that it is lacks sufficient specificity. For example, in the presence of severe calcification and in the absence of information on the hemodynamic significance of CAD, it could potentially lead to more referrals for additional stress imaging and invasive angiography. Patients in this scenario would actually receive more radiation, and care would be more costly. Because of this controversy, adoption of CTA into practice has been variable, as has been reimbursement policies for U.S. payers.

Accuracy of Cardiac Computed Tomography Angiography for Detection of Coronary Artery Disease

Over the past two decades, CT has rapidly evolved. State-of-the-art scanners acquire 64 to 320 cross sections per rotation, depicting vascular details with a spatial resolution of less than 0.5 mm. Fast scanner technology combined with heart rate–reducing medication now makes it possible to image the coronary arteries without motion artifacts in most patients. ECG-synchronized, contrast-enhanced images of the heart and coronary arteries can be acquired in one to five heart cycles. With that, CCTA has evolved into a robust and reliable technique for detection and assessment of coronary stenosis and atherosclerotic plaque. A wealth of single and multicenter trials have established CCTA as a noninvasive diagnostic test with excellent sensitivity (97.2%; 95% CI, 96.2% to 98.0%) and good specificity (87.4%; 95% CI, 84.5% to 89.8%) for the detection of more than 50% coronary artery stenosis compared with the gold standard of invasive coronary angiography.[23] The major strength of CCTA is its high negative predictive value (typically approaching 99%), and thus, CCTA permits confident exclusion of significant coronary stenosis. In addition, CCTA accurately detects nonobstructive calcified and noncalcified atherosclerotic plaque (accuracy, 92%; 95% CI, 90% to 93%) compared with the gold standard of intravascular ultrasound. The reproducibility of CCTA for both the detection of coronary plaque and stenosis is high (κ, 0.85 to 0.93).[24]

Observational Studies with Cardiac Computed Tomography Angiography in Evaluation of Acute Chest Pain

The ability to rapidly image coronary arteries with a noninvasive technique with strong performance characteristics is a potentially attractive option in the setting of evaluating patients with suspected ACS in the ED. With substantial technical developments and wide availability, CCTA has evolved into a viable alternative to standard of care (SOC) management in patients presenting to the ED with acute chest pain.

The prospective observational cohort ROMICAT (Rule Out Myocardial Infarction using Computer Assisted Tomography) trial, published in 2009, was the first large clinical trial that assessed the potential role of CCTA in the ED.[25] The ROMICAT trial had a unique blinded observational cohort study design. The trial included 368 patients with acute chest pain from the ED with an initial inconclusive assessment who underwent CCTA. Care providers were blinded to the CCTA results, and therefore, the diagnostic performance of CCTA for ACS and its association with other test findings could be studied in a truly unbiased fashion. Among the more notable findings of this study were the following: (1) the distribution of CAD in patients presenting with acute chest pain—50% had no evidence of CAD, 30% had nonobstructive plaque, and approximately 20% of patients had obstructive CAD; (2) the absence of CAD had 100% negative predictive value for ACS, whereas the presence of obstructive CAD (>50% luminal narrowing) only had 77% sensitivity (and 87% specificity) for ACS; and (3) not surprisingly, the presence and extent of coronary plaque and stenosis were superior in their discriminative capacity for ACS compared with clinical risk scores such as TIMI or Goldman.

Takakuwa and colleagues[26] performed a meta-analysis of available observational studies that evaluated the accuracy of CCTA to detect ACS in 1559 acute chest pain patients (42% women, mean age 52 years, low-to-intermediate likelihood of ACS) (Table 9-2). The pooled results confirmed the excellent negative predictive value (99.3%; 95% CI, 98.7% to 99.6%), but also confirmed a low positive predictive value (48.1%; 95% CI, 42.5% to 53.8%) of the presence of 50% stenosis to identify patients with ACS during the index hospitalization and major cardiovascular events during 30-day follow-up. Hence, the absence of CAD on CCTA may allow for immediate hospital discharge (Figure 9-e3).

However, the studies demonstrated that the mere detection of obstructive CAD by CCTA does not equate to a diagnosis of ACS (Figure 9-4). In the ROMICAT trial, only 20 of 34 patients with obstructive CAD were clinically diagnosed with ACS.[25] In the study by Hollander and colleagues, only 7 of 54 patients with obstructive CAD by CCTA had a stenosis confirmed by invasive coronary angiography (i.e., underwent invasive angiography on clinical grounds) or a major cardiovascular event within 30 days.[27] However, the low positive predictive value (35% to 50%) of obstructive CAD combined with the low prevalence of ACS (2% to 8%) represents a major challenge for the management of acute chest pain patients. Hence, a finding of 50% has similar importance as a finding that indicates an increased likelihood for future cardiovascular events and an indicator of an ACS.

Randomized Comparative Effectiveness Trials of Cardiac Computed Tomography Angiography versus Standard of Care

As a next step, several randomized trials measured the effectiveness of CCTA when implemented in clinical care (Table 9-3).[2,28,29] These studies were noncontrolled comparative effectiveness trials, in which decisions of care were made by caregivers, and thus, the results reflect common practice patterns. Although the CT-STAT trial compared

TABLE 9-2 Detection of Acute Coronary Syndrome Based on Coronary Computed Tomography Angiography in Observational Studies

STUDY	N	POPULATION	SCANNER	ACS DEFINITION	ACS RATE (MI RATE)	CT CRITERION	SENS	SPEC
Rubinshtein (2007)	58	Higher risk (including history of CAD)	64-CT	Positive troponins, or >50% stenosis by invasive angiography, or positive ischemia test	34%	Stenosis	100%	92%
Gallagher (2007)	92	Low-risk ED	64-CT	MI, UA	13%	Stenosis	86%	92%
ROMICAT I (2009)	368	Low-risk ED	64-CT*	MI (8), UA (23)	8.4% (2%)	Plaque Stenosis	100% 77%	54% 87%
Hansen (2010)	89	Low-risk ED	64-DSCT	MI	4% (4%)	Plaque Stenosis	100% 75%	41% 86%
Dedic (2013)	111	Any-risk ED (including low-positive troponins)	64-DSCT*	MI (13), UA (6)	17% (12%)	Calcium Plaque Stenosis	89% 100% 89%	41% 40% 79%

ACS, Acute coronary syndrome; *CAD*, coronary artery disease; *DSCT*, dual-source CT; *ED*, emergency department; *MI*, myocardial infarction; *Sens*, sensitivity; *Spec*, specificity; *UA*, unstable angina.
*Blinded cardiac CT examination, without affecting management.

Patients with acute chest pain but without known CAD, ECG signs of ischemia, or positive initial troponin

Evaluation for presence, extent, and composition of CAD and optional for resting perfusion and function by contrast enhanced CTA*

Identify high-risk coronary anatomy; identify lesions that could be the reason for the chest pain, and optionally validate this with proof of matching myocardial perfusion deficits and wall motion abnormalities

Normal CTA, low probabilty of ACS including no CAD or minimal <40%

↓

No further testing

Check for noncoronary (pericardial effusion) and noncardiac conditions such as pulmonary embolism and/or aortic dissection

Direct discharge from the ED after 2nd troponin (<6 hours)

Selected patients may need follow-up for myocarditis or vasoactive angina

Moderate CAD (40% – 70%)

Severe CAD (>70%)

Assess functional relevance of the anatomically defined lesions‡ either by including functional assessment into the CT for wall motion abnormalities and/or myocardial perfusion deficits (if desired) or by secondary functional testing

Identify whether CAD is incidental or related to symptoms and help to define the best medical management

Use complete information on troponin, ECG, symptoms, anatomy, and function to determine whether ACS is present

For ACS determine whether coronary revascularization or medical management is most beneficial

In those without ACS, optimize preventive medical therapy AND tailor medical therapy to presence and extent of CAD

*In the future, high-sensitivity troponin assays may permit improved selection of patients for imaging and improved diagnosis of ACS.

‡Assessing if a lesion is significant may be done with top technology scanners which have minimal additional radiation exposure or in the future by approximating fractional flow reserve.

FIGURE 9-4 **Combined multimodality algorithm based on the use of coronary computed tomographic angiography (CCTA) for acute chest pain evaluation.** *ACS*, Acute coronary syndrome; *CAD*, coronary artery disease; *CTA*, computed tomographic angiography; *ECG*, electrocardiogram; *ED*, emergency department.

TABLE 9-3 Contemporary Randomized Comparative Effectiveness Trials

STUDY	CT-STAT (2011)		ACRIN (2012)		ROMICAT II (2012)	
Population	699 TIMI risk score 0–4 MI 0.9%		1370 TIMI risk score 0–2 MI 1%		985 Low to intermediate risk MI 2.5%	
Randomization	1:1		2:1		1:1	
Control group	SPECT MPI		Usual care		Usual care	
	CTA	**Controls**	**CTA**	**Controls**	**CTA**	**Controls**
ACS diagnosis	1.1%	2.4%	1%	1%	9%	6%
ED discharge			**50%**	**23%**	**47%**	**12%**
ICA rate	8.0%	7.4%	5%	4%	12%	8%
Revascularization	4.3%	2.7%	3%	1%	6%	4%
Time to diagnosis, hr (median, range)	**2.9* (2.1–4.0)**	**6.3 (4–19)**				
Length of stay, hr (median, range)			**18.0 (8–27)**	**24.8 (19–31)**	**23.2***	**30.8**
1-mo MACE			**0%***	**0%**	0.4%	1.2%
6-mo MACE	0.8%	0.4%				
Cost (US$)	**2137†**	**3458**			4026‡	3874

ACS, Acute coronary syndrome; *CTA*, computed tomographic angiography; *ED*, emergency department; *ICA,* invasive coronary angiography; *MACE*, major adverse cardiovascular events; *MI*, myocardial infarction; *MPI*, myocardial perfusion imaging; *SPECT*, single-photon emission tomography; *TIMI*, Thrombolysis In Myocardial Infarction.
*Primary endpoint of the study.
†Represents only ED costs.
‡Index hospitalization, including angiograms and interventions.
Statistically significant results in bold.

coronary CTA with SPECT,[28] the ACRIN and ROMICAT II trials compared CTA with SOC.[2,29] Patients were predominantly enrolled at academic centers in the United States that performed in-patient functional testing, but which had no accelerated care protocol. The study cohorts were at low (ACRIN, CT-STAT) or low to intermediate risk for ACS (ROMICAT II) and represented between 10% and 15% of patients who presented with acute chest pain to the ED.

Taken together, the three trials had more than 3000 patients, and follow-up analysis demonstrated that based on the CTA results, not a single patient was discharged with a missed diagnosis of ACS. The ACRIN trial specifically demonstrated that CTA is safe in low-risk patients, with a 0% adverse event rate at 30 days (95%, CI 0% to 0.57%; primary endpoint). Another goal of these trials was to demonstrate the efficiency of CTA compared with SOC. This objective was primarily tested in the ROMICAT II trial, which demonstrated a reduction in length of stay, hospital admissions, and ED cost, whereas overall hospital costs remained similar to SOC, driven by a higher rate of invasive angiography and revascularizations. Across the trials, patients randomized to CTA more often underwent cardiac catheterization (8.4% vs. 6.3%) and percutaneous coronary intervention (4.6% vs. 2.6%). A major safety focus of these trials was on radiation exposure. The data demonstrated that CCTA had lower radiation exposure compared with SPECT MPI, but cumulative radiation exposure was higher with CTA because SOC included exercise testing or no testing of up to 30% of patients. Unfortunately, the trials were not powered to prove that increased revascularization rates resulted in improved clinical outcomes. However, the evidence provided by the three large randomized trials established cardiac CT as a viable alternative to functional testing for triage of low-risk patients with acute chest pain.

Prediction of Mid-term Outcome

Several studies demonstrated that CTA findings of nonobstructive CAD, obstructive CAD, and regional left ventricular wall motion abnormalities identify increasing risk of future adverse cardiovascular events (Table 9-4).[30–33] Importantly, patients without CAD remained virtually event-free over the next 2 years, which could result in a decrease of diagnostic testing at repeat ED presentations.[30]

Challenges to Implementation of Cardiac Computed Tomography in the Emergency Department

Although the potential diagnostic value of cardiac CT in the ED seems evident, there are practical obstacles that interfere with widespread implementation. CT equipment with sufficient cardiac imaging capabilities (minimally, a single-source 64-slice system), fully trained technologists, and experienced cardiac CT readers are essential. Not all patients are eligible for CCTA, including those with known CAD, cardiac arrhythmia, tachycardia, or severe obesity (typically body mass index of >40 kg/m^2). CT angiography is associated with risks caused by radiation exposure, although doses have decreased substantially over the past decade. Use of iodine-containing contrast media is contraindicated in cases of renal dysfunction or related allergies. The guidelines emphasize that the choice of test, whether CT or another modality, should be based on local expertise and individual characteristics that affect eligibility.[34] More advanced CT technology, dual-source CT systems, or wider detector arrays can improve image quality in somewhat less suitable patients. Presently, few centers have sufficient experienced personnel to offer cardiac CT around the clock. Guidelines on the practice of cardiac CT in the ED specify needs for certification and maintenance of certification for imaging centers, interpreting physicians, and medical staff.[35]

Appropriate Use Criteria, Guidelines, and Clinical Role

The ACCF/SCCT/ACR/AHA/ASE/ASNC/NASCI/SCAI/SCMR 2010 appropriate use criteria for cardiac computed tomography includes a section on the use of CCTA in acute chest pain.[36] These guidelines considered CCTA in patients with acute chest pain, negative electrocardiogram and biomarkers, and low or intermediate likelihood of obstructive CAD as appropriate. The ACCF/AHA guidelines for the management of patients with NSTEMI and unstable angina pectoris, which were formulated before completion of the most recent trials, do not provide a specific recommendation for the use of CCTA in patients with acute chest pain and suspected ACS.[34]

TABLE 9-4 Prognostic Value of Cardiac Computed Tomography in Acute Chest Pain

AUTHOR/YEAR	N	ACS RISK	FOLLOW-UP	EVENT DEFINITION	CT CRITERION (% TOTAL COHORT)	EVENTS
Rubinshtein (2007)	58	Avg TIMI 1.3	1 yr	Death, MI, revasc.	ED discharge (55%)	0
Hollander (2007)	588	TIMI 0-1	1 yr	Death, MI, revasc.	Stenosis <50% (82%)	0.2%
ROMICAT I (2011)	368	Low risk	2 yr	Death, MI, revasc.*	Normal (50%) <50% stenosis (32%) >50% stenosis (19%)	0 4.6% 30.3%
CT-STAT (2011)	361	Avg TIMI 1	6 mo	Death, MI, revasc.	(Nearly) normal (74%)	0.8%
Singer (2012)	507	Avg TIMI 1	6 mo	Death, revasc.	Stenosis <50% (96%)	0
Christiaens (2012)	175	Low-int. risk	6 mo	MACE (nonspecified)	Stenosis <50% (78%)	0

ACS, Acute coronary syndrome; *ED*, emergency department; *MACE*, major adverse cardiovascular events; *MI*, myocardial infarction; *TIMI*, Thrombolysis In Myocardial Infarction.

*Includes index events.

Based on the experience from large multicenter randomized trials, the available evidence suggests that CCTA use in the setting of low- and low-to-intermediate risk of ACS in acute chest pain patients in the ED may have a favorable impact on patient management, largely through speeding the direct discharge of those without CAD. Approximately half of patients studied in the three randomized trials had no evidence of CAD on CCTA. This type of patient, with no CAD on CCTA, can be safely discharged after CCTA, thus reducing the duration of the hospital stay and cost in this subgroup. Furthermore, patients with minimal nonobstructive CAD are also candidates for early discharge with arrangement of outpatient follow-up. On the other side of the spectrum are patients with a definite coronary stenosis. These patients require admission to the hospital, further evaluation, and guideline-directed therapies. An area of uncertainty involves patients with nondiagnostic CCTA or evidence of non-negligible coronary plaque, but who have no significant stenosis. These patients usually require observation with serial biomarkers and ECGs, and often a functional stress test for evaluation of ischemia. A suggested algorithm to incorporate CCTA in the management of ED patients with low-to-intermediate likelihood of ACS because of potential findings on CCTA is provided in Figure 9-4.

Beyond the Coronary Lumen: Anatomic and Functional Information

There are several techniques in active development that would integrate the potential functional impact of obstructive CAD as detected by CCTA with the potential to improve accuracy and efficiency of CCTA in patients with acute chest pain, including the assessment of global and regional left ventricular function,[37] evaluation of myocardial perfusion,[38,39] advanced high-risk coronary plaque analysis,[40–42] and noninvasive fractional flow reserve (FFR).[43,44] Figure 9-5 illustrates the complementary nature of anatomic and functional information (see also Figure 9-e4).

Myocardial Perfusion Imaging

Acute rest SPECT-MPI has high predictive value for ACS in the ED setting. Similarly, CCTA can take advantage of the fact that in patients with acute chest pain, myocardial ischemia or myocardial infarction can be identified on routine CTA as myocardial hypoenhancement during rest.[45] For the purpose of accurate myocardial perfusion assessment by CCTA, thick-slice (10 mm), short-axis datasets need to be reconstructed and should be visualized using a narrow window to increase the contrast. The presence of resting myocardial enhancement defects on CTA has a sensitivity and specificity of approximately 90% to identify patients with an MI.[39,46] Although chronic myocardial scar and acute hypoperfusion both show lower contrast enhancement on CCTA scans, chronic infarction can often be differentiated by wall thinning or lower attenuation values (below 0 HU) as a result of fat tissue within the scar.

More importantly, a subanalysis from ROMICAT I in 183 patients provided initial evidence that early rest perfusion CCTA provides incremental value beyond obstructive CAD to detect ACS (sensitivity for ACS increased from 77% [95% CI, 59% to 90%] for obstructive CAD to 90% [95% CI, 74% to 98%] with addition of rCTP [$P = .05$)] and is noninferior to a combination of CCTA for anatomy and stress SPECT-MPI for myocardial perfusion to discriminate ACS (area under the curve, 0.88 vs. 0.90; $P = .64$) using a noninferiority margin of 10%.[47] Hence, resting myocardial perfusion by CCTA provides important additional information, and in some cases (i.e., the occlusion of small branches) may provide the only hint for an ACS on CTA (Figure 9-6).

Coronary Computed Tomography Angiography–Derived Fractional Flow Reserve

The hemodynamic severity of CAD can also be estimated by calculation of the FFR from CT angiograms using computational fluid dynamics.[48] CTA-derived FFR can exclude hemodynamically significant CAD more confidently, with a correlation to invasively measure FFR between 0.7 and 0.8.

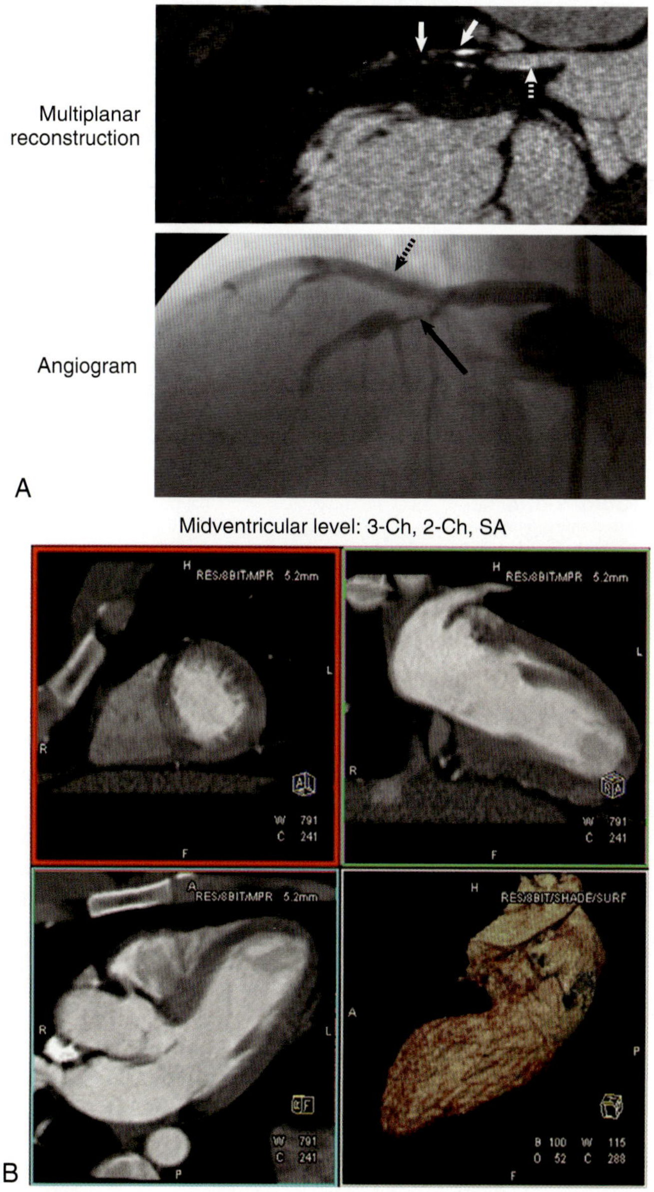

FIGURE 9-5 (**A**) *Upper level,* Multiplanar reconstructed CT image of the left anterior descending coronary artery, demonstrating a contrast-filled lumen at the beginning (*dashed white arrow*) of the procedure. After approximately 2 cm, the lumen over a long segment (*white solid arrows*) is filled with low attenuation material, representing either noncalcified plaque or acute thrombus. Because of the presentation of the patient, acute thrombotic subtotal occlusion is more likely. Partial reconstitution of the lumen occurs. Some wall calcifications are also visible. *Lower level,* invasive coronary angiogram of the left ascending coronary artery. Subtotal occlusion of the proximal left anterior descending artery as seen in CT (*solid black arrow*). Patent large first diagonal branch (*dashed black arrow*). (**B**) *Midventricular level,* Three- and two-chamber, and short-axis cine loops as well as a left ventriculogram. Hypokinesia by absence of wall thickening in systole of the septal and anterior wall is demonstrated. Left ventriculography shows that the contrast blood close to the anterior wall is not moving during the cardiac cycle.

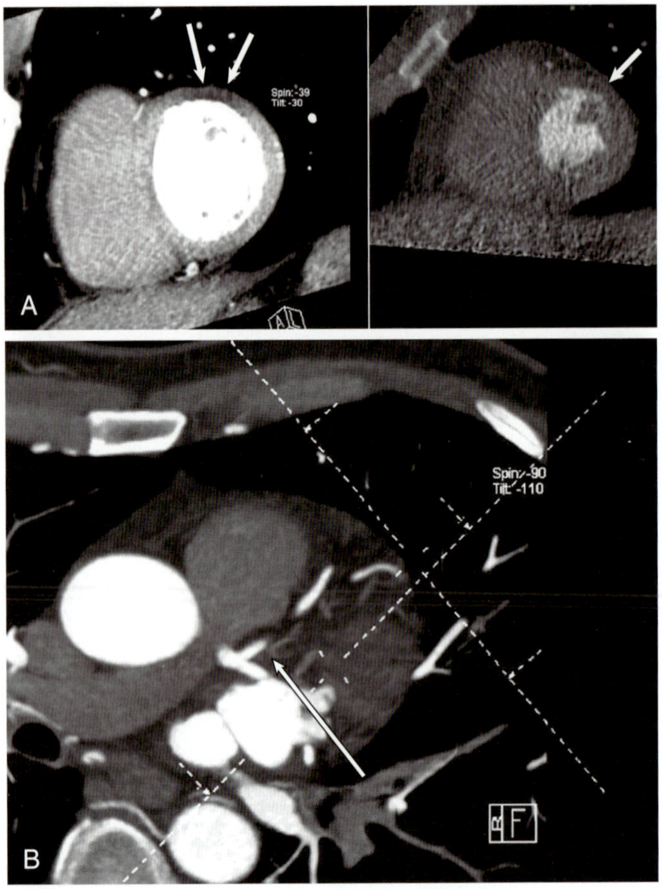

FIGURE 9-6 (**A**) Two-chamber, short-axis view with a narrow "contrast" window used to assess differences in myocardial tissue attenuation. In the anterior myocardial wall, there is a sharply delineated area of low attenuation, representing a perfusion deficit. In cine loops, this appeared to be associated with a hypokinesia by absence of wall thickening in systole of that segment. The patient ultimately developed an increase in cardiac troponin and was diagnosed with non–ST-elevation myocardial infarction (NSTEMI). NSTEMI is often based on occlusions of smaller diagonal or obtuse marginal branches. Hence, highly skilled interpretation of coronary CT angiography is needed to recognize these appropriately. (**B**) Contrast enhanced coronary CT angiograph displaying the bifurcation of the left main coronary artery. The proximal left anterior descending artery gives rise to a small first diagonal branch (*arrow*), which appears to be occluded. This finding is easy to miss, leaving myocardial perfusion defect as the sole evidence of an ongoing acute coronary syndrome. Subsequent invasive coronary angiography confirmed proximal occlusion of the first diagonal branch.

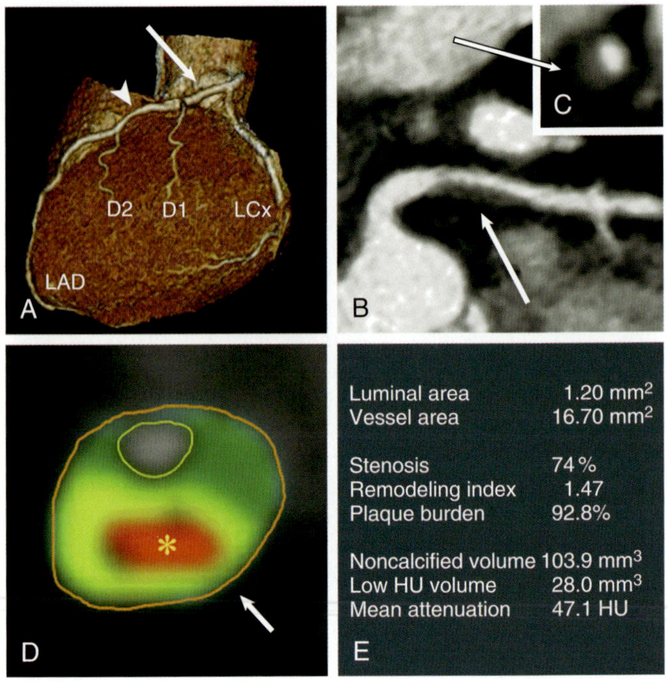

FIGURE 9-7 Example of advanced quantitative analysis of noncalcified plaque (NCP). (**A** to **C**) Identification of NCP. (**A**) Three-dimensional, volume-rendered image of the coronary tree. (**B**) Multiplanar reformatted long-axis and (**C**) short-axis images of the proximal left anterior descending artery area (*white arrows*) demonstrating NCP. (**D** and **E**) Proposed methods of quantification of NCP. (**D**) Cross section depicting central low attenuation core (*red*) with peripheral high attenuation (*green*) representing a napkin ring sign. (**E**) Output of quantitative analysis of NCP. *LAD*, left anterior descending artery; *LCx*, left circumflex artery.

In a trial of 251 patients, CTA-FFR had a sensitivity of 84% and a specificity of 86% to accurately detect invasive FFR positive and/or negative patients.[43] Thus, although this technique has not yet been investigated in patients with acute chest pain, it could reduce the need for further functional testing or invasive angiography. However, currently available CTA-FFR algorithms require processing on a powerful remote computer, and point-of-care CTA-FFR with a processing time of less than 1 hour as needed for ED use is not yet available.[49]

Calcium Imaging

Calcium imaging in acute chest pain remains controversial. Although the absence of calcium in low-risk acute chest pain indicates a low probability of ACS and good overall prognosis, a negative coronary calcium scan alone does not completely rule out ACS in patients with chest pain.[50]

High-risk Plaque Features

A unique feature of coronary CTA is the potential to noninvasively visualize and characterize coronary atherosclerotic plaque, both in stenotic and in nonobstructive lesions. CTA can classify plaque composition as calcified or noncalcified. More importantly, CTA can detect features associated with plaque instability, such as low attenuation (<30 HU), outward vessel remodeling, high total plaque burden, and spotty calcifications (Figure 9-7) with good correlation to intravascular imaging and histology.[51] Initial data suggest that these CTA-determined plaque features predict adverse events, independent of the angiographic stenosis severity (Table 9-5). In a subanalysis of the ROMICAT II trial cohort, the presence of high-risk plaque features on coronary CTA increased the likelihood of ACS, independent of the angiographic CAD severity and clinical risk assessment.[40] The role for these plaque features in individual clinical decisions requires further investigation.

Noncoronary Cardiovascular Emergencies

An advantage of CCTA may be that other life-threatening conditions that are differential diagnoses in acute chest pain, including pulmonary embolism, aortic dissection, pneumothorax and pericarditis, may be diagnosed. For example, in patients with suspected stroke, the thoracic aorta is imaged to exclude aortic dissection. Nongated images may suggest aortic dissection because pulsaton artifacts are seen. ECG gating resolves these artifacts (Figure 9-e5). In addition, masses or tumors may be discovered in patients with acute chest pain. Cine images can demonstrate the morphology and the motion of tumors during the cardiac cycle and can contribute to alternative diagnoses (Figure 9-e6). An ECG-synchronized thoracic CT scan with pulmonary and aortic contrast enhancement can rule out all of these conditions. However, a triple rule-out protocol is not recommended for routine use in suspected ACS because of the low incidence of noncoronary emergencies, the higher scan complexity, and the higher radiation and contrast medium dose.

Cardiac Computed Tomography in the Era of High-Sensitivity Troponin Assays

High-sensitivity assays for troponin (see Chapter 7) that allow more sensitive and earlier detection of MI[52] have profoundly affected the daily management of patients with acute chest pain in Europe. The identification of a low-risk group of patients by new biomarker assays may obviate the use of imaging in this select group. However, a challenge arises from the fact that more patients will have a measurable high-sensitivity troponin in the absence of acute coronary disease. The application of cardiac CT may develop as an effective means to rule out CAD in patients with minor troponin elevations. Initial work has shown that high-sensitivity troponin closely correlates with the presence and extent of CAD,[53] as well as the presence of myocardial perfusion abnormalities,[54] and suggests that baseline troponin will enable an improved and more efficient selection of patients for subsequent diagnostic testing. With the availability of high-sensitivity troponin and the development of functional CT applications, the role of cardiac CT may, in the future, shift from a rule-out test for low-risk patients to a more comprehensive and potentially therapy-guiding modality.

CARDIAC MAGNETIC RESONANCE IMAGING

CMR imaging has been explored only to a limited extent in the setting of acute chest pain. However, especially in patients with known CAD or previous MI, the strengths of CMR imaging, including the ability to comprehensively evaluate cardiac morphology, function, perfusion, and especially tissue characterization without radiation exposure, are particularly attractive in this setting (see also Chapter 33). However, CMR imaging is complex and requires substantial technical expertise to ensure high-quality diagnostic examinations and interpretation.

In the setting of acute chest pain, superb tissue characterization of the myocardium is the most attractive aspect of CMR. The key attributes of characterization of myocardial tissue include the ability to differentiate infarcted tissue (using the late gadolinium enhancement technique) and ischemic myocardium (rest perfusion defect without evidence of infarct) from normal myocardium, to diagnose MI before troponin elevation, to differentiate between new and old infarcts, and to determine prognosis.[55] CMR is a favorable approach in patients with known previous MI, a group of patients in whom the discrimination of new versus old infarction limits the usefulness of CCTA or MPI.

Observational Studies and Trials of Cardiac Magnetic Resonance

The usefulness of CMR in patients with previous events who present with a possible new MI was initially demonstrated by Kwong and colleagues.[56] In this resting protocol, an abnormal CMR study was defined by either a regional wall motion abnormality or an area of late gadolinium enhancement with or without matching perfusion defect. Among 161 patients, of whom 16% had a final diagnosis of ACS, CMR imaging had a sensitivity of 84% and a specificity of 85% for detecting ACS before troponin elevation. In a subsequent smaller study (n = 62), the incorporation of T2-weighted CMR imaging of myocardial edema improved specificity, positive predictive value, and overall accuracy to differentiate acute regional ischemia or infarction from chronic infarcts in the ED setting.[57]

Several relatively small single center trials were reported from centers with superb expertise in the acquisition and interpretation of CMR. These randomized trials aimed to define the value of stress CMR in patients with chest pain in the ED performed as part of an observation unit protocol, and demonstrated that such a strategy may reduce median costs, primarily driven by fewer cardiac-related ED visits, hospitalizations, and catheterizations, possibly because of the perceived more definitive diagnostic information provided initially by CMR.[58–60]

Although the available evidence suggests that CMR may be useful in the management of patients with known CAD who present with suspected acute MI, the administrative, technical and logistical challenges of performing CMR are barriers to routine use in patients with acute chest pain.

Identifying Alternative Causes for Apparent Acute Coronary Syndrome

See Chapter 33.

Appropriate Use Criteria, Guidelines, and Clinical Role

The 2006 ACCF/ACR/SCCT/SCMR/ASNC/NASCI/SCAI/SIR appropriateness criteria for cardiac CT and CMR imaging list the use of vasodilator or dobutamine stress CMR imaging as of "uncertain" appropriateness in patients in the aftermath of acute chest pain,[9] which in contemporary nomenclature would be considered as "may be appropriate." It is important to note that virtually all of the literature on the use of CMR in this setting has appeared after that document was prepared.

FUTURE DIRECTIONS

Technical advances in the existing modalities may foster continued evolution of how imaging is used in the ED setting. For SPECT MPI, high-speed and high-efficiency cameras are now available that allow high-quality imaging with lower radionuclide doses, reducing radiation exposure, and with protocols that are completed more quickly. In an observational study of more than 1400 ED patients who underwent CCTA or stress testing (with ECG or imaging with a high-efficiency SPECT camera), Duvall and colleagues reported that similar proportions of patients were directly discharged from the ED with either testing strategy, but the CCTA group had longer length of stay, higher mean effective radiation dose exposure, and more follow-up testing.[61] The higher efficiency SPECT cameras also enable the possibility of "stress only" imaging, which when combined with attenuation correction techniques for selected patients, significantly reduces the time and dose for radionuclide imaging.[62]

Other developments include the ability to image the "ischemic memory" by identifying metabolic abnormalities reflective of the previous ischemic event even many hours after symptoms have resolved. Beta-methyl-p-[123I]-iodophenyl-pentadecanoic acid (BMIPP) is a fatty acid

TABLE 9-5 High-Risk Plaque and Major Adverse Cardiovascular Events

FIRST AUTHOR, YEAR	STUDY DESIGN	CHARACTERISTICS OF STUDY POPULATION					MEDIAN FU (MOS)
			SYMPTOMATIC				
		Asymptomatic (%)	Acute (%)	Stable (%)	Known CAD (%)	Unknown Status	
Matsumoto, 2007	Retrospective cohort (n = 810)	Y (15%)	Y (61%)	—	Y	Y	35
Motoyama, 2009	Retrospective cohort (n = 1059)	—	—	—	Y	Y	27
Otsuka, 2013	Prospective cohort (n = 895)	Y (40%)	Y(60%)		Y	—	28
Yamamoto, 2013	Prospective cohort (n = 511)	Y (46%)	Y (54%)		Y (4.7 %)	—	40

ACS, Acute coronary syndrome; *Ca*, calcium; *CACS*, calcium score; *CAD*, coronary artery disease; *CCTA*, cardiac computed tomographic angiography; *CI*, confidence interval; *DM*, diabetes mellitus; *FU*, follow-up; *HLP*, hyperlipidemia; *HR*, hazard ratio; *HRPF*, high-risk plaque features; *HTN*, hypertension; *LAP*, low attenuation plaque with <30 HU; *MI*, myocardial infarction; *NRS*, napkin-ring sign; *PCI*, percutaneous coronary intervention; *PR*, positive remodeling; *UA*, unstable angina.

that is taken up in the myocardium and not significantly metabolized. Imaging of this agent, even up to 30 hours after the resolution of chest pain symptoms, allows for delayed detection of ischemic myocardium, which appears as a defect reflecting the reduced regional fatty acid metabolism. In practice, BMIPP imaging in ED patients may permit for accurate detection of myocardial ischemia as long as within 30 hours after chest pain resolution.[63] BMIPP has not yet been approved by the Food and Drug Administration for this purpose in the United States.

The technology to perform CCTA also continues to evolve. In an initial study, Achenbach and colleagues reported on using a new CT acquisition scan mode to achieve high quality CCTA imaging with acquisition times of approximately 4 minutes and radiation exposures of less than 1 mSv.[64] Min and colleagues have published a series of reports, including a multicenter trial, assessing the ability of the noninvasive CT images to evaluate FFR associated with a stenosis.[44] Once mature, this technology may attenuate the apparent increase in downstream catheterizations that have been observed in some CCTA studies, by enabling interrogation of the physiologic significance of a stenosis seen on CCTA.

Thus, the technologies involved in imaging patients in this setting continue to evolve toward a more personalized way of managing patients, carefully weighing which test and which diagnostic information may affect management of each patient in the most meaningful way. It is important to acknowledge that the evaluation of imaging techniques for ED patients with suspected ACS in clinical trials has been leading the way in setting an example of how to rigorously assess technology for clinical use, resulting in a high-level evidence base that can assist clinicians in selecting the right test for the right patient.

SUMMARY

Imaging, especially echocardiography and MPI, is well established in guiding triage and further management of patients presenting with acute chest pain. Stress imaging in the observation unit has become common clinical practice. CCTA and CMR expand the opportunities to image coronary atherosclerosis and assess salvageable myocardium. Because of the low prevalence of ACS among the ED population with chest pain, anatomic methods are attractive for their assessment, especially if tools currently under investigation (left ventricular function, perfusion, or CTA-FFR) ultimately prove to substantially increase the positive predictive value of noninvasive cardiac imaging. Imaging that provides myocardial tissue characterization is likely to be more useful in patients with known CAD because most management decisions require differentiation of old versus new infarcts. In the future, integrated testing using both CCTA and high-sensitivity cardiac troponin assays may enable even more effective early triage through more efficient selection of patients needing diagnostic testing.

HRPF ASSESSED	NO. AND TYPE OF OUTCOMES	INDEPENDENT ADJUDICATION OF EVENTS?	EVENT RATES	UNADJUSTED HR (95% CI)	ADJUSTED HR (95% CI)	GENERAL REMARKS
LAP (min HU <68)	n = 22 Cardiac death, nonfatal MI, or UA	Y	At 4 yrs: LAP (+) vs (−): 5.29 % vs. 1.9% ACS and 1.05% vs. 0.6% cardiac death	LAP: 2.9 (1.24–6.73)	2.53 (1.08–5.92) after adjusting for age, gender, HTN, HLP, DM, smoking, previous MI	10% underwent CCTA for evaluation of post-PCI status and 7% had previous MI.
PR (RI >1.1) and LAP (<30 HU)	n = 15 ACS	N	At 27 mos: 2 feature (PR and LAP) plaque: 22.2%; 1 feature plaque (PR or LAP) 3.7%; 0 feature plaque: 0.49%	Not reported	2 or 1 feature: 22.79 (6.91–75.17) after adjusting for HTN, HLP, previous MI	Cohort consists of patients with suspected or known CAD with no further explanation of "suspected."
PR (RI >1.1), LAP (<30 HU), NRS	n = 24 Cardiac death, nonfatal MI, or UA	N	Event rates not reported. Event rate in the entire population is 2.7% (2 yrs).	NRS: 5.5 (2.2–12.7); LAP: 3.75 (1.4–9.8); PR: 5.2 (2.2-12.7)	Not reported	20% had history of MI. The study basically evaluated NRS compared with other high-risk features. Per segment analysis, culprit segments of ACS compared with nonculprit segments; authors do not report controlling for clustering effect
LAP (<34 or 38 HU), PR (>1.05 or 1.2), spotty Ca (<2/3 vessel diameter)	n = 15 Cardiac death, nonfatal MI, UA	N	Annual hard event rate: 6.2% (LAP), 8.6% (PR), 4.5% (spotty Ca), 9.9% (LAP+PR)	LAP: 11.7 (3.73–51.3); PR: 10.2 (3.69–30.6); LAP+PR: 12.3 (4.42–36.6); spotty Ca: 3.74 (1.34–10.7)	LAP: 8.23 (2.41–37.7); PR: 8.3 (2.83–26.7); LAP+PR:11.2 (3.71–36.7); spotty Ca: 2.41 (0.80–7.51) adjusted for age, sex, and >50% stenosis	Patients w/ early revasc (<3 mos) excluded.

Classic References

Achenbach S, et al.: Detection of coronary artery stenoses by contrast-enhanced, retrospectively electrocardiographically-gated, multislice spiral computed tomography, *Circulation* 103:2535–2538, 2001.

Agatston AS, et al.: Quantification of coronary artery calcium using ultrafast computed tomography, *J Am Coll Cardiol* 15:827–832, 1990.

Fesmire FM, et al.: The Erlanger chest pain evaluation protocol: a one-year experience with serial 12-lead ECG monitoring, two-hour delta serum marker measurements, and selective nuclear stress testing to identify and exclude acute coronary syndromes, *Ann Emerg Med* 40:584–594, 2002.

Hoffmann U, et al.: Coronary multidetector computed tomography in the assessment of patients with acute chest pain, *Circulation* 114:2251–2260, 2006.

Kontos MC, et al.: Value of acute rest sestamibi perfusion imaging for evaluation of patients admitted to the emergency department with chest pain, *J Am Coll Cardiol* 30:976–982, 1997.

Motoyama S, et al.: Computed tomographic angiography characteristics of atherosclerotic plaques subsequently resulting in acute coronary syndrome, *J Am Coll Cardiol* 54:49–57, 2009.

References

1. Bhuiya FA, Pitts SR, McCaig LF: Emergency department visits for chest pain and abdominal pain: United States, 1999-2008, *NCHS Data Brief* 1–8, 2010.
2. Litt HI, et al.: CT angiography for safe discharge of patients with possible acute coronary syndromes, *N Engl J Med* 366:1393–1403, 2012.
3. Roe MT, et al.: Clinical and therapeutic profile of patients presenting with acute coronary syndromes who do not have significant coronary artery disease. The Platelet Glycoprotein IIb/IIIa in Unstable Angina: Receptor Suppression Using Integrilin Therapy (PURSUIT) Trial Investigators, *Circulation* 102:1101–1106, 2000.
4. Fishbein MC: The vulnerable and unstable atherosclerotic plaque, *Cardiovasc Pathol* 19:6–11, 2010.
5. Gibbons RJ, et al.: The quantification of infarct size, *J Am Coll Cardiol* 44:1533–1542, 2004.
6. Notghi A, Low CS: Myocardial perfusion scintigraphy: past, present and future, *Br J Radiol* 3:S229–236, 2011. 84 Spec No.
7. Tatum JL, et al.: Comprehensive strategy for the evaluation and triage of the chest pain patient, *Ann Emerg Med* 29:116–125, 1997.
8. Udelson JE, et al.: Myocardial perfusion imaging for evaluation and triage of patients with suspected acute cardiac ischemia: a randomized controlled trial, *JAMA* 288:2693–2700, 2002.
9. Hendel RC, et al.: American College of Cardiology Foundation Quality Strategic Directions Committee Appropriateness Criteria Working Group, American College of Radiology, Society of Cardiovascular Computed Tomography, Society for Cardiovascular Magnetic Resonance, American Society of Nuclear Cardiology, North American Society for Cardiac Imaging, Society for Cardiovascular Angiography and Interventions, Society of Interventional Radiology. ACCF/ACR/SCCT/SCMR/ASNC/NASCI/SCAI/SIR 2006 appropriateness criteria for cardiac computed tomography and cardiac magnetic resonance imaging: a report of the American College of Cardiology Foundation Quality Strategic Directions Committee Appropriateness Criteria Working Group, American College of Radiology, Society of Cardiovascular Computed Tomography, Society for Cardiovascular Magnetic Resonance, American Society of Nuclear Cardiology, North American Society for Cardiac Imaging, Society for Cardiovascular Angiography and Interventions, and Society of Interventional Radiology, *J Am Coll Cardiol* 48:1475–1497, 2006.
10. Priest VL, et al.: Cost-effectiveness of coronary computed tomography and cardiac stress imaging in the emergency department: a decision analytic model comparing diagnostic strategies for chest pain in patients at low risk of acute coronary syndromes, *J Am Coll Cardiol* 4:549–556, 2011.
11. Labovitz AJ, et al.: Focused cardiac ultrasound in the emergent setting: a consensus statement of the American Society of Echocardiography and American College of Emergency Physicians, *J Am Soc Echocardiogr* 23:1225–1230, 2010.
12. Stride E: Physical principles of microbubbles for ultrasound imaging and therapy, *Cerebrovasc Dis* 27(Suppl 2):1–13, 2009.
13. Lepper W, et al.: Myocardial contrast echocardiography, *Circulation* 109:3132–3135, 2004.
14. Wei K: Utility contrast echocardiography in the emergency department, *J Am Coll Cardiol* 3:197–203, 2010.
15. American College of Cardiology Foundation Appropriate Use Criteria Task Force, American Society of Echocardiography, American Heart Association, American Society of Nuclear Cardiology, Heart Failure Society of America, Heart Rhythm Society, Society for Cardiovascular Angiography and Interventions, Society of Critical Care Medicine, Society of Cardiovascular Computed Tomography, Society for Cardiovascular Magnetic Resonance, Douglas PS, et al.: ACCF/ASE/AHA/ASNC/HFSA/HRS/SCAI/SCCM/SCCT/SCMR 2011 appropriate use criteria for echocardiography. A report of the American College of Cardiology Foundation Appropriate Use Criteria Task Force, American Society of Echocardiography, American Heart Association, American Society of Nuclear Cardiology, Heart Failure Society of America, Heart Rhythm Society, Society for Cardiovascular Angiography and Interventions, Society of Critical Care Medicine, Society of Cardiovascular Computed Tomography, and Society for Cardiovascular Magnetic Resonance Endorsed by the American College of Chest Physicians, *J Am Coll Cardiol* 57:1126–1166, 2011.
16. Fesmire FM, et al.: The Erlanger chest pain evaluation protocol: a one-year experience with serial 12-lead ECG monitoring, two-hour delta serum marker measurements, and selective nuclear stress testing to identify and exclude acute coronary syndromes, *Ann Emerg Med* 40:584–594, 2002.
17. Lim SH, et al.: Stress myocardial perfusion imaging for the evaluation and triage of chest pain in the emergency department: a randomized controlled trial, *J Nucl Cardiol* 20:1002–1012, 2013.
18. Bholasingh R, et al.: Prognostic value of predischarge dobutamine stress echocardiography in chest pain patients with a negative cardiac troponin t, *J Am Coll Cardiol* 41:596–602, 2003.
19. Nucifora G, et al.: Comparison of early dobutamine stress echocardiography and exercise electrocardiographic testing for management of patients presenting to the emergency department with chest pain, *Am J Cardiol* 100:1068–1073, 2007.

20. Hendel RC, et al.: ACC/AHA/ACR/ASE/ASNC/HRS/NASCI/RSNA/SAIP/SCAI/ SCCT/SCMR/SIR 2008 key data elements and definitions for cardiac imaging: a report of the American College of Cardiology/American Heart Association task force on clinical data standards (writing committee to develop clinical data standards for cardiac imaging), *Circulation* 119:154–186, 2009.
21. Douglas PS, et al.: American College of Cardiology Foundation Appropriateness Criteria Task F, American Society of Echocardiography, American College of Emergency Physicians, American Heart Association, American Society of Nuclear Cardiology, Society for Cardiovascular Angiography and Interventions, Society of Cardiovascular Computed Tomography, Society for Cardiovascular Magnetic Resonance. ACCF/ASE/ACEP/AHA/ASNC/SCAI/SCCT/SCMR 2008 appropriateness criteria for stress echocardiography: a report of the American College of Cardiology Foundation Appropriateness Criteria Task Force, American Society of Echocardiography, American College of Emergency Physicians, American Heart Association, American Society of Nuclear Cardiology, Society for Cardiovascular Angiography and Interventions, Society of Cardiovascular Computed Tomography, and Society for Cardiovascular Magnetic Resonance: Endorsed by the Heart Rhythm Society and the Society of Critical Care Medicine, *Circulation* 117:1478–1497, 2008.
22. Patel MR, et al.: Low diagnostic yield of elective coronary angiography, *N Engl J Med* 362:886–895, 2010.
23. Schuetz GM, et al.: Meta-analysis: noninvasive coronary angiography using computed tomography versus magnetic resonance imaging, *Ann Intern Med* 152:167–177, 2010.
24. Maurovich-Horvat P, et al.: Methods of plaque quantification and characterization by cardiac computed tomography, *J Cardiovasc Comput Tomogr* 3(Suppl 2):S91–98, 2009.
25. Hoffmann U, et al.: Coronary computed tomography angiography for early triage of patients with acute chest pain: The ROMICAT (Rule Out Myocardial Infarction Using Computer Assisted Tomography) trial, *J Am Coll Cardiol* 53:1642–1650, 2009.
26. Takakuwa KM, et al.: A meta-analysis of 64-section coronary CT angiography findings for predicting 30-day major adverse cardiac events in patients presenting with symptoms suggestive of acute coronary syndrome, *Acad Radiol* 18:1522–1528, 2011.
27. Hollander JE, et al.: Coronary computed tomographic angiography for rapid discharge of low-risk patients with potential acute coronary syndromes, *Ann Emerg Med* 53:295–304, 2009.
28. Goldstein JA, et al.: The CT-STAT (Coronary Computed Tomographic Angiography for Systematic Triage of Acute Chest Pain Patients to Treatment) trial, *J Am Coll Cardiol* 58:1414–1422, 2011.
29. Hoffmann U, et al.: Investigators R-I. Coronary CT angiography versus standard evaluation in acute chest pain, *N Engl J Med* 367:299–308, 2012.
30. Schlett CL, et al.: Prognostic value of CT angiography for major adverse cardiac events in patients with acute chest pain from the emergency department: 2-year outcomes of the Romicat trial, *J Am Coll Cardiol* 4:481–491, 2011.
31. Hollander JE, et al.: One-year outcomes following coronary computerized tomographic angiography for evaluation of emergency department patients with potential acute coronary syndrome, *Acad Emerg Med* 16:693–698, 2009.
32. Singer AJ, et al.: Utilization of coronary computed tomography angiography for exclusion of coronary artery disease in ED patients with low- to intermediate-risk chest pain: a 1-year experience, *Am J Emerg Med* 30:1706–1711, 2012.
33. Christiaens L, et al.: Impact of 64-slice coronary CT on the management of patients presenting with acute chest pain: results of a prospective two-centre study, *European Radiology* 22:1050–1058, 2012.
34. Anderson JL, et al.: Writing Group Members, ACCF/AHA Task Force Members. 2011 ACCF/AHA focused update incorporated into the ACC/AHA 2007 guidelines for the management of patients with unstable angina/non-ST-elevation myocardial infarction: a report of the American College of Cardiology Foundation/American Heart Association task force on practice guidelines, *Circulation* 123:e426–579, 2011.
35. Raff GL, et al.: Society of Cardiovascular Computed Tomography Guidelines Committee. SCCT guidelines on the use of coronary computed tomographic angiography for patients presenting with acute chest pain to the emergency department: a report of the Society of Cardiovascular Computed Tomography Guidelines Committee, *J Cardiovasc Comput Tomogr* 8:254–271, 2014.
36. Taylor AJ, et al.: American College of Cardiology Foundation Appropriate Use Criteria Task F, Society of Cardiovascular Computed Tomography, American College of Radiology, American Heart Association, American Society of Echocardiography, American Society of Nuclear Cardiology, North American Society for Cardiovascular Imaging, Society for Cardiovascular Angiography and Interventions, Society for Cardiovascular Magnetic Resonance. ACCF/SCCT/ACR/AHA/ASE/ASNC/NASCI/SCAI/SCMR 2010 appropriate use criteria for cardiac computed tomography. A report of the American College of Cardiology Foundation Appropriate Use Criteria Task Force, the Society of Cardiovascular Computed Tomography, the American College of Radiology, the American Heart Association, the American Society of Echocardiography, the American Society of Nuclear Cardiology, the North American Society for Cardiovascular Imaging, the Society for Cardiovascular Angiography and Interventions, and the Society for Cardiovascular Magnetic Resonance, *Circulation* 122:e525–555, 2010.
37. Seneviratne SK, et al.: Incremental diagnostic value of regional left ventricular function over coronary assessment by cardiac computed tomography for the detection of acute coronary syndrome in patients with acute chest pain: From the ROMICAT trial, *Circ Cardiovasc Imaging* 3:375–383, 2010.
38. Bezerra HG, et al.: Incremental value of myocardial perfusion over regional left ventricular function and coronary stenosis by cardiac CT for the detection of acute coronary syndromes in high-risk patients: a subgroup analysis of the ROMICAT trial, *Journal of Cardiovascular Computed Tomography* 5:382–391, 2011.
39. Feuchtner GM, et al.: Evaluation of myocardial CT perfusion in patients presenting with acute chest pain to the emergency department: comparison with SPECT-myocardial perfusion imaging, *Heart (British Cardiac Society)* 98:1510–1517, 2012.
40. Puchner SB, et al.: High-risk plaque detected on coronary CT angiography predicts acute coronary syndromes independent of significant stenosis in acute chest pain: results from the ROMICAT-II trial, *J Am Coll Cardiol* 64:684–692, 2014.
41. Pflederer T, et al.: Characterization of culprit lesions in acute coronary syndromes using coronary dual-source CT angiography, *Atherosclerosis* 211:437–444, 2010.
42. Ferencik M, et al.: A computed tomography-based coronary lesion score to predict acute coronary syndrome among patients with acute chest pain and significant coronary stenosis on coronary computed tomographic angiogram, *Am J Cardiol* 110:183–189, 2012.
43. Norgaard BL, et al.: Group NXTTS. Diagnostic performance of noninvasive fractional flow reserve derived from coronary computed tomography angiography in suspected coronary artery disease: The NXT trial (Analysis of Coronary Blood Flow Using CT Angiography: Next Steps), *J Am Coll Cardiol* 63:1145–1155, 2014.
44. Min JK, et al.: Diagnostic accuracy of fractional flow reserve from anatomic CT angiography, *JAMA* 308:1237–1245, 2012.
45. Pattanayak P, Bleumke DA: Tissue characterization of the myocardium: state of the art characterization by magnetic resonance and computed tomography imaging, *Radiol Clin North Am* 53:413–423, 2015.
46. Schepis T, et al.: Prevalence of first-pass myocardial perfusion defects detected by contrast-enhanced dual-source CT in patients with non-ST segment elevation acute coronary syndromes, *Eur Radiol* 20:1607–1614, 2010.
47. Pursnani A, et al.: Early resting myocardial computed tomography perfusion for the detection of acute coronary syndrome in patients with coronary artery disease, *Circulation. Cardiovascular Imaging* 8, 2015. e002404.
48. Taylor CA, Fonte TA, Min JK: Computational fluid dynamics applied to cardiac computed tomography for noninvasive quantification of fractional flow reserve: scientific basis, *J Am Coll Cardiol* 61:2233–2241, 2013.
49. Coenen A, et al.: Fractional flow reserve computed from noninvasive CT angiography data: diagnostic performance of an on-site clinician-operated computational fluid dynamics algorithm, *Radiology* 274:674–683, 2015.
50. Pursnani A, et al.: Use of coronary artery calcium scanning beyond coronary computed tomographic angiography in the emergency department evaluation for acute chest pain: The ROMICAT II trial, *Circ Cardiovasc Imaging* 8, 2015. pii: e002225.
51. Maurovich-Horvat P, et al.: Comprehensive plaque assessment by coronary CT angiography, *Nat Rev Cardiol* 11:390–402, 2014.
52. Reichlin T, et al.: Early diagnosis of myocardial infarction with sensitive cardiac troponin assays, *N Engl J Med* 361:858–867, 2009.
53. Januzzi Jr JL, et al.: High-sensitivity troponin t concentrations in acute chest pain patients evaluated with cardiac computed tomography, *Circulation* 121:1227–1234, 2010.
54. Ahmed W, et al.: Single resting hsTNT level predicts abnormal myocardial stress test in acute chest pain patients with normal initial standard troponin, *J Am Coll Cardiol* 6:72–82, 2013.
55. Heydari B, Jerosch-Herold M, Kwong RY: Assessment of myocardial ischemia with cardiovascular magnetic resonance, *Prog Cardiovasc Dis* 54:191–203, 2011.
56. Kwong RY, et al.: Detecting acute coronary syndrome in the emergency department with cardiac magnetic resonance imaging, *Circulation* 107:531–537, 2003.
57. Cury RC, et al.: Cardiac magnetic resonance with t2-weighted imaging improves detection of patients with acute coronary syndrome in the emergency department, *Circulation* 118:837–844, 2008.
58. Miller CD, et al.: Stress CMR imaging observation unit in the emergency department reduces 1-year medical care costs in patients with acute chest pain: a randomized study for comparison with inpatient care, *J Am Coll Cardiol* 4:862–870, 2011.
59. Miller CD, et al.: Stress cardiac magnetic resonance imaging with observation unit care reduces cost for patients with emergent chest pain: a randomized trial, *Ann Emerg Med* 56:209–219, 2010. e202.
60. Miller CD, et al.: Provider-directed imaging stress testing reduces health care expenditures in lower-risk chest pain patients presenting to the emergency department, *Circ Cardiovasc Imaging* 5:111–118, 2012.
61. Duvall WL, et al.: A comparison of coronary CTa and stress testing using high-efficiency SPECT MPI for the evaluation of chest pain in the emergency department, *J Nucl Cardiol* 21:305–318, 2014.
62. Duvall WL, et al.: Stress-only Tc-99m myocardial perfusion imaging in an emergency department chest pain unit, *J Emerg Med* 42:642–650, 2012.
63. Yoshinaga K, et al.: Ischaemic memory imaging using metabolic radiopharmaceuticals: Overview of clinical settings and ongoing investigations, *Eur J Nucl Med Mol* 41:384–393, 2014.
64. Achenbach S, et al.: Coronary computed tomography angiography with a consistent dose below 1 msv using prospectively electrocardiogram-triggered high-pitch spiral acquisition, *Eur Heart J* 31:340–346, 2010.

10 Optical Coherence Tomography and Other Emerging Diagnostic Procedures for Vulnerable Plaque

Ik-Kyung Jang and Daniel S. Ong

INTRODUCTION

Outcomes after percutaneous coronary intervention (PCI) have improved significantly over the past few decades, in large part because of newer stent platforms, better implantation techniques, and improved adjunctive medical therapy. However, the risk of recurrent cardiac events after successful PCI remains high, and the culprit site for these events often differs from that of the index procedure.[1,2] Traditional clinical risk models, such as the Framingham risk score, are useful for predicting overall risk of atherosclerosis and coronary events. However, clinical risk indicators do not provide anatomic information, and angiographic parameters have poor predictive accuracy in identifying the specific high-risk lesions responsible for future coronary events.[3,4] Early angiographic studies suggested that the culprit lesions for these recurrent events were often only mildly stenotic at the time of index angiography, whereas pathological studies of patients with fatal cardiac events found that most acute occlusive thromboses occurred at sites with a large plaque burden and severe luminal narrowing.[5] Therefore, a significant amount of research has been devoted to exploring the risk factors for individual plaque progression and thrombosis. In this chapter, we explore the concept of plaque vulnerability as introduced by pathological studies (see Chapter 3), and the contribution of intravascular imaging, in particular, optical coherence tomography (OCT), toward extending our understanding of vulnerable plaques and facilitating their identification in vivo. The use of cardiac computed tomography and magnetic resonance imaging to characterize plaque composition in large arteries is discussed in Chapter 9 and Chapter 33. Molecular imaging applications are addressed in Chapter 32.

DEFINITION OF VULNERABLE PLAQUE

Vulnerable plaques have been defined as those at high risk for evolving into culprit lesions, including both plaques that are prone to provoking thrombosis and plaques at risk for rapid progression.[6] The framework for studying vulnerable plaque features was established by data from autopsy studies that examined the culprit lesions of patients with sudden coronary death (see also Chapter 3). These studies revealed three main patterns observed in thrombotic culprit lesions: plaque rupture, plaque erosion, and calcified nodules. Ruptured plaques are the most common, accounting for approximately 60% of cases, and are characterized by fibrous cap disruption with overlying thrombus that is in continuity with an underlying necrotic core. In contrast, eroded plaques are found in approximately 35% of cases and are characterized pathologically by coronary thrombus with an intact fibrous cap. The endothelial lining is commonly absent, exposing the intima, which is primarily composed of smooth muscle cells and proteoglycan. Calcified nodules include approximately 5% of cases and are identified pathologically by fibrous cap disruption and thrombus overlying a fractured calcified plate.[7]

Pathological studies are limited to the retrospective identification of features prevalent in culprit plaques, which are assumed to contribute to plaque vulnerability. However, the introduction and development of intravascular imaging modalities has enabled the study of these same features in vivo and prospectively, and multiple studies have sought to validate and extend the vulnerable plaque hypotheses generated by pathological studies. Although each of the intravascular imaging modalities has unique advantages and disadvantages, they can be broadly grouped into modalities that provide primarily anatomic or compositional information, such as OCT, intravascular ultrasound (IVUS), near-infrared spectroscopy (NIRS), and intravascular magnetic resonance imaging (IV-MRI), and modalities that provide functional or biomechanical information, such as thermography, elastography and/or palpography, and near-infrared fluorescence (NIRF) imaging. In addition, some modalities that provide primarily anatomic information may also indirectly facilitate functional assessment; for example, the identification of macrophages may serve as a marker of local inflammation. However, none of these imaging modalities independently provides physiologic information on coronary hemodynamics, which is better evaluated with techniques such as fractional flow reserve (see Chapter 17).

INTRAVASCULAR ASSESSMENT OF CORONARY PLAQUE ANATOMY OR COMPOSITION

Optical Coherence Tomography

OCT is a high-resolution intravascular imaging modality that enables the detailed characterization of plaque morphology in vivo.[8] In a manner analogous to the use of sound waves in ultrasonography, OCT technology measures the magnitude and time delay of backscattered light waves to produce images resembling an "optical biopsy," with 15- to 20-μm resolution. This represents a 10-fold improvement in resolution compared with IVUS and has allowed for the in vivo differentiation of fibrous, lipid, and calcific plaques (Figure 10-1). In addition, OCT can be used in the detection of intraluminal thrombus and the identification of plaque rupture, plaque erosion, and calcified nodules (Figure 10-2). The OCT definitions for these thrombosis mechanisms are based on the pathological definitions, with slight modifications to account for the possibility that luminal thrombus may dissolve or embolize distally, precluding its identification on in vivo imaging. Plaque rupture is identified on OCT imaging as lipid plaque with fibrous cap discontinuity and cavity formation inside the plaque. Because the coronary endothelial lining remains below the resolution of OCT imaging, OCT-defined plaque erosion is confirmed by the presence of attached thrombus overlying an intact and visualized plaque. Probable plaque erosion is identified by attached thrombus in the absence of underlying plaque or neighboring superficial lipid or calcium, or if there is culprit site luminal irregularity without an attached thrombus. Calcified nodules appear on OCT imaging as sites with fibrous cap disruption and underlying plaque characterized by protruding calcification, superficial calcium, and significant calcium adjacent to the lesion.[9]

The high resolution of OCT imaging has enabled the identification of many features suggested by pathological studies to be associated with plaque vulnerability. Because of the high prevalence of plaque rupture as the underlying mechanism for coronary thrombus formation, the features and risk factors associated with plaque vulnerability for rupture are the most commonly studied, and therefore, are the best understood. These features include large extracellular lipid pools, thin fibrous caps, small calcifications, macrophage accumulation, microchannels, and cholesterol crystals (Figure 10-3). However, these characteristics may differ from the features and risk factors associated with plaque erosion and calcified nodules.

Extracellular Lipid Pools

Autopsy studies have identified large lipid cores as a common feature of culprit plaques in patients with sudden coronary death. On OCT imaging, lipid appears as a homogeneous area with low-signal intensity (dark) and high-signal attenuation (significant shadowing) in contrast to fibrous tissue that appears as a homogeneous area with high-signal intensity (bright) and low-signal attenuation (no significant shadowing). Lipid-rich plaques are defined as those with a lipid arc of more than 90 degrees on cross-sectional imaging (see Figure 10-3A). OCT studies have shown that lipid-rich plaques are more prevalent in the culprit lesions of patients with acute unstable presentations such as ST-elevation myocardial infarction (STEMI) or non–ST-elevation MI (NSTEMI) compared with those presenting with stable angina pectoris (SAP).[10] Furthermore, lipid pools are associated with plaque progression. In a study of 53 patients with 69 nonculprit plaques (<50% luminal stenosis on angiography), OCT-identified lipid pools were significantly more prevalent in lesions that progressed on angiographic follow-up performed between 6 and 9 months later compared with lesions that did not progress (100% vs. 61%; $P = .02$).[11]

Thin-Cap Fibroatheroma

Thin-cap fibroatheroma (TCFA) are postulated to represent the vulnerable precursor lesion for plaque rupture because of their morphological similarity (see also Chapter 3). On pathological examination, most ruptured coronary plaques have fibrous caps measuring less than 65 μm, and therefore, this threshold has been used to define thick- versus thin-cap fibroatheroma. The sharp contrast in appearance between lipid and fibrous tissue on OCT imaging, coupled with its high resolution, make it an ideal intravascular imaging modality for measuring fibrous cap thickness, thereby identifying TCFA (see Figure 10-3B). Multiple OCT studies have shown a higher prevalence of TCFA at culprit sites in patients with acute or unstable clinical presentations compared with those with SAP.[12] Initially, nonculprit plaques with TCFA are more likely to show progression on angiographic follow-up than those without TCFA.[11] Moreover, statin therapy has been shown to increase fibrous cap thickness, suggesting that one of the mechanisms underlying the clinical benefit of statins is the stabilization of vulnerable TCFA plaques (Figure 10-4).[13,14]

Calcifications

Coronary artery calcium score, as assessed using cardiac computed tomography, has been shown to correlate with total atherosclerotic burden and risk for future events.[15] However, biomechanical models and pathological studies suggest that the pattern of vascular calcification may be a more important determinant of local plaque vulnerability than the total burden of calcium.[16] On OCT imaging, calcium deposits appear as heterogeneous areas of high- and low-signal intensity with low-signal attenuation and a sharp demarcating border. Spotty calcium deposits are defined as small calcifications with an arc ≤90 degrees on cross-sectional imaging (see Figure 10-3C). In contrast to ultrasound signals, which are highly attenuated by calcium, the light waves used in OCT imaging are able to penetrate calcium, thereby allowing for more detailed characterization of calcium deposits and better visualization of structures deep to those deposits than is possible with IVUS. In a study of 189 patients with coronary artery disease who underwent OCT imaging of culprit lesions, the number of spotty calcium deposits was significantly greater in patients presenting with acute MI and unstable angina (UA) compared with those presenting with SAP. In addition, these calcium deposits were more superficial in location in the MI and UA groups than in the SAP groups. Although all imaged lesions in this study were culprit lesions, plaque rupture as an underlying mechanism correlated positively with the number of spotty calcium deposits and inversely with the number of large calcium deposits.[17] Taken together, these results support the mechanistic hypothesis that small calcifications can increase plaque vulnerability for rupture.[18]

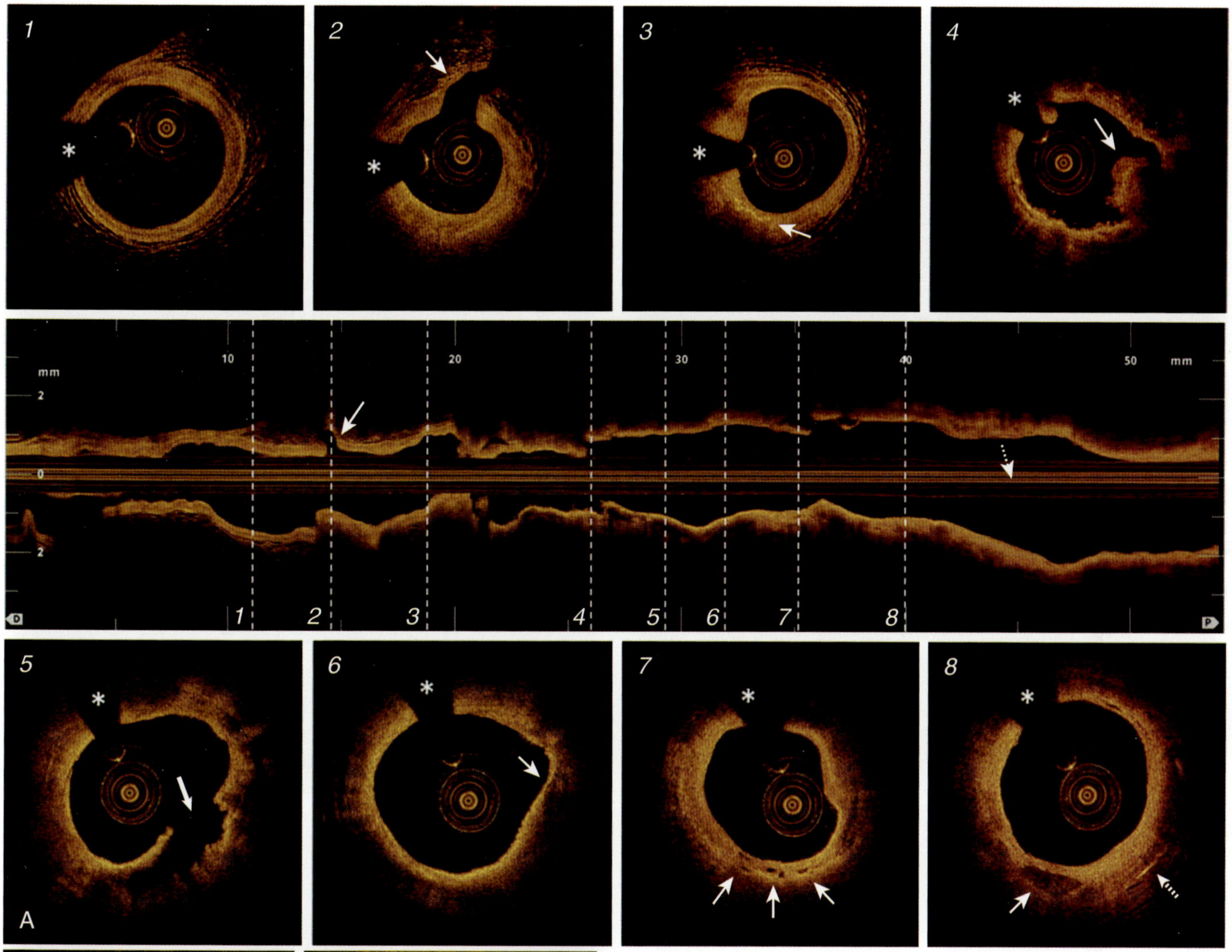

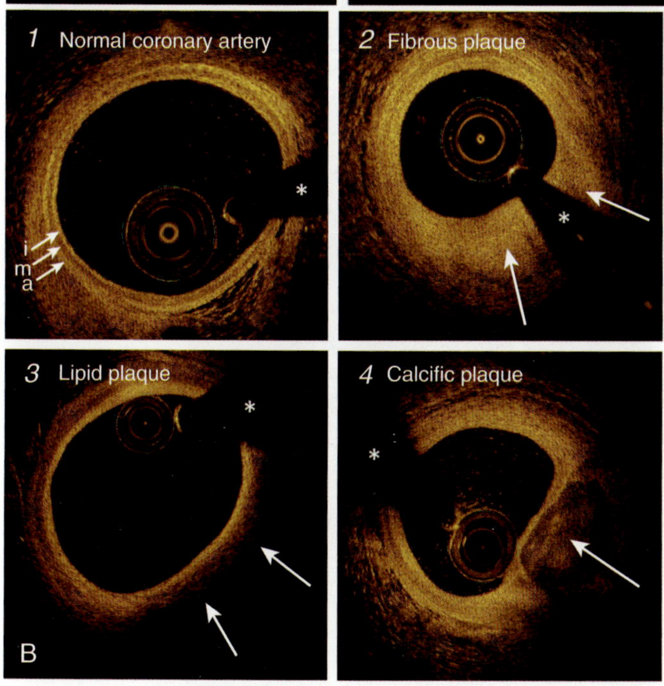

FIGURE 10-1 (A) An 80-year-old woman presented with ST-elevation myocardial infarction and, after undergoing thrombectomy, underwent optical coherence tomography imaging of the culprit left circumflex artery. The longitudinal view (*middle panel*) depicts pull-back imaging of a 54-mm segment of the vessel, with the distal vessel oriented toward the left and the proximal vessel oriented toward the right. The OCT catheter itself (*dotted arrow in middle panel*) runs across the center of the longitudinal image. Cross-sectional images (1 to 8) correspond to different points along the longitudinal view (*horizontal dotted lines*). The *asterisks* in each cross-sectional image denote guidewire shadow artifact. The most distal cross-section (*1*) shows the three-layered structure of a normal coronary artery segment. A small side branch can be seen on both cross-sectional imaging (*arrow in 2*) and on the longitudinal view (*arrow in middle panel*). Cross-sectional images reveal a ruptured plaque with fibrous cap disruption and cavity formation (*arrow in 5*) and multiple features associated with plaque vulnerability, including macrophage accumulation (*arrow in 3*), intracoronary thrombus (*arrow in 4*), lipid-rich plaque with a thin fibrous cap (*arrow in 6*), microchannels (*arrows in 7*), spotty calcium (*arrow in 8*), and cholesterol crystals (*dotted arrow in 8*). **(B)** Plaque characterization using optical coherence tomography. (*1*) Cross-sectional optical coherence tomography image of a normal coronary artery with a three-layered structure, corresponding to the intima (i), media (m), and adventitia (a). (*2*) Fibrous tissue (*arrows*) appears as a homogenous area with high-signal intensity and low-signal attenuation. (*3*) Lipid (*arrows*) appears as a homogenous area with low-signal intensity and high-signal attenuation. (*4*) Calcium (*arrow*) appears as a heterogeneous area of high- and low-signal intensity with low-signal attenuation and a sharp demarcating border. The *asterisks* denote guidewire shadow artifact.

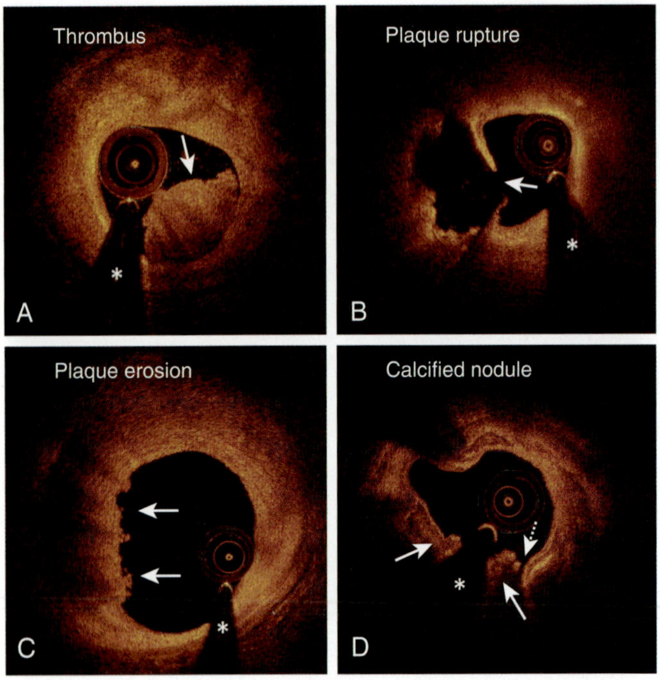

FIGURE 10-2 Acute coronary syndrome assessment using optical coherence tomography. (**A**) Thrombus (*arrow*) is identified as a protruding mass attached to the arterial wall. (**B**) Plaque rupture is identified as lipid plaque with fibrous cap discontinuity (*arrow*) and cavity formation inside the plaque. (**C**) Plaque erosion is confirmed by the presence of attached thrombus (*arrows*) overlying an intact and visualized plaque. (**D**) Calcified nodule appears on optical coherence tomography as a site with fibrous cap disruption (*dotted arrow*) and underlying plaque characterized by protruding calcification, superficial calcium, and significant calcium adjacent to the lesion (*arrows*). The *asterisks* denote guidewire shadow artifact. *(Adapted from Jia H, Abtahian F, Aguirre AD, et al: In vivo diagnosis of plaque erosion and calcified nodule in patients with acute coronary syndrome by intravascular optical coherence tomography.* J Am Coll Cardiol *62:1748–1758,2013.)*

Macrophages/Bright Spots

Inflammation plays an important role in the development of atherosclerosis. Pathological studies suggest that macrophages can also promote plaque vulnerability, because lipid-laden macrophages have been shown to constitutively produce extracellular matrix–degrading enzymes (see Chapter 3).[19] Macrophage accumulations have been identified on OCT imaging as a linear series of signal-rich (bright) spots with high-signal attenuation (see Figure 10-3D). The original technique used to objectively identify macrophages on OCT images, termed "normalized standard deviation," has recently been called into question because of methodological problems.[20] In response, a new algorithm has been developed to more objectively identify bright spots within an OCT image, correcting for differences in signal intensity caused by tissue depth, distance from the catheter, and signal-to-noise ratio. In a pathological validation study, OCT bright spots identified using this algorithm were poorly specific for macrophages, which were present in only 57% of bright spot–positive regions. Instead, OCT bright spots were correlated with the interface of plaque components with different optical indexes of refraction, including not only macrophages, but also cholesterol clefts in necrotic cores and the interfaces between old and new fibrous tissue, calcium and lipid or fibrous tissue, fibrous cap and lipid pools, or neovascularization and the media. In addition, not all macrophage accumulations identified histologically were visible on OCT imaging as bright spots, which may relate to differences in the backscattering properties of the different types of macrophages present (for example, M1 vs. M2 macrophages). Therefore, OCT bright spot density may be more reflective of plaque complexity than specific macrophage accumulation.[21]

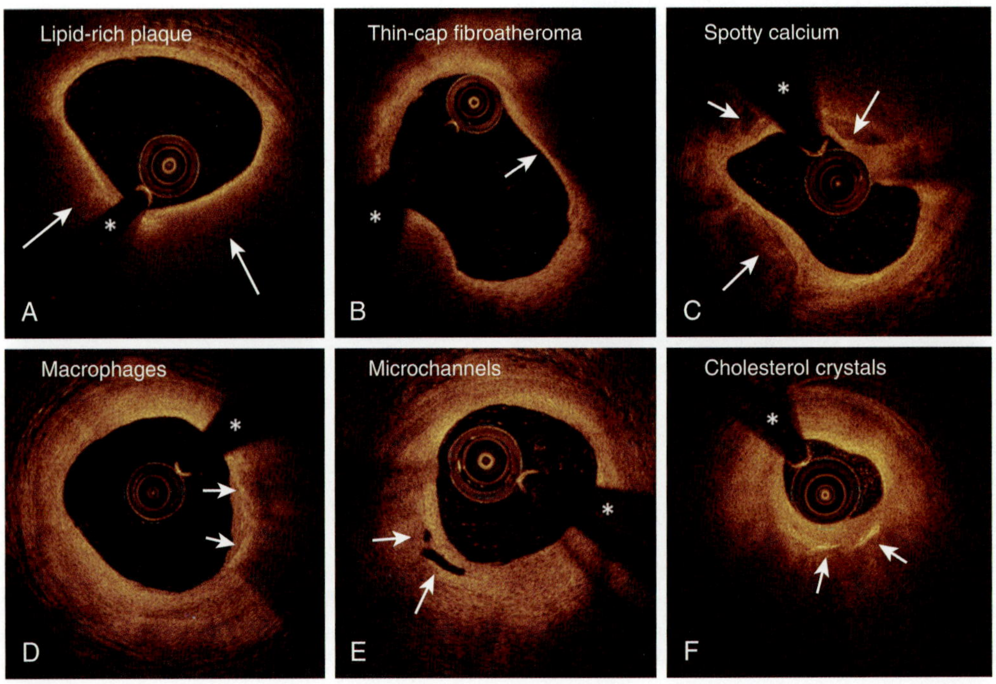

FIGURE 10-3 Vulnerable plaque features identified using optical coherence tomography. (**A**) Lipid-rich plaques are defined as those with a lipid arc of more than 90 degrees (*arrows*). (**B**) Thin-cap fibroatheroma are identified as lipid-rich plaque with an overlying fibrous cap measuring less than 65 μm (*arrow*). (**C**) Spotty calcium deposits are defined as small calcifications with an arc ≤90 degrees (*arrows*). (**D**) Macrophages and/or bright spots appear as a linear series of signal-rich (bright) spots with high-signal attenuation (*arrows*). (**E**) Microchannels and/or neovascularization are identified as small black holes or tubes (*arrows*) measuring 50 to 300 μm in diameter and spanning at least three consecutive cross-sectional frames on pull-back imaging. (**F**) Cholesterol crystals appear as thin, linear, signal-rich structures with low-signal attenuation (*arrows*). The *asterisks* denote guidewire shadow artifact.

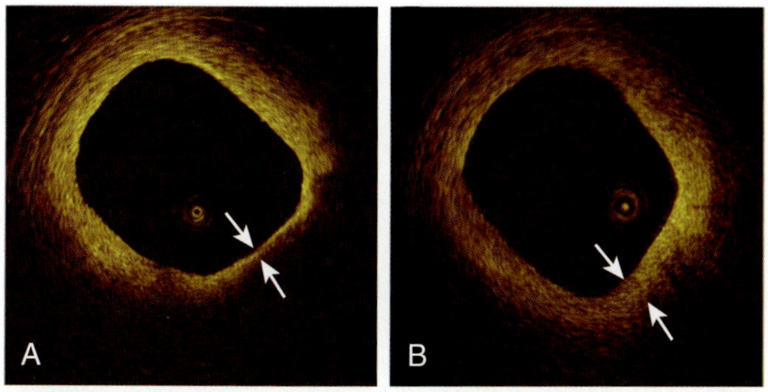

FIGURE 10-4 Matching optical coherence tomography cross-sections of a lipid-rich plaque at (**A**) baseline and (**B**) 12-month follow-up in a patient receiving 20 mg/day of atorvastatin, showing thickening of the fibrous cap (*arrows*). *(From Komukai K, Kubo T, Kitabata H, et al: Effect of atorvastatin therapy on fibrous cap thickness in coronary atherosclerotic plaque as assessed by optical coherence tomography: the EASY-FIT study.* J Am Coll Cardiol *64:2207–2217,2014.)*

Microchannels/Neovascularization

Mechanistically, the development of microchannels (neovascularization) within a plaque is believed to facilitate inflammatory cell infiltration and necrotic core formation. These factors, along with a greater risk of intraplaque hemorrhage, may contribute to more rapid plaque progression. On OCT imaging, microchannels are identified as small black holes or tubes measuring 50 to 300 μm in diameter and spanning at least three consecutive cross-sectional frames on pullback imaging (see Figure 10-3E). In one study (n = 53), OCT-identified microchannels were more prevalent in nonculprit plaques that showed progression on follow-up angiography than those without progression (77% vs. 14%; $P < .01$).[11] In another OCT study, among culprit lesions in patients with UA, plaques with microchannels had significantly thinner fibrous caps, greater lipid arcs, longer lipid lengths, and a greater prevalence of TCFA than those without microchannels.[22] Plaques with microchannels have been shown to respond less favorably to statin therapy in terms of fibrous cap thickening compared with plaques without microchannels, despite comparable reductions in serum cholesterol levels.[23] Moreover, OCT-identified microchannels have also been associated with coronary endothelial dysfunction. In a study of patients (n = 40) with early coronary artery disease, endothelial function testing with acetylcholine revealed significantly worse function in segments with microchannels compared with segments without microchannels. In addition, the segments with both OCT-identified microchannels and macrophage accumulation had even more severe endothelial dysfunction, compared with segments with only microchannels or only macrophage accumulation. The authors speculated that there was an incremental effect of inflammation and intimal neovascularization on atherogenesis, in which intimal neovascularization increased vascular wall blood flow and facilitated the penetration of inflammatory cells into the developing plaque, and activated macrophages to promote further angiogenesis and additional macrophage recruitment.[24]

Cholesterol Crystals

Cholesterol crystal content has been shown in pathological studies to be an independent predictor of thrombus formation and clinical events. Volume expansion during cholesterol crystallization is hypothesized to cause disruption and perforation of neighboring fibrous tissue, thereby contributing to plaque vulnerability for rupture.[25] On OCT imaging, cholesterol crystals appear as thin, linear, signal-rich structures with low-signal attenuation (see Figure 10-3F). Although few OCT studies have directly investigated the potential role of cholesterol crystals in plaque vulnerability, the presence of OCT-identified cholesterol crystals has been associated with a greater prevalence of other vulnerable plaque features, including lipid-rich plaque, spotty calcifications, and microchannels.[26]

Limitations of Optical Coherence Tomography

One of the limitations of OCT imaging is the need to image through a blood-free field, which is achieved by flushing the vessel with Ringer lactate, saline, or contrast during pullback imaging. Although improvements in image acquisition speed have eliminated the need for proximal balloon occlusion during this process, it nonetheless remains difficult to evaluate ostial lesions using OCT because of image artifacts created by residual blood in the ostial vessel lumen. In addition, the tissue penetration depth of OCT imaging is limited to approximately 3 mm, compared with the 8- to 10-mm depth of IVUS imaging. Penetration depth is important for the evaluation of plaque burden and arterial remodeling, because these parameters require measurement of the vessel area delineated by the external elastic membrane (see Chapter 3). Plaque area is calculated as the difference between vessel and lumen areas, and plaque burden is calculated as the proportion of vessel area composed of plaque. In addition, the direction and degree of arterial remodeling is determined by comparing the area bounded by the external elastic membrane at the culprit site with that of reference vessel segments. Because of the limited penetration of the OCT signal and its attenuation by lipid, OCT has not previously been used to assess plaque burden or remodeling. However, a recent study has explored the feasibility of measuring vessel area using OCT imaging of eccentric lipid-rich plaques by using the portion of the vessel circumference that is visible to extrapolate the remaining vessel contour that is not clearly identified because of excessive depth or shadowing by overlying lipid.[27]

Intravascular Ultrasonography

IVUS is an older, and therefore, a more extensively studied and widely available catheter-based imaging modality than OCT. Although IVUS produces images with significantly lower resolution compared with OCT, it does not require clearance of blood from the lumen and can therefore be used to evaluate ostial coronary segments. In addition, IVUS remains the most robust intravascular imaging modality for the assessment of plaque burden and arterial remodeling.

On gray-scale IVUS, echolucent plaque regions have been correlated with the presence of a lipid-rich core, and the combination of echolucency and high-signal attenuation in the absence of bright calcium has been defined as "attenuated plaque." In addition to positive remodeling, the presence of attenuated plaque is associated with increased plaque vulnerability.[28–30] Moreover, calcifications are readily identified on IVUS imaging as bright, signal-rich structures with high-signal attenuation, and the presence of small "spotty calcium" deposits have been more frequently identified in patients with unstable coronary presentations compared with those with SAP.[28]

The spatial resolution of gray-scale IVUS imaging is 100 to 200 μm, which is insufficient for the evaluation of TCFA,

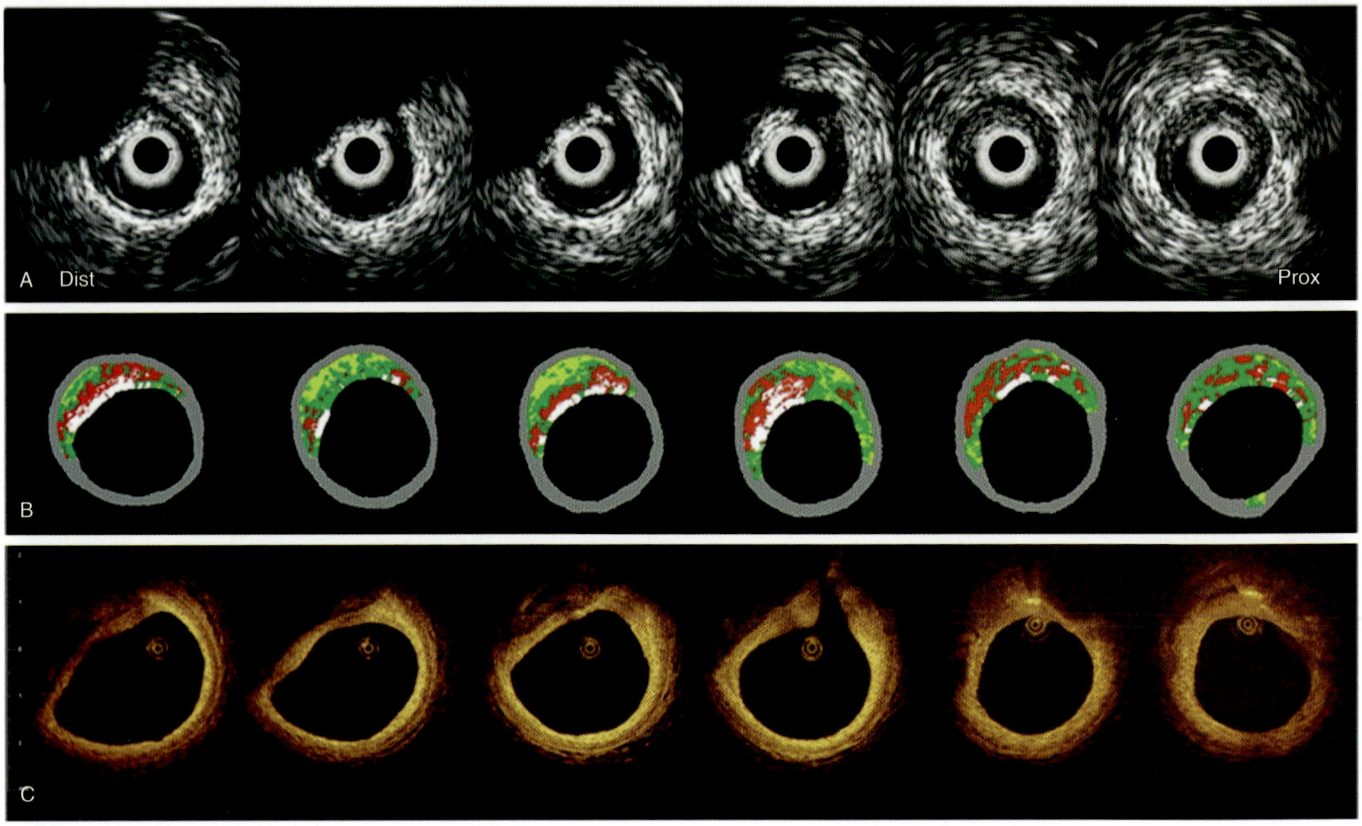

FIGURE 10-5 Matching cross sections of a calcific plaque, imaged using (**A**) gray-scale intravascular ultrasonography, (**B**) virtual histology intravascular ultrasonography (VH-IVUS), and (**C**) optical coherence tomography. VH-IVUS imaging depicts fibrous tissue as *green*, fibrofatty tissue as *light green*, necrotic core as *red*, and dense calcium as *white*. *Dist*, Distal cross sections; *Prox*, proximal cross sections. *(From Gonzalo N, Serruys PW, Barlis P, et al: Multi-modality intra-coronary plaque characterization: a pilot study.* Int J Cardiol *138:32–39,2010.)*

macrophages, microchannels, or cholesterol crystals. To facilitate more detailed plaque assessment, algorithms have been developed to perform spectral analysis of the raw IVUS radiofrequency backscatter signal, transforming this information into a color-coded representation of plaque composition. The most widely used method is virtual histology (VH)-IVUS, which depicts fibrous tissue as green, fibrofatty tissue as light green, the necrotic core as red, and dense calcium as white (Figure 10-5). VH-IVUS–identified TCFA have been defined as necrotic core-rich (≥10%) plaques, without evident overlying fibrous tissue, and with plaque volume ≥40% seen on at least three consecutive frames.[31]

In the landmark PROSPECT study, 697 patients with acute coronary syndrome (ACS) underwent three-vessel coronary angiography, gray-scale IVUS, and VH-IVUS imaging after PCI. Subsequent major adverse cardiac events (MACEs) were recorded over a median follow-up of 3.4 years, and these events were adjudicated as related to either the originally treated culprit lesion or an untreated nonculprit lesion. The 3-year cumulative rate of MACEs was 20.4%, with approximately one-half related to the initial culprit lesion and one-half related to an initially nonculprit lesion. Interestingly, no angiographic variables were strongly associated with subsequent events. Rather, the independent predictors of nonculprit lesion-related MACEs were the presence of TCFA by VH-IVUS, plaque burden ≥70%, and a minimum lumen area ≤4.0 mm^2 (Figure 10-6).[32] These findings were confirmed by the VIVA and ATHEROREMO-IVUS studies, which prospectively enrolled 170 and 581 patients, respectively, and included both ACS and SAP cases.[33,34]

IVUS has also been used to study the effects of statin therapy on plaque morphology and composition. Treatment with a high-intensity statin has been associated with plaque regression, as measured using serial gray-scale IVUS imaging as a decrease in percent atheroma volume, which is the proportion of vessel wall occupied by atherosclerotic plaque.[35] Moreover, high-intensity statin therapy has also been associated with an increase in plaque calcification over time, suggesting that statin-mediated plaque stabilization may also derive from the coalescence of spotty calcifications into larger calcifications that confer less vulnerability for plaque rupture.[36] Serial VH-IVUS imaging was performed in a subset of 71 patients with stable nonobstructive coronary disease enrolled in the SATURN trial, revealing that plaque regression with high-intensity statin therapy was associated with a decrease in fibrofatty tissue volume and an increase in dense calcium tissue volume.[37] In the IBIS-4 study of 103 patients with STEMI who were treated with a high-intensity statin, serial VH-IVUS imaging performed at baseline and 13 months of follow-up similarly showed an increase over time in the percent volume composed of dense calcium. However, no significant change was observed in the proportion of lipid-rich tissue components (fibrofatty or necrotic core) or the number of VH-IVUS–identified TCFA.[38]

Near-Infrared Spectroscopy

NIRS is an optical imaging modality that analyzes the absorbance spectra of a tissue sample to determine its chemical composition. For intracoronary imaging, it has been widely

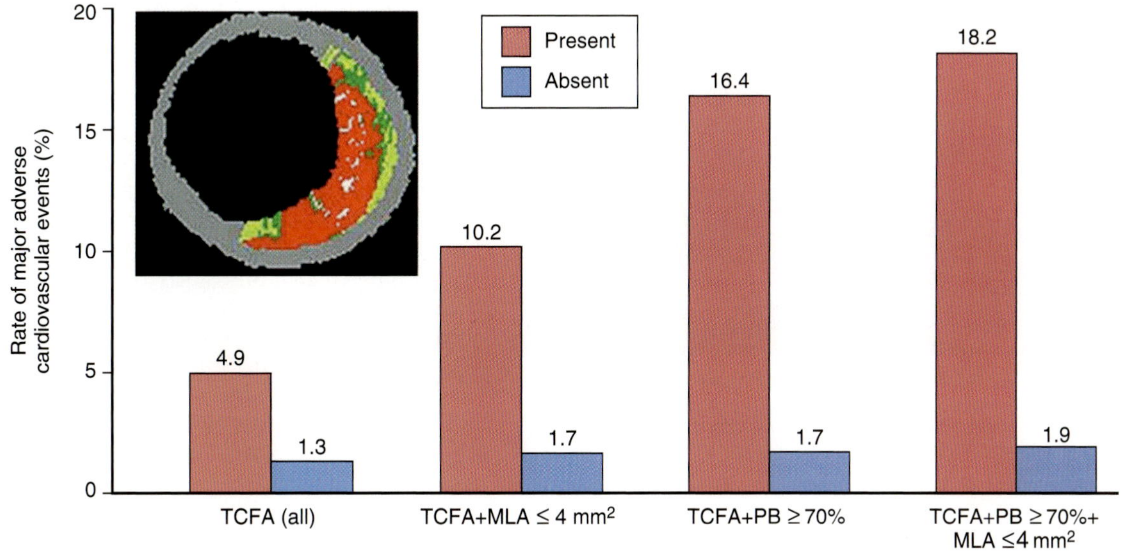

	TCFA (all)	TCFA+MLA ≤ 4 mm²	TCFA+PB ≥ 70%	TCFA+PB ≥ 70%+ MLA ≤4 mm²
Lesion hazard ratio (95% CI)	3.90 (2.25–6.76)	6.55 (3.43–12.51)	10.83 (5.55–21.10)	11.05 (4.39–27.82)
***P* value**	<0.001	<0.001	<0.001	<0.001
Prevalence (%)	46.7	15.9	10.1	4.2

FIGURE 10-6 In the PROSPECT study, the rate of major adverse cardiac events, at a median follow-up of 3.4 years, was higher for nonculprit lesions characterized by virtual histology intravascular ultrasonography (VH-IVUS) at baseline as thin-cap fibroatheromas (TCFA) compared with those that were not. In addition, even higher event rates were seen for TCFA with minimum luminal area (MLA) ≤4 mm², plaque burden (PB) ≥70%, or both, as characterized using gray-scale IVUS. The *inset* shows an example of a TCFA imaged by VH-IVUS. *CI*, Confidence interval. *(From Stone GW, Maehara A, Lansky AJ, et al: A prospective natural-history study of coronary atherosclerosis.* N Engl J Med *364:226–235,2011.)*

used to identify lipid core cholesterol, depicting its location and intensity in a "chemogram" and enabling the identification of lipid-rich plaques.[39] NIRS-identified, lipid-rich plaques have been shown to be more common in the culprit plaques of patients with ACS than in those with SAP.[40]

In the prospective ATHEROREMO-NIRS study, 203 patients who underwent coronary angiography for ACS or SAP had NIRS imaging performed in the proximal segment of a nonculprit coronary artery with more than 50% angiographic stenosis. A lipid core burden index (LCBI) score was calculated based on the fraction of pixels in the chemogram with a high probability for the presence of a lipid core, and the median LCBI score was used to categorize individual plaques into high versus low LCBI groups. Over 1 year of follow-up, the cumulative incidence of the primary endpoint (death, nonfatal ACS, stroke, and unplanned coronary revascularization, exclusive of events related to the culprit lesion at index angiography) was 10.4% in the entire study population and fourfold higher in the high LCBI group compared with the low LCBI group (16.7% vs. 4.0%; P = .003). LCBI, peripheral artery disease, and a history of stroke were the only predictors of the primary endpoint. Although this study supported a role for NIRS imaging in providing prognostic information, it is important to note its limitations with respect to the identification and characterization of the vulnerable plaque. NIRS imaging was performed only in the proximal segment of a single nonculprit vessel, and although the study was prospective, adverse events were not necessarily attributable to the imaged segment.[41]

NIRS imaging has also been used to evaluate statin therapy. In the prospective YELLOW trial, 87 patients with multivessel coronary artery disease, including at least one severely obstructive (fractional flow reserve ≤0.80) nonculprit lesion, were randomized to continuation of standard-of-care lipid-lowering therapy or intensive statin therapy with rosuvastatin 40 mg/day. Serial NIRS imaging was performed at baseline and after 7 weeks of therapy. The LCBI decreased significantly in the intensive statin therapy group, whereas there was no significant change in the standard therapy group. Although this pilot study suggests that intensive statin therapy can rapidly reduce the lipid content of obstructive lesions, no significant differences in clinical endpoints between the standard and intensive therapy groups could be detected because of the low number of adverse events and short follow-up period.[42]

Notable limitations to NIRS imaging include its exclusive evaluation of lipid content, the lack of a clear LCBI threshold that can be used to discriminate high- versus low-risk lesions, the lack of information on the depth of detected lipid, and the need for another imaging modality to provide complementary vascular structural information on which to superimpose the NIRS-derived chemogram (Figure 10-7). A combined NIRS-IVUS imaging system and catheter is already commercially available,[43] and a combined NIRS-OCT system is under development.[44]

Angioscopy

Coronary angioscopy uses a fiberoptic catheter and light source to facilitate direct visualization of the endoluminal surface color and morphology. Intraluminal thrombi and intimal disruption can be readily assessed, and neointimal strut coverage can be evaluated in stented coronary segments. Angioscopy has been studied for its potential usefulness in identifying vulnerable plaques, because the color of the endoluminal surface overlying a plaque may provide indirect information on its composition. Studies have correlated yellow coloration with an underlying lipid pool covered by a thin fibrous cap and white coloration with fibrous plaques or a lipid pool covered by a thick fibrous cap.[45]

The major limitation to the use of angioscopy in the evaluation of plaque vulnerability is its restriction to

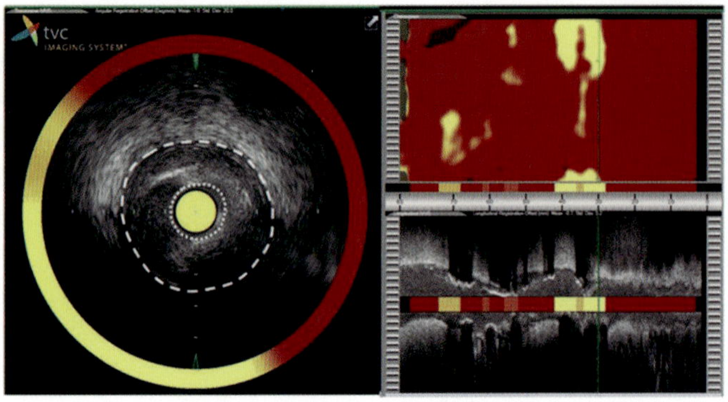

FIGURE 10-7 Near-infrared spectroscopy (NIRS) and intravascular ultrasonography (IVUS) images of the culprit lesion in a patient presenting with non–ST-elevation myocardial infarction. The longitudinal NIRS chemogram (*top right*) displays the lipid signal in *yellow* and can be superimposed onto the longitudinal IVUS image (*bottom right*), which provides complementary structural information. The *green vertical line* designates the lesion location along the artery that is depicted in the cross-sectional image (*left panel*), which reveals an IVUS-identified attenuated plaque between 3 and 10 o'clock with NIRS-identified lipid core plaque between 5 and 10 o'clock. The *dashed circle* demarcates the external elastic membrane, and the *dotted circle* demarcates the lumen–lesion interface. *(From Fenning RS, Wilensky RL: New insights into the vulnerable plaque from imaging studies.* Curr Atheroscler Rep *16:397, 2014.)*

surface morphology evaluation. Detailed plaque characterization or the assessment of plaque burden and arterial remodeling are not possible. Additional limitations to this technique include the need for proximal balloon occlusion to create a blood-free field and the subjective nature of plaque coloration grading, although continuous flush techniques that do not require proximal vessel occlusion and quantitative colorimetric methods have been proposed.[46]

Intravascular Magnetic Resonance Imaging

Conventional MRI could be a powerful tool in the evaluation of plaque vulnerability, because it enables detailed soft tissue characterization and may enable both anatomic and functional assessment. However, its usefulness for characterizing coronary plaques is significantly limited by cardiac and respiratory motion, as well as the deep location of arteries. Intravascular detector coils have been developed to improve the signal-to-noise ratio at the level of the coronary wall, thereby increasing spatial resolution. In preliminary studies using human autopsy samples and in vivo rabbit models, the combination of an external MRI scanner and intravascular MR detector enabled accurate measurement of vascular plaque fibrous cap thickness.[47] Limitations to this technique include the theoretical safety concern for local vascular heating with the use of intravascular detector coils and its impracticality for use during routine cardiac catheterization because of the need for an external MRI scanner.

A self-contained IV-MRI probe has been developed that integrates the magnets, detectors coils, and electronics into the tip of the catheter, which then does not require an external scanner. The self-diffusion of water molecules is analyzed in two separate zones (a superficial 100-μm zone and a deeper 100- to 250-μm zone) within a 60-degree sector of the arterial wall to determine the lipid fraction index (LFI) of each zone. Data acquisition takes 51 seconds for each sector, and the probe is manually rotated to interrogate additional sectors for more circumferential assessment. Lesions with increased lipid fraction in the superficial zone compared with the deeper zone have been correlated with TCFA.[48] The LFI can also be used to classify plaques as fibrous (<30% LFI), intermediate (31% to 55% LFI), or lipid-rich (>55% LFI). However, to eliminate motion artifacts and improve image resolution, the self-contained MRI probe must be stabilized against the arterial wall by inflating a partially occlusive balloon opposite the detector coil to oppose the probe over the arterial segment in question. This probe was tested in a first-in-man feasibility study of 28 patients, and 10 patients (36%) had transient electrocardiographic changes during side balloon inflation, although there were no MACEs over 30 days of follow-up.[49] Important limitations to the current technique include the potential for blind spots because of the imprecise nature of manual rotation of the probe and the limited 60-degree field of view analyzed during each interrogation.

INTRAVASCULAR ASSESSMENT OF FUNCTIONAL ACTIVITY OR BIOMECHANICS

Thermography

Inflammation plays a critical role in the development of atherosclerosis and the destabilization of coronary lesions. Intracoronary thermography was developed around the hypotheses that plaque temperature may serve as a marker for local inflammation and that the detection of thermal heterogeneity may therefore provide a functional assessment of plaque vulnerability. Studies have shown a correlation among measured temperature, macrophage density, and systemic inflammatory markers. In addition, in a study that explored the temperature difference between plaques and healthy vessel segments in individual patients, thermal heterogeneity was present in 67% of patients with acute MI, 40% of patients with unstable angina, and 20% of patients with SAP, in comparison with 0% of control subjects.[50]

Limitations to this technique include a significant overlap in the degree of thermal heterogeneity between patients with unstable versus stable presentations, making it difficult to identify a thermal parameter by which to identify vulnerable or "hot" plaques. In addition, because of the cooling effects of blood flow, perturbations to blood flow or pressure may confound thermal heterogeneity measurements in atherosclerotic vessels. Lastly, some temperature measuring techniques require direct contact between the thermal sensor and the vessel wall, introducing the potential risk of traumatizing a vulnerable rupture-prone plaque. Other temperature measuring techniques use infrared technology to measure temperature without contacting the vessel wall, although these systems measure the temperature of the blood within the lumen rather than the arterial plaque and/or wall itself.[50]

Elastography/Palpography

Plaque mechanics may be useful in the assessment of plaque vulnerability, because softer areas of tissue should deform to a greater degree in response to increased pressure than harder areas of tissue. Mechanical strain and local tissue deformation can be assessed by analyzing radiofrequency IVUS signals recorded at two different intraluminal

TABLE 10-1 Comparison of Intravascular Imaging Modalities for the Detection of Vulnerable Plaque Features

	THROMBUS	LIPID	FIBROUS CAP/TCFA	CALCIUM	MACROPHAGES/ INFLAMMATION	MICROCHANNELS/ NEOVASCULARIZATION	CHOLESTEROL CRYSTALS	PLAQUE BURDEN	ARTERIAL REMODELING	FUNCTIONAL DATA/ BIOMECHANICS
OCT	++	+++	+++	++	+	+	+	–	–	Indirect
GS-IVUS	+	+	–	+++	–	–	–	+++	+++	–
VH-IVUS	+	++	++	+++	–	–	–	+++	+++	–
NIRS	–	+++	–	–	–	–	–	–	–	–
Angioscopy	+++	++	+	–	–	–	–	–	–	–
IV-MRI	–	++	+	–	–	–	–	–	–	–
Thermography	–	–	–	–	+++	–	–	–	–	Direct
Elastography	–	–	–	–	–	–	–	–	–	Direct
NIRF	–	–	–	–	+++	–	–	–	–	Direct

GS-IVUS, Gray-scale intravascular ultrasonography; *IV-MRI*, intravascular magnetic resonance imaging; *NIRF*, near-infrared fluorescence; *NIRS*, near-infrared spectroscopy; *OCT*, optical coherence tomography; *TCFA*, thin-cap fibroatheroma; *VH-IVUS*, virtual histology intravascular ultrasonography.

pressures and using these data to derive strain maps for rupture-prone areas within a plaque (elastography) or at the luminal boundary (palpography).[51] Highly distensible plaques detected using this technique have been correlated with angioscopic yellow plaques, and a significantly higher prevalence of deformable plaques has been demonstrated in patients with unstable presentations compared with those with SAP.[52]

Near-Infrared Fluorescence

Intravascular NIRF is a novel technique that uses molecular imaging to assess specific molecular processes within a vessel. The functional assessment of inflammation, angiogenesis, and apoptosis holds significant promise in the identification and study of plaque vulnerability. Cysteine protease activity has been investigated as a measure of inflammation in rabbit models using an intravascular NIRF imaging catheter and a molecular agent that, when cleaved by cysteine proteases, generates fluorescence. Increased cysteine protease activity has been demonstrated in atherosclerosis and in the setting of vascular injury following stent implantation.[53] Importantly, NIRF imaging provides only functional information, which can only be localized when co-registered with complementary anatomic and/or structural information obtained with IVUS or OCT. Dual-modality NIRF-IVUS and NIRF-OCT have been developed and are under investigation.[54,55]

FUTURE POTENTIAL

The intravascular imaging modalities discussed in this chapter are unique in their ability to identify different features associated with plaque vulnerability (Table 10-1), and combination modality imaging catheters represent a promising area for future investigation and development. A combined OCT-IVUS imaging catheter has been tested in ex vivo coronary samples, capitalizing on the high resolution of OCT imaging and the deeper tissue penetration of IVUS imaging.[56] Because some intravascular imaging modalities provide anatomic and compositional information, whereas others provide information on plaque functional activity or biomechanics, hybrid catheters could integrate these potentially complementary imaging tools, facilitating the identification of vulnerable plaques with greater sensitivity and specificity.

Although stented coronary segments have not traditionally been included as potential vulnerable plaques, the mechanisms and risk factors underlying in-stent restenosis and stent thrombosis may be similar to those that drive rapid plaque progression and thrombosis in de novo coronary arteries. Intravascular imaging, and in particular, OCT, has been integral to the study of stents and their related complications, and many vulnerable plaque features have been identified in neoatherosclerotic lesions within coronary stents.[57]

Limitations to the Assessment of Plaque Vulnerability

Although intravascular imaging has significantly advanced our understanding of vulnerable plaques, the mechanisms underlying acute coronary events, and the effect of drug therapy on atherosclerotic disease, further research is needed before this information can be used in clinical decision-making. A significant limitation to the clinical applicability of these techniques is the high prevalence of intravascular imaging–detected vulnerable features or patterns in comparison to the timing and frequency of subsequent events. Clinically actionable parameters remain elusive, because only a fraction of identified vulnerable plaques will progress to form thrombus through rupture, erosion, or calcified nodules. Furthermore, those thrombotic events may be partially or fully occlusive, as well as symptomatic or clinically silent. An important concept in the study of individual plaque vulnerability is that it is not the only determinant of clinical events, because it does not account for patient or vessel vulnerability. For example, a vulnerable plaque may rupture, but the size and extent of the associated thrombus formation may be influenced by patient-related factors such as systemic inflammation and hypercoagulability. In addition, a small thrombus could be occlusive if the residual vessel lumen at the culprit site is highly stenotic or only partially occlusive, and possibly clinically silent if the culprit site lumen remains accommodatingly large.

The focus on individual lesion vulnerability has been criticized in favor of shifting our attention back to the assessment of the risk related to overall atherosclerotic burden.[58] The isolated assessment of local plaque vulnerability without consideration of the overall clinical context certainly runs the risk of "missing the forest for the trees." Therefore, future investigation should integrate the assessment of vulnerable plaque features by intravascular imaging with an assessment of vulnerable patient features, including clinical risk factors, systemic inflammation, and hypercoagulability. In addition, because of the invasive nature of intravascular imaging, its future clinical usefulness will require evidence from prospective natural history studies, without which it will be impossible to determine if pharmacologic- or device-based treatment of vulnerable plaques can improve clinical outcomes in a cost-effective manner.[59] For these reasons, at present, we do not use intravascular imaging for plaque vulnerability in our own clinical practice.

SUMMARY

Approximately one-half of recurrent events in patients with ACS are related to an initially nonculprit lesion. Intravascular imaging has advanced our understanding of the mechanisms underlying coronary events and the concept of the vulnerable plaque. The high resolution of OCT imaging make it a robust tool for identifying microscopic anatomic features associated with plaque vulnerability, although it has limited use in the assessment of plaque burden, arterial remodeling, and plaque functional activity or biomechanics. The presence of TCFA by VH-IVUS, plaque burden ≥70%, and a minimum lumen area ≤4.0 mm^2 assessed using gray-scale IVUS are independent predictors of future events related to initially nonculprit lesions. Hybrid imaging catheters are under development to take advantage of the complementary information provided by different intravascular imaging modalities, and there is a growing body of intravascular imaging data providing new insight into the development and associated risk of neoatherosclerotic lesions within stented coronary segments.

Classic References

Jang IK, Tearney GJ, MacNeill B, et al.: In vivo characterization of coronary atherosclerotic plaque by use of optical coherence tomography, *Circulation* 111(12):1551–1555, 2005.

Schaar JA, Muller JE, Falk E, et al.: Terminology for high-risk and vulnerable coronary artery plaques. Report of a meeting on the vulnerable plaque, June 17 and 18, 2003, Santorini, Greece, *Eur Heart J* 25:1077–1082, 2004.

Virmani R, Burke AP, Farb A, Kolodgie FD: Pathology of the vulnerable plaque, *J Am Coll Cardiol* 47(8 Suppl):C13–18, 2006.

Virmani R, Kolodgie FD, Burke AP, Farb A, Schwartz SM: Lessons from sudden coronary death: a comprehensive morphological classification scheme for atherosclerotic lesions, *Arterioscler Thromb Vasc Biol* 20(5):1262–1275, 2000.

References

1. Fleg JL, Stone GW, Fayad ZA, et al.: Detection of high-risk atherosclerotic plaque: report of the NHLBI Working Group on current status and future directions, *JACC Cardiovasc Imaging* 5(9):941–955, 2012.
2. Bortnick AE, Epps KC, Selzer F, et al.: Five-year follow-up of patients treated for coronary artery disease in the face of an increasing burden of co-morbidity and disease complexity (from the NHLBI Dynamic Registry), *Am J Cardiol* 113(4):573–579, 2014.
3. Bourantas CV, Garcia-Garcia HM, Farooq V, et al.: Clinical and angiographic characteristics of patients likely to have vulnerable plaques: analysis from the PROSPECT study, *JACC Cardiovasc Imaging* 6(12):1263–1272, 2013.
4. Chan KH, Ng MK: Is there a role for coronary angiography in the early detection of the vulnerable plaque? *Int J Cardiol* 164(3):262–266, 2013.
5. Fishbein MC: The vulnerable and unstable atherosclerotic plaque, *Cardiovasc Pathol* 19(1):6–11, 2010.
6. Naghavi M, Libby P, Falk E, et al.: From vulnerable plaque to vulnerable patient: a call for new definitions and risk assessment strategies: part I, *Circulation* 108(14):1664–1672, 2003.
7. Arbab-Zadeh A, Nakano M, Virmani R, Fuster V: Acute coronary events, *Circulation* 125(9):1147–1156, 2012.
8. Tearney GJ, Regar E, Akasaka T, et al.: Consensus standards for acquisition, measurement, and reporting of intravascular optical coherence tomography studies: a report from the International Working Group for Intravascular Optical Coherence Tomography Standardization and Validation, *J Am Coll Cardiol* 59(12):1058–1072, 2012.
9. Jia H, Abtahian F, Aguirre AD, et al.: In vivo diagnosis of plaque erosion and calcified nodule in patients with acute coronary syndrome by intravascular optical coherence tomography, *J Am Coll Cardiol* 62(19):1748–1758, 2013.
10. Abtahian F, Jang IK: Optical coherence tomography: basics, current application and future potential, *Curr Opin Pharmacol* 12(5):583–591, 2012.
11. Uemura S, Ishigami K, Soeda T, et al.: Thin-cap fibroatheroma and microchannel findings in optical coherence tomography correlate with subsequent progression of coronary atheromatous plaques, *Eur Heart J* 33(1):78–85, 2012.
12. Sinclair H, Bourantas C, Bagnall A, Mintz GS, Kunadian V: OCT for the identification of vulnerable plaque in acute coronary syndrome, *JACC Cardiovasc Imaging* 8(2):198–209, 2015.
13. Takarada S, Imanishi T, Kubo T, et al.: Effect of statin therapy on coronary fibrous-cap thickness in patients with acute coronary syndrome: assessment by optical coherence tomography study, *Atherosclerosis* 202(2):491–497, 2009.
14. Komukai K, Kubo T, Kitabata H, et al.: Effect of atorvastatin therapy on fibrous cap thickness in coronary atherosclerotic plaque as assessed by optical coherence tomography: the EASY-FIT study, *J Am Coll Cardiol* 64(21):2207–2217, 2014.
15. Alluri K, Joshi PH, Henry TS, Blumenthal RS, Nasir K, Blaha MJ: Scoring of coronary artery calcium scans: history, assumptions, current limitations, and future directions, *Atherosclerosis* 239(1):109–117, 2015.
16. Otsuka F, Sakakura K, Yahagi K, Joner M, Virmani R: Has our understanding of calcification in human coronary atherosclerosis progressed? *Arterioscler Thromb Vasc Biol* 34(4):724–736, 2014.
17. Mizukoshi M, Kubo T, Takarada S, et al.: Coronary superficial and spotty calcium deposits in culprit coronary lesions of acute coronary syndrome as determined by optical coherence tomography, *Am J Cardiol* 112(1):34–40, 2013.
18. Kelly-Arnold A, Maldonado N, Laudier D, Aikawa E, Cardoso L, Weinbaum S: Revised microcalcification hypothesis for fibrous cap rupture in human coronary arteries, *Proc Natl Acad Sci U S A* 110(26):10741–10746, 2013.
19. Medbury HJ, Williams H, Fletcher JP: Clinical significance of macrophage phenotypes in cardiovascular disease, *Clin Transl Med* 3(1):63, 2014.
20. Tearney GJ, Yabushita H, Houser SL, et al.: Quantification of macrophage content in atherosclerotic plaques by optical coherence tomography, *Circulation* 107(1):113–119, 2003.
21. Phipps JE, Vela D, Hoyt T, et al.: Macrophages and intravascular OCT bright spots: a quantitative study, *JACC Cardiovasc Imaging* 8(1):63–72, 2015.
22. Tian J, Hou J, Xing L, et al.: Significance of intraplaque neovascularisation for vulnerability: optical coherence tomography study, *Heart* 98(20):1504–1509, 2012.
23. Tian J, Hou J, Xing L, et al.: Does neovascularization predict response to statin therapy? Optical coherence tomography study, *Int J Cardiol* 158:469–470, 2012.
24. Choi BJ, Matsuo Y, Aoki T, et al.: Coronary endothelial dysfunction is associated with inflammation and vasa vasorum proliferation in patients with early atherosclerosis, *Arterioscler Thromb Vasc Biol* 34(11):2473–2477, 2014.
25. Abela GS, Aziz K, Vedre A, Pathak DR, Talbott JD, Dejong J: Effect of cholesterol crystals on plaques and intima in arteries of patients with acute coronary and cerebrovascular syndromes, *Am J Cardiol* 103(7):959–968, 2009.
26. Nakamura S, Inami S, Murai K, et al.: Relationship between cholesterol crystals and culprit lesion characteristics in patients with stable coronary artery disease: an optical coherence tomography study, *Clin Res Cardiol* 103:1015–1021, 2014.
27. Kubo T, Yamano T, Liu Y, et al.: Feasibility of optical coronary tomography in quantitative measurement of coronary arteries with lipid-rich plaque, *Circ J* 79(3):600–606, 2015.
28. Fujii K, Hao H, Ohyanagi M, Masuyama T: Intracoronary imaging for detecting vulnerable plaque, *Circ J* 77(3):588–595, 2013.
29. Hong YJ, Jeong MH, Choi YH, et al.: Positive remodeling is associated with vulnerable coronary plaque components regardless of clinical presentation: virtual histology-intravascular ultrasound analysis, *Int J Cardiol* 167(3):871–876, 2013.
30. Wu X, Maehara A, Mintz GS, et al.: Virtual histology intravascular ultrasound analysis of non-culprit attenuated plaques detected by grayscale intravascular ultrasound in patients with acute coronary syndromes, *Am J Cardiol* 105(1):48–53, 2010.
31. Kato K, Yasutake M, Yonetsu T, et al.: Intracoronary imaging modalities for vulnerable plaques, *J Nippon Med Sch* 78(6):340–351, 2011.
32. Stone GW, Maehara A, Lansky AJ, et al.: A prospective natural-history study of coronary atherosclerosis, *N Engl J Med* 364(3):226–235, 2011.
33. Calvert PA, Obaid DR, O'Sullivan M, et al.: Association between IVUS findings and adverse outcomes in patients with coronary artery disease: the VIVA (VH-IVUS in Vulnerable Atherosclerosis) Study, *JACC Cardiovasc Imaging* 4(8):894–901, 2011.
34. Cheng JM, Garcia-Garcia HM, de Boer SP, et al.: In vivo detection of high-risk coronary plaques by radiofrequency intravascular ultrasound and cardiovascular outcome: results of the ATHEROREMO-IVUS study, *Eur Heart J* 35(10):639–647, 2014.
35. Nicholls SJ, Ballantyne CM, Barter PJ, et al.: Effect of two intensive statin regimens on progression of coronary disease, *N Engl J Med* 365(22):2078–2087, 2011.
36. Puri R, Nicholls SJ, Shao M, et al.: Impact of statins on serial coronary calcification during atheroma progression and regression, *J Am Coll Cardiol* 65(13):1273–1282, 2015.
37. Puri R, Libby P, Nissen SE, et al.: Long-term effects of maximally intensive statin therapy on changes in coronary atheroma composition: insights from SATURN, *Eur Heart J Cardiovasc Imaging* 15(4):380–388, 2014.
38. Räber L, Taniwaki M, Zaugg S, et al.: Effect of high-intensity statin therapy on atherosclerosis in non-infarct-related coronary arteries (IBIS-4): a serial intravascular ultrasonography study, *Eur Heart J* 36(8):490–500, 2015.
39. Jaguszewski M, Klingenberg R, Landmesser U: Intracoronary near-infrared spectroscopy (NIRS) imaging for detection of lipid content of coronary plaques: current experience and future perspectives, *Curr Cardiovasc Imaging Rep* 6:426–430, 2013.
40. Madder RD, Smith JL, Dixon SR, Goldstein JA: Composition of target lesions by near-infrared spectroscopy in patients with acute coronary syndrome versus stable angina, *Circ Cardiovasc Interv* 5(1):55–61, 2012.
41. Oemrawsingh RM, Cheng JM, García-García HM, et al.: Near-infrared spectroscopy predicts cardiovascular outcome in patients with coronary artery disease, *J Am Coll Cardiol* 64(23):2510–2518, 2014.
42. Kini AS, Baber U, Kovacic JC, et al.: Changes in plaque lipid content after short-term intensive versus standard statin therapy: the YELLOW trial (reduction in yellow plaque by aggressive lipid-lowering therapy), *J Am Coll Cardiol* 62(1):21–29, 2013.
43. Roleder T, Kovacic JC, Ali Z, et al.: Combined NIRS and IVUS imaging detects vulnerable plaque using a single catheter system: a head-to-head comparison with OCT, *EuroIntervention* 10(3):303–311, 2014.
44. Fard AM, Vacas-Jacques P, Hamidi E, et al.: Optical coherence tomography–near infrared spectroscopy system and catheter for intravascular imaging, *Opt Express* 21(25):30849–30858, 2013.
45. Ueda Y, Ogasawara N, Matsuo K, et al.: Acute coronary syndrome: insight from angioscopy, *Circ J* 74(3):411–417, 2010.
46. Mizuno K, Wang Z, Inami S, et al.: Coronary angioscopy: current topics and future direction, *Cardiovasc Interv Ther* 26(2):89–97, 2011.
47. Qian D, Bottomley PA: High-resolution intravascular magnetic resonance quantification of atherosclerotic plaque at 3T, *J Cardiovasc Magn Reson* 14:20, 2012.
48. Schneiderman J, Wilensky RL, Weiss A, et al.: Diagnosis of thin-cap fibroatheromas by a self-contained intravascular magnetic resonance imaging probe in ex vivo human aortas and in situ coronary arteries, *J Am Coll Cardiol* 45(12):1961–1969, 2005.
49. Regar E, Hennen B, Grube E, et al.: First-in-man application of a miniature self-contained intracoronary magnetic resonance probe. A multi-centre safety and feasibility trial, *EuroIntervention* 2(1):77–83, 2006.
50. Larsen PK, Waxman S: Intracoronary thermography: utility to detect vulnerable and culprit plaques in patients with coronary artery disease, *Current Cardiovascular Imaging Reports* 2(4):300–306, 2009.
51. Puri R, Worthley MI, Nicholls SJ: Intravascular imaging of vulnerable coronary plaque: current and future concepts, *Nat Rev Cardiol* 8(3):131–139, 2011.
52. Suh WM, Seto AH, Margey RJ, Cruz-Gonzalez I, Jang IK: Intravascular detection of the vulnerable plaque, *Circ Cardiovasc Imaging* 4(2):169–178, 2011.
53. Jaffer FA, Calfon MA, Rosenthal A, et al.: Two-dimensional intravascular near-infrared fluorescence molecular imaging of inflammation in atherosclerosis and stent-induced vascular injury, *J Am Coll Cardiol* 57(25):2516–2526, 2011.
54. Ughi GJ, Verjans J, Fard AM, et al.: Dual modality intravascular optical coherence tomography (OCT) and near-infrared fluorescence (NIRF) imaging: a fully automated algorithm for the distance-calibration of NIRF signal intensity for quantitative molecular imaging, *Int J Cardiovasc Imaging* 31(2):259–268, 2015.
55. Dixon AJ, Hossack JA: Intravascular near-infrared fluorescence catheter with ultrasound guidance and blood attenuation correction, *J Biomed Opt* 18(5):56009, 2013.
56. Li BH, Leung AS, Soong A, et al.: Hybrid intravascular ultrasound and optical coherence tomography catheter for imaging of coronary atherosclerosis, *Catheter Cardiovasc Interv* 81(3):494–507, 2013.
57. Ong DS, Jang IK: Causes, assessment, and treatment of stent thrombosis–intravascular imaging insights, *Nat Rev Cardiol* 12:325–336, 2015.
58. Arbab-Zadeh A, Fuster V: The myth of the "vulnerable plaque": transitioning from a focus on individual lesions to atherosclerotic disease burden for coronary artery disease risk assessment, *J Am Coll Cardiol* 65(8):846–855, 2015.
59. Kaul S, Narula J: In search of the vulnerable plaque: is there any light at the end of the catheter? *J Am Coll Cardiol* 64(23):2519–2524, 2014.

11 Risk Stratification in Acute Myocardial Infarction

L. Kristin Newby, Amit N. Vora, and Christopher B. Granger

INTRODUCTION

Acute myocardial infarction (MI) is a leading cause of morbidity and mortality worldwide (see Chapter 2).[1] Although an estimated 157,000 patients will die each year in the United States as a result of an MI, this statistic belies the wide variability in the rate of mortality and recurrent ischemic events across the spectrum of patients with MI. Although patients presenting with ST-elevation MI (STEMI) are at higher risk for short-term mortality, patients with non–ST-elevation MI (NSTEMI) are at higher long-term risk, which is believed to be related to older age and comorbid medical conditions.

Risk stratification is an integral component of the management of patients presenting with acute MI. Prognostic information is important for appropriate triage and resource allocation to provide the appropriate intensity and location of care for MI patients. Patients and their families, when confronted with an acute MI, expect information about its severity and anticipated consequences. Although treatment for patients with STEMI is directed toward timely reperfusion of the occluded vessel with primary percutaneous coronary intervention (PCI) or fibrinolysis, accurate risk stratification is integral in providing appropriate monitoring and care after reperfusion is achieved (see Chapter 14). Moreover among patients with NSTEMI, risk stratification provides not only important prognostic information, but is also critical in deciding the most appropriate care pathway (see Chapter 16). Patients at high risk may be more likely to benefit from an early invasive strategy and timely revascularization, whereas an ischemia-driven strategy may be more appropriate for lower risk patients. In addition, many treatment options for patients with acute MI, including revascularization, dual antiplatelet therapy, glycoprotein IIb/IIIa inhibitors, or other anticoagulants, may carry significant bleeding risks. Risk stratification allows clinicians to weigh the benefits and risks of specific therapies when delineating a treatment plan, with the recognition that many (but not all) of the characteristics that portend increased ischemic risk are also contributors to bleeding risk.

Individualized risk assessment for acute MI involves the integration of multiple data points that are available at first medical contact and initially is composed of baseline demographic and clinical characteristics. Upon presentation, additional information gleaned during the initial evaluation, including physical examination findings, the electrocardiogram (ECG), and biomarkers of cardiomyocyte necrosis, is integrated. These data may then be combined into a validated risk model, such as the GRACE (Global Registry of Acute Coronary Events) Risk Score or the TIMI (Thrombolysis In Myocardial Infarction) Risk Score, to provide clear prognostic guidance on short- and long-term risks of death or major adverse cardiovascular events. Such risk scores may be combined with the measurement of additional biomarkers to provide incremental discrimination and potentially reclassify patients more accurately (see Chapter 8). Risk evolves in a dynamic way throughout the clinical course based on the therapies delivered, and risk assessment at discharge allows stratification of the likelihood of recurrent ischemic events, sudden cardiac death, and hospital readmission.

In this chapter, we provide an in-depth perspective on clinical risk prediction in acute MI. We begin with demographic and clinical risk factors and then incorporate information on the acute presentation, including symptoms, the physical examination, and the ECG. We then review the development, validation, and use of comprehensive, integrated risk models in clinical use, such as the GRACE Risk Score and the TIMI Risk Scores for STEMI and unstable angina (UA)-NSTEMI. We also discuss the value of ancillary novel biomarkers in conjunction with the integrated risk scores (see also Chapter 8). Finally, we describe the importance of postdischarge risk stratification for patients with acute MI.

DEMOGRAPHIC AND CLINICAL RISK PREDICTORS

Age

The incidence and prevalence of acute MI increases with each decade of age; the average age of the first MI is

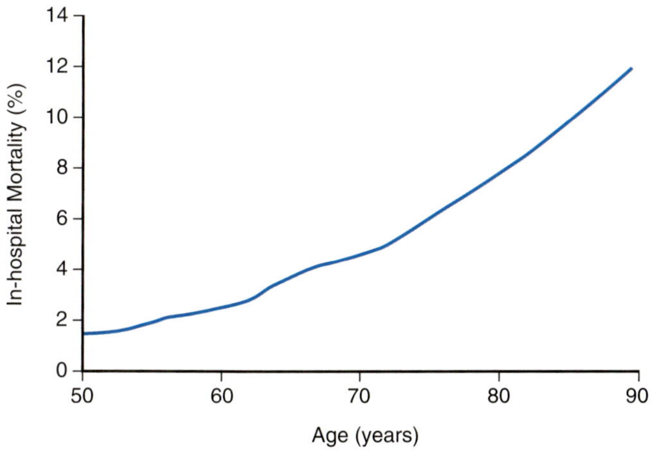

FIGURE 11-1 The relationship between age and in-hospital mortality in the CRUSADE Registry. *(From Alexander KP, et al: Evolution in cardiovascular care for elderly patients with non-ST-segment elevation acute coronary syndromes: results from the CRUSADE National Quality Improvement Initiative.* J Am Coll Cardiol *46:1479–1487, 2005.)*

approximately 65 years in men and 72 years among women.[2] Older patients are at increased risk of adverse outcomes after an acute MI (Figure 11-1).[3] In the derivation population of the TIMI Risk Score for STEMI (median age 62 years; interquartile range 52 to 70), the univariate odds of mortality were increased almost fivefold among patients older than 65 years (odds ratio [OR], 4.9; 95% confidence interval [CI], 4.2 to 5.7). In a substudy of STEMI patients from the GUSTO-IIb study, each decade of age increased the odds of death or MI by 1.32 (95% CI, 1.04 to 1.76).[4] From most datasets, age is the most important determinant of short-term adverse outcomes across the spectrum of acute coronary syndrome (ACS), although it is more pronounced among patients with acute MI than UA.

There are a number of reasons older patients may have worse outcomes following acute MI. First, older patients have more comorbid conditions, including renal dysfunction, and have a significant burden of multiple medications compared with younger patients. Older patients are more likely to present with atypical symptoms, but they are less likely to have diagnostic ECGs. Older patients are also less likely to receive guideline-recommended medical therapy and to undergo revascularization. Older patients are at significantly increased risk of bleeding,[5] which may be further compounded by inappropriate dosing of antithrombotic medications. Although there is benefit of revascularization for older patients—a benefit that in the population included in clinical trials may be even greater than for younger patients—the benefits of an early invasive strategy have to be balanced against bleeding risk. From the Treat Angina With Aggrastat and Determine the Cost of Therapy With an Invasive or Conservative Strategy (TACTICS)-TIMI 18 study, older patients experienced a greater absolute benefit of early invasive management, with lower rates short- and medium-term cardiovascular ischemic outcomes at the cost of an increased rate of major bleeding. In a patient-level meta-analysis of the Fast Revascularisation during InStability in Coronary artery disease (FRISC-II), Invasive versus Conservative Treatment in Unstable coronary Syndromes (ICTUS), and Randomized Intervention Trial of unstable Angina (RITA-III) trials, the incidence of adverse cardiovascular outcomes at 5 years was significantly lower among patients ages 65 to 74 years (hazard ratio [HR], 0.72; 95% CI, 0.58 to 0.90) and 75 years or older (HR, 0.71; 95% CI, 0.55 to 0.91) who underwent a routine invasive strategy compared with conservative management.[6]

Because of the importance of age in risk stratification among patients presenting with acute MI, it is incorporated in most common risk prediction tools. Despite the evidence that age is the most impactful single predictor of risk, the importance of age tends to be underappreciated by clinicians in their gestalt assessment of risk,[7] a fact that underscores the importance of using objective tools to assess risk.

Sex

Previous studies demonstrated that compared with men, women have a higher burden of comorbid conditions, more often have atypical chest symptoms,[8,9] present later after symptom onset,[10] and are more likely to be inappropriately discharged from the emergency department. From the CRUSADE (Can Rapid Risk Stratification of Unstable Angina Patients Suppress Adverse Outcomes With Early Implementation of the ACC/AHA Guidelines) Registry, women more frequently had traditional risk factors but were less likely to receive evidence-based therapies during the hospitalization and at discharge. Although women are at higher unadjusted risk for death and adverse cardiovascular outcomes, this higher risk is largely explained by differences in the underlying risk factors, such as age, comorbidities, and treatment.[11] In a pooled analysis of 11 randomized clinical trials that included 136,247 patients (28% women), women had significantly higher odds of in-hospital mortality (OR, 1.91; 95% CI, 1.83 to 2.00), although this relationship was not significant after multivariable adjustment (adjusted OR, 1.06; 95% CI, 0.99 to 1.15).[12] In a meta-analysis of eight randomized trials, an invasive strategy was preferred among women with high-risk features (OR, 0.67; 95% CI, 0.50 to 0.88), but the point estimate favored harm among low-risk women (OR, 1.35; 95% CI, 0.78 to 2.35); therefore, guidelines support a conservative approach for low-risk women.[13]

Diabetes

According to data from the National Health and Nutrition Examination Survey, diabetes mellitus (DM) affects approximately 28.2 million American adults. Across the spectrum of atherosclerosis and ischemic heart disease, DM is an established potent risk factor for increased mortality, stroke, and coronary artery disease.[1] Patients with diabetes are less likely to present with typical symptoms suggestive of ischemia and more likely to have a delay to presentation.[14] Patients with diabetes are also significantly more likely to have other cardiovascular risk factors, including hypertension and hypercholesterolemia.[14,15]

Approximately 25% of patients in the GRACE Registry had diabetes and had higher rates of heart failure, renal failure, cardiogenic shock, and in-hospital mortality than patients without diabetes across the spectrum of ACS. In a Finnish population-based study, the risk of first MI in a patient with diabetes was similar to the risk of recurrent MI in a patient without diabetes. From a pooled analysis of 62,036 patients (n = 46,577 with STEMI and n = 15,459 with UA-NSTEMI) from 11 TIMI trials, there was an approximate doubling of 30-day mortality among patients with diabetes compared with patients without diabetes in both UA-NSTEMI (2.1% vs 1.1%; $P < .001$; OR, 1.78; 95% CI, 1.24 to 2.56) and STEMI (8.5%

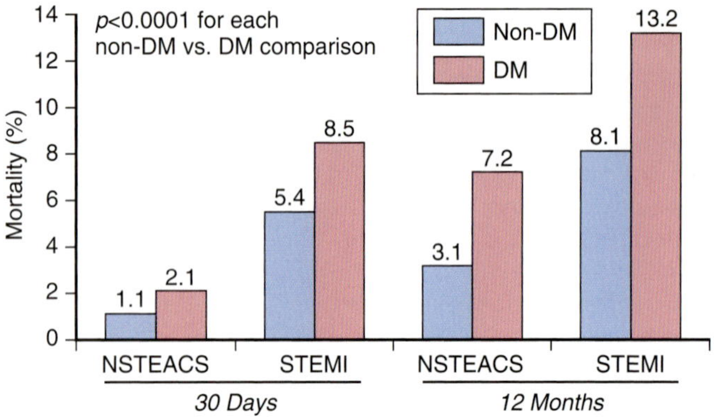

FIGURE 11-2 Thirty-day and 1-year mortality by type of acute coronary syndrome, stratified by presence or absence of diabetes mellitus (DM). *NSTEACS,* Non–ST-elevation acute coronary syndrome; *STEMI,* ST-elevation myocardial infarction. *(Data from a pooled analysis of 11 independent TIMI Study Group clinical trials.)*

vs. 5.4%; $P < .001$; OR, 1.40; 95% CI, 1.24 to 1.57) (Figure 11-2),[16] and subsequent analyses of many clinical trials have consistently demonstrated substantially increased risk of death and adverse cardiovascular outcomes among patients with diabetes. Although patients with diabetes are at higher risk of bleeding and other complications following PCI, an early invasive strategy has been associated with improved outcomes in this patient group. In addition, diabetes is a risk feature that seems to identify a population of patients with multivessel disease who derive particular benefit from coronary artery bypass surgery.[17,18]

Renal Disease

Patients with chronic kidney disease are at increased risk for adverse cardiovascular outcomes and bleeding (Figure 11-3).[19] In an analysis of 1.2 million patients, Go and colleagues[2] noted a stepwise, graded increase in death and cardiovascular outcomes among patients with worsening renal function, with an almost sixfold increase in adjusted all-cause mortality (adjusted HR, 5.9; 95% CI, 5.4 to 6.5) and a threefold increased risk of any cardiovascular event (adjusted HR, 3.4; 95% CI, 3.1 to 3.8). In an analysis of the VALIANT (Valsartan in Acute Myocardial Infarction Trial) study, even mild renal insufficiency was associated with a 10% increase in the risk of death and adverse cardiovascular outcomes for each 10 mL/min/1.73 m^2 reduction in the estimated glomerular filtration rate less than 81.0 mL/min/1.73 m^2. Worsening renal disease (estimated glomerular filtration rate <60 mL/min/1.73 m^2) remained an independent predictor of increased cardiovascular mortality in the A to Z Trial, even after adjustment for inflammation with C-reactive protein (CRP) (HR, 1.82; 95% CI, 1.1 to 2.97).

Assessment of renal function is critical in initial risk stratification, because patients with renal disease are not only at increased risk of bleeding,[20-23] but also may develop worsening renal dysfunction because of acute kidney injury following an invasive strategy. Worsening renal dysfunction after cardiac catheterization may be the result of direct renal injury from iodinated contrast, atheroemboli from aortic plaque, or both. Patients presenting with NSTEMI with renal dysfunction may be less likely to undergo an invasive strategy despite the benefit among patients with mild to moderate renal dysfunction.[24,25] Although providers routinely use either the Modification of Diet and Renal Disease or the Cockcroft-Gault methods to calculate estimated renal function, the Cockcroft-Gault method may be better in predicting mortality following acute MI, particularly among women, small patients (body mass index <25 kg/m^2), or the elderly.[26]

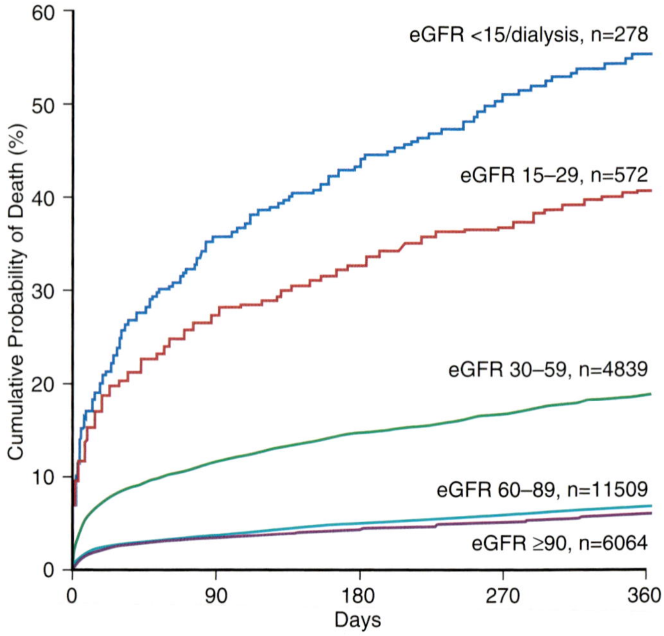

FIGURE 11-3 Renal function and 1-year mortality among NSTEMI patients in the SWEDEHEART Registry. *eGFR,* Estimated glomerular filtration rate. *(From Szummer K, et al: Influence of renal function on the effects of early revascularization in non-ST-elevation myocardial infarction: data from the Swedish Web-System for Enhancement and Development of Evidence-Based Care in Heart Disease Evaluated According to Recommended Therapies [SWEDEHEART].* Circulation *120:851–858, 2009.)*

Smoking

Although smoking is a traditional cardiovascular risk factor and the cause of an estimated 467,000 deaths annually in the United States,[2] a "smoker's paradox," in which smokers presenting with acute MI have better outcomes than nonsmokers, was first described in 1993 among patients presenting with STEMI who received fibrinolytic therapy. However, smokers were approximately 9 years younger than nonsmokers, and subsequent studies have attributed almost all of the improved outcomes among smokers to their younger age and the presence of fewer comorbidities, such as these patients presenting with MI at a younger age when they are better able to survive. In addition, the study that initially described the smoker's paradox focused on patients who underwent fibrinolytic therapy; subsequent studies that have evaluated patients who underwent invasive management have been conflicting. In an analysis of NSTE-ACS patients from the ACUITY (Acute Catheterization and Urgent Intervention Triage Strategy) trial, Robertson and colleagues reported similar short-term outcomes but worse 1-year outcomes among smokers; in addition, they noted that smokers and nonsmokers had similar anatomic extent of coronary artery disease, despite the fact that smokers were almost a decade younger than nonsmokers.[27] A subsequent analysis from the Synergy between Percutaneous Coronary Intervention with TAXUS and Cardiac Surgery (SYNTAX) trial also described worse clinical outcomes at 5 years among smokers.[28]

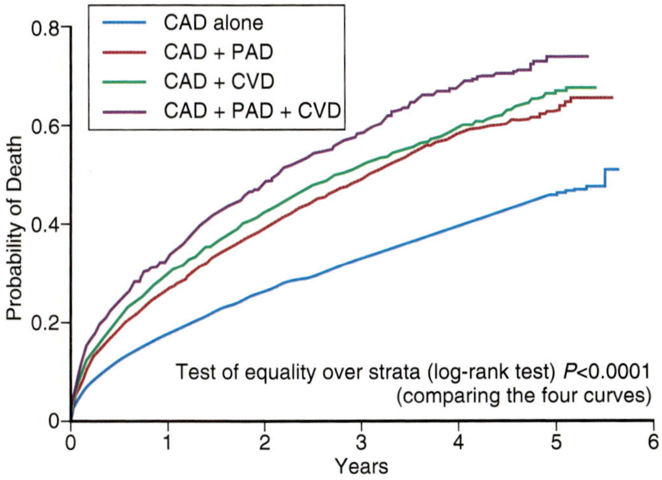

FIGURE 11-4 Long-term mortality following non–ST-elevation myocardial infarction among patients with polyvascular disease by previous vascular bed involvement in the CRUSADE Registry. *CAD*, Coronary artery disease; *CVD*, cerebrovascular disease; *PAD*, peripheral artery disease. *(From Subherwal S, et al: Polyvascular disease and long-term cardiovascular outcomes in older patients with non-ST-segment-elevation myocardial infarction.* Circ Cardiovasc Qual Outcomes *5:541–549, 2012.)*

Peripheral Artery Disease

The presence of peripheral artery disease (PAD) is also an established a marker of increased risk of adverse cardiovascular outcomes among patients presenting with acute MI. Among patients with ACS enrolled in the Oral Glycoprotein IIb/IIIa Inhibition With Orbofiban in Patients With Unstable Coronary Syndrome (OPUS)-TIMI 16 Study, patients with PAD were at higher risk of mortality (8.8% vs. 3.9%; adjusted HR, 1.39; 95% CI, 1.07 to 1.81) compared with patients without PAD.[29] From the CRUSADE Registry, Bhatt and colleagues observed an increasing odds of in-hospital ischemic outcomes with disease in multiple vascular beds (OR, 1.31 in patients with disease in three vascular beds; $P < .001$),[30] whereas Subherwal and colleagues described increased risk of long-term mortality among patients with extensive disease (adjusted HR, 1.49; 95% CI, 1.38 to 1.61) (Figure 11-4).[31] The presence of PAD remained an independent predictor of in-hospital mortality among acute MI patients who underwent PCI (OR, 2.2; 95% CI, 1.7 to 3.0).

Previous Aspirin Use

Although aspirin has been the cornerstone of medical therapy during and following acute MI,[32] previous studies have demonstrated worse outcomes among patients taking aspirin before the event, and previous aspirin use is included as an independent predictor in the TIMI Risk Score for UA-NSTEMI. Although the underlying pathophysiology for this phenomenon is unclear, the relationship may reflect a heighted risk associated with "failure" of therapy with aspirin or the presence of more severe disease in patients who were previously prescribed aspirin.[33,34]

INITIAL PRESENTATION

Quality of Angina

The nature, quality, and duration of chest discomfort are known to have prognostic implications, with typical anginal symptoms, defined by Braunwald and colleagues as (1) substernal chest discomfort with a characteristic quality and duration that is (2) provoked by exertion or emotional stress, and (3) relieved by rest or nitroglycerin,[35] conferring worse prognosis than atypical or noncardiac chest pain. The presence of severe angina symptoms, defined as two or more anginal episodes in the previous 24 hours, was incorporated into the TIMI Risk Score for UA-NSTEMI (see the section on Integrated Risk Models for Early Risk Assessment). Types of discomfort not characteristic of acute myocardial ischemia include extremely brief episodes of discomfort (less than a few seconds), pleuritic pain, middle and/or lower abdominal pain, localized pain (especially at the left ventricular apex or costochondral junction), pain reproduced with palpation or movement, or pain radiating to the lower extremities. However, atypical chest discomfort does not necessarily exclude the possibility of acute MI, because a significant proportion of patients in an older series with acute MI presented with atypical symptoms, including pleuritic pain and/or pain reproducible by palpation. In addition, improvement with either nitroglycerin or a gastrointestinal cocktail does not necessarily include or exclude acute MI.[36]

Hemodynamic Instability

A thorough physical examination, beginning with measurement of vital signs, may be helpful in eliciting signs of heart failure or cardiogenic shock, either as a result of severe left ventricular dysfunction or a mechanical complication of acute MI, such as chordal rupture of the mitral valve apparatus or ventricular wall rupture (see Chapter 25). Findings of tachycardia, hypotension, rales, a third heart sound, or a mitral regurgitation murmur are associated with a higher risk of adverse outcomes following MI. The Killip classification, first described in 1967, relied on physical examination findings only and demonstrated increased mortality with escalating signs of heart failure. Although initially described among patients with STEMI, the Killip classification was validated in a pooled analysis of 26,090 NSTEMI patients, with patients presenting with Killip class III/IV at a significantly increased risk of 30-day (HR, 2.35; 95% CI, 1.69 to 3.26) and 6-month mortality (HR, 2.12; 95% CI, 1.63 to 2.75).[37] Because of the importance of these physical examination findings, Killip class was incorporated into the TIMI Risk Score for STEMI and the GRACE Risk Score. Heart rate and blood pressure in and of themselves contain important prognostic information, such that higher heart rate and lower blood pressure at presentation are important risk predictors.

Electrocardiogram

The ECG is a critical component in both risk stratification and management in patients presenting with acute MI.[38] Current guidelines recommend that an ECG be performed within 10 minutes of presentation for all patients with chest pain concerning for acute ischemia.[36,39] Patients presenting with acute ST-segment elevation are directed along a rapid reperfusion pathway (see Chapter 13). Among patients without ST-segment elevation, even relatively minor ST-segment deviations have been correlated with adverse outcomes. Patients with ST-segment depression of even 0.05 mV (0.5 mm on a standard ECG) had higher rates of death or MI compared with patients with T-wave inversions only, even after multivariable adjustment (Figure 11-5). In addition, the

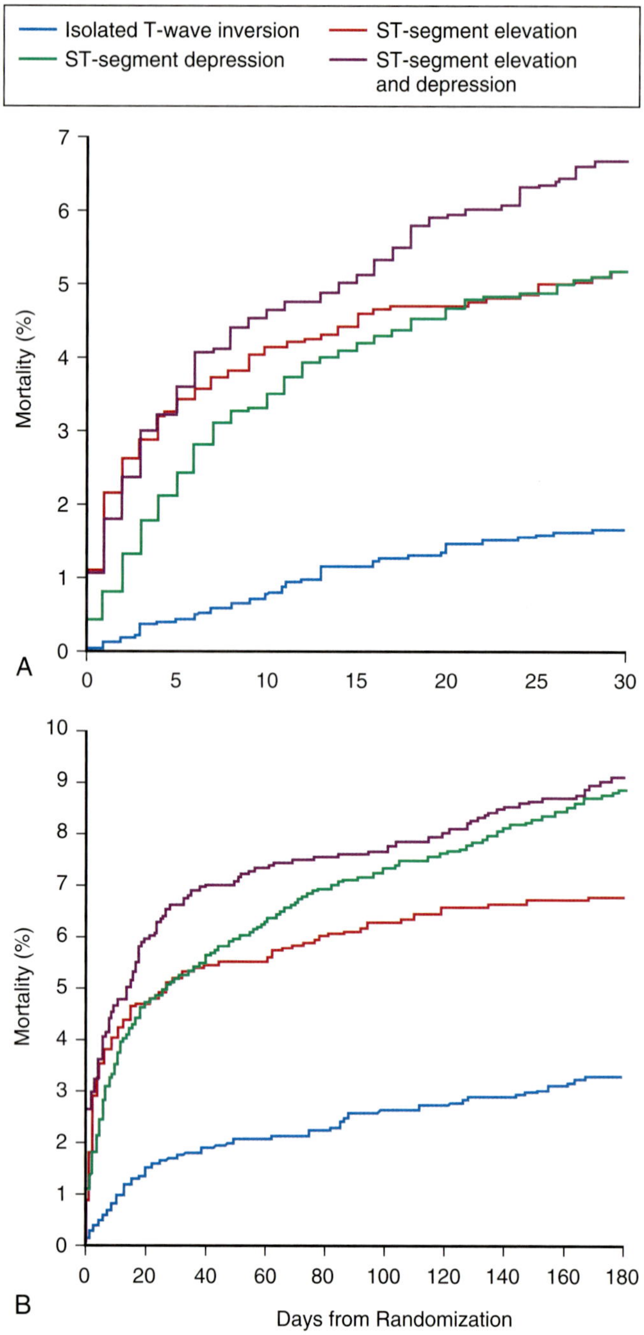

FIGURE 11-5 Kaplan-Meier mortality estimates at (**A**) 30 days and (**B**) 6 months by abnormal electrocardiographic finding in patients with an acute coronary syndrome. *(From Savonitto S, et al: Prognostic value of the admission electrocardiogram in acute coronary syndromes.* JAMA *1999;281:707–13, 1999.)*

degree of ST-segment deviation is also predictive of adverse outcomes. In an analysis of 7800 NSTE-ACS patients from the GUSTO-IV trial, ST-segment deviation of ≥0.2 mV was a stronger predictor of short- and long-term mortality than any other clinical factor or biomarker. Among patients with NSTE-ACS, there was an association between in-hospital revascularization and lower 4-year mortality, especially among patients with ST-segment depression of ≥0.1 mV on the presenting ECG.

Symmetrical T-wave inversions of ≥0.2 mV may be indicative of proximal left anterior descending ischemia; however, nonspecific T-wave inversions less than 0.2 mV may not be helpful from a clinical perspective.[36] It is also important to note that a normal ECG does not exclude acute MI in patients with concerning symptoms, because 2% to 6% of patients presenting with acute MI may have an initially normal or nonspecific ECG; however, patients with acute MI presenting with a normal or nonspecific ECG appear to have lower rates of in-hospital mortality than those with a diagnostic ECG.

Although most studies have evaluated use of the presentation ECG in risk assessment and treatment pathway, Carmo and colleagues evaluated the utility of 24-hour continuous ECG monitoring in 234 NSTE-ACS patients and reported limited incremental prognostic information, especially compared with the GRACE Risk Score.[40] Scirica and colleagues studied the use of 7-day continuous ECG monitoring, and among 6355 patients enrolled in the Metabolic Efficiency With Ranolazine for Less Ischemia in Non–ST-Elevation Acute Coronary Syndromes (MERLIN)-TIMI 36 Trial, they found that patients with one episode or more of ischemia (defined as ≥0.1 mV of ST-segment depression lasting ≥1 minute with a heart rate at the onset of the episode <100 beats/min) had an increased risk of adverse cardiovascular outcomes, even after multivariable adjustment (risk of death: 7.7% vs 2.7%; $P < .001$; adjusted HR, 2.46; 95% CI, 1.81 to 3.33).[41]

Markers of Cardiomyocyte Necrosis

Evidence of myocardial necrosis in the presence of symptoms concerning for acute ischemia is central to the diagnosis of acute MI. Although less specific markers of myocyte necrosis, including myoglobin, creatine kinase, and creatine kinase-myocardial band fraction, were used in previous decades, cardiac troponin measurements, both the I and T isoforms, are now the most sensitive and specific measures of myocyte necrosis (see Chapter 7) and have redefined the UA-NSTEMI spectrum of ACS (see Chapter 1).[42]

Biomarkers of necrosis consistently identify a graded relationship with the risk of death after presentation with MI. Importantly, the risk of recurrent ischemia and infarction is shown as an inverted U-shaped pattern, with highest risk in those with low to intermediate increases in biomarkers of necrosis. This presumably identifies patients with high-risk ACS in whom the culprit territory remains at risk. In the TIMI IIIB Trial, Antman and colleagues demonstrated a 1.8- to 7.8-fold increased mortality risk among patients with elevated cardiac troponin I, concordant with similar findings from the GUSTO IIA Trial.

Since these landmark publications, in more than 30 studies, including both clinical trials and community-based cohorts, cardiac troponin has independently predicted the risk of death and recurrent ischemic events among patients with ACS. In aggregate, patients presenting with suspected NSTE-ACS and an elevated concentration of troponin are at an approximately fourfold higher risk of death or recurrent infarction. In patients with STEMI, an elevated concentration of troponin at presentation is also associated with higher short-term mortality. This prognostic information obtained from measurement of cardiac troponin is complementary to the important clinical indicators of risk identified in this chapter, including patient age, ST deviation, and presence of heart failure.

With the development of high-sensitivity assays for cardiac troponin, it is possible to measure low concentrations of troponin and to characterize troponin distribution in healthy populations with greater precision (see Chapter 7). In this context, the recommended clinical decision limits have moved toward lower concentrations, raising questions regarding the clinical relevance of low or very low levels of troponin elevation. There are now multiple studies that have validated the heightened risk of patients with positive troponin results using high-sensitivity assays. As an example, in a study of more than 4600 patients, a high-sensitivity troponin assay identified patients at significantly higher 30-day risk of cardiovascular death or new MI using the guideline-based 99th percentile decision limit.[43] Importantly, the study identified a gradient of risk at the low end of concentration that was not reliably measured with previous generations of the same assay. Conversely, a troponin concentration less than the 99th percentile cut point identified a cohort of patients with a clinical diagnosis of NSTE-ACS who were at low risk for death or recurrent ischemic events over 30 days.

INTEGRATED RISK MODELS FOR EARLY RISK ASSESSMENT

GRACE Risk Score

The risk score for predicted in-hospital mortality from the GRACE trial remains one of the best validated and most widely used risk scores for early assessment of in-hospital predicted mortality risk. The score was initially developed in an unselected cohort of 11,389 patients (including 509 in-hospital deaths) who presented with ACS in 94 hospitals in 14 geographically diverse countries (Argentina, Australia, Austria, Belgium, Brazil, Canada, France, Germany, Italy, New Zealand, Poland, Spain, the United Kingdom, and the United States) from 1999 to 2001.

The initial model was developed using a multivariable logistic regression modeling technique in which a logistic regression model was used to examine the relationship between candidate variables (selected from clinical variables, expert opinion, and previous model results); a multivariable stepwise logistic regression was used to estimate in-hospital mortality. Eight independent risk factors accounted for almost 90% of the prognostic information and were the components of the final model: age (OR, 1.7 per decade; 95% CI, 1.55 to 1.85); Killip class (OR, 2.0 per class; 95% CI, 1.81 to 2.29); systolic blood pressure (OR, 1.4 per 20-mm Hg decrease; 95% CI, 1.27 to 1.45); ST-segment deviation (OR, 2.4; 95% CI, 1.90 to 3.00); cardiac arrest during presentation (OR, 4.3; 95% CI, 2.80 to 6.72); serum creatinine level at presentation (OR, 1.2 per 1 mg/dL increase; 95% CI, 1.15 to 1.35); positive cardiac biomarkers at presentation (OR, 1.6; 95% CI, 1.32 to 2.00); and heart rate (OR, 1.3 per 30 beats/min increase; 95% CI 1.16 to 1.48). An updated version of the risk score (found at http://www.gracescore.org) allows its use when Killip class and serum creatine are not available, and provides estimates of in-hospital, 6-month, 1- and 3-year death, and 1-year death or MI.

The final model displayed excellent discrimination ability with a c-statistic of 0.83 in the derivation cohort. Of note, univariable predictors of in-hospital mortality that were not found to be statistically significant in the multivariable model included sex, history of heart failure, and history of renal insufficiency. In addition, previous aspirin use (OR, 0.73; 95% CI, 0.58 to 0.91) and previous statin use (OR, 0.50; 95% CI, 0.34 to 0.97) were found to be significant in the multivariable model, but they only added marginally to the overall discriminatory ability (c-statistic = 0.85), and therefore, were not included in the final, simplified model (Figure 11-6).

The GRACE Risk Score has been well-validated in many subsequent cohorts and by the United Kingdom National Institute for Health and Care Excellence. It was initially validated in a continuation of the GRACE Registry among a subsequent sample of 3972 patients (including 215 deaths) who were enrolled after March 21, 2001 and performed well, with a c-statistic of 0.85. In the GUSTO-IIb cohort, which included 12,142 patients at 373 hospitals in 13 countries randomized to intravenous heparin or hirudin within 72 hours of presentation of ACS, the model performed well (c-statistic = 0.79), despite the fact that the most powerful predictor of mortality, cardiac arrest at presentation, was not collected in this dataset.

A complementary risk score was developed using the GRACE cohort to predict 6-month mortality among patients at discharge using stepwise Cox proportional hazards regression for candidate variables, then using a backward stepwise selection methodology to create the multivariable model with α value of less than 0.05. The final postdischarge to 6-month mortality model included the following nine variables: age (OR, 1.7 per 10-year increase; 95% CI, 1.63 to 1.84); history of MI (OR, 1.4; 95% CI, 1.20 to 1.59); history of congestive heart failure (OR, 2.1; 95% CI, 1.80 to 2.47); heart rate (OR, 1.3 per 30 beats/min increase; 95% CI, 1.23 to 1.47); systolic blood pressure (OR, 1.1 per 20-mm Hg decrease; 95% CI, 1.06 to 1.17); initial serum creatinine level (OR, 1.2 per 1 mg/dL increase; 95% CI, 1.12 to 1.23); initial cardiac biomarker elevation (OR, 1.5; 95% CI, 1.33 to 1.79); ST-segment depression (OR, 1.5; 95% CI, 1.29 to 1.69); and no in-hospital PCI (OR, 1.9; 95% CI, 1.30 to 1.88). This model also displayed good discrimination ability, with a c-statistic of 0.77 in the overall cohort (n = 22,645) (Figure 11-7).

A comprehensive model was subsequently developed using similar methodology to predict risk of mortality or recurrent MI from presentation to 6 months in a population of 43,810 patients through September 2005 from the GRACE Registry. The simplified model included the same eight independent predictors of the in-hospital mortality model and demonstrated good discrimination, with a c-statistic of 0.81 for predicting mortality and a c-statistic of 0.73 for death or recurrent MI to 6 months from MI presentation.

Although the GRACE Risk Scores were developed in the late 1990s and early 2000s, before the development of contemporary therapies for acute MI, such as drug-eluting stents, next-generation antiplatelet agents, and robust anticoagulants, their validity was demonstrated in an analysis of 5985 patients who presented with ACS in the MASCARA Spanish Registry. In this Registry, the GRACE Risk Scores demonstrated robust discrimination, with a c-statistic of 0.85 for predicted in-hospital mortality and a c-statistic of 0.81 for predicted 6-month mortality.[44]

The GRACE Risk Score has a number of advantages over previously developed risk models. First, it was developed using a general, unselected, global population of patients who underwent routine clinical care; other risk scores were derived using cohorts enrolled in randomized clinical trials. Next, it has excellent discriminatory capability, with a c-statistic of 0.83 in the initial model. Third, compared with other models that predict a composite endpoint, the GRACE risk models predict only hard outcomes; the initial model predicted in-hospital mortality, although subsequent models have predicted risk of death or recurrent MI to 6 months. Finally, a uniform model predicts risk across the ACS spectrum, from UA to STEMI.

1. Find points for each predictive factor:

Killip class	Points	SBP, mm Hg	Points	Heart rate, beats/min	Points	Age, years	Points	Creatinine level, mg/dL	Points
I	0	≤80	58	≤50	0	≤30	0	0–0.39	1
II	20	80–99	53	50–69	3	30–39	8	0.40–0.79	4
III	39	100–119	43	70–89	9	40–49	25	0.80–1.19	7
IV	59	120–139	34	90–109	15	50–59	41	1.20–1.59	10
		140–159	24	110–149	24	60–69	58	1.60–1.99	13
		160–199	10	150–199	38	70–79	75	2.00–3.99	21
		≥200	0	≥200	46	80–89	91	>4.0	28
						≥90	100		

Other risk factors	Points
Cardiac arrest at admission	39
ST-segment deviation	28
Elevated cardiac biomarker levels	14

2. Sum points for all predictive factors:

Killip class + SBP + Heart rate + Age + Creatinine level + Cardiac arrest at admission + ST-segment deviation + Elevated cardiac biomarker levels = Total points

3. Look up risk corresponding to total points

Total points	≤60	70	80	90	100	110	120	130	140	150	160	170	180	190	200	210	220	230	240	≥250
Probability of in-hospital death, %	≤0.2	0.3	0.4	0.6	0.8	1.1	1.6	2.1	2.9	3.9	5.4	7.3	9.8	13	18	23	29	36	44	≥52

For example, a patient has Killip class II, SBP of 100 mm Hg, heart rate of 100 beats/min, is 65 years of age, has serum creatinine level of 1 mg/dL, did not have a cardiac arrest at admission but did have ST-segment deviation and elevated enzyme levels.

His score would be 20 + 53 + 15 + 58 + 7 + 0 + 28 + 14 = 196.

This person would have an approximately 16% risk of having an in-hospital death.

Similarly, a patient with a Killip class I, SBP of 80 mm Hg, heart rate of 60 beats/min, is 55 years of age, has serum creatinine level of 0.4, and no risk factors would have the following score:

0 + 58 + 3 + 41 + 1 =103, which gives approximately a 0.9% risk of having an in-hospital death.

FIGURE 11-6 Initial GRACE Risk Score model nomogram. *SBP*, Systolic blood pressure. *(From Granger CB, et al: Predictors of hospital mortality in the global registry of acute coronary events.* Arch Intern Med *163:2345–2353,2003.)*

TIMI Risk Score for ST-Elevation Myocardial Infarction

The TIMI Risk Score for STEMI was constructed using the patient cohort from the inTIME (Intravenous nPA for Treatment of Infarcting Myocardium II) trial, which randomized 14,114 patients to either lanecteplase or alteplase. It comprised 8 predictors of increased 30-day mortality with variable weights for a total of 14 points: age; diabetes, hypertension, or angina; systolic blood pressure less than 100 mm Hg; heart rate more than 100 beats/min; Killip classes II to IV; weight less than 67 kg; new left bundle branch block or anterior ST-segment elevation; and time to fibrinolytic therapy of more than 4 hours (Figure 11-8). The model demonstrated good discriminatory ability (c-statistic = 0.78) and a significant gradation of risk of 30-day mortality, from 0.8% in patients with a risk score of 0% to 35.9% for patients with a risk score greater than 8. Although the TIMI STEMI Risk Score was derived in a population of patients who received fibrinolytic therapy, the score has subsequently been validated in patients who underwent reperfusion via primary PCI.[45] The main strength of the TIMI Risk Score is its ability to be calculated at the bedside as a simple integer score based on clinical history, ECG, and physical examination.

TIMI Risk Score for Unstable Angina: Non–ST-Elevation Myocardial Infarction

The TIMI Risk Score for UA and/or NSTEMI was initially derived using the heparin-only arm (n = 1957) of the TIMI-11B Trial, which evaluated the safety and efficacy of enoxaparin compared with unfractionated heparin in patients who presented with UA or NSTEMI. The risk score was validated using the enoxaparin arm (n = 1953) and both arms (n = 3171) from the similar ESSENCE (Efficacy and Safety of Subcutaneous Enoxaparin in Unstable Angina and Non-Q-Wave MI) trial, which also compared efficacy of subcutaneous enoxaparin with unfractionated heparin in patients with unstable angina or non–Q-wave MI. The model was developed using multivariable regression modeling techniques to assess the significance of candidate variables and then tested using a multivariate stepwise (backward elimination) regression model.

The multivariable model revealed seven independent predictors of the composite endpoint of death, recurrent MI, or recurrent ischemia that required urgent revascularization within 14 days: age 65 years or older (OR, 1.75; 95% CI, 1.35 to 2.25), at least three risk factors for coronary artery disease

Risk Calculator for 6-Month Postdischarge Mortality After Hospitalization for Acute Coronary Syndrome

Record the points for each variable at the bottom left and sum the points to calculate the total risk score. Find the total score on the x-axis of the nomogram plot. The corresponding probability on the y-axis is the estimated probability of all-cause mortality from hospital discharge to 6 months.

Medical History

① Age in years	Points
≤29	0
30–39	0
40–49	18
50–59	36
60–69	55
70–79	73
80–89	91
≥90	100

② History of congestive heart failure — 24

③ History of myocardial infarction — 12

Findings in Initial Hospital Presentation

④ Resting heart rate, beats/min	Points
≤49.9	0
50–69.9	3
70–89.9	9
90–109.9	14
110–149.9	23
150–199.9	35
≥200	43

⑤ Systolic blood pressure, mmHg	
≤79.9	24
80–99.9	22
100–119.9	18
120–139.9	14
140–159.9	10
160–199.9	4
≥200	0

⑥ ST-segment depression — 11

Findings During Hospitalization

⑦ Initial serum creatinine, mg/dL	Points
0–0.39	1
0.4–0.79	3
0.8–1.19	5
1.2–1.59	7
1.6–1.99	9
2–3.99	15
≥4	20

⑧ Eleveated cardiac biomarkers – 15

⑨ No in-hospital percutaneous coronary intervention — 14

Points

① ________

② ________

③ ________

④ ________

⑤ ________

⑥ ________

⑦ ________

⑧ ________

⑨ ________

Total risk score ________ (sum of points)

Mortality risk ________ (from plot)

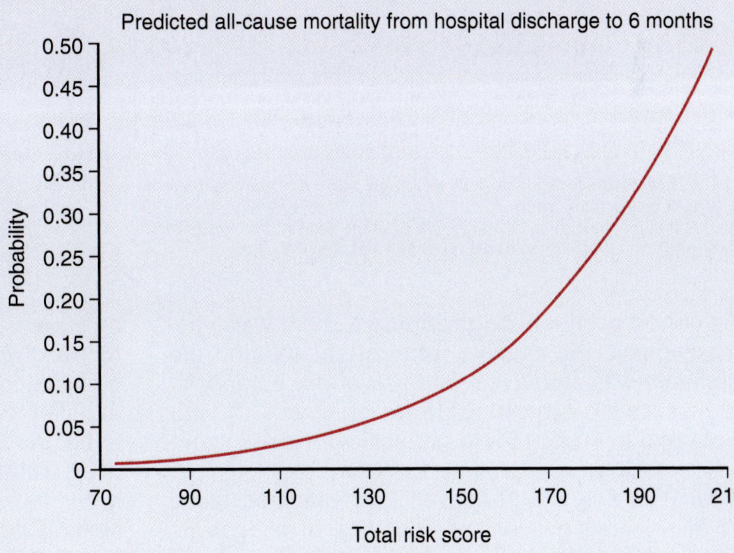

FIGURE 11-7 **GRACE Risk Score model risk calculator for 6-month postdischarge mortality after hospitalization for acute coronary syndrome.** *(From Eagle KA, et al: A validated prediction model for all forms of acute coronary syndrome: estimating the risk of 6-month postdischarge death in an international registry.* JAMA 291:2727–2733, 2004.*)*

(risk factors included family history of coronary artery disease, hypertension, hypercholesterolemia, diabetes, or current smoking status) (OR, 1.54; 95% CI, 1.16 to 2.06), previous coronary stenosis of ≥50% (OR, 1.70; 95% CI, 1.30 to 2.21), ST-segment deviation (OR, 1.51; 95% CI, 1.13 to 2.02), two or more anginal episodes in the previous 24 hours (OR, 1.53; 95% CI, 1.20 to 1.96), and elevated serum cardiac markers (either creatine kinase-MB or cardiac specific troponin) (OR, 1.56; 95% CI, 1.21 to 1.99). Because of the relatively similar prognostic weights, the final TIMI risk score was the sum of the individual predictors (range, 0 to 7).

The TIMI Risk Score showed modest discrimination in the derived cohort (c-statistic = 0.65) and in each of the initial validation cohorts (c-statistic = 0.63 in the combined

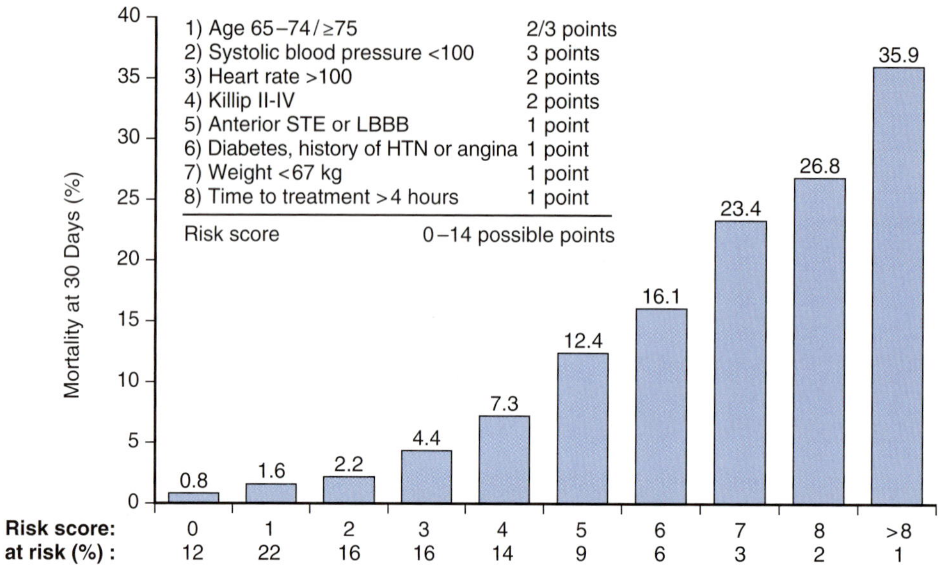

FIGURE 11-8 TIMI Risk Score for ST-elevation (STE) myocardial infarction and 30-day risk for mortality. *HTN,* Hypertension; *LBBB,* left bundle branch block. *(From Morrow DA, et al.: TIMI risk score for ST-elevation myocardial infarction: a convenient, bedside, clinical score for risk assessment at presentation: an intravenous nPA for treatment of infarcting myocardium early II trial substudy.* Circulation *102:2031–2037,2000.)*

Historical	**Points**
Age ≥65	1
≥3 CAD risk factors (FHx, HTN, ↑chol, DM, active smoker)	1
Known CAD (stenosis ≥50%)	1
ASA use in past 7 days	1
Presentation	
Recent (≤24 hour) severe angina	1
↑ Cardiac markers	1
ST deviation ≥0.05 mV	1
Risk Score = Total Points (0–7)	

Risk of cardiac events (%) by 14 days in TIMI 11B trial*

Risk Score	**Death or MI**	**Death, MI, or Urgent Revascularization**
0/1	3	5
2	3	8
3	5	13
4	7	20
5	12	26
6/7	19	41

*Entry criteria: UA or NSTEMI defined as ischemic pain at rest within past 24 hours, with evidence of CAD (ST segment deviation or + biomarker).

FIGURE 11-9 TIMI Risk Score for non–ST-elevation acute coronary syndromes and 14-day risk of death, myocardial infarction, or severe recurrent ischemia prompting urgent revascularization. *ASA,* Aspirin; *CAD,* coronary artery disease; *DM,* diabetes mellitus; *FHx,* family history; *HTN,* hypertension; *MI,* myocardial infarction; *NSTEMI,* non–ST-elevation myocardial infarction; *UA,* unstable angina. *(Data from Antman EM, et al: The TIMI risk score for unstable angina/non-ST elevation MI: A method for prognostication and therapeutic decision making.* JAMA *284:835–42,2000.)*

validation cohort as described previously). There was a linear increase in risk with a higher risk score. In addition, the TIMI Risk Score was able to predict risk of the composite endpoint over a wide range of risk, from less than 4.7% with a risk score of 0 to 1 to 40.9% in patients with a risk score of 6 to 7.

The TIMI Risk Score was derived and validated using a cohort of selected patients participating in a rigorous, well-designed randomized clinical trial and has been well-validated in subsequent clinical trial and contemporary practice populations. The composite endpoint incorporates clinically meaningful endpoints other than only mortality. In addition, although the different components of the GRACE Risk Score denote differential risk and must be weighted to achieve the final risk score, the relatively similar weights in the TIMI Risk Score allow for an arithmetic sum that can be calculated simply to facilitate risk stratification that directly relates to outcomes (Figure 11-9). Finally, although the c-statistic is lower compared with other validated risk models, some have questioned the use of the c-statistic as the only measure of a model's utility[46] and have favored other metrics instead, such as the proportion of patients that are reclassified using a particular model. Even more importantly, the TIMI Risk Score for UA and/or NSTEMI has been shown to be useful for guiding therapeutic decision-making, identifying patients with a greater potential for benefit from early invasive management and more potent antithrombotic therapies (Figure 11-10). Coupling the practical bedside application and the direct clinical relevance for treatment, the TIMI Risk Score remains one of the most widely used scores for clinical risk stratification.

Dynamic Risk Modeling

Although the GRACE Risk Score and the TIMI Risk Scores are among the most widely used for risk stratification in acute MI, both scores rely on data captured at a specific time point. However, in clinical practice, patient risk is continually variable and changes in response to delivered therapies and complications. For example, among patients treated with

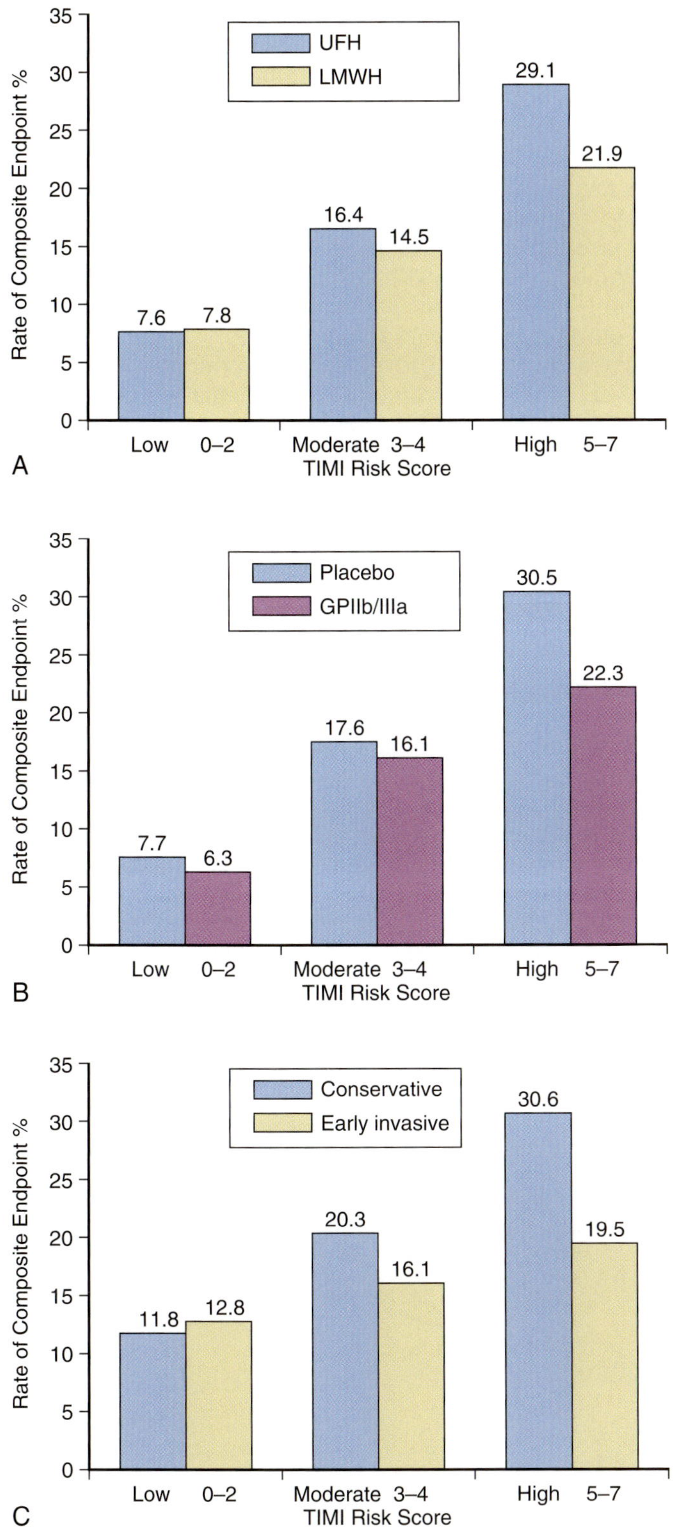

FIGURE 11-10 Relationship between the TIMI Risk Score for non–ST-elevation acute coronary syndromes and the benefit of selected therapies. Effective management strategies offer the greatest absolute benefit in patients with higher TIMI Risk Scores. Rate of the composite endpoints (%) is stratified by risk group and treatment allocation (see individual references for endpoint definitions). *GP*, Glycoprotein; *LMWH*, low-molecular-weight heparin; *UFH*, unfractionated heparin. *(Data from **[A]** Antman EM, et al: The TIMI risk score for unstable angina/non-ST elevation MI: a method for prognostication and therapeutic decision making.* JAMA *284:835–842,2000, **[B]** Morrow DM, et al: An integrated clinical approach to predicting the benefit of tirofiban in non-ST elevation acute coronary syndromes. Application of the TIMI Risk Score for UA/NSTEMI in PRISM-PLUS.* Eur Heart J *23:223–229,2002, and **[C]** Cannon CP, et al: Comparison of early invasive and conservative strategies in patients with unstable coronary syndromes treated with the glycoprotein IIb/IIIa inhibitor tirofiban.* N Engl J Med *344:1879–1887,2001)*

	Points
Baseline TIMI risk score for STEMI	0 to 14 possible points
Age (years)	
65 to 74	2
>75	3
DM/HTN/angina	1
Systolic blood pressure <100 mm Hg	3
Heart rate >100 bpm	2
Killip class II to IV	2
Weight <67 kg	1
Anterior STE or LBBB	1
Time to treatment >4 hours	1
Added index hospital events for dynamic score	
Recurrent MI	1
Stroke	5
Major bleed	1
CHF/Shock	3
Arrhythmia	2
Renal failure	3
Dynamic TIMI risk score	0 to 29 possible

Baseline TIMI risk score for STEMI has 0 to 14 possible points.

FIGURE 11-11 Dynamic TIMI Risk Score for ST-elevation myocardial infarction (STEMI). *CHF*, Congestive heart failure; *DM*, diabetes mellitus; *HTN*, hypertension; *LBBB*, left bundle branch block; MI, myocardial infarction. *(From Amin ST, et al: Dynamic TIMI risk score for STEMI.* J Am Heart Assoc *2:e003269, 2013.)*

fibrinolysis, continual assessment of treatment efficacy guides subsequent timing of angiography and potential rescue PCI. In addition, the development of heart failure or severe left ventricular systolic dysfunction are among the most potent predictors of future adverse cardiac outcomes, although they may not have been present in the initial evaluation, and therefore, would not be captured accurately using a static model.

The GRACE Risk Score includes a postdischarge model that incorporates some in-hospital events, but there have been few models that have systematically captured data at different time points to allow for most accurate risk prediction. Dynamic models in the NSTE-ACS populations that have incorporated data from multiple time points during a patient's hospitalization reported significant improvements in accuracy for 30-day mortality prediction.[36] Dynamic modeling of 90-day mortality using data captured at baseline and at 2, 24, and 96 hours after presentation among STEMI patients enrolled in the Assessment of Pexelizumab in Acute Myocardial Infarction (APEX-MI) trial was performed by Westerhout and colleagues, who reported that the importance of some characteristics, such as heart rate, Killip class, and creatinine declined, whereas the importance of in-hospital events, such as successful reperfusion or cardiogenic shock, became increasingly important. Overall, the final model provided improved discrimination (c-statistic improved from 0.819 at baseline to 0.847 at 96 hours) and more accurately predicted patients at low risk of 90-day mortality.[47] Similarly, Amin and colleagues created a dynamic TIMI Risk Score for STEMI, adding in-hospital events such as recurrent MI, stroke, major bleed, congestive heart failure and/or shock, arrhythmia, and renal failure to create a more comprehensive score with improved discrimination (Figure 11-11).[48] Therefore, dynamic risk modeling, which incorporates data captured at baseline but also at specific time points throughout the course of the hospitalization, may be an effective way to capture changes in overall risk.

Addition of Novel Biomarkers

The use of biomarkers other than cardiac troponin for risk stratification in MI is discussed in Chapter 8. Herein, we offer an additional perspective on the integration of these additional biomarkers into clinical risk stratification.

C-Reactive Protein

Synthesized by hepatocytes in response to chemokine stimulation (especially interleukin-6), the acute-phase systemic inflammatory marker CRP has been studied extensively among patients with atherosclerosis and acute MI, and there is evidence that CRP itself may be involved in the atherothrombotic cascade.[49] CRP levels are elevated in acute MI and generally peak about 72 hours after reperfusion is achieved.[50] Although there is a graded increase in mortality, a CRP level of more than 10 mg/L is associated with the highest risk of cardiovascular mortality. CRP has been used in conjunction with the GRACE Risk Score to predict mortality, but its incremental value is unclear; in one small study of 290 patients with ACS, elevated levels of high-sensitivity CRP were associated with increased in-hospital events, although the addition of high-sensitivity CRP to the GRACE model did not increase the c-statistic (0.705 to 0.718; $P = .46$) or increase net reclassification.[51] As such, although elevated levels of CRP at presentation may predict increased risk of cardiovascular events, its role in addition to well-validated integrated risk scores is unclear.

Natriuretic Peptides

Secreted by the ventricles in response to mechanical stretch and promoting natriuresis and reduction in systemic vascular resistance, B-type natriuretic peptide (BNP) and the N-terminal portion of the pro-BNP peptide (NT–pro-BNP) have been used extensively among patients with heart failure. These natriuretic peptides are also robust predictors of the risk of death and new heart failure across the spectrum of ACS (see Chapter 8). BNP also enhances risk prediction in combination with established risk scores. In an analysis of a French registry presenting with acute MI, older patients with above-median levels of NT–pro-BNP levels and GRACE Risk Scores had a 1-year cardiovascular mortality rate that approached 50%.[52] In a study of 600 patients who presented with NSTE-ACS, the addition of BNP to either the TIMI Risk Score for UA-NSTEMI or the GRACE Risk Score significantly improved discrimination for in-hospital mortality.[53] However, in another study that evaluated the use of BNP in addition to high-sensitivity cardiac troponin T among patients initially stratified by the GRACE Risk Score, BNP did not offer additional prognostic use for 1-year mortality,[54] although the c-statistics were greater than 0.85 for each model.

Growth-Differentiation Factor 15

Growth-differentiation factor 15 (GDF-15) is a cytokine in the transforming growth factor-β superfamily that has been shown in animal models to be upregulated in conditions such as acute myocardial ischemia, reperfusion injury, and heart failure. In an analysis of patients who presented with NSTE-ACS from the GUSTO-IV trial, elevated GDF-15 levels were associated with markedly increased 1-year mortality (14.1% in the highest tertile vs. 1.5% in the lowest tertile; $P < .001$). In addition, a GDF-15 level more than 1800 ng/L was a strong, independent discriminator for mortality (c-statistic = 0.757) and added prognostic information independent of traditional cardiovascular risk factors and biomarkers.[55] Multiple studies have validated the use of GDF-15 in conjunction with validated risk scores to improve mortality prediction after acute MI. Among patients with NSTE-ACS, GDF-15 added to the overall discriminatory capacity of the GRACE risk score for mortality at 5 years (Figure 11-12).[56] Eggers and colleagues found an improvement in discrimination from the GRACE score alone among 453 patients who presented with chest pain.[57] Widera and colleagues described significant improvements in both discrimination (c-statistic from 0.79 to 0.85; $P < .001$) and the net reclassification index (>0 of 0.58; $P = .002$) with the addition of GDF-15 to the GRACE Risk Score among patients who presented with NSTE-ACS.[58]

Suppression of Tumorigenicity 2

Suppression of tumorigenicity 2 (ST2) is a member of the interleukin-1 family, is upregulated during myocardial ischemic and mechanical stress, and is believed to play a role in ventricular remodeling following ischemic injury (see Chapter 8).[59] Plasma ST2 concentration is independently associated with increased mortality in patients with MI, but it is not associated with the risk of recurrent ischemia. Sabatine and colleagues demonstrated a complementary role for risk prediction using ST2 and NT–pro-BNP in addition to clinical risk factors, with an improvement in the c-statistic from 0.82 (95% CI, 0.77 to 0.87) to 0.86 (95% CI, 0.81 to 0.90).[60] Among 677 patients who presented with STEMI, Dhillon and colleagues showed that combining ST2 and NT–pro-BNP with the GRACE Risk Score significantly increased discrimination for 30-day mortality (c-statistic = 0.82 for GRACE Risk Score, 0.90).[60a]

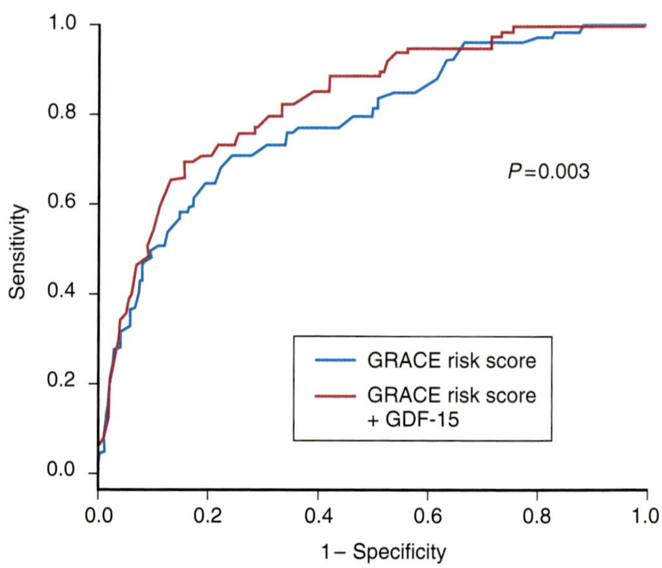

FIGURE 11-12 Receiver-operating characteristic curves demonstrating the incremental benefit of growth-differentiation factor 15 (GDF-15) in conjunction with the GRACE Risk Score for prediction of long-term mortality. *(From Eggers KM, et al: Improving long-term risk prediction in patients with acute chest pain: the Global Registry of Acute Coronary Events [GRACE] risk score is enhanced by selected nonnecrosis biomarkers.* Am Heart J *160:88–94, 2010.)*

Pro-Substance P

Pro-substance P, a more stable surrogate of the tachychinin substance P, has been evaluated in patients who presented with acute MI and was found to be an independent predictor of increased risk of major adverse cardiac events (HR, 1.42; 95% CI, 1.10 to 1.54) and death and/or repeat MI (HR, 1.42; 95% CI, 1.20 to 1.68). Interestingly, when used in conjunction with the GRACE Risk Score, it significantly reclassified patients, especially low-risk patients.[61]

Integrated Biomarker-Based Approaches

Just as combining various clinical and laboratory factors provides an integrated risk score that can accurately discriminate risk, combining biomarkers into a quantitative score would be expected to improve risk prediction. A multimarker approach used by Sabatine and colleagues demonstrated improved prediction of 6-month risk of death, MI, and/or heart failure among ACS patients in the OPUS-TIMI 16 and TACTICS-TIMI 18 Trials.[62,63] O'Malley and colleagues assessed the prognostic implications of a multimarker strategy using markers that have been associated with increased hemodynamic stress: C-terminal pro-vasopressin (copeptin), midregional pro-adrenomedullin, and midregional pro-atrial natriuretic peptide among patients presenting with NSTE-ACS in the MERLIN-TIMI 36 Trial; they found that high concentrations of each biomarker were associated with increased risk of cardiovascular death or heart failure, even after multivariable adjustment. In addition, each biomarker maintained an independent association with cardiovascular death and/or heart failure after adjusting for more commonly used biomarkers such as BNP, troponin I, ST2, pregnancy-associated plasma protein A (PAPP-A), and myeloperoxidase.[64]

Although several studies have demonstrated the feasibility of using a multimarker strategy in risk stratification following acute MI, few studies have demonstrated that such a strategy in conjunction with established risk scores provides clinically compelling improvements in discrimination or reclassifies patients better than a well-validated risk score alone.

Treatment Pathways Based on Early Risk Stratification

The integration of early risk stratification into clinical decision-making differs for STEMI versus NSTEMI. Among patients who present with STEMI, the goal of therapy is timely reperfusion of the occluded vessel. Primary PCI is the preferred method and the dominant form of reperfusion for STEMI (see Chapter 13 and Chapter 17). Nevertheless, fibrinolytic therapy may be reasonable in appropriate patients, especially among low- and intermediate-risk patients who are unable to receive timely primary PCI (see Chapter 14). Claeys and colleagues stratified 5295 patients by the TIMI Risk Score for STEMI and demonstrated a reduction in in-hospital mortality among patients at high risk (TIMI Risk Score ≥7) who underwent primary PCI (23.7% vs. 30.6%; P = .03), but they only found marginal benefit among intermediate-risk patients (2.9% vs. 3.1%; P = .30) and low-risk patients (0.3% vs. 0.4%; P = .60).[65] In the STREAM trial, which evaluated a fibrinolytic strategy among STEMI patients unable to undergo primary PCI within 60 minutes, there was no difference in the primary composite cardiovascular endpoint between the two strategies (HR, 0.86; 95% CI, 0.68 to 1.09). In addition, there was no interaction in the subgroup analysis after stratifying patients by TIMI Risk Score ($P_{interaction}$ = .71).[66]

Among patients with NSTEMI, initial risk stratification is critical in driving the initial management strategy (see Chapter 16). Patients with refractory angina, new or worsening heart failure or mitral regurgitation, hemodynamic instability, recurrent angina, or electrical instability should undergo immediate invasive therapy. However, for other patients who present with definite or likely NSTE-ACS, guidelines currently recommend either an early invasive strategy or an ischemia-driven strategy consisting of initial medical therapy and escalation if ineffective.[36]

Although multiple studies, including comprehensive meta-analyses, have demonstrated that a routine invasive strategy is generally superior to a selective invasive strategy or an ischemia-driven strategy, the latter may be appropriate in low-risk patients, who are defined as having a GRACE score less than 109 or a TIMI Risk Score for UA-NSTEMI of 0 to 1 (see Figure 11-10). Among patients undergoing an invasive strategy, the GRACE Risk Score may be helpful in deciding between an early (coronary angiography within 24 hours) or delayed invasive strategy. In the TIMACS (Timing of Intervention in Acute Coronary Syndrome) study, 3031 patients with NSTE-ACS were randomized to routine early intervention (coronary angiography within 24 hours) or delayed intervention (≥36 hours). Although there was no difference between groups with respect to the primary composite outcome of death, MI, or stroke at 6 months (HR, 0.85; 95% CI, 0.68 to 1.06), an early invasive strategy was superior in patients with a GRACE Risk Score of more than 140 (HR, 0.65; 95% CI, 0.48 to 0.89).[67] Therefore, current guidelines support an early invasive strategy among patients with a GRACE Risk Score of more than 140 (estimated risk of in-hospital death >3%), serial elevation in cardiac troponin, or new ST-segment depression. A delayed invasive strategy (coronary angiography within 25 to 72 hours) may be appropriate among patients with a GRACE Risk Score of 109 to 140 or a TIMI Risk Score ≥2, diabetes, renal insufficiency, recent PCI, previous coronary artery bypass graft surgery, or left ventricular systolic dysfunction.[36]

PREDISCHARGE RISK STRATIFICATION

Use of Noninvasive Testing for Ischemia

The use of noninvasive testing in patients following acute MI is discussed in Chapter 30. In 1979, Theroux and colleagues demonstrated that patients with an abnormal limited treadmill test 1 day before discharge following an MI had increased rates of angina and mortality at 1 year (P <.001), findings that have since been confirmed across the spectrum of ACS. Therefore, in STEMI patients, current guidelines offer a class I recommendation for noninvasive testing for ischemia before discharge among patients who have not undergone coronary angiography and do not have high-risk features for which angiography would be warranted, and a class IIb indication for noninvasive testing to identify the functional significance of a lesion detected at angiography and to guide a postdischarge exercise prescription.[39]

For patients who present with NSTEMI, noninvasive imaging may be a useful tool to identify patients at high risk for whom an invasive strategy may be more appropriate. Current guidelines support the use of noninvasive testing in

coronary artery disease and an unstable coronary lesion precipitating ACS. Although the presence of known coronary artery disease increases the probability of developing ACS, patients with stable coronary artery disease commonly present with nonischemic or even noncardiac causes of chest symptoms. Patients can have underlying asymptomatic coronary artery disease and present with symptomatic gastrointestinal reflux disease (GERD) symptoms. Thus, diagnosing the presence of coronary artery disease does not equate to a diagnosis of ACS—a mistake that is commonly made in both clinical practice and clinical investigation. The clinical scenario of presentation is essential to making the diagnosis of ACS.

Identifying the Low-Probability Patient

Although many different algorithms are available for defining a low probability for the presence of ACS, all classification systems incorporate elements of history, physical examination, electrocardiogram, and cardiac biomarkers (see also Chapter 6). Defining low probability is, in this sense, excluding those clinical features that identify a high-probability patient. Specifically, patients are considered to have a low probability for ACS if they do not have typical chest pain symptoms, including angina similar to previous angina, or chest and left arm pain or discomfort (see Figure 6-4). Low-probability patients tend to be younger and have fewer identifiable cardiovascular disease risk factors. Under this paradigm, it is difficult for example to categorize a patient older than 70 years of age with a history of diabetes as inherently having a low probability for ACS, regardless of the clinical scenario. On physical examination, the low-probability patient should be free of any evidence of volume overload or extracardiac vascular disease. Patients are considered to be in the low-probability group if their ECG is normal in terms of ischemic changes or demonstrates, at most, T-wave flattening or inversions of less than 0.1 mV. Perhaps most important, initial levels of biomarkers in a low-probability patient should be normal.

Epidemiology of Low-Probability Patients

A majority of patients who present with chest pain have either a low- or an intermediate-probability for presence of unstable coronary artery disease. It is difficult to accurately estimate the exact proportion of patients classified as low probability, because of variable definitions of low probability across clinical studies, which also span heterogeneous cohorts. With those caveats, between 25% and 40% of all patients presenting with chest pain appear to have a low probability for ACS.

ACCELERATED DIAGNOSTIC PROTOCOLS

Most strategies to identify and appropriately triage patients with a low probability for ACS are based on some type of accelerated diagnostic protocol. These protocols may be implemented in the ED, in dedicated chest pain units, and on inpatient wards. Current reimbursement in United States rewards shorter hospital stays, with the goal of more patients discharged directly from the ED and limiting in-hospital stays to less than 24 hours. Thus, the metrics of a successful algorithm, in addition to ensuring a very low rate of missed ACS cases, include time until discharge and need for subsequent testing.

Risk Scores

A variety of clinical risk scores have been proposed for the evaluation of patients with suspected ischemic symptoms. Some are specifically derived from broad populations of patients with chest pain, whereas others either implement or modify existing clinical risk scores that were originally derived in patients with established ACS. A key principle of such scores is that the chance of a final diagnosis of an MI is extremely small in a low-probability population. Comparison of the performance of one score versus another is challenging because of differences in the inclusion criteria between studies and which biomarker of necrosis was measured. For example, the same risk score tool will perform substantially differently if cTn is used instead of creatine kinase–myocardial biomarker (CK-MB) (see Chapter 1 and Chapter 7).

Goldman and colleagues proposed one of the earliest comprehensive algorithms three decades ago. Many of the subsequently developed algorithms have utilized risk scores such as Thrombolysis in Myocardial Infarction (TIMI) Risk Score, the Global Registry of Acute Coronary Events (GRACE) Risk Score, and the PURSUIT Risk Score,[3] which originally were derived and validated in clinical trials or registries of patients with confirmed ACS (see Chapter 11). By design, these risk scores predict major cardiovascular outcomes in patients with ACS and are neither sensitive nor specific enough alone to use for the *diagnosis* of ACS. Even modifying the TIMI risk score[4] by giving more weight to abnormal cTn levels or ECG changes may still not be sensitive enough at scores of 0 to allow early discharge.[5]

Other studies derived new scores with the specific goal of identifying the population of low-probability patients who could be discharged safely without subsequent testing; such scores have seen limitations to wide implementation, however, because the false-negative or "miss" rate has not consistently been demonstrated to be below the commonly accepted threshold of 1%. One of the most extensively validated risk scores for chest pain is the HEART Score, which evaluates patients on five domains—history, ECG, age, risk factors, and troponin— to generate a score from 0 to 10 (see Figure 6-6). In validation studies, the risk of a subsequent cardiac event was less than 1% in the roughly one third of patients with a low HEART Score (0 to 3).[6]

All of the diagnostic risk scores use a biomarker of cardiac necrosis. The inclusion of cTn improves the diagnostic performance of all risk scores, but as discussed further on in this chapter, a single measurement of cTn is not always sufficiently sensitive to exclude a diagnosis of ACS.

A dynamic risk score is one that will incorporate additional data collected after the initial presentation. Most algorithms for identifying low- or intermediate-probability patients need to be dynamic, because no single test or algorithm is sufficiently sensitive or specific when based on the initial clinical and biochemical assessment alone.

"Rule Out Myocardial Infarction"

Historically, patients presenting with suspected ischemic syndromes were given the classic diagnosis of "rule out MI" ("R/O MI"), which was actually a diagnostic strategy rather than a diagnosis. The strategy included serial ECGs and biomarker measurements 8 hours apart (usually a total of three), followed by an exercise stress test. With the transition from CK-MB to cTn, many institutions now omit the third biomarker assessment and shorten the interval between measurements to 3 to 6 hours (see Chapter 7). Even with a reduced number of biomarker measurements and shorter time intervals, the evaluation may require 18 to 36 hours, depending on the availability of a stress testing protocol. Accordingly, efforts have now focused on identifying better algorithms that will facilitate the early triage and discharge of patients with a low probability for ACS.

Shortening the interval between repeat biomarker assessments is one of the easiest ways to accelerate a dynamic protocol, but the question of how short the interval can be remains controversial (see also Chapter 7). With earlier generations of biochemical assays, poor analytic performance and relatively high diagnostic cutpoints limited the detection of an early rise in biomarkers or low levels of cardiac injury. This shortcoming was partially overcome in the original R/O MI protocols by requiring 6 to 8 hours between CK-MB assays. Even early cTn assays, although superior to CK-MB assays, lacked the sensitivity to detect necrosis early after event onset, and use of serial measurements at similar intervals was required to maintain adequate sensitivity. With the introduction of newer-generation assays for cTn (not including the high-sensitivity assays discussed further on), troponin testing can be done at reduced intervals of 0 and 3 hours, with some algorithms using 2-hour intervals.

Integrated Algorithms

Most contemporary chest pain algorithms incorporate an assessment of probability based on clinical presentation combined with two sequential cTn measurements. One relatively simple algorithm, the North American Chest Pain Rule (see Figure 6-6), accurately identified a low-probability population by combining just one troponin assay with three clinical features in patients 40 years of age or younger, with use of two sequential troponin measurements for patients 40 to 50 years of age.[7] Unfortunately, this algorithm did not perform well in patients older than 60 years, highlighting the problems of excluding ACS in patients with higher pretest probability of disease.

The HEART Score, which used data from clinical presentation, was updated into the HEART Pathway by integrating serial troponin measurements at 0 and 3 hours[8] (Figure 12-2). Patients deemed to have a low probability for ACS based on the Heart Pathway (HEART Score 0 to 3 and negative serial cTn assays), who accounted for roughly 50% of the population studied, were discharged home from the ED without further testing. In a randomized trial compared with standard care, the HEART Pathway decreased the frequency of cardiac testing, lowered length of hospital stay by 12 hours, and increased the proportion of patients discharged early. No patients within the low-risk group experienced a subsequent cardiac event.

At our institution, we have integrated the HEART Score into a dynamic algorithm for the diagnosis of suspected ACS. In our algorithm, patients with a low HEART Score at admission can be discharged if symptom onset was more than 6 hours before presentation. Because we do not utilize a high-sensitive troponin assay, if a patient presents within 6 hours of symptom onset, we order a second cTn at 3 hours. If that value is also below the 99th percentile, then the patient can be discharged home without further testing (Figure 12-3).

Several studies have evaluated an accelerated diagnostic protocol using 0- and 2-hour conventional cTn assays in combination with the TIMI Risk Score. The observational Asia-Pacific Evaluation of Chest Pain Trial (ASPECT) study included 3582 patients who presented with at least 5 minutes of chest pain and without ST-segment elevation. Among the 352 patients (9.8%) classified as having a low probability for ACS—a TIMI Risk Score of 0, no new ischemic ECG changes, and negative 0- and 2-hour troponin measurements—only 3 (0.9%) patients had a subsequent cardiac event. The major limitation of this protocol is that most patients with chest pain in this cohort (approximately 90%) did not fulfill the strict criteria for early discharge without subsequent testing, thus limiting its overall utility.[9] The ASPECT accelerated diagnostic protocol was prospectively evaluated in a randomized pilot study. The accelerated protocol doubled the number of patients discharged within 6 hours compared with the standard algorithm of troponin assays at 6 to 12 hours after the onset of pain, although this study was too small to definitively ascertain whether this algorithm maintained an acceptable "false" rate.[10] Another, larger study evaluated the same protocol in a cohort of patients from North America. Overall, almost 50% of the patients fit the low-probability criteria, and in this population, only 5 patients (0.9%) experienced a major cardiac event within the next 30 days. Because this study was embedded within a trial specifically designed to enroll only low- to intermediate-probability patients in evaluating the role of CT angiography (CTA), the proportion of low-probability patients is likely to be artificially high; however, the subsequent event rate of 0.9% also may be falsely elevated, because four of the five cardiac events were associated with revascularization procedures, whose clinical significance is difficult to interpret in that CTA, rather than symptoms, drove the decision for coronary revascularization.[11]

TROPONIN IN THE LOW-PROBABILITY PATIENT

Cardiac troponin is the preferred marker for myocardial necrosis and constitutes a cornerstone of laboratory evaluation in patients with suspected ischemic symptoms (see Chapter 7). Many hospitals have "retired" the CK assay, except to detect postrevascularization necrosis or to detect reinfarction when troponin is still elevated from the initial event.

High-Sensitivity Assays for Cardiac Troponin

The introduction of more sensitive troponin assays has significantly altered the approach to the patient with a low probability for ischemia. Multiple studies have now demonstrated that more sensitive assays for cTn are able to (1) detect myocardial damage at levels well below those for conventional assays, thus shifting the diagnosis of unstable angina to MI (see Chapter 1)[12]; and (2) identify necrosis earlier than older assays (Figure 12-4). Thus, high-sensitivity assays for troponin (hsTn) further improve the ability to identify those patients with the lowest probability for ACS. The concurrent increase in the proportion of patients without ACS who have elevated values of hsTn is discussed in Chapter 7. The gain in sensitivity for identifying myocardial necrosis (of any type) necessarily diminishes specificity for the diagnosis of ACS. Similarly, a nondetectable hsTn level increases the sensitivity for ruling out ACS,

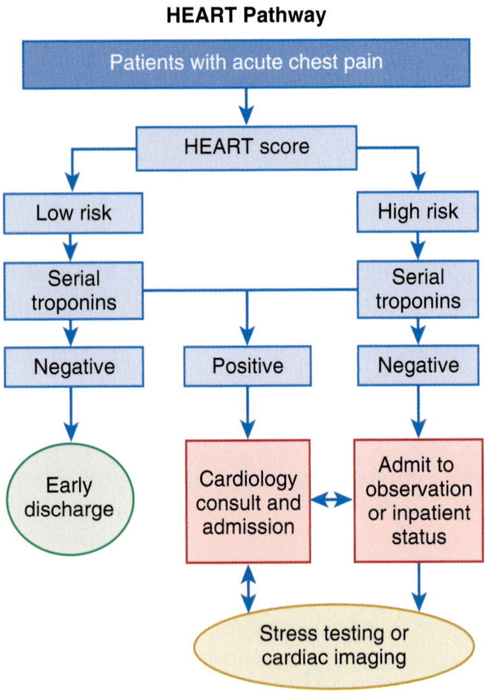

Patient ID __________
☐ Initial Assessment
☐ Second Assessment

HEART Score:

History:

High-Risk Features:
- Middle- or left-sided
- Heavy chest pain
- Diaphoresis
- Radiation
- Nausea/vomiting
- Exertional
- Relief of symptoms by sublingual nitrates

Low-Risk Features:
- Well localized
- Sharp pain
- Nonexertional
- No diaphoresis
- No nausea/vomiting

☐ Highly suspicious	**2 points**	**Mostly high-risk features**
☐ Moderately suspicious	**1 point**	**Mixture of high-risk and low-risk features**
☐ Slightly suspicious	**0 points**	**Mostly low-risk features**

ECG:

☐ New ischemic changes	**2 points**	• Ischemic ST-segment depression • New ischemic T-wave inversions
☐ Nonspecific changes	**1 point**	• Repolarization abnormalites • Nonspecific T wave changes • Nonspecific ST-segment depression or elevation • Bundle branch blocks • Pacemaker rhythms • Left ventricular hypertrophy • Early repolarization • Digoxin effect
☐ Normal	**0 points**	**• Completely normal**

Age:

☐ ≥65	**2 points**
☐ 45–64	**1 point**
☐ <45	**0 points**

Risk Factors:

☐ Obesity (BMI ≥30)
☐ Current or recent (≤90 days) smoker
☐ Currently treated diabetes mellitus
☐ Family history of CAD (1st degree relative <55 years)
☐ Diagnosed and/or treated hypertension
☐ Hypercholesterolemia

☐ Three or more risk factors listed above **OR** any of the following: ☐ Known CAD ☐ Prior stroke ☐ Peripheral arterial disease	**2 points**
☐ 1–2 risk factors	**1 point**
☐ No risk factors	**0 points**

Troponin (initial)

☐ >0.120 ng/mL	**2 points**	NB: The troponin cut-points listed are specific to the assay used by this hospital and must be determined for each assay.
☐ 0.041–0.120 ng/mL	**1 point**	
☐ 0–0.040 ng/mL	**0 points**	

HEART Score (total points) ________ Add points from each category above

Serial 3-Hour Troponin Measurement:
☐ Normal
☐ Positive

HEART Pathway:
☐ High Risk = HEART score 4 or more, or any positive troponin
☐ Low Risk = HEART score 0–3 and negative troponins at 0 and 3 hours

Attending Signature:______________________________ Date: ____________

Attending Name:______________________________

FIGURE 12-2 **HEART Pathway algorithm *(left)* and HEART Pathway assessment form *(right)*.** *BMI,* Body mass index; *CAD,* coronary artery disease; *ECG,* electrocardiogram. *(From Mahler SA, Miller CD, Litt HI, et al: Performance of the 2-hour accelerated diagnostic protocol within the American College of Radiology Imaging Network PA 4005 cohort.* Acad Emerg Med *22:452-460, 2015.)*

although at the price of identifying fewer patients in this low-probability category. Because hsTn assays are not commercially available in the United States, most of the "real world" data on hsTn comes from Europe, where it has been used in clinical practice for years and has now been advocated for use in a 1-hour rule-out approach in the European Society of Cardiology guidelines for the management of NSTE-ACS.[13]

When used alone, hsTn assays have negative predictive values ranging from 92% to 100%. The diagnostic accuracy is lower when measured early after the onset of symptoms (less than 2 hours) but is still superior to that of conventional cTn assays.[14,15] The variability in negative predictive values between studies is due to the differences in the study populations, the timing of testing in relationship to symptoms, analytic properties of the assay, and most important, the cutpoint used. For example, using a cutpoint of the lower level of detection (e.g., below 3 ng/L for the Roche hsTnT assay) gives a much higher negative predictive value than using the 99th percentile cutpoint (14 ng/L). The tradeoff of using the lower threshold is that fewer patients will be categorized as low probability.[16]

SCAMPs Data Form
Attending Physician: ___________________
Combined Chest Pain SCAMP: Emergency Department

PATIENT IDENTIFICATION AREA

MRN: ______________________

Name: ______________________

Date: ______________________

Presentation highly concerning for ACS:
☐ STEMI ☐ Unstable angina
☐ Definite NSTEMI ☐ Rest angina
☐ Dynamic ECG changes ☐ New-onset angina
☐ Increasing angina

☐ YES → ☐ Admit to cardiology ☐ Admit to cath lab (form complete)

☐ NO ↓

Admitting or discharging patient for diagnosis unrelated to cardiac chest pain

☐ YES →

Cardiac
☐ Heart failure
☐ Arrhythmia
☐ Other noncoronary cardiac disease __________
Noncardiac
☐ Musculoskeletal
☐ Gastrointestinal
☐ Pulmonary
☐ Other:__________

→ Best clinical judgment for management (form complete)

☐ NO ↓

HEART Score for Chest Pain	2 points	1 point	0 points	Total
History:	☐ Highly suspicious	☐ Moderately suspicious	☐ Slightly or nonsuspicious	
ECG:	☐ Significant ST-depression	☐ Nonspecific repolarization disturbance	☐ Normal	
Age:	☐ ≥65 years	☐ >45–<65 years	☐ ≤45 years	
Risk factors: (diabetes mellitus, current smoker, hypertension, hypercholesterolemia, family history of CAD)	☐ ≥3 risk factors, or history of atherosclerotic disease	☐ 1 or 2 risk factors	☐ No risk factors known	
Troponin:	☐ ≥0.03 ng/mL	☐ ≥0.01 to <0.03ng/mL	☐ <assay	
			HEART Score:	

☐ 7–10 points → **SCAMP Probability: High**

SCAMP recommendation:

Admit to Cardiology

SCAMP Recommends: Consult patient's cardiologist

☐ Patient's cardiologist: ☐ BWH ☐ Outside
What action did you take:
☐ I spoke with cardiologist
☐ I did not attempt to contact cardiologist
☐ I was unable to reach cardiologist
☐ Patient does not have a cardiologist

YOUR PLAN OF CARE:

☐ Admit to the hospital as an inpatient:
☐ Cardiology
☐ Medicine/Other, because:__________
____

☐ Assign to ED Observation, because:
☐ Recommendation of cardiologist
☐ Other: __________
____

☐ Discharge home, because:
☐ Recommendation of cardiologist
☐ Other: __________
____

☐ Consult Cardiology, because:
☐ Other: __________

☐ 4–6 points → **SCAMP Probability: Intermediate**

SCAMP recommendation:

Assign to ED Observation Unit for 8 hours

SCAMP Recommends: Consult patient's cardiologist

☐ Patient's cardiologist: ☐ BWH ☐ Outside
What action did you take:
☐ I spoke with cardiologist
☐ I did not attempt to contact cardiologist
☐ I was unable to reach cardiologist
☐ Patient does not have a cardiologist

YOUR PLAN OF CARE:

☐ Assign to ED Observation Unit

☐ Admit to the hospital as an inpatient:
☐Cardiology ☐ Medicine/Other
REASON:
☐ ED Observation is full
☐ Recommendation of cardiologist
☐ Other: __________

☐ Keep in ED (not assigned to Observation): (CONTINUE ON BACK)
Additional troponin at:
☐ 3 hours ☐ 6 hours ☐ Other:__________
REASON:
☐ ED Observation is full
☐ Other: __________

☐ Discharge home without 2nd troponin, because:
☐ Recommendation of cardiologist
☐ Other: __________

☐ 0–3 points → **SCAMP Probability: Low**

SCAMP recommendation:
>6 hours since last episode → discharge patient
≤6 hours since last episode of pain → Order 3-hour troponin

SCAMP Recommends: Consult patient's cardiologist

☐ Patient's cardiologist: ☐ BWH ☐ Outside
What action did you take:
☐ I spoke with cardiologist
☐ I did not attempt to contact cardiologist
☐ I was unable to reach cardiologist
☐ Patient does not have a cardiologist

YOUR PLAN OF CARE:

☐ Order additional troponin in ED (CONTINUE ON BACK)
☐ 3 hours ☐ 6 hours, because:__________

☐ Admit to the hospital as an inpatient:
☐Cardiology ☐ Medicine/Other
REASON:
☐ ED Observation is full
☐ Patient's nursing care needs
☐ Recommendation of cardiologist
☐ Other: __________

☐ Assign to ED Observation, because:
☐ Recommendation of cardiologist
☐ Other: __________

☐ Discharge home without 2nd troponin, because:
☐ >6 hours since last episode of pain
☐ Recommendation of cardiologist
☐ Other: __________

FIGURE 12-3 Brigham and Women's Hospital (BWH) Evaluation of Chest Pain Algorithm. This practice pathway, designated a Standardized Clinical Assessment and Management Plan (SCAMP) (Institute for Relevant Clinical Data Analytics, Inc., Boston, MA; http://www.scamps.org), uses the HEART Score to categorize patients into low-, intermediate-, and high-probability categories. For low-probability patients, if symptoms started earlier than 6 hours before presentation and the initial troponin assay is negative, they can be discharged home immediately. If symptom onset was at 6 hours or less before presentation, another troponin level is measured 3 hours later, and if the result is negative, the patient is discharged home. Intermediate-probability patients are admitted to the emergency department for further observation or testing. The recommendation of the algorithm is to arrange for outpatient noninvasive testing whenever feasible to expedite discharge. *ACS,* Acute coronary syndrome; *CAD,* coronary artery disease; *ED,* emergency department; *ECG,* electrocardiogram; *NSTEMI,* non–ST-elevation myocardial infarction; *PCP,* primary care provider; *STEMI,* ST-elevation myocardial infarction.

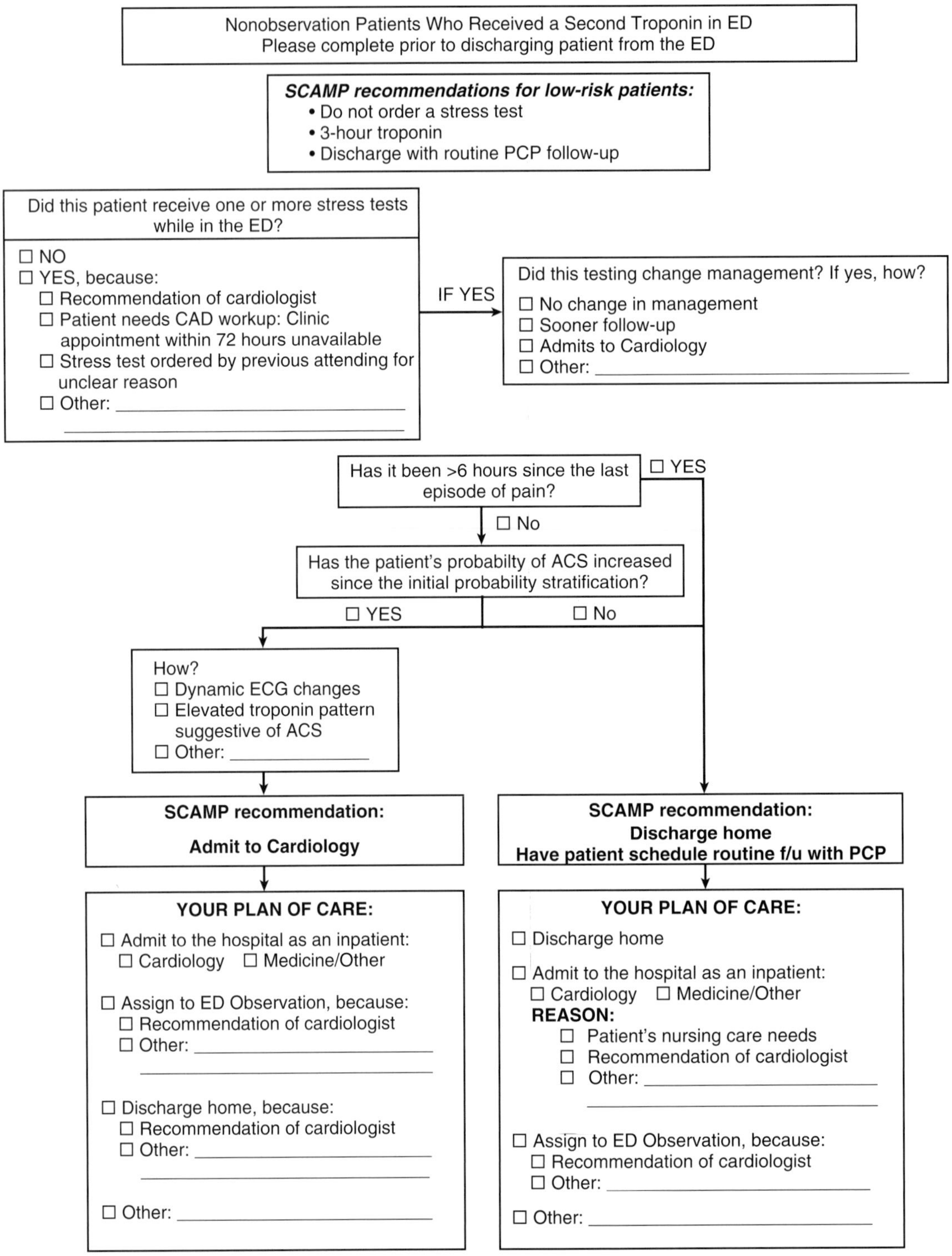

FIGURE 12-3, Cont'd

However, a test with a negative predictive value less than 99% typically is not acceptable in the early identification of patients who can be safely discharged from the ED after just one measurement. Therefore, most studies using hsTn either incorporate other clinical data such as ECG findings or propose rapid reassessment of hsTn with serial measurements. One large cohort study of 14,636 subjects found a 99.8% negative predictive value in patients presenting with chest discomfort who had a very low level of hsTnT (less than 5 ng/L) and no ischemic changes on the ECG.[17] Of the 39 patients with hsTnT levels below 5 ng/L who eventually were diagnosed with an MI, 24 had ischemic ECG changes. Thus, the ECG should always remain central to the evaluation of these patients, even with the use of hsTn. Other groups have advocated using higher hsTn level cutpoints (below 14 ng/L) but with a more detailed clinical assessment (e.g., modified Goldman criteria) and a normal ECG pattern to identify a larger proportion of patients who can be safely discharged early (Table 12-1). The goal is to try to improve specificity of the algorithm over that of hsTn alone, which has very high sensitivity (approximately 100%) but relatively low specificity for ACS. Using this algorithm, the proportion of patients who could be safely discharged at the initial hsTn increased from 7.9% and 29.3% using cutpoints of 3 and 5 ng/L, respectively, to 39.8%.[18]

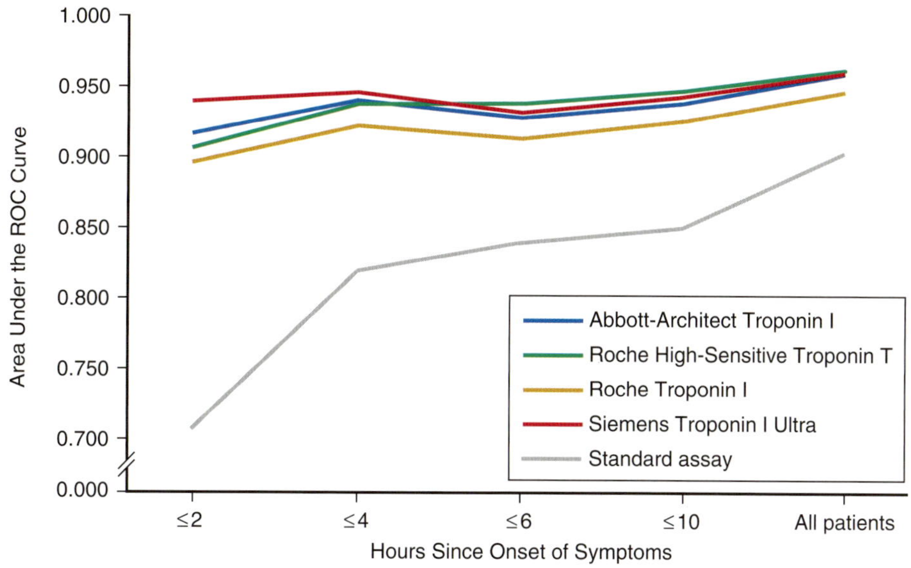

FIGURE 12-4 Diagnostic accuracy of different troponin assays according to time since symptom onset. The sensitivity for identifying patients with a myocardial infarction is less than 70% in patients with symptom onset less than 2 hours earlier and is still less than 90% at 10 hours. By contrast, the sensitivity of new-generation assays is greater than 90% at 2 hours. The area under the receiver-operating-characteristic (ROC) curve is shown, according to time since the onset of chest pain, for the four sensitive cardiac troponin assays and the standard assay performed on blood samples obtained at presentation for the diagnosis of acute myocardial infarction. *(From Reichlin T, Hochholzer W, Bassetti S, et al: Early diagnosis of myocardial infarction with sensitive cardiac troponin assays.* N Engl J Med *361:858-867, 2009.)*

TABLE 12-1 The Modified Goldman Score and the TRUST Accelerated Diagnostic Protocol (ADP)

Modified Goldman Score	
RISK FACTOR	**SCORING (1 POINT FOR EACH VARIABLE PRESENT)**
Typical new-onset chest pain at rest	
Pain the same as previous myocardial infarction	
Pain not relieved by glyceryl trinitrate (GTN) spray within 15 minutes	
Pain lasting more than 60 minutes	
Pain occurring with increasing frequency	
Hypotension (systolic blood pressure <100 mm Hg)	
Acute shortness of breath	
Pain within 6 weeks of a myocardial infarction or revascularization procedure	
Modified Goldman score total	*(0-8)*
TRUST ADP	
CATEGORY	**DIAGNOSTIC CRITERIA**
Low risk* (suitable for discharge)	Modified Goldman score ≤1 Nonischemic ECG pattern Presentation high-sensitivity troponin T <14 ng/L
Not low risk	Modified Goldman score >1 Ischemic ECG changes Presentation high-sensitivity troponin T ≥14 ng/L

**Safety point*: Protocol not validated in patients 80 years of age and older.
ECG, Electrocardiogram; *TRUST*, Triage Rule-out Using High-Sensitivity Troponin.
From Carlton EW, Cullen L, Than M, et al: A novel diagnostic protocol to identify patients suitable for discharge after a single high-sensitivity troponin. Heart *101:1041-1046, 2015.*

Other investigations have proposed more rapid diagnostic protocols using a second serial hsTnT measurement 1 or 2 hours apart. In a study using hsTnI, the negative predictive value for an acute coronary event was 100% in the 20% to 25% of the cohort who met low-probability criteria based on two undetectable hsTnI measurements and a TIMI score of 0. Using a TIMI risk score of 0-1 included approximately 50% more patients in the low-probability group, and the negative predictive value fell to only 99.7%.[19] In another cohort of 1042 patients, use of an hsTnI level of 6 ng/L or less at 0 and 1 hours had a negative predictive value of 99.7% and identified almost 40% of the patients for potential rapid discharge.[20]

Another strategy employs the change in hsTnT over a short period of observation. In a study of 1665 patients, the combination of an initial hsTnT level below 12 ng/L and an absolute change in hsTnT of less than 3 ng/L at 1 hour after presentation maintained a 100% negative predictive value (see Figure 7-4).[21] This approach was validated in another cohort of 1320 patients, achieving a negative predictive value of 99.9% (i.e., there was one missed MI case)[22] (Figure 12-e1). Findings from this group support that using an absolute change criterion, rather than a relative change, is more accurate in identifying the patients with a low probability for ACS.[23] The use of such 1-hour "rule-out" strategies has now been recommended for incorporation in European professional society guidelines[13] but has not yet achieved consensus among experts in the United States (see Chapter 7).

NONINVASIVE TESTING

In view of the high negative predictive value of many of the accelerated diagnostic protocols that utilize newer-generation or hsTn assays, the benefit of additional testing in low-probability patients is questionable. What additional test, for example, can improve on a negative predictive value of greater than 99%? The elimination of confirmatory functional or anatomic testing from the algorithm for managing patients with suspected ischemic symptoms would be a natural evolution in care, but such revision represents a major shift in the diagnostic paradigm for the evaluation of ACS.

Two categories of tests are available to confirm that the patient does not have ACS. Functional, or "provocative" testing, is just that—a test to provoke ischemia. The exercise treadmill test (ETT), the classic functional test, is considered "positive" if it generates typical reproducible symptoms, ST-segment depression, or a drop in blood pressure. In a patient with an unstable coronary syndrome, presumably with little ischemic reserve, one would expect the symptoms to begin at a low workload. Reconciling the diagnosis of an ACS with chest pain precipitated only in stage 4 of a standard Bruce protocol is challenging, and such chest pain is more likely to represent stable coronary disease in a patient with noncardiac symptoms at rest. A pharmacologic vasodilatory stress test poses a similar problem because it cannot identify "low-level" ischemia. Imaging studies, either myocardial perfusion imaging (MPI), echocardiography, or magnetic resonance imaging, typically improve the sensitivity and specificity of a standard ETT; however, the additional imaging should be used in patients with abnormal baseline ECG findings and in those unable to exercise.

Of the functional tests, rest myocardial imaging, which uses either radiopharmaceutical labeling or echocardiography to identify ischemic areas at rest in patients with active pain, is the most intuitively rational test to exclude ACS (see Chapter 9). In studies of patients with acute chest pain rest MPI has a negative predictive value of 99% to 100%; in practice, however, mobilizing the resources to perform the test while the patient is experiencing chest pain is challenging. Moreover, most of the studies of rest MPI or echo were done before the widespread use of sensitive cTn assays.[1]

The use of computed tomography angiography (CTA) as "anatomic" noninvasive testing is discussed in detail in Chapter 9. Together, the completed studies of patients with suspected ischemic pain indicate that a strategy using CTA significantly reduces time to discharge from the ED but increases downstream testing, including invasive testing, and radiation exposure.[24-26] Totally normal findings on CTA are reassuring in terms of excluding a diagnosis of ACS; however, the detection of a coronary lesion does not in itself indicate whether it is the "culprit" lesion or just an asymptomatic stenosis unrelated to the presenting symptoms. Perhaps more than any other noninvasive test, careful patient selection is critical to the utility of CTA in diagnosing ACS.

When Should Additional Noninvasive Testing Be Performed?

The earliest chest pain algorithms observed patients for 48 hours for "stabilization" before any provocative testing. With time, intervals between cTn testing have progressively shortened, but even the most recent consensus statements still recommend performing a treadmill ECG with or without imaging in patients with normal serial ECGs and biomarkers. In the past, it was felt that this provocative test must be completed before discharge, although now the guidelines allow that it can be performed as an outpatient procedure, within 72 hours of discharge.[27] Current recommendations from the American Heart Association/American College of Cardiology (AHA/ACC) are presented in Table 12-2. Reflective of the uncertainty surrounding the best management of these patients is the class of recommendation (IIa) and the level of evidence (mostly B or C). Moreover, these recommendations speak of "possible ACS," which is more consistent with a clinical category of intermediate probability rather than low probability. The argument for eliminating the subsequent testing after a negative result for an accelerated diagnostic protocol (ADP) rests on the fact that if the pretest probability ACS is low (in this case, less than 1%, based on the literature reviewed earlier), then the value of an additional test, no matter how sensitive or specific, is minimal.

The results of noninvasive diagnostic testing are most likely to influence subsequent decisions when the pretest probability of ACS is in the intermediate range. In the patient whose diagnosis is uncertain after the initial assessment, such as a 50-year-old patient with typical chest pain and several risk factors for or known coronary disease but normal ECG or biomarker levels, noninvasive testing would helpful for establishing or excluding the diagnosis of ACS. If this patient's pretest probability of ACS was approximately 50%, an early positive stress test result would increase the likelihood of ischemia (posttest probability of approximately 85%), whereas a negative result on exercise testing dramatically reduces the likelihood (posttest probability less than 10%). By contrast, an abnormal result on exercise testing in a 35-year-old woman with atypical chest pain and normal ECG and biomarker levels (pretest probability of ACS of 1%) is likely to represent a false positive, prompting the use of unnecessary medications or invasive diagnostic testing; a negative result would simply support a low index of clinical suspicion for coronary heart disease (CHD). Therefore, noninvasive testing in such a low-risk patient would not be helpful (see Figure 12-1).

Even the value of testing in the intermediate-probability patients has been challenged. A recent observational study identified 4181 patients admitted to an observational unit with acute chest pain who also, per protocol, underwent a functional study (ETT or MPI). Almost three fourths of the patients were classified as having an intermediate probability (10% to 90%) for CAD, and less than 20% had a very low or low probability. Routine provocative cardiac testing showed ischemia in 470 patients (11.2%). Of the 123 who subsequently underwent angiography, 63 (1.5%) had a new diagnosis of obstructive disease, and only 28 (0.7%) had lesions that warranted revascularization. Only 1.5% of intermediate-probability patients and 0.75% of very-low- or low-probability patients had obstructive coronary disease.[28]

TABLE 12-2 Discharge from the Emergency Department or Chest Pain Unit: Class IIa Recommendations

1. It is reasonable to observe patients with symptoms consistent with ACS without objective evidence of myocardial ischemia (nonischemic initial ECG and normal cardiac troponin) in a chest pain unit or telemetry unit with serial ECGs and cardiac troponin measurements at 3- to 6-hour intervals (*level of evidence*: B).
2. It is reasonable for patients with possible ACS who have normal serial ECGs and cardiac troponin levels to have a treadmill ECG (*level of evidence*: A), stress myocardial perfusion imaging, or stress echocardiography before discharge or within 72 hours after discharge (*level of evidence*: B).
3. In patients with possible ACS and a normal ECG, normal cardiac troponins, and no history of CAD, it is reasonable to initially perform (without serial ECGs and troponin assays) coronary CT angiography to assess coronary artery anatomy (*level of evidence*: A) or at-rest myocardial perfusion imaging with a technetium-99m radiopharmaceutical to exclude myocardial ischemia (*level of evidence*: B).
4. It is reasonable to give low-risk patients who are referred for outpatient testing daily aspirin, short-acting nitroglycerin, and other medication if appropriate (e.g., beta blockers), with instructions about activity level and clinician follow-up (*level of evidence*: C).

ACS, Acute coronary syndrome; *CAD*, coronary artery disease; *ECG*, electrocardiogram.
From Amsterdam EA, Wenger NK, Brindis RG, et al: 2014 AHA/ACC Guideline for the Management of Patients with Non-ST-Elevation Acute Coronary Syndromes: A report of the American College of Cardiology/American Heart Association Task Force on Practice Guidelines. J Am Coll Cardiol *64:e139-e228, 2014.*

Further supporting the concept of discharging patients with a low probability for presence of ACS without any testing are the results of one of the CTA studies that measured hsTnT and found that in patients with undetectable hsTnT, the median calcium score was 0. Only 11% had evidence of any atherosclerosis, and none had stenosis greater than 50%.[29] With use of the less sensitive conventional troponin assay, however, 12.5% of patients with an undetectable level of troponin had stenosis with greater than 70% occlusion.

Subsequent diagnostic testing still may play a role in the evaluation of "intermediate-probability" patients, many of whom will not require hospital admission but can be managed within the ED and/or in observation units, thereby preventing hospital admissions and additional health care costs. In addition, as emphasized in the most recent guidelines, even intermediate-probability patients can be discharged home with planned outpatient testing within 72 hours.[27] The most challenging component of a strategy of discharge before testing is establishing a system of care that ensures that the discharged patient will receive appropriate follow-up care. The transfer of responsibility from the physician providing the initial care to the outpatient physician is the critical link.

SUMMARY

Considering the number of patients presenting with suspected MI, the magnitude of associated health care resources, and the decades of research into ACS, the management and evaluation of patients with acute chest pain have remained very much an "art," relying as much on clinical suspicion as on objective data. Moreover, entrenched practice patterns, designed to prevent any missed cases of MI, are slow to change in response to newer assays of myocardial necrosis, which, together with simple clinical criteria, can identify a large population of patients who can be discharged home safely with the reassurance that they are at extremely low risk for subsequent ischemic events. Changing practice culture, especially one so intertwined with divergent incentives (e.g., principle of beneficence, medicolegal issues, reimbursement rules), is challenging. A collaborative, integrated approach (Figure 12-5) that leverages ED, cardiology, and outpatient follow-up evaluation offers the greatest potential to expedite the investigation of chest pain, minimize unnecessary testing, and identify those patients who require urgent management of ACS.

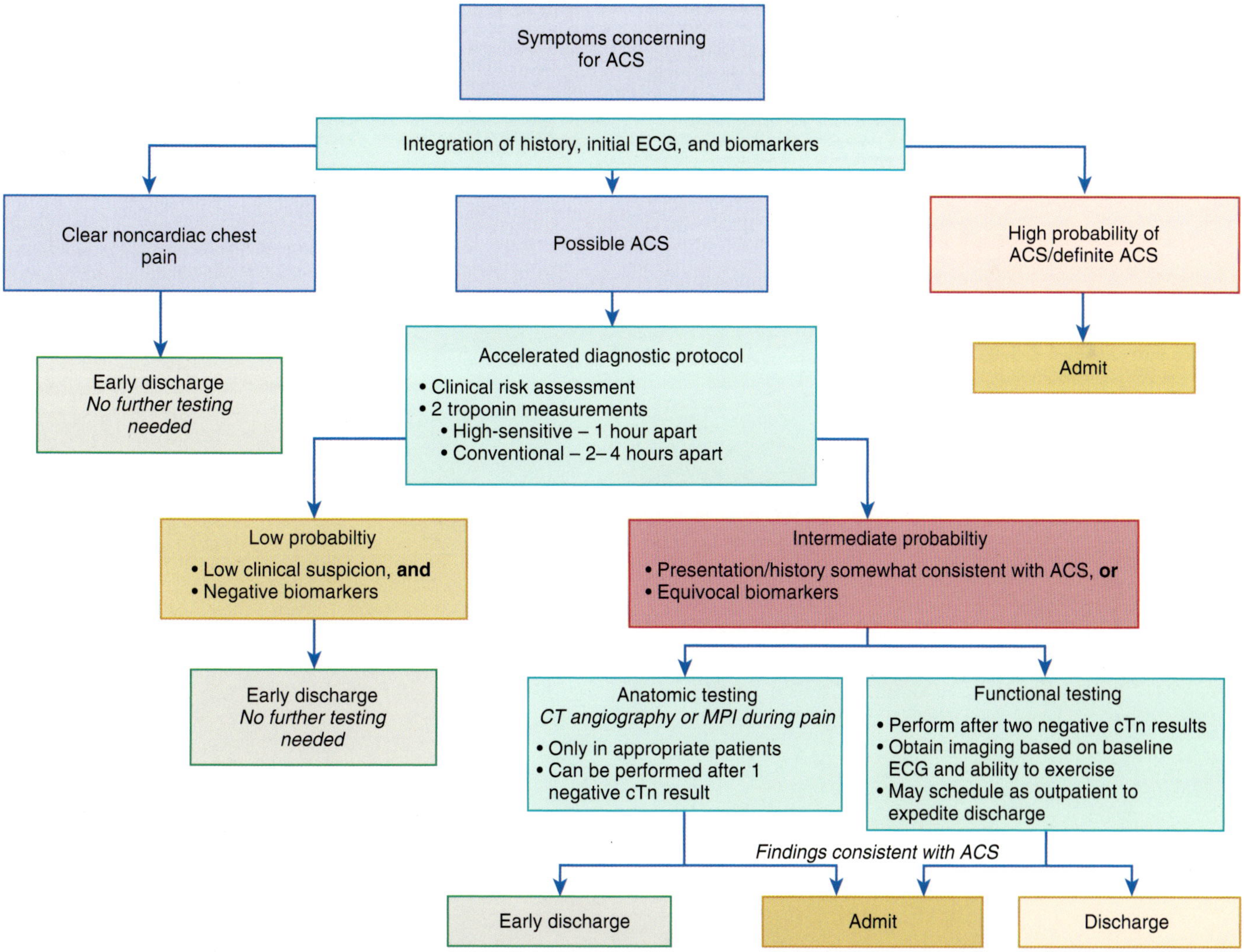

FIGURE 12-5 Integrated schema for the evaluation of patients with symptoms suggestive of acute coronary syndrome (ACS). All patients with suspected acute coronary ischemia should receive a thorough history and physical examination and have an initial electrocardiogram (ECG) performed and troponin measured. Patients with clearly noncardiac chest pain can be discharged immediately, and those with high probability for ACS or a clear-cut diagnosis of ACS are admitted to the cardiology unit. Patients with possible ACS (i.e., with a low to intermediate probability of having ACS) should undergo an accelerated diagnostic protocol (ADP) that includes a second biomarker measurement. Patients with negative troponin assays and low clinical risk can be discharged immediately with no further testing. Patients with either a presentation that is somewhat consistent with ACS in the setting of negative or equivocal results on serial troponin assays may benefit from subsequent noninvasive testing. In selected patients, a computed tomography (CT) coronary angiogram can be done early in the evaluation and may prompt early discharge. Functional testing can be performed on an inpatient basis, but in patients without further symptoms and normal troponin measurements, outpatient testing is appropriate. *cTn,* Cardiac troponin; *MPI,* myocardial perfusion imaging.

Classic References

Antman EM, Cohen M, Bernink PJ, et al.: The TIMI risk score for unstable angina/non-ST elevation MI: A method for prognostication and therapeutic decision making, *JAMA* 284(7):835–842, 2000.

Boersma E, Pieper KS, Steyerberg EW, et al.: Predictors of outcome in patients with acute coronary syndromes without persistent ST-segment elevation. Results from an international trial of 9461 patients. The PURSUIT Investigators, *Circulation* 101(22):2557–2567, 2000.

Eagle KA, Lim MJ, Dabbous OH, et al.: A validated prediction model for all forms of acute coronary syndrome: Estimating the risk of 6-month postdischarge death in an international registry, *JAMA* 291(22):2727–2733, 2004.

Goldman L, Cook EF, Brand DA, et al.: A computer protocol to predict myocardial infarction in emergency department patients with chest pain, *N Engl J Med* 318(13):797–803, 1988.

Sanchis J, Bodi V, Nunez J, et al.: New risk score for patients with acute chest pain, non-ST-segment deviation, and normal troponin concentrations: A comparison with the TIMI risk score, *J Am Coll Cardiol* 46:443–449, 2005.

References

1. Amsterdam EA, Kirk JD, Bluemke DA, et al.: Testing of low-risk patients presenting to the emergency department with chest pain: A scientific statement from the American Heart Association, *Circulation* 122(17):1756–1776, 2010.
2. Bhuiya FA, Pitts SR, McCaig LF: Emergency department visits for chest pain and abdominal pain: United States, 1999-2008, *NCHS Data Brief* Sep(43):1–8, 2010.
3. Lee B, Chang AM, Matsuura AC, et al.: Comparison of cardiac risk scores in ED patients with potential acute coronary syndrome, *Crit Pathways Cardiol* 10(2):64–68, 2011.
4. Hess EP, Perry JJ, Calder LA, et al.: Prospective validation of a modified thrombolysis in myocardial infarction risk score in emergency department patients with chest pain and possible acute coronary syndrome, *Acad Emerg Med* 17(4):368–375, 2010.
5. Macdonald SP, Nagree Y, Fatovich DM, Brown SG: Modified TIMI risk score cannot be used to identify low-risk chest pain in the emergency department: A multicentre validation study, *Emerg Med J* 31(4):281–285, 2014.
6. Backus BE, Six AJ, Kelder JC, et al.: Chest pain in the emergency room: A multicenter validation of the HEART Score, *Crit Pathways Cardiol* 9(3):164–169, 2010.
7. Hess EP, Brison RJ, Perry JJ, et al.: Development of a clinical prediction rule for 30-day cardiac events in emergency department patients with chest pain and possible acute coronary syndrome, *Ann Emerg Med* 59(2):115–125.e111, 2012.
8. Mahler SA, Riley RF, Hiestand BC, et al.: The HEART Pathway randomized trial: Identifying emergency department patients with acute chest pain for early discharge, *Circ Cardiovasc Qual Outcomes* 8(2):195–203, 2015.
9. Than M, Cullen L, Reid CM, et al.: A 2-h diagnostic protocol to assess patients with chest pain symptoms in the Asia-Pacific region (ASPECT): A prospective observational validation study, *Lancet* 377(9771):1077–1084, 2011.
10. Than M, Aldous S, Lord SJ, et al.: A 2-hour diagnostic protocol for possible cardiac chest pain in the emergency department: a randomized clinical trial, *JAMA Intern Med* 174(1):51–58, 2014.
11. Mahler SA, Miller CD, Litt HI, et al.: Performance of the 2-hour accelerated diagnostic protocol within the American College of Radiology Imaging Network PA 4005 cohort, *Acad Emerg Med* 22(4):452–460, 2015.
12. Braunwald E, Morrow DA: Unstable angina: is it time for a requiem? *Circulation* 127(24): 2452–2457, 2013.
13. Roffi M, Patrono C, Collet JP, et al.: 2015 ESC guidelines for the management of acute coronary syndromes in patients presenting without persistent ST-segment elevation: Task Force for the Management of Acute Coronary Syndromes in Patients Presenting without Persistent ST-Segment Elevation of the European Society of Cardiology (ESC), *Eur Heart J* 37(3):267–315, 2016.
14. Keller T, Zeller T, Ojeda F, et al.: Serial changes in highly sensitive troponin I assay and early diagnosis of myocardial infarction, *JAMA* 306(24):2684–2693, 2011.
15. Rubini Gimenez M, Twerenbold R, Reichlin T, et al.: Direct comparison of high-sensitivity-cardiac troponin I vs. T for the early diagnosis of acute myocardial infarction, *Eur Heart J* 35(34): 2303–2311, 2014.
16. Body R, Carley S, McDowell G, et al.: Rapid exclusion of acute myocardial infarction in patients with undetectable troponin using a high-sensitivity assay, *J Am Coll Cardiol* 58(13):1332–1339, 2011.
17. Bandstein N, Ljung R, Johansson M, Holzmann MJ: Undetectable high-sensitivity cardiac troponin T level in the emergency department and risk of myocardial infarction, *J Am Coll Cardiol* 63(23):2569–2578, 2014.
18. Carlton EW, Cullen L, Than M, et al.: A novel diagnostic protocol to identify patients suitable for discharge after a single high-sensitivity troponin, *Heart* 101(13):1041–1046, 2015.
19. Cullen L, Mueller C, Parsonage WA, et al.: Validation of high-sensitivity troponin I in a 2-hour diagnostic strategy to assess 30-day outcomes in emergency department patients with possible acute coronary syndrome, *J Am Coll Cardiol* 62(14):1242–1249, 2013.
20. Neumann JT, Sorenson NA, Schwemer T, et al.: *Accurate and rapid diagnosis of myocardial infarction using a high-sensitivity troponin I 1-hour algorithm*, London, UK, 2015, European Society of Cardiology. https://www.escardio.org/static_file/Escardio/Press-media/Press%20releases/2015/Congress/westermann-bacc.pdf.
21. Reichlin T, Cullen L, Parsonage WA, et al.: Two-hour algorithm for triage toward rule-out and rule-in of acute myocardial infarction using high-sensitivity cardiac troponin T, *Am J Med* 128(4): 369–379, 2015. e364.
22. Reichlin T, Twerenbold R, Wildi K, et al.: Prospective validation of a 1-hour algorithm to rule-out and rule-in acute myocardial infarction using a high-sensitivity cardiac troponin T assay, *CMAJ* 187(8):E243–E252, 2015.
23. Reichlin T, Irfan A, Twerenbold R, et al.: Utility of absolute and relative changes in cardiac troponin concentrations in the early diagnosis of acute myocardial infarction, *Circulation* 124(2):136–145, 2011.
24. Hoffmann U, Truong QA, Schoenfeld DA, et al.: Coronary CT angiography versus standard evaluation in acute chest pain, *N Engl J Med* 367(4):299–308, 2012.
25. Litt HI, Gatsonis C, Snyder B, et al.: CT angiography for safe discharge of patients with possible acute coronary syndromes, *N Engl J Med* 366(15):1393–1403, 2012.
26. Hulten E, Goehler A, Bittencourt MS, et al.: Cost and resource utilization associated with use of computed tomography to evaluate chest pain in the emergency department: the Rule Out Myocardial Infarction using Computer Assisted Tomography (ROMICAT) study, *Circ Cardiovasc Qual Outcomes* 6(5):514–524, 2013.
27. Amsterdam EA, Wenger NK, Brindis RG, et al.: 2014 AHA/ACC guideline for the management of patients with non-ST-elevation acute coronary syndromes: A report of the American College of Cardiology/American Heart Association Task Force on Practice Guidelines, *J Am Coll Cardiol* 64(24):e139–e228, 2014.
28. Hermann LK, Newman DH, Pleasant WA, et al.: Yield of routine provocative cardiac testing among patients in an emergency department-based chest pain unit, *JAMA Intern Med* 173(12): 1128–1133, 2013.
29. Januzzi JL, Sharma U, Zakroysky P, et al.: Sensitive troponin assays in patients with suspected acute coronary syndrome: Results from the Multicenter Rule Out Myocardial Infarction Using Computer Assisted Tomography II trial, *Am Heart J* 169(4):572–578 e571, 2015.

SECTION III

TREATMENT

13 Management Principles in Myocardial Infarction

Keith A. A. Fox

INTRODUCTION

The key principles that underlie management of myocardial infarction (MI) are based on the pathophysiology of the condition and the time course of irreversible myocardial injury. The fundamental goals of managing acute MI include (1) minimizing the duration of exposure of myocardium to ischemia, (2) rapidly establishing effective reperfusion, (3) preventing recurrent ischemia and re-occlusion, (4) managing arrhythmic and mechanical complications, and (5) modifying underlying atherosclerosis toward the aim of long-term secondary prevention (Figure 13-1). The targets for therapy are the molecular, cellular, and anatomic features in the onset, evolution, and complications of MI.

The most prevalent precursor of MI is rupture or erosion of an atheromatous plaque in the coronary artery, with thrombotic occlusion and embolization of thrombotic fragments into the distal territory of the affected coronary artery (type 1 MI), together with changes in vascular tone (Figure 13-2 and Video 13-1; also see Chapter 3). Oxygen supply–demand imbalance can also lead to infarction (type 2 MI) without coronary occlusion. The management of type 2 MI focuses on correction of the cause of the imbalance (e.g., anemia, tachycardia, heart failure). These pathobiological insights form the basis for therapies aimed at contributors to coronary thrombosis at the time of presentation (see the section on Emergency In-Hospital Management), during the initial hospitalization (see the section on Recurrent Ischemia), and over the long-term (see the section on Secondary Prevention and Rehabilitation).

The clinical manifestations and complications of MI are dependent on the extent and duration of ischemia and the volume of myocardium affected. This tight temporal relationship with outcomes frames the initial management objectives for acute MI (see the sections on Prehospital Management and Emergency In-Hospital Management) and the importance of developing systems of care that achieve these objectives (see Chapter 5). Acute myocardial ischemia may manifest clinically as ST-elevation MI (STEMI), as non–ST-elevation MI (NSTEMI), or if there is no detectable injury, as unstable angina (see Chapter 1). Despite substantial progress in the acute management of STEMI, approximately 15% to 20% of patients still present too late for reperfusion (especially older adults and those with major comorbidities), and internationally, many healthcare systems fail to achieve the standards set out in professional guidelines (see the section on Early Recognition of Myocardial Infarction). However, multiple reports demonstrate that the guideline targets are achievable and are associated with improved cardiovascular outcomes after STEMI.[1] Prompt reperfusion of a greater proportion of eligible STEMI patients would achieve greater overall healthcare gains than have been made possible by incremental advances in hospital care (e.g., emergence of newer reperfusion strategies).

This chapter provides an overview of these essential general principles of managing acute MI, including initial reperfusion, as well as the ischemic, thrombotic, electrical, and mechanical complications of MI. The chapter constructs a scaffold on which the subsequent chapters in this section

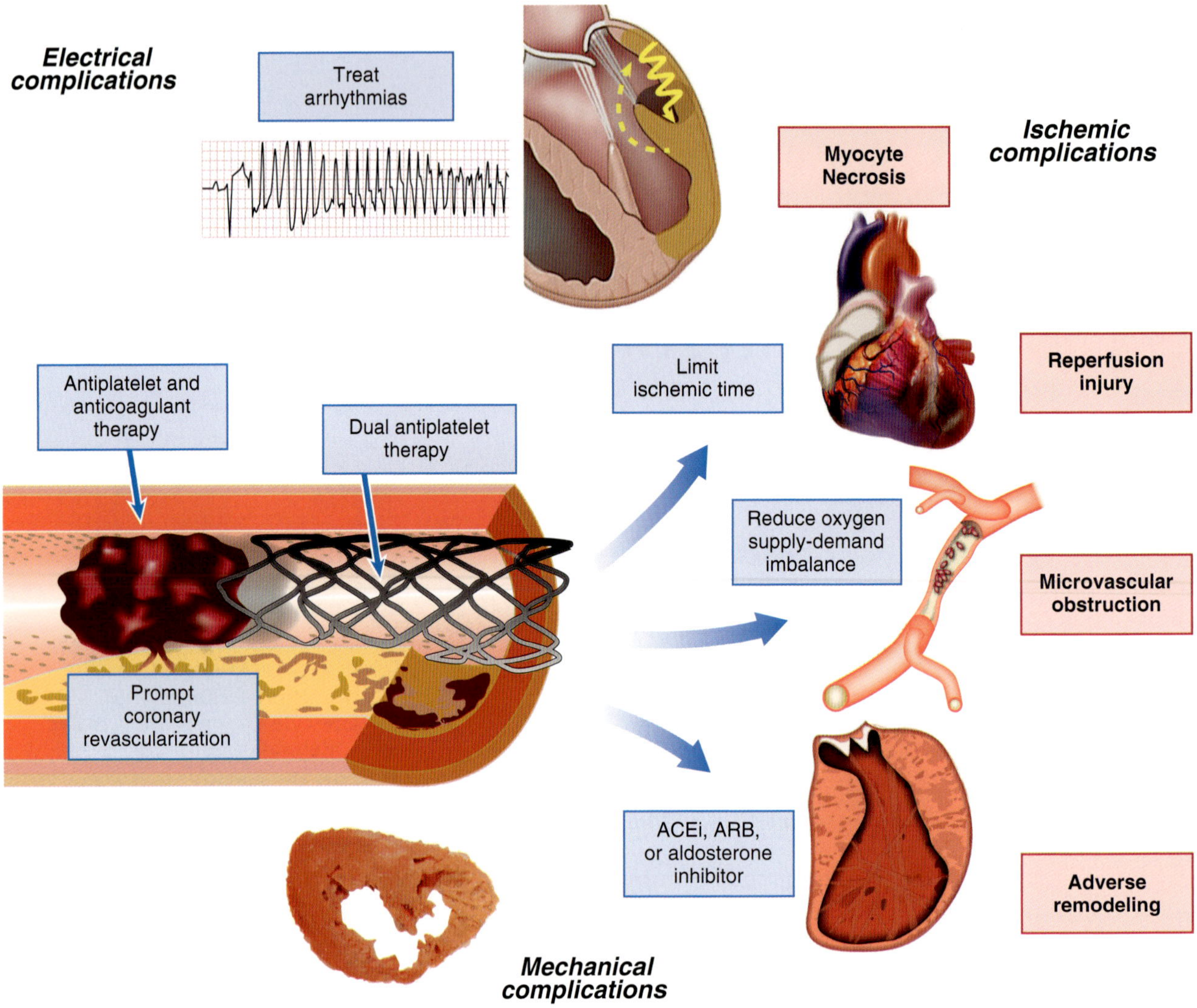

FIGURE 13-1 The major complications of myocardial infarction and targets for therapy. A coronary artery of a patient who has had plaque rupture and coronary occlusion with subsequent therapeutic stent implantation. Key principles of management are to treat arrhythmic complications, to minimize ischemic time before reperfusion, to use antithrombotic therapy to inhibit thrombus propagation and embolization, to improve oxygen supply–demand imbalance, to inhibit adverse remodeling, and to treat mechanical complications. *ACEi*, Angiotensin-converting enzyme inhibitors; *ARB*, angiotensin receptor blocker.

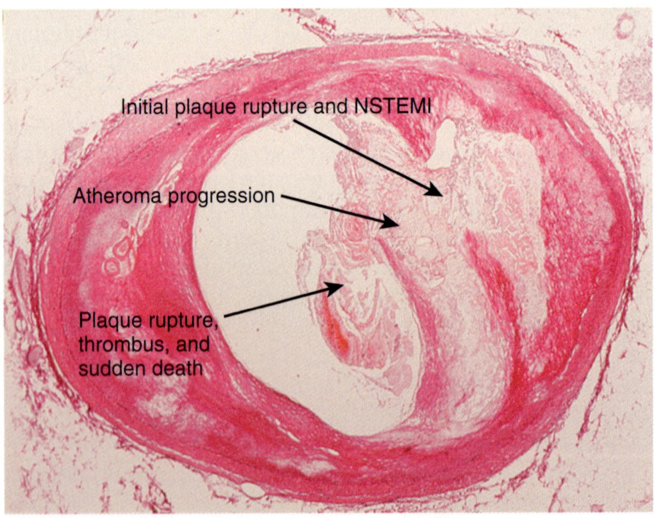

FIGURE 13-2 Cross section of a pathology specimen of coronary artery of a patient who died after a second plaque rupture event. The first plaque rupture precipitated and non–ST-elevation myocardial infarction (NSTEMI), but without an obstructive coronary lesion, and the patient was treated without revascularization. Progressive atheroma development and plaque growth occurred despite secondary prevention therapy. The patient experienced a second plaque rupture and arrhythmic death before reaching the hospital (thrombus on the lesion and evidence of distal embolization). *(Adapted from Fox KAA: What are the pharmacological approaches to treat the vulnerable plaque? Dialog Cardiovasc Med 19[1]:41-48,2014. ©2014, Les Laboratoires Servier.)*

build the details of treatment. The pathobiology of atherothrombosis, ischemic injury, myocardial healing, and remodeling are described in Chapter 3, Chapter 4, and Chapter 36, respectively. The diagnosis of MI is discussed in Chapter 6 and Chapter 7.

PREHOSPITAL MANAGEMENT

Early Recognition of Myocardial Infarction

Key challenges in the early management of MI require recognition by the patient that the symptoms merit emergency evaluation, and then actions that lead to prompt presentation to emergency medical systems (together this interval constitutes "patient delay") (Box 13-1 and Figure 14-1). Some patients experience prodromal unstable angina followed by progression to infarction (with or without complete coronary occlusion). Many patients fail to recognize the symptoms of MI and may delay presentation because of atypical symptoms, or fear and denial that they are experiencing a heart attack. Public awareness campaigns can trigger a spate of false alarms in the short term, but improved public education has led to a shortening of the time to presentation in many healthcare systems. Women tend to present later than men, as well as older adults, some ethnic groups (e.g., Hispanics, African Americans, those of South Asian ancestry), and the socioeconomically disadvantaged. Patients presenting with MI for the second time tend to delay more than first presenters, implicating a possible role of denial and fear.

Prehospital approaches to facilitate rapid diagnosis of MI once the patient has made a first medical contact are described in Chapter 5.

Cardiac Arrest

Epidemiological studies demonstrate that 60% to 73% of deaths associated with STEMI occur out of hospital, mainly within the first 1 to 2 hours after onset. These early deaths are mainly the result of cardiac arrest caused by ventricular fibrillation. Interrupting the link between acute MI and sudden cardiac death is a critical goal in the management of MI (Box 13-2). Despite major advances in in-hospital care of MI, there is little evidence for a decline in the rates of prehospital mortality. However, ongoing initiatives in many communities are aiming to address this deficiency; for example, Chain of Survival campaigns,[2] which promote the availability of trained individuals to initiate cardiopulmonary resuscitation (CPR) and to use automatic external defibrillators, are designed to reduce prehospital mortality caused by cardiac arrest (see Chapter 5). Educational initiatives have increased awareness of CPR and have increased the proportion of patients with cardiac arrest receiving CPR.[3] For patients successfully resuscitated after ventricular fibrillation complicating MI, current guidelines recommend emergency angiography and prompt primary percutaneous revascularization.[4,5]

BOX 13-1 Principles of Management: Prehospital

Early Recognition of Myocardial Infarctions

- Public education challenges: "false alarms;" slow responders, including older adults, the frail, certain ethnic groups; slower responses among women versus men.
- Availability of rapid response emergency medical systems with integrated cardiac networks of care and direct access to "Heart Attack (percutaneous coronary intervention [PCI] capable) Centers."
- ST-elevation myocardial infarction (STEMI): avoiding interhospital transfers; prehospital diagnosis (e.g., electrocardiography telemetry to cardiac center); bypassing hospitals without direct PCI capability unless none available.
- STEMI: prehospital fibrinolysis if no PCI-capable hospital is <60 min away.

BOX 13-2 Principles of Management: Cardiac Arrest

Sudden Cardiac Death and Resuscitation

- Prehospital cardiac arrests and sudden deaths account for most early deaths from acute myocardial infarction.
- Success of resuscitation is critically time dependent (after each minute of ventricular fibrillation survival diminishes 7%–10%).
- Bystander cardiopulmonary resuscitation (CPR) increases survival by approximately 30%.
- Regions with well-developed CPR training and availability of automated external defibrillators (AEDs) have two- to three-fold greater survival rates from out-of-hospital cardiac arrests.

Systems Development for Rapid Reperfusion

Governmental health systems, professional societies, hospitals, and individual providers for patients with MI have focused substantial attention on in-hospital delays (door-to-needle or door-to-balloon time); yet, prehospital delays are the largest contributor to ischemic time. Therefore, systems-based approaches are needed to deliver effective integrated management with shortened overall ischemic time. The overall systems goal of limiting ischemic time (ideally ≤120 minutes),[4,5] challenges in meeting current targets,[6] and operational approaches to achieve these goals are discussed comprehensively in Chapter 5. Development of well-organized systems for MI care is possible, and achievement of such targets for time to treatment are realistic. In this context, comprehensive national[7–11] and international registries (e.g., GRACE) have demonstrated important temporal trends of diminishing mortality and decreasing incidence of new-onset heart failure (see Chapter 2).[12,13]

EMERGENCY IN-HOSPITAL MANAGEMENT

The emergency management of patients with suspected MI is rooted in rapid diagnosis and swift restoration of flow in the culprit artery. Critical concepts in the emergency management of MI are listed in Box 13-3 and reviewed in the following section. The initial diagnostic assessment of patients with suspected acute MI is discussed in Chapter 6, and the related use of cardiac biomarkers and imaging methods are detailed in Chapter 7, Chapter 8, and Chapter 9.

Rapid Reperfusion

Minimizing the delay to reperfusion in patients with STEMI is critical to salvage ischemic myocardium, to limit residual injury, to reduce the risk of subsequent heart failure, and to improve survival (see Chapter 14 and Chapter 36). The impact of time delay is not linear (Figure 13-3); the most effective salvage of myocardium is achieved with reperfusion within 60 to 90 minutes of ischemic onset. The term "golden hour" has been applied to the first 60 minutes of infarction because restoring myocardial function is best achieved within this period, and some patients even experience aborted infarction without evolving electrocardiographic (ECG) changes of MI and without measurable mechanical deficit (see Figure 13-3).

The clinical manifestations of MI are a function of the severity and duration of ischemia and the consequent volume of myocardium with irreversible cellular injury. Therefore, the

BOX 13-3 Principles of Emergency Management of ST-Elevation Myocardial Infarction

- Reperfusion and revascularization are critical to reduce ischemic time.
- The goals include: emergency medical service response times within <10 min, transfer to percutaneous coronary intervention capable center <30 min, first medical contact to reperfusion <90 min.
- Electrocardiography telemetry and bypassing of emergency room for confirmed myocardial infarction.
- Prehospital fibrinolysis if transfer times prolonged.
- Adjunctive therapies to reduce recurrent ischemia and to manage arrhythmias and heart failure.

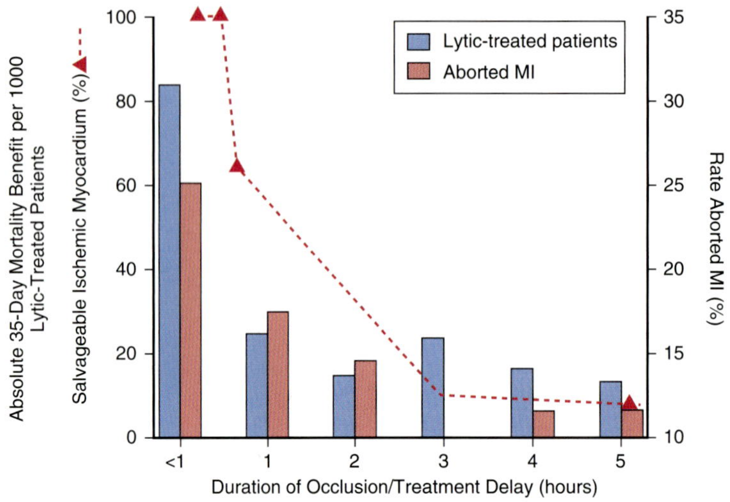

FIGURE 13-3 The relationship between elapsed time (ischemic time) and myocardial salvage, lives saved, and frequency of aborted myocardial infarction (MI) with reperfusion therapy. *Solid blue bars* represent number of lives saved per 1000 patients treated with fibrinolysis according to time from symptom onset. *Red bars* represent the proportion of aborted myocardial infarctions (MI) in fibrinolytic-treated patients according to time from symptom onset. *(Adapted from Armstrong PW, Westerhout CM, Welsh RC: Duration of symptoms is the key modulator of the choice of reperfusion for ST-elevation myocardial infarction.* Circulation *119:1293, 2009.)*

initial care of the patient with STEMI is targeted at initiating therapy to restore flow in the infarct-related artery as rapidly as possible. The selection of the approach to reperfusion therapy, including the choice of administration of a fibrinolytic agent versus primary percutaneous coronary intervention (PCI), and related decisions regarding interhospital transfer, are addressed in Chapter 14. Fibrinoytic therapy for STEMI is discussed comprehensively in Chapter 15, and the approach to primary PCI is detailed in Chapter 17.

Although more attention has focused on the timing of reperfusion in patients with STEMI, patients with NSTEMI may also develop major complications, including heart failure, hypotension, and arrhythmias as a consequence of prolonged ischemia. Patients with NSTEMI, particularly those at high risk, should also be considered for emergency revascularization to resolve ongoing or intermittent ischemia (see the section on Initial Risk Assessment and Chapter 16).

Fibrinolysis

Administration of a fibrinolytic agent was the cornerstone of reperfusion therapy before the development of primary PCI, and still constitutes important therapy in settings where primary PCI is not available or not available expeditiously (see Chapter 14). The oldest fibrinolytic agents (streptokinase and urokinase) are still widely used in some parts of the world because of cost. Subsequent evolution of fibrinolytic therapy has aimed to improve ease and rapidity of administration, as well as the balance of fibrinolytic efficacy versus bleeding. In comparison to streptokinase, later generation fibrinolytics, including alteplase, reteplase, and tenecteplase, have amplified effects at the sites of thrombus formation (see Chapter 15).

Despite the similarities in the early mechanisms of STEMI and acute coronary syndromes (ACSs) without ST-elevation, and the key role of thrombosis in both, fibrinolysis failed to demonstrate benefit in early studies of the treatment of unstable angina. Because those studies included low-risk patients, some experts have questioned whether there could be a role for coronary administration of modern fibrinolytic agents in high-risk NSTEMI. Nevertheless, because of the absence of established benefit and a clear increased risk of serious bleeding, professional society guidelines do not recommend administration of fibrinolytic agents to patients with NSTEMI.

Pathways of Care: ST-Elevation Myocardial Infarction

Pathways of care for patients with STEMI are aimed at minimizing the duration of ischemia and triage of patients to the optimal environment for management of the complications of MI (see Chapter 5). Timely primary PCI is preferred whenever it is available and provided by experienced STEMI teams, and has become the dominant approach to reperfusion therapy in most countries (Figure 13-4). Critical elements of pathways of care for STEMI include prompt recognition by the patient of the need to call emergency medical systems, rapid dispatch and arrival of emergency providers (<10 minutes), in-ambulance diagnosis of suspected STEMI, administration of analgesia and antithrombotic agents, rapid transfer to a PCI-capable center (<30 minutes), and mobilization for timely PCI (Figure 13-5). Direct admission to the catheterization laboratory avoids the delays involved in emergency department evaluation. When prehospital transfers are prolonged because of distance from the PCI center, or traffic and adverse weather, the option of prehospital administration of fibrinolysis is needed (see Chapter 14). Even after apparently successful fibrinolysis, transfer to a PCI-capable center is needed to treat the underlying stenosis, to minimize risks of reocclusion, and to consider revascularization of nonculprit coronary stenoses (see the section on Recurrent Ischemia and Chapter 14).

Pathways of Care: Non–ST-Elevation Myocardial Infarction

The clinical presentation of NSTEMI is more insidious than that of STEMI and may be preceded by new-onset exertional angina, deteriorating or unstable angina, or no previous symptoms. Unlike STEMI, autonomic features do not usually accompany the onset of NSTEMI. Because of the pattern of onset, the patient may misinterpret the symptoms as gastrointestinal or musculoskeletal in nature, and presentation is frequently to nonemergency medical services (primary care or internal medicine, or

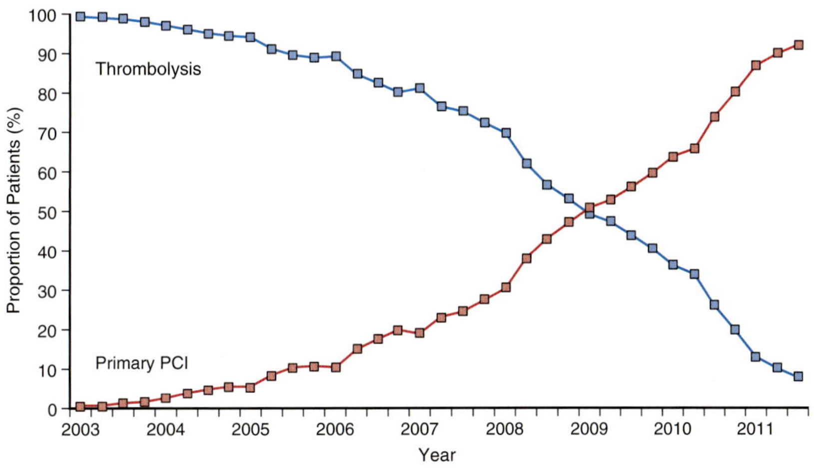

FIGURE 13-4 Frequency of fibrinolysis and primary percutaneous coronary intervention (PCI) in the United Kingdom, over time. The Myocardial Infarction National Audit Program records treatments and outcomes for all patients with MI, admitted to all hospitals in England and Wales and demonstrates the replacement of fibrinolysis with primary PCI.[10] *(Source: Myocardial Ischaemia National Audit Project.* www.ucl.ac.uk/nicor/audits/minap.*)*

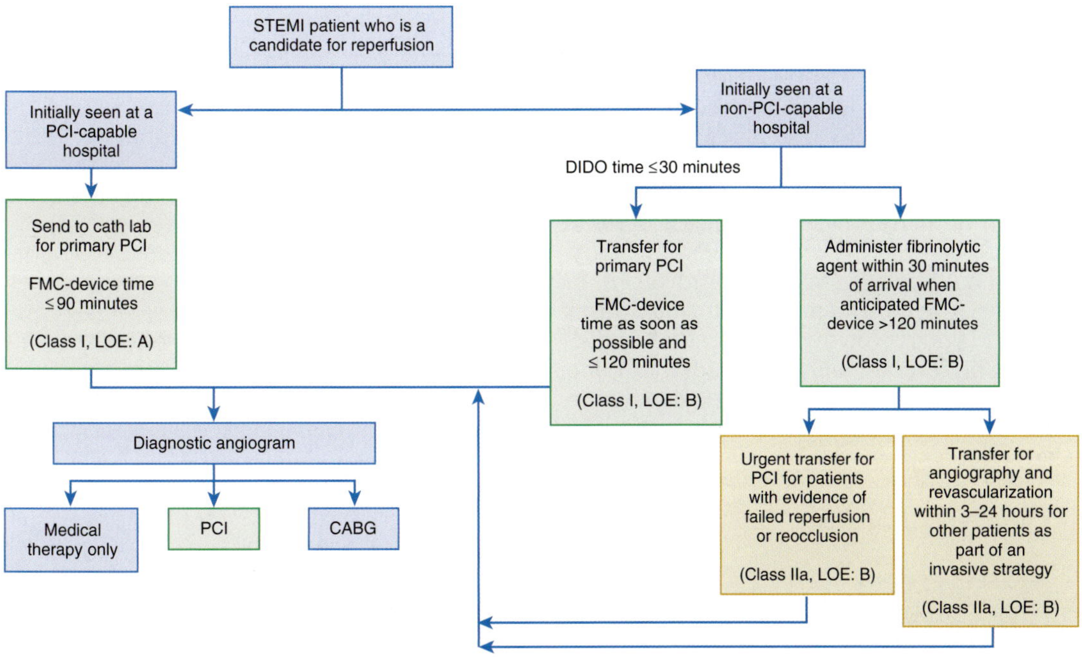

FIGURE 13-5 The American College of Cardiology Foundation/American Heart Association guidelines depicts the flow of decision-making for reperfusion strategies in ST-elevation myocardial infarction (STEMI). *CABG*, Coronary artery bypass graft; *DIDO*, door-in-door-out; *FMC*, first medical contact; *LOE*, level of evidence; *PCI*, percutaneous coronary intervention. *(From O'Gara PT, et al: 2013 ACCF/AHA guideline for the management of ST-elevation myocardial infarction: a report of the American College of Cardiology Foundation/American Heart Association Task Force on Practice Guidelines.* J Am Coll Cardiol *61:e78, 2013.)*

to nonemergency chest pain clinics). The diagnosis is based on the clinical syndrome plus ECG findings of ischemia, but without persistent ST-elevation (see Chapter 1 and Chapter 6) and sensitive biomarkers of necrosis (e.g., high-sensitivity troponin; see Chapter 7). However, the diagnosis can be challenging in the presence of minor nonspecific ECG abnormalities and biomarkers of necrosis that may be elevated by supply–demand imbalance (type 2 MI) or myocyte necrosis in the absence of coronary occlusion (e.g., in heart failure or pulmonary embolism).[14] Particular care is needed to identify patients with evolving infarction but who do not have ST-elevation at the time of first presentation. Repeated ECG analysis or continuous ST monitoring is important for this reason. Once the diagnosis of NSTEMI is established, antithrombotic therapies should be initiated while consideration of invasive evaluation is undertaken (see the section on Initial Risk Assessment).

Other Medical Therapy at Presentation

A schematic overview of the management of MI is provided in Figure 13-6. The rationale for use of anticoagulant and antiplatelet agents are addressed later in this chapter, as are agents to mitigate myocardial oxygen supply–demand mismatch (see the section on Recurrent Ischemia).

Analgesics

Relief of pain is important, not only to relieve distress, but also to avoid the consequences of sympathetic simulation on the heart, including increases in afterload and arrhythmogenesis (see Chapter 28). Intravenous opioid analgesia is the most commonly used therapy and should be carefully titrated, and is often administered with antiemetics. For example, intravenous morphine sulfate at a dose of 2 to 8 mg repeated at intervals of 5 to 15 minutes has been recommended, until the pain is relieved or side effects (e.g., hypotension, depression of respiration, or severe vomiting) emerge. The reduction of anxiety with successful analgesia diminishes the patient's restlessness and the activity of the autonomic nervous system, with a consequent reduction of the heart's metabolic demands. Morphine may also provide favorable effects in patients with pulmonary edema caused by peripheral arterial and venous dilation, reduction of the work of breathing, and slowing of heart rate secondary to combined withdrawal of sympathetic tone and augmentation of vagal tone. Observational studies have identified an association between administration of morphine and adverse outcomes in patients with ACS; however, it is challenging to disentangle this observation from confounding by indication.

Nitrates

Nitrates are commonly given in acute MI, and they may relieve vasospasm and reduce pain. By virtue of their ability to enhance coronary blood flow by coronary vasodilation and to decrease ventricular preload by increasing venous capacitance, sublingual nitrates have been recommended for the initial treatment of patients with MI. At present, the only groups of patients with STEMI in whom sublingual nitroglycerin should not be given are those with suspected right ventricular infarction or marked hypotension (e.g., systolic pressure <90 mm Hg), especially if accompanied by bradycardia. The patient should be observed for improvement in symptoms or change in hemodynamics. Even small doses can produce sudden hypotension and bradycardia, a reaction that can usually be reversed with intravenous atropine. Long-acting oral nitrate preparations should be avoided in the early course of STEMI because of the frequently changing hemodynamic status of the patient. In patients with a prolonged period of waxing and waning chest pain, intravenous nitroglycerin may help to control symptoms and correct ischemia, but requires frequent monitoring of blood pressure. Initiation of a reperfusion strategy in patients with STEMI should not be delayed while assessing the patient's response to sublingual or intravenous nitrates. Despite the strong pathobiological rationale, administration of nitrates has not been shown to improve clinical outcomes compared with placebo in patients with MI (see the section on Other Medical Therapies to Reduce Ischemia).

Oxygen

Treating all patients hospitalized with MI with oxygen for at least 24 to 48 hours is common practice on the basis of the empirical assumption of hypoxia and evidence that increased oxygen in the inspired air may protect ischemic myocardium. However, the evidence to support its use in those without heart failure or hypoxia is lacking.[15] In patients with hypoxia (oxygen saturation below ~94%), hypoxia can be corrected by oxygen delivery using a face mask. However, for those with more profound hypoxia associated with heart failure, ventilation and circulation support may be required (see Chapter 25). Conversely, in a small study comparing oxygen and air administration for those with oxygen saturations more than 94%, there was no evidence of benefit and a trend toward harm (6-month infarct size) in those given supplemental oxygen.

RECURRENT ISCHEMIA

Complete and durable relief of ischemia, alleviation of symptoms, and prevention of recurrent coronary thrombotic complications are core management goals for the

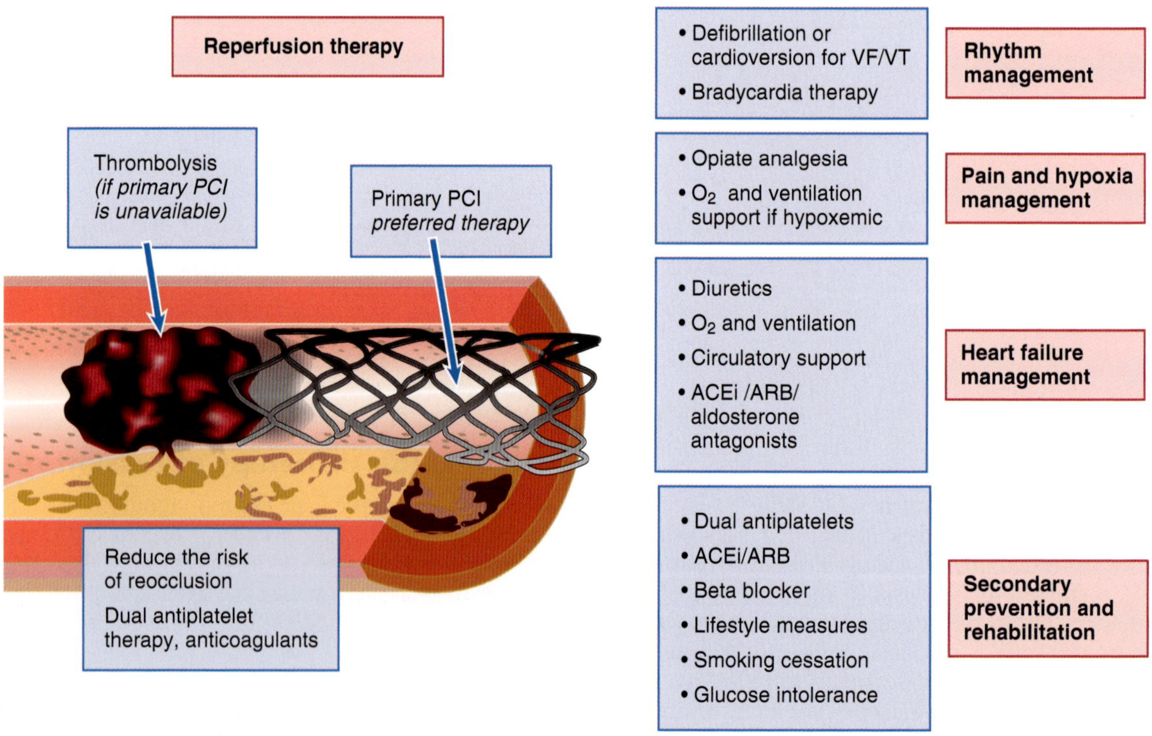

FIGURE 13-6 The key therapeutic approaches and the main classes of therapy following ST-elevation myocardial infarction (STEMI) and reperfusion therapy. *ACEi*, Angiotensin-converting enzyme inhibitor; *ARB*, angiotensin receptor blocker; O_2, oxygen; *PCI*, percutaneous coronary intervention; *VF*, ventricular fibrillation; *VT*, ventricular tachycardia.

care of patients with MI (Box 13-4). Early recurrent ischemia and reinfarction are important complications of acute MI; although their rate has declined with routine coronary revascularization (see Chapter 23). Fibrinolysis is an option for initial dissolution of completely obstructive thrombus in patients with STEMI, if timely primary PCI is not available (see the section on Rapid Reperfusion and Chapter 15). Antiplatelet and anticoagulant therapy are important to reduce the extension of thrombus or reocclusion, and coronary revascularization is critically important to relieve coronary artery obstruction. These are the mainstays of therapy to address coronary occlusions in most patients with STEMI. For patients with NSTEMI and patients with STEMI who have residual coronary disease after culprit vessel reperfusion, therapies to improve myocardial oxygen supply–demand mismatch are a cornerstone of therapy and are used in conjunction with antithrombotic therapy (Figure 13-7). Because of the risks of progression of infarction and the development of complications, including heart failure, arrhythmias, and cardiogenic shock, with ongoing or recurrent ischemia, management by a team with ACS expertise and appropriate facilities is necessary. Careful and systematic assessment of the risk of death and recurrent ischemic events is central to the appropriate selection of management strategies and triage to the best care environment (see also Chapter 11).

BOX 13-4 Principles of Emergency Management of Non–ST-Elevation Myocardial Infarction

- Key principles are to relieve ischemia, alleviate symptoms, and to prevent coronary thrombotic complications.
- High-sensitivity biomarkers of necrosis to rule out myocardial infarction (MI).
- Elevated biomarkers of necrosis in type 2 MI, "supply–demand imbalance."
- Risk assessment, including use of risk scores (TIMI, GRACE), is critical in identifying patients for emergency and urgent revascularization.
- Dual antiplatelet and anticoagulant strategies to reduce thrombotic complications.
- Minimizing bleeding risk (patient selection, vascular access route, choice of antithrombotic agents).
- Adjunctive therapies to reduce ischemia and to manage arrhythmias and heart failure.

Initial Risk Assessment

In STEMI, the default management is emergency reperfusion unless the patient has risk features that preclude it or has experienced prolonged ischemic time. There are few absolute contraindications to primary PCI, and the key contraindication to thrombolysis is the risk of cerebral hemorrhage. The critical-related decision in the emergency setting is whether comorbidities and bleeding risks are sufficient to outweigh the advantages of reperfusion. Thus, emergency risk assessment is commonly based on clinical evaluation, and risk assessment tools are mainly used to guide triage and later therapeutic choices, with the aim of reducing complications.

In patients with NSTEMI, the pivotal early decision is whether to proceed to emergency, urgent, or early elective angiography, with a view to revascularization (see Chapter 16). Randomized trials have demonstrated the

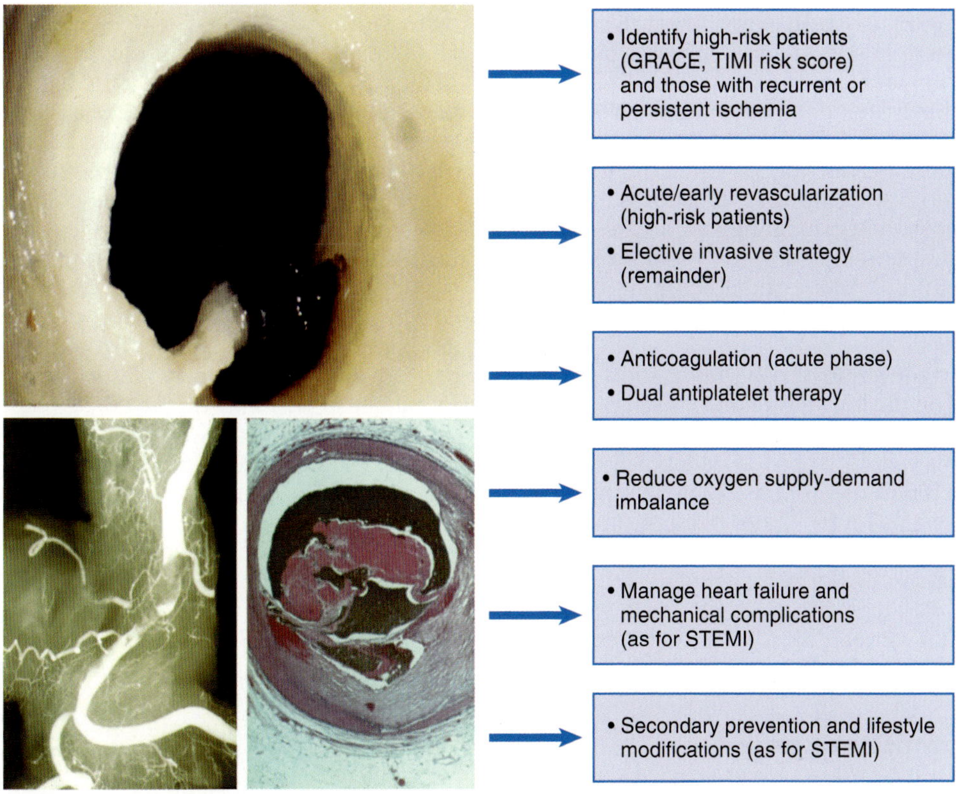

FIGURE 13-7 Strategies for preventing recurrent ischemia in patients with non–ST-elevation myocardial infarction (NSTEMI). Partial occlusion of a coronary artery (angiogram and pathology section) and plaque rupture and thrombus attachment in a patient with NSTEMI. The principles of management are to identify high-risk patients for early revascularization based on clinical findings and use of a risk score (GRACE or TIMI score), to inhibit thrombus propagation and embolization, to address oxygen supply–demand imbalance, to treat heart failure and mechanical complications, and to initiate secondary prevention and lifestyle measures to reduce the risk of recurrence.

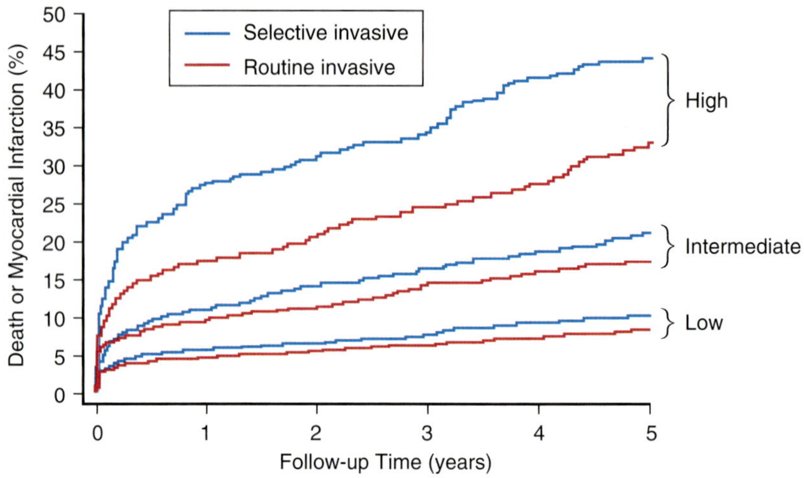

Selective invasive	2746	2452	2351	2178	2077	2005
Routine invasive	2721	2485	2410	2235	2166	2079

FIGURE 13-8 The impact of an initial conservative or an interventional strategy on the subsequent rate of death or myocardial infarction. Those in the upper third of baseline risk had an absolute benefit of 11 per 100 with revascularization, in the intermediate group 3.8 and in the lower risk group 2.0 showing most benefit, per patient treated, among higher risk patients. *(From the Task Force on Myocardial Revascularization of the European Society of Cardiology [ESC] and the European Association for Cardio-Thoracic Surgery [EACTS]: Guidelines on revascularization.* Eur Heart J *31:2501, 2010; and Fox KAA, et al., for the FIR Collaboration: Long-term outcome of a routine versus selective invasive strategy in patients with non–ST-Segment elevation acute coronary syndrome: a meta-analysis of individual patient data.* J Am Coll Cardiol *55:2435, 2010.)*

most benefit in the prevention of future death, myocardial infarction, and rehospitalization in higher risk patients with ACS, and an angiographic strategy is recommended in the guidelines for such patients (Figure 13-8). Although some high-risk patients are evident clinically, based on continuing signs and symptoms of ischemia (e.g., widespread ST depression on the ECG) or complications of ischemia like heart failure and arrhythmia, many others are less evident. Risk assessment tools have been derived and validated (e.g., TIMI risk score, GRACE risk score).[16,17] In practice, a "treatment-risk paradox" exists, in which lower risk patients rather than higher risk patients are more likely to be treated with revascularization and more aggressive antithrombotic therapies.[17,18] It is likely that clinicians in practice tend to underestimate the potential for benefit and overestimate the potential for harm, especially in older patients and those with comorbidities. Composite risk scores provide a rapid and robust method of estimating risk; hence, they are a key method to guide therapy and are recommended in all the major guidelines.[19,20] Many healthcare systems now incorporate risk assessment into the triage and early management of NSTEMI.

As an example of the value of risk stratification for decision-making, based on the long-term randomized trials of an interventional strategy in NSTEACS, the absolute risk reduction in deaths or MIs was 11.1 per 100 patients in the high-risk category, 4 per 100 in medium-risk patients, and only 2 per 100 in the low-risk patients.[21] It has been estimated that if clinicians applied the rates of intervention achieved in the randomized trials in higher risk patients, in contrast to the rates observed in large-scale registries, there would be between 30 and 80 fewer cardiovascular deaths or MIs for each 10,000 patients with non–STE-ACS.[17]

Thrombotic Complications

Thrombotic mechanisms are central to the progression from early plaque disruption to coronary occlusion and to the consequences of embolic occlusions in the territory of the affected artery (see Chapter 3). Although there has been much debate about the contributions of systemic upregulation of thrombotic and inflammatory risk ("vulnerable blood"), and the contributions of local mechanical and biological stimuli in the disrupted plaque ("vulnerable plaque"), current evidence suggests that both mechanisms are important and that there is an interplay between the local and systemic stimuli. For these reasons, antiplatelet and anticoagulant therapies should be administered systemically to all patients with type 1 MI, with the aim of inhibiting thrombosis locally at the site of plaque disruption.

Although reducing recurrent thrombosis is a central goal of therapy, this objective should be balanced against the risk of serious bleeding (see Chapter 29). The results of trials of potent antithrombotic therapy for ACS have suggested that minimizing bleeding can also reduce morbidity. Moreover, lower bleeding rates have been associated with lower risks of death and recurrent MI. Early studies of anticoagulants used high dosages, with the aim of reducing thrombotic complications, but bleeding risks were high (see Chapter 18). The complications of major bleeding are not only those directly associated with the bleeding event, but there are also indirect adverse consequences later after the bleeding event. These late events may be the consequence of management changes following bleeding, like stopping antithrombotic therapy or the adverse consequences of transfusion (see Chapter 29). In consequence, an important contemporary principle of anticoagulant management is that "less may be more," with the aim of achieving a minimum effective concentration of anticoagulant therapy.

Antiplatelet Therapies

The principles of antiplatelet therapy are introduced here, and the therapies are discussed in detail in Chapter 19 and Chapter 20. Experimental and pathological studies have established the pivotal role of the platelet in coronary thrombosis, and subsequent clinical trials have conclusively demonstrated that antiplatelet therapies are effective in reducing the recurrent thrombotic complications of MI. The generation of platelet aggregates at the site of plaque disruption amplifies further platelet aggregation and precipitates thrombus formation. Activated platelets and platelet microparticles stimulate the coagulation cascade via thrombin activation, and in turn, thrombin is a potent activator of platelets. Consequently, management is directed toward inhibition of activated platelets and inhibition of thrombin. However, a key balance of platelet activation and parenteral anticoagulation is required; this balance must be sufficient to inhibit thrombosis, but insufficient to precipitate major bleeding. The clinical aims of antiplatelet therapy are to inhibit the propagation of thrombus, to minimize thrombotic complications, including distal embolization, occlusion, or reocclusion at the site of plaque disruption, and stent thrombosis.

Aspirin

Pivotal early studies established a role for antiplatelet agents in ACS by demonstrating the benefit of aspirin in the RISK study and several modest-sized trials among patients with NSTE-ACS,[22] and in the large ISIS-2 study in patients with STEMI (see Chapter 19). Together, the NSTEMI trials included 2448 patients, a modest number by today's standards, but they demonstrated an approximate halving of the risk of death or MI and established antiplatelet therapy as a key part of the management of ACS.

$P2Y_{12}$ Receptor Inhibition

Platelets have multiple redundant pathways for activation. Inhibition of platelet pathways complementary to aspirin has proven to offer incremental benefit in the management of patients with MI (see Chapter 19). Dual antiplatelet therapy was first tested using a second-generation thienopyridine, clopidogrel, plus aspirin versus aspirin alone, among patients with NSTE-ACS and resulted in an approximate 20% improvement in the composite of death, MI, and stroke.[22] Subsequent studies have extended evidence for benefit to patients with STEMI (see Chapter 19).[4] Moreover, mechanistic studies have subsequently demonstrated hyporesponsiveness to clopidogrel ("resistance") in some patients and linked these observations to adverse clinical outcomes (see Chapter 20). In this context, more potent adenosine diphosphate (ADP) receptor antagonists have been developed and tested in large randomized clinical trials, with the results demonstrating further reduction in recurrent atherothrombotic events with the third-generation $P2Y_{12}$ inhibitors, prasugrel and ticagrelor (see Chapter 19).[23,24]

Glycoprotein IIb/IIIa Inhibitors

These agents block the final common pathway, the binding of fibrinogen or von Willebrand factor to the platelet IIb/IIIa integrin receptor (see Chapter 19). They were introduced early in the development of percutaneous revascularization for ACSs to minimize thrombotic, microvascular, and periprocedural complications. At that time, the standard of care was single antiplatelet therapy, usually aspirin. The influential studies were conducted before the current era of potent dual antiplatelet therapy and current interventional therapy. For these reasons, current guidelines have downgraded the use of glycoprotein IIb/IIa inhibitors, reserving them for use in the context of PCI, as a bailout for patients with complex procedures and thrombotic complications. Thus, glycoprotein IIb/IIIa inhibitors are not recommended for use in all patients, nor are they recommended for systematic use before angiography.

Anticoagulant Therapy

Anticoagulants are administered in patients with MI with the goal of inhibiting the generation and propagation of "red thrombus" at sites where a nidus of platelet aggregation has initiated thrombus formation ("white thrombus" contains mainly platelet aggregates). Although anticoagulants remain a core element in the management of acute MI, changes to antiplatelet therapy and enhancement of interventional devices and techniques have resulted in evolution of anticoagulant therapy in acute MI. Early interventional techniques (balloon angioplasty and first-generation stents) were highly thrombogenic, and high doses of parenteral anticoagulants were commonly used, but these had significant bleeding complications. As techniques have improved, especially with the latest generation of stents, instrumentation, and effective dual antiplatelet therapy (aspirin plus ticagrelor or prasugrel), much less anticoagulation appears to be needed, and bleeding complications have been reduced (for example, using bivalirudin in place of heparin plus a glycoprotein IIb/IIIa inhibitor; see Chapter 18).

Unfractionated Heparin

The most widely used anticoagulant around the world remains unfractionated heparin (UFH). Notably, the initial trials testing UFH were small in size, and the benefit was demonstrated only in a pooled analysis (see Chapter 18). The optimal dosage of UFH has not been defined, and older studies tended to use higher dosages (e.g., bolus of 140 U/kg) and were associated with higher rates of bleeding than reported in modern studies using lower dosages (e.g., bolus of 60 U/kg).

Low–Molecular-Weight Heparins

Because treatment with UFH leads to unpredictable anticoagulation, requiring careful monitoring and dose adjustment, anticoagulants that act more predictably via inhibition upstream of UFH in the coagulation cascade have been developed and tested for clinical use (see Chapter 18). Studies of low-molecular-weight heparins (LMWHs) demonstrate lower rates of death and/or MI weighed against an increase in bleeding. LMWH regimens are given subcutaneously and without the need for monitoring and repeated dose adjustments, and are, therefore, simpler to administer than UFH. In the context of predominantly conservative management strategies for ACS, several studies showed greater efficacy of the LMWH regimen compared with UFH (see Chapter 18). However, when used as part of an invasive strategy, LMWH regimens do not appear to offer clear benefit and are associated with increased bleeding.

Factor Xa Inhibitor

Analogously to LMWH, direct anti-Factor Xa inhibitors act higher up the coagulation cascade than agents acting on thrombin (IIa inhibitors); therefore, they are effective at inhibiting thrombin generation, but they do not act against thrombin in clots (see Chapter 18). The parenteral pentasaccharide, fondaparinux, is a factor Xa inhibitor tested against the LMWH enoxaparin.[25] In these trials, the objective was to test the minimum effective dosage of fondaparinux against the standard of care using enoxaparin LMWH, with the aim of minimizing bleeding complications, but with similar efficacy. In OASIS 5, fondaparinux met the criteria for noninferiority (at 9 days), demonstrated half the rate of major bleeding, and showed decreased mortality at 30 days and 6 months compared with LMWH (see Chapter 18). However, there was evidence of an increased rate of catheter-related thrombosis. Fondaparinux does not block factor IIa and is less effective than UFH at blocking catheter-related contact activation. Administration of a low dose of UFH in conjunction with fondaparinux appears necessary to prevent catheter-related thrombosis, but this approach has not been validated in large-scale studies. Fondaparinux has gained acceptance, where it is approved for clinical use in ACS outside of the United States, for use in community hospital settings, and in those selected for noninvasive management because of the lower rates of bleeding and the logistic advantage that it is simple to administer. However, patients transferred for interventions are usually converted to another anticoagulant, commonly UFH.

Direct Thrombin Inhibitors

The direct thrombin inhibitors (hirudin, agatroban, bivalirudin) do not require cofactors for their activation; they directly inhibit existing thrombin, but they do not inhibit factors higher up the coagulation cascade. The use of bivalirudin in patients with MI is discussed in Chapter 18.

Other Medical Therapies to Reduce Ischemia

In addition to the therapies designed to restore vascular patency and to prevent thrombotic and arrhythmic complications, adjunctive therapies aim to alleviate supply–demand mismatch, and ischemic symptoms.

Nitrates

The potential benefits of nitrates include dilation of large coronary arteries and arterioles, and this may improve perfusion of ischemic zones. Nitrates dilate the venous system and decrease preload and ventricular volume, and they reduce pulmonary capillary wedge pressure. They also produce systemic arterial dilation, which decreases afterload. In combination, these changes lower wall stress and oxygen consumption, and reduce angina. Despite these potential favorable effects in patients with acute ischemia, routine use of nitrates has not been shown to improve major cardiovascular outcomes in two mega-trials compared with placebo. Nitrates are only indicated in the acute phase to manage hypertension or heart failure, or for the relief of anginal symptoms. There is no clear benefit to empirical long-term nitrates in the asymptomatic patient, and nitrates, in general, are not indicated beyond the first 48 hours, unless angina or ventricular failure is present.

Calcium Channel Blockers

Calcium antagonists are not routinely recommended in acute MI because the summation of evidence does not show benefit, but a trend toward harm.

Beta-Adrenergic Blockers

The effects of beta blockers in the treatment of patients with MI can be divided into those that are immediate (early in the course of infarction) and those that are long term. The immediate intravenous administration of beta blockers reduces the cardiac index, heart rate, and blood pressure with a net reduction in myocardial oxygen consumption. Despite this favorable effect of early administration of intravenous beta blockers, there are potentially detrimental effects in some patients, which have led present guidelines to omit early administration of intravenous beta blockers for most patients.

More than 52,000 patients were randomized in clinical trials that studied β-adrenergic blockade in acute MI. However, these trials were conducted mainly in the pre-reperfusion era, and in many, beta blockers were administered in the convalescent phase after MI. The available data in the pre-reperfusion era suggested there were favorable trends toward a reduction in mortality, reinfarction, and cardiac arrest. However, in the reperfusion era, the addition of an intravenous beta blocker to fibrinolytic therapy was not associated with a reduction in mortality, but they did reduce the rate of recurrent ischemic events. In a large trial that randomized 45,852 patients within 24 hours of MI to metoprolol, which was given as sequential intravenous boluses of 5 mg up to 15 mg followed by 200 mg/day orally, or to placebo, there was no difference in the rate of the composite endpoint of death, reinfarction, or cardiac arrest in the metoprolol group compared with the placebo group. However, significant reductions occurred in reinfarction and episodes of ventricular fibrillation in the metoprolol group, translating into 5 fewer events for each of these endpoints per 1000 patients treated. However, there were 11 more episodes of cardiogenic shock in the metoprolol group per 1000 patients treated. The risk of developing cardiogenic shock was greatest in patients presenting with moderate to severe left ventricular dysfunction (Killip class II or greater).

Therefore, although robust evidence supports the use of beta blockers for the management of patients with chronic heart failure, the evidence for their routine use in all patients with MI is less clear.[26] Nonetheless, because of the aggregate evidence of benefits of early beta blocker administration in MI, current professional guidelines recommend the administration of oral beta blockers within the first 24 hours in patients without a contraindication. It is also reasonable to administer intravenous beta blockers to MI patients if a tachyarrhythmia or hypertension is present, in the absence of signs of heart failure and/or low output, increased risk of developing shock, indicators of high risk of developing shock, or other relative contraindications to beta blockers. Moreover, patients who initially have contraindications to a beta blocker (e.g., heart failure) should be re-evaluated with respect to their candidacy for an oral beta blocker after 24 hours. Beta blockers may be especially helpful in patients with significant residual unrevascularized coronary artery disease and evidence of recurrent ischemia or tachyarrhythmias early after the onset of infarction.

Therefore, beta blockers are recommended in professional guidelines for early use in the setting of acute MI, except where contraindicated, and then for secondary prevention. However, there remains no clear evidence-based recommendation in the current guidelines regarding the appropriate duration of treatment with beta blockers in post-MI patients with normal left ventricular ejection fractions who are not experiencing angina or who do not require beta blockers for hypertension or dysrhythmia.

Coronary Revascularization

The goals of coronary revascularization are to restore perfusion to ischemic myocardium and to reduce the risks of subsequent occlusion at sites of stenosis and plaque rupture. In STEMI, emergency revascularization aims to limit ischemic injury and to minimize complications of infarction (see Chapter 17). The primary goal is to treat the occluded culprit lesion, and there is debate and ongoing studies concerning the treatment of nonculprit lesions. Many patients have additional lesions at other sites in the coronary tree. Current guidelines recommend revascularizing only the culprit lesion at the time of primary PCI, but a recent modest sized study suggests that complete revascularization may improve outcomes (CvLPRIT trial).[27] The much larger COMPLETE trial (NCT01740479), which is testing a staged revascularization strategy for nonculprit lesions, is ongoing.

Selection of patients for acute revascularization after NSTEMI is based on the identification of higher risk individuals (Figure 13-8; see Chapter 16), and the emergency treatment of those with ongoing ischemia and ischemic complications. The remaining patients may undergo a nonacute angiographic strategy or the identification of occult ischemia using imaging (see the section on Identification of Occult Ischemia and Chapter 30).

Identification of Occult Ischemia

In addition to treatment of the culprit lesion, prevention of recurrent ischemia related to disease in other coronary vessels is a key aspect of overall management of patients with MI. Invasive identification of untreated coronary lesions and assessment of their significance, or use of noninvasive testing, may be useful to reveal areas of ischemia for subsequent treatment. These approaches are not mutually exclusive. However, a more conservative strategy of "watchful waiting," based on symptoms and exercise testing, has been shown to be inferior to angiography and revascularization in NSTEMI.[21]

Invasive Detection of Occult Ischemia

Fractional flow reserve across a coronary stenosis can be measured using a flow-sensitive guidewire to determine the functional significance of coronary stenosis, and this approach is superior to an angiographically guided strategy and superior to a medical strategy.[28,29] High-resolution magnetic resonance imaging can also provide estimates of coronary flow, but large-scale clinical validation is still yet to be done (see Chapter 33).[30]

Noninvasive Detection of Occult Ischemia

Several noninvasive approaches are available to detect occult ischemia based on echocardiography with perfusion imaging (see Chapter 31), nuclear imaging (see Chapter 32), and magnetic resonance imaging (see Chapter 33). These approaches have been extensively studied, but mainly in patients with stable coronary disease.[31] Each of these imaging techniques is superior to the previously accepted practice of treadmill exercise testing, which has relatively poor sensitivity and suboptimal specificity (see Chapter 30).

ELECTRICAL AND MECHANICAL COMPLICATIONS

Management of acute complications of MI begins in the prehospital phase and continues through in-hospital care. The key principles of management rest upon the therapies to mitigate the risk of developing major mechanical complications, and the prevention and rapid treatment of life-threatening arrhythmias (Box 13-5). Once major complications have developed (e.g., severe heart failure, reduced cardiac output and cardiogenic shock, subacute rupture), there may be limited scope to reverse severe myocardial compromise.

BOX 13-5 Principles of Management of Electrical and Mechanical Complications

- Inhibition of the maladaptive pathways of neurohormonal activation to mitigate heart failure and adverse remodeling.
- Identification and management of arrhythmias (including sustained ventricular arrhythmias and atrial fibrillation).
- Adjunctive therapies to alleviate symptoms.
- Device therapy for mechanical dysfunction and heart failure.
- Management of hyperglycemia and hyperlipidemia.
- Identification and management of occult ischemia.
- Secondary prevention and rehabilitation.

Arrhythmias

Ventricular fibrillation is the major cause of sudden death in the early hours after infarction; therefore, there is a need for rapid identification of those with evolving MI and access to physicians who are trained and equipped to perform CPR (see Chapter 5). The epidemiology is challenging because early deaths are excluded from hospital-based studies. Community epidemiology studies demonstrate that 60% to 73% of deaths associated with STEMI occur out of hospital, mainly within the first 1 to 2 hours after onset. Interrupting the link between acute MI and sudden cardiac death is a critical goal in the management of MI. The key elements of early treatment involve rapid prehospital resuscitation and defibrillation. Later arrhythmias (ventricular tachycardia, ventricular fibrillation, and atrial fibrillation) may be the consequence of extensive infarction and muscle injury; therefore, effective and prompt reperfusion is critical for their prevention. For those that sustain muscle injury and impaired systolic function, implantable cardiac devices for treatment can be useful (see Chapter 28). Ventricular arrhythmias in the later phase of infarction are markers of continuing ischemia, mechanical dysfunction, and heart failure, and are indicators of adverse outcome.

Other arrhythmias and conduction disturbances are commonly seen in the acute phase of infarction, especially in those with impaired ventricular function, and the most frequent is new-onset atrial fibrillation, followed by nonsustained ventricular tachycardia and conduction defects (see Chapter 28).[32] High-degree atrioventricular block is a more powerful predictor of cardiac death than tachyarrhythmias in patients with impaired ventricular function.[32]

Mechanical Complications

Despite the currently available therapies, many patients sustain sufficient myocardial injury that produces systolic mechanical dysfunction and its associated complications. Specific mechanical complications, such as myocardial rupture and acute dysfunction of the mitral valve, are discussed in Chapter 26. In addition, impairment of ventricular contractile function because of ischemic stunning (see Chapter 24) and adverse remodeling of the ventricle are important consequences of increased wall stress associated with ventricular enlargement and mechanical dysfunction of the ventricle. Neuroendocrine activation occurs and is associated with changes in gene expression, alterations in calcium handling, myocyte cell death, and hypertrophy in nonischemic myocardium, and it is also associated with dilation of the affected myocardium. In consequence, there is further mechanical dysfunction and wall stress, and the development of a viscous cycle, leading to maladaptive or pathological remodeling (see Chapter 36).

The most common manifestation of adverse remodeling is heart failure (see Chapter 25), and substantial progress has been made in reducing the impact of heart failure over the longer term (see Chapter 36). Several stages of intervention may be beneficial in mitigating the risk of heart failure in patients with acute MI. First, minimizing the extent of myocardial injury by prompt revascularization is, again, the central tenet of management. Second, amelioration of reperfusion injury may diminish the size of the final territory of infarction, and novel therapies to limit reperfusion injury are under investigation (see Chapter 24). Third, the promotion of myocardial healing and prevention of adverse remodeling of the injured ventricle has been proven to reduce heart failure. In particular, inhibition of the maladaptive pathways of neurohormonal activation has provided a revolutionary advance in management. The role and application of renin-angiotensin and aldosterone antagonists, which have markedly improved outcomes and quality of life for patients with MI at risk for or complicated by heart failure, are discussed in detail elsewhere (see Chapter 25 and Chapter 36). In patients with markers of increased risk of heart failure as a result of MI, prioritization of these agents over the introduction of early beta blockers is reasonable. Nonetheless, although not recommended in the early phase of MI in such patients, beta-adrenergic blockers have a key role in the long-term management of heart failure caused by ischemic cardiomyopathy after MI (see Chapter 25).

Ventricular assist devices were initially developed to support cardiac output and to stabilize the acutely failing patient as a bridge to definitive therapy, usually cardiac transplantation. Major challenges remain with mechanical assist devices, including the risk of infection, bleeding, and stroke, but future developments may allow miniaturized devices to be implanted over the longer term, as "destination therapy" (see Chapter 27).

ADJUNCTIVE THERAPIES IN THE ACUTE PHASE

Lipid-Lowering Agents

The long-term benefits of lipid lowering for secondary prevention have been demonstrated unequivocally, and statin therapy has a class 1 recommendation in the guidelines.[33,34] Moreover, in pooled analyses, more intensive therapy results in fewer subsequent infarctions, ischemic strokes, and revascularizations, and a lower rate of cardiovascular death compared with moderate low-intensity statin therapy.[33] Initiation of lipid-lowering therapy during the initial hospitalization for acute MI appears to improve adherence to therapy and thus is recommended for all patients with MI in the absence of contraindications. In addition, early statin therapy may contribute to reducing plaque vulnerability and complications of revascularization to provide additional early clinical benefits. The use of lipid-lowering therapy for long-term secondary prevention is discussed in Chapter 34.

Management of Hyperglycemia

Hyperglycemia is commonly seen in the acute phase of STEMI and NSTEMI, and is a strong predictor of adverse long-term outcome, both in patients with and without diabetes. Although glucose elevation occurs acutely in the early phase of infarction, in response to catecholamine and other stimuli, it is also a marker of unrecognized diabetes and impaired glucose metabolism. The first manifestation of diabetes and glucose intolerance may occur during the course of infarction. Guidelines recommend measuring fasting glucose and glycosylated hemoglobin in all those showing early hyperglycemia, and performing oral glucose tolerance tests when diabetes is suspected.[5] Correction of hyperglycemia using insulin has shown benefit in clinical trials, but there have also been some conflicting results.[35]

Infusion of a combination of glucose, insulin, and potassium has failed to show benefit in two large-scale trials, and intensive insulin therapy may result in hypoglycemia-related complications in critically ill patients. Despite the absence of definitive proof from large-scale studies, guidelines recommend a strategy of careful but moderate control of hyperglycemia and avoiding hypoglycemia.[4,5]

SECONDARY PREVENTION AND REHABILITATION

Atherothrombosis is a chronic disease with a natural history that is punctuated by periods of instability and of relative quiescence over time. Patients may leave the hospital with the misimpression that they have been cured by successful coronary revascularization after presentation with an acute MI. However, patients with MI have a more than twofold higher risk of major cardiovascular events than individuals without a previous MI. For this reason, several of the pharmacological secondary prevention measures are initiated during the in-hospital phase and continued after discharge. These include the management of antithrombotic risk, lipid lowering, and modifications of the neurohormonal system (see Chapter 34).

Duration of Therapy

Atherothrombosis is a chronic disease that commonly diffusely involves the arterial tree, with multiple nonobstructive lesions. Nevertheless, these nonobstructive lesions can give rise to future obstructions (approximately 50% of the subsequent events in a longitudinal study of patients with coronary disease were caused by nonculprit lesions[36]; see Chapter 10). For these reasons, there is a strong rationale for long-term secondary preventive therapy in patients after acute MI.

The duration of treatment is life-long for lipid-lowering therapy, for aspirin and for angiotensin-converting enzyme inhibitors, angiotensin receptor blockers, and renin antagonists. However, for dual antiplatelet therapy, the balance of benefit and risk should be weighed for each patient beyond the first year of treatment after MI, taking into account thrombotic risk, bleeding risk, cost, and availability (see Chapter 35).[37,38]

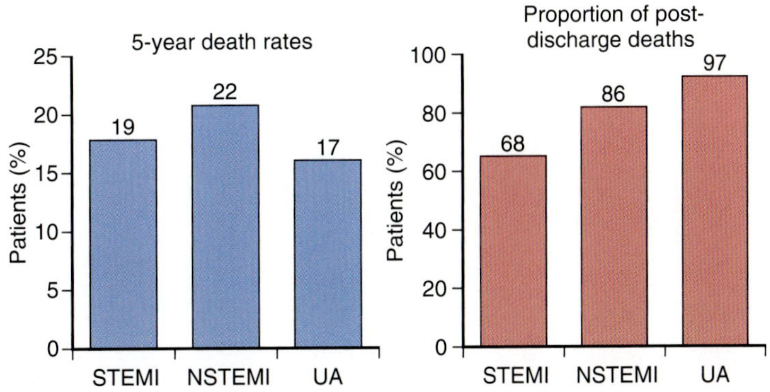

FIGURE 13-9 Five-year event rates after hospitalization with ST-elevation myocardial infarction (STEMI), non–ST-elevation myocardial infarction (NSTEMI), or unstable angina (UA) with documented evidence of coronary disease from the large multinational GRACE registry. Overall, approximately 1 in 5 patients will have died by 5 years, and the majority of the events occur after hospital discharge. *(From Fox KAA, et al: Underestimated and under-recognized: the late consequences of acute coronary syndrome [GRACE UK—Belgian Study].* Eur Heart J *31:2755, 2010.)*

Lifestyle Changes and Cardiac Rehabilitation

The long-term consequences following MI are influenced not only by the index event and the extent of myocardial injury, but also by the totality of risk factors affecting the patient. The cumulative impact of the long-term risks after MI is frequently under-recognized. For example, for patients with an NSTEMI who reach a hospital, more than 80% of their 5-year risk of death or MI is beyond the time of hospital discharge (Figure 13-9).[39]

Lifestyle changes to reduce cardiovascular risk are challenging to implement, and even more challenging to sustain. Quality improvement programs for monitoring smoking cessation and engagement in rehabilitation programs are examples of interventions to support secondary prevention. Key lifestyle interventions include smoking cessation, blood pressure control, dietary and glycemic modification, weight reduction, and exercise programs. Unfortunately, many affected patients fail to make the initial changes, and among those who take up the programs, only a minority complete them. Patient adherence to secondary preventive therapies is a critical target for long-term prevention.[5]

Obesity is a major problem in almost all industrialized communities, and simply providing dietary advice has limited effectiveness. More recently, the role of bariatric surgery has been investigated in severely obese patients and those with type 2 diabetes mellitus. It has been shown to not only reduce weight, but also to reverse glucose intolerance.[40] However, such surgical approaches are not applicable to most patients after an ACS event.

Exercise-based rehabilitation programs have been shown to not only improve health-related quality of life, but also to reduce the risk of subsequent cardiovascular events (see Chapter 34).[4,5]

FUTURE PERSPECTIVES

Current therapeutic interventions have radically improved outcomes following MI, at least for patients who survive to reach medical care. Case fatality has progressively fallen, and this is temporally associated with the uptake of the key evidence-based therapies. However, much remains to be done, especially in reducing prehospital mortality and in reducing the long-term risks after MI.

A key, and as yet unrealized principle in the management of MI, consists of early identification of patients with disrupted plaques to prevent thrombotic and occlusive complications, and hence, prevent progression to MI. Plaque disruption without major coronary vessel occlusion occurs more frequently and more widely than disruption, followed by clinically manifest MI (see Chapter 3). Angioscopic, intravascular ultrasound studies (with "virtual histology") and postmortem analyses have revealed that plaque rupture events may occur at multiple sites in the coronary (and systemic) arterial system, and that many of the plaque rupture events occur silently and without clinically manifest complications. These plaque ruptures may repair without detectable thrombotic complications, but can contribute to the progression of atheromatous coronary lesions (see Chapter 10).[41,42] If susceptible plaques could be identified and treated, this would revolutionize management of MI.[43]

Current research efforts are focused on the early identification of plaques susceptible to rupture, the so-called "vulnerable plaques," but as yet, identification and treatment of such plaques is beyond the scope of current management.[44] For example, positron emission tomography combined with computed tomography (Figure 13-10)[45] may be used to identify high-risk plaque. Identification of vulnerable patients is an ongoing challenge, but recent developments in biomarkers of inflammation, repair, and myocyte injury have opened the door to future changes in treatment and prevention of MI (see Chapter 8) and an emerging investigational paradigm in the principles of management of MI.

In acute cardiology, there is already an abundance of trial evidence and a consistency of international guidelines. However, for pharmacological treatments, there are multiple options and challenges for emergency care clinicians and acute care cardiologists. There are important gaps in the uptake of evidence-based therapies, especially among those with comorbidities, the frail, and in some ethnic and socioeconomic groups. From a societal perspective, there are larger potential gains from treating all those potentially eligible for class 1 guideline-recommended treatments than from choosing among therapeutic options in those selected for treatment. This problem requires robust quality improvement programs, organizational changes, and adequate funding.[40] Considerable challenges and room for further advances lie ahead.

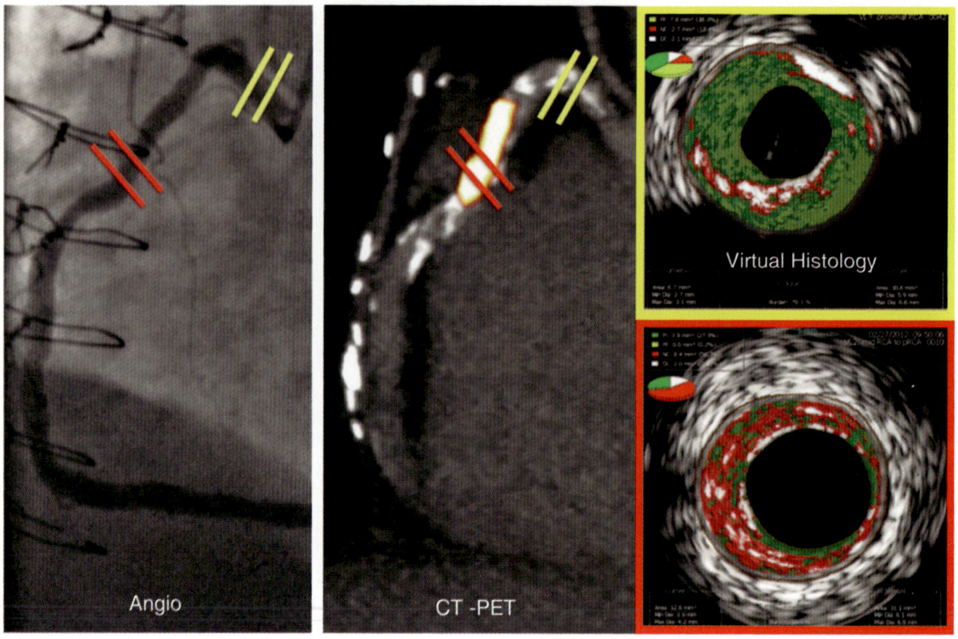

FIGURE 13-10 Coronary angiogram (*left panel*) showing evidence of diffuse disease but no obstructive lesions. Combined positron emission tomography-computed tomography (PET-CT) showing macrocalcification (dense white lesions) and two atheromatous lesions. Virtual histology using intravascular ultrasound (IVUS) of the 18F-NaF negative plaque (*yellow and upper*) shows mainly fibrofatty tissue (*green*) with some calcification (*white*) but little necrosis. 18F-NaF positive plaque (*red and lower*) demonstrates microcalcification (*white*) and a large necrotic core (*red*). 18F-NaF positive plaques were identified at sites of plaque rupture after presentation with an acute coronary syndrome. *(From Joshi NV, et al: 18F-fluoride positron emission tomography for identification of ruptured and high-risk coronary atherosclerotic plaques: a prospective clinical trial.* Lancet *383:705, 2014.)*

Classic References

Eikelboom JW, et al.: Adverse impact of bleeding on prognosis in patients with acute coronary syndromes, *Circulation* 114:774, 2006.

The Clopidogrel in Unstable Angina to Prevent Recurrent Events Trial Investigators: Effects of clopidogrel in addition to aspirin in patients with acute coronary syndromes without ST-segment elevation, *N Engl J Med* 345:494, 2001.

ISIS-2 (Second International Study of Infarct Survival) Collaborative Group: Randomised trial of intravenous streptokinase, oral aspirin, both, or neither among 17,187 cases of suspected acute myocardial infarction: ISIS-2 (Second International Study of Infarct Survival) Collaborative Group, *Lancet* 2:349, 1988.

The Risk Group: Risk of myocardial infarction and death during treatment with low dose aspirin and intravenous heparin in men with unstable coronary artery disease, *Lancet* 336:827, 1990.

Salomaa V, et al.: Decline in out-of-hospital coronary heart disease deaths has contributed the main part to the overall decline in coronary heart disease mortality rates among persons 35 to 64 years of age in Finland. The FINAMI Study, *Circulation* 108:691, 2003.

References

1. Jollis JG, et al.: Systems of care for ST-segment-elevation myocardial infarction: a report from the American Heart Association's mission: lifeline, *Circ Cardiovasc Qual Outcomes* 5:423, 2012.
2. Weisfeldt DT, et al.: Survival after application of automatic external defibrillators before arrival of the emergency medical system, *J Am Coll Cardiol* 55:1713, 2010.
3. Lloyd-Jones D, et al.: Executive summary: Heart disease and stroke statistics – 2010 update: a report from the American Heart Association, *Circulation* 121:948, 2010.
4. O'Gara PT, et al.: 2013 ACCF/AHA Guideline for the management of ST-elevation myocardial infarction: executive summary: a report of the American College of Cardiology Foundation/ American Heart Association Task Force on Practice Guidelines, *Circulation* 127:529, 2013.
5. Steg PG, et al.: Guidelines for the management of acute myocardial infarction in patients presenting with ST-segment elevation, *Eur Heart J* 33:2569, 2012.
6. Fox KAA, Huber KA: European perspective on improving acute systems of care in STEMI: we know what to do but how can we do it? *Nat Clin Pract Cardiovasc Med* 5:708, 2008.
7. Roe MY, et al.: Treatments, trends and outcomes of acute myocardial infarction and percutaneous coronary intervention, *J Am Coll Cardiol* 56:254, 2010.
8. Desta L, Jernberg T, Löfman I: Incidence, temporal trends, and prognostic impact of heart failure complicating acute myocardial infarction: the SWEDEHEART Registry (Swedish Web-System for Enhancement and Development of Evidence-Based Care in Heart Disease Evaluated According to Recommended Therapies): a study of 199,851 patients admitted with index acute myocardial infarctions, 1996 to 2008, *J Am Coll Cardiol Heart Failure* 3:234, 2015.
9. Lamberts M, et al.: Oral anticoagulation and antiplatelets in atrial fibrillation patients after myocardial infarction and coronary intervention, *J Am Coll Cardiol* 62:981, 2013.
10. Myocardial Ischaemia National Audit Project (MINAP) UK: How the NHS cares for patients with heart attack. Annual Public Report April 2013–May 2014. http://www.ucl.ac.uk/nicor/audits/minap/documents/annual_reports/minap-public-report-2014.
11. Hanssen M, et al.: French Registry on acute ST-elevation and non ST-elevation myocardial infarction 2010. FAST-MI 2010, *Heart* 98:699, 2012.
12. Schiele F, et al.: Reperfusion strategy in Europe: temporal trends in performance measures for reperfusion therapy in ST-elevation MI, *Eur Heart J* 31:2614, 2010.
13. Gale CP, et al.: Resolving inequalities in care? Reduced mortality in the elderly after acute coronary syndromes. The Myocardial Ischaemia National Audit Project 2003 – 2010, *Eur Heart J* 33:630, 2011.
14. Thygesen K, et al.: the Writing Group on behalf of the Joint ESC/ACCF/AHA/WHF Task Force for the Universal Definition of Myocardial Infarction. Third universal definition of myocardial infarction, *Eur Heart J* 233:2551, 2012.
15. Cabello JB, et al.: Oxygen therapy for acute myocardial infarction, *Cochrane Database Syst Rev* 16:CD007160, 2010.
16. Amin ST, et al.: Dynamic TIMI risk score for STEMI, *J Am Heart Assoc* 2:e003269, 2013.
17. Fox KAA, et al.: Should patients with acute coronary disease be stratified for management according to their risk? Derivation, external validation and outcomes using the updated GRACE risk score, *BMJ Open* 21:4, 2014.
18. Fox KAA, on behalf of the GRACE Investigators, et al.: Intervention in acute coronary syndromes: do patients undergo intervention on the basis of their risk characteristics? The Global Registry of Acute Coronary Events (GRACE), *Heart* 93:177, 2007.
19. Amsterdam EA, et al.: AHA/ACC guideline for the management of patients with non-ST-elevation acute coronary syndromes: a report of the American College of Cardiology/American Heart Association Task Force on Practice Guidelines, *J Am Coll Cardiol* 64:e139, 2014.
20. Hamm CW, et al.: ESC guidelines for the management of acute coronary syndromes in patients presenting without persistent ST-segment elevation. The Task Force for the management of acute coronary syndromes (ACS) in patients presenting without persistent ST-segment elevation of the European Society of Cardiology (ESC), *Eur Heart J* 32:2999, 2011.
21. Fox KAA, for the FIR Collaboration, et al.: Long-term outcome of a routine versus selective invasive strategy in patients with non–ST-segment elevation acute coronary syndrome: a meta-analysis of individual patient data, *J Am Coll Cardiol* 55:2435, 2010.
22. Jneid H, et al.: 2012 ACCF/AHA focused update of the guideline for the management of patients with unstable angina/non-ST-Elevation Myocardial Infarction (Updating the 2007 Guideline Cardiology Foundation/American Heart Association Task Force on Practice Guidelines and Replacing the 2011 Focused Update) : A Report of the American College of Cardiology Foundation/American Heart Association Task Force on Practice Guidelines, *Circulation* 126:875, 2012.
23. Wiviott SD, et al.: Prasugrel versus clopidogrel in patients with acute coronary syndromes, *N Engl J Med* 357:200, 2007.
24. Wallentin L, et al.: Ticagrelor versus clopidogrel in patients with acute coronary syndromes, *N Engl J Med* 361:1045, 2009.
25. Mehta SR, et al.: Antithrombotic therapy with fondaparinux in relation to interventional management strategy in patients with ST and non-ST segment elevation acute coronary syndromes. An individual patient-level combined analysis of the Fifth and Sixth Organization to Assess Strategies in Ischemic Syndromes (OASIS 5 and 6) Randomized Trials, *Circulation* 118:2038, 2008.
26. Bangalore S, et al.: Clinical outcomes with β-blockers for myocardial infarction: a meta-analysis of randomized trials, *The American Journal of Medicine* 127:939, 2014.
27. Gershlick AH, et al.: Randomized Trial of Complete Versus Lesion-Only Revascularization in Patients Undergoing Primary Percutaneous Coronary Intervention for STEMI and Multivessel Disease: The CvLPRIT Trial, *J Am Coll Cardiol* 65:963, 2015.
28. Tonino PAL, et al.: Fractional flow reserve versus angiography for guiding percutaneous coronary intervention, *N Engl J Med* 360:213, 2009.
29. De Bruyne B, et al.: Fractional flow reserve–guided PCI versus medical therapy in stable coronary disease, *N Engl J Med* 367:991, 2012.
30. Chiribiri A, et al.: Assessment of coronary artery stenosis severity and location: quantitative analysis of transmural perfusion gradients by high-resolution MRI versus FFR, *J Am Coll Cardiol Img* 6:600, 2013.
31. Garcia-Garcia HM, et al.: Imaging plaques to predict and better manage patients with acute coronary events, *Circ Res* 114:1904, 2014.
32. Bloch Thomsen PE, et al.: Long-term recording of cardiac arrhythmias with an implantable cardiac monitor in patients with reduced ejection fraction after MI, *Circulation* 122:1258, 2010.
33. Reiner Z, et al.: ESC/EAS Guidelines for the management of dyslipidaemias. The Task Force for the management of dyslipidaemias of the European Society of Cardiology (ESC) and the European Atherosclerosis Society (EAS), *Eur Heart J* 32:1769, 2011.
34. Stone NJ, et al.: 2013 ACC/AHA guideline on the treatment of blood cholesterol to reduce atherosclerotic cardiovascular risk in adults. A report of the American College of Cardiology/American Heart Association Task Force on Practice Guidelines, *Circulation* 129:S1, 2014.
35. De Caterina R, et al.: Glycaemic control in acute coronary syndromes: prognostic value and therapeutic options, *Eur Heart J* 31:1557, 2010.
36. Stone GW, et al.: A prospective natural-history study of coronary atherosclerosis, *N Engl J Med* 364:226, 2011.

37. Colombo A, Chieffo A: Dual antiplatelet therapy after drug-eluting stents — how long to treat? *N Engl J Med* 371:2225, 2014.
38. Bonaca MP, et al.: Long-term use of ticagrelor in patients with prior myocardial infarction, *N Engl J Med* 373:1274, 2015.
39. Fox KAA, et al.: Underestimated and under-recognized: the late consequences of acute coronary syndrome (GRACE UK – Belgian Study), *Eur Heart J* 31:2755, 2010.
40. Ricci C, et al.: Early impact of bariatric surgery on type II diabetes, hypertension, and hyperlipidemia: a systematic review, meta-analysis and meta-regression on 6,587 patients, *Obes Surg* 4:522, 2014.
41. Baber U, et al.: Prevalence, impact and predictive value of detecting subclinical coronary and carotid atherosclerosis in asymptomatic adults: The Bioimage study, *J Am Coll Cardiol* 65:1065, 2015.
42. Uchida Y: Recent advances in coronary angioscopy, *J Cardiol* 57:18, 2011.
43. Finn AV, et al.: Concept of vulnerable/unstable plaque, *Arterioscler Thromb Vasc Biol* 30:1282, 2010.
44. Jo JA, et al.: Simultaneous morphological and biochemical endogenous optical imaging of atherosclerosis, *Eur Heart J Cardiovasc Imaging* 16:910, 2015.
45. Joshi NV, et al.: 18F-fluoride positron emission tomography for identification of ruptured and high-risk coronary atherosclerotic plaques: a prospective clinical trial, *Lancet* 383:705, 2014.

14

Clinical Practice/Controversy

Selection of Reperfusion Therapy and Transfer Strategies for Patients with ST-Elevation Myocardial Infarction

Kevin R. Bainey and Paul W. Armstrong

CASE PRESENTATION

A 57-year-old man presents to a community hospital without capability for primary percutaneous coronary intervention (PPCI) in the early morning (4 AM) with a 1.5-hour history of severe chest pain. His medical history is significant for hypertension. His wife called 911, and at the time of first medical contact by paramedics, he was hemodynamically stable. On cardiac examination, his jugular venous pressure is elevated to 7 cm above the sternal angle, and a third heart sound is noted. Respiratory examination revealed basilar crackles in the lower lung fields. His electrocardiogram (ECG), which was recorded within 10 minutes of arrival, shows an anterior ST-elevation myocardial infarction (STEMI) with a large territory of myocardium at risk without baseline Q waves. Emergency medical service (EMS) transfer times to a PCI-capable hospital for PPCI are estimated to be 60 minutes, notwithstanding the harsh winter conditions. Tenecteplase (TNK) is readily available to administer at the presenting hospital site.

INTRODUCTION

In the current era of evidence-based therapy, morbidity and mortality from STEMI have remarkably declined (see Chapter 2). This trend has been accompanied by infarct size reduction and improvement in left ventricular function, largely mediated by timely and effective reperfusion therapy (see Chapter 13). Furthermore, enhanced public education leading to earlier patient presentation, rapid emergency response from well-trained and equipped paramedical personnel, improved treatment in the field, and application of the best reperfusion strategy for the right patient, at the right time, in the right place—all integrated with streamlined triage—have enhanced the care of STEMI patients (see Chapter 5).

The appreciation that early risk assessment informs diagnosis and guides use of appropriate contemporary pharmacologic and/or invasive strategies are key components of optimal patient-based care (see Chapter 11). However, in many jurisdictions, the prevailing clinical belief is that PPCI is not only the preferred reperfusion strategy as supported by a class I guideline recommendation (provided PPCI can be delivered expeditiously in a skilled 24/7 facility), but that it should be the only strategy. Although timely PPCI can now generally be accomplished in those patients presenting to a PPCI center, the feasibility of achieving this goal in the majority of STEMI patients (i.e., those presenting to a non–PCI-capable center, such as featured in the previously described case) is much more challenging. Placing the large majority of STEMI patients in the context of their geographic location, access to timely and expert 24/7 PPCI, transfer logistics, and the total elapsed ischemic time (defined as the delay from symptom onset to effective reperfusion therapy) unmasks the stark reality of significant management challenges. Because the key modulator of STEMI outcome is total ischemic time, yet widespread evidence exists that this recommended temporal window is consistently exceeded in a large number of patients transferred for PPCI, alternate strategies need to be explored. A pharmacoinvasive (PI) strategy has now emerged as a legitimate alternative.

Our aim in this chapter is to provide insights with regard to the selection of reperfusion strategies in STEMI patients who require transfer to a PCI-capable hospital. As first articulated in the 2004 American College of Cardiology Foundation (ACCF)/American Heart Association (AHA) STEMI guidelines, these insights align with the four key components of the recommended approach to STEMI, namely, evaluation of (1) baseline attributable risk from the STEMI, (2) the risk of fibrinolytic therapy, (3) the time from first medical contact, and (4) the time required to reliably achieve expert PPCI.

ELEMENTS THAT INFLUENCE REPERFUSION DELAY FOR PRIMARY PERCUTANEOUS CORONARY INTERVENTION IN TRANSFER PATIENTS

Primary PCI performed expeditiously in a high-volume expertise center has excellent outcomes. However, patients without ready access to PCI sites are particularly sensitive to delays that may offset these clinical benefits (Figure 14-1; see also Chapter 5).

Patient Delay

Despite global public education efforts, many patients still do not seek medical attention for approximately 1 to 2 hours following symptom presentation.[1,2] A profile of those patients who are most likely to delay activation of health care service has emerged and indicates they are more likely to be older adults, women, have diabetes, be African American, or of lower socioeconomic status.[3,4] Clinical trial data from nearly 6000 STEMI patients who underwent PPCI within 6 hours of symptom onset emphasized the growing importance of older adults; whereas only 17% of this cohort was aged older than 65 years, they accounted for 64% of the deaths.[5] An additional issue relates to patient choice of transportation to a health care facility. Because at least 50% of patients do not use the EMS system, they self-present as "walk-ins" to the nearest emergency room[6] and are subject to further delays in diagnostic recognition and therapy (see Figure 5-12). Results from the Acute Coronary Treatment and Intervention Outcomes Network–Get With The Guideline (ACTION-GWTG) registry (>37,000 patients) found that only 60% of patients with STEMI activated EMS. The self-transport patients were more likely to be younger, men, hemodynamically stable, and have less co-morbid conditions. Longer ischemic times and extended treatment delays were noted, subjecting these patients to adverse outcomes.[7]

Prehospital System Delay

In patients who directly activate EMS, continued challenges exist regarding transport to PCI-capable hospitals. Efforts have been made to bypass non-PCI sites and proceed to regional STEMI referral centers; however, 80% of such patients still do not achieve PPCI within 90 minutes (see Chapter 5).[8] Despite major national efforts to reduce treatment times for PPCI, an analysis of more than 12,000 STEMI patients in the ACTION-GWTG registry (including patients from the "Mission: Lifeline" program [2008 to 2011]) found emergency department bypass occurred infrequently (10.5%) and occurred primarily during usual working hours only. Shorter first medical contact to device times were noted in patients who bypassed the emergency department, but these shorter times were associated with marginal improvements in adjusted in-hospital mortality (odds ratio [OR], 0.69; 95% confidence interval [CI], 0.45 to 1.03; $P = .07$).[9]

In a key observational registry of 6209 Danish patients with STEMI transported by EMS for PPCI (35% who were transferred prehospital direct to a PCI center, with the remaining patients transferred from a non–PCI-capable hospital), long-term mortality (median 3.4 years, interquartile range [IQR], 1.8 to 5.2) increased with system delays (see Figure 5-9).[10] Hence, the impact of total ischemic time is critically important and prognostically relevant as represented

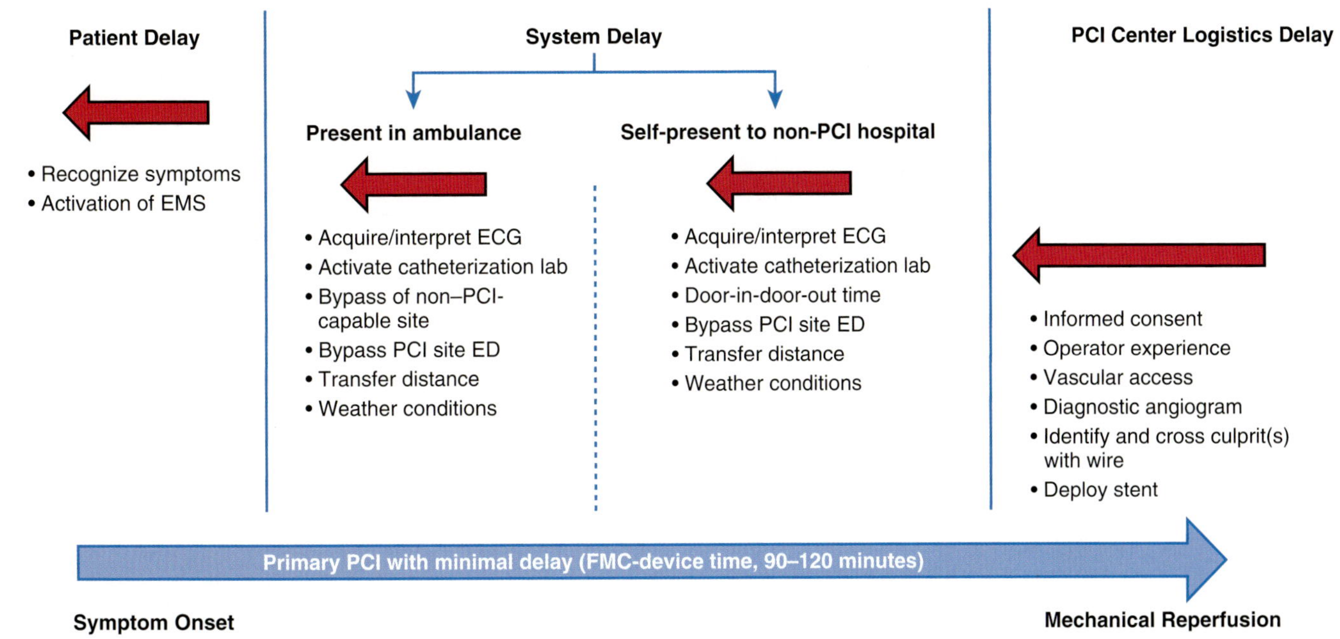

FIGURE 14-1 Components of delays in transfer of ST-elevation myocardial infarction (STEMI) for primary percutaneous coronary intervention (PCI). Patients presenting by ambulance are encouraged to bypass non-PCI hospitals and proceed directly to a PCI site. However, transfer logistics may still result in ambulance transport to a non–PCI-capable hospital, which then introduces further delays. *ECG*, Electrocardiogram; *ED*, emergency department; *EMS*, emergency medical services; *FMC*, first medical contact.

by the system delay (i.e., first medical contact to procedure) when considering transfer for PPCI. These data are especially noteworthy because (1) they demonstrate the inability to provide timely PPCI for most of the patients in the small country of Denmark, where drive times are short and PPCI facilities are abundant; (2) Denmark has substantial experience in conducting trials of transfer strategies that strongly influenced the movement towards PPCI; and (3) short-term mortality (in-hospital, 30 day, or even 1 year) is a blunt instrument to assess the longer term implications of delayed reperfusion. This issue is explored further in the section on Future Perspectives.

Interhospital System Delay

In the United States, most STEMI patients do not present to a PCI-capable site because the majority (approximately 80%) of health care institutions across the country are community hospitals without PPCI capability. For those patients who self-present to a non–PCI-capable facility and who require transfer, door-to-balloon times remain well above the targeted recommendation (transfer door to balloon ≤90 minutes) to improve timely access to care (7.6% in 2007 to 18.7% in 2009).[8] Using the National Cardiovascular Data Registry (NCDR)-CathPCI Registry data between 2005 and 2007, Wang and colleagues assessed more than 115,000 STEMI patients who underwent PPCI at 790 hospitals across the United States.[11] Of these, 25% of patients presented to non-PCI hospitals. Treatment of STEMI patients who had to be transferred significantly exceeded the guideline limits, with longer median door-to-balloon times than those who presented directly to PPCI centers (median 149 minutes vs. 79 minutes). Only 10% of transfer patients achieved a door-to-balloon time within 90 minutes of presentation. The ACTION Registry–GWTG reviewed more than 20,000 fibrinolysis-eligible STEMI patients who presented to a non–PCI-capable center with interhospital drive times of 30 to 120 minutes.[12] Of these, most patients (70.5%) were transferred to a PCI-capable facility for PPCI. Disappointingly, only 51.3% were able to achieve ACC/AHA guideline-recommended first medical contact to reperfusion time within 120 minutes. Figure 14-2 highlights the proportion of patients who achieved successful mechanical reperfusion times, stratified according to drive times for transfer. Of note, only 52.7% of patients with a drive time longer than 60 minutes received fibrinolysis (see Figure 14-2). Hence, this persistent delay in achieving timely PPCI in those patients transferred from other institutions is still unacceptably high and does not meet current guideline metrics for STEMI.[13]

Door-in-Door-out Time

Because of the delays that occur at the referral site (i.e., awaiting transport and emergency department delay), increased efforts have been initiated to reduce the delay between arrival to a non-PCI hospital and transfer to a PCI facility.[14] Termed as door-in-door-out (DIDO) time, the 2008 ACC/AHA Clinical Performance Measures for Acute Myocardial Infarction recommended a DIDO time of less than 30 minutes.[15] This quality metric was evaluated in nearly 15,000 STEMI patients who participated in the NCDR ACTION-GWTG registry who were initially seen in a non–PCI-capable hospital and subsequently transferred. The median DIDO was 68 minutes (IQR 43 to 120 minutes), with a DIDO time of ≤30 minutes achieved in only 11% of patients (see Figure 5-10). Predictors of longer

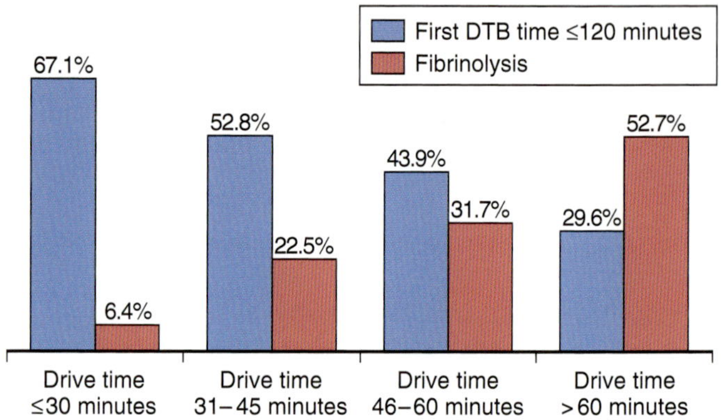

FIGURE 14-2 Proportion of door-to-balloon (DTB) times ≤120 minutes (*blue bars*) achieved versus percentage of patients with fibrinolysis administered (*red bars*) stratified by interhospital drive time among patients requiring transfer for ST-elevation myocardial infarction (STEMI). A report from the US National Cardiovascular Data Registry. *(Data from Vora AN, et al: Fibrinolysis use among patients requiring interhospital transfer for ST-segment elevation myocardial infarction care: A report from the US National Cardiovascular Data Registry.* JAMA Intern Med *175:207–215, 2015.)*

DIDO times included older age, female gender, off-hour presentation, and non-EMS arrival to the referring hospital.[16]

Mode of Transfer

Transfer times are also dependent on geographic constraints. Even in a well-developed STEMI transfer system of care, first door-to-device (D2D) times of 90 to 120 minutes can only be achieved for those hospitals located within a 30-minute transfer drive time (median D2D time of 93 minutes for drive times ≤30 minutes, 117 minutes for drive times of 31 to 45 minutes, and 121 minutes for drive times >45 minutes).[17] Air transport has been explored to help expedite transport of STEMI patients, but without consistent success. In a study of 140 patients transported from 16 hospitals by helicopter service within a 150-mile radius to 6 PCI-capable centers in Cincinnati, Ohio for PPCI, 111 ultimately underwent PCI, with 97% of cases exceeding a D2D time of 90 minutes (median 131 minutes).[18] Compared with ground transport, helicopter transport delayed D2D times irrespective of the distance-associated transfer drive time (helicopter transfer median D2D time 125 minutes for drive times of 31 to 45 minutes and 138 minutes for drive times >45 minutes).[17]

Primary Percutaneous Coronary Intervention Center Logistics Delay

Even if rapid transfer of patients to a PPCI-capable facility can be achieved, obstacles to delivering timely PPCI still exist. In an observational study of approximately 83,000 STEMI patients in the NCDR CathPCI Registry (2009 to 2011), delays to PPCI occurred in 14.7% of patients because of informed consent, concerns about obtaining vascular access, and difficulties crossing the infarct-related artery. Not surprisingly, the in-hospital mortality was substantially higher in patients with a delay compared with patients without a PPCI center logistics delay even after adjustment for baseline risk (15.1% vs. 2.5%; $P < .01$).[19] This observation reinforces the importance of the skill set developed in a high-volume experienced PPCI center[20] and constitutes a cautionary reminder about the propensity to build low-volume PPCI centers in areas already well served by such facilities. Strategies to develop systems to minimize such delays in an ideal STEMI system are discussed in detail in Chapter 5.

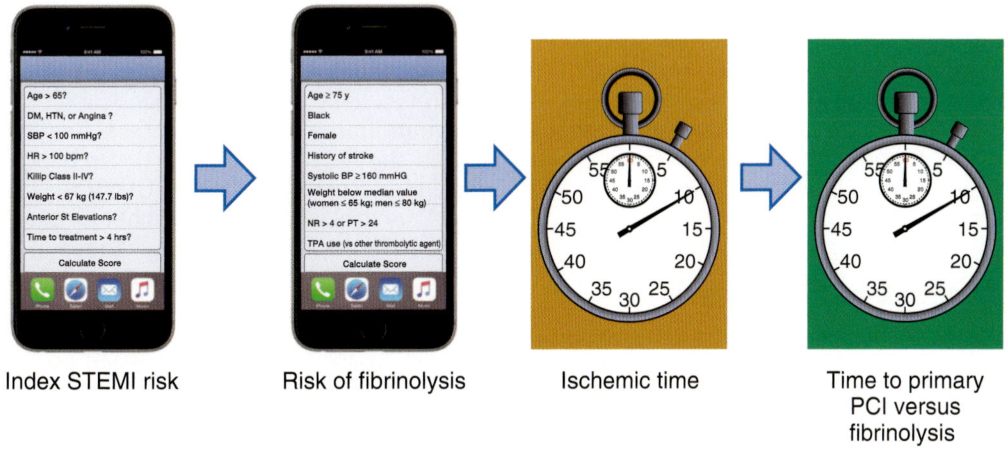

FIGURE 14-3 The four key factors to be considered when selecting a reperfusion strategy in ST-elevation myocardial infarction (STEMI) patients who require transfer to a percutaneous coronary intervention (PCI)-capable hospital.

CHOICE OF REPERFUSION STRATEGY IN TRANSFER PATIENTS

A "one-size-fits-all" approach does not adequately address the needs of patients with STEMI who require transfer to a health care facility, whether it be in an ambulance or to a community hospital. Although the particular approach requires sensitivity and understanding of regional realities and resources, the time-honored admonition formulated first in the 2004 ACC/AHA STEMI guidelines remains central to best practice, that is, "the appropriate and timely use of some form of reperfusion therapy is likely more important than the choice of therapy. Greatest emphasis is to be placed on the delivery of reperfusion therapy to the individual patient as rapidly as possible." For that reason, application of evidence-based reperfusion choices to promote and sustain high-quality reperfusion, limit myocardial damage, prevent unfavorable left ventricular remodeling, and reduce mechanical complications of myocardial infarction (MI) are key responsibilities of the front-line clinician (see Chapter 13). This responsibility to the STEMI patient is best discharged by integrating the factors illustrated in Figure 14-3.

Influence of Index ST-Elevation Myocardial Infarction Risk

Because baseline risk strongly intersects with time from symptom onset to reperfusion in modulating reperfusion strategies, an appreciation for the wide spectrum of STEMI risk is paramount. Morrow and colleagues demonstrated that most of the STEMI patients in the National Registry of Myocardial Infarction (NRMI)-3 registry were at a low risk (i.e., Thrombolysis In Myocardial Infarction [TIMI] risk score <5).[21] Ten years later, this finding was substantiated by registry data in Belgium that demonstrated that only 18.5% of patients had a high-risk TIMI profile.[22] Although no difference in survival between those treated with PPCI versus fibrinolysis was observed in most of the patients, that is, those at low risk (0.3% vs. 0.4%; adjusted $P = .60$) or intermediate risk (2.9% vs. 3.1%; adjusted $P = .30$), in-hospital survival was improved with PPCI compared with fibrinolysis in the TIMI high-risk patients (23.7% vs. 30.6%; adjusted $P = .03$).[22] These data are well aligned with the 3-year follow-up from the Danish Multicentre Randomized Study of Fibrinolytic Therapy vs. Primary Angioplasty in Acute Myocardial Infarction (DANAMI)-2 trial, which stratified STEMI patients according to baseline risk using the TIMI risk score (low risk TIMI 0 to 4; high risk TIMI ≥5).[23] Only high-risk patients experienced a survival benefit from PPCI compared with fibrinolysis (25.3% vs. 36.2%; $P = .02$) (Figure 14-4), whereas, once again, most of the low-risk STEMI patients (74%) showed no survival benefit with PPCI (8.0% vs. 5.6%).

Although the high-risk TIMI score patients derived clinical benefit with PPCI, other high-risk cohorts deserve further clarification. In patients who presented with hemodynamic compromise, secondary analyses from the Should We Emergently Revascularize Occluded Coronaries for Cardiogenic Shock (SHOCK) trial demonstrated benefit with early coronary angiography and emergent revascularization (PCI or coronary artery bypass graft [CABG]) compared with medical stabilization and delayed invasive assessment. Approximately 50% of the patients randomized to emergent revascularization received fibrinolysis before the procedure.[24] In the SHOCK Trial Registry, a combination of fibrinolytic therapy and intra-aortic balloon pump counterpulsation appeared to reduce in-hospital mortality.[25] Thus, for hospitals without revascularization capabilities and long transfer times to a PCI-capable hospital, fibrinolysis may be a reasonable alternative with immediate transfer to a PCI-capable site.

Notwithstanding the key influence of baseline risk, none of the previous studies addressed the intersection between this key variable and total ischemic time. Arguably, the early presenting patient with a large territory of myocardium at risk has the highest mortality compared with the later presenting patient who has outlived the time period with the greatest risk of death. This survival bias effect was well demonstrated in the prefibrinolytic era, in which 88% of patients who presented within 1 hour of symptoms (compared with 43% of patients who presented after 1 hour of symptoms) died either before or during hospital admission.[26,27] Hence, there is growing acceptance from previous registry data of the need to also account for the myocardial territory at risk in choosing a reperfusion strategy and a greater imperative for shorter delay from first medical contact to reperfusion in early presenting (<2 to 3 hours) patients. Based on the NRMI registry analysis of Pinto and colleagues, a young patient with an anterior STEMI (i.e., a large territory of myocardium at risk) who presents early with symptoms should be considered for fibrinolysis because of the equipoise with PPCI (Figure 14-5).[28] In this regard, the 2012 European Society of Cardiology (ESC) STEMI guidelines indicate a preferred target of less than 90 minutes from first medical contact for reperfusing such patients. This recommendation has now been supported by an analysis of the Strategic Reperfusion Early After Myocardial Infarction (STREAM) trial, which randomized patients to a PI versus PPCI strategy in early presenting STEMI patients and demonstrated similar rates of the composite of death, shock heart failure, and reoccurrence of MI between randomized treatment groups irrespective of ischemic area at risk (defined by the baseline electrocardiogram).[28a]

Influence of the Risk of Fibrinolysis

A cardinal decision point in the choice of acute reperfusion therapy is prompt evaluation of the risk of fibrinolysis. Contraindications to fibrinolysis, including a heightened risk of intracranial hemorrhage (ICH), are summarized in Chapter 15 (see Table 15-5). The overall incidence of ICH with contemporary fibrinolysis agents is approximately 1%[29] and must be incorporated into the risk–benefit analysis of pharmacologic reperfusion using predictors identified from previous fibrinolytic studies (see Chapter 15). For example, in the Global Utilization of Streptokinase and TPA for Occluded Coronary Arteries (GUSTO)-1 trial, patients with a previous stroke or transient ischemic attack were at heightened risk of ICH (5% to 7%).[30] Independent predictors of ICH formulated from more than 30,000 Medicare patients in the Cooperative Cardiovascular Project who received fibrinolytic therapy between 1994 and 1995 (overall risk of ICH was 1.43%) were incorporated into a risk model that revealed a range from 0.69% (risk score 0 to 1) to 4.11% (risk score ≥5) (Table 14-1).[31]

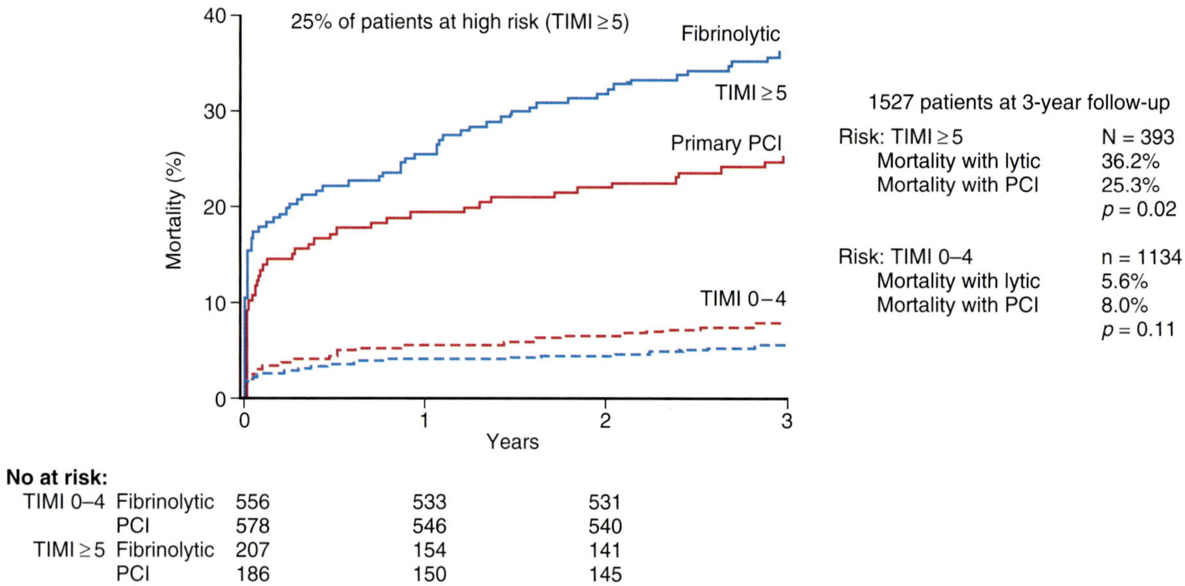

FIGURE 14-4 Three-year follow-up data from DANAMI-2. Mortality outcomes partitioned according to baseline Thrombolysis In Myocardial Infarction (TIMI) risk score. Note for the 25% of patients with TIMI risk ≥5, primary percutaneous coronary intervention (PCI) demonstrated an advantage, whereas for 75% of the population, the reverse tended to be true. Patients with TIMI risk 0 to 4 are indicated with *dotted lines*, those with TIMI risk ≥5 are indicated with *solid lines*. *(Adapted from Thune JJ, et al: Simple risk stratification at admission to identify patients with reduced mortality from primary angioplasty.* Circulation *112:2017–2021, 2005; Figure 1.)*

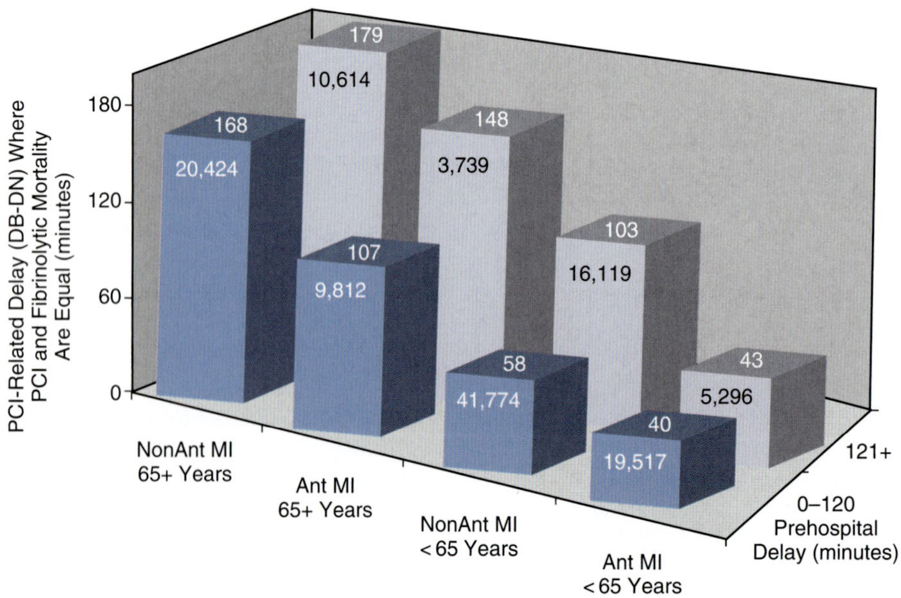

FIGURE 14-5 Influence of infarct location, age, and ischemic time on percutaneous coronary intervention (PCI)-related delay in which PCI and fibrinolytic mortality are equal. Note the narrow PCI-related delay window for a young patient with an anterior (Ant) ST-elevation myocardial infarction. *DB-DN*, Door-to-balloon, door-to-needle time. *(From Pinto DS, et al: Hospital delays in reperfusion for ST-elevation myocardial infarction: implications when selecting a reperfusion strategy.* Circulation *114:2019–2025, 2006; Figure 4.)*

Table 15-5 distinguishes between absolute and relative contraindications; in the former, PPCI is the only legitimate option, whereas in the latter situation, the use of fibrinolytic therapy needs to be weighed against the risk of the MI and the cost of a major delay to PPCI. The risk of non-ICH bleeding should also be considered, but its overall incidence is comparable or less than that found with PPCI.[29,32]

However, even when patients are considered eligible for fibrinolysis, a preoccupation with door-to-balloon times and PPCI tends to dominate, which could result in unforeseen consequences.[33] In a large NCDR registry study of 22,481 STEMI patients who were eligible for fibrinolysis, who presented to a non-PCI hospital, and who required transfer, only 29.5% received fibrinolytic therapy.[12] Moreover, the door-to-needle times appeared to be longer in high-volume PPCI facilities, which suggested "skill atresia" for a simple bolus fibrinolysis approach.[34,35] This fundamental skill set, particularly among young clinicians (many of whom have never administered fibrinolytic therapy for STEMI), is waning, but it is imperative to maintain competence and proficiency in treating all STEMI patients.

Influence of Ischemic Time

From the original canine experiments of Jennings and Reimer,[36] ischemic necrosis begins in the subendocardium within 20 minutes of coronary occlusion and proceeds in a transmural wavefront of cell death, culminating within 3 to 6 hours. Reperfusion within the first hour salvages almost two-thirds of the myocardium at risk, but thereafter salvage abruptly declines. Moreover, the Fibrinolytic Therapy Trialists' (FTT) Collaborative Group demonstrated maximum survival benefit (35-day mortality) in patients who received fibrinolytic therapy within 60 minutes of symptom onset (see Figure 13-3).[37] Cardiac magnetic resonance findings by Francone and colleagues examined different total ischemic time intervals to PPCI and found that myocardial salvage markedly decreased in tandem with increased microvascular obstruction when symptom onset to balloon time exceeded 90 minutes (Figure 14-6).[38] Hence, the success of either form of reperfusion therapy is unequivocally time dependent.

TABLE 14-1 Risk Score for Predicting Intracranial Hemorrhage with Fibrinolysis

RISK FACTOR*	RISK SCORE	RATE OF ICH (%)
Age ≥75 yrs	0–1	0.69
Black race	2	1.02
Female gender	3	1.63
History of stroke	4	2.49
SBP ≥160 mmHg	≥5	4.11
Weight ≤65 kg for women or ≤80 kg for men		
INR >4 or PT >24		
Use of alteplase		

ICH, Intracranial hemorrhage; *INR*, international normalized ratio; *PT*, prothrombin time; *SBP*, systolic blood pressure.
*Each risk factor is worth 1 point if present, 0 points if absent.

Early Presenters

The impact of ischemic time on choice of reperfusion strategy has largely been overlooked in contemporary management. By exploring the temporal relationships between fibrinolysis and PPCI, the slope of efficacy over time is shallower for PPCI compared with fibrinolysis; this relationship is related in part to the more successful pharmacologic lysis of younger thrombi versus the more consistent, less time-sensitive PPCI efficacy of opening occluded vessels. In a meta-analysis of more than 50,000 patients who received fibrinolysis for STEMI, the benefit was greatest in those patients who received therapy within 2 hours; thereafter, a linear decline in mortality was noted.[39] In a combined analysis of the Comparison of primary Angioplasty and Pre-hospital fibrinolysis In acute Myocardial infarction (CAPTIM) and Which Early ST-Elevation Myocardial Infarction Therapy (WEST) trials, which were aimed at early treated patients who presented within 2 hours of symptom onset, a temporal interaction demonstrated that those who received early fibrinolysis (and frequent timely coronary co-intervention) demonstrated improved 1-year survival compared with PPCI (2.8% vs. 6.9%; HR 0.43; 95% CI, 0.20 to 0.91; $P = .021$). This reinforced the importance of attenuating total ischemic time in early presenting patients with STEMI. This finding may be related to a lesser frequency of cardiogenic shock and heart failure, and a greater propensity for "aborting" MI (see Figure 13-3).

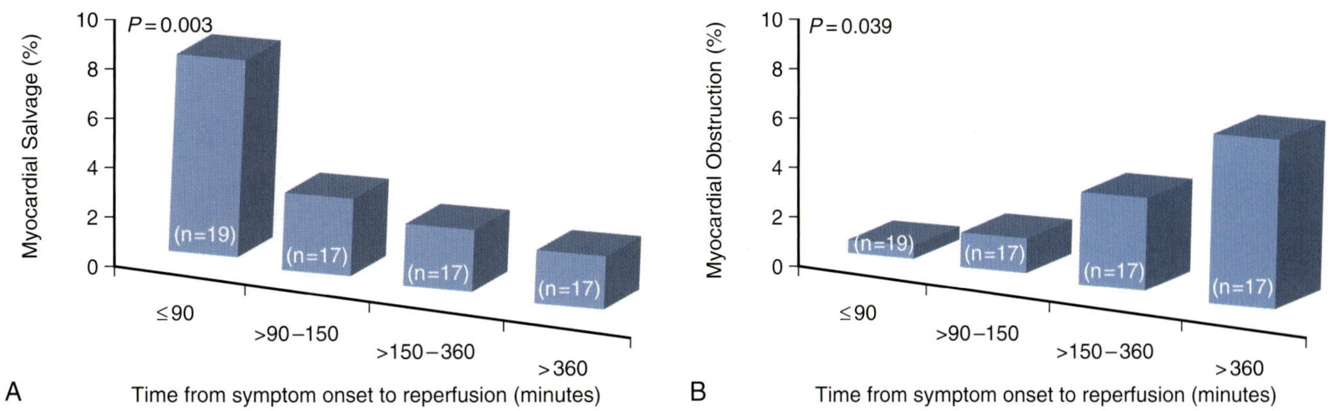

FIGURE 14-6 Relationship between (**A**) myocardial salvage and (**B**) microvascular obstruction, with time from symptom onset to reperfusion in 70 consecutive patients with first ST-elevation myocardial infarction (STEMI) undergoing primary percutaneous coronary intervention (PPCI) within 12 hours of symptom onset at a single center. As time to PPCI increases beyond 90 minutes, the extent of myocardial salvage declines and frequency of microvascular obstruction rises. *(Adapted from Francone M, et al: Impact of primary coronary angioplasty delay on myocardial salvage, infarct size, and microvascular damage in patients with ST-segment elevation myocardial infarction: Insight from cardiovascular magnetic resonance.* J Am Coll Cardiol *54:2145–2153, 2009.)*

In the Assessment of the Safety and Efficacy of a New Thrombolytic (ASSENT)-3 fibrinolytic trial, one in four patients treated within the first hour of symptom onset exhibited complete resolution of their initial ST elevation with minimal or no myocardial necrosis.[40] This pattern was also evident in a prespecified analysis from the STREAM trial (patients were randomized <3 hours after symptoms), in which aborted MI was more frequent with early fibrinolysis compared with PPCI (11.1% vs. 6.9%; P <.01). Aborted MI was associated with improved clinical outcomes at 30 days (death, cardiogenic shock, congestive heart failure, and/or recurrent MI: 7.0% vs. 12.5%; P = .042); the patients who had early fibrinolysis aborted had a lower composite endpoint (5.1% vs. 12.0%; P = .038).[41] There was good temporal alignment between the ischemic time, experimental myocardial salvage (see Figure 14-6), and lives saved from early fibrinolytic therapy and a propensity for aborted MI with prompt reperfusion therapy (see Figure 13-3).

Late Presenters

Those STEMI patients who present more than 3 to 4 hours after symptom onset fall into a time period with a shallower slope of the survival curve versus the time-to-reperfusion curve for fibrinolytic therapy; therefore, the impact of total ischemic time may be less relevant. These patients should be especially considered for PPCI because of the improved efficacy of reperfusion. In many STEMI patients, the time of symptom onset is difficult to ascertain and largely dependent on patient recollection; this challenge is especially true in older patients, women, patients with diabetes, and heart failure patients.[42] Assessment of the baseline Q wave in the distribution of the baseline ST elevation may provide additional insight into the status of MI evolution, and has been shown to be associated with reduced myocardial perfusion and adverse clinical outcomes, surpassing the time of symptom onset as a prognostic marker.[43] This relationship appears to be especially relevant to women with STEMI.[44] Hence, when a Q wave is already formed, less potential for salvaging myocardium is expected (despite total ischemic time), and consideration for PPCI with a transfer to a PCI-capable facility may be warranted. In this respect, it is of interest to compare the ECG in our Case Presentation with those in two patients who presented early with anterior MI (~2 hours); despite similar times and extent of ST elevation, there was a well-formed Q wave on the baseline ECG from the patient on the right (Figure 14-7). The additional insight provided by the ECG into the state of evolution of the STEMI may be useful in modulating the reperfusion pathway.

Influence of Transfer Time to Primary Percutaneous Coronary Intervention versus Fibrinolysis

Several randomized trials have suggested the benefit of a transfer strategy for PPCI in patients who present to a non-PCI capable hospital. The PRimary Angioplasty in patients transferred from General community hospitals to specialized PTCA Units with or without Emergency thrombolysis (PRAGUE)-2 trial randomized 850 patients with STEMI in the Czech Republic to either in-hospital fibrinolysis (with PCI according to routine clinical indication) or immediate transfer for PPCI (see Figure 5-e7). The time from randomization to balloon in the PCI group was remarkably short (97 ± 27 minutes), suggesting efficient transport with minimal system delays. In this context, a trend toward reduced 30-day mortality was observed with a transfer PPCI approach compared with fibrinolysis (6.8% vs. 10.0%; P = .12). However, in patients who presented early (<3 hours), no difference in mortality was seen, taking into consideration the use of a nonfibrin specific agent (streptokinase) (7.3% vs. 7.4%).[45]

Similarly, the Danish DANAMI-2 investigators randomized 1771 patients to early fibrinolysis versus PPCI, and in the 1129

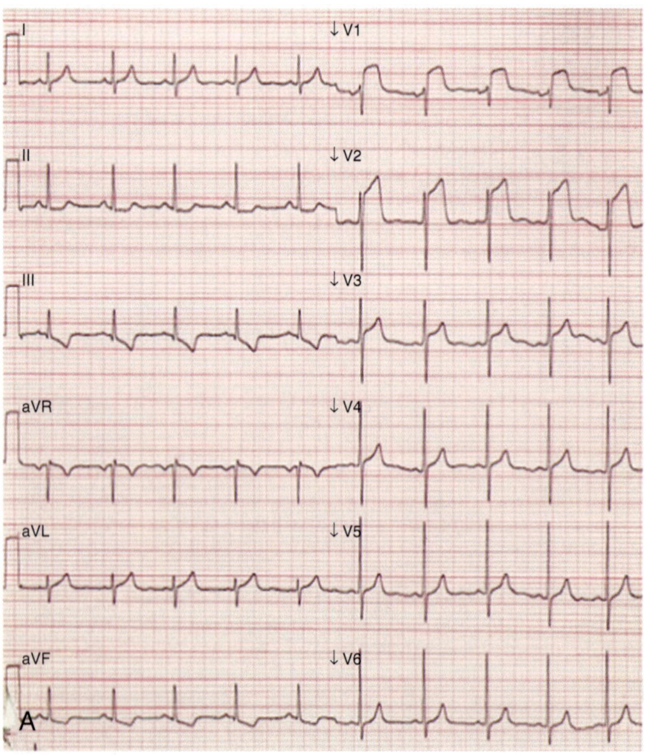

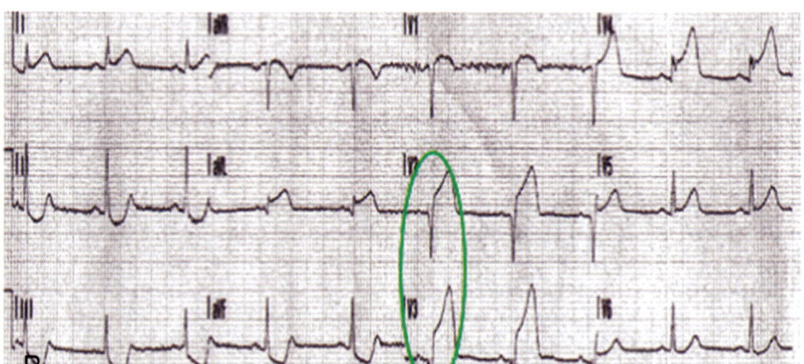

FIGURE 14-7 Twelve-lead electrocardiograms from two anterior ST-elevation myocardial infarction (STEMI) patients presenting at the same time from symptom onset (2 hours). Note the patient in the *left panel* has no baseline Q-wave, whereas the patient on the *right* already has a well-formed Q-wave.

patients randomized at a non–PCI-capable hospital, clinical benefit (death, clinical evidence of reinfarction, or disabling stroke) was seen with a transfer PPCI approach (8.5% vs. 14.2%; $P = .002$) (see Figure 5-e8). Again, system delays were minimal in these patients because randomization to treatment was a median of 90 minutes (IQR, 74 to 108 minutes). Furthermore, benefits were mainly driven by a reduction in reinfarction (1.6% vs. 6.3%; $P < .001$), in which routine coronary angiography for fibrinolysis patients was not mandated (and repeat fibrinolysis was recommended for failed reperfusion). No differences in death (6.6% vs. 7.8%; $P = .35$) or stroke (1.1% vs. 2.0%; $P = .15$) were observed.[46] As described previously, and unlike subsequent "real-world" registry data that examine transfer times, the system delays were short in both these studies, which contributed to the success of PPCI for those patients who presented to a non–PCI-capable hospital. More specifically, it should be noted that there was a remarkably short time difference in the initiation of reperfusion therapy (28 minutes) between the fibrinolytic strategy and PPCI in DANAMI 2.

Most recently, the STREAM trial (n = 1892) tested an early fibrinolysis strategy coupled with timely co-intervention (PI approach) compared with PPCI in patients who presented within 3 hours of symptom onset who were not able to obtain timely PCI within 60 minutes (most commonly because of the need for transfer to a PCI-capable facility). No difference in the 30-day primary endpoint of death, shock, congestive heart failure, or reinfarction was seen between the two groups (12.4% for PI vs. 14.3% for PPCI; relative risk [RR], 0.86; 95% CI, 0.68 to 1.09).[29] In addition, no difference in mortality was noted at 1 year.[47] Hence, this study, which amended the fibrinolytic dose by one-half in patients aged 75 years or older after 20% of patients were enrolled because of safety concerns, provided support for using the PI approach as a legitimate alternative for the large cohort of STEMI patients who cannot undergo timely PCI. It is especially noteworthy that the STEMI patients were reperfused much earlier than in many other STEMI randomized studies during the time when opportunities for salvage were most opportune (Figure 14-8).

Percutaneous Coronary Intervention–Related Delay

Establishing the juncture at which similar mortality rates occur when balancing ischemic wait times in transfer patients for PPCI compared with the option of administering fibrinolysis has been the subject of ongoing debate. Nallamothu and colleagues undertook a weighted meta-regression analysis of 23 randomized trials of PPCI versus fibrinolysis in 7739 patients with STEMI and found similar 4- to 6-week survival with a PCI-related delay of 62 minutes.[48] In the NRMI registry study,[28] Pinto and colleagues calculated PCI-related delays in more than 192,000 STEMI patients from 645 NCDR hospitals. The time observed in which the odds of in-hospital death were equal (true equipoise) between either reperfusion strategy was at a PCI-related delay of approximately 114 minutes (nearly one-half the patients in the analysis had transfer delays of more than 120 minutes). However, these results are based on an observational analysis in which confounding factors likely contributed to extended PCI-related delays. An additional prespecified STREAM analysis, which was stratified by delays in PPCI, indicated that the early fibrinolysis approach was similar to PPCI at 50 to 60 minutes, but that superiority over PPCI emerged if the PCI-related delay extended beyond 90 minutes (Figure 14-9).[49]

Summary of Considerations for Selection of Reperfusion Therapy

Taking into consideration these four key components modulating the choice of reperfusion noted in Figure 14-3, an overview of reperfusion options for the clinician treating STEMI patients is provided in Figure 14-10. In our view, fibrinolysis is preferred in early presenting patients particularly when accompanied by a large myocardial territory at risk because of the potential for major salvage or even aborting the MI. This decision is best made at the point of first medical contact and ideally in the ambulance or the emergency department of a non–PCI-capable hospital. An additional metric that appears to reflect the state of evolution of the infarction

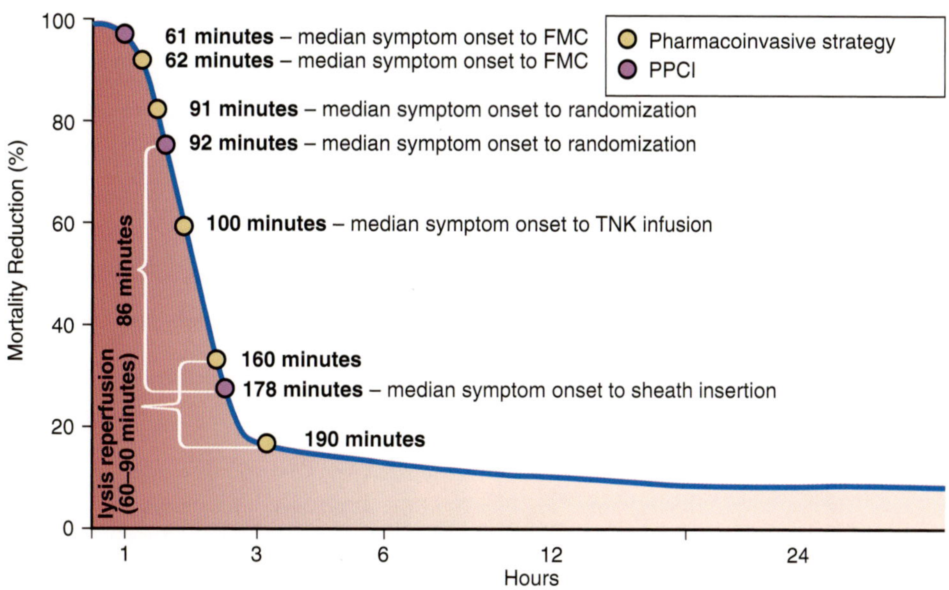

FIGURE 14-8 **Schema to reflect critical relationship between mortality reduction (and presumed myocardial salvage) and elapsed time from symptom onset.** The key times from symptom onset through first medical contact (FMC) to commencing the differing reperfusion therapies used in the STREAM trial are depicted. Note that reperfusion began on the early and steep portion of this curve. *PPCI*, Primary percutaneous coronary intervention; *TNK*, tenecteplase. *(Adapted from Gersh BJ, et al: Pharmacological facilitation of primary percutaneous coronary intervention for acute myocardial infarction: is the slope of the curve the shape of the future?* JAMA *293:979–986, 2005; and Armstrong PW, et al: Fibrinolysis or primary PCI in ST-segment elevation myocardial infarction.* N Engl J Med *368:1379–1387, 2013.)*

is the absence of a baseline Q wave in the region of ST elevation on the presenting ECG. This indicator has proven to be incrementally predictive of outcome over time from symptom onset and may be especially useful when time from symptom onset is difficult to ascertain.[43]

The time to reliably achieve PPCI in an expert 24/7 facility is exceedingly difficult to predict. Generally, however, if it is anticipated that a delay of more than 90 minutes (or 60 minutes in early presenters) to achieve PPCI is likely, then fibrinolysis should be administered. Primary PCI is favored for high-risk STEMI and/or unstable patients in whom reliable restoration of infarct-related artery patency is imperative to ensure clinical stability. Patients who present with prolonged ischemic times (>3 hours) and/or a baseline Q wave are also better served with PPCI because of the lesser efficacy of fibrinolysis and an attenuated likelihood of salvaging the myocardium. Primary PCI should be also be favored when the diagnosis of STEMI is in doubt (i.e., a masquerading MI) or contraindications to fibrinolysis exist.

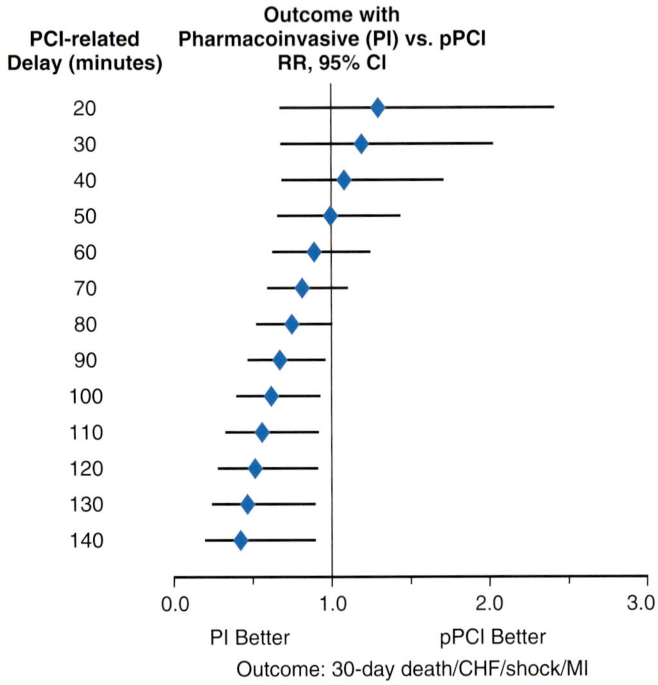

FIGURE 14-9 Relative association of continuous primary percutaneous coronary intervention (PPCI)-related delay (minutes) and study treatment with 30-day death, congestive heart failure (CHF), shock, and/or myocardial infarction (MI) from the STREAM study. Relative risks (RRs) and 95% confidence intervals (CIs) are presented (pharmacoinvasive [PI] vs. PPCI). Equipoise between treatments appears at approximately 50 to 60 minutes and an advantage for PI therapy occurs by 80 to 90 minutes of PPCI-related delay. *(From Gershlick AH, Westerhout CM, Armstrong PW, et al: Impact of a pharmacoinvasive strategy when delays to primary PCI are prolonged.* Heart *101:692–698, 2015.)*

KEY ELEMENTS OF A SUCCESSFUL PHARMACOINVASIVE APPROACH

Prehospital Fibrinolysis

The success of fibrinolytic therapy is largely dependent on the age of the coronary thrombus with a fresh clot in early presenters having the highest reperfusion rates (see Chapter 13). Because of the persistent delays incumbent with in-hospital therapy, prehospital fibrinolysis was advocated to further improve clinical outcomes. The potential advantage of prehospital fibrinolysis was first demonstrated in the early 1990s in an observational study in which patients who received prehospital thrombolytics less than 1.5 hours after symptoms (compared with 1.5 to 4 hours after symptoms) demonstrated reduced MI size and preserved left ventricular function.[50] In a subsequent meta-analysis of 6 randomized trials (6434 patients), prehospital fibrinolysis compared with in-hospital fibrinolysis shortened times to administer fibrinolysis (104 minutes vs. 162 minutes), with a commensurate reduced all-cause in-hospital mortality (OR, 0.83; 95% CI, 0.70 to 0.98) that translated into an absolute reduction of 2%, saving 1 life for every 62 patients treated.[51] Prehospital fibrinolysis has now been integrated into STEMI care pathways and networks in several locales.

Rescue Intervention

Resolution of ischemic chest pain, restoration of hemodynamic stability, emergence of an accelerated idioventricular

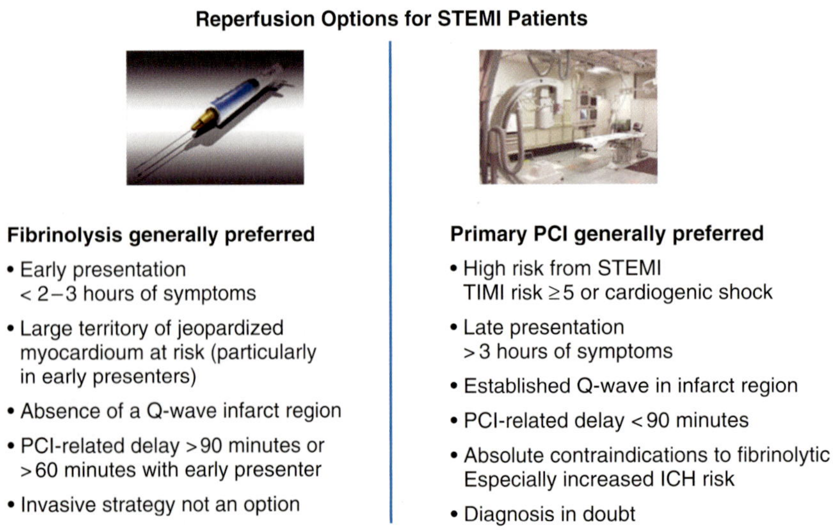

FIGURE 14-10 Considerations for selecting among reperfusion options in ST-elevation myocardial infarction (STEMI). *ICH*, Intracranial hemorrhage; *PCI*, percutaneous coronary intervention. *(Adapted from Antman EM, et al: ACC/AHA guidelines for the management of patients with ST-elevation myocardial infarction: A report of the American College of Cardiology/American Heart Association Task Force on Practice Guidelines [Committee to Revise the 1999 Guidelines for the Management of Patients with Acute Myocardial Infarction].* J Am Coll Cardiol *44:E1–E211, 2004.)*

rhythm, and, most importantly, resolution of the initial ST-segment elevation by at least 50% of its original height at 60 to 90 minutes after fibrinolysis are useful signs of successful reperfusion (see Chapter 23). However, failure to achieve reperfusion with fibrinolysis occurs in at least one-third of STEMI patients and prompts both the obligation and need to proceed with timely coronary co-intervention. The Rescue Angioplasty Versus Conservative Therapy or Repeat Thrombolysis (REACT) trial demonstrated superiority with this approach compared with conservative therapy or repeat fibrinolysis.[52] The benefits of rescue intervention have also been confirmed in two large meta-analyses.[53,54] Applying this approach in both the CAPTIM and WEST studies, as well as in STREAM trial, appears to reflect their favorable outcomes.

Routine Mechanical Co-Intervention

Using a combined adjunctive strategy of coronary angiography routinely with fibrinolysis has subsequently become an attractive reperfusion strategy, yet the optimal timing of cardiac catheterization following fibrinolysis in patients in whom reperfusion is successful has been controversial. Based on a series of previous trials, including ASSENT 4PCI and Facilitated Intervention with Enhanced Reperfusion Speed to Stop Events (FINESSE), a strategy of using pharmacologic therapy (either full-dose fibrinolytic therapy or one-half dose with concomitant glycoprotein IIb/IIIa therapy) followed by immediate mechanical intervention (facilitated PCI) has been largely been abandoned because of an excessive risk of bleeding and failure to improve outcomes during PCI.[55,56] Caution regarding the rapid systematic use of PCI following fibrinolysis is also suggested by data derived from the French registry of Acute ST-elevation or non-ST-elevation Myocardial Infarction (FAST MI).[57]

Other studies have explored a wider window for co-intervention to mitigate this risk. Randomized data from the GRupo de Análisis de la Cardiopatía Isquémica Aguda (GRACIA) study (500 patients randomized within 12 hours of symptom onset) found that those who underwent early catheterization at 6 to 24 hours after successful fibrinolysis had a lower rate of death, reinfarction, or revascularization at 12 months compared with an ischemia-guided conservative approach (9% vs. 21%; RR, 0.44; 95% CI, 0.28 to 0.70; $P = .0008$).[58] The Combined Abciximab REteplase Stent Study in Acute Myocardial Infarction (CARESS-in-AMI) trial, which examined a one-half dose fibrinolytic therapy with abciximab, found that immediate PCI in approximately 2.3 hours (as opposed to standard therapy with catheterization only when rescue PCI was indicated) led to a reduction in death, reinfarction, or refractory angina at 30 days (4.4% vs. 10.7%; hazard ratio [HR], 0.40; 95% CI, 0.21 to 0.76; $P = .004$).[59] A meta-analysis of seven randomized clinical trials (including the two aforementioned ones) conducted between 2003 and 2010 included 2961 patients randomized to early PCI after fibrinolysis (within 24 hours) versus standard fibrinolytic therapy (with variable rates of rescue PCI and invasive therapy). In this meta-analysis, a strategy of early coronary angiography led to a reduction in 30-day combined death and/or reinfarction (OR, 0.65; 95% CI, 0.49 to 0.88; $P = .004$) and recurrent ischemia (OR, 0.25; 95% CI, 0.13 to 0.49; $P < .001$), with no increase in major bleeding (OR, 0.93; 95% CI, 0.67 to 1.34; $P = .70$) or stroke (OR, 0.63; 95% CI, 0.31 to 1.26; $P = .21$). Moreover, maintenance of benefits at 6 to 12 months (death and/or reinfarction 0.71; 95% CI, 0.52 to 0.97; $P = .03$) were also evident.[60] These data are in concert with the Minnesota observational registry experience of Larson and colleagues who observed the safety and efficacy of a PI strategy (one-half dose fibrinolytic) in patients with STEMI, with expected delays because of long distance transfers.[61]

Transfer After Fibrinolysis

The Trial of Routine ANgioplasty and Stenting after Fibrinolysis to Enhance Reperfusion in Acute Myocardial Infarction (TRANSFER AMI) studied 1059 patients who presented to a non–PCI-capable hospital, who received full-dose fibrinolytic therapy (TNK), and who were randomized to receive either routine early PCI, which was constructed as urgent transfer to a PCI-capable hospital with a goal of performing PCI within 6 hours of fibrinolysis (median 2.8 hours) or standard treatment. Standard treatment consisted of transfer only for rescue PCI and otherwise remaining at the non–PCI-capable hospital for 24 hours with nonurgent cardiac catheterization encouraged (median 32.5 hours). Patients randomized to routine early PCI found improvement in the composite of death, reinfarction, recurrent ischemia, new or worsening congestive heart failure, or cardiogenic shock at 30 days (11.0% vs. 17.2%; HR, 0.64; 95% CI, 0.47 to 0.87; $P = .004$).[62] However, the rates of death and shock were numerically higher in the early transfer group and opposite to the direction of the less severe endpoints of reinfarction and recurrent ischemia in this study. In 266 STEMI patients aged 75 years or younger who presented within 6 hours, the NORwegian study on DIstrict treatment of STEMI (NORDISTEMI) trial tested the strategy of immediate routine transfer for PCI compared with ischemia-driven PCI after fibrinolysis in patients with long transfer times to a PCI-capable facility. Although no difference in the primary endpoint of death, reinfarction, stroke, or new ischemia at 12 months was noted, the incidence of death, recurrent infarction, or stroke was reduced with immediate transfer for PCI (6% vs. 16%; HR, 0.36; 95% CI, 0.16 to 0.81; $P = .01$).[63] This result was largely influenced by fewer reinfarctions and somewhat surprisingly by stroke.

Until further evidence is available, we support the current guideline recommendation for routine transfer for patients receiving fibrinolysis to a PCI-capable facility as part of a PI strategy, with the aim of performing angiography within 24 hours, and avoiding mechanical co-intervention within 2 to 3 hours after fibrinolysis (unless mandated by the need for rescue intervention) (Figure 14-11; see also the section on What Do the Guidelines Recommend).

However, logistical constraints and financial barriers may preclude such a strategy for all STEMI patients treated with fibrinolysis. When circumstances dictate a more selective approach, a focus on high-risk cohorts becomes warranted. Hence, patients with a large area of jeopardized myocardium or other high-risk features, as well as those who develop cardiogenic shock or acute severe heart failure, should be transferred to a PCI-capable hospital immediately following fibrinolysis for coronary angiography and emergent revascularization (PCI or CABG).[24,60] Also, patients in whom fibrinolytic therapy has failed or who demonstrate re-occlusion require transfer for rescue intervention at a PCI-capable site.[54] However, in the stable patient 24 to 48 hours without recurrent ischemia following fibrinolysis who is not transferred to a PCI-capable facility, the benefits

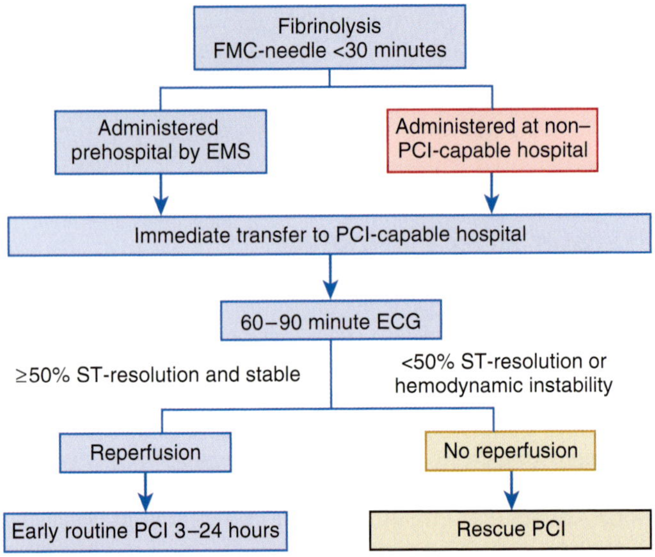

FIGURE 14-11 Transfer and evaluation algorithm following fibrinolysis for ST-elevation myocardial infarction. *ECG*, Electrocardiogram; *EMS*, emergency medical services; *FMC*, first medical contact; *PCI*, percutaneous coronary intervention.

of routine transfer to a PCI-capable facility for mechanical co-intervention are less clear, especially when the initial territory at risk is small. The ESC (class I) and ACC/AHA (class IIa) guidelines provide somewhat differing recommendations for routine transfer for PCI after fibrinolysis in stable patients. Because of the uncertainty around this issue, we contend that in such circumstances, an ischemia-driven cardiac catheterization approach is a reasonable alternative. Further support for an ischemia-driven approach in these patients exists in the Occluded Artery Trial (OAT) of 2166 clinically stable patients who did not have evidence of ischemia despite an occluded infarct-related artery at 3 to 28 days after MI, among whom optimal medical therapy versus PCI resulted in similar 4-year rates of death, reinfarction, and heart failure.[64,65]

ADJUNCTIVE THERAPIES TO REPERFUSION IN TRANSFER PATIENTS

For patients receiving fibrinolysis, adjunctive antithrombotic therapy must be administered concomitantly. For antiplatelets (see Chapter 19), both a loading dose of aspirin (162 to 325 mg)[66] and clopidogrel (300 mg for patients 75 years or younger; 75 mg for patients older than 75 years)[67,68] should be given before or with the fibrinolytic.[68] The use of more potent $P2Y_{12}$ inhibitors has not been prospectively established and cannot be recommended with fibrinolysis. The use of intravenous glycoprotein IIb/IIIa receptor antagonists should be avoided because of the detrimental risk of major bleeding during fibrinolysis.[56,69] For anticoagulation (see Chapter 18), enoxaparin given as an intravenous bolus (30 mg for patients 75 years or younger; no bolus for patients older than 75 years), followed by a weight-based subcutaneous dose (1 mg/kg twice daily for those 75 years or younger; 0.75 mg/kg for those older than 75 years) is favored over unfractionated heparin (weight-based intravenous bolus followed by an infusion to maintain a partial thromboplastin time of 50 to 70 seconds).[70]

In patients transferred for PPCI (see also Chapter 17), a loading dose of both aspirin (162 to 325 mg)[66] and a $P2Y_{12}$ inhibitor should be given as early as possible before mechanical reperfusion. Options for the loading dose include clopidogrel (600 mg),[71] ticagrelor (180 mg),[72] or prasugrel (60 mg).[73] Anticoagulant strategies to support PPCI are discussed in Chapter 17 and Chapter 18.

ST-ELEVATION MYOCARDIAL INFARCTION NETWORKS

Even with one of the world's highest occurrence rates for PCIs, less than 20% of United States hospitals have facilities for expert 24/7 PPCI. Therefore, regionalization of care for STEMI, with options of dual modes to reperfusion (PPCI reperfusion when feasible, and alternatively, PI reperfusion), along with the development of effective transfer strategies remains a key consideration. Organization of such networks allows for optimal reperfusion to limit total ischemic time, ensuring that all eligible patients receive therapy efficiently for STEMI (Figure14-12).[74] The rationale, organization, and implementation of such regional systems are discussed in Chapter 5. Successful implementation of STEMI networks have resulted in improved clinical outcomes. Protocols for several of these programs are outlined in Table 14-e1. Within Canada, the Northern Alberta Vital Heart Response network (built on the foundation of the WEST trial[75]) is an example of a mixed, dual reperfusion STEMI system of care serving a large metropolitan city (Edmonton; approximately 1 million people) and rural Northern Alberta (approximately 400,000 km^2). In-hospital outcomes demonstrate low in-hospital mortality, with a PI approach appearing to be safe and effective in patients in whom delay to mechanical reperfusion is anticipated (i.e., rural patients).[76]

Despite the successes of well-designed regional systems, they are subject to geographic diversity, altered weather patterns, variation in transportation modes and times, availability of resources and infrastructure, and characteristics and/or features of the health care system (universal, two-tier, private, and so on). These issues are not infrequent (7% to 25%) despite having an established STEMI network, and can result in altered survival if PPCI is relied upon as the only default mode for reperfusion.[8,10,33,77–79]

WHAT DO THE GUIDELINES RECOMMEND?

The updated 2013 ACCF/AHA STEMI guidelines emphasize advances in reperfusion therapy, organization of regional systems of care, transfer algorithms, antithrombotic and medical therapies, and subsequent secondary prevention strategies to optimize patient outcome (see Figure 13-5). In patients who present less than 12 hours with symptoms, PPCI is favored if it can be performed in a timely fashion with experienced operators (class I, level of evidence [LOE] A). EMS should transfer patients to a PCI-capable hospital (i.e., bypass non-PCI sites) for PPCI if a first medical contact to device time of within 90 minutes can be achieved (class I, LOE B). If a patient presents to a facility not capable of PCI, immediate transfer to a PCI site for PPCI should be considered with a first medical contact to device time of within 120 minutes (class 1, LOE B). If this goal cannot be achieved, in the absence of contraindications, timely fibrinolysis should be administered (class I, LOE A) within 30 minutes (class I, LOE B).[80]

Similarly, the 2012 European Society of Cardiology (ESC) guidelines on the management of STEMI highlight the importance of timely reperfusion, but these guidelines

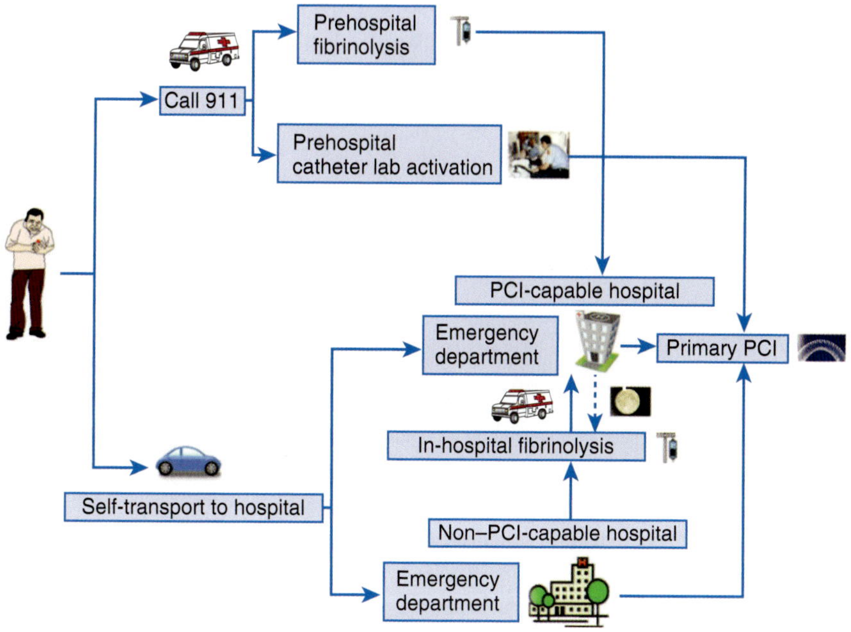

FIGURE 14-12 **A successful ST-elevation myocardial infarction network construct governed by the four key factors influencing reperfusion options.** *PCI*, Percutaneous coronary intervention. *(Adapted from Welsh RC, et al: Canadian Society Working Group: Providing a perspective on the 2007 focused update of the American Heart Association 2004 guidelines for the management of ST elevation myocardial infarction.* Can J Cardiol *25:25–32, 2009).*

focus on access to prehospital care (regional STEMI networks), where ambulance teams are trained and equipped to recognize STEMI and deliver reperfusion therapy expeditiously (including fibrinolysis). If fibrinolysis is selected, therapy should be administered within 30 minutes of first medical contact. In patients who present to an EMS or non–PPCI-capable hospital, PPCI is recommended over fibrinolysis if immediate transfer to a PCI center can occur and PPCI can be performed by an experienced team within 120 minutes of first medical contact (class I, LOE A), otherwise fibrinolysis should be performed. However, in patients who present early (<2 hours after symptom onset) with a large area of myocardium at risk, fibrinolysis should be considered if timely PPCI cannot be performed within 60 minutes of first medical contact (class I, LOE B).[81]

RECOMMENDED APPROACH TO ST-ELEVATION MYOCARDIAL INFARCTION CARE USING A DUAL REPERFUSION STRATEGY

The concept that PPCI is the only reperfusion strategy for STEMI is simply neither evidence-based nor logical because of the abundant evidence that STEMI patients face long transfer times, with unfavorable outcomes. Moreover, the premise that longer reperfusion delays for PPCI is acceptable cannot be justified in the current era in which the new reperfusion paradigm and appropriate focus is on reducing total ischemic time. Recognizing the importance of both reperfusion strategies and the complementary role within a STEMI network will ensure optimal care for patients. A shift toward recognizing the early presenting patient is paramount, because prompt reperfusion will salvage myocardium and enhance clinical outcome (i.e., reduce infarct size, heart failure, and lower mortality). Therefore, improvements at the public health level must occur to ensure earlier prehospital diagnosis, treatment, and triage for patients who present with STEMI. However, one must also consider environmental and patient modulators when choosing a reperfusion strategy (Figure 14-13). We provide a suggested algorithm for selection of reperfusion therapy for patients presenting in the ambulance or to a non-PCI hospital who require transfer for STEMI care (Figure 14-14).

RETURN TO THE CASE

After careful deliberation with the on-call interventional cardiologist, dual antiplatelet therapy (162 mg aspirin/300 mg clopidogrel) and parenteral enoxaparin (30 mg intravenously followed by 1 mg/kg subcutaneously) were administered. Shortly after, 40 mg of TNK (70 kg male) was given as a bolus intravenous injection (reconstituted in 8 mL) over 5 seconds, with a door-to-needle time of 25 minutes. Immediate transfer to a PCI-capable hospital was arranged, and the patient arrived at the coronary care unit 80 minutes later. Upon arrival, there was symptomatic relief, and the 90-minute ECG showed complete ST-segment resolution without Q-wave development. Later that day (at approximately 5 hours), routine coronary angiography using a transradial approach was performed. An isolated 80% proximal stenosis in the left anterior descending artery was identified, with normal anterograde flow. A bolus of intravenous enoxaparin (35 mg) was administered, and PCI was performed with a drug-eluting stent. On post-admission day 2, troponin I levels were minimally elevated, and subsequent cardiac magnetic resonance imaging showed a left ventricular ejection fraction of 50% with subtle anterior wall hypokinesis and myocardial edema. On day 4, he was discharged with an angiotensin-converting enzyme inhibitor, β-blocker, high-dose statin therapy, and dual antiplatelet therapy (aspirin and clopidogrel).

FUTURE PERSPECTIVES

The remarkable progress in STEMI care over the past decade constitutes a challenge to evaluating future advances. It seems clear that future quality metrics of timely reperfusion must focus on total ischemic time and incorporate risk assessment.

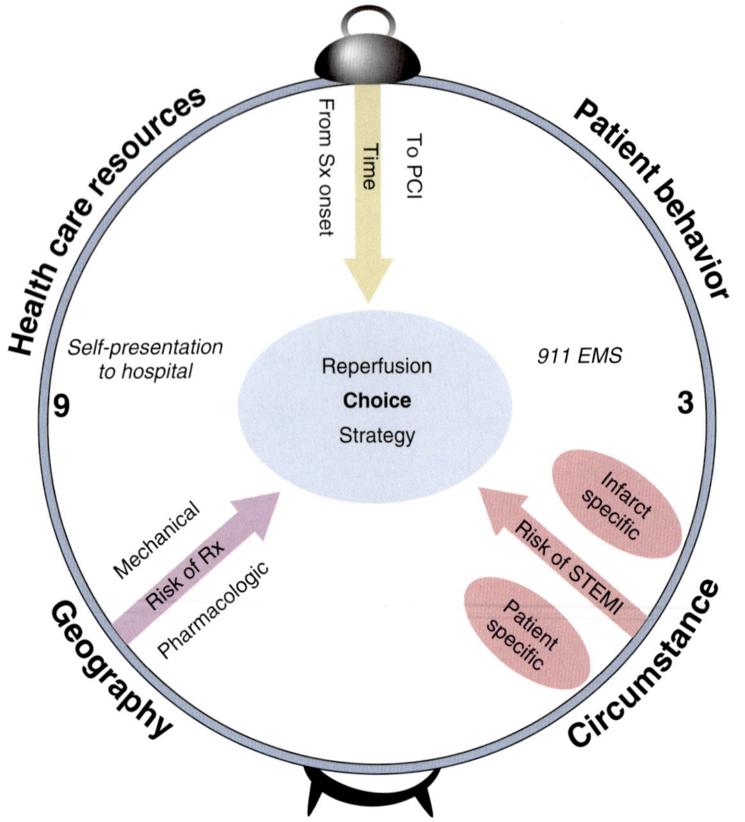

FIGURE 14-13 Conceptual model of ST-elevation myocardial infarction (STEMI) nexus modulating choice of reperfusion strategy. The factors that compose the external environmental framework surround the model. Patient-, infarct-, and risk-of-reperfusion–specific factors converge with both time from symptom onset and the expected time to achieve percutaneous coronary infarction (PCI) in this model. *EMS,* emergency medical services; *Rx,* treatment; *Sx,* symptoms. *(From Armstrong PW, et al: Duration of symptoms is the key modulator of the choice of reperfusion for ST-elevation myocardial infarction.* Circulation *119:1293–1303, 2009.)*

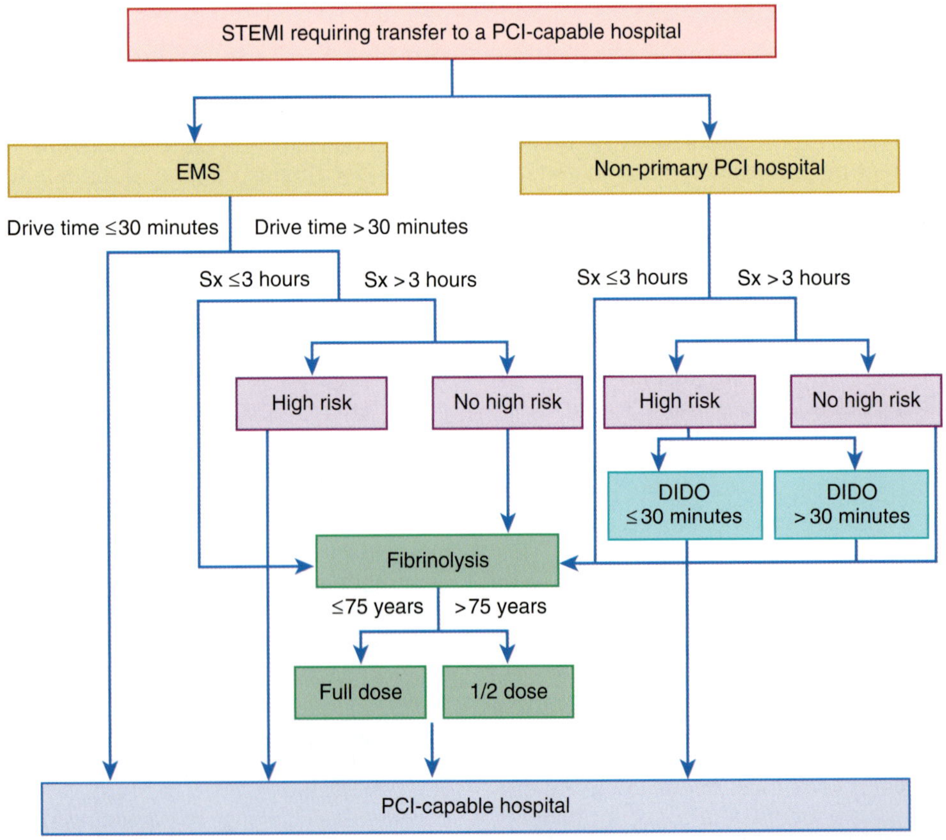

FIGURE 14-14 Authors' recommended treatment algorithm for transfer patients with ST-elevation myocardial infarction (STEMI) using both reperfusion options. *DIDO,* Door-in-door-out; *EMS,* emergency medical services; *PCI,* percutaneous coronary intervention; *Sx,* symptoms.

As mortality declines to unprecedented low rates, it has become apparent that this metric is a blunt measurement, especially if measured in the short term. The move toward measuring composite endpoints, although understandable, is fraught with hazards because of the differing clinical significance of the components of such endpoints and the realization that they do not always behave in a symmetrical fashion. One attractive option is to count all of the events each patient experiences (as opposed to just the first one) and to prespecify the relative weights of each component according to its clinical significance. This approach can be informed by input from both clinical investigators and patients.[82,83] There also may be opportunities to introduce new endpoints into future studies, such as the occurrence of aborted MI.

As the frequency of STEMI increases in many of the developing countries, greater uptake of a PI approach seems probable and is already evident in a number of regions. Because of the emergence of more powerful oral $P2Y_{12}$ platelet inhibitors, their role as concomitant therapy in the milieu of fibrinolytic therapy requires further study. The optimal dosing of fibrinolytics also needs further study, as demonstrated by data in the older adult patient cohort of the STREAM study (see Chapter 15).

Finally, an open question exists as to whether routine cardiac catheterization is necessary in all patients who receive fibrinolytic therapy. Low-risk patients without recurrent ischemia after successful reperfusion may fall into this category; at routine catheterization several hours after treatment, a proportion of such patients are found to have open coronary vessels with excellent perfusion and have been successfully managed medically. Further study will be required to address this issue and others in the ongoing care of STEMI patients.

References

1. Goldberg RJ, et al.: Prehospital delay in patients with acute coronary syndromes (from the Global Registry of Acute Coronary Events [GRACE]), *Am J Cardiol* 103:598–603, 2009.
2. Spencer FA, et al.: Delay to reperfusion in patients with acute myocardial infarction presenting to acute care hospitals: an international perspective, *Eur Heart J* 31:1328–1336, 2010.
3. Canto JG, et al.: Prevalence, clinical characteristics, and mortality among patients with myocardial infarction presenting without chest pain, *JAMA* 283:3223–3229, 2000.
4. Gibler WB, et al.: Persistence of delays in presentation and treatment for patients with acute myocardial infarction: the GUSTO-I and GUSTO-III experience, *Ann Emerg Med* 39:123–130, 2002.
5. Gharacholou SM, et al.: Age and outcomes in ST-segment elevation myocardial infarction treated with primary percutaneous coronary intervention: findings from the APEX-AMI trial, *Arch Intern Med* 171:559–567, 2011.
6. Canto JG, et al.: Use of emergency medical services in acute myocardial infarction and subsequent quality of care: observations from the National Registry of Myocardial Infarction 2, *Circulation* 106:3018–3023, 2002.
7. Mathews R, et al.: Use of emergency medical service transport among patients with ST-segment-elevation myocardial infarction: findings from the National Cardiovascular Data Registry Acute Coronary Treatment Intervention Outcomes Network Registry-Get With The Guidelines, *Circulation* 124:154–163, 2011.
8. Roe MT, et al.: Treatments, trends, and outcomes of acute myocardial infarction and percutaneous coronary intervention, *J Am Coll Cardiol* 56:254–263, 2010.
9. Bagai A, et al.: Emergency department bypass for ST-segment-elevation myocardial infarction patients identified with a prehospital electrocardiogram: a report from the American Heart Association Mission: Lifeline program, *Circulation* 128:352–359, 2013.
10. Terkelsen CJ, et al.: System delay and mortality among patients with STEMI treated with primary percutaneous coronary intervention, *JAMA* 304:763–771, 2010.
11. Wang TY, et al.: Door-to-balloon times for patients with ST-segment elevation myocardial infarction requiring interhospital transfer for primary percutaneous coronary intervention: a report from the National Cardiovascular Data Registry, *Am Heart J* 161:76–83 e71, 2011.
12. Vora AN, et al.: Fibrinolysis use among patients requiring interhospital transfer for ST-segment elevation myocardial infarction care: a report from the US National Cardiovascular Data Registry, *JAMA Intern Med* 175:207–215, 2015.
13. Ranasinghe I, et al.: Comparative effectiveness of population interventions to improve access to reperfusion for ST-segment-elevation myocardial infarction in Australia, *Circ Cardiovasc Qual Outcomes* 5:429–436, 2012.
14. Miedema MD, et al.: Causes of delay and associated mortality in patients transferred with ST-segment-elevation myocardial infarction, *Circulation* 124:1636–1644, 2011.
15. Krumholz HM, et al.: ACC/AHA 2008 performance measures for adults with ST-elevation and non-ST-elevation myocardial infarction: a report of the American College of Cardiology/American Heart Association Task force on performance measures (writing committee to develop performance measures for ST-elevation and non-ST-elevation myocardial infarction): Developed in collaboration with the American Academy of Family Physicians and the American College of Emergency Physicians: Endorsed by the American Association of Cardiovascular and Pulmonary Rehabilitation, Society for Cardiovascular Angiography and Interventions, and Society of Hospital Medicine, *Circulation* 118:2596–2648, 2008.
16. Wang TY, et al.: Association of door-in to door-out time with reperfusion delays and outcomes among patients transferred for primary percutaneous coronary intervention, *JAMA* 305: 2540–2547, 2011.
17. Munoz D, et al.: Transport time and care processes for patients transferred with ST-segment-elevation myocardial infarction: the reperfusion in acute myocardial infarction in Carolina emergency rooms experience, *Circ Cardiovasc Interv* 5:555–562, 2012.
18. McMullan JT, et al.: Reperfusion is delayed beyond guideline recommendations in patients requiring interhospital helicopter transfer for treatment of ST-segment elevation myocardial infarction, *Ann Emerg Med* 57:213–220 e211, 2011.
19. Swaminathan RV, et al.: Nonsystem reasons for delay in door-to-balloon time and associated in-hospital mortality: a report from the National Cardiovascular Data Registry, *J Am Coll Cardiol* 61:1688–1695, 2013.
20. Canto JG, et al.: The volume of primary angioplasty procedures and survival after acute myocardial infarction. National Registry of Myocardial Infarction 2 Investigators, *N Engl J Med* 342: 1573–1580, 2000.
21. Morrow DA, et al.: Application of the TIMI risk score for ST-elevation MI in the National Registry of Myocardial Infarction 3, *JAMA* 286:1356–1359, 2001.
22. Claeys MJ, et al.: Contemporary mortality differences between primary percutaneous coronary intervention and thrombolysis in ST-segment elevation myocardial infarction, *Arch Intern Med* 171:544–549, 2011.
23. Thune JJ, et al.: Simple risk stratification at admission to identify patients with reduced mortality from primary angioplasty, *Circulation* 112:2017–2021, 2005.
24. Hochman JS, et al.: One-year survival following early revascularization for cardiogenic shock, *JAMA* 285:190–192, 2001.
25. Sanborn TA, et al.: Impact of thrombolysis, intra-aortic balloon pump counterpulsation, and their combination in cardiogenic shock complicating acute myocardial infarction: a report from the SHOCK trial registry. Should we emergently revascularize occluded coronaries for cardiogenic shock? *J Am Coll Cardiol* 36:1123–1129, 2000.
26. Lowel H, Lewis M, Hormann A: (Prognostic significance of prehospital phase in acute myocardial infarct. Results of the Augsburg Myocardial Infarct Registry, 1985-1988), *Dtsch Med Wochenschr* 116:729–733, 1991.
27. The pre-hospital management of acute heart attacks: Recommendations of a task force of the European Society of cardiology and the European Resuscitation Council, *Eur Heart J* 19: 1140–1164, 1998.
28. Pinto DS, et al.: Hospital delays in reperfusion for ST-elevation myocardial infarction: implications when selecting a reperfusion strategy, *Circulation* 114:2019–2025, 2006.
28a. Bainey KR, et al.: Implications of ischaemic area at risk and mode of reperfusion in ST-elevation myocardial infarction, *Heart*. Epub ahead of print, 2016.
29. Armstrong PW, et al.: Fibrinolysis or primary PCI in ST-segment elevation myocardial infarction, *N Engl J Med* 368:1379–1387, 2013.
30. Gore JM, et al.: Stroke after thrombolysis. Mortality and functional outcomes in the GUSTO-I trial. Global Use of Strategies to Open Occluded Coronary Arteries, *Circulation* 92:2811–2818, 1995.
31. Brass LM, et al.: Intracranial hemorrhage associated with thrombolytic therapy for elderly patients with acute myocardial infarction: results from the Cooperative Cardiovascular Project, *Stroke* 31:1802–1811, 2000.
32. Keeley EC, Boura JA, Grines CL: Primary angioplasty versus intravenous thrombolytic therapy for acute myocardial infarction: a quantitative review of 23 randomised trials, *Lancet* 361:13–20, 2003.
33. Armstrong PW, Boden WE: Reperfusion paradox in ST-segment elevation myocardial infarction, *Ann Intern Med* 155:389–391, 2011.
34. Nallamothu BK, et al.: Relation between hospital specialization with primary percutaneous coronary intervention and clinical outcomes in ST-segment elevation myocardial infarction: National Registry of Myocardial Infarction-4 analysis, *Circulation* 113:222–229, 2006.
35. Nallamothu BK, et al.: Times to treatment in transfer patients undergoing primary percutaneous coronary intervention in the United States: National Registry of Myocardial Infarction (NRMI)-3/4 analysis, *Circulation* 111:761–767, 2005.
36. Jennings RB, Reimer KA: Factors involved in salvaging ischemic myocardium: effect of reperfusion of arterial blood, *Circulation* 68:I25–I36, 1983.
37. Indications for fibrinolytic therapy in suspected acute myocardial infarction: Collaborative overview of early mortality and major morbidity results from all randomised trials of more than 1000 patients. Fibrinolytic Therapy Trialists' (FTT) Collaborative Group, *Lancet* 343:311–322, 1994.
38. Francone M, et al.: Impact of primary coronary angioplasty delay on myocardial salvage, infarct size, and microvascular damage in patients with ST-segment elevation myocardial infarction: insight from cardiovascular magnetic resonance, *J Am Coll Cardiol* 54:2145–2153, 2009.
39. Boersma E, et al.: Early thrombolytic treatment in acute myocardial infarction: reappraisal of the golden hour, *Lancet* 348:771–775, 1996.
40. Taher T, et al.: Aborted myocardial infarction in patients with ST-segment elevation: insights from the assessment of the safety and efficacy of a new thrombolytic regimen-3 trial electrocardiographic substudy, *J Am Coll Cardiol* 44:38–43, 2004.
41. Dianati Maleki N, et al.: Aborted myocardial infarction in ST-elevation myocardial infarction: insights from the strategic reperfusion early after myocardial infarction trial, *Heart* 100:1543–1549, 2014.
42. Canto AJ, et al.: Differences in symptom presentation and hospital mortality according to type of acute myocardial infarction, *Am Heart J* 163:572–579, 2012.
43. Armstrong PW, et al.: Baseline Q-wave surpasses time from symptom onset as a prognostic marker in ST-segment elevation myocardial infarction patients treated with primary percutaneous coronary intervention, *J Am Coll Cardiol* 53:1503–1509, 2009.
44. Kaul P, et al.: Relative prognostic value of baseline Q wave and time from symptom onset among men and women with ST-elevation myocardial infarction undergoing percutaneous coronary intervention, *Am J Cardiol* 110:1555–1560, 2012.
45. Widimsky P, et al.: Long distance transport for primary angioplasty vs immediate thrombolysis in acute myocardial infarction. Final results of the Randomized National Multicentre Trial–PRAGUE-2, *Eur Heart J* 24:94–104, 2003.
46. Andersen HR, et al.: A comparison of coronary angioplasty with fibrinolytic therapy in acute myocardial infarction, *N Engl J Med* 349:733–742, 2003.
47. Sinnaeve PR, et al.: ST-segment-elevation myocardial infarction patients randomized to a pharmaco-invasive strategy or primary percutaneous coronary intervention: Strategic Reperfusion Early After Myocardial Infarction (STREAM) 1-year mortality follow-up, *Circulation* 130: 1139–1145, 2014.
48. Nallamothu BK, Bates ER: Percutaneous coronary intervention versus fibrinolytic therapy in acute myocardial infarction: is timing (almost) everything? *Am J Cardiol* 92:824–826, 2003.
49. Gershlick AH, et al.: Impact of a pharmacoinvasive strategy when delays to primary PCI are prolonged, *Heart* 101:692–698, 2015.
50. Linderer T, et al.: Prehospital thrombolysis: beneficial effects of very early treatment on infarct size and left ventricular function, *J Am Coll Cardiol* 22:1304–1310, 1993.
51. Morrison LJ, et al.: Mortality and prehospital thrombolysis for acute myocardial infarction: a meta-analysis, *JAMA* 283:2686–2692, 2000.
52. Gershlick AH, et al.: Rescue angioplasty after failed thrombolytic therapy for acute myocardial infarction, *N Engl J Med* 353:2758–2768, 2005.
53. Collet JP, et al.: Percutaneous coronary intervention after fibrinolysis: a multiple meta-analyses approach according to the type of strategy, *J Am Coll Cardiol* 48:1326–1335, 2006.
54. Wijeysundera HC, et al.: Rescue angioplasty or repeat fibrinolysis after failed fibrinolytic therapy for ST-segment myocardial infarction: a meta-analysis of randomized trials, *J Am Coll Cardiol* 49:422–430, 2007.

55. Assessment of the Safety and Efficacy of a New Treatment Strategy with Percutaneous Coronary Intervention (ASSENT-4 PCI) Investigators. Primary versus tenecteplase-facilitated percutaneous coronary intervention in patients with ST-segment elevation acute myocardial infarction (ASSENT-4 PCI): randomised trial, *Lancet* 367:569–578, 2006.
56. Ellis SG, et al.: Facilitated PCI in patients with ST-elevation myocardial infarction, *N Engl J Med* 358:2205–2217, 2008.
57. Danchin N, et al.: Comparison of thrombolysis followed by broad use of percutaneous coronary intervention with primary percutaneous coronary intervention for ST-segment-elevation acute myocardial infarction: data from the French Registry on Acute ST-elevation Myocardial Infarction (FAST-MI), *Circulation* 118:268–276, 2008.
58. Fernandez-Aviles F, et al.: Routine invasive strategy within 24 hours of thrombolysis versus ischaemia-guided conservative approach for acute myocardial infarction with ST-segment elevation (GRACIA-1): a randomised controlled trial, *Lancet* 364:1045–1053, 2004.
59. Di Mario C, et al.: Immediate angioplasty versus standard therapy with rescue angioplasty after thrombolysis in the combined abciximab reteplase stent study in acute myocardial infarction (CARESS-in-AMI): an open, prospective, randomised, multicentre trial, *Lancet* 371:559–568, 2008.
60. Borgia F, et al.: Early routine percutaneous coronary intervention after fibrinolysis vs. standard therapy in ST-segment elevation myocardial infarction: a meta-analysis, *Eur Heart J* 31:2156–2169, 2010.
61. Larson DM, et al.: Safety and efficacy of a pharmaco-invasive reperfusion strategy in rural ST-elevation myocardial infarction patients with expected delays due to long-distance transfers, *Eur Heart J* 33:1232–1240, 2012.
62. Cantor WJ, et al.: Routine early angioplasty after fibrinolysis for acute myocardial infarction, *N Engl J Med* 360:2705–2718, 2009.
63. Bohmer E, et al.: Efficacy and safety of immediate angioplasty versus ischemia-guided management after thrombolysis in acute myocardial infarction in areas with very long transfer distances results of the NORDISTEMI (Norwegian Study on District Treatment of ST-Elevation Myocardial Infarction), *J Am Coll Cardiol* 55:102–110, 2010.
64. Hochman JS, et al.: Coronary intervention for persistent occlusion after myocardial infarction, *N Engl J Med* 355:2395–2407, 2006.
65. Hochman JS, et al.: Long-term effects of percutaneous coronary intervention of the totally occluded infarct-related artery in the subacute phase after myocardial infarction, *Circulation* 124:2320–2328, 2011.
66. Antithrombotic Trialists' Collaboration: Collaborative meta-analysis of randomised trials of antiplatelet therapy for prevention of death, myocardial infarction, and stroke in high risk patients, *BMJ* 324:71–86, 2002.
67. Sabatine MS, et al.: Addition of clopidogrel to aspirin and fibrinolytic therapy for myocardial infarction with ST-segment elevation, *N Engl J Med* 352:1179–1189, 2005.
68. Chen ZM, et al.: Addition of clopidogrel to aspirin in 45,852 patients with acute myocardial infarction: randomised placebo-controlled trial, *Lancet* 366:1607–1621, 2005.
69. Assessment of the Safety and Efficacy of a New Thrombolytic Regimen (ASSENT)-3 Investigators: Efficacy and safety of tenecteplase in combination with enoxaparin, abciximab, or unfractionated heparin: The ASSENT-3 randomised trial in acute myocardial infarction, *Lancet* 358:605–613, 2001.
70. Antman EM, et al.: Enoxaparin versus unfractionated heparin with fibrinolysis for ST-elevation myocardial infarction, *N Engl J Med* 354:1477–1488, 2006.
71. Mehta SR, et al.: Double-dose versus standard-dose clopidogrel and high-dose versus low-dose aspirin in individuals undergoing percutaneous coronary intervention for acute coronary syndromes (CURRENT-OASIS 7): a randomised factorial trial, *Lancet* 376:1233–1243, 2010.
72. Wallentin L, et al.: Ticagrelor versus clopidogrel in patients with acute coronary syndromes, *N Engl J Med* 361:1045–1057, 2009.
73. Wiviott SD, et al.: Prasugrel versus clopidogrel in patients with acute coronary syndromes, *N Engl J Med* 357:2001–2015, 2007.
74. Armstrong PW, Westerhout CM, Welsh RC: Duration of symptoms is the key modulator of the choice of reperfusion for ST-elevation myocardial infarction, *Circulation* 119:1293–1303, 2009.
75. Armstrong PW: A comparison of pharmacologic therapy with/without timely coronary intervention vs. primary percutaneous intervention early after ST-elevation myocardial infarction: The WEST (Which Early ST-elevation Myocardial Infarction Therapy) study, *Eur Heart J* 27:1530–1538, 2006.
76. Shavadia J, et al.: Bridging the gap for nonmetropolitan STEMI patients through implementation of a pharmacoinvasive reperfusion strategy, *Can J Cardiol* 29:951–959, 2013.
77. Huber K, et al.: Enhancing the efficacy of delivering reperfusion therapy: a European and North American experience with ST-segment elevation myocardial infarction networks, *Am Heart J* 165:123–132, 2013.
78. Huber K, Goldstein P, Danchin N, Fox KA: Network models for large cities: the European experience, *Heart* 96:164–169, 2010.
79. Lambert L, et al.: Association between timeliness of reperfusion therapy and clinical outcomes in ST-elevation myocardial infarction, *JAMA* 303:2148–2155, 2010.
80. O'Gara PT, et al.: 2013 ACCF/AHA guideline for the management of ST-elevation myocardial infarction: a report of the American College of Cardiology Foundation/American Heart Association Task Force on Practice Guidelines, *J Am Coll Cardiol* 61:e78–e140, 2013.
81. Steg PG, et al.: ESC guidelines for the management of acute myocardial infarction in patients presenting with ST-segment elevation, *Eur Heart J* 33:2569–2619, 2012.
82. Bakal JA, et al.: Evaluation of early percutaneous coronary intervention vs. standard therapy after fibrinolysis for ST-segment elevation myocardial infarction: contribution of weighting the composite endpoint, *Eur Heart J* 34:903–908, 2013.
83. Stafinski T, et al.: Incorporating patient preferences into clinical trial design: results of the opinions of patients on treatment implications of new studies (options) project, *Am Heart J* 169: 122–131 e122, 2015.

15 Fibrinolytic Therapy for Patients with ST-Elevation Myocardial Infarction

Peter R. Sinnaeve and Frans Van de Werf

INTRODUCTION

A ST-segment myocardial infarction (STEMI) is caused by the occlusion of a major epicardial coronary artery and is generally triggered by rupture of a vulnerable plaque, with subsequent formation of an occlusive thrombus. Rapid restoration of coronary blood flow is essential in preventing myocardial necrosis, and early reperfusion of the infarct-related artery limits infarct size and improves outcome (see also Chapter 13). Therefore, achieving the shortest possible delay between symptom onset and reperfusion is one of the most critical factors in the management of STEMI (see Chapter 5). Effective reperfusion of the infarct-related artery can be achieved by mechanical reperfusion, using primary percutaneous coronary intervention (PCI) (see Chapter 17) or by pharmacological reperfusion using fibrinolytic agents. Unfortunately, only a minority of hospitals worldwide have immediate access to a catheterization facility. Moreover, hospitals with a catheterization laboratory often do not offer primary PCI during nonoffice hours. In contrast, fibrinolysis is universally available without the need for advanced logistics (Table 15-1). Thus, despite the impressive benefit and increasing use of primary PCI (see Figure 13-4), fibrinolysis remains the only option for reperfusion for many STEMI patients worldwide. In the past few decades, remarkable progress has been made in improving fibrinolytic therapies, in identifying patients who benefit from this treatment, and in identifying patients at risk of bleeding. In addition, in the past several years, studies have provided answers on to how to fit fibrinolytic therapy into contemporary hospital networks, especially when and how to plan angiography and PCI in successfully reperfused patients after fibrinolysis (see Chapter 14).

A BRIEF HISTORICAL OVERVIEW

Sudden thrombotic occlusion of an epicardial coronary artery was identified as the trigger for MI by James Herrick as early as 1912, but this pathophysiological mechanism was largely ignored in subsequent decades.[1] In a postmortem study in the 1960s of 176 "fresh" infarctions, Kagan and colleagues found evidence of a thrombotic coronary occlusion in only 87 patients, versus a "nonthrombotic" occlusion in an additional 43 patients. Interest in thrombolysis for MI did not accelerate until more than a decade later in 1980, after DeWood and colleagues provided strong angiographic evidence of a total occlusion in STEMI patients who presented early after onset of symptoms.

Pharmacological reperfusion for patients with an MI was investigated as early as the 1950s by Fletcher and colleagues. In the 1960s and 1970s, several studies of intravenous and intracoronary thrombolytic therapy showed conflicting results, mainly because of small sample sizes, and different treatment protocols and endpoint analyses. In addition, bleeding risk was often deemed to be unacceptably high. Nevertheless, a pivotal European trial in 1971, coordinated by Verstraete (n = 764), demonstrated a significant benefit of intravenous streptokinase versus heparin with respect to in-hospital mortality (18.5% vs. 26.3%; $P = .011$) in STEMI patients.[1a] In 1981, a pilot trial by Markis and colleagues with nine patients treated with an intracoronary infusion of streptokinase showed that local lytic therapy had the potential of salvaging jeopardized myocardium, especially in early presenters. Another trial, the Western Washington study (n = 250), also demonstrated an almost threefold reduction in 30-day mortality among patients treated with intracoronary streptokinase, a benefit that persisted at 1-year follow-up.[1b] Because of the logistic challenges associated with intracoronary administration and the lack of a perceived benefit of intracoronary versus systemic administration, later studies used simpler intravenous dosing schemes. A meta-analysis from 1985 that included 33 trials confirmed a significant beneficial effect of thrombolytic agents on outcome.[2] The era of fibrinolysis in STEMI had finally dawned. In 1986, the first large-scale trial to show a significant reduction in mortality with a fibrinolytic agent was the landmark Gruppo Italiano per lo Studio della Streptochinasi nell'Infarto Miocardio (GISSI-1) trial (see the section on Clinical Trials of Streptokinase).

Role of Fibrinolysis in Contemporary Care

Is fibrinolysis still relevant in the 21st century, now that guidelines and advocacy groups unequivocally recommend

TABLE 15-1 Comparison of Advantages and Disadvantages of Fibrinolysis versus Primary Percutaneous Coronary Intervention

FIBRINOLYSIS	PRIMARY PCI
Advantages	
Universally available	More efficient reperfusion and better outcome
Independent of physician's experience and can be used by trained paramedics	Less risk of reinfarction or residual ischemia
Can be administered in prehospital setting or community hospitals	Less risk of systemic and intracranial hemorrhage
Disadvantages	
Higher risk of systemic and intracranial bleeding	Dependent of experience of team and on availability of 24/7 facilities
Reperfusion in 60% of patients	PCI-related time delays can be long
Not efficient in patients presenting late	

PCI, Percutaneous coronary intervention.

primary PCI (PPCI) as the preferred reperfusion strategy? Compared with fibrinolysis, PPCI achieves higher patency rates and is associated with fewer intracranial bleeding complications (see Chapter 17). PPCI also immediately deals with the underlying lesion or ruptured plaque, and easily gauges the extent of coronary disease (Table 15-1). In aggregate, PPCI is better than lytic therapy in terms of outcome,[3] but only if it can be done within 120 minutes after first medical contact by an experienced catheterization team (see Chapter 5 and Chapter 14). Achieving such rapid implementation of PPCI is not possible in a considerable proportion of STEMI patients worldwide, depending on geography and the healthcare organization. As a consequence, fibrinolysis remains an important option for many patients. For example, in the contemporary international long-tErm follow-uP of anti-thrombotic management patterns In acute COronary syndrome patients (EPICOR) registry, fibrinolytic agents were used in 14% to 33% of STEMI patients, depending on the region.[4] Also, in the most recent European survey, the rate of fibrinolysis varied greatly among the 37 participating countries, from being almost nonexistent in the Czech Republic to more than 80% (300 per 1 million inhabitants) of patients who received reperfusion therapy in the Ukraine (Figure 15-1).[5]

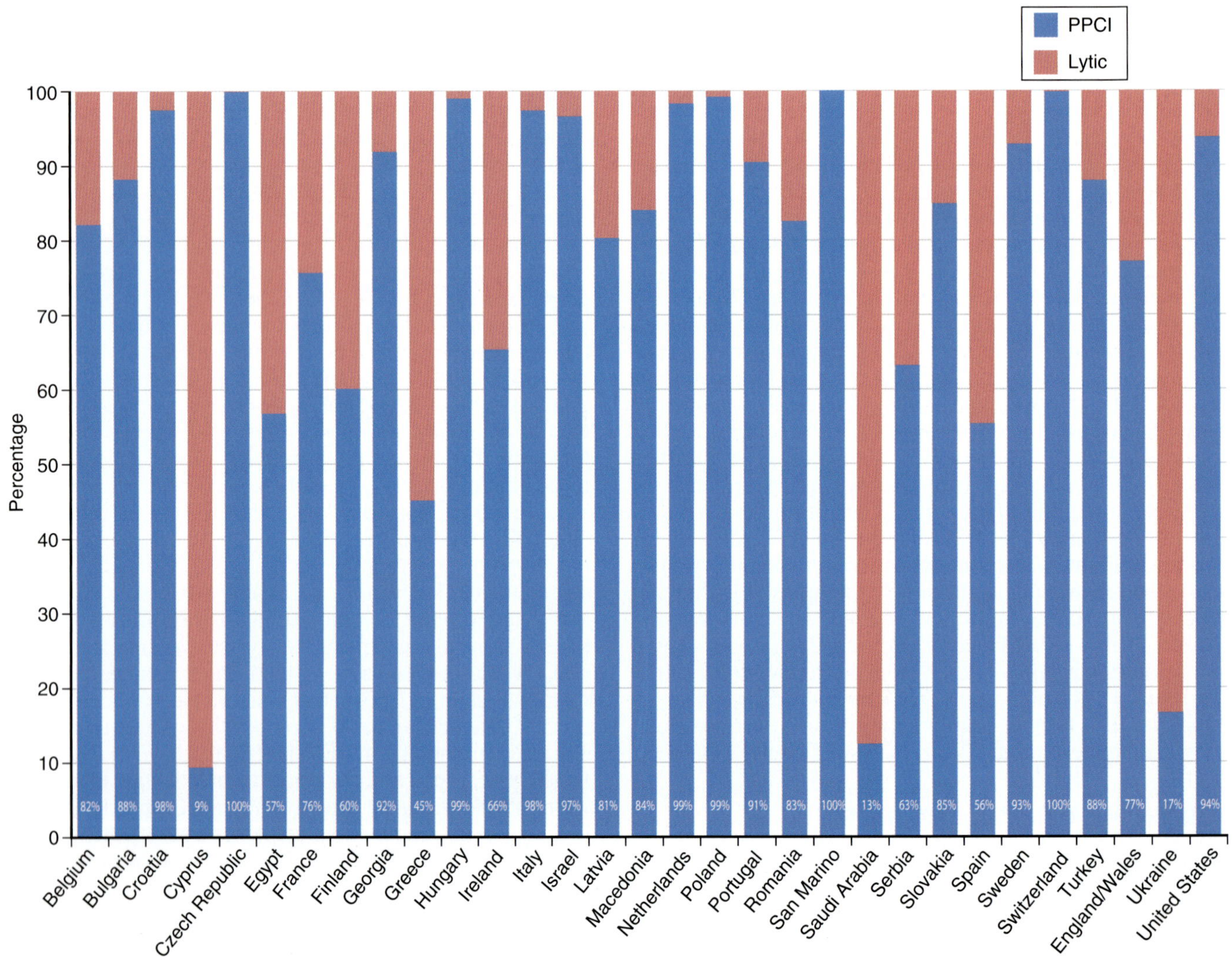

FIGURE 15-1 Relative proportion of patients with ST-elevation myocardial infarction who received reperfusion therapy and who were treated with fibrinolytic or primary percutaneous coronary intervention (PPCI) in Europe and the United States (data from 2010 to 2011). *(Data from Kristensen SD, et al: Reperfusion therapy for ST elevation acute myocardial infarction 2010/2011: current status in 37 ESC countries.* Eur Heart J *2014;35:1957; and Morrow DA, personal communication, July 28, 2015.)*

It is clear that in remote or sparsely populated areas, fibrinolysis is often the only option to expedite reperfusion.[6] Structural and unexpected interhospital transfer delays are often underestimated in urban areas as well. Once a STEMI patient is committed to be sent to a PPCI-capable center, but unanticipated delays occur, an opportunity for early reperfusion is lost. Such patients are likely to have benefited from early fibrinolysis in the absence of contraindications. Transfer-related delays in PPCI are common, and as door-to-balloon delays increase, the outcome advantage of PPCI over fibrinolysis clearly diminishes (see Chapter 14).[7] In a large American registry (n = 115,316), only one-half of the STEMI patients referred for PPCI achieved the guideline-recommended first door-to-balloon time of less than 120 minutes. More specifically, less than half of the patients with an estimated transfer delay greater than 30 minutes were treated within 120 minutes.[8] In contrast, only half of the STEMI patients with an estimated drive time exceeding 60 minutes were treated with fibrinolysis. In essence, although efforts to reduce transfer times and optimize STEMI networks for prompt referral are obviously needed, a substantial proportion of patients with STEMI might still benefit from lytic therapy. For example, in a recent systematic registry performed in Belgium (a small country with a high density of catheterization laboratories), the shift of fibrinolytic therapy in non–PCI-capable hospitals to referring for PPCI has resulted in longer overall treatment delays and no change in overall outcome.[9] In most STEMI networks, fibrinolysis is not isolated from PCI.[6] The optimal combination of fibrinolysis and PCI (rescue or planned) is still being investigated, and is the subject of a separate chapter (see Chapter 14). In addition, interest in local intracoronary administration of lytics has attracted renewed interest, especially as an alternative for PPCI patients with a large thrombotic burden.[10] For these reasons, fibrinolysis in well-established networks is still relevant today.[11]

HOW DO FIBRINOLYTIC AGENTS WORK?

The goal of administering a fibrinolytic agent is to dissolve the clot that impedes blood flow in a coronary artery. This dissolution of thrombus is achieved pharmacologically by activating the fibrinolytic system. Fibrinolytic agents convert the inactive proenzyme plasminogen to its active state, plasmin (Figure 15-2). Plasmin then degrades fibrin, a major constituent of thrombi, to soluble fibrin-degradation products, ultimately resulting in clot dissolution. Fibrinolytic agents are traditionally categorized as fibrin-selective versus nonselective agents, depending on whether they lyse clots in the absence of systemic plasminogen activation (Table 15-2).

Streptokinase, anistreplase, and urokinase are nonfibrin-selective fibrinolytic agents, and indiscriminately activate both circulating and clot-bound plasminogen to plasmin. This activity not only causes local dissolution of a thrombus, but also causes systemic degradation of circulating fibrinogen. In contrast, alteplase and its derivatives, as well as staphylokinase, digest clot-bound fibrinogen relatively selectively and tend not to deplete systemic coagulation factors as much as streptokinase. Fibrin-selective drugs are more efficient in dissolving thrombi. However, the selective nature of fibrin-specific lytic agents does have some unwanted side effects; their lack of systemic fibrinogen depletion might increase the risk of rethrombosis and reocclusion (see Chapter 23). Subsequent derivatives of alteplase have been aimed at providing more practical bolus delivery at the same time as potential improvements in the risk–benefit balance caused by the enhanced fibrin specificity of some derivatives.

Several circulating factors suppress the activation of plasminogen, most notably plasminogen activator inhibitor (PAI)-1 (see Figure 15-2). Active plasmin is inhibited by α_2-antiplasmin. Resistance or lack of resistance to PAI-1 partially characterizes the potency of the different fibrinolytic agents. Consequently, PAI-1 is a major determinant of the resistance of platelet-rich thrombi to lysis by fibrinolytic agents.

SPECIFIC FIBRINOLYTIC AGENTS

Streptokinase

Streptokinase is a nonfibrinogen-specific fibrinolytic agent that indirectly activates plasminogen (Tables 15-3 and 15-4).

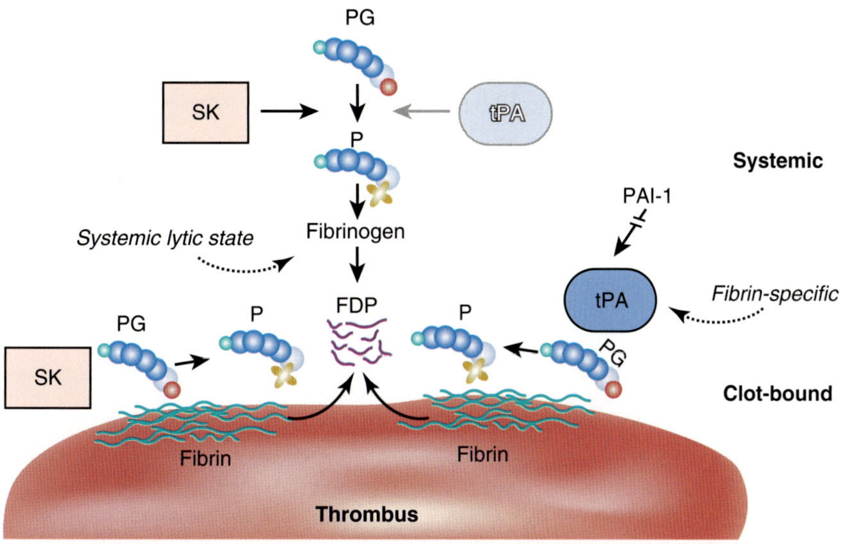

FIGURE 15-2 Mechanism of fibrinolytic agents: tissue plasminogen activator (tPA) (alteplase) predominantly activates plasminogen bound to the clot's surface, whereas streptokinase activates clot-bound and fluid-phase plasminogen indiscriminately. *FDP*, Fibrin degradation products; *P*, plasmin; *PAI-1*, plasminogen activator inhibitor 1; *PG*, plasminogen; *SK*, streptokinase.

TABLE 15-2 Fibrinolytic Agents

NONFIBRIN-SPECIFIC AGENTS	FIBRIN-SPECIFIC AGENTS
Streptokinase	Alteplase and derivatives
Saruplase	Reteplase
APSAC (anistreplase)	Tenecteplase Lanoteplase Amediplase Monteplase Pametiplase
	Staphylokinase

APSAC, Anisoylated plasminogen streptokinase activator complex.

TABLE 15-3 Characteristics of Lytic Agents

	FIBRIN SPECIFICITY	HALF-LIFE (MIN)	PAI-1 RESISTANCE
Streptokinase	–	18–23	–
APSAC	–	40–90	–
Alteplase	↑	3–4	–
Reteplase	↓	15–18	–
Tenecteplase	↑↑	20–24	↑
Lanoteplase	↓	30–45	↑
Pametiplase	↑	30–47	–
Monteplase	↑	23	↑
Staphylokinase (PEG)	↑↑↑	13	–

APSAC, Anisoylated plasminogen streptokinase activator complex; *PAI-1*, plasminogen activator inhibitor 1; *PEG*, polyethylene glycol.

Streptokinase is a single-chain, 414-amino acid long protein that resembles serine proteases, but it does not have enzymatic activity on its own. Plasminogen is activated after forming a complex with streptokinase, exposing its active site, which catalyzes the conversion to plasmin. This complex is more resistant against inactivation by α_2-antiplasmin than free-circulating plasmin.

In STEMI, 1.5 million units of streptokinase is usually given in a 1-hour infusion. However, because of its lack of fibrin specificity, streptokinase generates active plasmin in the circulation and induces a systemic lytic state, when α_2-antiplasmin becomes exhausted. Circulating fibrinogen levels decrease well below 20% of baseline within the first 60 minutes after infusion.[12] As a consequence, additional anticoagulants are not always recommended in combination with streptokinase or other nonfibrin-specific fibrinolytics (see Chapter 18). Whether there is a benefit in adding intravenous heparin is still a matter of debate.

Because streptokinase is produced by hemolytic streptococci, patients who receive streptokinase invariably develop antistreptococcal antibodies. This immunological reaction often causes fever, but would also completely neutralize a new dose of streptokinase in the first 3 months after administration, effectively precluding early re-administration. In some patients, high neutralizing antibody titres persist for years after their treatment. In addition, preexisting anti-streptokinase antibodies are relatively common and can impede reperfusion after treatment with streptokinase in patients with acute MI. However, hypotension, a frequent but often transient side effect of streptokinase, is more likely the result of bradykinin release than being caused by an acute allergic reaction.

TABLE 15-4 Dosing Regimens of Frequently Used Fibrinolytic Agents

Streptokinase
1.5 million IU/1 h
Alteplase
15-mg bolus
90-min infusion
• 0.75 mg/kg over 30 min (max 50 mg) • 0.50 mg/kg over next hour (max 35 mg) • Total dose not to exceed 100 mg
Reteplase
Initial 10 U bolus, followed by second 10 U bolus 30 min later
Tenecteplase
Weight-adjusted single bolus: • 30 mg if <60 kg • 35 mg if 60–69 kg • 40 mg if 70–79 kg • 45 mg if 80–89 kg • 50 mg if ≥90 kg
Half-dose if age >75 yrs*

*Not indicated in the label.

Clinical Trials of Streptokinase

In the GISSI-1 study, 11,806 patients with STEMI presenting within 12 hours of symptom onset were randomized to either intravenous streptokinase or control therapy. In-hospital mortality was 10.7% in patients treated with intravenous streptokinase versus 13.1% in control patients, indicating 23 lives saved per 1000 patients treated. This benefit in mortality was preserved after 1- and 10-year follow-up (Figure 15-3). Another landmark trial, ISIS-2 (Second International Study of Infarct Survival), clearly showed a benefit of adding aspirin to streptokinase; 17,187 patients received 1.5-MU streptokinase, 160-mg/day aspirin for 1 month, both treatments, or neither. Treatment with aspirin or streptokinase alone resulted in a significant reduction in mortality (23% and 24%, respectively), with a much greater benefit with a combined administration. Aspirin significantly reduced nonfatal reinfarction and was not associated with any significant increase in intracranial hemorrhages (ICHs) (see Chapter 19). The reinfarction rate was higher when streptokinase was used alone, an effect that was abolished when aspirin was added.

Tissue-Type Plasminogen Activator

Recombinant tissue-type plasminogen activator (rt-PA; alteplase) is a single-chain, tissue-type plasminogen activator molecule, manufactured by recombinant DNA technology (see Tables 15-3 and 15-4). Alteplase is a relatively weak plasminogen activator in the absence of fibrin. However, the presence of fibrin at the surface of a clot considerably boosts alteplase's activation rate of plasminogen by forming a ternary complex. As a consequence, it has considerably greater fibrin specificity than streptokinase, but it induces mild systemic fibrinogen depletion.[13] Plasmin formed at the surface of fibrin is also more resistant to inactivation by α_2-antiplasmin. The effectiveness of alteplase is also offset to some extent by PAI-1. Alteplase requires a continuous intravenous infusion because of its short half-life. It also needs concomitant anticoagulant therapy, because fibrin-specific

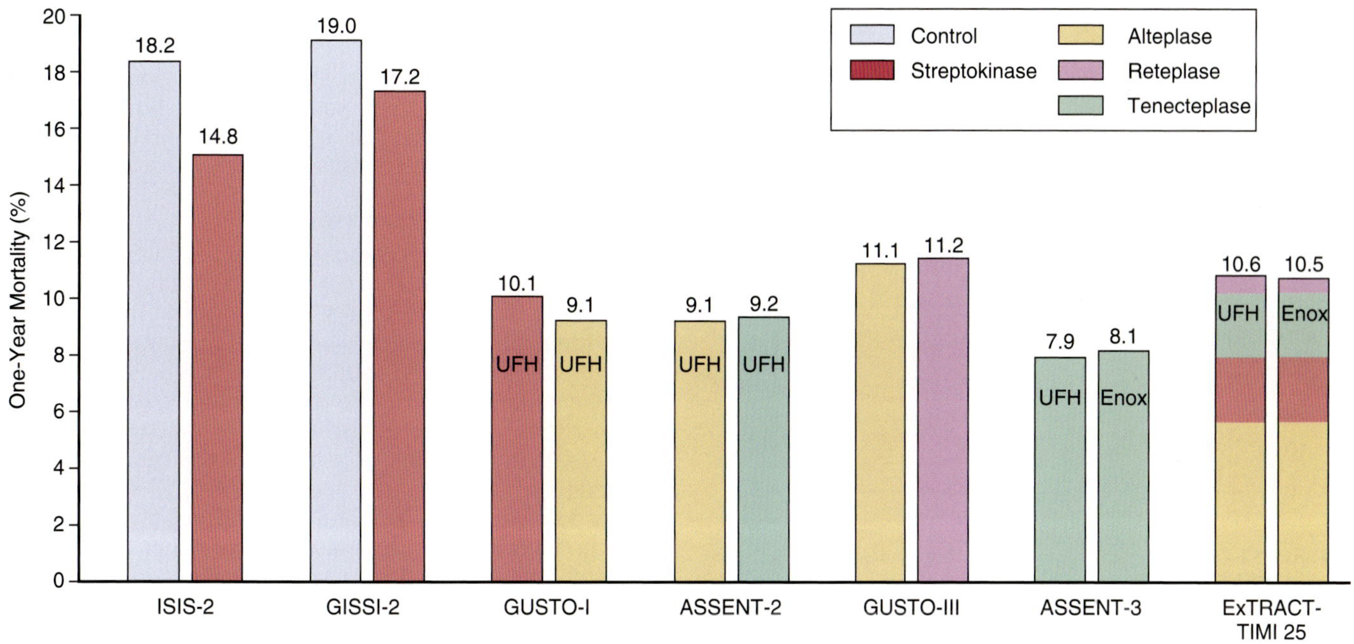

FIGURE 15-3 One-year mortality rates in key fibrinolytic trials. *Enox*, Enoxaparin; *UFH*, unfractionated heparin.

agents increase the risk of reocclusion by a factor of two in the absence of a generalized systemic lytic state.

Clinical Trials of Tissue-Plasminogen Activator

The initial experience with alteplase in STEMI patients confirmed its thrombolytic potency and its fibrin specificity. Before settling on the current front-loaded dosing, a variety of alteplase dosing schemes were tested in several studies. In one of the first large-scale study with alteplase, the ASSET (Anglo-Scandinavian Study of Early Thrombolysis) trial in 1988, an unusually long administration of alteplase was used. This first trial showed a 26% mortality reduction compared with placebo, despite the absence of aspirin in this study. Alteplase, given in a 3-hour dosing regimen, was subsequently shown to achieve significantly better patency scores than streptokinase, although in two large-scale trials, ISIS-3 (n = 41,299, with duteplase)[14] and GISSI-2–International (n = 12,490, with alteplase),[15] a similar tPA regimen resulted in the same mortality rates as streptokinase.

The question which of the two, streptokinase or alteplase, is the most effective in terms of mortality reduction was finally settled in 1993 in the first Global Utilization of Streptokinase and Tissue Plasminogen Activator for Occluded Coronary Arteries (GUSTO) trial.[16] In this trial, which included more than 40,000 patients, a shorter 90-minute dosing regimen of alteplase was used and was shown to achieve higher patency rates than the 3-hour scheme. Thirty-day mortality was 6.3% in patients who received alteplase and intravenous heparin compared with 7.4% in patients treated with streptokinase and intravenous heparin ($P = .001$), which was driven by a significantly higher Thrombolysis In Myocardial Infarction (TIMI) flow grade 3 at 90 minutes (54% vs. 32%, with streptokinase).[17] Early reocclusion was not uncommon in the era before systematic planned angiography and angioplasty after lytic therapy (see Chapter 23), in part because of the paradoxical procoagulant and platelet-activating side effects of fibrinolytic agents, and was associated with a high 30-day mortality—12% compared with 1.1% in patients with early and persistently patent coronary arteries.[18] In the end, GUSTO-1 convincingly settled the discussion whether successful early vessel patency associated with fibrinolysis, as observed in the earlier phase II studies, directly translated into improved outcome, often referred to as the "open artery theory," or whether fibrinolysis improved outcome by mechanisms other than early coronary reperfusion. The 30-day mortality differences between the four fibrinolytic strategies compared in the main GUSTO-I trial (all 41,021 patients) were predicted accurately from differences in the 90-minute TIMI grade 3 flow rates in the angiographic substudy.[19] This close match between mortality differences predicted from early patency data and actual mortality supported the paradigm that early, complete, and sustained epicardial coronary artery reperfusion is an essential mechanism underlying the life-saving potential of fibrinolytic therapy.

Reteplase

After the identification of the molecular structure of tissue plasminogen activator, several attempts were made at improving its properties by targeted mutations and deletions (see Tables 15-3 and 15-4). In general, these efforts focused on improving fibrin specificity and resistance to PAI-1, and especially on prolonging its half-life. Reteplase, a second-generation thrombolytic agent, was a first attempt to improve on the shortcomings of alteplase. It is a mutant of alteplase in which the finger, the kringle-1 domain, and epidermal growth factor domains are removed. This results in a decreased plasma clearance with a longer half-life than alteplase (see Table 15-3), allowing administration as bolus injection. However, the removal of the finger domain diminishes fibrin specificity, although inactivation by PAI-1 remains similar to alteplase.

Clinical Trials of Reteplase

In two open-label randomized pilot trials, different doses of reteplase were evaluated in patients with acute MI. In two studies (Reteplase [r-PA] vs Alteplase Patency Investigation During Acute Myocardial Infarction [RAPID] I and II)

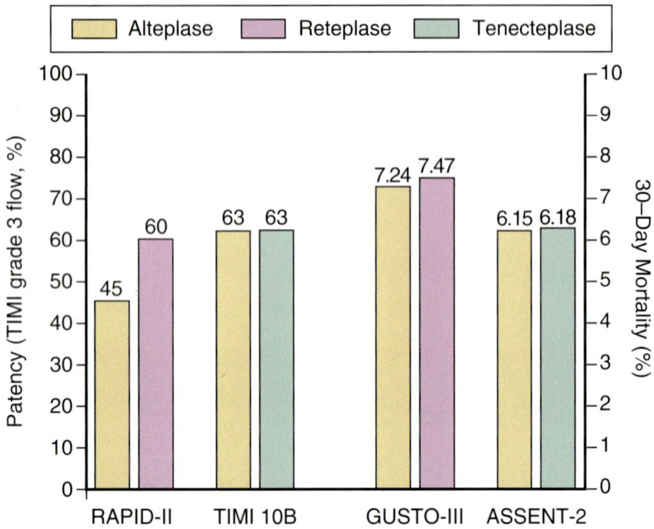

FIGURE 15-4 Patency versus outcome in the landmark reteplase and tenecteplase trials.

patients treated with two boluses of 10 U reteplase, given 30 minutes apart, had significantly higher rates of TIMI grade 3 flow compared with patients treated with either the 3-hour or front-loaded infusion of alteplase (Figure 15-4). Encouraged by these favorable early patency rates, reteplase was evaluated in two large outcome trials. In the double-blind International Joint Efficacy Comparison of Thrombolytics (INJECT) trial, 6010 patients with acute MI within 12 hours of symptom onset were randomized to either double-bolus reteplase (10 U), given 30 minutes apart, or streptokinase. INJECT did not find any difference in 35-day mortality between double-bolus reteplase and streptokinase. The percentage of patients with complete ST-segment resolution was significantly higher with reteplase in a substudy of INJECT, but this did not translate into improved outcome.[20] In the GUSTO-III trial, which was designed as a superiority trial, 15,059 patients were randomized to double-bolus reteplase or front-loaded alteplase.[21] Like the INJECT study, mortality at 30 days was again similar for both treatment arms (7.47% vs. 7.24%), as was the incidence of hemorrhagic stroke (0.91% vs. 0.93%) or other major bleeding complications. Similar mortality rates were maintained for both treatment groups at 1-year follow-up (see Figure 15-3) and remained consistent among various subgroups, including older adults and patients presenting early after symptom onset. Thus, higher patency rates at 90 minutes with reteplase did not translate into lower short- or intermediate-term mortality rates. This discordance between initial patency and outcomes might be explained in part by increased platelet activation and surface receptor expression, and subsequent reocclusion, with reteplase compared with alteplase. Reteplase is still available and in clinical use today.

Tenecteplase

Tenecteplase is bioengineered from alteplase with mutations at three places (T103, N117, KHRR296-299), which increases its plasma half-life (T103, 20 minutes), improves fibrin binding and fibrin specificity, and increases resistance to PAI-1 (N117 and KHRR296-299). Its slower clearance allows convenient single-bolus administration (see Tables 15-3 and 15-4). The higher fibrin specificity of tenecteplase is the result of reduced efficiency of plasminogen activation in the presence of fibrinogen and fibrin degradation products, whereas efficiency in the presence of fibrin remains equivalent. As a result, tenecteplase leads to faster recanalization compared with alteplase. Tenecteplase also has higher thrombolytic potency on platelet-rich clots than its parent molecule.

Clinical Trials of Tenecteplase

Efficacy of different doses of tenecteplase with respect to establishing angiographic patency was initially evaluated in the TIMI 10A and 10B trials. Taken together, patency rates were identical after a single-bolus administration of 40-mg tenecteplase compared with alteplase (63%). A 50-mg dose of tenecteplase had to be discontinued early because of an excess of ICHs in the TIMI 10B trial (Figure 15-5). Concomitantly, the safety of single-bolus administration of tenecteplase was evaluated in the ASSENT (Assessment of the Safety and Efficacy of a New Thrombolytic) 1 study; 3325 patients received a single bolus of either 30- or 40-mg tenecteplase. Mortality or severe bleeding complications, including ICHs, occurred in a low proportion of patients, without significant differences among the treatment groups.

In the double-blind ASSENT-2 trial, 16,949 patients were randomized to a single-bolus, weight-adjusted tenecteplase or weight-adjusted front-loaded alteplase.[22] Specifically designed as an equivalency trial, this study showed that tenecteplase and alteplase were equivalent for 30-day mortality (6.18% vs. 6.15%; 90% confidence interval [CI], 0.917 to 1.104). The two treatments did not differ significantly in any subgroup analysis, except for a lower 30-day mortality with tenecteplase in patients treated after 4 hours of symptom onset. Although the rates of ICH were similar for tenecteplase (0.93%) and rt-PA (0.94%), women, patients older than 75 years, and patients weighing less than 67 kg tended to have lower rates of ICH after treatment with tenecteplase. Noncerebral bleeding complications occurred less frequently in the tenecteplase group, a difference that was even more apparent in high-risk women. Thus, the increased fibrin specificity of tenecteplase may induce both a better outcome in late-treated patients and fewer bleeding complications in high-risk patients.

After the ASSENT trials, different doses of tenecteplase were used in real-world practice and in clinical trials. In the pharmaco-invasive Strategic Reperfusion Early After Myocardial Infarction (STREAM) study (see Chapter 14), the dose of tenecteplase was reduced by 50% in patients older than 75 years of age, after enrolling approximately 20% of the ultimate study population, because of an excess of bleeding complications, including ICH in older adults.[23] After implementing the age-adjusted dose, no more ICHs were seen in patients 75 years of age or older assigned to the lytic arm. This observation suggests that older adult patients might have a more favorable balance of benefit and risk using only one-half dose of tenecteplase; however, formal professional society recommendations have not been made to support this regimen.

Lanoteplase

Lanoteplase is of historical interest, but it ended development before coming to clinical use. Lanoteplase is a deletion mutant of alteplase by deleting its fibronectin fingerlike and epidermal growth factor domains and mutating Asn to Gln at residue 117 in the kringle domain (see Tables 15-3 and 15-4). Lanoteplase can be given as a single-bolus injection, with decreased plasma clearance (30 minutes) allowing administration.

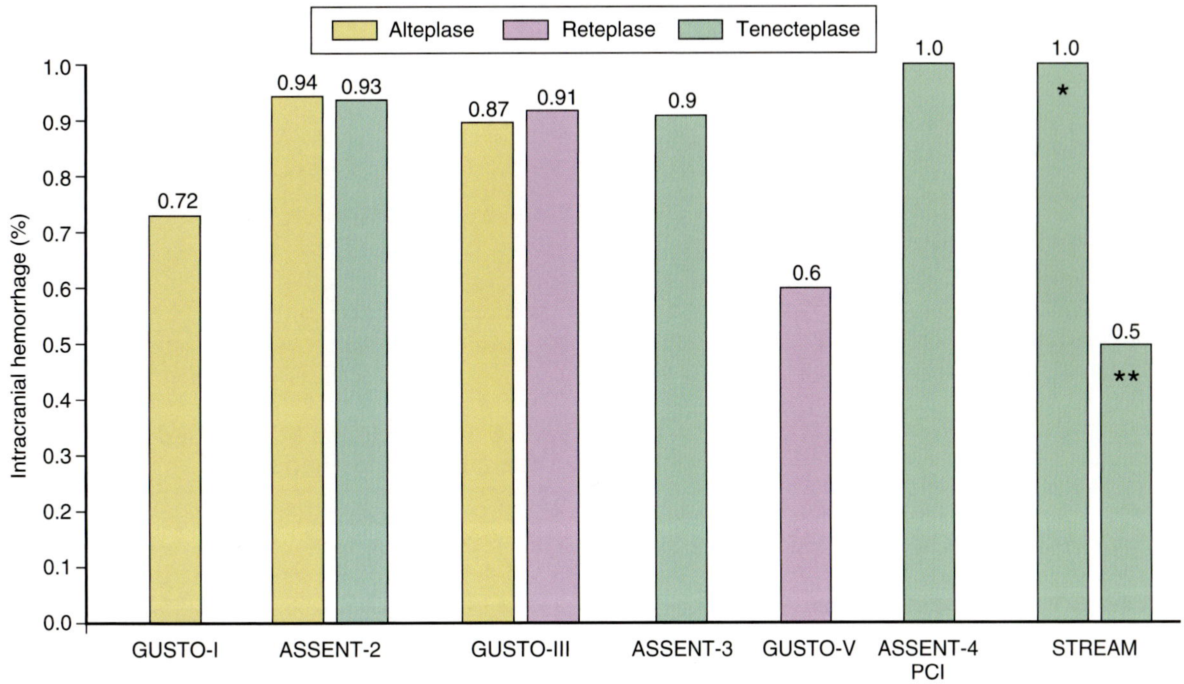

FIGURE 15-5 Intracranial hemorrhage rates in randomized fibrinolytic studies. For ASSENT-4 PCI and STREAM, only the rates in the lytic arms are shown (*before and **after an amendment in STREAM that halved the dose of tenecteplase in patients 75 years of age and older).

In the Intravenous nPA for Treatment of Infarcting Myocardium Early (InTIME)-2-trial, 15,078 patients were randomized in a 2:1 ratio to single-bolus lanoteplase (120 kU/kg) or front-loaded alteplase. Thirty-day mortality was equivalent for both groups (6.75% vs. 6.61%).[24] Unfortunately, the rate of hemorrhagic strokes was significantly higher in patients treated with lanoteplase (1.12% compared with 0.64% for alteplase). The increased rate of ICH and minor bleeding with lanoteplase was believed to be related to the relatively high dose and the lower fibrin specificity. The InTIME-2 trial highlighted the importance of adequately sized phase II trials for dose selection and also revealed lower rates of bleeding with reduced dosing of intravenous heparin, supporting the trend toward lower dosing regimens of anticoagulant therapy during fibrinolysis (see Chapter 18).

Fibrinolytics of Historical Interest

Staphylokinase

Recombinant staphylokinase has only limited use in some countries and is described briefly here for completeness. Although staphylokinase, a bacterial profibrinolytic agent, was discovered in 1908, its clinical use in STEMI only regained interest and momentum in the last decade of the 20th century (see Tables 15-3 and 15-4). This delay, in contrast to the rapid uptake of streptokinase, was caused by the presence of antibody-related neutralizing activity in serum samples of test subjects and massive bleeding in staphylokinase-treated dogs in the 1960s. In retrospect, the choice of this animal model was unfortunate, because staphylokinase lacks fibrin specificity in dogs, in contrast to other species.[25]

Staphylokinase has a high thrombolytic potency and is effective in dissolving platelet-rich thrombi, and it possesses high fibrin specificity in human plasma. In the Recombinant Staphylokinase (STAR) trial, the effects of staphylokinase versus front-loaded and weight-adjusted alteplase on early coronary artery patency were evaluated in 100 STEMI patients. TIMI-3 flow at 90 minutes was reached in 58% of patients treated with alteplase and in 62% of patients treated with staphylokinase. Staphylokinase proved to be highly fibrin specific, preserving circulating fibrinogen, plasminogen, and α_2-antiplasmin levels, whereas alteplase caused a significant drop in fibrinogen, plasminogen, and α_2-antiplasmin. Although wild-type staphylokinase induces an antibody response, engineered variants with reduced antigenicity have been shown to decrease the occurrence and magnitude of inactivating antibodies.

Saruplase

Saruplase or prourokinase is infrequently used in STEMI patients, but it is not approved in Europe or the United States.[26] Saruplase is a single-chain recombinant urokinase-type plasminogen activator without immunogenicity. Although not fibrin specific, it has a plasma half-life of 9 minutes. In the COMPASS (Comparison Trial of Saruplase and Streptokinase) trial, 3089 patients were randomized to saruplase or streptokinase. Thirty-day mortality was numerically lower in the saruplase group (5.7% vs 6.7% for streptokinase). ICHs were higher with saruplase (0.9% vs 0.3% for streptokinase), although only a limited number of older adult patients were included in this trial. In another study, the BASE (Bolus Administration of Saruplase in Europe) trial, several dosing regimens were tested. Although the highest dose, a double bolus of 40/40 mg, resulted in the highest patency, it also had the highest complication rate.

Amediplase

Amediplase is a chimeric fusion protein consisting of the kringle 2 domain of t-PA and the catalytic domain of urokinase-PA. It is fibrin-specific, nonimmunogenic, and can be given as a single bolus. In vitro, it appears to be somewhat more potent than prourokinase or tenecteplase. In two angiographic studies (2k2 and 3k2), TIMI flow grade 3 was obtained in more than 50% of the patients in a dose of ±1 mg/kg with a good safety profile. Amediplase was not further developed after these initial studies.

CLINICAL USE, INDICATIONS, AND CONTRAINDICATIONS FOR FIBRINOLYTIC THERAPY

Indications for Fibrinolytic Therapy

Traditionally, patients with typical chest pain of up to 12-hour duration presenting with electrocardiographic ST-segment elevations or presumed new bundle branch block are eligible for fibrinolytic therapy. The clot-lysing efficacy of fibrinolytic therapy is clearly time-dependent, working best on newly formed clots. In addition, early in the course of STEMI, the thrombus may be smaller and thus faster and easier to lyse. Consequently, treatment delays are associated with less successful ST-segment recovery after fibrinolysis and lead to higher long-term mortality rates. Although administering fibrinolytic agents up to 12 hours after the onset of symptoms may be beneficial in terms of outcome, and the most recent American Heart Association (AHA)/American College of Cardiology (ACC) and European Society of Cardiology (ESC) guidelines recommend this time window[27,28]; every minute that reperfusion is postponed will inevitably result in more extensive necrosis. The relative mortality reduction following fibrinolytic therapy was found to be more than twice as high in patients treated within 2 hours versus in those treated later.[29]

The usual electrocardiographic criterion for administration of fibrinolytic therapy is at least 0.1 mV of ST-segment elevation in two or more contiguous leads (see Chapter 6). Because mortality is significantly higher in patients with complete left bundle branch block, administration of a fibrinolytic agent is also recommended in this population.

Contraindications to Fibrinolysis

Contraindications to fibrinolysis are in essence precautions to avoid excessive risk of hemorrhage (Tables 15-5 and 15-6). In these patients, especially those with a history of stroke or recent major surgery or bleeding, PPCI should be considered even when this would be associated with a significant treatment delay.

Registries have suggested that there is a mortality disadvantage in fibrinolysis-treated patients who are older than 75 years of age, possibly because of an excess of major bleeding complications. This excessive mortality might also be explained in part by negative selection, because fitter older adult patients might have been more likely amenable for PPCI. However, mortality rates in these observational studies are in contrast to findings from large randomized trials. In the Senior Primary Angioplasty in Myocardial Infarction (SENIOR PAMI) trial, PPCI was not found to be superior to fibrinolytics in 481 older patients (≥70 years of age). Furthermore, data from the FTT (Fibrinolytic Therapy Trialists) group in 3300 STEMI patients older than age 75 years showed a significant absolute mortality reduction by fibrinolytic therapy that was even greater than that in younger patients (34 patients vs. 16 patients per 1000 randomized patients).[30] An ongoing concern is the risk of ICH with lytic therapy, especially in older adults (Figure 15-5). Recently, results from trials, including STREAM and registries, have suggested that reduced-dose fibrinolysis might be a safe and effective alternative for older adults. However, the trade-off between safety and benefit of reduced fibrinolysis in a contemporary setting of standard upfront dual antiplatelet therapy and planned PCI needs to be addressed prospectively.

TABLE 15-5 Contraindications for Fibrinolysis

ABSOLUTE	RELATIVE
Previous hemorrhagic stroke at any time	Transient ischemic attack <6 mo
Nonhemorrhagic stroke <6 mo	Uncontrolled or refractory hypertension
CNS malformation, neoplasm or damage	Traumatic cardiopulmonary resuscitation or prolonged CPR
Recent surgery or significant trauma within 2–4 weeks	Current use of anticoagulants
Active (uncontrolled) bleeding	Recent bleeding (2–4 weeks)
Gastrointestinal bleeding within last month	Pregnancy
Known bleeding disorder	
Suspected aortic dissection	

CNS, Central nervous system; *CPR*, cardiopulmonary resuscitation.

TABLE 15-6 Patients at Increased Risk for Intracranial Hemorrhage

- History of cerebrovascular disease, including cerebrovascular accident and transient ischemic attack
- Age >75 yrs
- Female gender
- Low body weight
- High blood pressure or pulse pressure on admission

ASSESSMENT OF REPERFUSION

The early efficacy trials used 60- or 90-minute patency of the infarct-related vessel on angiography as the most important demonstration of successful fibrinolysis. A TIMI flow grade of less than 3 in the infarct-related artery is associated with poor functional recovery of the left ventricle and increased mortality. However, angiography at best presents a snapshot view of the dynamic process of coronary occlusion and recanalization. Myocardial tissue reperfusion correlates better with outcome than epicardial coronary artery patency, but restored epicardial blood flow does not adequately reflect reperfusion at the tissue level.[31] Restoration of reperfusion at the tissue level can be assessed noninvasively with contrast echocardiography (see Chapter 31), magnetic resonance imaging (see Chapter 33), or ST-segment monitoring. ST-segment resolution, which reflects myocardial reperfusion, has been shown to be associated with better short- and long-term mortality. In contrast, even in patients with TIMI grade 3 flow after lytic therapy, failure to achieve early ST-segment recovery is associated with a worse outcome. In contemporary practice and clinical trials, ST-segment resolution of 50% or more at 90 minutes after lytic therapy is also used to assess early success reperfusion. A rescue PCI should be considered in case of signs of failed reperfusion, such as insufficient ST-segment resolution, as well as hemodynamic or electrical instability or ongoing chest pain (see Chapter 14). In contrast, angiography and PCI should only be planned between 3 and 24 hours after successful lytic therapy to avoid periprocedural thrombotic complications.

Concomitant Therapies

Because the formation and lysis of a coronary thrombus results from a complex interplay of different pathways involving platelets and the coagulation system, the additional use of agents that target each of these separate components beyond lytic therapy potentially optimizes clot lysis and prevents reocclusion. A major drawback of fibrinolytic therapy is its procoagulant side effect caused by increased thrombin generation. Therefore, better as well as safer inhibition of thrombin and platelets improves the efficacy of fibrinolysis. The use of anticoagulants and antiplatelet therapy is described in detail in Chapter 18 and Chapter 19, respectively, and is discussed briefly here.

Anticoagulation with Fibrinolysis

Unfractionated Heparin

Intravenous unfractionated heparin (UFH) has been a standard adjunctive antithrombotic therapy with fibrin-specific fibrinolytics since the first GUSTO trial. UFH does not necessarily improve early patency rates, but improves patency rates at later time points by preventing rethrombosis. It took several large trials and over a decade to settle on the most optimal UFH dosing regimen, balancing bleeding risk versus thrombosis. Giugliano and colleagues analyzed different heparin dosing schemes and monitoring regimens in several studies.[32] In three of these trials (TIMI 9, GUSTO II, and TIMI 10B), heparin doses were reduced during the course of the trial, resulting in lower rates of ICH. The current recommended dosing scheme that was used in the ASSENT-3 trial also includes an early measurement of the activated partial thromboplastin time after 3 hours.[33]

The use of UFH has significant drawbacks. The level of anticoagulation with UFH is highly variable in patients because of low bioavailability and variable clearance, requiring frequent activated partial thrombin time monitoring. UFH is also relatively ineffective in inhibiting clot-associated thrombin and factor X, and does not reduce the generation of thrombin associated with fibrinolysis. These properties can result in rebound activation of the coagulation cascade after cessation of an infusion, increasing the risk of reocclusion (see Chapter 23). UFH has been largely replaced by low–molecular-weight heparin (LMWH) as an adjunct to lytic therapy.

Low–Molecular-Weight Heparins and Pentasaccharides

LMWH has several advantages over conventional UFH, including greater bioavailability, better resistance to inhibition by activated platelets, and a lower incidence of heparin-induced thrombocytopenia. Also, a better anti-Xa:IIa ratio than that of UFH more efficiently promotes the inhibition of thrombin generation. LMWHs are much easier to administrate, and have a more stable and predictable anticoagulant response that eliminates the need for activated partial thrombin time monitoring. Subcutaneous administration and a longer half-life significantly facilitate prehospital and in-hospital administration compared with UFH.

Studies have shown a reduction in reinfarction rates and enhanced late patency with the use of LMWH in acute coronary syndromes. Compared with UFH, patency rates after alteplase administration tended to be higher with dalteparin or enoxaparin in the ASSENT PLUS and HART II (Heparin Aspirin Reperfusion Trial II) trials. In the ENTIRE-TIMI (Enoxaparin and Tenecteplase with or without Glycoprotein IIb/IIIa Inhibitor as Reperfusion strategy in ST elevation MI–Thrombolysis in Myocardial Infarction) 23 trial, enoxaparin plus full-dose tenecteplase achieved similar TIMI 3 flow rates compared with UFH plus tenecteplase at 60 minutes.[34]

In the ASSENT-3 study, enoxaparin (30-mg intravenous bolus followed by 1 mg/kg immediately and every 12 hours subcutaneously for 7 days) was compared with UFH in combination with tenecteplase.[33] Enoxaparin significantly reduced the risk for ischemic complications at 30 days (see Figure 15-3). Enoxaparin in combination with tenecteplase was also evaluated in the prehospital setting in the ASSENT-3 PLUS trial. A nonsignificant reduction in ischemic complications with enoxaparin was observed, at the expense of an increase in ICH in older adult patients. However, by using an age-adjusted dose (no bolus and 75% of the maintenance dose), enoxaparin still increased the risk of major bleeding by 50%, but not the risk of ICH after fibrinolytic therapy, while it still reduced the risk of ischemic complications in the Enoxaparin and Thrombolysis Reperfusion for Acute Myocardial Infarction Treatment–Thrombolysis In Myocardial Infarction (ExTRACT-TIMI)-25 study. Two meta-analyses of trials that compared LMWH to UFH confirmed that LMWH reduced the risk of death and reinfarction, but were associated with a higher risk of major bleeding complications (odds ratio, 1.45, 95% CI, 1.24 to 1.91).[35,36] In the current guidelines, enoxaparin, in the age- and weight-adjusted ExTRACT dose, is recommended over UFH (class IA recommendation).[27,28]

Fondaparinux, a synthetic pentasaccharide, is a selective antithrombin-dependent factor Xa inhibitor. As with LMWH, fondaparinux is less biologically variable and does not need monitoring of its anticoagulant effect. In the Organization to Assess Strategies for Ischemic Syndromes (OASIS)–6 trial, fondaparinux was compared with UFH or placebo in 12,092 patients with STEMI.[37] Lytic therapy was used in 45% of patients (n = 5436), most of whom received a nonfibrin-specific agent. In these patients, fondaparinux was associated with a significant 21% lower risk of death or MI compared with standard heparin or placebo. In addition, the risk of bleeding, including ICH, was considerably lower with fondaparinux, irrespective of the type of fibrinolytic agent. Guidelines recommend fondaparinux as adjunctive therapy to all fibrinolytics (AHA/ACC, class IB) or to streptokinase only (ESC, class IIaA).[27,28]

Direct Thrombin Inhibitors

In contrast to UFH, which only inhibits fluid-phase thrombin, direct thrombin inhibitors inhibit both fibrin-bound and circulating thrombin. Because inadequately inactivated thrombin at the site of the thrombus is in part responsible for the procoagulant side effect of fibrinolysis, direct inhibition of thrombin might reduce the occurrence of ischemic complications after reperfusion. Thrombin inhibitors like hirudin or bivalirudin only appear to interact favorably with streptokinase, not with alteplase. In the HERO-2 (Hirulog and Early Reperfusion or Occlusion) trial, 17,073 patients with STEMI were randomized to streptokinase and UFH or streptokinase and bivalirudin.[38] Mortality at 30 days was not different between both regimens, although the reinfarction rate within 96 hours was significantly lower in the bivalirudin group, suggesting that early and more efficient inhibition of thrombin might prevent reocclusion. However, mild to moderate bleeding complications were higher in the bivalirudin group. Direct thrombin and factor Xa inhibitors have not been studied with fibrin-specific agents.

Antiplatelet Agents with Fibrinolysis

In the landmark ISIS-2 study, aspirin was clearly beneficial when given to STEMI patients. In addition, the reinfarction

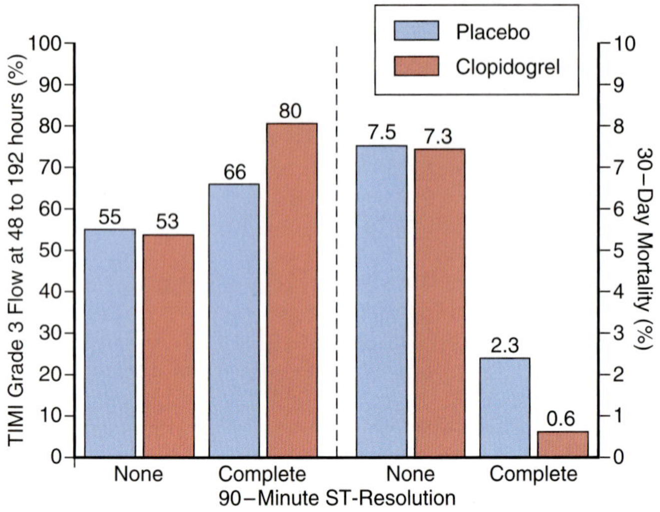

FIGURE 15-6 TIMI grade 3 flow rates at angiography performed 48 to 192 hours after the start of study medication (*left bars*) and outcome (*right bars*) versus early (90-minute) ST-segment resolution in patients randomized to placebo or clopidogrel in the CLARITY-TIMI 28 study.

rate was lower than when streptokinase was used alone. Since then, aspirin has been standard therapy with fibrinolysis.

Adenosine Diphosphate Receptor Antagonists

Despite use of aspirin in lytic-treated patients, reocclusion and reinfarction after successful pharmacological reperfusion continues to be a problem, especially when a planned early (3 to 24 hour) PCI is not possible. The CLARITY (Clopidogrel as Adjunctive Reperfusion Therapy) trial examined whether clopidogrel, a $P2Y_{12}$ receptor inhibitor (300 mg bolus followed by 75 mg/day), was associated with higher rates of infarct-related artery patency in patients treated with a fibrinolytic agent and aspirin.[39] Clopidogrel appears to improve patency rates by preventing reocclusion rather than through facilitating early reperfusion (Figure 15-6). At angiographic follow-up at least 2 days after fibrinolytic therapy, clopidogrel was associated with significantly better patency rates in CLARITY. No increased risk of bleeding complications, including ICHs, with clopidogrel was observed. However, because no patients older than 75 years of age were included in CLARITY, it remains uncertain whether upfront dual antiplatelet therapy is safe in older adults treated with lytic therapy. In contemporary practice, most lytic-treated patients receive early coronary angiography (see Chapter 14). When using fibrinolysis in patients who cannot undergo primary PCI, but who still have access to PCI facilities in a STEMI network, it appears to be sensible to load clopidogrel upfront, at the time of starting lytic therapy and not to wait until the intervention. Clopidogrel's benefit in CLARITY appeared to be irrespective of additional glycoprotein (GP) IIb/IIIa inhibitors given at the time of PCI, suggesting that starting clopidogrel upfront at the time of fibrinolysis could reduce the need for additional antithrombotic agents at the time of rescue or planned early PCI. In the ASSENT-4 PCI study, clopidogrel was only started per protocol when a PCI was deemed necessary; the delay of clopidogrel administration might have been one of the reasons why the patency rate with tenecteplase was lower than expected. In contrast, in the STREAM study, comparing fibrinolysis with rescue or planned PCI versus primary PCI in patients unable to undergo PPCI within 60 minutes, a loading dose of 300-mg clopidogrel was given upfront, followed by a daily dose of 75 mg.[40] However, in patients older than 75 years of age, no loading dose was given because of a lack of safety data. Ultimately, both strategies appeared to be similar in terms of outcomes.[23,40]

A recent mechanistic study has suggested that two-thirds of patients still have unacceptably high residual platelet reactivity after clopidogrel and fibrinolysis, when measured 3 to 48 hours after initiation but before their planned angiography or PCI.[41] Switching to ticagrelor versus reloading with 600-mg clopidogrel was associated with a significantly lower platelet reactivity rate. The efficacy and safety of switching to ticagrelor or upfront ticagrelor with fibrinolysis has not been assessed in adequately sized clinical trials. In addition, there are no data on the efficacy or safety of prasugrel administered acutely together with fibrinolysis. However, anecdotal evidence suggests that clopidogrel can be safely switched to prasugrel at the time of PCI in selected lytic-treated patients.[42]

Glycoprotein IIb/IIIa Antagonists

The addition of GP IIb/IIIa inhibitors to fibrinolytic regimens was long believed to overcome some of the drawbacks of fibrinolytic therapy. The combination of a half-dose lytic and a GP IIb/IIIa inhibitor was shown to induce less systemic plasminogen activation and to reverse the platelet-activating effect of fibrinolytic drugs, which resulted in a reduction in angiographically evident thrombus. The efficacy and safety of abciximab in combination with reduced-dose fibrinolysis was evaluated in GUSTO-V and ASSENT-3.[33,43] Taken together, combination therapy with fibrinolysis and abciximab resulted in a reduction in ischemic complications after acute MI, but this benefit was clearly offset by an increased risk of bleeding complications, particularly in older adults. As a consequence, abciximab is not routinely used with fibrinolytic therapies.

PREHOSPITAL FIBRINOLYSIS

Time lost between symptom onset and treatment initiation remains a crucial contributor to treatment delay in STEMI and might be especially problematic in rural or sparsely inhabited regions. Because mortality rates in randomized fibrinolytic trials are consistently lower when patients are treated within 2 hours of symptom onset, prehospital treatment is one attractive approach to improve early reperfusion and outcome with fibrinolysis. The convenience of administering a single bolus fibrinolytic agent (e.g., tenecteplase) along with a simple dose of enoxaparin has undoubtedly facilitated prehospital reperfusion protocols. This combination was investigated in the prehospital setting in the ASSENT-3 PLUS trial. Initiation of the lytic agent in the ambulance rather than in the emergency room resulted in a time gain of 47 minutes, significantly increasing the fraction of patients treated within 2 hours after symptom onset from 29% in ASSENT-3 to 52% in ASSENT-3 PLUS. These patients had a lower mortality rate than those who were treated more than 2 hours after symptom onset. A meta-analysis confirmed that the time gained with prehospital treatment resulted in a significant 17% mortality reduction compared with in-hospital fibrinolysis.[44] The question whether prehospital fibrinolysis compares favorably to transport to a center with interventional facilities for PPCI was addressed in the CAPTIM (Comparison of Angioplasty and Prehospital Thrombolysis in Acute Myocardial Infarction) trial.[45] PPCI was not found to be superior to prehospital fibrinolysis in terms of outcome, even at 5-year follow-up. However, rescue PCI after lysis was frequent, and this might have contributed to the favorable outcomes in the prehospital group. A report from the French Registry on Acute ST-Elevation Myocardial Infarction (FAST-MI) showed that the 5-year outcome with prehospital fibrinolysis in a contemporary pharmaco-invasive setting was associated with excellent outcomes, compared with those after PPCI.[46] Likewise, prehospital fibrinolysis followed by planned PCI compared favorably to transport for PPCI in the STREAM trial, provided that the dose of tenecteplase was halved in patients older than 75 years of age.[23]

SUMMARY

Despite the proven benefit and increasing use of PPCI worldwide, fibrinolysis remains relevant as a treatment option for STEMI patients. It significantly improves outcome, and is the preferred reperfusion therapy in absence of PCI facilities or when a timely PPCI is not possible. For many STEMI patients, especially in rural or remote areas, it often is the only option for immediate reperfusion. Ideally, single-bolus fibrinolysis is started in the prehospital setting within established STEMI networks, is accompanied by enoxaparin and clopidogrel in the absence of contraindications, and is followed by early invasive management (see Chapter 14). The optimal dose of tenecteplase in the elderly still needs to be assessed prospectively, but the favorable balance between benefit and bleeding risk in recent studies suggests that a half bolus might be the preferred regimen in this population.

Classic References

DeWood MA, et al.: Prevalence of total coronary occlusion during the early hours of transmural myocardial infarction, *N Engl J Med* 303:897, 1980.

Effectiveness of intravenous thrombolytic treatment in acute myocardial infarction: Gruppo Italiano per lo Studio della Streptochinasi nell'Infarto Miocardico (GISSI), *Lancet* 1:397, 1986.

Fletcher A, et al.: Treatment of of patients suffering from early myocardial infarction with massive and prolonged streptokinase therapy, *Trans Assoc Am Physicians* 71:287–296, 1958.

Herrick JB: Landmark article (JAMA 1912). Clinical features of sudden obstruction of the coronary arteries. By James B. Herrick, *JAMA* 250:1757, 1983.

Kagan A, Livsic AM, Sternby N, Vihert AM: Coronary-artery thrombosis and the acute attack of coronary heart-disease, *Lancet* 2:1199, 1968.

Markis JE, et al.: Myocardial salvage after intracoronary thrombolysis with streptokinase in acute myocardial infarction, *N Engl J Med* 305:777, 1981.

References

1. Van de Werf FJ, Topol EJ, Sobel BE: The impact of fibrinolytic therapy for ST-segment-elevation acute myocardial infarction, *J Thromb Haemost* 7:14, 2009.

1a. Streptokinase in recent myocardial infarction: a controlled multicentre trial. European working party, *Br Med J* 3:325–331, 1975.

1b. Kennedy JW, et al.: The western Washington randomized trial of intracoronary streptokinase in acute myocardial infarction:a 12-month follow-up report, *N Engl J Med* 312:1073–1078, 1985.

2. Yusuf S, et al.: Intravenous and intracoronary fibrinolytic therapy in acute myocardial infarction: overview of results on mortality, reinfarction and side-effects from 33 randomized controlled trials, *Eur Heart J* 6:556, 1985.

3. Keeley EC, Boura JA, Grines CL: Primary angioplasty versus intravenous thrombolytic therapy for acute myocardial infarction: a quantitative review of 23 randomised trials, *Lancet* 361:13, 2003.

4. Bueno H, et al.: Opportunities for improvement in anti-thrombotic therapy and other strategies for the management of acute coronary syndromes: insights from EPICOR, an international study of current practice patterns, *Eur Heart J Acute Cardiovasc Care* 5:3–12, 2016.

5. Kristensen SD, et al.: Reperfusion therapy for ST elevation acute myocardial infarction 2010/2011: current status in 37 ESC countries, *Eur Heart J* 35:1957, 2014.

6. Halvorsen S: STEMI treatment in areas remote from primary PCI centres, *EuroIntervention* (8 Suppl P)P44, 2012.

7. Pinto DS, et al.: Benefit of transferring ST-segment-elevation myocardial infarction patients for percutaneous coronary intervention compared with administration of onsite fibrinolytic declines as delays increase/clinical perspective, *Circulation* 124:2512, 2011.

8. Vora AN, et al.: Fibrinolysis use among patients requiring interhospital transfer for ST-segment elevation myocardial infarction care: a report from the US National Cardiovascular Data Registry, *JAMA Internal Medicine* 175:207, 2015.

9. Claeys MJ, et al.: Contemporary mortality differences between primary percutaneous coronary intervention and thrombolysis in ST-segment elevation myocardial infarction, *Arch Intern Med* 171:544, 2011.

10. Boscarelli D, et al.: Intracoronary thrombolysis in patients with ST-segment elevation myocardial infarction presenting with massive intraluminal thrombus and failed aspiration, *Eur Heart J Acute Cardiovasc Care* 3:229, 2014.

11. Henry TD, Jacobs AK, Granger CB: Regional systems of care for ST-elevation myocardial infarction: do they save lives? *Am Heart J* 166:389, 2013.

12. Collen D, et al.: Analysis of coagulation and fibrinolysis during intravenous infusion of recombinant human tissue-type plasminogen activator in patients with acute myocardial infarction, *Circulation* 73:511, 1986.

13. Van de Werf F, et al.: Coronary thrombolysis with intravenously administered human tissue-type plasminogen activator produced by recombinant DNA technology, *Circulation* 69:605, 1984.

14. ISIS-3: a randomised comparison of streptokinase vs tissue plasminogen activator vs anistreplase and of aspirin plus heparin vs aspirin alone among 41,299 cases of suspected acute myocardial infarction. ISIS-3 (Third International Study of Infarct Survival) Collaborative Group, *Lancet* 339:753, 1992.

15. GISSI-2: a factorial randomised trial of alteplase versus streptokinase and heparin versus no heparin among 12,490 patients with acute myocardial infarction. Gruppo Italiano per lo Studio della Sopravvivenza nell'Infarto Miocardico, *Lancet* 336:65, 1990.

16. An international randomized trial comparing four thrombolytic strategies for acute myocardial infarction. The GUSTO investigators, *N Engl J Med* 329:673, 1993.

17. The effects of tissue plasminogen activator, streptokinase, or both on coronary-artery patency, ventricular function, and survival after acute myocardial infarction. The GUSTO Angiographic Investigators, *N Engl J Med* 329:1615, 1993.

18. Reiner JS, et al.: Early angiography cannot predict postthrombolytic coronary reocclusion: observations from the GUSTO angiographic study. Global Utilization of Streptokinase and t-PA for Occluded Coronary Arteries, *J Am Coll Cardiol* 24:1439, 1994.

19. Simes RJ, et al.: Link between the angiographic substudy and mortality outcomes in a large randomized trial of myocardial reperfusion. Importance of early and complete infarct artery reperfusion. GUSTO-I Investigators, *Circulation* 91:1923, 1995.

20. Schroder R, et al.: Extent of early ST segment elevation resolution: a strong predictor of outcome in patients with acute myocardial infarction and a sensitive measure to compare thrombolytic regimens. A substudy of the International Joint Efficacy Comparison of Thrombolytics (INJECT) trial, *J Am Coll Cardiol* 26:1657, 1995.

21. A comparison of reteplase with alteplase for acute myocardial infarction: The Global Use of Strategies to Open Occluded Coronary Arteries (GUSTO III) Investigators, *N Engl J Med* 337:1118, 1997.

22. Assessment of the Safety and Efficacy of a New Thrombolytic Investigators: Single-bolus tenecteplase compared with front-loaded alteplase in acute myocardial infarction: the ASSENT-2 double-blind randomised trial, *Lancet* 354:716, 1999.

23. Sinnaeve PR, et al.: STEMI patients randomized to a pharmaco-invasive strategy or primary PCI: The STREAM 1-year mortality follow-up, *Circulation* 130:1139, 2014.

24. InTime II Investigators: Intravenous NPA for the treatment of infarcting myocardium early; InTIME-II, a double-blind comparison of single-bolus lanoteplase vs accelerated alteplase for the treatment of patients with acute myocardial infarction, *Eur Heart J* 21:2005, 2000.

25. Collen D, et al.: Recombinant staphylokinase variants with altered immunoreactivity. III: Species variability of antibody binding patterns, *Circulation* 95:455, 1997.

26. Han YL, et al.: The efficacy and safety of pharmacoinvasive therapy with prourokinase for acute ST-segment elevation myocardial infarction patients with expected long percutaneous coronary intervention-related delay, *Cardiovascular Therapeutics* 31:285, 2013.

27. O'Gara PT, et al.: 2013 ACCF/AHA guideline for the management of ST-elevation myocardial infarction: a report of the American College of Cardiology Foundation/American Heart Association Task Force on Practice Guidelines, *Circulation* 127:e362, 2013.

28. Steg PG, et al.: ESC Guidelines for the management of acute myocardial infarction in patients presenting with ST-segment elevation, *Eur Heart J* 33:2569, 2012.

29. Boersma E, et al.: Early thrombolytic treatment in acute myocardial infarction: reappraisal of the golden hour, *Lancet* 348:771, 1996.

30. White HD: Thrombolytic therapy in the elderly, *Lancet* 356:2028, 2000.

31. Ross AM, et al.: Extended mortality benefit of early postinfarction reperfusion. GUSTO-I Angiographic Investigators. Global Utilization of Streptokinase and Tissue Plasminogen Activator for Occluded Coronary Arteries Trial, *Circulation* 97:1549, 1998.

32. Giugliano RP, et al.: Lower-dose heparin with fibrinolysis is associated with lower rates of intracranial hemorrhage, *Am Heart J* 141:742, 2001.

33. Assessment of the Safety and Efficacy of a New Thrombolytic Regimen (ASSENT)-3 Investigators: Efficacy and safety of tenecteplase in combination with enoxaparin, abciximab, or unfractionated heparin: the ASSENT-3 randomised trial in acute myocardial infarction, *Lancet* 358:605, 2001.

34. Antman EM, et al.: Enoxaparin as adjunctive antithrombin therapy for ST-elevation myocardial infarction: results of the ENTIRE-Thrombolysis in Myocardial Infarction (TIMI) 23 Trial, *Circulation* 105:1642, 2002.

35. Eikelboom JW, et al.: Unfractionated and low-molecular-weight heparin as adjuncts to thrombolysis in aspirin-treated patients with ST-elevation acute myocardial infarction: a meta-analysis of the randomized trials, *Circulation* 112:3855, 2005.

36. Murphy SA, et al.: Efficacy and safety of the low-molecular weight heparin enoxaparin compared with unfractionated heparin across the acute coronary syndrome spectrum: a meta-analysis, *Eur Heart J* 28:2077, 2007.

37. Yusuf S, et al.: Effects of fondaparinux on mortality and reinfarction in patients with acute ST-segment elevation myocardial infarction: the OASIS-6 randomized trial, *JAMA* 295:1519, 2006.

38. White H: Thrombin-specific anticoagulation with bivalirudin versus heparin in patients receiving fibrinolytic therapy for acute myocardial infarction: the HERO-2 randomised trial, *Lancet* 358:1855, 2001.

39. Sabatine MS, et al.: Addition of clopidogrel to aspirin and fibrinolytic therapy for myocardial infarction with ST-segment elevation, *N Engl J Med* 352:1179, 2005.

40. Armstrong PW, et al.: Fibrinolysis or primary PCI in ST-segment elevation myocardial infarction, *N Engl J Med* 368(15):1379, 2013.

41. Alexopoulos D, et al.: Ticagrelor versus high dose clopidogrel in ST-segment elevation myocardial infarction patients with high platelet reactivity post fibrinolysis, *J Thromb Thrombolysis* 40:261, 2015.

42. Almendro-Delia M, et al.: Safety and efficacy of in-hospital clopidogrel-to-prasugrel switching in patients with acute coronary syndrome: an analysis from the 'real world.', *J Thromb Thrombolysis* 39:499, 2015.

43. Topol EJ: Reperfusion therapy for acute myocardial infarction with fibrinolytic therapy or combination reduced fibrinolytic therapy and platelet glycoprotein IIb/IIIa inhibition: the GUSTO V randomised trial, *Lancet* 357:1905, 2001.

44. Morrison LJ, et al.: Mortality and prehospital thrombolysis for acute myocardial infarction: A meta-analysis, *JAMA* 283:2686, 2000.

45. Bonnefoy E, et al.: Primary angioplasty versus prehospital fibrinolysis in acute myocardial infarction: a randomised study, *Lancet* 360:825, 2002.

46. Danchin N, et al.: Five-year survival in patients with ST-segment-elevation myocardial infarction according to modalities of reperfusion therapy: the French Registry on Acute ST-Elevation and Non-ST-Elevation Myocardial Infarction (FAST-MI) 2005 Cohort, *Circulation* 129:1629, 2014.

16 Revascularization in Non–ST-Elevation Acute Coronary Syndrome: For Whom, When, and How?

Stefan James, Daniel Lindholm, and Christoph Varenhorst

INTRODUCTION

A non–ST-elevation acute coronary syndrome (NSTE-ACS) is caused by a severe flow-limiting stenosis or acute thrombotic obstruction of a coronary artery (see Chapter 13). In the absolute majority of cases, levels of myocardial markers also are elevated, indicating myocardial damage related to thrombotic obstruction at the site of the culprit coronary lesion, as well as to downstream embolization of thrombotic material from the lesion. The thrombotic component of the disease can be influenced by treatment with anticoagulant and antiplatelet agents (see Chapter 18 and Chapter 19). Most often, however, one or more severe coronary stenoses remain, with consequent high risk for recurrent events during or after withdrawal of the initially intense antithrombotic treatment. Intervention to improve coronary flow is the rationale for early use of coronary angiography and revascularization.[1]

Elimination or bypass of the flow-limiting lesions by means of percutaneous coronary intervention (PCI) or coronary artery bypass grafting (CABG) complements medical therapy for rapid initial as well as long-term stabilization of the patient's condition.[2] The benefits and risks are related not only to lesion characteristics but also to patient characteristics that affect the progression of atherothrombosis and the risk of complications with these invasive procedures (see Chapter 17). Early risk stratification (see Chapter 11) is important to identify patients at high immediate- and long-term risk for death and cardiovascular events, in whom an early invasive strategy with adjunctive medical therapy may reduce that risk.[1,2]

CORONARY ANGIOGRAPHY

Invasive coronary angiography, followed by coronary revascularization, is performed in a majority of patients hospitalized with NSTE-ACS in geographic regions with well-developed health care systems. The decision for an invasive strategy should carefully weigh the risks of invasive diagnostics and the potential benefits. The decision to proceed with coronary revascularization, once the anatomy is defined by angiography, takes into account the risk in terms of morbidity and mortality associated with the proposed procedure (PCI or CABG) and the benefits in terms of short- and long-term prognosis, symptom relief, quality of life, and duration of hospital stay.

In the vast majority of cases, coronary angiography allows clinicians to achieve the following:

- Confirm the diagnosis of ACS related to obstructive epicardial coronary artery disease (CAD) (or rule out epicardial CAD as the origin of chest pain).
- Guide subsequent antithrombotic treatment or avoid unnecessary exposure to antithrombotic agents.
- Identify the culprit lesion(s).
- Establish an indication for coronary revascularization and assess the suitability of coronary anatomy for PCI and CABG.
- Stratify the patient's short- and long-term risk.

Angiographic patterns of CAD in patients with NSTE-ACS are diverse, ranging from a normal appearance of epicardial coronary arteries to a severely and diffusely diseased coronary artery tree. In patients with a clinical diagnosis of ACS, approximately 10% will be found to have disease of the left main artery, 25% will have three-vessel disease, 25% will have two-vessel disease, 25% will have one-vessel disease, and 15% will have no significant CAD at coronary angiography. Risk indicators such as age, male gender, diabetes mellitus, previous myocardial infarction (MI), previous severe angina, renal dysfunction, left ventricular dysfunction (manifesting as elevated B-type natriuretic peptide), ST-segment depression, elevated troponins, elevated growth differentiation factor 15 (GDF15), and higher risk response on stress testing are associated with a higher likelihood of multivessel or left main coronary artery disease (see Chapter 11).[3] However, the correlations between the extent of CAD and these risk indicators are rather weak.

Identification of the Culprit Lesion

In patients with NSTE-ACS, it is important to try to identify the culprit lesion on angiography. Such lesions typically are seen as intraluminal filling defects, consistent with thrombus, plaque ulceration, plaque irregularity, dissection, or impaired flow. Multiple vulnerable plaques may coexist, mostly as thin-cap fibroatheroma, within the coronary tree of a patient with NSTE-ACS (see Chapter 3). Nearly one fourth of patients with NSTE-ACS present with an acute occluded coronary artery, and two thirds of the occlusions are already collateralized at the time of angiographic examination. As a consequence, differentiation between an acute or subacute and chronic occlusion may sometimes be challenging, and identification of the culprit lesion based solely on angiography findings may not be possible.

ROUTINE INVASIVE VERSUS SELECTIVE INVASIVE MANAGEMENT

Multiple clinical trials and meta-analyses[4,5] have compared a routine invasive versus selective invasive management strategy in patients with NSTE-ACS. Compared with a selective invasive strategy, a routine invasive strategy improves clinical outcomes and reduces rates of recurrent ACS, subsequent rehospitalization, and revascularization (Figure 16-1A-C).[6] The FRISC-2, TACTICS-TIMI 18, and the RITA-3 trials were the first three trials in which patients received contemporary antithrombotic therapy, and most of the revascularization procedures were either PCI with routine stenting or CABG. All three trials demonstrated a reduction in the composite of death, MI, and recurrent severe angina, with a routine invasive strategy compared with a primarily conservative (selective invasive) treatment. Although an early hazard with more procedure-related MIs during hospitalization was noted for FRISC-2 and TACTICS-TIMI 18, a reduction of death and MI was seen in the intermediate term on follow-up evaluation at 6 months. In long-term follow-up extending to 5 years, other benefits

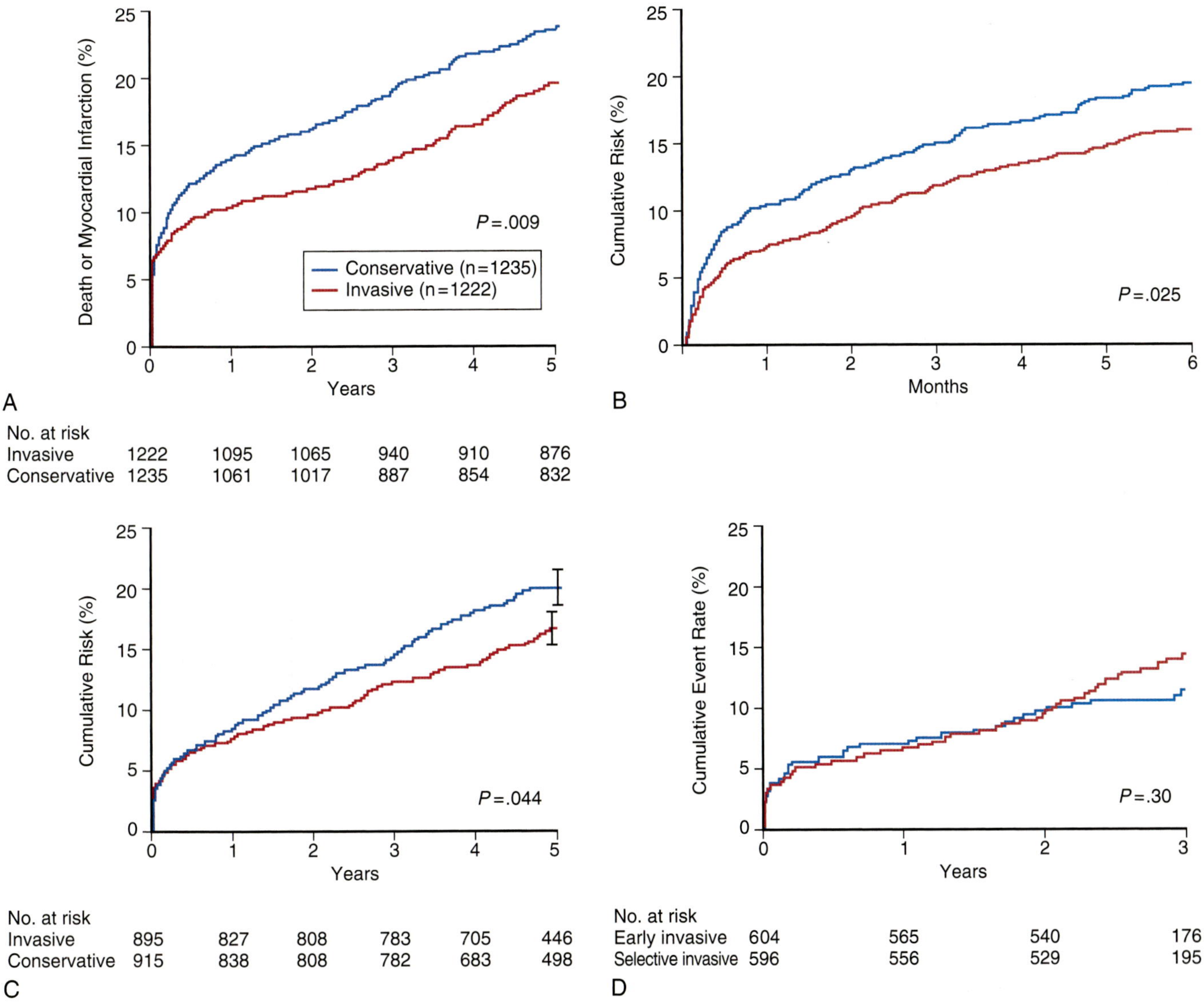

FIGURE 16-1 Longest-term outcome of the four large prospective randomized trials in non–ST-elevation acute coronary syndrome. A, Five-year outcome for the primary endpoint—death or myocardial infarction—in the FRISC-2 trial. **B,** Six-month outcome for the primary endpoint—death, myocardial infarction, and rehospitalization for acute coronary syndrome—for the TACTICS-TIMI 18 trial. **C,** Average 5-year outcome for the composite endpoint of death, myocardial infarction in the RITA-3 trial. **D,** Average 3-year outcome for the composite endpoint of death and spontaneous myocardial infarction in the ICTUS trial. (***A,*** *From Lagerqvist B, Husted S, Kontny F, et al: 5-year outcomes in the FRISC-II randomised trial of an invasive versus a non-invasive strategy in non-ST-elevation acute coronary syndrome: A follow-up study.* Lancet *368:998-1004, 2006.* ***B,*** *From Cannon CP, Weintraub WS, Demopoulos LA, et al. Comparison of early invasive and conservative strategies in patients with unstable coronary syndromes treated with the glycoprotein IIb/IIIa inhibitor tirofiban.* N Engl J Med *344:1879-1887, 2001.* ***C,*** *From Fox KA, Poole-Wilson P, Clayton TC, et al: 5-year outcome of an interventional strategy in non-ST-elevation acute coronary syndrome: The British Heart Foundation RITA 3 randomised trial.* Lancet *366:914-920, 2005.* ***D,*** *From Hirsch A, Windhausen F, Tijssen JG, et al: Long-term outcome after an early invasive versus selective invasive treatment strategy in patients with non-ST-elevation acute coronary syndrome and elevated cardiac troponin T (the ICTUS trial): A follow-up study.* Lancet *369:827-835, 2007.)*

included persistent reduction in the composite of death and MI and a trend toward improved overall survival (see Figure 16-1A-C).

Somewhat surprisingly, the ICTUS trial, performed in a population of patients with troponin-positive NSTE-ACS, demonstrated no advantage with an early invasive approach over a more selective approach with revascularization only in those with ischemia at rest or exercise (see Figure 16-1D). However, the differing outcome in this trial compared with that in the other two is likely to be explained by a substantial crossover of 44% of patients receiving the noninvasive management to an invasive intervention.

Across the multiple trials of early invasive versus conservative management, the proportion of patients undergoing revascularization in the different trials varied markedly. In some trials, less than 50% of patients in the invasive arm underwent early revascularization procedures, compared with a 35% to 45% early revascularization rate in the noninvasive arm (Figure 16-2). Consequently, the ability to demonstrate a mortality benefit with routine revascularization may depend on the difference in revascularization rate between randomized arms (Figure 16-3).

Furthermore, the true benefit of a routine invasive treatment shown in trials probably is underestimated—not only because revascularization was allowed when patients deteriorated while on medical therapy (crossover) but also because trials excluded those with very-high-risk features and did not include consecutive patients. When the ICTUS trial began enrolling patients, the availability of results from previous trials might have increased the likelihood of excluding high-risk patients from the trial by sending them directly to invasive treatment.

Meta-Analyses

The first meta-analysis, by Mehta and colleagues, reported an overall benefit of routine invasive treatment, with reductions in the composite of death and MI, and in MI alone (Table 16-1). There was, however, an early (in-hospital) risk of ischemic events in patients in the routine invasive treatment group. During the time span of enrollment in studies included in this meta-analysis (1994 to 2005), several aspects of the management of NSTE-ACS patients changed, including the use of thienopyridines and glycoprotein GPIIb/IIIa inhibitors, as well as the evolution of interventional technology, such as placement of coronary stents. In a stratified analysis, the reduction in ischemic events was more pronounced in studies published after 1999, as compared with those published earlier. In a subanalysis of the three studies with troponin results available, substantial benefit

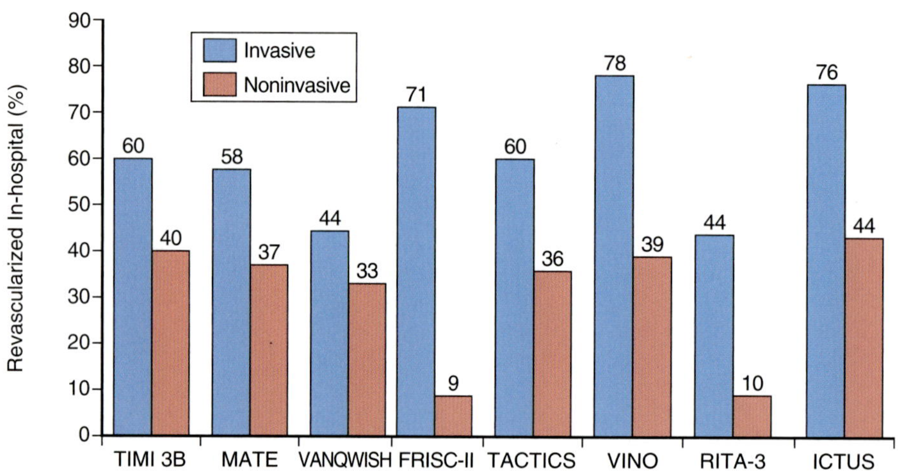

FIGURE 16-2 **Proportion of cardiac tissue revascularized in hospital in prospective randomized trials of an early invasive compared with a noninvasive approach in non–ST-elevation acute coronary syndrome.**

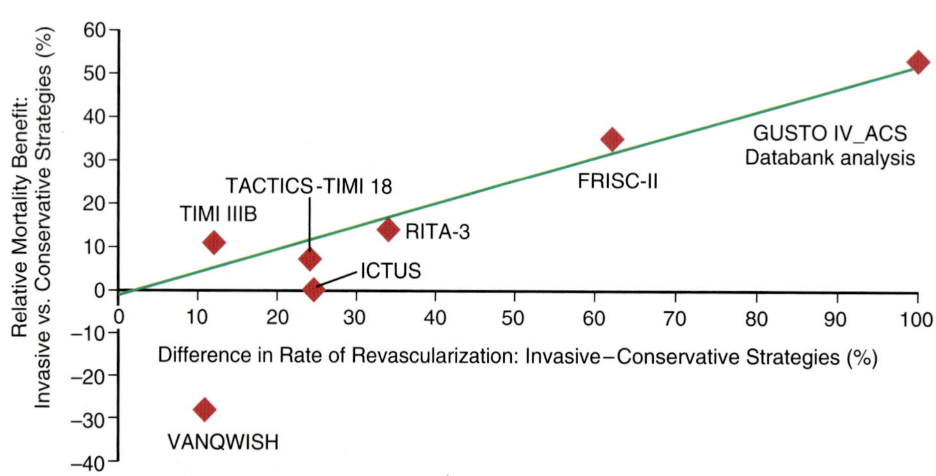

FIGURE 16-3 **The ability to demonstrate relative mortality benefit with the revascularization strategy depends on the gradient in rates of revascularization between both randomization arms.** *(From Task Force for Diagnosis and Treatment of Non-ST-Segment Elevation Acute Coronary Syndromes of European Society of Cardiology, Bassand JP, Hamm CW, et al: Guidelines for the diagnosis and treatment of non-ST-segment elevation acute coronary syndromes.* Eur Heart J *28:1598-1660, 2007.)*

was seen among patients with elevated troponin, with no apparent benefit for a routine invasive management strategy in patients with no elevation in troponin level. An analysis of all included studies using any biomarker of myocardial damage (i.e., creatine kinase, creatine kinase–MB fraction, or troponin) revealed similar results.

O'Donoghue and colleagues included all studies included in the previous analysis conducted by Mehta and associates, along with one additional study (ICTUS), and also extracted gender-specific information (see Table 16-1). After addition of data for the neutral ICTUS trial, no statistically significant difference was evident in the endpoints of death/MI and MI alone; however, routine invasive management reduced the composite endpoint of death, MI, and rehospitalization. This benefit was greatest in patients with elevated risk (as reflected in elevated levels of biomarkers of myocardial damage), for both men and women. Among women with negative biomarker assay results, a routine early invasive strategy provided no apparent benefit. Analogously, in a meta-analysis of data for women included in FRISC-II, RITA-3, ICTUS, and OASIS-5, a routine invasive management strategy offered no benefit over that of a selective invasive approach and appeared to result in higher mortality.[5] In the meta-analysis performed by Bavry and colleagues,[6] one requirement for inclusion was the availability of GPIIb/IIIa inhibitors and thienopyridines. Also, studies that included fibrinolysis were excluded. As a consequence, the earliest trials were not included (see Table 16-1). Routine invasive management reduced both mortality and subsequent MI; as well, the early hazard of MI and mortality previously described with this approach was not apparent, with similar reductions in ischemic events at 1 month and later during follow-up.

Long-Term Outcomes

Five-year outcomes (as opposed to up to 1 year in the preceding three meta-analyses) with a routine invasive versus selective invasive strategy were assessed in a patient-level meta-analysis of the FRISC-II, RITA-3, and ICTUS trial data. A routine invasive strategy was consistently associated with lower rates for the composite endpoint of death and MI, and for MI alone, when compared with a selective invasive strategy, and with a hazard ratio (HR) of 0.90 (CI, 0.77 to 1.05) for mortality alone.[4] In a patient-pooled analysis of individual data from the FRISC-II, ICTUS, and RITA-2 trials, the effect of age on long-term outcomes with a routine or selective invasive strategy was assessed. The long-term, 5-year benefit of the routine invasive strategy was attenuated in patients younger than 65 years of age, as well as in women.[7] The more recently published 10-year results of the RITA-3 trial showed that the survival advantage afforded by a routine approach attenuated after 5 years and disappeared at 10 years regardless of patient risk.[8] The rates of all-cause and cardiovascular death were similar for the routine approach and the selective invasive strategy groups (all-cause death: 25.1% versus 25.4%; $P = 0.94$; and cardiovascular death: 15.1% versus 16.1%; $P = 0.65$) for routine and selective invasive treatment, respectively). However, an interaction between treatment and time associated with lower all-cause mortality was evident during the first 5 years, but this rate was higher during the second 5 years for routine than for selective invasive treatment.

The significant treatment effect from the initial studies, the widespread clinical uptake of the findings, and guideline recommendations are likely to have caused the shift in clinical practice toward more routine invasive care.

Patient Selection

An early invasive strategy is recommended in a majority of patients with ACS, both to identify all severe coronary lesions and to improve clinical outcomes by early revascularization.[1,9,10] Although the vast majority of data support a routine invasive strategy, guidelines also highlight the importance of risk stratification in the decision-making process (Figure 16-4; Table 16-2). Both European Society of Cardiology (ESC) and American Heart Association/American College of Cardiology (AHA/ACC) guidelines state that an early invasive strategy is not recommended in patients with extensive comorbidity, in whom the risks associated with revascularization and the comorbid conditions are likely to outweigh the benefits of

TABLE 16-1 Meta-Analyses of Randomized Trials Evaluating Routine Invasive versus Selective Invasive Management for Non–ST-Elevation Acute Coronary Syndrome

			META-ANALYSIS			
TRIAL/STUDY	YEAR PUBLISHED	*N*	Mehta et al. (2005)	Bavry et al. (2006)	O'Donoghue et al. (2008)	Fox et al. (2010)
TIMI-IIIB	1994	1473	x		x	
VANQWISH	1998	920	x		x	
MATE	1998	201	x		x	
FRISC-II	1999	2457	x	x	x	x
TRUCS	2000	148		x		
TACTICS-TIMI 18	2001	2220	x	x	x	
VINO	2002	131	x	x	x	
RITA-3	2002	1810	x	x	x	x
ISAR-COOL	2003	410		x		
ICTUS	2005	1200		x	x	x
Outcome						
Death/MI			OR, 0.82 (0.72-0.93)	Not reported	OR, 0.92 (0.69-1.23)	HR, 0.85 (0.75-0.96)
Death			OR, 0.92 (0.77-1.09)	RR, 0.75 (0.63-0.90)	OR, 0.97 (0.71-1.32)	HR, 0.90 (0.77-1.05)
MI			OR, 0.75 (0.65-0.88)	RR, 0.83 (0.72-0.96)	OR, 0.84 (0.64-1.12)	HR, 0.77 (0.65-0.90)

HR, Hazard ratio; *OR*, odds ratio; *RR*, relative risk.

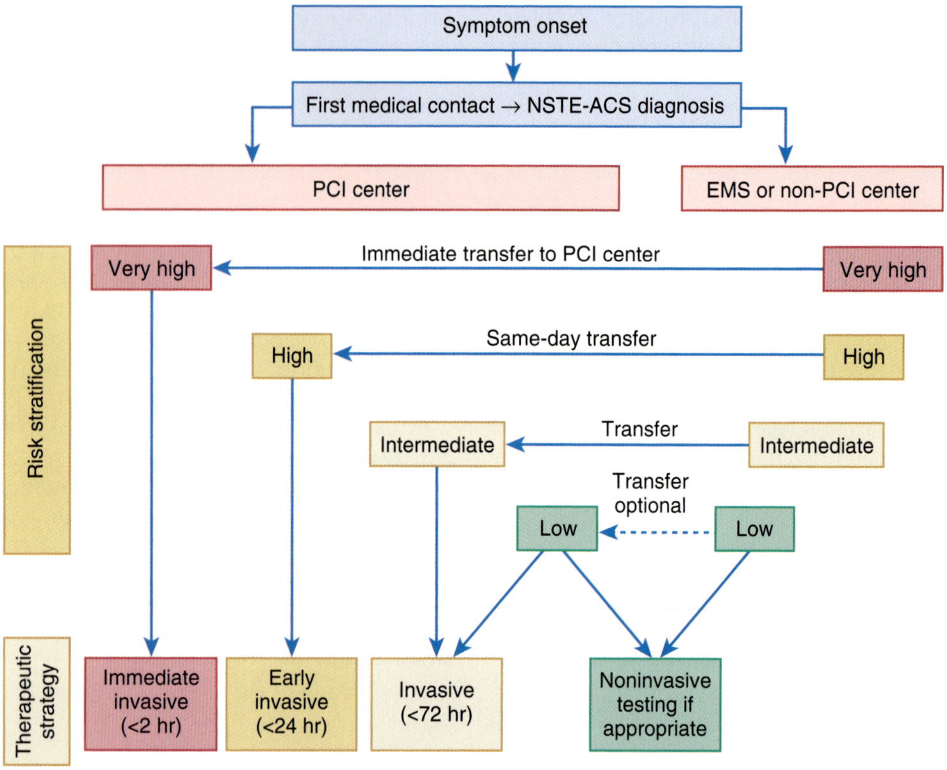

FIGURE 16-4 **Selection of non–ST-elevation acute coronary syndrome (NSTE-ACS) treatment strategy and timing according to initial risk stratification.** *EMS,* Emergency medical services; *PCI,* percutaneous coronary intervention. *(From Roffi M, et al: 2015 ESC guidelines for the management of acute coronary syndromes in patients presenting without persistent ST-segment elevation: Task Force for the Management of Acute Coronary Syndromes in Patients Presenting without Persistent ST-Segment Elevation of the European Society of Cardiology,* Eur Heart J *37:267–315, 2016.)*

TABLE 16-2 Risk Criteria for Invasive Therapy in Patients with Non–ST-Elevation Acute Coronary Syndrome

Very-High-Risk Criteria
Hemodynamic instability or cardiogenic shock
Recurrent or ongoing chest pain refractory to medical treatment
Life-threatening arrhythmias or cardiac arrest
Mechanical complications of MI
Acute heart failure
Recurrent dynamic ST-T wave changes, particularly with intermittent ST-segment elevation
High-Risk Criteria
Rise or fall in cardiac troponin compatible with MI
Dynamic ST- or T-wave changes (symptomatic or silent)
GRACE risk score >140
Intermediate-Risk Criteria
Diabetes mellitus
Renal insuffiency (eGFR <60 mL/min/1.73 m^2)
LVEF <40% or congestive heart failure
Early postinfarction angina
Previous PCI
Previous CABG
GRACE risk score >109 and <140
Low-Risk Criteria
Any characteristic not mentioned above

CABG, Coronary artery bypass grafting; *eGFR,* estimated glomerular filtration rate; *LVEF,* left ventricular ejection fraction; *MI,* myocardial infarction; *PCI,* percutaneous coronary intervention.

invasive treatment. Furthermore, patients with acute chest pain and a low likelihood of ACS who are troponin assay–negative are not likely to benefit from routine invasive strategy.

Approximately 10% of patients with NSTE-ACS have nonobstructive CAD.[10] Compared with patients with obstructive CAD, this group of patients is more likely to be of younger age and female and less likely to have diabetes mellitus or a history of previous MI or PCI. Data regarding outcomes in patients in whom revascularization is not feasible owing to a diffuse or very severe CAD are sparse. For these patients, sometimes pharmacologic treatment, to reduce long-term risk and address refractory angina, remains the only option. An invasive evaluation, and if indicated a revascularization procedure, is sometimes not offered because of the treating physician's appreciation of a negative balance between benefit (ischemic risk reduction) and risk (related to the procedure). Other patients sometimes withheld from an invasive strategy are those who are very elderly or frail, with comorbid conditions such as dementia or cancer, or those at high risk for bleeding complications.

TIMING OF REVASCULARIZATION

Although a routine invasive management intervention is recommended for high-risk patients with NSTE-ACS, the optimal timing of angiography and revascularization is still a matter of some debate.

Candidates for Immediate Invasive Evaluation

Very-high-risk patients with NSTE-ACS, defined as those having at least one very-high-risk criterion, generally have been excluded from randomized controlled trials (RCTs). These very-high-risk criteria include the following:

- Hemodynamic instability or cardiogenic shock
- Recurrent or ongoing chest pain refractory to medical treatment

TABLE 16-3 Meta-Analyses of Randomized Trials and Observational Studies Evaluating Early versus Delayed Invasive Management of Non–ST-Elevation Acute Coronary Syndrome

			META-ANALYSIS	
TRIAL/STUDY	**YEAR PUBLISHED**	***N***	**Katritsis et al. (2011)**	**Navarese et al. (2013)**
RCTs				
ISAR-COOL	2003	410	x	x
ELISA	2003	220	x	x
ABOARD	2009	352	x	x
OPTIMA	2009	142		x
TIMACS	2009	3031	x	x
Zhang et al.	2010	815		x
LIPSIA-NSTEMI	2012	602		x
Observational				
ACUITY*	2010	7749		x
SYNERGY*	2007	10,027		x
CRUSADE	2005	56,352		x
GRACE	2005	8853		x
Outcomes				
RCTs				
Death/MI			Not reported	
Death			RR 0.85 (0.64-1.11)	OR 0.83 (0.64-1.09)
MI			RR 0.94 (0.61-1.45)	OR 1.15 (0.65-2.01)
Observational				
Death/MI				
Death				OR 0.80 (0.63-1.02)
MI				OR 0.86 (0.69-1.08)

*Although SYNERGY and ACUITY were RCTs, they were not conducted primarily to assess timing of invasive procedures. Hence, they are considered observational in this context.
MI, Myocardial infarction; *RCTs,* randomized controlled studies.

- Life-threatening arrhythmias or cardiac arrest
- Mechanical complications of MI
- Acute heart failure with refractory angina or ST-segment deviation
- Recurrent dynamic ST- or T-wave changes, particularly with intermittent ST-segment elevation

For these patients, a poor short- and long-term prognosis can be expected in the absence of appropriate treatment. An additional risk is the possibility of misclassifying the patient as having NSTE-ACS, when in fact the causative lesion is an acutely occluded artery. An immediate invasive strategy (i.e., within 2 hours from hospital admission, analogous to ST-elevation myocardial infarction [STEMI] management) with intent to establish the diagnosis and perform revascularization is recommended, irrespective of ECG or biomarker findings. Centers without STEMI programs should transfer such very-high-risk patients immediately.

Randomized Trials

An early invasive versus a delayed invasive approach has been tested in several relatively small randomized trials,[11-14] and in one larger trial (TIMACS)[15] (Table 16-3). In a meta-analysis performed by Katritsis and colleagues[16] comprising four RCTs (including TIMACS), no difference was found between an early invasive and a delayed invasive management strategy in terms of all-cause mortality or MI. However, the risk of recurrent ischemia and the duration of hospitalization were reduced with an early invasive strategy. The median time from randomization/admission to coronary angiography ranged between 1.16 and 14 hours in the early invasive treatment group and between 20.8 and 86 hours in the delayed treatment group.

An updated meta-analysis, which included an additional three RCTs, observational data from two registries, and post-hoc analyses from two RCTs, demonstrated similar results. There was no apparent difference in mortality or MI with an early invasive approach (defined as less than 20 hours in the analysis of RCTs and less than 24 hours for the observational studies).[17]

In a (prespecified) subgroup analysis of TIMACS, outcomes were assessed in relation to ischemic risk, as calculated by the GRACE score. High-risk patients, i.e. those with GRACE score above 140, had a substantial benefit of revascularization within 24 hours, with a relative risk reduction of 35% (absolute risk reduction 7.1%) in the composite endpoint of death, MI, or stroke; whereas no significant difference was seen in patients with GRACE score higher than 140[15] (Figure 16-5).

Professional Guidelines

Accordingly, the ESC guidelines on myocardial revascularization state that in NSTE-ACS, "An early invasive strategy (<24 hours) is recommended in patients with at least one primary high-risk criterion," where rise/fall in troponin, dynamic ST-T changes, and GRACE score higher than 140 are considered primary high-risk criteria (see Figure 16-4 and Table 16-2).[2]

Primary outcome

Characteristic	No. of Patients	Early (%)	Delayed (%)	Hazard Ratio for Event (95% CI)	*P* Value for Interaction
Overall	3031	9.6	11.3	0.85 (0.68–1.06)	
Age					0.46
<65 yr	1293	6.4	6.4	0.98 (0.64–1.52)	
≥65 yr	1736	12.2	14.6	0.83 (0.64–1.07)	
Sex					0.53
Female	1052	9.6	12.3	0.77 (0.53–1.12)	
Male	1976	9.6	10.7	0.89 (0.68–1.18)	
ST-segment deviation					0.71
No	1523	7.5	8.5	0.88 (0.62–1.26)	
Yes	1508	11.6	14.2	0.81 (0.61–1.07)	
Elevated cardiac marker					0.43
No	668	10.4	10.4	1.00 (0.62–1.60)	
Yes	2363	9.4	11.5	0.81 (0.63–1.04)	
GRACE score					0.01
0–140	2070	7.6	6.7	1.12 (0.81–1.56)	
≥141	961	13.9	21.0	0.65 (0.48–0.89)	

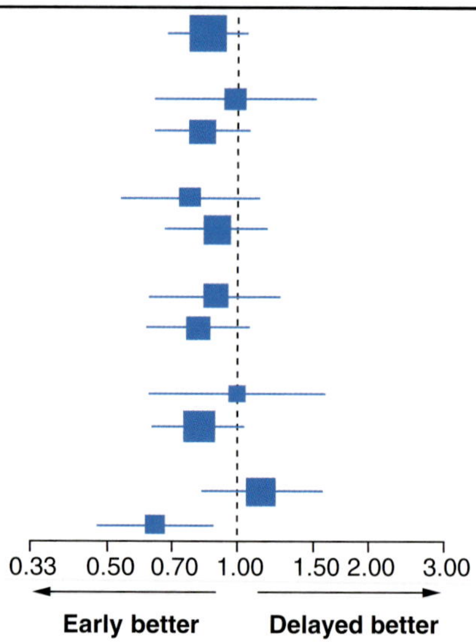

A

Secondary outcome

Characteristic	No. of Patients	Early (%)	Delayed (%)	Hazard Ratio for Event (95% CI)	*P* Value for Interaction
Overall	3031	9.5	12.9	0.72 (0.58–0.89)	
Age					0.86
<65 yr	1295	6.0	8.3	0.70 (0.46–1.06)	
≥65 yr	1736	12.3	16.2	0.74 (0.58–0.95)	
Sex					0.69
Female	1052	9.9	14.3	0.68 (0.48–0.97)	
Male	1978	9.2	12.2	0.74 (0.56–0.97)	
ST-segment deviation					0.86
No	1523	7.0	10.0	0.69 (0.49–0.98)	
Yes	1508	11.9	16.0	0.72 (0.55–0.94)	
Elevated cardiac marker					0.22
No	666	11.8	12.9	0.92 (0.59–1.41)	
Yes	2365	8.8	13.0	0.67 (0.52–0.85)	
GRACE score					0.15
0–140	2049	7.5	8.8	0.83 (0.61–1.12)	
≥141	982	13.7	21.6	0.62 (0.45–0.83)	

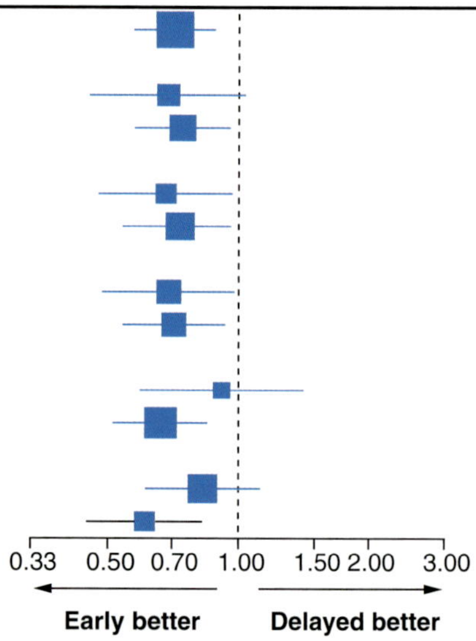

B

FIGURE 16-5 Hazard ratios for the primary and secondary outcomes in prespecified subgroups in the Timing of Intervention in Acute Coronary Syndromes (TIMACS) trial. A shows hazard ratios for the composite primary outcome of death, myocardial infarction, or stroke in the early intervention group, as compared with the delayed-intervention group, in selected subgroups of patients. **B** shows hazard ratios for the composite secondary outcome of death, myocardial infarction, or refractory ischemia in the same subgroups. The size of the squares is proportional to the size of the corresponding subgroup. *GRACE,* Global Registry of Acute Coronary Events. *(From Mehta SR, et al: Early versus delayed invasive intervention in acute coronary syndromes,* N Engl J Med *360:2165–2175, 2009.)*

Also AHA/ACC guidelines recommend an early invasive strategy in patients with NSTE-ACS who have refractory angina or hemodynamic or electrical instability (without serious comorbidity or contraindications to such procedures).[9]

REVASCULARIZATION IN SUBSETS OF PATIENTS WITH NON–ST-ELEVATION ACUTE CORONARY SYNDROME

Chronic Kidney Disease

Impaired kidney function affects 25% to 30% of patients admitted with ACS. Moreover, chronic kidney disease (CKD) is associated with a substantial increase in mortality. Patients with CKD frequently have comorbid conditions that increase both bleeding and ischemic risk. Despite the advantage with invasive treatment, revascularization is underused in patients with CKD.[18] Consistent results from several observational studies indicate that an early invasive therapy is associated with lower mortality in patients with mild to moderate renal insufficiency. In patients with end-stage renal disease, the benefit seems to be attenuated and, therefore, the advantage of early invasive therapy is less certain in these patients.

Since patients with CKD are commonly excluded from RCTs, there is little evidence regarding the effect of early invasive management in patients with mild to moderate CKD and NSTE-ACS. In the FRISC-II trial, where subjects with creatinine levels greater than 150 μmol/L (1.7 mg/dL)

were excluded, the absolute risk reduction in death/MI was higher in patients with impaired kidney function.[6] Patients with creatinine levels above 221 µmol/L (2.5 mg/dL) were excluded in the TACTICS-TIMI 18 trial, but found similar reductions in patients with mild to moderate kidney disease and those with normal kidney function.[19]

Contrast-induced nephropathy (CIN) is an important complication associated with the routine invasive strategy. The most important predictor of CIN is CKD. Patients with CKD have a 20-fold higher risk than that for a healthy individual of developing CIN.[20] In a study of 8000 patients undergoing PCI, a CIN risk score based on certain risk factors was developed. Important risk factors included in this score are hypotension, intraaortic balloon pump, congestive heart failure, CKD, age older than 75 years, anemia, and volume of contrast. High-risk patients are those with a score above 16, corresponding to a 57.3% risk of CIN and 12.6% risk of dialysis, whereas low-risk patients are those with a score less than 5 associated with a 7.5% risk of CIN and 0.04% risk of dialysis.[21]

In an observational study from a large cohort of patients with end-stage renal disease, CABG was suggested to be preferable to PCI for multivessel coronary revascularization. Compared with PCI, CABG was associated with lower risk of death or MI.[22] Nonetheless, in the most fragile patients, the least invasive approach seems preferable.

Elderly Patients

In the United States, the proportion of the population 65 years of age and older (13%) is expected to reach approximately 20% by 2050. With changing demographics, the interest in studying ACS outcomes in older adults has increased, as have efforts to delineate the differences between older men and older women undergoing revascularization. Older adults (older than 75 years) are underrepresented in ACS clinical trials. Among ACS subtypes, compared with patients with STEMI, those with NSTE-ACS are on average older. Because older people are underrepresented in clinical trials, they are less likely to receive treatment according to guidelines.

It has been suggested that older women benefit less than older men from an early invasive approach. Older women are less likely to undergo revascularization at time of hospitalization than older men. Whether this difference is related to bias or an appropriate case selection remains unsettled. A meta-analysis of data from three trials assessing routine invasive strategy versus selective invasive strategy in NSTE-ACS (FRISC-II, ICTUS, and RITA-3) showed a larger early risk and less long-term benefit in women than in men regardless of age.[23] The After Eighty study randomly assigned patients with NSTE-ACS who were older than 80 years of age to either an invasive or a conservative strategy. The overall age was 84 years, and approximately one half of all patients were female. The invasively treated patients demonstrated a 47% reduction in ischemic outcomes compared with the group of patients who received conservative (medical) treatment.[24]

Gender and Selection of Invasive Treatment

In the FRISC-2 and the RITA-3 trials, a significantly greater effect of the invasive strategy was observed in men than in women.[25] This observation might be explained partly by the lower proportion of women undergoing revascularization in the invasive group consequent to a lower rate of significant epicardial coronary lesions in females than in males. Another reason might be a raised risk for periprocedural complications in women undergoing coronary artery bypass surgery, especially among those with diabetes mellitus and older age. However, these gender-related differences in the effects of early invasive treatment were not observed in either the TACTICS-TIMI 18[25] or the ICTUS trial. In a meta-analysis of data on all published prospective randomized trials, no significant sex-related difference was found in the overall benefit of routine invasive management. In women as well as in men, the benefits were confined to those at higher risk, that is, with elevated troponin and/or ST-segment depression.

For proper evaluation of women with ACS, it seems preferable to use the same indications for diagnostic coronary angiography in both sexes—that is, a moderate to high risk for subsequent events. In the selection of the most appropriate treatment, however, the better long-term prognosis and the higher periprocedural risks in women compared with men should be taken into consideration. Finally, because of the uncertainties of the balance between benefits and risks in women, new prospective trials comparing an early invasive against a conservative strategy focusing on women are warranted.

REVASCULARIZATION STRATEGY: PERCUTANEOUS CORONARY INTERVENTION VERSUS CORONARY ARTERY BYPASS GRAFTING

Revascularization with CABG has been performed for more than 50 years and PCI for more than 35 years. Both revascularization techniques have undergone continued advances. The progressing technology has resulted in a steady decline of periprocedural adverse events, resulting in excellent outcomes with both revascularization techniques. Notwithstanding, the differences between the two revascularization strategies should be recognized. In CABG, bypass grafts are placed to the mid-coronary vessel beyond the culprit lesion(s), offering protection against the consequences of further proximal obstructive disease. By contrast, optimally placed coronary stents will restore normal blood flow of the native coronary vasculature through local treatment of obstructive lesions without offering protection against new disease proximal to the stent. Myocardial revascularization has been subject to more RCTs than almost any other intervention.

The main objectives of coronary angiography and revascularization are improvement of prognosis and symptom relief. Although the reperfusion treatment of choice for most patients with STEMI is primary PCI (see Chapter 14), the rudiments for revascularization in NSTE-ACS involve selection of patients suitable for a diagnostic catheterization followed by revascularization by either PCI or CABG. No specific randomized clinical trials have compared PCI with CABG in NSTE-ACS. The current evidence supports the use of both revascularization strategies (PCI and CABG), and the selection of procedure type in the individual patient with NSTE-ACS depends on several factors.

In stabilized patients with NSTE-ACS, the revascularization strategy should be chosen using similar considerations as for patients with stable coronary artery disease[2] (Table 16-4). In single-vessel disease (present in approximately 30% of cases of NSTE-ACS), PCI is the treatment of choice for most patients. In approximately 50% of patients, more than one vessel is

TABLE 16-4 Recommendations for Revascularization (CABG versus PCI) in Stabilized Patients with Non–ST-Elevation Acute Coronary Syndrome and with Suitable Coronary Anatomy for Both Procedures and Low Predicted Surgical Mortality

RECOMMENDATION ACCORDING TO EXTENT OF CAD	CLASS OF RECOMMENDATION*	
	CABG	PCI
One- or two-vessel disease without proximal LAD stenosis	IIB	I
One-vessel disease with proximal LAD stenosis	I	I
Two-vessel disease with proximal LAD stenosis	I	I
Left main artery disease with SYNTAX score ≤22	I	I
Left main artery disease with SYNTAX score 23-32	I	IIa
Left main artery disease with SYNTAX score >32	I	III
Three-vessel disease with SYNTAX score ≤22	I	I
Three-vessel disease with SYNTAX score 23-32	I	III
Three-vessel disease with SYNTAX score >32	I	III

Adapted from Windecker S, Kolh P, Alfonso F, et al: 2014 ESC/EACTS guidelines on myocardial revascularization: The Task Force on Myocardial Revascularization of the European Society of Cardiology (ESC) and the European Association for Cardio-Thoracic Surgery (EACTS). Developed with the special contribution of the European Association of Percutaneous Cardiovascular Interventions (EAPCI). Eur Heart J *35(37):2541-2619, 2014.*

CABG, Coronary artery bypass grafting; *CAD,* coronary artery disease; *LAD,* left anterior descending (artery); *PCI,* percutaneous coronary intervention.

*I: Evidence and/or general agreement that a given treatment or procedure is beneficial, useful, effective; IIa: conflicting evidence, but weight of evidence/opinion is in favor of usefulness/efficacy; IIb: conflicting evidence, and usefulness/efficacy is less well established by evidence/opinion; III: evidence or general agreement that the given treatment or procedure is not useful/effective and in some cases may be harmful.

diseased, and a decision between culprit vessel PCI, multivessel PCI (ad hoc or staged), or CABG needs to be made. In these patients, a multidisciplinary approach, such as "heart team" consultation involving the noninvasive cardiologist, the invasive cardiologist, and the cardiac surgeon, is advised to determine revascularization strategy integrating patient preferences.[2]

The choice of revascularization strategy depends largely on the extent and severity of CAD. For left main artery disease, CABG has historically been regarded as the treatment of choice, but observational studies have shown that PCI can be performed with good results. Left main artery disease often involves the bifurcation, which in turn increases restenosis and stent thrombosis risk. If multivessel disease is present, CABG has been associated with better survival compared with PCI, independent of the presence of left main artery disease.[26] Recent evidence suggests that PCI provides results similar to those with CABG in the treatment of at least lower-severity left main artery stenosis, with comparable rates of death and MI up to 5 years after the procedure.[27] In the SYNTAX (Synergy between Percutaneous Coronary Intervention with TAXUS and Cardiac Surgery) trial, 1800 patients with stable ischemic heart disease and three-vessel or left main artery disease were randomly assigned to undergo CABG or PCI.[28] In the overall study population, death and MI rates were similar at 1 year, but stroke rates were increased in the CABG group, and repeat revascularizations were more frequent in the PCI group.

The SYNTAX score was a grading tool developed to evaluate the coronary angiography and determine the complexity of coronary artery disease based on the sum of points allocated to the identified lesions found in the coronary angiography. A SYNTAX score above 32 identifies a group of patients with an especially high risk, whereas scores below 22 denotes a low risk. Of importance, in the patient groups with low SYNTAX scores, rates of major adverse events were similar for PCI and CABG, with lower stroke rates for PCI. In recent years, an increase in the use of drug-eluting stents (DESs) has been associated with lower restenosis risk and decreased need for repeat revascularization. Accordingly, the benefit of CABG in studies conducted before widespread use of DESs may be overestimated. For more severe three-vessel disease, findings from randomized and observational studies are consistent regarding the survival advantage for CABG versus PCI.

Apart from the severity and complexity of coronary artery disease as assessed during coronary angiography, the revascularization treatment decision also needs to be based on the patient's preferences, left ventricular function, and comorbidity and on the overall estimated procedure risk.

SUMMARY

NSTE-ACS is the most frequent manifestation of unstable CAD and the most frequent indication for coronary angiography and revascularization. Early identification of the culprit lesion and potentially other flow-limiting stenoses is important for confirmation of the diagnosis, risk stratification, and selection of the mode of revascularization. Patients at very high risk for progression of infarction and death or with a high likelihood of occlusion of a coronary artery should undergo emergent coronary angiography. Most patients with NSTE-ACS should have their coronary anatomy investigated in the following 1 to 2 days to reduce the risk of ischemic complications, limit the duration of potent antithrombotic therapy, and minimize the duration of hospitalization. The mode of revascularization should be decided in consensus by a multidisciplinary team consisting of noninvasive and invasive cardiologists and a cardiothoracic surgeon.

Classic References

Bavry AA, Kumbhani DJ, Rassi AN, et al.: Benefit of early invasive therapy in acute coronary syndromes: A meta-analysis of contemporary randomized clinical trials, *J Am Coll Cardiol* 48(7):1319–1325, 2006.

Boden WE, O'Rourke RA, Crawford MH, et al.: Outcomes in patients with acute non-Q-wave myocardial infarction randomly assigned to an invasive as compared with a conservative management strategy. Veterans Affairs Non-Q-Wave Infarction Strategies in Hospital (VANQWISH) Trial Investigators, *N Engl J Med* 338(25):1785–1792, 1998.

Cannon CP, Weintraub WS, Demopoulos LA, et al.: Comparison of early invasive and conservative strategies in patients with unstable coronary syndromes treated with the glycoprotein IIb/IIIa inhibitor tirofiban, *N Engl J Med* 344(25):1879–1887, 2001.

de Winter RJ, Windhausen F, Cornel JH, et al.: Early invasive versus selectively invasive management for acute coronary syndromes, *N Engl J Med* 353(11):1095–1104, 2005.

Effects of tissue plasminogen activator and a comparison of early invasive and conservative strategies in unstable angina and non-Q-wave myocardial infarction: Results of the TIMI IIIB Trial. Thrombolysis in Myocardial Ischemia, *Circulation* 89(4):1545–1556, 1994.

Fox KA, Poole-Wilson PA, Henderson RA, et al.: Interventional versus conservative treatment for patients with unstable angina or non-ST-elevation myocardial infarction: The British Heart Foundation RITA 3 randomised trial. Randomized Intervention Trial of unstable Angina, *Lancet* 360(9335):743–751, 2002.

Invasive compared with non-invasive treatment in unstable coronary-artery disease: FRISC II prospective randomised multicentre study. FRagmin and Fast Revascularisation during InStability in Coronary artery disease (FRISC II) Investigators, *Lancet* 354(9180):708–715, 1999.

McCullough PA, O'Neill WW, Graham M, et al.: A prospective randomized trial of triage angiography in acute coronary syndromes ineligible for thrombolytic therapy. Results of the medicine versus angiography in thrombolytic exclusion (MATE) trial, *J Am Coll Cardiol* 32(3):596–605, 1998.

Mehta SR, Cannon CP, Fox KAA, et al.: Routine vs selective invasive strategies in patients with acute coronary syndromes: a collaborative meta-analysis of randomized trials, *JAMA* 293(23):2908–2917, 2005.

Michalis LK, Stroumbis CS, Pappas K, et al.: Treatment of refractory unstable angina in geographically isolated areas without cardiac surgery. Invasive versus conservative strategy (TRUCS study), *Eur Heart J* 21(23):1954–1959, 2000.

Neumann FJ, Kastrati A, Pogatsa-Murray G, et al.: Evaluation of prolonged antithrombotic pretreatment ("cooling-off" strategy) before intervention in patients with unstable coronary syndromes: A randomized controlled trial, *JAMA* 290(12):1159–1593, 2003.

O'Donoghue M, Boden WE, Braunwald E, et al.: Early invasive vs conservative treatment strategies in women and men with unstable angina and non-ST-segment elevation myocardial infarction: A meta-analysis, *JAMA* 300(1):71–80, 2008.

Spacek R, Widimský P, Straka Z, et al.: Value of first day angiography/angioplasty in evolving non-ST segment elevation myocardial infarction: An open multicenter randomized trial. The VINO Study, *Eur Heart J* 23(3):230–238, 2002.

References

1. Roffi M, Patrono C, Collet JP, et al.: 2015 ESC guidelines for the management of acute coronary syndromes in patients presenting without persistent ST-segment elevation: Task Force for the Management of Acute Coronary Syndromes in Patients Presenting without Persistent ST-Segment Elevation of the European Society of Cardiology, *Eur Heart J* 37(3):267–315, 2016.
2. Windecker S, Kolh P, Alfonso F, et al.: 2014 ESC/EACTS guidelines on myocardial revascularization: The Task Force on Myocardial Revascularization of the European Society of Cardiology (ESC) and the European Association for Cardio-Thoracic Surgery (EACTS). Developed with the special contribution of the European Association of Percutaneous Cardiovascular Interventions (EAPCI), *Eur Heart J* 35(37):2541–2619, 2014.
3. Wallentin L, Lindholm D, Siegbahn A, et al.: Biomarkers in relation to the effects of ticagrelor in comparison with clopidogrel in non-ST-elevation acute coronary syndrome patients managed with or without in-hospital revascularization: A substudy from the Prospective Randomized Platelet Inhibition and Patient Outcomes (PLATO) trial, *Circulation* 129(3):293–303, 2014.
4. Fox KA, Clayton TC, Damman P, et al.: Long-term outcome of a routine versus selective invasive strategy in patients with non-ST-segment elevation acute coronary syndrome: A meta-analysis of individual patient data, *J Am Coll Cardiol* 55(22):2435–2445, 2010.
5. Swahn E, Alfredsson J, Afzal R, et al.: Early invasive compared with a selective invasive strategy in women with non-ST-elevation acute coronary syndromes: A substudy of the OASIS 5 trial and a meta-analysis of previous randomized trials, *Eur Heart J* 33(1):51–60, 2012.
6. Hoenig MR, Aroney CN, Scott IA: Early invasive versus conservative strategies for unstable angina and non-ST elevation myocardial infarction in the stent era, *Cochrane Database Syst Rev*(3), 2010. CD004815.
7. Damman P, Clayton T, Wallentin L, et al.: Effects of age on long-term outcomes after a routine invasive or selective invasive strategy in patients presenting with non-ST segment elevation acute coronary syndromes: A collaborative analysis of individual data from the FRISC II-ICTUS-RITA-3 (FIR) trials, *Heart* 98(3):207–213, 2012.
8. Henderson RA, Jarvis C, Clayton T, et al.: 10-year mortality outcome of a routine invasive strategy versus a selective invasive strategy in non–ST-segment elevation acute coronary syndrome: The British Heart Foundation RITA-3 randomized trial, *J Am Coll Cardiol* 66:511–520, 2015.
9. Amsterdam EA, Wenger NK, Brindis RG, et al.: 2014 AHA/ACC guideline for the management of patients with non–ST-elevation acute coronary syndromes: A report of the American College of Cardiology/American Heart Association Task Force on Practice Guidelines, *Circulation* 130(25):e344–e426, 2014.
10. De Ferrari GM, Fox KA, White JA, et al.: Outcomes among non-ST-segment elevation acute coronary syndrome patients with no angiographically obstructive coronary artery disease: Observations from 37,101 patients, *Eur Heart J Acute Cardiovasc Care* 3:37–45, 2014.
11. Montalescot G, Cayla G, Collet JP, et al.: Immediate vs delayed intervention for acute coronary syndromes: a randomized clinical trial, *JAMA* 302(9):947–954, 2009.
12. Riezebos RK, Ronner E, Bals Ter E, et al.: Immediate versus deferred coronary angioplasty in non-ST-segment elevation acute coronary syndromes, *Heart* 95(10):807–812, 2009.
13. Zhang J, Qiao SB, Zhu J: Chinese Cooperative Group of the Timing of Intervention in Acute Coronary Syndrome: [Outcome of patients with non-ST segment elevation acute coronary syndrome undergoing early or delayed intervention], *Zhonghua Xin Xue Guan Bing Za Zhi* 38(10):865–869, 2010.
14. Thiele H, Rach J, Klein N, et al.: Optimal timing of invasive angiography in stable non-ST-elevation myocardial infarction: The Leipzig Immediate versus early and late PercutaneouS coronary Intervention triAl in NSTEMI (LIPSIA-NSTEMI Trial), *Eur Heart J* 33(16):2035–2043, 2012.
15. Mehta SR, Granger CB, Boden WE, et al.: Early versus delayed invasive intervention in acute coronary syndromes, *N Engl J Med* 360(21):2165–2175, 2009.
16. Katritsis DG, Siontis GCM, Kastrati A, et al.: Optimal timing of coronary angiography and potential intervention in non-ST-elevation acute coronary syndromes, *Eur Heart J* 32(1):32–40, 2011.
17. Navarese EP, Gurbel PA, Andreotti F, et al.: Optimal timing of coronary invasive strategy in non-ST-segment elevation acute coronary syndromes: A systematic review and meta-analysis, *Ann Intern Med* 158(4):261270, 2013.
18. Szummer K, Lundman P, Jacobson SH, et al.: Influence of renal function on the effects of early revascularization in non-ST-elevation myocardial infarction: Data from the Swedish Web-System for Enhancement and Development of Evidence-Based Care in Heart Disease Evaluated According to Recommended Therapies (SWEDEHEART), *Circulation* 120(10): 851–858, 2009.
19. G1 Marenzi, Cabiati A, Assanelli E: Chronic kidney disease in acute coronary syndromes, *World J Nephrol* 1(5):134–145, 2012.
20. Nicola R, Shaqdan KW, Aran K, et al.: Contrast-induced nephropathy: Identifying the risks, choosing the right agent, and reviewing effective prevention and management methods, *Curr Probl Diagn Radiol* 44(6):501–504, 2015.
21. National Clinical Guideline Centre: *Acute kidney injury: Prevention, detection and management up to the point of renal replacement therapy*, London, UK, 2013, Royal College of Physicians (UK); National Institute for Health and Clinical Excellence: Guidance.
22. Chang TI, Shilane D, Kazi DS, et al.: Multivessel coronary artery bypass grafting versus percutaneous coronary intervention in ESRD, *J Am Soc Nephrol* 23(12):2042–2049, 2012.
23. Damman P, et al.: Effects of age on long-term outcomes after a routine invasive or selective invasive strategy in patients presenting with non-ST segment elevation acute coronary syndromes: a collaborative analysis of individual data from the FRISC II-ICTUS-RITA-3 (FIR) trials, *Heart* 98:207–213, 2012.
24. Tegn N, et al.: Invasive versus conservative strategy in patients aged 80 years or older with non-ST-elevation myocardial infarction or unstable angina pectoris (After Eighty study): an open-label randomised controlled trial, *Lancet* 387:1057–1065, 2016.
25. Dolor RJ, Melloni C, Chatterjee R, Allen LaPointe NM, editors: *Treatment strategies for women with coronary artery disease*, Rockville, Md, 2012, Agency for Healthcare Research and Quality.
26. Park SJ, Kim YH, Park DW, et al.: Randomized trial of stents versus bypass surgery for left main coronary artery disease, *N Engl J Med* 364(18):1718–1727, 2011.
27. Morice MC, Serruys PW, Kappetein AP, et al.: Outcomes in patients with de novo left main disease treated with either percutaneous coronary intervention using paclitaxel-eluting stents or coronary artery bypass graft treatment in the Synergy Between Percutaneous Coronary Intervention with TAXUS and Cardiac Surgery (SYNTAX) trial, *Circulation* 121(24):2645–2653, 2010.
28. Serruys PW, Morice MC, Kappetein AP, et al.: Percutaneous coronary intervention versus coronary-artery bypass grafting for severe coronary artery disease, *N Engl J Med* 360(10):961–972, 2009.

17 Approach to Percutaneous Coronary Intervention in Myocardial Infarction

Deepak L. Bhatt and Jeremiah P. Depta

INTRODUCTION

Percutaneous coronary intervention (PCI) is the dominant strategy used for coronary revascularization in acute myocardial infarction (MI). In the United States, approximately 600,000 patients are discharged from the hospital with a principal diagnosis of acute MI (see Chapter 2), which includes a substantial percentage of the primary indications for PCI of the estimated 954,000 PCIs performed annually.[1] This chapter reviews the evidence and practical considerations for PCI in patients with acute MI, including both ST-elevation MI (STEMI) and non–ST-elevation MI (NSTEMI). Selection among the options for reperfusion therapy for STEMI is addressed in Chapter 14, and selection among strategies for management of NSTEMI is discussed in Chapter 16. Antiplatelet therapy is discussed in Chapter 19, and anticoagulant therapy is discussed in Chapter 18.

TIMING OF PERCUTANEOUS CORONARY INTERVENTION

ST-Elevation Myocardial Infarction Strategies for Reducing Time to Treatment

If performed in a timely fashion by experienced operators, primary PCI is the recommended method for reperfusion in patients presenting with STEMI.[2] The benefit of reperfusion therapy is greatest in the first 3 hours after symptom onset (see Chapter 13). The development of regional systems for STEMI care and reperfusion therapy to limit the total ischemic time and meet time-to-treatment goals is detailed in Chapter 5. Regardless of the recommended time-to-treatment goals, reperfusion should always be established as rapidly as possible for any individual patient. It is estimated that 90% of STEMI patients presenting to a PCI-capable hospital achieve the door-to-device time goal of ≤90 minutes in the absence of a clinical reason for delay.[3] A checklist (Table 17-1) was developed by the American College of Cardiology (ACC)/American Heart Association (AHA) with practical system strategies to minimize door-to-device time.[2]

Non–ST-Elevation Myocardial Infarction: Timing of Angiography

In patients with NSTEMI, the timing of diagnostic angiography with intent to perform PCI is driven by risk stratification, clinical stability, and patient preferences (see Chapter 16). Patients treated using an early invasive strategy will undergo angiography, whereas those managed with the ischemia-guided strategy will typically receive angiography after medical treatment has failed, with objective evidence of ischemia on noninvasive stress testing or with a very high risk for mortality or morbidity.[4] The timing of angiography in the invasive strategy is stratified based on clinical risk assessment (Table 17-2) into urgent (<2 hours), early (<24 hours), and delayed (25 to 72 hours). Patients with refractory symptoms, severe heart failure, or electrical and/or hemodynamic instability should undergo immediate invasive evaluation (see Chapter 16).

TABLE 17-1 Checklist for Reducing Door-to-Device Times in ST-Elevation Myocardial Infarction

Time-to-Treatment Goals
PCI-Capable Hospital
Goal: FMC-to-device time <90 min
Non–PCI-Capable Hospital
Goal: Transfer to PCI-capable hospital with FMC-to-device time of <120 min (door-in-door-out <30 min) If anticipated FMC-to-device is >120 min, administer fibrinolytic within 30 minutes of arrival.
Checklist for Reducing Door-to-Device Times
☐ Pre-hospital ECG to diagnose STEMI and activate PCI team ☐ Emergency room physicians activate the PCI team ☐ A single call to a central paging system activates the PCI team ☐ PCI team arrival to the catheterization laboratory within 20 min ☐ Timely analysis and feedback of time-to-treatment metrics by the STEMI care team

ECG, Electrocardiogram; *FMC*, first medical contact; *PCI*, percutaneous coronary intervention; *STEMI*, ST-elevation myocardial infarction.
Adapted from O'Gara PT, et al. 2013 ACCF/AHA guideline for the management of ST-elevation myocardial infarction: a report of the American College of Cardiology Foundation/American Heart Association Task Force on Practice Guidelines. Circulation *127:e362, 2013.*

TABLE 17-2 Timing of Angiography in the Early Invasive Strategy or Ischemia-Guided Strategy in Patients with Non–ST-Elevation Myocardial Infarction

Ischemia-Guided Strategy
• Low-risk score (e.g., TIMI [0 or 1], GRACE [<109]) • Low-risk troponin-negative female patients • Patient or clinician preference in the absence of high-risk features
Immediate Invasive (within 2 h)
• Refractory angina • Signs or symptoms of heart failure • New or worsening mitral regurgitation • Hemodynamic instability • Recurrent angina or ischemia at rest or with low-level activities despite intensive medical therapy • Sustained VT or VF
Early Invasive (within 24 h)
• None of the above, but GRACE risk score >140 • Temporal change in troponin • New or presumably new ST depression
Delayed Invasive (within 25–72 h)
• None of the above, but diabetes mellitus • Renal insufficiency (GFR <60 mL/min/1.73 m^2) • Reduced LV systolic function (EF <0.40) • Early postinfarction angina • PCI within 6 months • Previous CABG • GRACE risk score 109–140; TIMI score >2

CABG, Coronary artery bypass graft; *EF*, ejection fraction; *GFR*, glomerular filtration rate; *LV*, left ventricular; *PCI*, percutaneous coronary intervention; *VF*, ventricular fibrillation; *VT*, ventricular tachycardia.
Adapted from Amsterdam EA, et al: 2014 AHA/ACC guideline for the management of patients with non–ST-elevation acute coronary syndromes: A report of the American College of Cardiology/American Heart Association Task Force on Practice Guidelines. Circulation *130:e344, 2014.*

An early invasive strategy did not improve survival or reduce recurrent MI compared with a delayed invasive strategy in a meta-analysis of seven randomized trials and four observational studies that included 82,869 patients with non–ST-elevation acute coronary syndrome (NSTE-ACS).[5] In the TIMACS (Timing of Intervention in Patients with Acute Coronary Syndromes) trial, high-risk patients (GRACE [Global Registry of Acute Coronary Events] risk score >140) who underwent an early invasive strategy had a 38% reduction in death, MI, and stroke at 6 months compared with a delayed invasive strategy.[6] An early invasive strategy is advocated in patients at higher risk for adverse clinical events (see Table 17-2).

VASCULAR ACCESS

Vascular access is vitally important for the success of PCI. Femoral access is the most common approach used for PCI in the United States. Radial access has gained significant popularity and is preferred by many patients and operators. Importantly, bleeding is the most common PCI-related complication, and it is also associated with higher rates of mortality.

Performing Vascular Access

Femoral

Retrograde puncture of the femoral artery (Figure 17-1) is required for femoral access during diagnostic coronary angiography and PCI.[7] The common femoral artery is used because of its larger size and its ability to compress against the femoral head during manual compression. Patients should receive sedation and a local anesthetic before arterial cannulation. Because of the variability in body habitus, several landmarks should be noted before choosing an arteriotomy site. A line drawn between the anterior

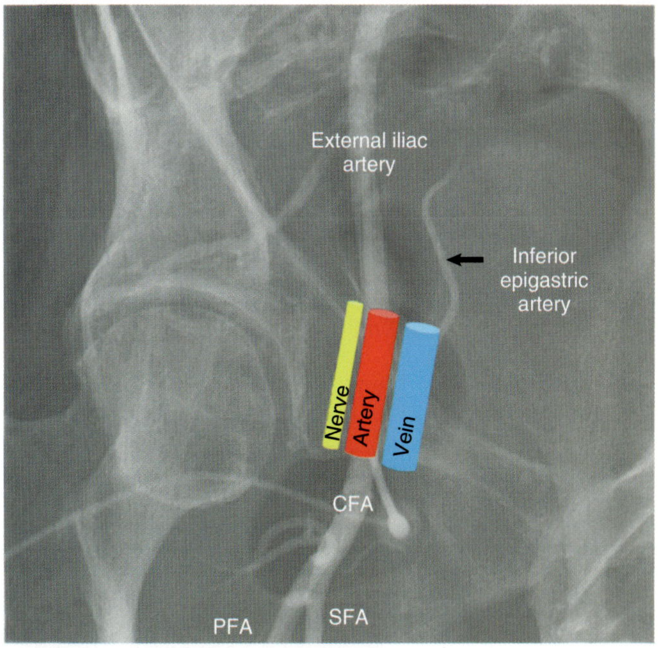

FIGURE 17-1 Anatomy of the femoral artery. Femoral angiography of the right femoral artery in a right anterior oblique view. The common femoral artery should be entered below the inguinal ligament in the middle one-third of the femoral head to avoid a low (i.e., at or below the femoral bifurcation) or high stick (i.e., above the inferior epigastric artery). *CFA*, Common femoral artery; *PFA*, profunda femoris artery; *SFA*, superficial femoral artery. *(From Bangalore S, Bhatt DL: Femoral arterial access and closure.* Circulation *124:e147–156, 2011.)*

superior iliac spine and pubis demarcates the inguinal ligament. The inguinal crease should not be used to approximate the inguinal ligament, especially in obese patients. Fluoroscopy should be used to mark the femoral head. The common femoral should be entered at a 30- to 45-degree angle approximately 1 to 2 cm below the inguinal ligament, which is typically at the center of the femoral head. A "low stick" can result in cannulation of the superficial femoral artery, which increases the risk of hematoma, dissection, arterial occlusion, or formation of a pseudoaneurysm or arteriovenous fistula. Conversely, a "high stick" above the inguinal ligament or above the inferior epigastric artery on angiography does not allow for effective manual compression against the femoral head, and significantly increases the risk for retroperitoneal hemorrhage. Before administering therapeutic anticoagulation for PCI, limited angiography through the femoral sheath at an oblique ipsilateral angle should be performed to determine the arteriotomy site in relationship to the femoral head, inferior epigastric artery, and femoral bifurcation, which could modify the timing of PCI and/or choice to use a vascular access closure device.

Two commonly used techniques to reduce vascular complications during femoral access include use of a micropuncture needle (Cook Medical, Bloomington, Ind.)[8] or guidance using ultrasound.[9] Traditionally, an 18-gauge wide open-bore needle has been used for arterial cannulation. A smaller micropuncture 21-gauge needle can be used to access the common femoral artery. After placement of a 0.018-inch wire into the artery, limited angiography can be used to localize the site of cannulation through the needle or inner dilator, and if acceptable, the 4F micropuncture sheath can be advanced over the wire. If the arteriotomy site is too low or high, then femoral access at an alternative site can be reattempted, and the needle or inner dilator removed, with minimal risks of bleeding. Real-time ultrasound guidance has also been used for femoral access and allows for visualization of needle entrance into the femoral artery. It can also determine the femoral bifurcation to facilitate cannulation of the common femoral artery above the bifurcation.

Radial

The learning curve for radial access is typically longer compared with femoral access. It should not be used in patients with forearm arteriovenous fistulas. Assessment for collateral ulnar circulation via the ulno-palmar arterial arch is advocated. However, failure to demonstrate dual circulation to the hand (i.e., incomplete palmar arch) is not an absolute contraindication.[10] Assessment is performed using either the modified Allen's or plethysmo-oxymetric test, the latter of which has a higher specificity. Any abnormal Allen's test should be confirmed by plethysmo-oxymetric testing. When attempting radial access, a smaller amount of lidocaine (1 to 2 mL) should be administered to minimize the risk of local vasospasm or obscuring the radial pulse. A micropuncture needle is used to access the radial artery and for placement of a hydrophilic radial arterial sheath over a 0.021- to 0.025-inch guidewire (Videos 17-1, 17-2, and 17-3). Ultrasound can also be used to minimize the number of attempts needed for arterial cannulation. Vasospasm can be a significant limitation in radial access. Intra-arterial administration of an antispasmolytic drug (e.g., nitroglycerin, diltiazem, verapamil) is mandatory. A number of single agents or "cocktail" regimens have been used to prevent vasospasm. Most operators use verapamil (2.5 to 5 mg) and/or nitroglycerin (100 to 200 μg). Anticoagulation should be initiated after radial artery cannulation to minimize the risk for radial artery occlusion. Low-dose unfractionated heparin (e.g., 2000 to 3000 IU or 50 IU/kg) can be administered and converted to therapeutic dosing upon placement of the guide catheters in the ascending aorta or with coronary cannulation. Access via the left radial may be advantageous over the right radial because of the higher prevalence of right-handed individuals; the aortic path approximates a transfemoral approach, which allows for easier coronary cannulation with standard Judkin's guide catheters and easier access to the left internal mammary artery in coronary artery bypass graft (CABG) patients.

Advantages and Disadvantages of Radial versus Femoral Access

When considering vascular access, operators should consider important differences between femoral and radial access (Table 17-3).[11] In the United States, rates of radial access for PCI had been less than 2% because of unfamiliarity with the radial approach and a concern for increased procedure length and radiation exposure. However, rates in the United States have increased to approximately 15% to 20% and are expected to increase over the next decade.

Current Evidence: Radial versus Femoral

Radial access is associated with a lower rate of vascular complications and major bleeding in comparison to femoral access, and in some studies, a lower rate of adverse cardiac

TABLE 17-3 Comparison of Femoral and Radial Access for Percutaneous Coronary Intervention

	FEMORAL	RADIAL
Anatomic		
Vessel size	6–10 mm	2–3 mm
Vascular course	Less variable	Highly variable
Vessel location	Variable because of body habitus	Superficial
Nearby neurovascular	Yes	No
Procedural		
Procedural success	Marginally higher	Marginally lower
Procedural time	Comparable	Comparable
Contrast load	Comparable	Comparable
Fluroscopy time	Marginally lower	Marginally higher
Choice of sheath size	Unrestricted	Restricted (typically 6F)
Learning curve	Shorter	Longer (typically 50 cases)
Patient Care		
Preference	Lower	Higher
Time to ambulation	Typically 2–6 h	Immediate
Length of stay	Longer	Shorter
Complications		
Access site bleeding	Higher	Lower
Vessel occlusion	Rare	0–10%
Pseudoaneurysm	1–5%	Rare

Adapted from Byrne RA, et al: Vascular access and closure in coronary angiography and percutaneous intervention. Nat Rev Cardiol *10:27–40, 2013.*

events. In the RIVAL (Radial vs. Femoral Access for Coronary Intervention) trial, no difference was observed in the composite rate of death, MI, stroke, or non-CABG major bleeding in patients who presented with ACS without ST-segment elevation and who were randomized to femoral versus radial access. However, vascular complications were significantly lower with radial access.[12] Patients who presented with STEMI in the RIFLE-STEACS (Radial Versus Femoral Randomized Investigation in ST-Elevation Acute Coronary Syndrome) and STEMI-RADIAL (ST Elevation Myocardial Infarction Treated by Radial or Femoral Approach) trials demonstrated a significant reduction in bleeding and vascular complications,[13,14] which translated into shorter hospital stays and lower mortality compared with the femoral approach.[13] The lower mortality in STEMI with radial catheterization was also demonstrated in a meta-analysis and observational data from the National Cardiovascular Data Registry.[15,16] More recently, the MATRIX (Minimizing Adverse Haemorrhagic Events by Transradial Access Site and Systemic Implementation of AngioX) trial also showed fewer major bleeding complications with a radial versus a femoral approach and lower mortality in ACS patients with or without STEMI.[17]

Considerations for Radial Approach in ST-Elevation Myocardial Infarction

Despite evidence that the radial approach reduces vascular complications, major bleeding, and mortality in STEMI patients, its use is paradoxically lower in this population than in patients with NSTEMI. One concern is that the increased time required for the radial approach may prolong the time-to-treatment goal in STEMI. However, a door-to-device delay of 83 minutes would be required to offset the mortality benefit of radial PCI over femoral PCI in STEMI.[18] Because of the higher risk for cardiogenic shock, the groin of a patient with STEMI should always be prepped for immediate venous access or additional arterial access for hemodynamic support.

Vascular Closure Devices: When to Consider Use

Vascular closure devices were initially designed to improve safety of PCI by reducing access site bleeding and vascular complications. However, clinical trials and meta-analyses have demonstrated that vascular closure devices do not lower bleeding or vascular complications compared with manual compression.[19] To this end, current ACC/AHA guidelines do not recommend routine use of vascular closure.[20]

When manual compression (i.e., 3 minutes per sheath French size [e.g., 6F = 18 minutes]) is used, femoral arterial sheaths can typically be pulled when the activated clotting time (ACT) is less than 160 to 180 seconds with heparin use or 2 hours after bivalirudin is stopped without checking the ACT. Manual compression can be performed digitally or using a manual compression assist device (e.g., FemoStop, St. Jude Medical, St. Paul, Minnesota). Vascular closure devices achieve faster hemostasis, which allows for earlier ambulation, improved patient satisfaction, and possibly shorter hospital length of stay. In the absence of a radial approach, obese patients, whose body habitus may limit effective manual compression, or individuals who cannot tolerate prolonged periods in a supine position, should undergo closure using a vascular closure device. Arteriotomy sites at the femoral bifurcation, in the superficial femoral artery, or in a smaller femoral artery (<5 mm) are associated with a higher risk for device failure, and potentially, arterial occlusion; thus, in general, vascular closure devices would not be recommended. A number of devices are currently approved and available with different mechanisms used for closure.[7] No sizeable randomized trial comparing the safety and efficacy of each device has been conducted.

Management of Vascular Complications

Vascular complications are the most common adverse event following PCI and are associated with an increase in cost, length of stay, morbidity, and mortality. The two most common complications are hematoma and pseudoaneurysm, whereas less common complications include dissection, arteriovenous fistula, arterial occlusion, retroperitoneal hemorrhage, femoral nerve damage, and infection. A hematoma is typically managed conservatively with local compression and rarely requires blood transfusion. The presence of a palpable bruit or pulsatile mass should prompt evaluation with an ultrasound. Small pseudoaneurysms (<3 cm) can be followed with serial ultrasounds. Pseudoaneurysms larger than 3 cm can be treated with ultrasound-guided thrombin injection. Retroperitoneal hemorrhage (RPH) should be suspected in any patient with a sudden onset of hypotension and flank pain ipsilateral to the vascular access site.[21] Prompt recognition with concomitant volume and blood support is essential for the management of a suspected RPH. Anticoagulation reversal or platelet infusion may also be necessary, despite the theoretical risks for stent thrombosis. Early computed tomography may be useful, but should not delay aggressive supportive measures or involve transport of an unstable patient. Most RPHs can be managed conservatively, and endovascular or open surgical treatment should only be considered in patients who cannot be stabilized hemodynamically. Arterial occlusion should be suspected in any patient with sudden onset of leg pain, paresthesia, decreased or absent pulses, and a cool and/or cyanotic limb. Suspected arterial occlusion is a vascular emergency and should be treated with intravenous (IV) anticoagulation and emergent endovascular or surgical repair.

INTERVENTIONAL PHARMACOTHERAPY

Procedural Sedation

PCI is typically performed under minimal to moderate sedation. The usual goal is for patients to be comfortable with depressed consciousness and the ability to follow verbal commands. Patients should receive supplemental oxygen during PCI as needed. Because of the potential risk for respiratory depression leading to hypoxia and/or hypercarbia, all patients should be assessed for a history of or clinical predictors for difficult intubation (e.g., obesity). If present, anesthesiology can be consulted to consider the need for monitored anesthesia care. Typically, an IV sedative and analgesic are administered in small incremental dosages during PCI. The two most common agents used are midazolam (0.5 to 1 mg IV boluses) as a sedative and fentanyl (25 to 50 μg IV bolus) as an analgesic. Both have a rapid onset of action (2 to 5 minutes), are rapidly metabolized within 30 to 60 minutes after administration, and are reversible with flumazenil and naloxone, respectively.

Oral Antiplatelet Therapy

Antiplatelet therapy is essential for PCI in acute MI (see Chapter 19 and Chapter 20). In this section, we focus on the practical aspects of oral antiplatelet therapy for operators performing PCI. All patients should receive a loading dose of aspirin (i.e., 325 mg) or a 600-mg rectal suppository if unable to swallow or if they are vomiting. Most patients with STEMI and NSTEMI should receive a loading dose of an adenosine diphosphate (ADP) $P2Y_{12}$ inhibitor (although the exact timing of administration is a matter of debate, especially in NSTEMI).

When to Preload with Oral Adenosine Diphosphate $P2Y_{12}$ Inhibitors

When possible, pretreatment with a loading dose of an oral ADP $P2Y_{12}$ inhibitor in patients with acute MI is recommended, with administration as early as possible after a diagnosis of STEMI. In a meta-analysis, clopidogrel pretreatment reduced mortality in STEMI and major coronary events in both STEMI and NSTE-ACS compared with no pretreatment.[22] The PLATO (Study of Platelet Inhibition and Patient Outcomes Clopidogrel) trial led to the approval of ticagrelor for patients with ACS.[23] All the patients in PLATO were pretreated with ticagrelor before PCI. Delayed administration of ticagrelor has not been formally tested against pretreatment in NSTEMI. Prasugrel is not currently recommended for use as upstream therapy in NSTEMI.[4] In the TRITON-TIMI 38 (Trial to Assess Improvement in Therapeutic Outcomes by Optimizing Platelet Inhibition with Prasugrel-Thrombolysis in MI) trial, prasugrel was administered at the time of PCI after coronary angiography. However, current ACC/AHA guidelines do advocate for prasugrel pretreatment when possible in STEMI.[2]

Anticoagulation Strategies

Anticoagulant therapy must be administered to all patients undergoing PCI. Selecting an initial agent will be discussed in detail in a subsequent chapter (see Chapter 18). In STEMI, unfractionated heparin or bivalirudin are the two agents recommended for anticoagulation; most operators will also use either agent for PCI in NSTEMI. Fondaparinux should never be used alone as an anticoagulant because of the risk of catheter thrombosis. In patients on therapeutic enoxaparin (i.e., 1 mg/kg every 12 hours), unfractionated heparin or bivalirudin is not recommended during PCI. If the last dose of enoxaparin was more than 8 to 12 hours before PCI or if the dosage was subtherapeutic, an IV dose of 0.3 mg/kg should be administered.

Practical Aspects of Monitoring Anticoagulation

ACTs are the standard method used to monitor the therapeutic effect of anticoagulation during PCI. In the balloon angioplasty era, higher levels of ACTs were associated with lower rates of periprocedural ischemic events, but also increased the risk of bleeding. However, this association has not been consistent in coronary stent trials. ACTs are routinely checked throughout the PCI procedure after administration of unfractionated heparin. A bolus of unfractionated heparin (70 to 100 U/kg) is administered, and the ACT is checked approximately 5 minutes later. Traditionally, a minimum therapeutic ACT level is more than 250 seconds without a glycoprotein IIb/IIIa inhibitor (GPI). If a GPI is also administered, an ACT level should be more than 200 seconds. The range of ACT levels may vary based on the complexity of the PCI, but typically should not exceed 350 seconds. If bivalirudin (0.75 mg/kg followed by a 1.75 mg/kg per hour IV infusion) is used, monitoring of ACT levels is not required. However, most operators will check one ACT level to determine that bivalirudin has been administered through a "working" peripheral IV line. In addition, low-molecular-weight heparin does not require any monitoring during PCI. Fondaparinux requires co-administration of heparin during PCI, for which an ACT can be checked to ensure therapeutic levels of anti-IIa activity.

Current Evidence: Bivalirudin versus Heparin in ST-Elevation Myocardial Infarction

Significant controversy has arisen about the safety and efficacy of bivalirudin in primary PCI during STEMI. The HORIZONS-AMI (Harmonizing Outcomes with Revascularization and Stents in Acute MI) trial showed that bivalirudin lowered mortality (all-cause and cardiac) in STEMI compared with heparin plus a GPI.[24] Bivalirudin was associated with a significantly higher rate of acute (i.e., <24 hours of primary PCI) stent thrombosis in the HORIZONS-AMI trial.[25] It was theorized that the risk of stent thrombosis surrounding PCI may be caused by discontinuation of bivalirudin after PCI, with clopidogrel (i.e., a less potent and slower onset ADP $P2Y_{12}$ agent) as the predominant antiplatelet therapy.

In the EUROMAX (European Ambulance ACS Angiography) trial, bivalirudin lowered net adverse events and major bleeding compared with unfractionated or low-molecular-weight heparin plus provisional GPI at 30 days.[26] This trial was designed to overcome the limitations of HORIZONS-AMI by using more potent oral ADP $P2Y_{12}$ inhibitors (i.e., prasugrel and ticagrelor). In addition, a reduced dose of bivalirudin (0.25 mg/kg per hour) was continued for several hours after PCI. Despite these differences, a higher rate of acute stent thrombosis was still observed in EUROMAX with bivalirudin. A subsequent open-label trial in consecutive STEMI patients who underwent primary PCI (HEAT-PPCI [How Effective are Antithrombotic Therapies in Primary PCI]) demonstrated that heparin with the use of bailout GPIs reduced all-cause mortality, stroke, reinfarction, or unplanned revascularization and stent thrombosis without any differences in the rates of major bleeding compared with bivalirudin.[27]

The BRIGHT (Bivalirudin in Acute Myocardial Infarction vs. Heparin and GPI Plus Heparin Trial) study was designed to overcome the limitations of HORIZONS-AMI by continuing bivalirudin at the standard dose (1.75 mg/kg per hour) for a median of 3 hours after PCI in acute MI patients, of whom 88% presented with STEMI.[28] In BRIGHT, a significant reduction in bleeding was seen in patients treated with clopidogrel and bivalirudin compared with heparin, with and without a GPI. No differences were observed between the groups in the rates of major adverse cardiac or cerebral events, including acute stent thrombosis. It is postulated that a prolonged infusion of standard dose bivalirudin abrogated the risk of acute stent thrombosis seen in the HORIZONS-AMI and EUROMAX trials. A meta-analysis comparing bivalirudin and heparin confirmed the higher rate of acute stent thrombosis with bivalirudin compared with heparin.[29] Prolonged infusion of bivalirudin may eliminate this risk, but this strategy should be confirmed in additional studies. Bleeding is lower with bivalirudin compared with heparin and GPI; yet, in the absence of routine GPIs and with radial access, the benefit appears to be less striking.

Intravenous Antiplatelet Therapy

When to Use a Glycoprotein IIb/IIIa Inhibitor?

GPI use was established predominantly in the era that predated the use of oral dual antiplatelet therapy (DAPT).[30] The use of GPIs reduces ischemic events during PCI, but it also increases the risk of bleeding. Currently, GPIs should be used provisionally during PCI for acute MI. Routine use with bivalirudin is not recommended. Provisional GPIs can be considered in patients with a large thrombus burden, patients with stent thrombosis while on DAPT, or patients with an inadequate loading of an ADP $P2Y_{12}$ inhibitor (e.g., poor gastrointestinal absorption in the setting of vomiting or cardiogenic shock). If used, abciximab (0.25 mg/kg IV bolus, then 0.125 μg/kg per minute [maximum 10 μg/min]), double-bolus eptifibatide (two 180 μg/kg IV boluses within 10 minutes and 2 μg/kg/min after the first bolus), or high-dose bolus tirofiban (25 μg/kg IV bolus, then 0.15 μg/kg/min) can be used. Intracoronary abciximab bolus (same dosing) may also be considered in patients with a large STEMI or clot burden, although there is no proven benefit over IV abciximab.[2]

Role for Intravenous Adenosine Diphosphate $P2Y_{12}$ Inhibitors?

In acute MI, an IV ADP $P2Y_{12}$ may be useful in selected patients. Cangrelor is a reversible, IV ADP $P2Y_{12}$ receptor antagonist that potently inhibits platelets within 3 to 6 minutes with complete platelet recovery after 60 minutes after discontinuation.[31] Cangrelor was initially studied in the CHAMPION (Cangrelor versus Standard Therapy to Achieve Optimal Management of Platelet Inhibition)-PCI and CHAMPION-PLATFORM trials, which compared cangrelor against a 600-mg loading dose of clopidogrel initiated before or after PCI. Both trials were stopped early because of no differences in the rates of the primary efficacy endpoint at 48 hours. A pooled analysis of these trials, which used the universal definition of MI (removing approximately 60% of clinical endpoints, namely, periprocedural MI), demonstrated a reduction in the composite of death, MI, or ischemia-driven revascularization and stent thrombosis without any increase in severe bleeding in patients randomized to cangrelor compared with clopidogrel.[32] Subsequently, the CHAMPION-PHOENIX trial was conducted; it randomized patients (44% with ACS, including 18% with STEMI) to cangrelor or a clopidogrel loading dose (300 to 600 mg) before elective or urgent PCI, which demonstrated that cangrelor reduced the primary efficacy endpoint (death, MI, ischemia-driven revascularization, or stent thrombosis) and the individual endpoints of stent thrombosis and intraprocedural stent thrombosis without any increase in bleeding.[33,34] Cangrelor may be useful as an agent to guarantee platelet inhibition in acute clinical situations like STEMI or NSTEMI, in which oral ADP $P2Y_{12}$ inhibition is inadequate or cannot be administered.

Practical Considerations for Patients on Oral Anticoagulation

Approximately 5% to 8% of patients are on an oral anticoagulant at admission for conditions such as atrial fibrillation, venous thromboembolism, or mechanical heart valves.[35] Interrupting therapy can lead to a higher rate or thromboembolism[36]; however, bridging strategies increases the risk of bleeding and adverse ischemic events.[37] If patients are on therapeutic oral anticoagulation and undergoing PCI for acute MI, a radial approach should be used, if possible, to minimize the risks of bleeding. Anticoagulation during PCI with either IV unfractionated heparin (dosed according to baseline ACT) or bivalirudin (without dose adjustment) is needed, regardless of the timing of the last dose of oral anticoagulation. GPIs should be avoided in these patients during PCI because of the higher risk of bleeding, other than for bailout indications.

Following PCI, the optimal antithrombotic regimen is not known.[35] Alternatives are discussed in Chapter 21. The WOEST (What Is the Optimal Antiplatelet and Anticoagulant Therapy in Patients with OAC and Coronary Stenting) study randomized patients who underwent PCI (n = 573) with an indication for oral anticoagulation to triple antithrombotic therapy (aspirin/clopidogrel/warfarin) or clopidogrel and warfarin.[38] Both groups had similar ischemic event rates at 12 months, but bleeding was significantly higher with the triple antithrombotic therapy. Somewhat analogously, the ISAR-TRIPLE (Intracoronary Stenting and Antithrombotic Regimen–Testing of a 6-Week Versus a 6-Month Clopidogrel Treatment Regimen in Patients With Concomitant Aspirin and Oral Anticoagulant Therapy Following Drug-Eluting Stenting) trial found that 6 months of triple therapy was not superior to 6 weeks of triple therapy, although there was less bleeding with the shorter duration of triple therapy.[39,40] Expert opinion on the management of patients on oral anticoagulation who are undergoing PCI is suggested in Table 17-4.[35]

PERCUTANEOUS CORONARY INTERVENTION

PCI is the treatment of choice for patients with STEMI and most patients who present with NSTEMI. The evolution of coronary intervention from balloon angioplasty to stenting to drug-eluting stents (DESs) has improved cardiac care and led to reductions in the morbidity associated with acute MI.

Rationale for Stenting

Stents were designed to overcome the limitations of balloon angioplasty, namely, acute recoil, abrupt vessel closure, and restenosis. Bare metal stents (BMSs) are made of stainless steel or cobalt chromium alloys (Table 17-5). In primary PCI, BMSs reduce target vessel revascularization compared with balloon angioplasty, but do not reduce mortality or recurrent MI.

When Is Balloon Angioplasty Alone Sufficient?

Balloon angioplasty alone is rarely performed in acute MI. It may be considered in patients at a high risk of bleeding or those that cannot take DAPT at all because of noncompliance, intolerance, or anticipated surgery. However, a BMS can often be used in these circumstances, if DAPT can be administered for 4 to 6 weeks. The smallest available stent is 2.00 mm. If the reference vessel diameter is less than 2.00 mm, balloon angioplasty may be an acceptable alternative.

ST-Elevation Myocardial Infarction: Direct Stenting versus Predilation

STEMI results from acute thrombotic occlusion secondary to plaque disruption, often with a large amount of thrombus and plaque burden. Conventional stenting involves predilating the lesion to allow for full stent expansion to attain the largest stent diameter that approximates the reference vessel diameter. Predilation is often necessary to "prep" stenotic

TABLE 17-4 Suggested Management of Patients on Oral Anticoagulation Undergoing Percutaneous Coronary Intervention in Acute Myocardial Infarction

TIMING	VKA	NOAC
Periprocedural Management: STEMI		
Anticoagulation	Uninterrupted	Uninterrupted
Additional IV UFH (dose)	Yes (reduced: 50 U/kg)	Yes (reduced: 50 U/kg)
IV bivalirudin (no dose adjustment)	May be considered, especially if bleeding risk high	May be considered, especially if bleeding risk high
Vascular access site	Radial	Radial
Type of stent	New-generation DES*	New generation DES*
Antiplatelet therapy	ASA 325 mg and clopidogrel LD (300–600 mg)	ASA 325 mg and clopidogrel LD (300–600 mg)
Adjunct GPI	No	No
Periprocedural Management: NSTEMI		
Anticoagulation	Uninterrupted	Discontinuation (24 h in advance without bridging)
Additional IV UFH (dose)	Yes (reduced: 50 U/kg)	Yes (reduced: 50 U/kg or standard 70–100 U/kg, depending on last dose)
IV bivalirudin (no dose adjustment)	May be considered, especially if bleeding risk high	May be considered, especially if bleeding risk high
Vascular access site	Radial	Radial
Type of stent	New-generation DES*	New-generation DES*
Antiplatelet therapy	ASA 325 mg and clopidogrel LD (300–600 mg)	ASA 325 mg and clopidogrel LD (300–600 mg)
Adjunct GPI	No	Provisional
Antithrombotic Management: 0–12 mos		
Initital therapy	Triple therapy (ASA 81 mg/day, clopidogrel, VKA)	Triple therapy (ASA 81 mg/day, clopidogrel, NOAC)
Duration of triple therapy	6 mos	6 mos
Intensity of OAC during triple therapy	Reduced (goal INR 2–2.5)	Reduced (lower dose of NOAC: dabigatran 110 mg bid; rivaroxaban 15 mg/day; apixaban 2.5 mg bid)
Monitoring during triple therapy	INR every 2 weeks	Hemoglobin and kindey function every 4 wks
Gastric protection	Yes (PPI)	Yes (PPI)
Antithrombotic management after triple therapy	VKA (goal INR 2–3) + single antiplatelet therapy (ASA 81 mg/day or clopidogrel)	NOAC (standard dosing) + single antiplatelet therapy (ASA 81 mg/day or clopidogrel)
Antithrombotic Management: > 12 mos		
Antithrombotic management	VKA monotherapy (+ ASA 81 mg/day or clopidogrel)†	NOAC monotherapy (+ ASA 81 mg/day or clopidogrel)†

ASA, Aspirin; *DES*, drug-eluting stent; *GPI*, glycoprotein IIb/IIIa inhibitors; *INR*, international normalized ratio; *IV*, intravenous; *LD*, loading dose; *NOAC*, nonvitamin K antagonist; *NSTEMI*, non–ST-elevation MI; *OACs*, oral anticoagulants; *PPI*, proton pump inhibitor; *STEMI*, ST-elevation MI; *UFH*, unfractionated heparin; VKA, vitamin K antagonists.
*Bare metal stents may be considered in patients at a highly increased risk of bleeding or when unavoidable surgery is planned within 6 months.
†Indefinite combination with either low-dose ASA (75 to 100 mg/day) or clopidogrel (depending on the individual risk of bleeding, especially gastrointestinal and stent thrombosis) may be considered in special situations (e.g., left main and/or last remaining vessel stenting, history of stent thrombosis and/or recurrent cardiac events, diffuse coronary artery disease), when bleeding risk is low.
Adapted from Rubboli A, et al: The optimal management of patients on oral anticoagulation undergoing coronary artery stenting. The 10th anniversary overview. Thromb Haemost *112:1080–1087, 2014.*

lesions that are fibrotic or calcified before stent deployment. In STEMI, most patients will have a diameter stenosis greater than 50%. Predilation has the potential to embolize thrombus and/or plaque to the distal coronary circulation, which can lead to dysfunction or injury of the microvasculature, resulting in impaired reperfusion or no-reflow. Direct stenting not only minimizes distal embolization, but it also reduces procedural time and costs. One randomized trial of 206 STEMI patients demonstrated that direct stenting improved reperfusion and ST-segment resolution compared with predilation. A post hoc analysis of HORIZONS-AMI and a large observational registry analysis showed similar improvements in reperfusion, but a lower mortality was also observed with direct stenting that persisted up to 1 year after stenting.[41,42] Direct stenting appears safe, effective, and should be considered in STEMI patients with thrombus-laden lesions that do not require predilation (e.g., noncalcified plaque).

Drug-Eluting Stents versus Bare Metal Stents

Rationale for Drug-Eluting Stent Development

As stent technology evolved, rates of acute stent thrombosis were significantly reduced (<1%), and in-stent

TABLE 17-5 Currently Available Coronary Stents in the Unites States

STENT NAME (MANUFACTURER)	STENT PLATFORM	DRUG	POLYMER
BMS			
Integrity (Medtronic)	Cobalt chromium	—	—
REBEL (Boston Scientific)	Platinum chromium	—	—
VeriFLEX (Boston Scientific)	Stainless steel	—	—
Vision (Abbott)	Cobalt chromium	—	—
DES			
Endeavour (Medtronic)	Cobalt chromium	Zotarolimus	Phosphoryl choline
Promus Element or Premier (Boston Scientific)	Platinum chromium	Everolimus	PMBA/PVDF-HFP
Resolute (Medtronic)	Cobalt chromium	Zotarolimus	Biolinx
Synergy (Boston Scientific)	Platinum chromium	Everolimus	Bioabsorbable PLGA
Taxus Ion (Boston Scientific)	Platinum chromium	Paclitaxel	SIBS
Xience V, Prime, Premier, Alpine (Abbott)	Cobalt chromium	Everolimus	PMBA/PVDF-HFP

BMS, Bare metal stent; *DES*, drug-eluting stent;*PBMA*, poly n-butyl methacrylate; *PEVA*, polyethylene-co-vinyl acetate; *PLGA*, poly-lactide-co-glycolide; *PVDF-HFP*, poly (vinylidene fluoride-hexafluoropropylene); *SIBS*, poly(styrene-b-isobutylene-b-styrene).

restenosis emerged as a major limitation of coronary stenting.[43] Coronary stents increase the acute gain compared with balloon angioplasty, primarily because of less recoil and larger acute luminal diameters. However, vascular injury and response to stent implantation exaggerates neointimal hyperplasia. Despite this adverse response, net gain is still significantly improved compared with balloon angioplasty. Angiographic restenosis after BMS implantation occurs in approximately 30% of patients in the first year, with only half of the patients presenting with symptoms. DESs are comprised of a stent, pharmacologic agent, and a polymer to control the pharmacokinetics of drug delivery. DESs maintain the mechanical advantages of BMSs, but also deliver antirestenotic therapy to the sites of vascular injury. The pharmacologic agents that were used in first-generation DESs were paclitaxel or rapamycin (i.e., sirolimus). Paclitaxel interferes with microtubule depolymerization, inhibiting cellular replication and cytokine-mediated smooth muscle cell proliferation and/or migration. Sirolimus inhibits mammalian target of rapamycin, which blocks the cell cycle transition from G_1 to S and impairs vascular smooth muscle cell proliferation. A number of rapamycin analogues have been developed and are currently used in second-generation DESs (e.g., everolimus, zotarolimus, biolimus).

Evidence in Acute Myocardial Infarction

The initial evidence comparing first-generation DESs to BMSs demonstrated a significant reduction in target vessel revascularization, without any differences in death, MI, or stent thrombosis in the first 2 years following PCI.[44] Two major trials have compared newer generation DESs to BMSs in STEMI. In the EXAMINATION (Everolimus-Eluting Stents Versus Bare-Metal Stents in ST Segment Elevation Myocardial Infarction) trial, everolimus-eluting stents (EESs) significantly reduced target vessel revascularization and stent thrombosis compared with BMSs at 2-year follow-up in STEMI.[45–47] No differences were observed in death and MI between EESs and BMSs. Similar reductions in target vessel revascularization were also seen in the COMFORTABLE AMI (Comparison of Biolimus Eluted From an Erodible Stent Coating With Bare Metal Stents in Acute ST-Elevation Myocardial Infarction) trial, which randomized STEMI patients to a biolimus-eluting stent or a BMS.[48]

Practical Considerations

DESs provide superior outcomes compared with BMSs, primarily with a reduction in target vessel revascularization. It can be challenging to determine if patients can tolerate or comply with prolonged DAPT (i.e., ≥12 months) with primary PCI in STEMI. DES placement should be avoided in patients who cannot tolerate (e.g., elevated bleeding risk or anticipated invasive or surgical procedures) or cannot comply with a prolonged DAPT course because of social or financial barriers.[2] DES should be considered in patients with lesions with a higher risk for restenosis. These high-risk indicators include both anatomic factors (e.g., long lesions, small vessel size, aorto-ostial lesions, restenotic lesions, previous stenting, lesions with higher complexity) and clinical factors (e.g., female sex, diabetes mellitus, chronic kidney disease, or multivessel coronary artery disease [CAD]).

Current Drug-Eluting Stent Platforms

The DESs available (see Table 17-5) in the United States vary by platforms, pharmacologic agent, and polymer type. In general, the efficacy and safety of the newer generation DESs are similar and do not strongly favor use of one individual stent type over the others.

Emerging Stent or Balloon Platforms

Limitations of DESs include restenosis and the risk for late (>30 days) or very late (>12 months) stent thrombosis. DAPT is currently recommended for a minimum of 12 months after DES placement to reduce the risk of stent thrombosis. Currently approved DESs (see Table 17-5) have a durable polymer that remains on the stent after the drug is eluted, which can act as a nidus for inflammation or delay endothelialization that leads to restenosis or stent thrombosis, respectively. Several newer stent designs are being investigated to reduce or eliminate the inflammatory stimulus from the stent polymer and/or scaffold. Bioresorbable polymer DESs contain a polymer that is completely or partially absorbed, and leaves a BMS behind without a polymer, which theoretically should lower the risk for restenosis and stent thrombosis. The Synergy DES (Boston Scientific, Marlborough, Mass.) was recently approved in the United States, and outcomes with these stents are comparable with second-generation DESs, although these outcomes are not better.[49] Polymer-free stents are also currently being developed that can elute a pharmacologic agent over the period of time needed to inhibit restenosis. Bioresorbable stents have been developed to be fully biodegradable, in which the stent platform or scaffold is completely reabsorbed after a period of time after implantation. Because restenosis is unlikely in the first 9 to 12 months after stent implantation, the need for a permanent vascular scaffold diminishes over time and may contribute to late restenosis or stent thrombosis. In addition, the requirement for long-term DAPT after DES could be minimized.

Trials are currently ongoing to assess the safety and efficacy of bioresorbable stents compared with current DESs. Drug-coated balloons have also been studied for PCI, but the results compared with DESs have not demonstrated similar efficacy for de novo CAD.[50] Finally, the MGuard (InspireMD, Tel Aviv, Israel) stent has been designed as a BMS with a polyethylene terephthalate micronet mesh to cover, trap, and exclude debris that could embolize to the distal circulation and which could potentially have a role in thrombus-laden lesions in STEMI. Initial evidence demonstrated that the MGuard stent improved ST-segment resolution and epicardial flow[51]; however, the clinical significance of these findings is not yet known.

ADJUNCTIVE DIAGNOSTIC AND THERAPEUTIC DEVICES

Practical Use of Intravascular Imaging

Coronary angiography is a two-dimensional image that has certain limitations, namely, that it is a "luminogram" that accurately describes the vessel lumen, but it provides limited information about plaque composition, size, and distribution. Intravascular imaging allows for real-time assessment of coronary stenoses, which can be used at various times during PCI. Two devices, intravascular ultrasound (IVUS) and optical coherence tomography (OCT), are the most commonly used intravascular imaging devices in clinical practice. Near-infrared spectroscopy may be useful at detecting the lipid composition and potential vulnerability of a plaque, but it is not commonly used to support PCI. Each of these devices is discussed in Chapter 10.

Evidence for use of intravascular imaging during PCI has been studied predominantly with IVUS in BMSs.[52] Overall, the results have been conflicting. The largest prospective study of IVUS use (n = 8583; 38% underwent IVUS) during PCI demonstrated that IVUS was associated with a significant reduction in major adverse cardiac events, MI, and stent thrombosis within the first 12 months after DES implantation.[53] Interestingly, this effect was strongest in patients who presented with STEMI.

IVUS and OCT are used at various stages of PCI. Before PCI, intravascular imaging can be used to determine plaque composition, size, location, and distribution. Lesion composition can change interventional strategies. For example, if a lesion is heavily calcified (e.g., circumferential calcium demonstrated on IVUS/OCT), rotational atherectomy may be used to prepare the lesion before balloon angioplasty. In addition, plaque location and distribution can significantly alter the stenting strategy of bifurcation lesions, especially in left main lesions.[54] Another important use of intravascular imaging is to determine the cause of stent failure in stent thrombosis or in-stent restenosis (Figure 17-e1). OCT may be the preferred imaging modality for this purpose because it can accurately assess endothelial coverage of the stent struts (i.e., a potential cause of late and very late stent thrombosis) or detect neoatherosclerosis, an emerging cause of late stent failure.[52]

When to Use Fractional Flow Reserve in Acute Myocardial Infarction?

Coronary angiography does not always accurately predict the hemodynamic significance of a coronary lesion.[55] Only angiographic stenoses of more than 80% to 90% can accurately predict a hemodynamically significant lesion by fractional flow reserve (FFR) of less than 0.80. FFR measures the hemodynamic significance of a coronary lesion by measuring the distal mean coronary and aortic pressures during maximal hyperemia, typically IV adenosine. In stable disease, FFR-guided revascularization improves clinical outcomes compared with angiography alone.[56,57] FFR is not a useful tool for determining the culprit vessel in STEMI, thus limiting its use during primary PCI. However, FFR may be an important diagnostic tool for assessing the ischemic potential of a nonculprit lesion in STEMI. In NSTEMI, it may be particularly difficult to determine the culprit lesion in patients with multivessel CAD by angiography alone. FFR can be used to guide revascularization of lesions with an FFR of less than 0.80. FFR may also be particularly useful to assess the ischemic potential of intermediate left main coronary stenoses (i.e., 50% to 70%).

Aspiration Thrombectomy

Thrombectomy can be performed by manual aspiration catheters or a rheolytic thrombectomy catheter system (e.g., Angiojet; Boston Scientific, Marlborough, Massachusetts), the latter of which uses a dedicated device that dissolves thrombus by a high-speed saline jet and aspirates surrounding blood and thrombus. Rheolytic thrombectomy has a higher risk of device-related vessel trauma. Manual aspiration catheters are simple to use, have a lower profile, and are preferred by many operators. In STEMI, manual aspiration has been used routinely by approximately half of operators.[2,20,58]

A meta-analysis of 11,321 patients from 20 randomized controlled trials demonstrated that major adverse cardiac events, including stent thrombosis, were significantly reduced in STEMI patients using aspiration thrombectomy before primary PCI compared with primary PCI alone.[59] However, randomized evidence from adequately sized trials of cardiovascular outcomes does not support its routine use. The TASTE (Thrombus Aspiration in ST-Elevation Myocardial Infarction in Scandinavia) trial did not show any reduction in death, MI, and stent thrombosis in STEMI patients (n = 7244) randomized to manual aspiration compared with primary PCI alone.[60] The TOTAL (Trial of Routine Aspiration Thrombectomy with PCI versus PCI Alone in Patients with STEMI) trial of 10,732 STEMI patients who underwent primary PCI randomized to bailout or upfront routine manual aspiration thrombectomy did not find any clinical benefit at 180 days with routine aspiration thrombectomy; moreover, a higher rate of stroke at 180 days was observed with routine aspiration thrombectomy compared with primary PCI alone (Figure 17-2).[61] In STEMI, manual aspiration thrombectomy should not be performed as a routine procedure, but may be considered in patients with a large thrombus burden or as bailout following primary PCI.

Distal Embolic Protection

Embolic protection devices have the potential to capture any atherosclerotic debris or thrombus that may be embolized during PCI. A number of embolic protection devices have been developed that use either proximal occlusion or a distal filter to catch embolic debris. The proximal occlusion device is no longer available in the United States. Thus, the filter-based devices (Figure 17-3) can be used for PCI and can capture debris that is more than 120 μm. One advantage to this device is that anterograde flow is maintained throughout PCI. Currently, embolic protection devices should be used for PCI of saphenous vein grafts (SVGs), which typically contain more friable atherosclerotic debris.[20] In the absence of an SVG, embolic protection is not indicated in PCI for MI, including STEMI. In a randomized trial of STEMI patients, distal embolic protection did not improve clinical outcomes or infarct size compared with primary PCI alone.[62]

LESION-SPECIFIC PERCUTANEOUS CORONARY INTERVENTION STRATEGIES

Bifurcation Lesions

Coronary bifurcation lesions occur at or near a division of a major coronary artery and are found in up to 20% of PCIs.[63] In STEMI, bifurcation lesions comprise approximately 10% of target lesions in primary PCI.[64] Procedural and clinical outcomes associated with PCI of bifurcation lesions remain suboptimal, because of the complexity of anatomy and the dynamic changes that occur to the lesion during revascularization. Selection of the optimal PCI strategy to manage bifurcation lesions is controversial. When considering bifurcation PCI, it is important to carefully assess the distribution of atherosclerotic disease, the relative size of the proximal and distal main branch and side branch, and the bifurcation angle of the main and side branches. During main branch stenting, side branch compromise that requires stenting may be required in 2% to 51% of PCIs of bifurcation lesions.[65] Dynamic changes can occur during stenting of the main branch that can compromise coronary blood flow to a side branch, including plaque or a carina shift, bifurcation angle change, vessel spasm, dissection, stent strut protrusion, and conformational changes to the side branch ostium.

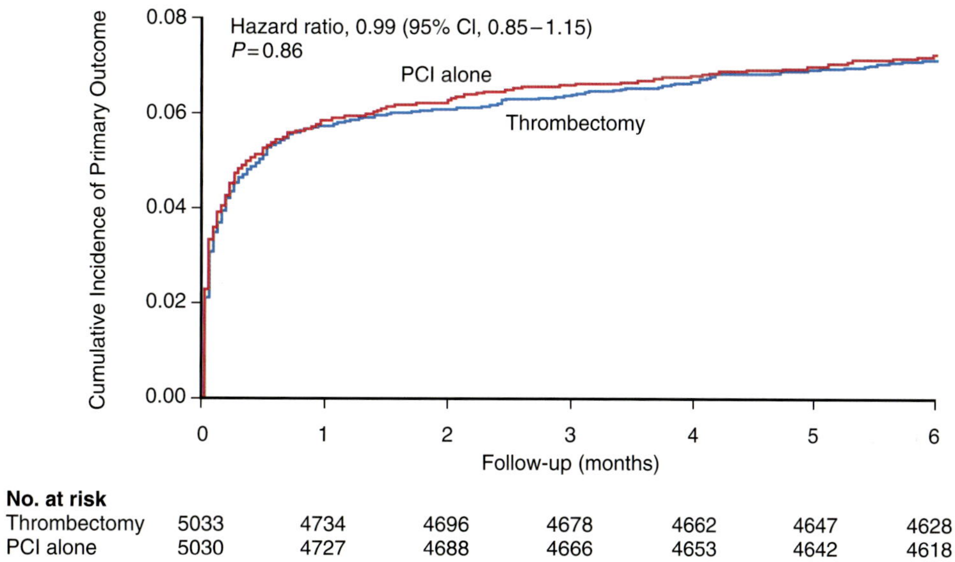

A

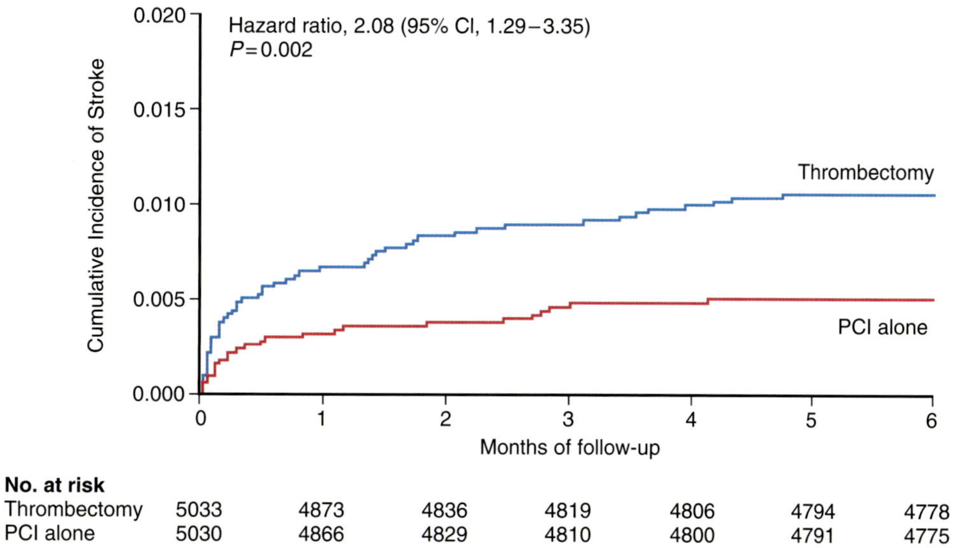

B

FIGURE 17-2 Kaplan-Meier estimates for clinical outcomes at 180 days in the TOTAL trial. (**A**) No difference was observed in the rate of the primary outcome (cardiovascular death, myocardial infarction, cardiogenic shock, or New York Heart Association class IV heart failure) between ST-elevation myocardial infarction patients (n =10,732) who underwent primary PCI randomized to upfront routine manual aspiration thrombectomy versus percutaneous coronary angiography (PCI) alone with bailout manual aspiration. (**B**) A significantly higher rate of stroke was observed in the routine thrombectomy group at 180 days compared with PCI alone with bailout thrombectomy. *CI*, Confidence interval. *(Adapted from Jolly SS, et al: Randomized trial of primary PCI with or without routine manual thrombectomy.* N Engl J Med *372:1389–1398, 2015.)*

The Medina classification is the most widely accepted scheme used (Figure 17-4). A "true" bifurcation lesion contains a significant (>50%) stenosis in both the main and side branches (i.e., Medina 1,1,1; 1,0,1; or 0,1,1). IVUS can also be used to assess the distribution of plaque in a bifurcation lesion, and will frequently reclassify lesions compared with angiographic classification.[54] During bifurcation PCI, it is important to determine a priori if a bifurcation lesion will be approached using a one-stent (i.e., provisional) or two-stent approach (Figure 17-e2). In a one-stent approach, the main branch is stented and the side branch is provisionally stented if clinical symptoms and/or angiographic (e.g., Thrombolysis in Myocardial Infarction [TIMI] <3 flow) or adjunctive measurements (e.g., FFR <0.80) warrant intervention.

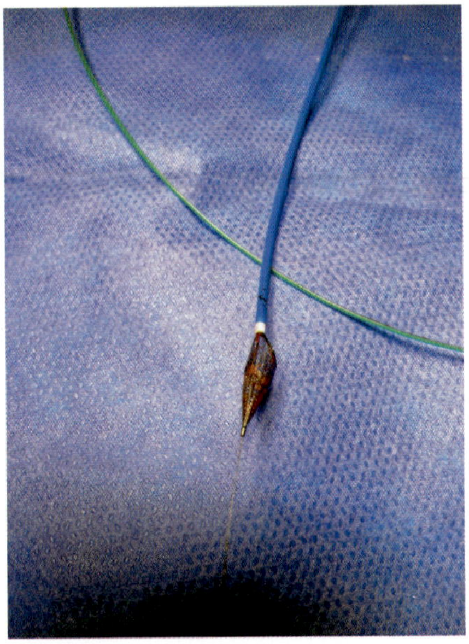

FIGURE 17-3 Filter embolic protection device. Atherosclerotic debris that was captured using a filter-based embolic protection device following percutaneous coronary intervention of a saphenous vein graft.

A two-stent approach involves stenting both the main and side branches. Randomized and observational data suggest that provisional side branch stenting compared with planned side branch stenting (i.e., two-stent approach) have similar clinical outcomes, except procedural time and contrast volume are reduced with a provisional approach. A meta-analysis of 9 randomized trials that included 2569 patients with coronary bifurcation lesions randomly selected to undergo PCI with either provisional or elective side branch stenting using DES demonstrated that the risk for MI was significantly higher with a two-stent approach compared with provisional side branch stenting.[66] However, the generalizability of this evidence to all bifurcation lesions is controversial, and strategies for PCI should be tailored for each lesion.

True bifurcation lesions with side branch disease that extends beyond the ostium may often be treated with a two-stent approach (see Figure 17-e2). A number of stenting strategies have been developed for the two-stent approach, including culotte, double-kissing crush, mini-crush, simultaneous "kissing" stents, T-stenting, and V-stenting. Regardless of the bifurcation stenting strategy, final kissing balloon inflation in the main and side branches should be performed. DESs are preferred in bifurcation PCI because of a lower rate of restenosis compared with BMSs. Dedicated bifurcation stents have been developed, but are not currently available in the United States.

Left Main Coronary Artery

Strategies used for left main coronary artery (LMCA) PCI will depend on the plaque distribution (i.e., ostium, body, distal), LMCA length and size, and the bifurcation angle. Focal LMCA stenoses at the ostium or body that do not involve the distal left main artery can often be treated with a short single stent. However, the same strategies used to perform bifurcation PCI also apply to LMCA disease that involves the distal left main and/or ostium of the left anterior descending or left circumflex arteries. Because of the limitations of angiography, IVUS use

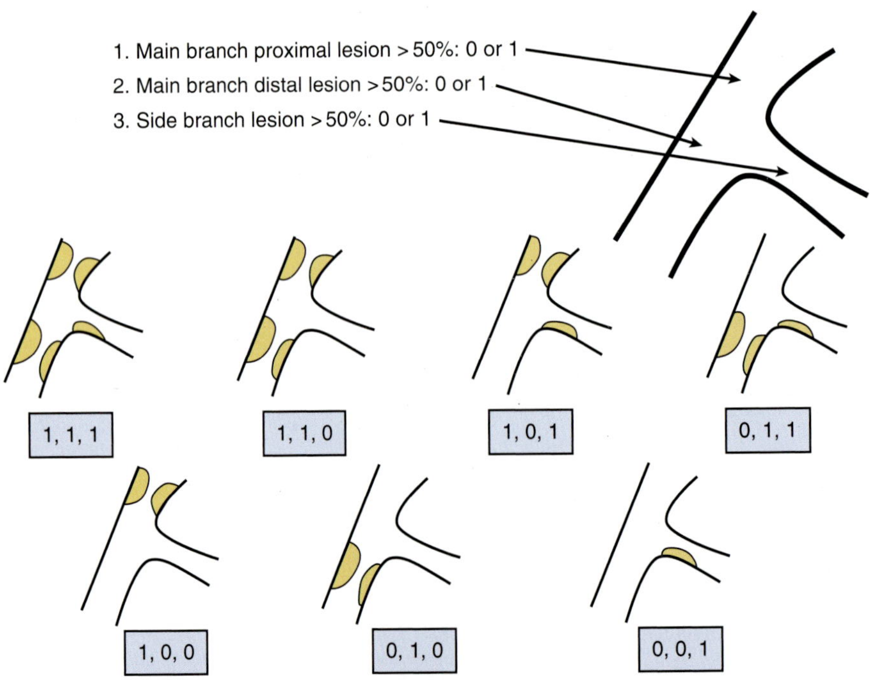

FIGURE 17-4 Medina classification of bifurcation lesions. *(Redrawn from Latib A, Colombo A: Bifurcation disease: what do we know, what should we do?* JACC Cardiovasc Interv *1:218–26, 2008.)*

should be considered when technically feasible to accurately assess distribution of plaque in the LMCA and its branches. In STEMI, if the LMCA is the culprit vessel, then PCI should be considered in patients with TIMI grade <3 flow.[20] In NSTEMI, the decision to treat LMCA disease with PCI or CABG should undergo a prompt evaluation using a heart team approach to assess the complexity of coronary disease (i.e., SYNTAX [Synergy Between Percutaneous Coronary Intervention with TAXUS and Cardiac Surgery] score), surgical risk (i.e., STS [Society of Thoracic Surgery] score), and other co-morbidities to determine the best revascularization strategy using local expertise and patient preferences.[20] In general, clinical outcomes comparing PCI and CABG are similar, with a higher rate of revascularization with PCI and increased risk of stroke with CABG.[20] In patients with a high syntax score (>33), diabetes mellitus, or multivessel CAD, CABG is typically preferred over PCI, and PCI is favored in patients with a low SYNTAX score (<22) or a high surgical risk (STS >5%).

Aorto-Ostial Lesions

Aorto-ostial lesions are typically defined as a lesion within 3 mm of the vessel origin (i.e., left main, right coronary artery, or anomalous coronary vessel). Aorto-ostial disease may be difficult to diagnose with angiography alone, and a high suspicion for its presence should be considered with dampening of the pressure waveform with coronary catheter engagement. IVUS and FFR are useful for determining the degree of stenosis or hemodynamic significance, respectively, in lesions that are intermediate or indeterminate on angiography. IVUS can also be used to assess plaque distribution, vessel size, and mark the ostium during stent deployment.[67] It is important to rule out catheter-induced spasm from engagement of the coronary ostium; spasm will typically resolve with intracoronary administration of nitroglycerin (100 to 200 μg). Aorto-ostial disease can be resistant to angioplasty and stenting because of recoil from the muscular and elastic layers of the aorta. DESs are preferred in aorto-ostial lesions over BMSs because of a lower rate of restenosis.[20]

Saphenous Vein Graft

PCI of SVGs is associated with a significantly higher rate of periprocedural MI and acute complications because of atheroembolization and release of vasoactive substances to the downstream microcirculation, which can lead to no-reflow. SVGs are more friable than native coronary disease and prone to distal embolization with manipulation during PCI. In STEMI, approximately 2% to 3% of patients have a history of CABG and approximately half of previous CABG patients will have an SVG that is the culprit vessel.[68,69] Primary PCI of patients with a history of CABG has a significant delay in door-to-device times (i.e., reperfusion), worse angiographic outcomes, and higher rates of adverse clinical outcomes, including death.[68,69] As mentioned previously, embolic protection devices should be considered during SVG PCI to improve clinical outcomes. DESs are preferred in SVG PCI compared with BMSs because of a reduction in adverse clinical outcomes and repeat revascularization.[70]

Calcified Lesions

Calcified lesions are less likely to cause ACS with or without ST-segment elevation compared with plaque rupture or erosion.[71] However, a subset of patients with a heavily calcified culprit lesion will present with an MI. During PCI, extensive calcification can be technically challenging. It can be difficult to deliver guidewires, balloons, or stents in calcified arteries because of their rigidity. Calcification can also be incredibly resistant to high-pressure balloon dilation, which can lead to stent underexpansion (i.e., a predictor of acute stent thrombosis). Rotational atherectomy should be used for calcified arteries when balloon dilation is inadequate or there is an inability to cross a lesion with a balloon or stent.[20] The most commonly used atherectomy device is the Rotablator rotational atherectomy device (Boston Scientific, Marlborough, Massachusetts), which removes plaque using a rapidly rotating (150,000 to 160,000 rpm) atherectomy burr with diamond chips embedded on the surface. Most operators will use a single smaller (1.5 or 1.75 mm) burr for plaque modification to allow for effective balloon dilation and complete stent expansion.

NONCULPRIT REVASCULARIZATION

An area of significant controversy in PCI in acute MI, primarily in patients with STEMI, is to consider revascularization or "preventive stenting" of nonculprit lesions.[72] In acute MI, patients with multivessel CAD have a significantly higher rate of adverse cardiac events, including death and reinfarction compared with patients with single-vessel CAD. During MI, it has been suggested that the pathophysiologic derangements leading to plaque rupture of the culprit vessel are generalized throughout the entire coronary vasculature, leading to plaque destabilization and vulnerability in nonculprit territories.[72]

Observational data and prospective studies have been inconclusive on the efficacy and safety of multivessel revascularization in STEMI. In the multicenter PRAMI (Preventive Angioplasty in Acute Myocardial Infarction) trial, patients (n = 465) with STEMI underwent culprit-lesion PCI and were randomized to nonstaged preventive PCI of any angiographically significant lesions (≥50% diameter stenosis) versus no further intervention.[73] At a mean follow-up of 23 months, preventive PCI significantly reduced a composite of cardiac death, nonfatal MI, and refractory angina compared with no preventive PCI (Figure 17-5A). The benefit of preventive stenting was still present when limited to cardiac death or nonfatal MI, and no differences were observed between the rates of stent thrombosis between the two groups. Unlike previous studies of multivessel revascularization in STEMI, PRAMI did not allow for staged PCI. Thus, a comparison between PRAMI and the previous published literature is difficult. In CvLPRIT (Complete versus Lesion-only Primary PCI trial), STEMI patients (n = 296) were randomized to in-hospital complete versus culprit-vessel only PCI; 64% of patients in the complete revascularization group underwent nonculprit vessel PCI at the time of primary PCI.[74,75] The composite primary endpoint of all-cause mortality, recurrent MI, heart failure, and ischemia-driven revascularization was significantly reduced at 12 months in patients who underwent complete in-hospital revascularization compared with PCI of the culprit vessel alone (see Figure 17-5B). In observational studies, complete revascularization appears to be beneficial in patients who present with NSTE-ACS.[76,77] Additional evidence on nonculprit revascularization is forthcoming in trials of STEMI and NSTE-ACS patients, which should further clarify the efficacy and safety of nonculprit PCI in acute MI.

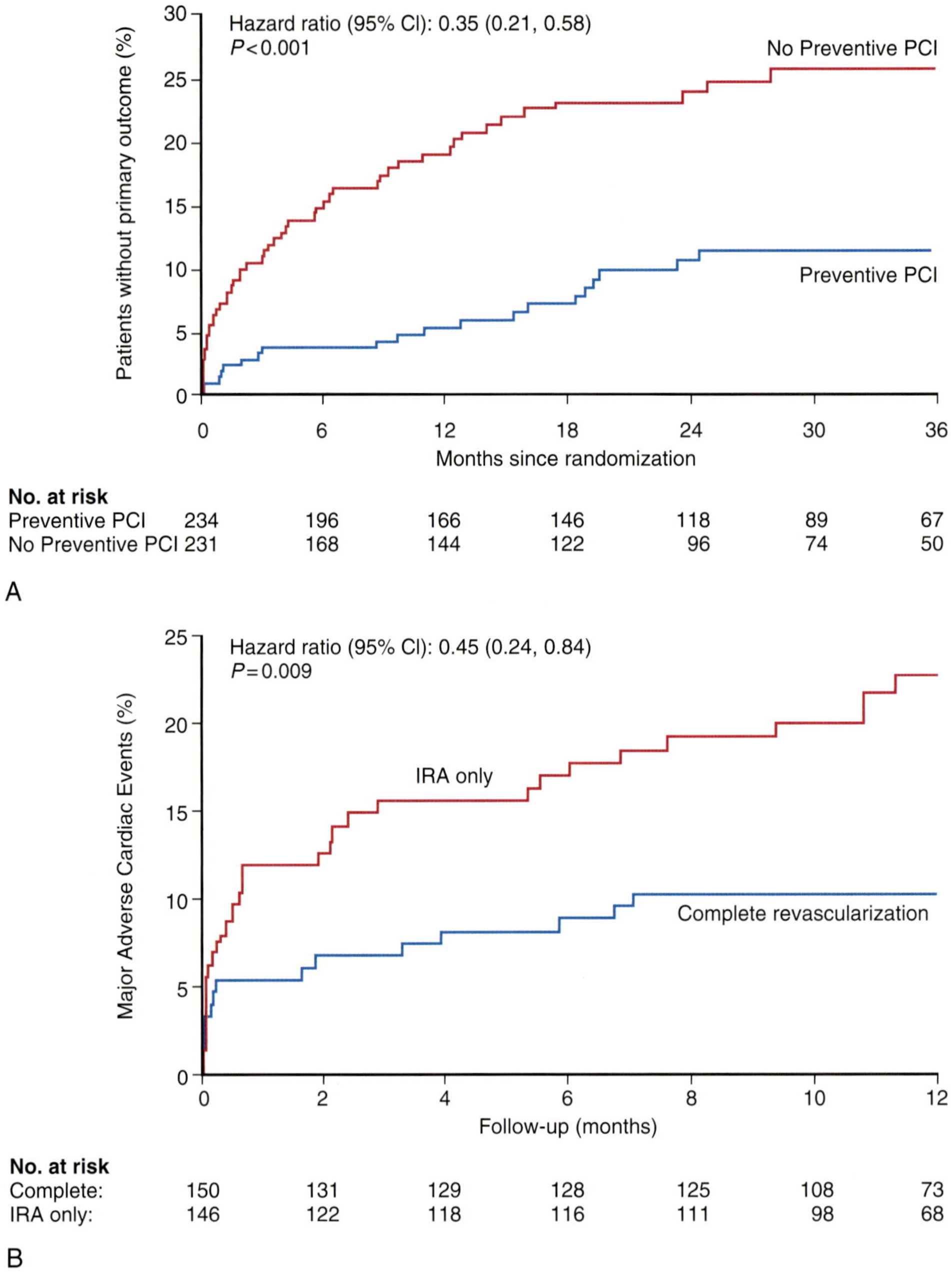

FIGURE 17-5 Kaplan-Meier estimates for clinical outcomes in the PRAMI and CvLPRIT trials. (**A**) In the PRAMI trial, patients (n = 465) with ST-elevation of myocardial infarction (STEMI) who were randomized to nonstaged preventive percutaneous coronary intervention (PCI) had significantly lower rates of the primary outcome (cardiac death, nonfatal myocardial infarction [MI], and refractory angina) compared with no preventive PCI (i.e., culprit vessel only) with a mean follow-up of 23 months.) (**B**) In CvLPRIT, complete revascularization significantly reduced major adverse cardiac events (all-cause mortality, recurrent MI, heart failure, and ischemia-driven revascularization) at 12 months in STEMI patients (n = 296) compared with PCI of the culprit vessel alone. *CI*, Confidence interval. *(Adapted from Wald DS, et al: Randomized trial of preventive angioplasty in myocardial infarction.* N Engl J Med *369:1115–23, 2013; and Gershlick AH, et al: Randomized trial of complete versus lesion-only revascularization in patients undergoing primary percutaneous coronary intervention for STEMI and multivessel disease: the CvLPRIT trial.* J Am Coll Cardiol *65:963–72, 2015.)*

ST-ELEVATION MYOCARDIAL INFARCTION: WHEN IS CORONARY ARTERY BYPASS GRAFTING NEEDED?

Emergent or urgent CABG (<1%) is rarely needed in patients who present with STEMI. CABG should be considered in patients with suitable anatomy for CABG if: (1) PCI cannot be performed or is unsuccessful, and there is persistent ischemia and/or hemodynamic instability; (2) for surgical repair of a postinfarction mechanical complication; or (3) for a life-threatening ventricular arrhythmia caused by ischemia and left main stenosis (>50%), or three-vessel CAD.[78] CABG should not be performed for persistent angina and a small area of viable myocardium in hemodynamically stable patients or PCI complicated by no-reflow.[78] In stable patients with coronary anatomy that is unsuitable for PCI and a patent infarct-related artery (i.e., TIMI 3 flow), CABG may also be considered if a large area of myocardium is at risk.

PERCUTANEOUS HEMODYNAMIC SUPPORT

Percutaneous hemodynamic assist devices provide superior circulatory support compared with pharmacotherapy. Benefits include (1) maintenance of organ perfusion, (2) prevention of systemic shock, (3) reduction of intracardiac

TABLE 17-6 Ellis Classification of Coronary Perforations

PERFORATION TYPE (%)	DESCRIPTION	DEATH	MI	TAMPONADE	EMERGENCY CARDIAC SURGERY
Type I (21%)	Extraluminal crater without myocardial blush, extravasation, or evidence of dissection	0%	0%	8%	15%
Type II (50%)	Myocardial or pericardial blush without extravasation	0%	14%	13%	10%
Type III (29%)	Extravasation through a >1-mm perforation or cavity spilling	19%	50%	63%	66%

MI, Myocardial infarction.
Adapted from Ellis SG, et al: Increased coronary perforation in the new device era. Incidence, classification, management, and outcome. Circulation *90:2725, 1994.*

filling pressures to relieve pulmonary congestion, and (4) reduced left ventricular end-diastolic volumes and improved myocardial perfusion.[79] The available devices, their indications, and complications are discussed in Chapter 27. In STEMI, mechanical circulatory support should be started before PCI in patients with cardiogenic shock refractory to medical therapy, despite the delay in door-to-device time. Mechanical circulatory support may also be used in patients undergoing high-risk PCI,[80] and it may be considered in patients with LMCA disease, severe multivessel CAD, or a last remaining conduit with an ejection fraction of less than 35% undergoing challenging or prolonged PCI.[79]

CORONARY COMPLICATIONS AND MANAGEMENT

No-Reflow

No-reflow is a known complication of PCI and defined as reduced coronary blood flow or perfusion despite reestablishing epicardial patency. In acute MI, the incidence of no-reflow is 2.3% and occurs more frequently in older patients, STEMI, prolonged delay from symptom onset to presentation, cardiogenic shock, longer lesion length, complex lesions (type C), bifurcation lesions, or TIMI less than grade 3 flow before revascularization.[81] No-reflow is associated with a significantly higher risk of in-hospital mortality (odds ratio 2.20; $P < .001$).[81] It can also occur during PCI of SVG lesions or use of rotational atherectomy. The mechanisms responsible for no-reflow are multifactorial and include ischemia–reperfusion injury, microcirculatory injury and dysfunction, and distal embolization (see Chapter 24).[82] Despite inconclusive results on the clinical efficacy of thrombus aspiration during primary PCI, aspiration thrombectomy reduces the risk of no-reflow and may be useful in STEMI patients with a large thrombus burden.[82] A number of pharmacologic agents have been studied for the prevention or treatment of no-reflow, including adenosine, calcium channel blockers (e.g., verapamil), epinephrine, GPIs, nitroglycerin, nitroprusside, and thrombolytics.[82] Evidence favoring a definitive pharmacologic agent or regimen for prevention or treatment of no-reflow is lacking. When no-reflow occurs, a reasonable approach would be to use adenosine, nitroprusside, or verapamil. GPIs and manual aspiration can be used if no-reflow occurs in the setting of a large residual thrombus burden.

Coronary Perforation

During PCI, coronary perforation occurs in 0.2% to 0.6% of patients and is higher in patients with complex lesions or with the use of rotational atherectomy. Most coronary perforations are self-limited, can be classified according to the Ellis criteria (Table 17-6), and are managed based on severity. Immediate recognition of any coronary perforation and prompt balloon occlusion proximal to the area of contrast extravasation in the perforated vessel is paramount. Prolonged balloon inflations are typically required (>10 minutes), which should stop blood flow into the pericardium. During this time, patients can be stabilized hemodynamically. The decision to perform emergent pericardiocentesis should be dictated by the patient's hemodynamics. If available, a perfusion balloon catheter can be used to provide distal blood flow beyond the site of balloon occlusion to perfuse the myocardium during prolonged balloon inflations. Subsequent management will depend on its severity, location, and response to balloon occlusion. Small perforations may be completely sealed with balloon inflation alone. Distal coronary perforation from coronary guidewires can be managed with balloon occlusion or microcatheter aspiration to collapse the distal vessel, but if bleeding persists, then embolization can be considered with the use of coils, vascular plugs, thrombus, subcutaneous fat, or fibrin glue. One caveat to distal embolization is that it typically will result in an occluded vessel at the site of embolization. If bleeding persists despite prolonged balloon occlusion, a polytetrafluoroethylene-covered stent can be placed. Type III coronary perforations usually result in cardiac tamponade, and a covered stent should be implanted for this type of perforation. Reversal of intraprocedural anticoagulation should be avoided in patients undergoing covered stenting (i.e., because of the risk of stent thrombosis when anticoagulation is fully reversed). In certain patients (e.g., previous CABG surgery), a hemorrhagic effusion may be focal and can self-tamponade the perforation. Emergency cardiac surgery should be considered for persistent bleeding and/or hemodynamic compromise despite pericardiocentesis.

Stent Thrombosis: Intraprocedural and Acute

The Academic Research Consortium standardized the definition of stent thrombosis into definite, probable, or possible.[83] Timing of stent thrombosis is defined as intraprocedural (before completion of PCI), acute (<24 hours), subacute (24 hours to 30 days), late (>30 days to 1 year), or very late (>1 year). The incidence of stent thrombosis in the first year is approximately 1%, with most occurring within the first 30 days. In acute MI, the risk for stent thrombosis increases incrementally in patients undergoing PCI in the setting of NSTEMI and STEMI.[84,85] In a large Dutch registry analysis of 21,009 patients who underwent PCI, the proportion of stent thrombosis that was acute, subacute, late, and very late was 32%, 41%, 13%, and 14%, respectively.[86] Clinical predictors associated with stent thrombosis include clinical, anatomic, and procedural factors (Table 17-7), with discontinuation of DAPT being a major contributing factor for stent thrombosis.

Development of intraprocedural stent thrombosis (i.e., new or increasing thrombus in or near a recently deployed stent before the end of PCI) is a major concern and risk for serious adverse clinical events. Acute MI, large thrombus burden, no-reflow, and bifurcation lesions increase the risk for intraprocedural stent thrombosis. Most cases of intraprocedural stent thrombosis occur in patients undergoing PCI for acute MI. If intraprocedural or acute stent thrombosis occurs, acute occlusion of the stented vessel occurs and should be managed accordingly. If intraprocedural stent thrombosis occurs, it is important to check the ACT to determine if subtherapeutic anticoagulation may have contributed to the event. Manual aspiration of thrombus is usually required with stent thrombosis. Intravascular imaging is key to determining if a mechanical issue led to stent thrombosis (e.g., flow-limiting dissection), which will dictate treatment strategies. Additional pharmacotherapy including GPIs may be useful. If stent thrombosis occurs on clopidogrel, and compliance has been verified, switching to a more potent ADP $P2Y_{12}$ inhibitor is often advised. One important consideration in preventing stent thrombosis in patients who present with MI complicated by cardiogenic shock is the potential for poor gastrointestinal absorption of oral medications. In these cases, it may be necessary to give a prolonged infusion of a GPI or cangrelor to ensure adequate platelet inhibition until oral intake of medications is adequate.

TABLE 17-7 Predictors Associated with Stent Thrombosis

Clinical Variables
• Acute MI (STEMI >> NSTEMI)
• Clopidogrel noncompliance or discontinuation
• Decreased clopidogrel bioavailability
• Diabetes mellitus
• Renal failure
• Congestive heart failure, especially left ventricular dysfunction
• Previous brachytherapy
• Malignancy
• Cocaine use
Anatomic Variables
• Long lesions
• Smaller vessels
• Multivessel disease
• Bifurcation lesions
Procedural Factors
• Side branch stenting
• Stent underexpansion
• Incomplete wall apposition (for late or very late stent thrombosis)
• Residual inflow and outflow disease
• Persistent dissection
• Crush technique
• Overlapping stent
• Residual thrombus
• Subtherapeutic anticoagulation during PCI
• Post-PCI TIMI flow <3
• No aspirin before PCI

MI, Myocardial infarction; *NSTEMI*, non–ST-elevation myocardial infarction; *PCI*, percutaneous coronary intervention; *STEMI*, ST-elevation myocardial infarction; *TIMI*, Thrombolysis in Myocardial Infarction.
Adapted from Mauri L, Bhatt DL: Percutaneous coronary intervention. In Mann DL, Zipes DP, Libby P, Bonow RO, eds: Braunwald's heart disease: a textbook of cardiovascular medicine. *ed 10. Philadelphia: Saunders, 2015 , p 1258.*

Optimal Duration of Dual Antiplatelet Therapy after Percutaneous Coronary Intervention: Prevention of Stent Thrombosis

Guidelines have recommended that DAPT should be continued for 12 months following PCI and/or acute MI.[2,4,20] Evidence suggests that second-generation DESs have lower rates of stent thrombosis than first-generation DESs.[87] Considerations that guide the duration of DAPT in patients with acute MI, including those treated with PCI, are detailed in Chapter 35. A careful discussion of the risks, benefits, and alternative therapies when considering the type of stent and DAPT duration in candidates for PCI is essential.

PRACTICAL HOSPITAL FOLLOW-UP AFTER PRIMARY PERCUTANEOUS CORONARY INTERVENTION

Assessment the Day after Percutaneous Coronary Intervention

Following PCI after MI, the site(s) of vascular access should be closely examined for complications. Patients should be encouraged to ambulate in the hospital to assess for symptom recurrence and for any femoral vascular access complications that can be exacerbated with ambulation. Importantly, a review of the current medications is vital, especially a discussion of use and adverse effects of the antiplatelet medications used for prevention of stent thrombosis. In addition, it is important to have a discussion on what to expect after discharge, with plans for an initial follow-up visit (see Chapter 34).

Biomarker Assessment

Routine assessment of cardiac biomarkers following revascularization is not recommended after PCI. Most patients will have elevated cardiac biomarkers at the time of PCI in acute MI. The clinical use of routinely checking cardiac biomarkers following successful revascularization in PCI is minimal and should only be used for patients with recurrent symptoms before discharge. It is difficult to assess for reinfarction using cardiac biomarkers in the acute infarct period after PCI, especially with cardiac troponins, which can remain elevated for 14 days after an acute MI (see Chapter 23).[4] One exception is in the setting of a coronary complication, where cardiac biomarkers are routinely measured.

Management of Recurrent Chest Pain

Approximately 30% to 40% of patients develop chest pain following PCI. The cause can range from noncardiac to life-threatening (e.g., stent thrombosis). Initial assessment should include an electrocardiogram (ECG) and cardiac biomarkers, and evaluation of use of anti-ischemic medications, predominantly nitroglycerin. The ECG should be assessed carefully for any new or worsening ischemic changes or other causes of chest pain in MI (e.g., postinfarction pericarditis). It can be difficult to assess for reinfarction on an ECG in patients with MI, especially STEMI (see Chapter 23). All patients should get an ECG immediately post-PCI, regardless of clinical presentation, which can be useful for comparison in patients with recurrent chest pain. If ST-segment elevations are worse or new following PCI, coronary angiography should be performed immediately to rule out stent thrombosis. Despite the frequency of recurrent chest pain, most patients will not have any new ECG changes. If chest pain is severe and refractory to medical treatment, one should also consider repeat coronary angiography. In patients with recurrent chest pain, it is important to review the PCI films, which may reveal a missed coronary complication or potential unrevascularized territories that could account for ischemic symptoms. Patients may also develop pain from local vascular injury to the vessel (i.e., stretch pain), which is typically benign.

Monitoring for Renal Dysfunction

Acute kidney injury (or contrast-induced nephropathy) occurs in approximately 7% of patients following PCI, and 0.3% of these patients will require hemodialysis.[88] Importantly, the risk for in-hospital mortality is 10% and 34% in patients with acute kidney injury or hemodialysis, respectively.[88] STEMI, cardiogenic shock, and severe baseline chronic kidney disease (glomerular filtration rate [GFR] <30 mL/min per 1.73 m^2) are strong independent predictors of acute kidney injury.[88] Renal function does not have to be monitored routinely following PCI, but should be assessed in patients with chronic kidney disease (GFR <60 mL/min per 1.73 m^2) or who received a large contrast volume (milliliter of contrast/GFR >2).[89]

When Is It Safe to Discharge Following ST-Elevation Myocardial Infarction Treated with Primary Percutaneous Coronary Intervention?

Evidence on the safety of early discharge following STEMI is lacking. In the United States, the median length of stay in the current era of primary PCI as the dominant approach to reperfusion therapy is approximately 3 days for STEMI patients, which is significantly shorter compared with other countries.[90] A registry analysis examined the 30-day clinical outcomes following primary PCI in STEMI patients aged older than 65 years.[91] Discharge at 48 hours following primary PCI had similar rates of mortality and major adverse cardiac events compared with hospital lengths of stay of 4 to 5 days, but the analysis did show that discharge on the same day or the following day after primary PCI was associated with a lower survival and worse clinical outcomes. This study suggests that discharge after 48 hours following STEMI is safe in selected patients.

SUMMARY

PCI is the principal treatment strategy for STEMI and most NSTEMI patients. The innovations in vascular access, equipment, stent design, adjunctive diagnostic and therapeutic devices, and intravascular imaging have improved the safety and efficacy of PCI in MI. The pharmacotherapy used during and after PCI is continuously evolving to reduce ischemic events and minimize bleeding. As new technologies emerge, PCI will continue to evolve as the treatment of choice for acute MI.

References

1. Mozaffarian D, et al.: Heart disease and stroke statistics-2015 update: a report from the American Heart Association, *Circulation* 131:e29–e322, 2015.
2. O'Gara PT, et al.: 2013 ACCF/AHA guideline for the management of ST-elevation myocardial infarction: a report of the American College of Cardiology Foundation/American Heart Association Task Force on Practice Guidelines, *Circulation* 127:e362–425, 2013.
3. Bradley EH, et al.: National efforts to improve door-to-balloon time results from the Door-to-Balloon Alliance, *J Am Coll Cardiol* 54:2423–2429, 2009.
4. Amsterdam EA, et al.: 2014 AHA/ACC Guideline for the management of patients with non-ST-elevation acute coronary syndromes: a report of the American College of Cardiology/American Heart Association Task Force on Practice Guidelines, *Circulation* 130:e344–426, 2014.
5. Navarese EP, et al.: Optimal timing of coronary invasive strategy in non-ST-segment elevation acute coronary syndromes: a systematic review and meta-analysis, *Ann Intern Med* 158:261–270, 2013.
6. Mehta SR, Granger CB, Boden WE, et al.: Early versus delayed invasive intervention in acute coronary syndromes, *N Engl J Med* 360:2165–2175, 2009.
7. Bangalore S, Bhatt DL: Femoral arterial access and closure, *Circulation* 124:e147–156, 2011.
8. Cilingiroglu M, et al.: Fluoroscopically-guided micropuncture femoral artery access for large-caliber sheath insertion, *J Invasive Cardiol* 23:157–161, 2011.
9. Seto AH, et al.: Real-time ultrasound guidance facilitates femoral arterial access and reduces vascular complications: FAUST (Femoral Arterial Access With Ultrasound Trial), *JACC Cardiovasc Interv* 3:751–758, 2010.
10. Valgimigli M, et al.: Transradial coronary catheterization and intervention across the whole spectrum of Allen test results, *J Am Coll Cardiol* 63:1833–1841, 2014.
11. Byrne RA, et al.: Vascular access and closure in coronary angiography and percutaneous intervention, *Nat Rev Cardiol* 10:27–40, 2013.
12. Jolly SS, et al.: Radial versus femoral access for coronary angiography and intervention in patients with acute coronary syndromes (RIVAL): a randomised, parallel group, multicentre trial, *Lancet* 377:1409–1420, 2011.
13. Romagnoli E, et al.: Radial versus femoral randomized investigation in ST-segment elevation acute coronary syndrome: the RIFLE-STEACS (Radial Versus Femoral Randomized Investigation in ST-Elevation Acute Coronary Syndrome) study, *J Am Coll Cardiol* 60:2481–2489, 2012.
14. Bernat I, et al.: ST-segment elevation myocardial infarction treated by radial or femoral approach in a multicenter randomized clinical trial: the STEMI-RADIAL trial, *J Am Coll Cardiol* 63:964–972, 2014.
15. Karrowni W, et al.: Radial versus femoral access for primary percutaneous interventions in ST-segment elevation myocardial infarction patients: a meta-analysis of randomized controlled trials, *JACC Cardiovasc Interv* 6:814–823, 2013.
16. Baklanov DV, et al.: The prevalence and outcomes of transradial percutaneous coronary intervention for ST-segment elevation myocardial infarction: analysis from the National Cardiovascular Data Registry (2007 to 2011), *J Am Coll Cardiol* 61:420–426, 2013.
17. Valgimigli M, et al.: Radial versus femoral access in patients with acute coronary syndromes undergoing invasive management: a randomised multicentre trial, *Lancet* 385:2465–2476, 2015.
18. Wimmer NJ, et al.: Delay in reperfusion with transradial percutaneous coronary intervention for ST-elevation myocardial infarction: might some delays be acceptable? *Am Heart J* 168:103–109, 2014.
19. Schulz-Schupke S, et al.: Comparison of vascular closure devices vs manual compression after femoral artery puncture: the ISAR-CLOSURE randomized clinical trial, *JAMA* 312:1981–1987, 2014.
20. Levine GN, et al.: 2011 ACCF/AHA/SCAI guideline for percutaneous coronary intervention. A report of the American College of Cardiology Foundation/American Heart Association Task Force on Practice Guidelines and the Society for Cardiovascular Angiography and Interventions, *J Am Coll Cardiol* 58:e44–122, 2011.
21. Ellis SG, et al.: Correlates and outcomes of retroperitoneal hemorrhage complicating percutaneous coronary intervention, *Catheter Cardiovasc Interv* 67:541–545, 2006.
22. Bellemain-Appaix A, et al.: Association of clopidogrel pretreatment with mortality, cardiovascular events, and major bleeding among patients undergoing percutaneous coronary intervention: a systematic review and meta-analysis, *JAMA* 308:2507–2516, 2012.
23. Wallentin L, et al.: Ticagrelor versus clopidogrel in patients with acute coronary syndromes, *N Engl J Med* 361:1045–1057, 2009.
24. Mehran R, et al.: Bivalirudin in patients undergoing primary angioplasty for acute myocardial infarction (HORIZONS-AMI): 1-year results of a randomised controlled trial, *Lancet* 374:1149–1159, 2009.
25. Brener SJ, et al.: Intra-procedural stent thrombosis: a new risk factor for adverse outcomes in patients undergoing percutaneous coronary intervention for acute coronary syndromes, *JACC Cardiovasc Interv* 6:36–43, 2013.
26. Steg PG, et al.: Bivalirudin started during emergency transport for primary PCI, *N Engl J Med* 369:2207–2217, 2013.
27. Shahzad A, et al.: Unfractionated heparin versus bivalirudin in primary percutaneous coronary intervention (HEAT-PPCI): an open-label, single centre, randomised controlled trial, *Lancet* 384:1849–1858, 2014.
28. Han Y, et al.: Bivalirudin vs heparin with or without tirofiban during primary percutaneous coronary intervention in acute myocardial infarction: the BRIGHT randomized clinical trial, *JAMA* 313:1336–1346, 2015.
29. Cavender MA, Sabatine MS: Bivalirudin versus heparin in patients planned for percutaneous coronary intervention: a meta-analysis of randomised controlled trials, *Lancet* 384:599–606, 2014.
30. Bhatt DL, Topol EJ: Current role of platelet glycoprotein IIb/IIIa inhibitors in acute coronary syndromes, *JAMA* 284:1549–1558, 2000.
31. Depta JP, Bhatt DL: New approaches to inhibiting platelets and coagulation, *Annu Rev Pharmacol Toxicol* 55:373–397, 2015.
32. White HD, et al.: Reduced immediate ischemic events with cangrelor in PCI: a pooled analysis of the CHAMPION trials using the universal definition of myocardial infarction, *Am Heart J* 163:182–190 e4, 2012.
33. Bhatt DL, et al.: Effect of platelet inhibition with cangrelor during PCI on ischemic events, *N Engl J Med* 368:1303–1313, 2013.
34. Genereux P, et al.: Impact of intraprocedural stent thrombosis during percutaneous coronary intervention: insights from the CHAMPION PHOENIX Trial (Clinical Trial Comparing Cangrelor to Clopidogrel Standard of Care Therapy in Subjects Who Require Percutaneous Coronary Intervention), *J Am Coll Cardiol* 63:619–629, 2014.
35. Rubboli A, et al.: The optimal management of patients on oral anticoagulation undergoing coronary artery stenting. The 10th Anniversary Overview, *Thromb Haemost* 112:1080–1087, 2014.
36. Ruiz-Nodar JM, et al.: Anticoagulant and antiplatelet therapy use in 426 patients with atrial fibrillation undergoing percutaneous coronary intervention and stent implantation implications for bleeding risk and prognosis, *J Am Coll Cardiol* 51:818–825, 2008.
37. Steinberg BA, et al.: Use and outcomes associated with bridging during anticoagulation interruptions in patients with atrial fibrillation: findings from the Outcomes Registry for Better Informed Treatment of Atrial Fibrillation (ORBIT-AF), *Circulation* 131:488–494, 2015.
38. Dewilde WJ, et al.: Use of clopidogrel with or without aspirin in patients taking oral anticoagulant therapy and undergoing percutaneous coronary intervention: an open-label, randomised, controlled trial, *Lancet* 381:1107–1115, 2013.

39. Fiedler KA, et al.: Duration of triple therapy in patients requiring oral anticoagulation after drug-eluting stent implantation: The ISAR-TRIPLE Trial, *J Am Coll Cardiol* 65:1619–1629, 2015.
40. Bhatt DL: When is a double better than a TRIPLE? Stenting in patients with atrial fibrillation, *J Am Coll Cardiol* 65:1630–1632, 2015.
41. Mockel M, et al.: Comparison of direct stenting with conventional stent implantation in acute myocardial infarction, *Am J Cardiol* 108:1697–1703, 2011.
42. Dziewierz A, et al.: Impact of direct stenting on outcome of patients with ST-elevation myocardial infarction transferred for primary percutaneous coronary intervention (from the EUROTRANSFER registry), *Catheter Cardiovasc Interv* 84:925–931, 2014.
43. Bavry AA, Bhatt DL: Appropriate use of drug-eluting stents: balancing the reduction in restenosis with the concern of late thrombosis, *Lancet* 371:2134–2143, 2008.
44. Brar SS, et al.: Use of drug-eluting stents in acute myocardial infarction: a systematic review and meta-analysis, *J Am Coll Cardiol* 53:1677–1689, 2009.
45. Sabate M, et al.: Everolimus-eluting stent versus bare-metal stent in ST-segment elevation myocardial infarction (EXAMINATION): 1 year results of a randomised controlled trial, *Lancet* 380: 1482–1490, 2012.
46. Bhatt DL: EXAMINATION of new drug-eluting stents–top of the class!, *Lancet* 380:1453–1455, 2012.
47. Sabate M, et al.: Comparison of newer-generation drug-eluting with bare-metal stents in patients with acute ST-segment elevation myocardial infarction: a pooled analysis of the EXAMINATION (clinical Evaluation of the Xience-V stent in Acute Myocardial INfArcTION) and COMFORTABLE-AMI (Comparison of Biolimus Eluted From an Erodible Stent Coating With Bare Metal Stents in Acute ST-Elevation Myocardial Infarction) trials, *JACC Cardiovasc Interv* 7:55–63, 2014.
48. Raber L, et al.: Effect of biolimus-eluting stents with biodegradable polymer vs bare-metal stents on cardiovascular events among patients with acute myocardial infarction: the COMFORTABLE AMI randomized trial, *JAMA* 308:777–787, 2012.
49. Natsuaki M, et al.: Two-year outcome of a randomized trial comparing second-generation drug-eluting stents using biodegradable or durable polymer, *JAMA* 311:2125–2127, 2014.
50. Byrne RA, et al.: Drug-coated balloon therapy in coronary and peripheral artery disease, *Nat Rev Cardiol* 11:13–23, 2014.
51. Stone GW, et al.: Prospective, Randomized, Multicenter Evaluation of a Polyethylene Terephthalate Micronet Mesh-Covered Stent (MGuard) in ST-Segment Elevation Myocardial Infarction: The MASTER Trial, *J Am Coll Cardiol* 60:1975–1984, 2012.
52. Mintz GS: Clinical utility of intravascular imaging and physiology in coronary artery disease, *J Am Coll Cardiol* 64:207–222, 2014.
53. Witzenbichler B, et al.: Relationship between intravascular ultrasound guidance and clinical outcomes after drug-eluting stents: the assessment of dual antiplatelet therapy with drug-eluting stents (ADAPT-DES) study, *Circulation* 129:463–470, 2014.
54. Oviedo C, et al.: Intravascular ultrasound classification of plaque distribution in left main coronary artery bifurcations: where is the plaque really located? *Circ Cardiovasc Interv* 3:105–112, 2010.
55. Tonino PA, et al.: Angiographic versus functional severity of coronary artery stenoses in the FAME study fractional flow reserve versus angiography in multivessel evaluation, *J Am Coll Cardiol* 55:2816–2821, 2010.
56. Tonino PA, et al.: Fractional flow reserve versus angiography for guiding percutaneous coronary intervention, *N Engl J Med* 360:213–224, 2009.
57. De Bruyne B, et al.: Fractional flow reserve-guided PCI versus medical therapy in stable coronary disease, *N Engl J Med* 367:991–1001, 2012.
58. Chiang A, et al.: Procedural variation in the performance of primary percutaneous coronary intervention for ST-elevation myocardial infarction: a SCAI-based survey study of US interventional cardiologists, *Catheter Cardiovasc Interv* 83:721–726, 2014.
59. Kumbhani DJ, et al.: Aspiration thrombectomy in patients undergoing primary angioplasty: totality of data to 2013, *Catheter Cardiovasc Interv* 84:973–977, 2014.
60. Frobert O, et al.: Thrombus aspiration during ST-segment elevation myocardial infarction, *N Engl J Med* 369:1587–1597, 2013.
61. Jolly SS, et al.: Randomized trial of primary PCI with or without routine manual thrombectomy, *N Engl J Med* 372:1389–1398, 2015.
62. Stone GW, et al.: Distal microcirculatory protection during percutaneous coronary intervention in acute ST-segment elevation myocardial infarction: a randomized controlled trial, *JAMA* 293:1063–1072, 2005.
63. Latib A, Colombo A: Bifurcation disease: what do we know, what should we do? *JACC Cardiovasc Interv* 1:218–226, 2008.
64. Dudek D, et al.: Impact of bifurcation target lesion on angiographic, electrocardiographic, and clinical outcomes of patients undergoing primary percutaneous coronary intervention (from the Harmonizing Outcomes With Revascularization and Stents in Acute Myocardial Infarction [HORIZONS-AMI] trial), *Eurointervention* 9:817–823, 2013.
65. Singh J, et al.: A modified provisional stenting approach to coronary bifurcation lesions: clinical application of the "jailed-balloon technique.", *J Interv Cardiol* 25:289–296, 2012.
66. Gao XF, et al.: Stenting strategy for coronary artery bifurcation with drug-eluting stents: a meta-analysis of nine randomised trials and systematic review, *EuroIntervention* 10:561–569, 2014.
67. Patel Y, et al.: Impact of intravascular ultrasound on the long-term clinical outcomes in the treatment of coronary ostial lesions, *Catheter Cardiovasc Interv* 87:232–240, 2016.
68. Welsh RC, et al.: Prior coronary artery bypass graft patients with ST-segment elevation myocardial infarction treated with primary percutaneous coronary intervention, *JACC Cardiovasc Interv* 3:343–351, 2010.
69. Nikolsky E, et al.: Comparison of outcomes of patients with ST-segment elevation myocardial infarction with versus without previous coronary artery bypass grafting (from the Harmonizing Outcomes With Revascularization and Stents in Acute Myocardial Infarction [HORIZONS-AMI] trial), *Am J Cardiol* 111:1377–1386, 2013.
70. Mehilli J, et al.: Drug-eluting versus bare-metal stents in saphenous vein graft lesions (ISAR-CABG): a randomised controlled superiority trial, *Lancet* 378:1071–1078, 2011.
71. Dong L, et al.: Comparison of plaque characteristics in narrowings with ST-elevation myocardial infarction (STEMI), non-STEMI/Unstable Angina Pectoris and Stable Coronary Artery Disease (from the ADAPT-DES IVUS Substudy), *Am J Cardiol* 115:860–866, 2015.
72. Pollack A, et al.: Preventive stenting in acute myocardial infarction, *JACC Cardiovasc Interv* 8:131–138, 2015.
73. Wald DS, et al.: Randomized trial of preventive angioplasty in myocardial infarction, *N Engl J Med* 369:1115–1123, 2013.
74. Gershlick AH, et al.: Randomized trial of complete versus lesion-only revascularization in patients undergoing primary percutaneous coronary intervention for STEMI and Multivessel Disease: the CvLPRIT trial, *J Am Coll Cardiol* 65:963–972, 2015.
75. Bhatt DL: Do we really know the CvLPRIT in myocardial infarction? Or just stent all lesions? *J Am Coll Cardiol* 65:973–975, 2015.
76. Shishehbor MH, et al.: In unstable angina or non-ST-segment acute coronary syndrome, should patients with multivessel coronary artery disease undergo multivessel or culprit-only stenting? *J Am Coll Cardiol* 49:849–854, 2007.
77. Zapata GO, et al.: Culprit-only or multivessel percutaneous coronary stenting in patients with non-ST-segment elevation acute coronary syndromes: one-year follow-up, *J Interv Cardiol* 22:329–335, 2009.
78. Hillis LD, et al.: 2011 ACCF/AHA guideline for coronary artery bypass graft surgery. A report of the American College of Cardiology Foundation/American Heart Association Task Force on Practice Guidelines. Developed in collaboration with the American Association for Thoracic Surgery, Society of Cardiovascular Anesthesiologists, and Society of Thoracic Surgeons, *J Am Coll Cardiol* 58:e123–210, 2011.
79. Rihal CS, et al.: 2015 SCAI/ACC/HFSA/STS clinical expert consensus statement on the use of percutaneous mechanical circulatory support devices in cardiovascular care: endorsed by the American Heart Assocation, the Cardiological Society of India, and Sociedad Latino Americana de Cardiologia Intervencion; Affirmation of Value by the Canadian Association of Interventional Cardiology-Association Canadienne de Cardiologie d'intervention, *J Am Coll Cardiol* 65:e7–e26, 2015.
80. Myat A, et al.: Percutaneous circulatory assist devices for high-risk coronary intervention, *JACC Cardiovasc Interv* 8:229–244, 2015.
81. Harrison RW, et al.: Incidence and outcomes of no-reflow phenomenon during percutaneous coronary intervention among patients with acute myocardial infarction, *Am J Cardiol* 111:178–184, 2013.
82. Niccoli G, et al.: No-reflow: again prevention is better than treatment, *Eur Heart J* 31:2449–2455, 2010.
83. Cutlip DE, et al.: Clinical end points in coronary stent trials: a case for standardized definitions, *Circulation* 115:2344–2351, 2007.
84. Aoki J, et al.: Early stent thrombosis in patients with acute coronary syndromes treated with drug-eluting and bare metal stents: the Acute Catheterization and Urgent Intervention Triage Strategy trial, *Circulation* 119:687–698, 2009.
85. Wiviott SD, et al.: Intensive oral antiplatelet therapy for reduction of ischaemic events including stent thrombosis in patients with acute coronary syndromes treated with percutaneous coronary intervention and stenting in the TRITON-TIMI 38 trial: a subanalysis of a randomised trial, *Lancet* 371:1353–1363, 2008.
86. van Werkum JW, et al.: Predictors of coronary stent thrombosis: the Dutch Stent Thrombosis Registry, *J Am Coll Cardiol* 53:1399–1409, 2009.
87. Tada T, et al.: Risk of stent thrombosis among bare-metal stents, first-generation drug-eluting stents, and second-generation drug-eluting stents: results from a registry of 18,334 patients, *JACC Cardiovasc Interv* 6:1267–1274, 2013.
88. Tsai TT, et al.: Contemporary incidence, predictors, and outcomes of acute kidney injury in patients undergoing percutaneous coronary interventions: insights from the NCDR Cath-PCI registry, *JACC Cardiovasc Interv* 7:1–9, 2014.
89. Gurm HS, et al.: Renal function-based contrast dosing to define safe limits of radiographic contrast media in patients undergoing percutaneous coronary interventions, *J Am Coll Cardiol* 58:907–914, 2011.
90. Kociol RD, et al.: International variation in and factors associated with hospital readmission after myocardial infarction, *JAMA* 307:66–74, 2012.
91. Swaminathan RV, et al.: Hospital length of stay and clinical outcomes in older STEMI patients after primary PCI: A report from the National Cardiovascular Data Registry, *J Am Coll Cardiol* 65:1161–1171, 2015.

18

Clinical Practice/Controversy

Selection of Initial Anticoagulant Therapy

Johanne Silvain, Lee Nguyen, and Gilles Montalescot

INTRODUCTION

Myocardial infarction (MI) includes patients presenting with ST-elevation MI (STEMI) and those without ST-segment MI (NSTEMI), and although these types of MI share a common physiopathology and principles of treatment (see Chapter 13), the approaches to management of anticoagulant therapy for these conditions differ by MI type and overall management strategy (invasive vs. conservative).

Rationale for Anticoagulant Therapy in Acute Coronary Syndrome

The rationale for administering anticoagulant therapy acutely in STEMI patients is strong and includes the following treatment goals[1,2]:

1. Establishing and maintaining patency of the infarct-related artery whatever the reperfusion strategy used (fibrinolysis, primary angioplasty, or no reperfusion therapy).
2. Prevention of ventricular thrombus formation and cerebral embolization.
3. Prevention of complications related to percutaneous coronary intervention (PCI), such as catheter thrombosis, distal embolization of fragmented thrombus, slow or no flow post-PCI, ischemic stroke, abrupt vessel closure, and acute stent thrombosis.

Other objectives are common to acute medical conditions and bed rest, such as prevention of deep venous thrombosis and possible consequent pulmonary embolism.

In NSTEMI, the objectives are similar, although the artery is rarely fully occluded[3]:

1. Maintaining patency of the infarct-related artery whatever strategy is decided by the treating physician (invasive strategy or medical therapy).
2. Prevention of PCI-related complications.
3. Prevention of complications or bed rest.

Containing Thrombus Formation and Propagation

Successful and durable myocardial reperfusion is the goal of the initial antithrombotic therapy, including anticoagulation and antiplatelet therapy (see Chapter 19). After the initial disruption or rupture of vulnerable plaque (see Chapter 3), the common pathophysiological substrate of acute coronary syndrome (ACS), the damaged endothelium, and the exposition of the lipid core leads to platelet adhesion and aggregation, followed almost instantly by activation of the coagulation cascade and formation of an initial platelet-rich thrombus (Figure 18-1A).

A key step in this process is the activation of prothrombin to thrombin (factor IIa), which transforms the circulating fibrinogen into fibrin fibers, forming the scaffold of the coronary thrombus and leading to its stabilization (see Figures 18-1B and 18-1C). The evolution of the thrombus may culminate in resolution with asymptomatic healing, a subtotal coronary artery occlusion leading to a NSTEMI, or to fully occlusive thrombus presenting as a STEMI. As a result, initial anticoagulant therapy is indicated in all patients with MI, in the absence of contraindications. The class of anticoagulant and dose regimen depends on the type of MI and whether the anticoagulant is to be used as an adjunct to PCI or fibrinolysis.

Although treatment with heparin, as the prototypical parenteral anticoagulant, has a strong pathobiological rationale and has become entrenched in the clinical management of MI, the evidence from clinical studies directly demonstrating the efficacy of heparin in MI is modest. However, the rationale for use of anticoagulants in MI has been bolstered by subsequent trials of newer anticoagulants, such as the low–molecular-weight heparins (LMWHs).

OVERVIEW OF AVAILABLE ANTICOAGULANT DRUGS

Although adjuvant anticoagulant therapy may result in a small improvement in initial restoration of flow in the

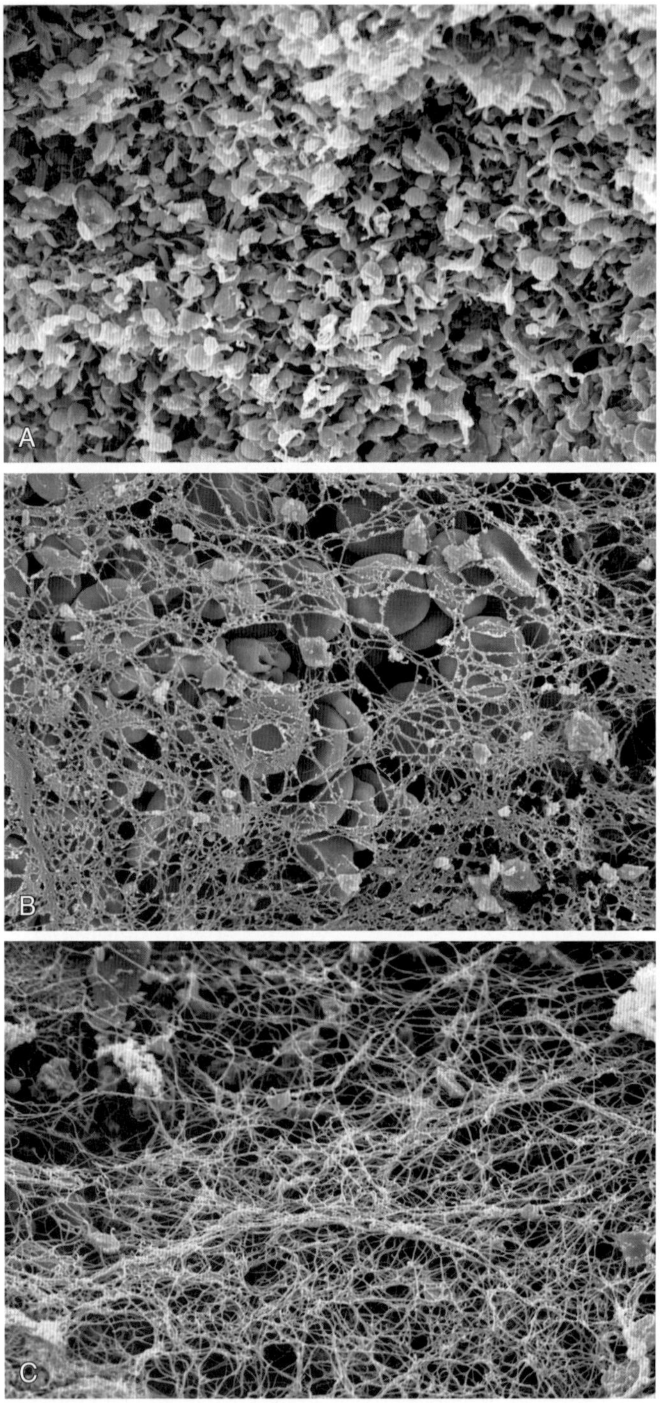

FIGURE 18-1 Coronary thrombus retrieved during acute myocardial infarction and observed with scanning electron microscopy. (**A**) Platelet-rich thrombus. (**B**) Stabilization of thrombus with fibrin fibers. (**C**) Fibrin-rich thrombus. *(From Silvain J, et al: Composition of coronary thrombus in acute myocardial infarction.* J Am Coll Cardiol *57:1359–1367,2011.)*

thrombotic coronary artery, its main roles are maintaining patency after successful reperfusion, preventing reocclusion, and reducing the risk of thrombotic complications of PCI. The options for initial anticoagulant therapy include four main drugs: unfractionated heparin (UFH), the LMWHs (e.g., enoxaparin), fondaparinux, and bivalirudin. UFH and enoxaparin are the most frequently used anticoagulants worldwide. They are both biological products that are derived from mucosal tissues (e.g., porcine or bovine intestines). Inherent drawbacks led to the development of synthetic anticoagulants, such as fondaparinux and bivalirudin. The mechanism of action of each of these four agents is illustrated in Figure 18-2 and compared in Table 18-1.

Unfractionated Heparin

UFH was the first anticoagulant used in the treatment of MI. UFH is a heterogeneous mixture of mucopolysaccharides, with a molecular weight ranging from 2000 to 30,000 Da (mostly 15,000 to 18,000), that bind and activate antithrombin, greatly increasing the inhibitory effects of antithrombin on thrombin. Activated antithrombin inhibits several coagulation factors, including factor Xa, resulting in an anticoagulant effect. Because its actions are via binding to antithrombin, UFH is classified as an indirect thrombin inhibitor (see Figure 18-2). Because UFH is poorly absorbed when injected via the subcutaneous (SC) route, intravenous (IV) administration is the preferred route of administration.

A major drawback of UFH is the significant variability of its therapeutic response. The heterogeneous composition and variable elimination of UFH through the endoplasmic reticulum results in marked interpatient therapeutic response variability and necessitates close monitoring of anticoagulant intensity with activated clotting time (ACT) or with activated partial thromboplastin time (aPTT). UFH can also cause an immunologically mediated thrombocytopenia, also known as heparin-induced thrombocytopenia (HIT), which is rare (2% to 3% of patients), but potentially life-threatening. Other drawbacks of UFH include an increase in platelet activation and aggregation, a dependency on antithrombin for inhibition of thrombin activity, a sensitivity to platelet factor 4, and an inability to inhibit clot-bound thrombin.

Even with standardized weight-based dosing nomograms, less than one-third of initial aPTT measurements are within the therapeutic range. The anticoagulant effect of UFH dissipates rapidly, within a few hours after interruption. During the first 24 hours after heparin cessation, there is a risk of reactivation of the coagulation process, and therefore, a transiently increased risk of recurrent ischemic events despite adjunctive aspirin treatment. A desire to overcome the disadvantages of UFH has stimulated interest in the development of alternative anticoagulants.

Historically, high doses of UFH were used in fibrinolysis or PCI to overcome thrombotic complications; however, studies showed that these higher doses were associated with a higher rate of bleeding without an effect on the ischemic endpoints, and that efficacy was preserved at the lower doses. The initial doses of UFH used in PCI (up to 175 UI/kg) were gradually lowered to 140, 100, 85, 70, 60, and 50 UI/kg in the latest trials when glycoprotein IIb/IIIa receptor inhibitors (GPIs) were used. A similar pattern was shown with the target ACT for the optimal ranging of UFH efficacy, suggesting that the therapeutic window for UFH is relatively narrow.

Low–Molecular-Weight Heparins

LMWHs are a class of heparin-derived compounds with molecular weights ranging from 2000 to 10,000 Da (Table 18-2). By virtue of enhanced binding of LMWH-antithrombin to factor Xa, LMWHs have a balanced anti-Xa and anti-IIa activity, with the relative activity against factor Xa versus IIa depending on the molecular weight of the molecule; the heavier the LMWH

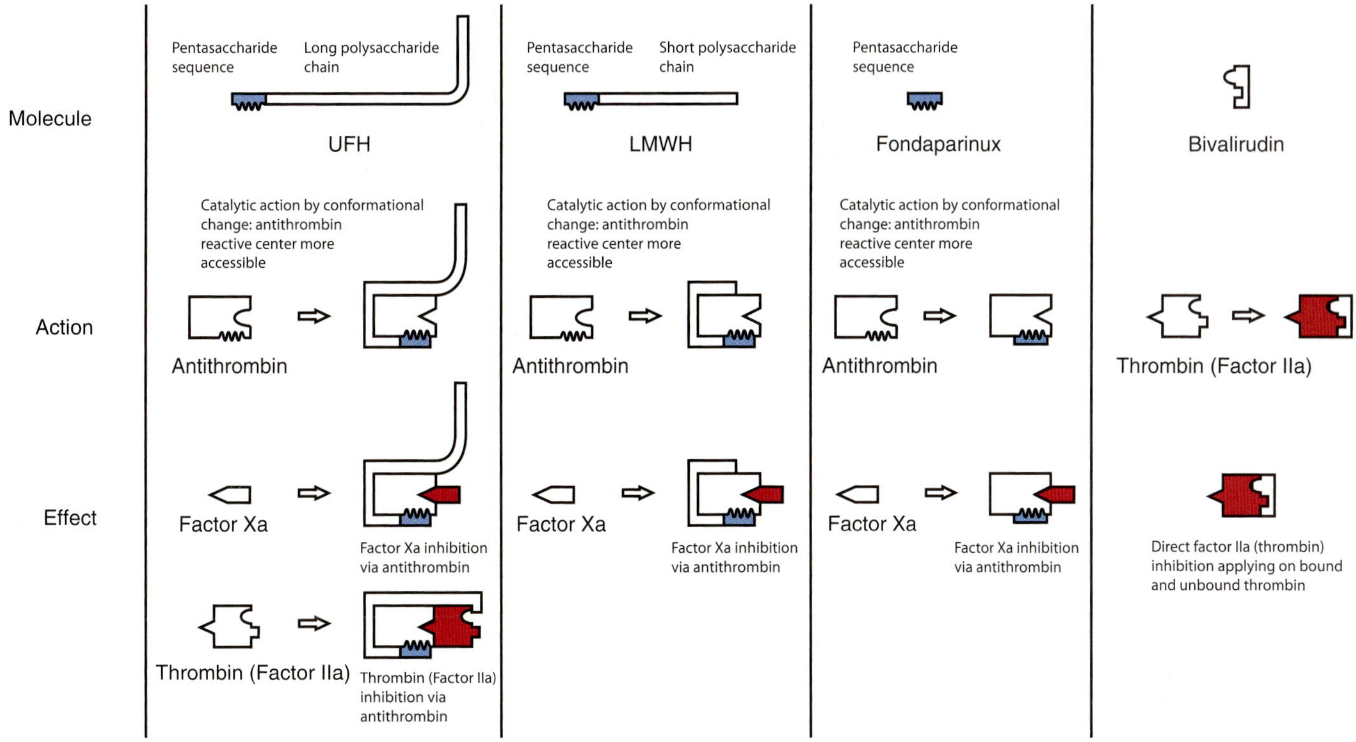

FIGURE 18-2 Action of available anticoagulants. By virtue of a greater proportion of short polysaccharide chains, which catalyze only inhibition of FXa, LMWHs have a greater relative acitivity against FXa. However, longer chains in LMWHs also inhibit FIIa.*LMWH*, Low–molecular weight heparin; *UFH*, unfractionated heparin.

TABLE 18-1 Pharmacological Properties of Parenteral Anticoagulants

MEDICATION	UFH	ENOXAPARIN	FONDAPARINUX	BIVALIRUDIN
Mechanism	AT mediated factor Xa and thrombin inhibitor	AT mediated factor Xa and thrombin inhibitor	Indirect factor Xa inhibitor	Direct thrombin inhibitor, reversible
Route of administration	IV–SC	IV–SC	SC	IV
Half-life	1–2 h	5–7 h	17–21 h	25 min
Molecular weight	3–30 kDa	2–10 kDa	1.7 kDa	2.2 kDa
Metabolism	Hepatic	Hepatic	Excreted largely as unchanged drug	Plasma proteases
Elimination	Extra-renal	Renal	Renal	Renal
Onset	Immediate (IV)	Immediate (IV) 3–5 h (SC)	2–3 h (SC)	Immediate
Notes	Inactive on clot-associated thrombin	Inactive on clot-associated thrombin More factor sXa selectivity	Inactive on clot-associated thrombin	Inhibits clot-associated thrombin
Incidence of HIT	1%–3%	≤0.2%	Negligible	None
Antidote	Protamine	Protamine (partial)	None	None

AT, Activated thrombin; *HIT* heparin-induced thrombocytopenia; *IV*, intravenous; *SC*, subcutaneous; *UFH*, unfractionated heparin.

is, the greater relative anti-IIa activity it has (see Figure 18-2). Enoxaparin is the most studied and widely used LMWH for the treatment of ACS. LMWHs are approximately one-third of the molecular weight of UFH, conferring greater bioavailability that enables administration via the SC route. Other advantages of enoxaparin include a stable and reliable anticoagulant effect without any need for monitoring, provided that weight-based dosing is used and renal failure is absent.

Once bound to antithrombin, enoxaparin provides a greater specificity for factor Xa compared with UFH, producing an enhanced blockade of the coagulation cascade upstream of thrombin generation. The ratio of inhibition of factor Xa/IIa varies between agents, and is 3 to 1 for enoxparin. HIT is 20 times less common with enoxaparin than with UFH, but it can still occur. On top of these anticoagulant actions, enoxaparin may have some anti-inflammatory properties and does not activate platelets.

The main drawback of enoxaparin is its renal elimination, which in the presence of renal dysfunction, can result in accumulation over time with repeated injections (>3 injections). Similarly to UFH, enoxaparin was used at high doses in the first phase II trials, such as TIMI 11A (Thrombolysis In Myocardial Infarction), which demonstrated that doses higher than 1.0 mg/kg should not be used because of excess bleeding.

Fondaparinux

Fondaparinux is a synthetic pentasaccharide that was developed to have a chemical structure similar to the antithrombin-binding active site domain of heparin (see Figure 18-2).

This highly selective drug induces conformational changes, leading to a potent inhibition of factor Xa, and thus, reducing thrombin generation. Unlike UFH and LMWH, fondaparinux has no inhibitory effect on thrombin (factor IIa) itself. Fondaparinux inhibits factor Xa by binding reversibly, with a high affinity to antithrombin. Like LMWH, but in a more selective manner, it targets this upstream step in the coagulation cascade of thrombin generation (Figure 18-3).

Advantages of fondaparinux include 100% bioavailability after SC injection and a long half-life of 15 to 17 hours, which allows for once daily administration. Fondaparinux is eliminated mainly by the kidneys and is contraindicated if creatine clearance is less than 30 mL/min. It has a predictable anticoagulant effect with no requirement for monitoring, and no cross reactivity with antibodies associated with HIT. Fondaparinux is insensitive to inactivation by platelet-released heparin neutralization proteins. Therefore, monitoring the platelet count is unnecessary, as is monitoring of anti-Xa activity. Phase II trials evaluated different doses of intravenous fondaparinux (2.5 and 5.0 mg) compared with UFH, and the lower dose of 2.5 mg was selected because of its good safety profile.

TABLE 18-2 Comparison of Low–Molecular-Weight Heparin Preparations*

GENERIC NAME (TRADE NAME OR SYNONYM)	MEAN MOLECULAR WEIGHT (Da)	ANTI-Xa: ANTI-IIa RATIO	FDA INDICATION FOR ACS
Enoxaparin (Lovenox, Clexane)	4200	3.8	Yes
Nadroparin (Fraxiparine, Sleparina)	4500	3.6	Yes
Reviparin (Clivaparine)	4000	3.5	No
Dalteparin (Fragmin)	6000	2.7	Yes
Parnaparin (Fluxum, Minidalton)	4500–5000	2.4	No
Ardeparin (Normiflo)	6000	1.9	No
Tinzaparin (Innohep, Logiparin)	4500	1.9	No
Certoparin (Alphaparin, Sandoparin, Embolex)	4200–6200		N/A

ACS, Acute coronary syndrome; *Da,* dalton; *FDA,* Food and Drug Administration.
*In descending order of relative anti-Xa:anti-IIa activity.

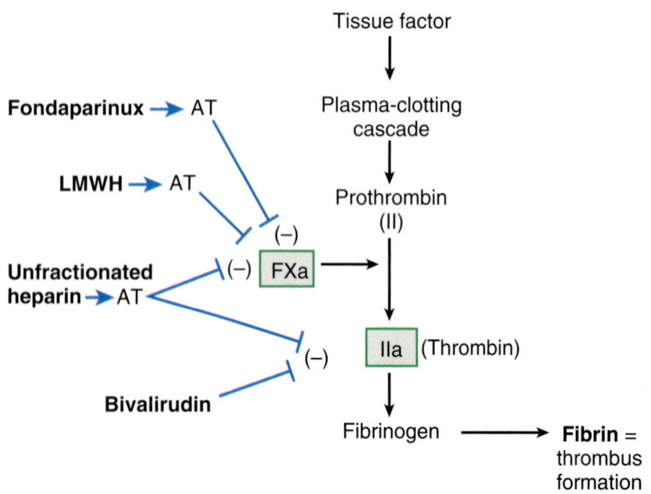

FIGURE 18-3 Anticoagulation targets. *AT,* Antithrombin; *FXa,* activated factor X; *IIa,* activated Factor II; *LMWH,* low–molecular-weight heparin.

Bivalirudin

Bivalirudin and hirudin are synthetic drugs that are direct thrombin (IIa) inhibitors. Several direct thrombin inhibitors have been tested over time, but only bivalirudin reached clinical use in PCI and ACS settings. Unlike UFH and LMWH, bivalirudin inactivates both fluid-phase thrombin and clot-bound thrombin, with less activation of platelets. Because it does not bind to plasma proteins, the anticoagulant effect of bivalirudin is more predictable. Bivalirudin is eliminated by the kidney. The effect of bivalirudin can be followed with routine coagulation tests (aPTT and ACT).

Initial phase II studies tested different regimens of the drug, starting with low bolus doses of 0.5 and 0.75 mg/kg, which were considered insufficient for PCI, and the first large trial used higher doses (bolus dose of 1.0 mg/kg followed by a 4-hour infusion of 2.5 mg/kg per hour and a 14- to 20-hour infusion of 0.2 mg/kg per hour) compared with high doses of UFH (175 UI/kg) for PCI. Subsequently, both the bolus and the infusion doses were lowered (0.75-mg/kg bolus plus 1.75 mg/kg per hour for the duration of PCI) with uncertainty about the optimal duration of infusion after PCI.

Other Parenteral Anticoagulants

Other parenteral anticoagulation therapies have been developed and tested in clinical trials. Otamixaban is a synthetic intravenous direct factor Xa inhibitor, with rapid onset and/or offset, linear kinetics, and no significant renal elimination. However, compared with UFH and eptifibatide, the drug failed to show a benefit in the large phase III Treatment of Acute Coronary Syndromes with Otamixaban (TAO) trial (n = 13,229 patients) of ACS and planned early PCI.[4]

REG-1, first of its class, was composed of two components, the first being a specific and synthetic factor IX inhibitor, pegnivacogin, and the second an injectable and specific antidote to the active drug, anivamersen.[5] Although such a combination seems ideal for emergency situations, allergic reactions to the drug led to a cessation of development of this molecule. The factor XI antisense oligonucleotide (ISIS 416858) that specifically reduces factor XI levels compared favorably against enoxaparin in the prevention of thrombosis after knee arthroplasty.

Monitoring of Available Anticoagulant Therapy

Biological monitoring of the anticoagulant effect of the various available drugs is not mandatory for all agents. For UFH, the therapeutic window is narrow; thus, it requires frequent monitoring of its anticoagulant activity. Two different biomarkers are commonly used to monitor the activity of UFH. One is aPTT, which can be obtained at less than 1 hour, has an optimal target of 50 to 75 seconds, and corresponds to 1.5 to 2.5 times the upper limit of normal. Above these values, the risk of bleeding complications increases, without further antithrombotic benefits; below these values, the antithrombotic effect is insufficient. The second biomarker available is ACT, which can be used for monitoring of UFH during PCI, but has not been linked to an improved prognosis.

Enoxaparin can reliably be monitored by assessing the anti-Xa activity level in a standard chromogenic laboratory assay. Although data showed that with a standard protocol adjusted for weight and renal function (more than 90% of patients are in the therapeutic window), insufficient levels of anti-Xa during PCI of patients with ACS have been linked to an increased risk of death and ischemic events in the periprocedural period. There is no easy bedside approach to monitoring of enoxaparin. ACT is not discriminant enough for monitoring LMWH therapy. Tests (e.g., the Hemonox bedside test) were developed and validated in a cohort of patients,[6] but these tests have not been adopted into routine use in practice because the enoxaparin level is within the therapeutic window in 95% of patients.

Fondaparinux has no significant influence on the usual variables that monitor anticoagulant activity, such as aPTT, ACT, prothrombin, and thrombin times, and requires an adapted anti-Xa assay that uses an appropriate standard curve.

Bivalirudin plasma concentration correlates well with coagulation tests (aPTT and ACT), which can be used to monitor the anticoagulant activity of bivalirudin in the same manner as UFH. In the Randomized Evaluation in PCI Linking Angiomax to Reduced Clinical Events (REPLACE)-2 trial, it was mandated to check the ACT after the initial bivalirudin bolus, with an additional bolus in case of a low ACT. However, the pharmacokinetics and pharmacodynamics of bivalirudin are such that low ACTs were only found in 2% to 3% of the patients, and therefore, there is no need to routinely monitor the degree of anticoagulation for short-term use as an adjunct to PCI.

In summary, the only anticoagulant that routinely requires monitoring is UFH. However, meta-analyses have shown that the available bedside test for ACT has a poor correlation with ischemic or bleeding complications.

Reversal of Anticoagulant Therapy

Because bleeding remains an important complication of anticoagulation therapy, availability of an antidote is important to the physician. Protamine sulfate can be used in an equimolar concentration to inhibit UFH, and to a lesser degree, it inhibits the anticoagulant effect of enoxaparin. Protamine has no effect on fondaparinux or bivalirudin. Because of the short half-life of bivalirudin, waiting until the end of its effect after drug cessation is reasonable. In the case of fondaparinux, there is currently no available specific antidote. Recombinant factor VIIa has been recommended, but it is associated with an increased risk of thrombotic complications.

INITIAL ANTICOAGULANT THERAPY

ST-Elevation Myocardial Infarction Treated with Primary Percutaneous Intervention

Although extensively studied, anticoagulation during primary PCI remains controversial (see also Chapter 17). Patients undergoing primary PCI should receive a combination of dual antiplatelet therapy (see Chapter 19) with the combination of a parenteral anticoagulant. Fondaparinux carries a possible hazard related to catheter thrombosis, is not recommended as an anticoagulant in this setting, and is not discussed in this section. Three options are used to support primary PCI: UFH, bivalirudin, or enoxaparin, all administered intravenously. Professional society guidelines for anticoagulant therapy in STEMI treated with primary PCI are summarized in Table 18-3.

Unfractionated Heparin During Primary Percutaneous Coronary Intervention

An intravenous UFH bolus adapted to the concomitant use of a GPI and titrated to an appropriate ACT time is a familiar and well-tested strategy for initial anticoagulant therapy at the time of primary PCI for STEMI. UFH has a class I recommendation in both the American College of Cardiology Foundation (ACCF)/American Heart Association (AHA) and European Society of Cardiology (ESC) guidelines,[7] but it also has a level of evidence C because of the absence of placebo-controlled trials evaluating UFH in primary PCI. Dosing should follow standard recommendations for PCI (initial bolus 70 to 100 U/kg when no GPI is planned or 50 to 60 U/kg when the use of GPI is expected).

TABLE 18-3 Initial Anticoagulant Therapy Recommended to Support Primary Percutaneous Coronary Intervention

ANTICOAGULANT	AHA		ESC	
	COR	LOE	COR	LOE
UFH				
With GP IIb/IIIa inhibitor planned: 50–70 U/kg	I	C	I	C
Without GP IIb/IIIa inhibitor planned: 70–100 U/kg	I	C	I	C
Bivalirudin				
0.75 mg/kg IV bolus, then 1.75 mg/kg/h infusion with or without previous treatment by UFH. An additional bolus of 0.3 mg/kg can be given if needed. Reduce infusion to 1 mg/kg/h with estimated CrCl <30 mL/min.	I	B	IIa	A
Preferred over UFH with GP IIb/IIIa inhibitor in patients at high risk of bleeding	IIa	B		
Enoxaparin				
0.5 mg/kg IV bolus with or without GP IIb/IIIa inhibitor			IIa	B
Fondaparinux				
Not recommended as sole anticoagulant for primary PCI	III	B	III	B

COR, Class of recommendation; *CrCl*, creatinine clearance; *GP*, glycoprotein; *IV*, intravenous; *LOE*, level of evidence; *PCI*, percutaneous coronary intervention; *UFH*, unfractionated heparin.

Enoxaparin versus Unfractionated Heparin for Primary Percutaneous Coronary Intervention

Enoxaparin is generally not used in the United States as adjunctive therapy for primary PCI. Nevertheless, intravenous enoxaparin (0.5 mg/kg followed by prophylactic 40 mg SC) has been suggested by several nonrandomized studies and an international open-label randomized trial (ATOLL [Acute Myocardial Infarction Treated with Primary Angioplasty and Intravenous Enoxaparin or Unfractionated Heparin to Lower Ischaemic and Bleeding Events at Short- and Long-term Follow-up]) to possibly be more predictable and reliable than UFH in primary PCI.[8] The primary composite endpoint of 30-day death, complication of MI, procedural failure, and major bleeding was not significantly reduced (relative risk reduction 17%; p = .063). Prespecified exploratory analyses showed reductions in the main secondary endpoint of death, recurrent MI, or ACS or urgent revascularization, and in other secondary composite endpoints such as death, or resuscitated cardiac arrest, death, or complication of MI. Importantly, bleeding was not increased with enoxaparin versus UFH. In the exploratory per-protocol analysis of the ATOLL trial,[9] which was pertinent to more than 87% of the study population, IV enoxaparin was superior to UFH in reducing the primary endpoint (relative risk [RR], 0.76; 95% confidence interval [CI], 0.62 to 0.94; $P = .012$), ischemic endpoints, mortality (RR, 0.36; 95% CI, 0.18 to 0.74; $P = .003$), and major bleeding (RR, 0.46; 95% CI, 0.21 to 1.01; $P = .050$), which contributed to the improvement of the net clinical benefit (RR, 0.46; 95% CI, 0.3 to 0.74; $P = .0002$) in patients who underwent primary PCI.

In a systematic review and meta-analysis of enoxaparin versus UFH in PCI,[10] which regrouped nonrandomized studies, post hoc analysis of randomized trials, and the ATOLL randomized trial, 10,243 patients underwent primary PCI for STEMI with either enoxaparin or UFH (Figure 18-4). In this meta-analysis, enoxaparin was associated with a significant 48% RR reduction of mortality with an enoxaparin relative reduction (RR, 0.52; 95% CI, 0.42 to 0.64; $P < .001$), a reduction of death or MI (RR, 0.61; 95% CI, 0.47 to 0.79; $P < .001$), a reduction of complications of MI (RR, 0.70; 95% CI, 0.62 to 0.80; $P < .001$), and also a reduction in the incidence of major bleeding (RR, 0.72; 95% CI, 0.56 to 0.93; $P = .01$). Such results were corroborated by others.[11,12] In another meta-analysis, the combination of LMWH with a GPI was considered the first choice for efficacy and the third choice for safety behind bivalirudin and UFH (Table 18-4).[13] Authors also mentioned that the bleeding risk could be reduced by using a high-rate radial approach, as was used in ATOLL and in routine practice in most European countries (see also Chapter 17). This combination was considered by the authors of the meta-analysis to be the best approach, balancing efficacy with preserved safety (Figure 18-e1).[14]

Based on these considerations and on the clinical experience with enoxaparin in other PCI settings, enoxaparin is recommended as a reasonable alternative anticoagulant during primary PCI in the ESC guidelines (class IIa) and may be preferred over UFH (see Table 18-3). However, in the ACCF/AHA guidelines, enoxaparin does not appear as a choice for anticoagulation during STEMI treated with primary PCI (see Table 18-3).

Bivalirudin versus Unfractionated Heparin for Primary Percutaneous Coronary Intervention

Multiple randomized trials have evaluated bivalirudin in the primary PCI setting (Figure 18-5). After the initial findings of the HORIZONS-AMI (Harmonizing Outcomes with Revascularization and Stents in Acute Myocardial Infarction) trial (see Chapter 17),[15] bivalirudin was given a class I recommendation in international guidelines. Notably, bivalirudin was observed to have similar results in terms of ischemic events, an increase in early stent thrombosis, and a reduction of the primary endpoint because of the reduction of major bleeding compared with UFH, along with routine use of a GPI (Figures 18-6A and 18-6B). Subsequent trials have included control groups with contemporary $P2Y_{12}$ antagonists and without routine use of a GPI.

The open-label EUROMAX (European Ambulance Acute Coronary Syndrome Angiography) trial[16] compared a strategy of prehospital bivalirudin with heparin (mostly UFH) with a

Study	No. needed to treat	No. of events/No. in group: Enoxaparin	No. of events/No. in group: Unfractionated heparin	Relative risk (95% CI) random	P value	Cochran Q for heterogeneity
All PCIs						
Death	60	278/13,943	622/17,023	0.66 (0.57 to 0.76)	<0.001	0.46
Death or MI	50	836/11,924	1351/14,968	0.68 (0.57 to 0.81)	<0.001	0.42
Complications of MI	66	765/13,943	1135/17,023	0.75 (0.66 to 0.85)	<0.001	0.55
Major bleeding	83	295/13,852	564/16,923	0.80 (0.68 to 0.95)	0.009	0.58
Minor bleeding	-	718/13,150	793/13,669	0.92 (0.74 to 1.14)	0.45	0.21
Primary PCI for STEMI						
Death	34	112/3590	401/6653	0.52 (0.42 to 0.64)	<0.001	0.53
Death or MI	28	139/3590	499/6653	0.56 (0.42 to 0.76)	<0.001	0.50
Complications of MI	68	96/3590	275/6653	0.76 (0.60 to 0.96)	0.022	0.80
Major bleeding	53	92/3499	298/6553	0.72 (0.56 to 0.93)	0.01	0.69
Minor bleeding	-	138/3216	177/4372	0.94 (0.60 to 1.47)	0.78	0.56

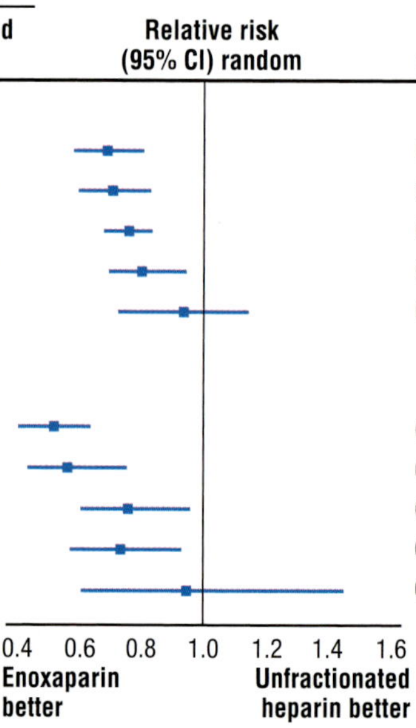

FIGURE 18-4 **Meta-analysis of enoxaparin versus unfractionated heparin in percutaneous coronary intervention (PCI) in all settings and in ST-elevation myocardial infarction (STEMI).** *CI,* Confidence interval. *(From Silvain J, et al: Efficacy and safety of enoxaparin versus unfractionated heparin during percutaneous coronary intervention: systematic review and meta-analysis.* BMJ *344:e553,2012.)*

lower use of GPIs (69%) in the heparin group. Bivalirudin was associated with a 40% reduction in death after non–coronary artery bypass graft (CABG) major bleeding at 30 days, but the mortality benefit observed in the HORIZONS-AMI trial was not confirmed by EUROMAX, and an excess of stent thrombosis was confirmed despite prolonged infusion of bivalirudin and the use of novel $P2Y_{12}$ inhibitors in more than one-half of the patients. The increase in acute stent thrombosis was paralleled by a trend toward a higher rate of reinfarction (1.7% vs. 0.9%, respectively; RR, 1.93; 95% CI, 0.90 to 4.14; $P = .08$).

A third randomized trial, HEAT-PCI (How Effective are Antithrombotic Therapies in PPCI) compared bivalirudin and UFH in all comers with STEMI who were scheduled to undergo primary PCI.[17] The study was representative of contemporary practice, with symmetrical and low use of GPIs in both arms (15%), frequent use of novel $P2Y_{12}$ inhibitors (89%), and a high rate of radial approach to lower procedure-related major bleeding events. In this trial, UFH was superior to bivalirudin with respect to the primary composite of all-cause mortality, stroke, recurrent infarction, and unplanned target lesion revascularization, with higher ischemic events in the bivalirudin group compared with the UFH group (8.7% vs. 5.7%, respectively; hazard ratio [HR], 1.52; 95% CI, 1.09 to 2.13; $P = .01$), including an increase in stent thrombosis (3.4% vs. 0.9%; RR, 3.91; 95% CI, 1.61 to 9.52; $P = .001$). Major bleeding was not reduced by bivalirudin (3.5% vs. 3.1%; $P = .59$).

The BRAVE (Bavarian Reperfusion Alternatives Evaluation 4) randomized trial[18] examined whether a strategy of prasugrel plus bivalirudin was superior to a strategy with clopidogrel plus UFH in primary PCI patients. No differences were found in the primary endpoint because the trial was interrupted because of slow patient recruitment. In the Chinese Bivalirudin in Acute Myocardial Infarction vs Heparin and GPI Plus Heparin Trial (BRIGHT) trial (n = 2194 patients), three arms were compared, bivalirudin with a post-PCI infusion of 1.75 mg/kg per hour for a median duration of 3 hours (n = 735), heparin alone (n = 729), or heparin plus tirofiban with a post-PCI infusion (n = 730). At 30 days, bivalirudin resulted in a decrease in major adverse coronary events (MACE) compared with both heparin alone and heparin plus tirofiban (8.8% vs. 13.2% vs. 17%, respectively), primarily because of a reduction in bleeding events, including minor bleeding with bivalirudin (4.1% vs. 7.5% vs. 12.3%, respectively) without significant differences in major adverse cardiac cerebral events, or stent thrombosis.[19]

Lastly, the Minimizing Adverse Haemorrhagic Events by Transradial Access Site and Systemic Implementation of AngioX: Bivalirudin vs. Heparin (MATRIX) trial (n = 7213 patients) found that bivalirudin was not statistically superior to UFH at 30 days for both co-primary endpoints of death, MI, or stroke (MACE) and net adverse clinical events (death, MI, or stroke and non-CABG bleeding). Several secondary endpoints, including major bleeding (1.4% vs. 2.5%; $P = .001$) and all-cause death (1.7% vs. 2.3%; $P = .042$) favored bivalirudin. Ultimately, GPI was administrated to 4.6% of the bivalirudin group and to 25.8% of the UFH group. However, definite stent thrombosis was more common in the bivalirudin-treated patients (1.0% vs. 0.6%; $P = .048$). In MATRIX, bivalirudin was dosed according to drug labeling, which included a prolonged infusion according to operator discretion.

Thus, when all the trials and various meta-analyses are put into perspective, bivalirudin without a GPI is associated with an increased risk of stent thrombosis and subsequent MI, but it has a reduction in bleeding that is most apparent compared with UFH plus routine use of GPIs.[20] The resulting effect on mortality is inconsistent. The ESC and European Association for Cardio-Thoracic Surgery downgraded the recommendation for bivalirudin from class I to IIa in patients with STEMI undergoing PCI in the 2014 guidelines on myocardial revascularization. The 2013 ACCF/AHA guidelines for management of STEMI provide a class I recommendation for bivalirudin as an alternative for anticoagulation during primary PCI (see Table 18-3).

ST-Elevation Myocardial Infarction Treated with Fibrinolysis

The potential benefits of acute therapy with anticoagulants in STEMI treated with fibrinolysis are multiple, including facilitating more rapid and durable patency of the infarct-related artery, and prevention of venous thromboembolism. Nevertheless, the data from clinical trials have engendered debate over the clinical benefit of anticoagulants as part of acute therapy. In particular, as reperfusion therapy has evolved, the relevance of data from previous clinical trials has become less certain. However, placebo-controlled data

TABLE 18-4 Ranking for Efficacy and Safety of Different Anticoagulant Regimens

ANTICOAGULANT PRACTICE	2013 ACC/AHA Guidelines	2014 ESC Guidelines	RANKING FOR EFFICACY OR SAFETY		
			MACE	Major Bleeding	Considerations for Current
Unfractionated heparin + GPI	COR I	COR I	Second	Fourth	Likely worse bleeding with newer $P2Y_{12}$ inhibitors. Bleeding risk somewhat mitigated with transradial procedure.
LMWH + GPI	None	COR IIa	First	Third	Likely worse bleeding with newer $P2Y_{12}$ inhibitors. Bleeding risk somewhat mitigated with transradial procedure.
Unfractionated heparin without GPI	COR I	COR I	Fourth	Second	Likely improved MACE with newer $P2Y_{12}$, but may negate bleeding advantage.
Bivalirudin	COR I	COR IIa	Third	First	Likely improved MACE with newer $P2Y_{12}$ inhibitors, but may negate bleeding advantage. Preferred over unfractionated heparin + GPI in those at high risk of bleeding (COR IIa).
Fondaparinux	COR III	COR III	Fifth	Fifth	Should not be recommend based on current data.

COR, Class of recommendation; *GPI*, glycoprotein IIb/IIIa inhibitor; *LMWH*, low–molecular-weight heparin; *MACE*, major adverse cardiovascular event.
From Bangalore S, et al: Anticoagulant therapy during primary percutaneous coronary intervention for acute myocardial infarction: a meta-analysis of randomized trials in the era of stents and P2Y12 inhibitors. BMJ *349:g6419, 2014.*

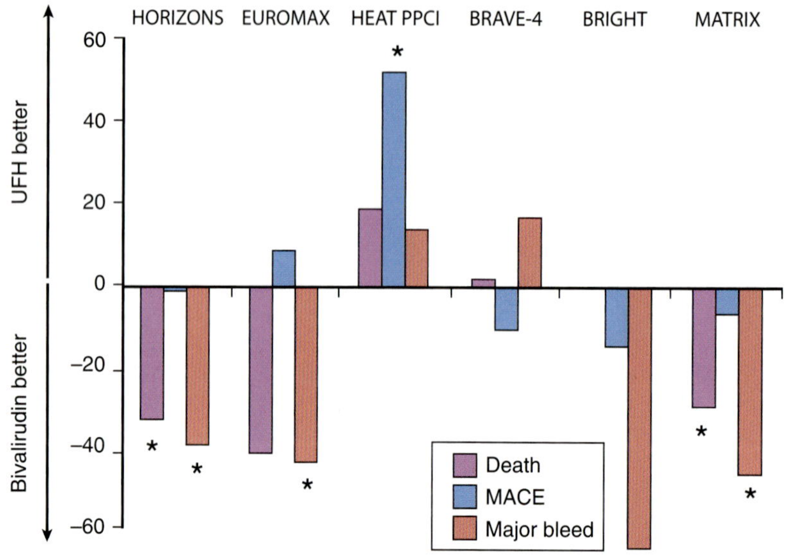

FIGURE 18-5 Summary of clinical trials of bivalirudin. *Significant result. *Bars* indicate relative differences. For the BRIGHT trial, only the comparison between unfractionated heparin (UFH) and bivalirudin alone was used. *MACE*, Major adverse cardiovascular events.

with LMWHs used as an adjunct to contemporary reperfusion regimens have provided additional support for acute administration of anticoagulants in patients with STEMI treated with fibrinolytics. As such, current professional society guidelines recommend that adequate anticoagulation therapies need to be administered during and after fibrinolysis to optimize patency, and should preferably be given until revascularization (if performed) (Tables 18-5 and 18-6). Anticoagulation should be given for at least 48 hour after fibrinolysis for a maximum of 1 week.

Unfractionated Heparin as an Adjunct to Fibrinolysis

In trials performed before the introduction of fibrinolytic therapy or the widespread and routine use of acetylsalicylic acid, early administration of IV UFH reduced venous thromboembolic events, stroke, and re-infarction. Subsequent trials in the reperfusion era are challenging to interpret in light of the important differences regarding the use of aspirin, the type of fibrinolytic used, and the dose of UFH administered. Meta-analyses of randomized trials in which patients received fibrinolysis have failed to show a clear benefit of UFH compared with placebo for the reduction of reinfarction or death. Nonetheless, overall, data from clinical trials at least raise the possibility that adjunctive therapy with UFH may enhance late patency after the administration of fibrin-specific fibrinolytics. In the absence of randomized clinical trials designed to detect differences in clinical events, expert guidelines have concluded (class IIa) that it is judicious to use heparin for ≥48 hours with fibrin-specific fibrinolytics.

If used, the recommended dose of UFH is an IV bolus of 60 U/kg (maximum of 4000 IU) followed by an IV infusion of 12 U/kg (maximum of 1000 U/h for 24 to 48 hours). If administered during fibrinolysis, careful dosing and close monitoring is mandatory (at 3, 6, 12, and 24 hours), with a target aPTT of 50 to 70 seconds, because high values of aPTT (>70 seconds) need to be avoided because they are associated with a higher likelihood of bleeding, reinfarction, and death.

Low–Molecular-Weight Heparin as an Adjunct to Fibrinolysis

In contrast to the uncertain evidence with UFH, trials of LMWHs have demonstrated a clear benefit compared with placebo and UFH, and have supported LMWHs as the treatment of choice for adjunctive anticoagulant therapy with fibrinolytics. Specifically, placebo-controlled studies with LMWH have confirmed the importance of an adjuvant anticoagulant strategy in fibrinolysis therapy with improvement of patency, ST-segment resolution, and composite endpoints of death, reinfarction and recurrent angina, or stroke weighed against an increase of major bleeding.

In the ASSENT 3 (Assessment of the Safety and Efficacy of a New Thrombolytic 3) trial, enoxaparin compared with UFH resulted in a similar rate of reperfusion of the infarct artery, but it reduced rates of reocclusion, reinfarction, or recurrent ischemic events. In the Enoxaparin and Thrombolysis Reperfusion for Acute Myocardial Infarction Treatment Thrombolysis in Myocardial Infarction (ExTRACT-TIMI)-25 trial (n = 20,475 patients), enoxaparin significantly reduced death or reinfarction balanced against an increase in major bleeding events. The benefits of enoxaparin over UFH are evident, regardless of the type of fibrinolytic administered (streptokinase or fibrin-specific), and the benefits can reach a wide range of patient subgroups. The recommended dose is a 30-mg IV bolus followed 15 minutes later by 1 mg/kg SC twice daily (with a maximum of 100 mg for the first two doses) until hospital discharge for a maximum of 8 days; however, a lower dose of enoxaparin needs to be given to patients older than 75 years of age (no bolus and 0.75 mg/kg SC twice daily, with a maximum of 75 mg for the first two doses) and to those with impaired renal function (estimated creatinine clearance <30 mL/min) with SC doses given only once every 24 hours.

Fondaparinux as an Adjunct to Fibrinolysis

Fondaparinux reduces the rate of reocclusion of the infarct-related artery. Moreover, in the large OASIS 6 trial (n = 12,092 patients), fondaparinux was superior to placebo with respect to the rate of death or reinfarction (HR, 0.79; 95% CI, 0.68 to 0.92) and was not superior to UFH in fibrinolytic-treated patients (HR, 0.96; 95% CI, 0.81 to 1.13). Nevertheless, the trial established the efficacy of an antithrombin, and compared with UFH, fondaparinux offered an attractive alternative with the convenience of once-daily SC injections (2.5 mg once daily for up to 8 days). However, its use is complicated by the need for co-administration of an additional

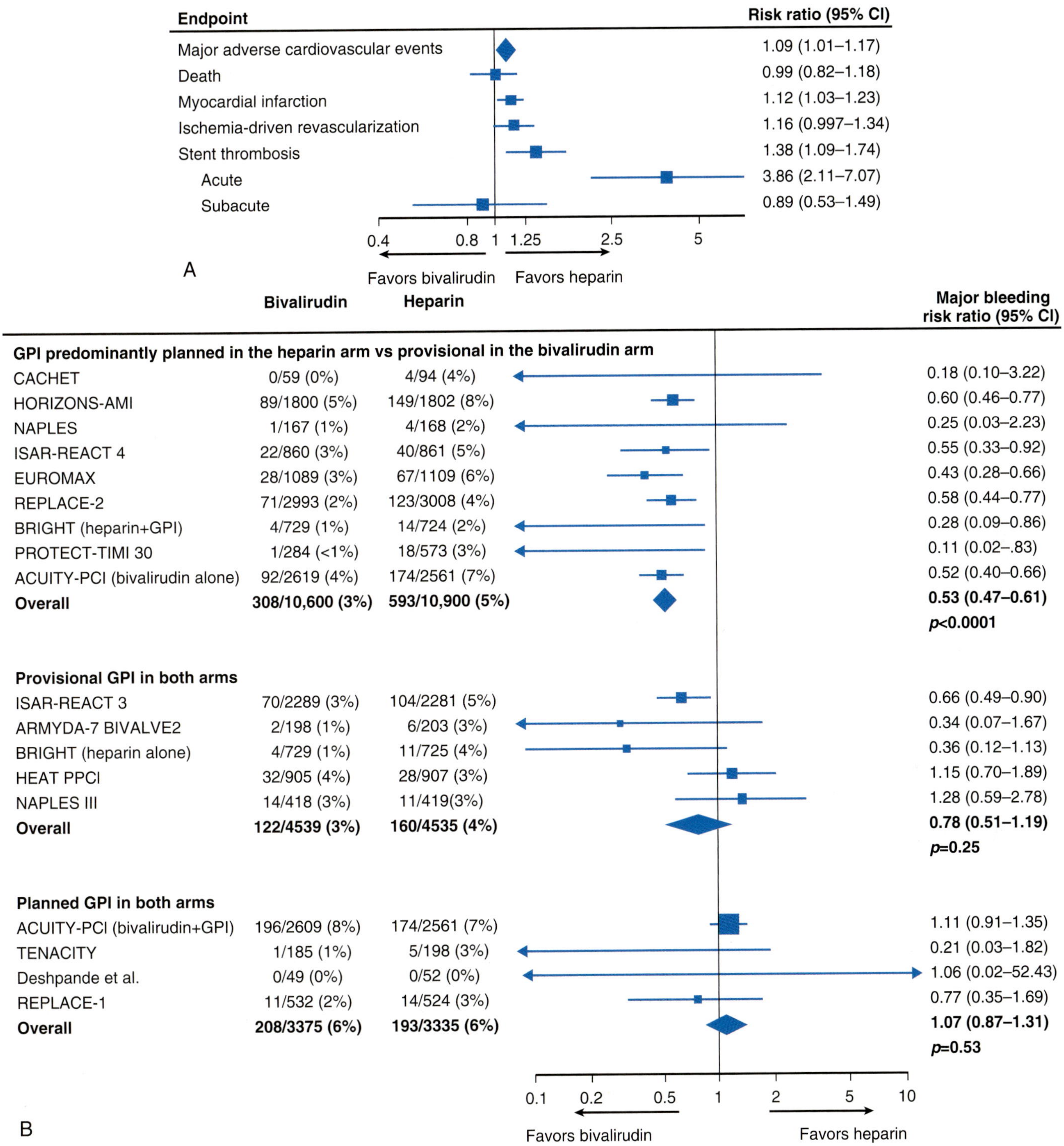

FIGURE 18-6 (**A**) Meta-analysis of studies of bivalirudin versus unfractionated heparin (UFH) on major cardiovascular events. (**B**) Meta-analysis of studies of bivalirudin versus UFH on major bleeding stratified by the use of platelet glycoprotein IIb/IIIa inhibitors (GPI) in the control arm. *CI*, Confidence interval. *(From Cavender MA, Sabatine MS: Bivalirudin versus heparin in patients planned for percutaneous coronary intervention: a meta-analysis of randomized controlled trials.* Lancet *384:599–606, 2014.)*

antithrombin with anti-IIa activity if PCI is to be performed. Fondaparinux should not be given as the sole anticoagulant to patients referred for PCI and is contraindicated for patients with a creatinine clearance of less than 30 mL/min.

Bivalirudin as an Adjunct to Fibrinolysis

The direct thrombin inhibitors hirudin and bivalirudin were compared with UFH in several randomized trials of patients with STEMI who underwent fibrinolysis (GUSTO IIb, n = 2274; HIT-4, n = 1208; and HERO-2, n = 17,073), all of which showed a reduction in the incidence of recurrent MI by 25% to 30% compared with UFH without improving mortality. In GUSTO IIb, hirudin lowered 30-day death and/or reinfarction (8.6% vs. 14.4%; $P = .004$) in conjunction with streptokinase, but it did not confer a benefit in patients treated with tissue-type plasminogen activator. In addition, at the doses studied, both hirudin and bivalirudin resulted in higher rates of major bleeding, including intracranial bleeding, versus UFH when

TABLE 18-5 Initial Anticoagulant Therapy to Support Reperfusion with Fibrinolytic Therapy

ANTICOAGULANT	AHA COR	AHA LOE	ESC COR	ESC LOE
Enoxaparin • If age <75 yrs, 30-mg IV bolus followed in 15 min by 1 mg/kg subcutaneously every 12 h (max 100 mg for the first 2 doses) • If age >75 yrs, no bolus, 0.75 mg/kg subcutaneously every 12 h (max 75 mg for the first 2 doses) • Regardless of age, if CrCl <30 mL/min, 1 mg/kg subcutaneously every 24 h • Duration: for the index hospitalization, up to 8 days or until revascularization	I	A	I	A
UFH • IV bolus of 60 U/kg (max, 4000 U) followed by infusion of 12 U/kg/h (max 1000 U) initially, adjusted to maintain aPTT at 1.5–2.0 times control for 48 h or until revascularization	I	C	I	C
Fondaparinux • Initial dose 2.5 mg IV, then 2.5 mg subcutaneously daily starting the following day, for the index hospitalization, up to 8 days or until revascularization • Contraindicated if CrCl <30 mL/min	I	B	IIa	B

aPTT, Activated partial prothrombin time; *COR*, class of recommendation; *CrCl*, creatinine clearance; *IV*, intravenous; *LOE*, level of evidence; *UFH*, unfractionated heparin.

TABLE 18-6 Adjunctive Antithrombotic Therapy to Support Rescue Percutaneous Coronary Intervention after Fibrinolytic Therapy

ANTICOAGULATION THERAPY	AHA COR	AHA LOE
Enoxaparin Continue through PCI • No additional drug if last dose was within previous 8h • 0.3 mg/kg IV bolus if last dose was 8 to 12 h earlier	I	B
UFH Continue through PCI, administering IV boluses as needed to maintain therapeutic ACT depending on use of GP IIb/IIIa receptor antagonist	I	C
Fondaparinux As sole anticoagulant for PCI	III	C

ACT, Activated clotting time; *COR*, class of recommendation; *GP*, glycoprotein; *IV*, intravenous; *LOE*, level of evidence; *PCI*, percutaneous coronary intervention; *UFH*, unfractionated heparin.

used in conjunction with fibrinolytic agents. Bivalirudin has not been studied with fibrin-specific agents.

In patients with a known history of HIT, it is possible to consider bivalirudin as a useful alternative to heparin to be used in conjunction with streptokinase (class IIa recommendation). Dosing according to the HERO 2 regimen (a bolus of 0.25 mg/kg followed by an IV infusion of 0.5 mg/kg per hour for the first 12 hours and 0.25 mg/kg per hour for the subsequent 36 hours) is recommended, but with a reduction in the infusion rate if the aPTT is longer than 75 seconds within the first 12 hours.

Anticoagulant Therapy in Non–ST-Elevation Myocardial Infarction

In addition to antiplatelet therapy, an anticoagulant should be added in patients with NSTEMI as soon as possible after presentation.[21,22] Anticoagulation is effective in addition to platelet inhibition, and the combination of the two is more effective than either treatment alone.[23,24] Several options are available (class I recommendation) for the treatment of NSTEMI (UFH, enoxaparin, fondaparinux, and bivalirudin). Selections of the optimal regimen are based on considerations of the strategy used (invasive or medical conservative), the ease of use, and the cost. Importantly, pretreatment with an anticoagulant should not delay angiography and revascularization. A general rule is to avoid crossover between antithrombins (with the exception of adding UFH to fondaparinux), especially between UFH and LMWH, and to discontinue anticoagulation after PCI in most cases. An overview of the anticoagulation therapy in NSTEMI is summarized in Figure 18-7, and professional society recommendations for anticoagulation in NSTEMI are summarized in Table 18-7.

Unfractionated Heparin in Treatment of Non–ST-Elevation Myocardial Infarction

Anticoagulation, traditionally with UFH, has been a cornerstone of therapy for patients with NSTEMI. A meta-analysis that re-grouped six trials comparing UFH versus placebo or untreated controls showed a 33% risk reduction in death and MI (odds ratio [OR], 0.67; 95% CI, 0.45 to 0.99; $P = .04$),[24] with a reduction in MI accounting for practically all of the beneficial effect. The benefit was observed at the cost of an increased risk of bleeding. In initial therapy, a recommend weight-adjusted bolus of UFH (60 U/kg) followed by continued infusion of 12 U/kg per hour is recommended, with frequent monitoring (every 6 hours until the target range is reached and every 12 to 24 hours thereafter) and adjustment of dose if necessary.

In the PCI setting, UFH is given as an IV bolus either under ACT guidance (ACT in the range of 250 to 350 seconds) or in a weight-adjusted manner (usually 70 to 100 IU/kg). Doses need to be lower if GPIs are used. Because of marked variability in UFH bioavailability, ACT-guided dosing is necessary and recommended, especially for prolonged procedures, when additional dosing may be required. Monitoring of the anticoagulant response by aPTT can also be made according to a standardized nomogram, aiming for an aPTT of 50 to 70 seconds or 1.5 to 2.5 times control. If the patient is already treated with an ongoing IV infusion of UFH, an additional IV bolus of UFH should be adapted according to the ACT values. HIT is particularly high in patients with use of UFH and more common with longer durations of treatment.

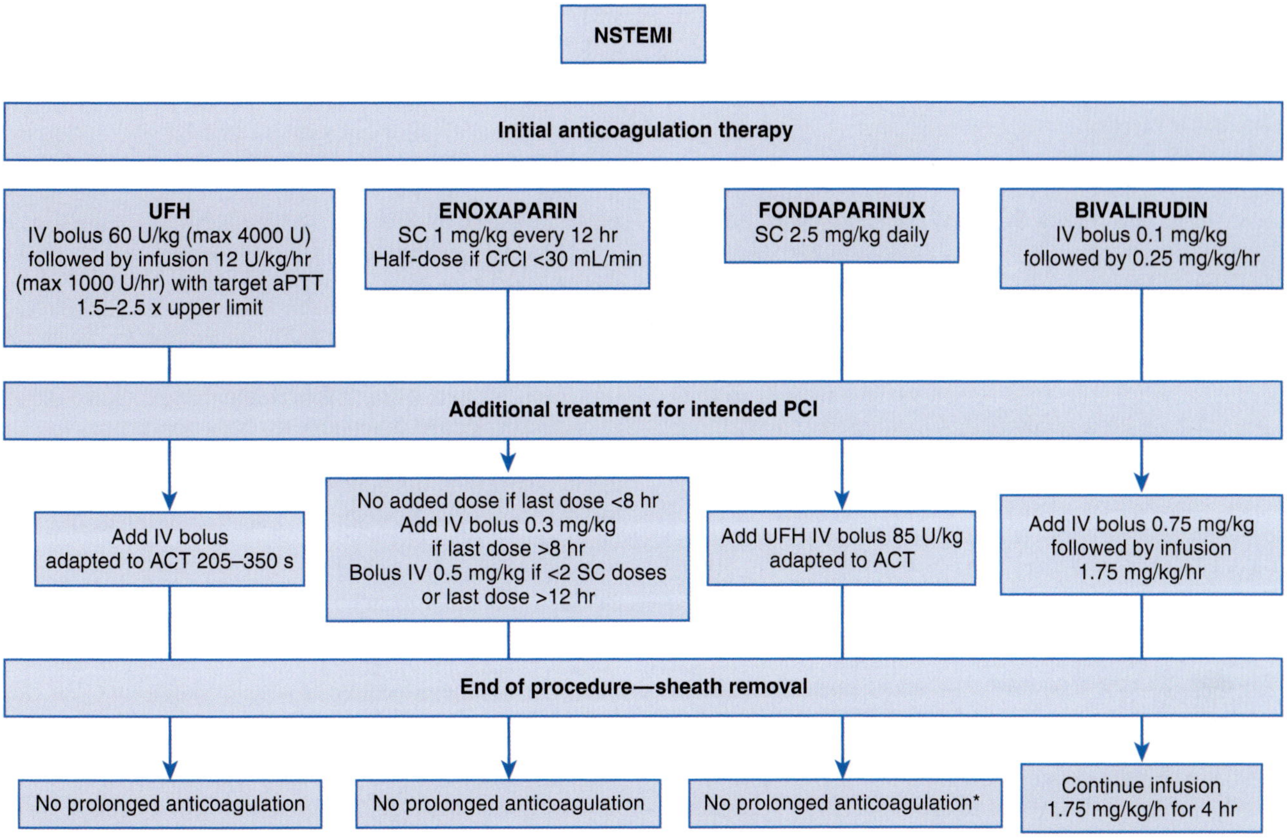

*In OASIS 5 fondaparinux was continued for 5 days in average

FIGURE 18-7 **Summary of the administration of anticoagulation therapy in non–ST-elevation myocardial infarction (NSTEMI).** *ACT*, Activated coagulation time; *aPTT*, activated partial thromboplastin time; *CrCl*, creatinine clearance; *IV*, intravenous; *PCI*, percutaneous coronary intervention; *SC*, subcutaneous; *UFH*, unfractionated heparin.

TABLE 18-7 Recommended Anticoagulant Therapy in Non–ST-Elevation Myocardial Infarction

ANTICOAGULANT THERAPY IN PATIENTS WITH NSTE-ACS UNDERGOING PCI	ACC		ESC	
	COR	LOE	COR	LOE
Anticoagulation is recommended for all patients in addition to antiplatelet therapy during PCI	I	C	I	A
Anticoagulation is selected according to both ischemic and bleeding risks, and according to the efficacy–safety profile of chosen agent			I	C
IV UFH is useful in patients with NSTE-ACS undergoing PCI	I	C		
Bivalirudin (0.75 mg/kg bolus, followed by 1.75 mg/kg/h for up to 4 hr after procedure) is recommended as alternative to UFH + GPI during PCI	I	B	I	A
UFH is recommended as anticoagulant in patients undergoing PCI who did not receive any anticoagulant			I	B
In patients with NSTE-ACS undergoing PCI who are at high risk of bleeding, it is reasonable to use bivalirudin monotherapy in preference to UFH + GPI	IIa	B		
In patients on fondaparinux (2.5 mg/day daily SC), a single bolus UFH (85 U/kg, or 60 U/kg in the case of concomitant use of GPI) is indicated during PCI	I	B	I	B
An additional dose of 0.3 mg/kg IV enoxaparin should be administered at the time of PCI to patients with NSTE-ACS who have received <2 therapeutic SC doses or received last SC dose 8–12 hr before PCI	I	B		
Enoxaparin should be considered as anticoagulant for PCI in patients pretreated with subcutaneous enoxaparin	IIb	B	IIa	B
Discontinuation of anticoagulation should be considered after an invasive procedure unless otherwise indicated	I	C	IIa	C
Fondaparinux should not be used as the sole anticoagulant to support to PCI in patients with NSTE-ACS because of an increased risk of catheter thrombosis	III	B		
Crossover of UFH and LMWH is not recommended			III	B

COR, Class of recommendation; *GPI*, glycoprotein IIa/IIIb inhibitors; *IV*, intravenous; *LMWH*, low-molecular-weight heparin; *LOE*, level of evidence; *NSTE-ACS*, non–ST-elevation-acute coronary syndrome; *PCI*, percutaneous coronary intervention; *SC*, subcutaneous; *UFH*, unfractionated heparin.

Both monitoring and safety (bleeding and HIT) are the major drawbacks of this traditional anticoagulant therapy.

Low–Molecular-Weight Heparin in Non–ST-Elevation Myocardial Infarction

LMWHs, including enoxaparin, have proven effective in the medical management of NSTEMI. The standard dose of enoxaparin is 1 mg/kg SC every 12 hours, with adaptation to once daily for patients with a creatinine clearance of less than 30 mL/min. When added to aspirin, enoxaparin leads to a 66% reduction in death or MI. In a meta-analysis of 21,945 NSTE-ACS patients, enoxaparin yielded a statistically significant 10% reduction in the odds of death or MI at 30 days compared with UFH (OR, 0.90; 95% CI, 0.81 to 0.99; P = .043).[25] In a meta-analysis that examined only patients managed invasively (n = 30,966), enoxaparin reduced death (RR, 0.66; 95% CI, 0.57 to 0.76; P < .001), the composite of death or MI (RR, 0.68; 95% CI, 0.57 to 0.81; P < .001), complications of MI (RR, 0.75; 95% CI, 0.6 to 0.85; P < .001), and the incidence of major bleeding (RR, 0.80; 95% CI, 0.68 to 0.95; P = .009). However, in the largest trial (SYNERGY; N = 9978) to evaluate enoxaparin among patients with NSTE-ACS who were managed invasively, enoxaparin was not superior to UFH, but it was noninferior (RR, 0.96; 95% CI, 0.86 to 1.06). Enoxaparin was a safe and effective alternative to UFH, with a modest excess of major bleeding. In light of these data, enoxaparin is an alternative for anticoagulation in all patients with NSTEMI (see Table 18-7) and is favored in the ACCF/AHA guidelines for patients who are managed noninvasively.

Pharmacodynamics of Enoxaparin and the Invasive Strategy

Enoxaparin pharmacology was well studied and is quite predictable because of its pharmacological proprieties and its renal elimination. The IV use of enoxaparin has a different pharmacokinetic or pharmacodynamic profile from SC use (Figure 18-e2). The doses tested in clinical trials were generally lower than SC doses (0.5 and 0.75 mg/kg) and reached the same peak of anti-Xa activity than the SC injection, but this occurred within 3 minutes for a duration of 2 hours in comparison with 2 hours for the SC dose, which lasts for 8 to 12 hours. IV enoxaparin was tested in the STEEPLE (Safety and Efficacy of Intravenous Enoxaparin in Elective Percutaneous Coronary Intervention: an International Randomized Evaluation) study (n = 3528 patients), which showed lower bleeding rates with 0.5 and 0.75 mg/kg compared with UFH in non-ACS patients. The trial was not powered to detect a difference in efficacy between enoxaparin groups, but the lower dose of 0.5 mg/kg exhibited a lower rate of bleeding and is the dose adopted in clinical practice in centers where enoxaparin is used. In NSTE-ACS patients pretreated with enoxaparin, no additional enoxaparin is recommended during PCI if the last SC enoxaparin injection was administered less than 8 hours before PCI. An additional 0.3 mg/kg IV bolus is recommended if the last SC enoxaparin injection was administered more than 8 hours before PCI. A full dose of enoxaparin 0.5 mg/kg IV is recommended if the last dose was more than 12 hours before, if the patients did not receive two SC doses, or if the delays are unknown.

Fondaparinux in Non–ST-Elevation Myocardial Infarction

In ACS, a 2.5-mg fixed daily dose of fondaparinux is an alternative (class I) as the initial anticoagulation therapy. In the OASIS 5 trial (n = 20,078) of NSTE-ACS patients, fondaparinux was compared with SC enoxaparin 1 mg/kg twice daily for a maximum of 8 days (average 5.2 days vs. 5.4 days, respectively), which is unusually long. The primary efficacy outcome (death, MI, or refractory ischemia at 9 days) was similar in both groups (5.7% for enoxaparin vs. 5.8% for fondaparinux; HR, 1.01; 95% CI, 0.90 to 1.13), fulfilling the criteria for noninferiority. Compared with enoxaparin, fondaparinux reduced major bleeding by 48% (2.2% vs. 4.1%; HR, 0.52; 95% CI, 0.44 to 0.61; P < .001). A reduction in mortality with fondaparinux at 30 days (2.9% vs. 3.5%; HR, 0.83; 95% CI, 0.71 to 0.97; P = .02) and at 6 months (5.8% vs. 6.5%; HR, 0.89; 95% CI, 0.80 to 1.00; P = .05) has been ascribed to the reduction in major bleeding. Of note with respect to the design of the comparator (enoxaparin) in the trial, it is possible that excessive dosing of enoxaparin occurred because no dose adjustment was made in the older adults or in patients with renal failure. Moreover, a full dose of UFH was administered in the catheter laboratory for PCI; this was a strategy associated with more bleeding in another trial (SYNERGY).

Despite the demonstrated efficacy for medical therapy, fondaparinux is associated with a higher rate of abrupt vessel closure and unexpected angiographic thrombus than UFH or enoxaparin. In the PCI population in OASIS-5, catheter thrombus occurred more frequently with fondaparinux (0.9%) than with enoxaparin (0.4%). This excess appears to be avoided by a bolus of UFH at the time of PCI. As a consequence, professional guidelines recommend that fondaparinux should not be used as a sole anticoagulant for patients undergoing PCI. The optimal dose of UFH to be administered during PCI in patients initially treated with fondaparinux was investigated in the FUTURA/OASIS-8 (Fondaparinux Trial With Unfractionated Heparin During Revascularization in Acute Coronary Syndromes) trial (n = 2026 patients), and the standard dose was found to be 85 IU/kg adjusted by ACT.[28]

Direct Thrombin Inhibitors

Overall, bivalirudin offers similar efficacy while significantly lowering the risk of major bleeding compared with heparin plus systematic GPIs for patients with NSTE-ACS who are undergoing PCI. In NSTE-ACS patients, bivalirudin is recommended at a low dose of 0.1 mg/kg IV bolus, followed by an infusion of 0.25 mg/kg per hour until PCI, and the dose must be changed for urgent or elective PCI to a 0.75 mg/kg IV bolus followed by 1.75 mg/kg per hour infusion. ACUITY was an open-label trial that tested bivalirudin specifically in the setting of NSTE-ACS (n = 13,819) planned for an invasive strategy. There was no significant difference between standard heparin plus systematic GPIs and the combination of bivalirudin plus systematic GPIs for the composite ischemia endpoint at 30 days (7.3% vs. 7.7%, respectively; RR, 1.07; 95% CI, 0.92 to 1.23; P = .39) or for major bleeding (5.7% vs. 5.3%; RR, 0.93; 95% CI, 0.78 to 1.10; P = .38). An arm of the trial with bivalirudin alone was noninferior to heparin plus systematic GPIs with respect to the composite ischemia endpoint (7.8% vs. 7.3%; RR, 1.08; 95% CI, 0.93 to 1.24; P = .32), but it was associated with a significantly lower rate of major bleeding (3.0% vs. 5.7%; RR, 0.53; 95% CI, 0.43 to 0.65; P < .001), which translated into better 30-day net clinical outcome (combining efficacy and bleeding endpoints).

However, in patients who were not pretreated with clopidogrel before PCI, a significant excess of ischemic endpoints was observed (9.1% vs. 7.1%; RR, 1.29; 95% CI, 1.03 to 1.63) with bivalirudin alone compared with heparin and GPI. The ISAR-REACT 3 trial (n = 4750 stable and unstable patients) compared UFH and bivalirudin in patients who had received 600 mg of clopidogrel. A reduced rate of major bleeding with bivalirudin was offset by an increase in ischemic events. However, patients in the heparin group received a bolus of 140 U/kg of heparin, which is twice the current recommended dose. For NSTEMI patients who underwent PCI, the ISAR-REACT 4 trial presented additional evidence in favor of the safety of bivalirudin in terms of bleeding compared with a combination of UFH and GPIs (abciximab).[26] It should be noted that most of the evidence in support of bivalirudin is derived from trials in which the comparator was either high doses of UFH or UFH plus systematic use of GPIs, which is a combination that is no longer routinely applied.

Myocardial Infarction Treated Without Reperfusion Therapy

In OASIS-6, fondaparinux was superior to UFH in a subgroup of 1641 STEMI patients who did not receive reperfusion therapy, which demonstrated a reduction of the composite of death or recurrent MI without an increase in severe bleeding.[27] In the TETAMI study (n = 1224) enoxaparin showed a similar nonsignificant trend compared with UFH. Therefore, anticoagulation with fondaparinux and enoxaparin in patients with nonreperfused MI (STEMI or non-STEMI) is a reasonable option. If PCI is needed in a patient receiving fondaparinux, IV UFH should be administered during the procedure, using the same doses as for primary PCI, to minimize the risk of catheter thrombosis.[28]

HIGH-RISK POPULATIONS

Dose Adjustment in Older Adult Patients

Despite the high proportion of older adult patients in registries, theses patients are often excluded from trials of NSTE-ACS. Even when older adult patients are recruited into clinical trials, those randomized have substantially less comorbidities than the patients encountered in daily clinical practice. Thus, the applicability of findings from clinical trials to older adult patients encountered in routine clinical practice may be questionable. Older adult patients are at a higher risk of bleeding with antiplatelet agents and anticoagulants; however, they have the largest benefit, in terms of both relative and absolute risk reductions.[29] Moreover, because of more prevalent renal dysfunction in older adult patients, they are more frequently exposed to excessive doses of antithrombotic drugs with renal excretion (enoxaparin, fondaparinux, and bivalirudin). Patients in whom an invasive strategy was chosen should be scheduled for rapid angiography to avoid drug accumulation and shorten exposure time. Another safe alternative is to use the IV bolus of enoxaparin, which avoids accumulation.

Renal Insufficiency

Renal dysfunction is present in 30% to 40% of patients with ACS. Chronic kidney disease (CKD) is an independent predictor of short- and long-term mortality and of major bleeding in patients with ACS. Such high-risk patients benefit even more than non-CKD patients from optimal pharmacotherapy.[30,31] However, caution is needed because they also carry a high bleeding risk because of comorbidities and antithrombotic overexposure. Anticoagulants (including enoxaparin, fondaparinux, and bivalirudin) with exclusive or substantial renal elimination need to be down-titrated or might even be contraindicated in CKD patients. In the case of severe renal failure (clearance <30 mL/min), when fondaparinux or enoxaparin are contraindicated, UFH should be used. However, in the GRACE registry, an increase in the risk of bleeding with declining renal function was observed with UFH, similar to that observed with LMWH.

Heparin-Induced Thrombocytopenia

In patients with a history of HIT, neither UFH nor LMWH should be used, because of concerns about cross reactivity. In these cases, bivalirudin is the best option for anticoagulation; other possible options are fondaparinux, argatroban, hirudin, lepirudin, and danaparoid.

SUMMARY

The critical role of the coagulation cascade in acute ischemic heart disease draws attention as a target for therapeutic intervention. Supported by a modest base of evidence from clinical trials and a strong pathobiological rationale, UFH has been a foundation of care for patients with MI. LMWHs are supported by a more robust and consistent body of clinical evidence for the acute medical management of MI. Placebo-controlled trials of LMWHs have contributed additional valuable support for the benefit of heparins in ACS, and randomized trials against UFH have shown similar (dalteparin, nadroparin) or superior (enoxaparin) efficacy. LMWHs appear to offer the greatest advantage over UFH in patients being managed without early PCI and are thus favored for those undergoing conservative therapy, as is fondaparinux. Bivalirudin is an alternative for adjunctive therapy for primary PCI and has the greatest potential advantage in patients at high risk of bleeding.

Classic References

Antman EM, et al.: ExTRACT-TIMI 25 Investigators. Enoxaparin versus unfractionated heparin with fibrinolysis for ST-elevation myocardial infarction, *N Engl J Med* 354:1477–1488, 2006.

Assessment of the Safety and Efficacy of a New Thrombolytic Regimen (ASSENT)-3 Investigators: Efficacy and safety of tenecteplase in combination with enoxaparin, abciximab, or unfractionated heparin: the ASSENT-3 randomised trial in acute myocardial infarction, *Lancet* 358:605–613, 2001.

Bittl JA, et al.: Treatment with bivalirudin (hirulog) as compared with heparin during coronary angioplasty for unstable or postinfarction angina. Hirulog Angioplasty Study Investigators, *N Engl J Med* 333:764–769, 1995.

Brener SJ, et al.: Relationship between activated clotting time and ischemic or hemorrhagic complications: analysis of 4 recent randomized clinical trials of percutaneous coronary intervention, *Circulation* 110:994–998, 2004.

Eikelboom JW, et al.: Unfractionated and low-molecular-weight heparin as adjuncts to thrombolysis in aspirin-treated patients with ST-elevation acute myocardial infarction: a meta-analysis of the randomized trials, *Circulation* 112:3855–3867, 2005.

Fifth Organization to Assess Strategies in Acute Ischemic Syndromes Investigators; Yusuf S, et al.: Comparison of fondaparinux and enoxaparin in acute coronary syndromes, *N Engl J Med* 354:1464–1476, 2006.

Montalescot G, et al.: Anti-Xa activity relates to survival and efficacy in unselected acute coronary syndrome patients treated with enoxaparin, *Circulation* 110:392–398, 2004.

References

1. O'Gara PT, et al.: 2013 ACCF/AHA guideline for the management of ST-elevation myocardial infarction: a report of the American College of Cardiology Foundation/American Heart Association Task Force on Practice Guidelines, *J Am Coll Cardiol* 61:e78–140, 2013.
2. Bhatt DL, et al.: Antiplatelet and anticoagulation therapy for acute coronary syndromes, *Circ Res* 114:1929–1943, 2014.
3. Amsterdam EA, et al.: American College of Cardiology; American Heart Association Task Force on Practice Guidelines; Society for Cardiovascular Angiography and Interventions; Society of Thoracic Surgeons; American Association for Clinical Chemistry. 2014 AHA/ACC Guideline for the management of patients with non-ST-elevation acute coronary syndromes: a report of the American College of Cardiology/American Heart Association Task Force on Practice Guidelines, *J Am Coll Cardiol* 64:e139–228, 2014.
4. Steg PG, et al.: TAO Investigators. Anticoagulation with otamixaban and ischemic events in non-ST-segment elevation acute coronary syndromes: the TAO randomized clinical trial, *JAMA* 310:1145–1155, 2013.
5. Cohen MGL, et al.: First clinical application of an actively reversible direct factor IXa inhibitor as an anticoagulation strategy in patients undergoing percutaneous coronary intervention, *Circulation* 122:614–622, 2010.

6. Silvain J, et al.: Enoxaparin anticoagulation monitoring in the catheterization laboratory using a new bedside test, *J Am Coll Cardiol* 55:617–625, 2010.
7. Authors/Task Force members Windecker S, et al.: 2014 ESC/EACTS Guidelines on myocardial revascularization: The Task Force on Myocardial Revascularization of the European Society of Cardiology (ESC) and the European Association for Cardio-Thoracic Surgery (EACTS) developed with the special contribution of the European Association of Percutaneous Cardiovascular Interventions (EAPCI), *Eur Heart J* 35:2541–2619, 2014.
8. Montalescot G, et al.: ATOLL Investigators. Intravenous enoxaparin or unfractionated heparin in primary percutaneous coronary intervention for ST-elevation myocardial infarction: the international randomised open-label ATOLL trial, *Lancet* 378:693–703, 2011.
9. Collet JP, et al.: ATOLL Investigators. A direct comparison of intravenous enoxaparin with unfractionated heparin in primary percutaneous coronary intervention (from the ATOLL trial), *Am J Cardiol* 112:1367–1372, 2013.
10. Silvain J, et al.: Efficacy and safety of enoxaparin versus unfractionated heparin during percutaneous coronary intervention: systematic review and meta-analysis, *BMJ* 344:e553, 2012.
11. Navarese EP, et al.: Low-molecular-weight heparins vs. unfractionated heparin in the setting of percutaneous coronary intervention for ST-elevation myocardial infarction: a meta-analysis, *J Thromb Haemost* 9:1902–1915, 2011.
12. Lavi S, et al.: Efficacy and safety of enoxaparin compared with unfractionated heparin in the pharmacoinvasive management of acute ST-segment elevation myocardial infarction: insights from the TRANSFER-AMI Trial, *American Heart Journal* 163:176–181, 2012. e2.
13. Bangalore S, et al.: Anticoagulant therapy during primary percutaneous coronary intervention for acute myocardial infarction: a meta-analysis of randomized trials in the era of stents and P2Y12 inhibitors, *BMJ* 349:g6419, 2014.
14. Iqbal Z, et al.: ATOLL Investigators. Safety and efficacy of adjuvant glycoprotein IIb/IIIa inhibitors during primary percutaneous coronary intervention performed from the radial approach for acute ST segment elevation myocardial infarction, *Am J Cardiol* 111:1727–1733, 2013.
15. Stone GW, et al.: HORIZONS-AMI Trial Investigators. Bivalirudin during primary PCI in acute myocardial infarction, *N Engl J Med* 358:2218–2230, 2008.
16. Steg PG, et al.: EUROMAX Investigators. Bivalirudin started during emergency transport for primary PCI, *N Engl J Med* 369:2207–2217, 2013.
17. Shahzad A, et al.: HEAT-PPCI trial investigators. Unfractionated heparin versus bivalirudin in primary percutaneous coronary intervention (HEAT-PPCI): an open-label, single centre, randomised controlled trial, *Lancet* 384:1849–1858, 2014. Erratum in *Lancet*. 2014;384:1848.
18. Schulz S, et al.: Bavarian Reperfusion Alternatives Evaluation (BRAVE) 4 Investigators. Prasugrel plus bivalirudin vs. clopidogrel plus heparin in patients with ST-segment elevation myocardial infarction, *Eur Heart J* 35:2285–2294, 2014.
19. Han Y, et al.: BRIGHT Investigators. Bivalirudin vs heparin with or without tirofiban during primary percutaneous coronary intervention in acute myocardial infarction: the BRIGHT randomized clinical trial, *JAMA* 313:1336–1346, 2015.
20. Cavender MA, Sabatine MS: Bivalirudin versus heparin in patients planned for percutaneous coronary intervention: a meta-analysis of randomized controlled trials, *Lancet* 384:599–606, 2014.
21. Amsterdam EA, et al.: American College of Cardiology; American Heart Association Task Force on Practice Guidelines; Society for Cardiovascular Angiography and Interventions; Society of Thoracic Surgeons; American Association for Clinical Chemistry. 2014 AHA/ACC guideline for the management of patients with non-ST-elevation acute coronary syndromes: a report of the American College of Cardiology/American Heart Association Task Force on Practice Guidelines, *J Am Coll Cardiol* 64:e139–228, 2014.
22. Hamm CW, et al.: ESC Committee for Practice Guidelines. ESC guidelines for the management of acute coronary syndromes in patients presenting without persistent ST-segment elevation: The Task Force for the management of acute coronary syndromes (ACS) in patients presenting without persistent ST-segment elevation of the European Society of Cardiology (ESC), *Eur Heart J* 32:2999–3054, 2011.
23. Harrington RA, et al.: Antithrombotic therapy for non-ST-segment elevation acute coronary syndromes: American College of Chest Physicians evidence-based clinical practice guidelines (8th edition), *Chest* 133:670S–707S, 2008.
24. Eikelboom JW, et al.: Unfractionated heparin and low-molecular-weight heparin in acute coronary syndrome without ST elevation: a meta-analysis, *Lancet* 355:1936–1942, 2000.
25. Murphy SA, et al.: Efficacy and safety of the low-molecular weight heparin enoxaparin compared with unfractionated heparin across the acute coronary syndrome spectrum: a meta-analysis, *Eur Heart J* 28:2077–2086, 2007.
26. Ndrepepa G, et al.: Bivalirudin versus heparin plus a glycoprotein IIb/IIIa inhibitor in patients with non-ST-segment elevation myocardial infarction undergoing percutaneous coronary intervention after clopidogrel pretreatment: pooled analysis from the ACUITY and ISAR-REACT 4 Trials, *Circ Cardiovasc Interv* 5:705–712, 2012.
27. Cohen M, Catalin B, Mateen A: Therapy for ST-segment elevation myocardial infarction patients who present late or are ineligible for reperfusion therapy, *J Am Coll Cardiol* 55:1895–1906, 2010.
28. FUTURA/OASIS-8 Trial Group Steg PG, et al.: Low-dose vs standard-dose unfractionated heparin for percutaneous coronary intervention in acute coronary syndromes treated with fondaparinux: the FUTURA/OASIS-8 randomized trial, *JAMA* 304:1339–1349, 2010.
29. Kolte D, et al.: Early invasive versus initial conservative treatment strategies in octogenarians with UA/NSTEMI, *Am J Med* 126:1076–1083, 2013. e1.
30. James S, et al.: Ticagrelor versus clopidogrel in acute coronary syndromes in relation to renal function: results from the Platelet Inhibition and Patient Outcomes (PLATO) trial, *Circulation* 122:1056–1067, 2010.
31. Montalescot G, Silvain J: Ticagrelor in the renal dysfunction subgroup: subjugated or substantiated? *Circulation* 122:1049–1052, 2010.

19 Overview of Antiplatelet Therapy for Myocardial Infarction

Dominick J. Angiolillo and Francesco Franchi

INTRODUCTION

Atherosclerotic plaque rupture followed by arterial thrombosis is the major determinant that leads to an acute coronary syndrome (ACS).[1,2] Platelet adhesion, activation, and aggregation have a pivotal role in the cascade of events that lead to arterial thrombosis, and therefore, antiplatelet therapy is essential in the treatment of patients with ACS.[3,4] Multiple platelet signaling pathways are involved in thrombus formation, which represent potential targets for antiplatelet agents.[3,4] Currently, several classes of antiplatelet therapies are clinically available for both oral and intravenous administration for the treatment of patients with ACS, including unstable angina, non–ST-elevation myocardial infarction (NSTEMI), and ST-elevation MI (STEMI).[5–10] This chapter provides an overview of these antiplatelet therapies used in the setting of acute MI, including describing the rationale for use, pharmacological principles, pivotal clinical trial data, and guidance for selecting the initial antiplatelet regimen in the early phase of management. Decisions regarding antiplatelet therapy for long-term secondary prevention are discussed in Chapter 35.

RATIONALE FOR USE OF ANTIPLATELET THERAPY

The pathobiology of atherothrombosis is discussed in Chapter 3, and the fundamental principles underlying the rationale for antiplatelet therapy are described in Chapter 13. Injury to the arterial vessel wall (e.g., plaque rupture, fissure, or erosion) exposes the subendothelial layer and leads to recruitment and activation of platelets, as well as generation of excessive levels of thrombin. These events ultimately result in the formation of a fibrin-rich thrombus (Animation 19-1).[1–4]

Platelet-mediated thrombosis follows three principal steps: (1) platelet adhesion, (2) activation and additional recruitment, and (3) aggregation (Figure 19-1).[3,4] Adhesion of platelets to the subendothelium during the rolling phase is mediated by the interaction between the glycoprotein (GP) Ib/V/IX receptor complex located on the platelet surface and the von Willebrand factor (vWf) and between the collagen exposed at the site of the vascular injury and the platelet collagen receptors.[3,4] After adhesion, binding of collagen to these receptors triggers intracellular mechanisms that shift platelet integrins to a high-affinity state and induce the release of activating factors that enhance the interactions among adherent platelets and promote further recruitment and activation of circulating platelets (see Animation 19-1).[3,4] Activating factors include thromboxane A_2 (TXA_2), adenosine diphosphate (ADP), serotonin, epinephrine, and thrombin.[3,4] Platelet activation by these mediators leads to changes in platelet shape, expression of proinflammatory molecules (e.g., soluble CD40 ligand and P-selectin) and expression of platelet procoagulant activity.[3,4] The final pathway for all agonists is the conversion of the platelet GP IIb/IIIa receptor, the main receptor that mediates platelet aggregation, into its active form.[3,4] Activated GP IIb/IIIa receptors bind to soluble adhesive substrates, including fibrinogen and vWf, which lead to platelet aggregation and thrombus formation mediated by platelet–platelet interactions.[3,4]

Vascular injury also exposes subendothelial tissue factor, which activates the clotting cascade leading to thrombin generation.[3,4,11,12] However, only a modest amount of thrombin is produced as a result of the coagulation cascade.[3,4,11,12] Thrombin is one of the most potent platelet activators, and the surface of activated platelets is the main source of circulating thrombin.[3,4,11,12] During arterial thrombosis, thrombin converts fibrinogen to fibrin, generating a fibrin-rich clot, and it further activates platelets by binding to protease-activated receptors (PARs) on the platelet membrane.[3,4,11,12] Therefore, pathogenic thrombosis is a complex interplay between cellular (i.e., platelets) and plasma (i.e., coagulation factors) components, which interact in an auto-amplified process (see Figure 19-1).

Multiple receptors and signaling pathways are involved in arterial thrombosis. Therefore, several antiplatelet agents have been developed to target different components of this complex process, as described in the following section (Figure 19-2).

ANTIPLATELET THERAPIES IN MYOCARDIAL INFARCTION

Several classes of antiplatelet agents, which are available for both oral and intravenous administration, are currently approved for clinical use in the management of patients with acute MI. These include (1) cyclooxygenase (COX)-1 inhibitors (aspirin), (2) ADP $P2Y_{12}$ receptor antagonists (ticlopidine, clopidogrel, prasugrel, ticagrelor, and cangrelor), (3) GP IIb/IIIa receptor inhibitors (abciximab, eptifibatide, and tirofiban), and (4) a PAR-1 receptor inhibitor (vorapaxar)

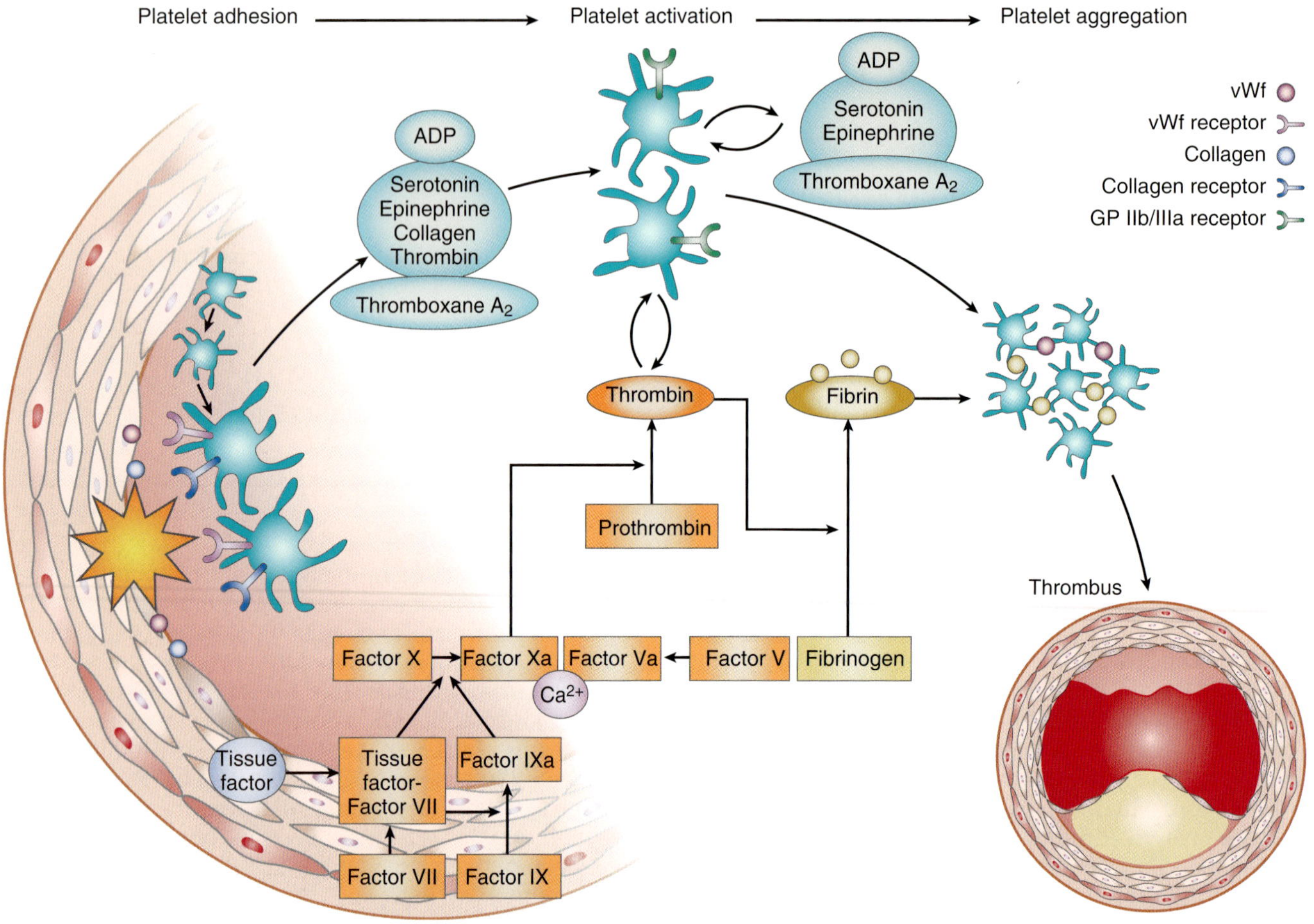

FIGURE 19-1 Mechanism of thrombus formation with platelets-thrombin-coagulation interaction. Plaque rupture exposes the subendothelium components. Platelet adhesion during the rolling phase is mediated by the interaction between the von Willebrand factor (vWf) and the glycoprotein (GP) Ib/V/IX receptor complex located on the platelet surface, and between the platelet collagen receptors (GP VI and GP Ia) and collagen exposed at the site of vascular injury. Binding of collagen to GP VI receptor triggers intracellular mechanisms that induce the release of activating factors (adenosine diphosphate [ADP], thromboxane A_2, serotonin, epinephrine, and thrombin), which enhance the interactions among adherent platelets and promote further recruitment and activation of circulating platelets. Platelet activation by these factors and collagen leads to change in platelet shape, expression of proinflammatory molecules (e.g., P-selectin and soluble CD40 ligand), expression of platelet procoagulant activity, and the conversion of the platelet integrin, GP IIb/IIIa (αIIbβ3) into its active form. The activated GP IIb/IIIa receptors bind to the extracellular ligands fibrinogen and vWf, leading to platelet aggregation and thrombus formation mediated by platelet–platelet interactions. Vascular injury also exposes subendothelial tissue factor (TF), which forms a complex with factor VIIa. TF-VIIa complex activates factor IX and factor X. Factor V is slowly activated by factor Xa. Factor Xa then binds to factor Va and calcium (Ca^{2+}) and forms the prothrombinase complex, which initiates conversion of prothrombin to thrombin (factor IIa). Only a modest amount of thrombin is produced as a result of the coagulation cascade, and its main source within a platelet plug is the surface of activated platelets. Thrombin converts fibrinogen to fibrin, generating a fibrin-rich clot, and further activates platelets, binding to the protease-activated receptor (PAR)-1 and PAR-4. *(Adapted from Franchi F, Angiolillo DJ: Novel antiplatelet agents in acute coronary syndrome.* Nat Rev Cardiol *12:30, 2015.)*

that is approved for secondary prevention in patients after an MI (see Chapter 35).[5–10] Details on the pharmacology and clinical trial development of these classes of antiplatelet agents are provided in the following sections.

Aspirin

Aspirin exerts its antiplatelet effects by irreversibly blocking the COX-1 enzyme by using acetylation; this enzyme is responsible for the generation of TXA_2 from arachidonic acid. Through inhibition of COX-1, aspirin decreases platelet activation mediated by the G-coupled thromboxane and prostaglandin endoperoxide receptors (see Figure 19-2).[13,14] Aspirin is rapidly absorbed in the upper gastrointestinal tract. The plasma half-life of aspirin is approximately 20 minutes, and peak plasma levels are achieved 30 to 40 minutes after ingestion of uncoated aspirin. In contrast, it can take up to 3 to 4 hours for peak plasma levels to occur after the administration of enteric-coated formulations.[13,14] Because the blockade of COX-1 induced by aspirin is irreversible, TXA_2-mediated aggregation is prevented for the entire life span of the platelet (approximately 7 to 10 days). Daily administration of 30 mg of aspirin results in virtually complete suppression of platelet TXA_2 production after 1 week. In clinical practice, standard regimens of aspirin range from 75 to 325 mg/day. Higher doses of aspirin are required to block COX-2, which has anti-inflammatory and analgesic effects, through inhibition of the vascular PGI2 (prostacyclin), which is a platelet inhibitor and a vasodilator.[13,14]

In the ISIS-2 (International Study of Infarct Survival-2) trial, aspirin therapy was associated with a significant reduction in vascular mortality in patients with suspected acute MI who were randomized to receive either aspirin, streptokinase, both agents, or placebo.[14] Other trials consistently demonstrated an important 40% to 50% reduction in cardiovascular events with aspirin treatment in MI patients.[14] The clinical benefit of aspirin is achieved at low doses (75 to 100 mg/day), with no additional benefit provided by higher doses. In contrast, a dose-dependent increase in the risk of bleeding has been shown, in particular, for upper gastrointestinal bleeding.[14,15] Despite the therapeutic benefit of aspirin, some patients who receive long-term therapy are at risk of thrombotic events because of the insufficient inhibition of platelets, giving rise to the term "aspirin resistance."[13,14] However, the association between

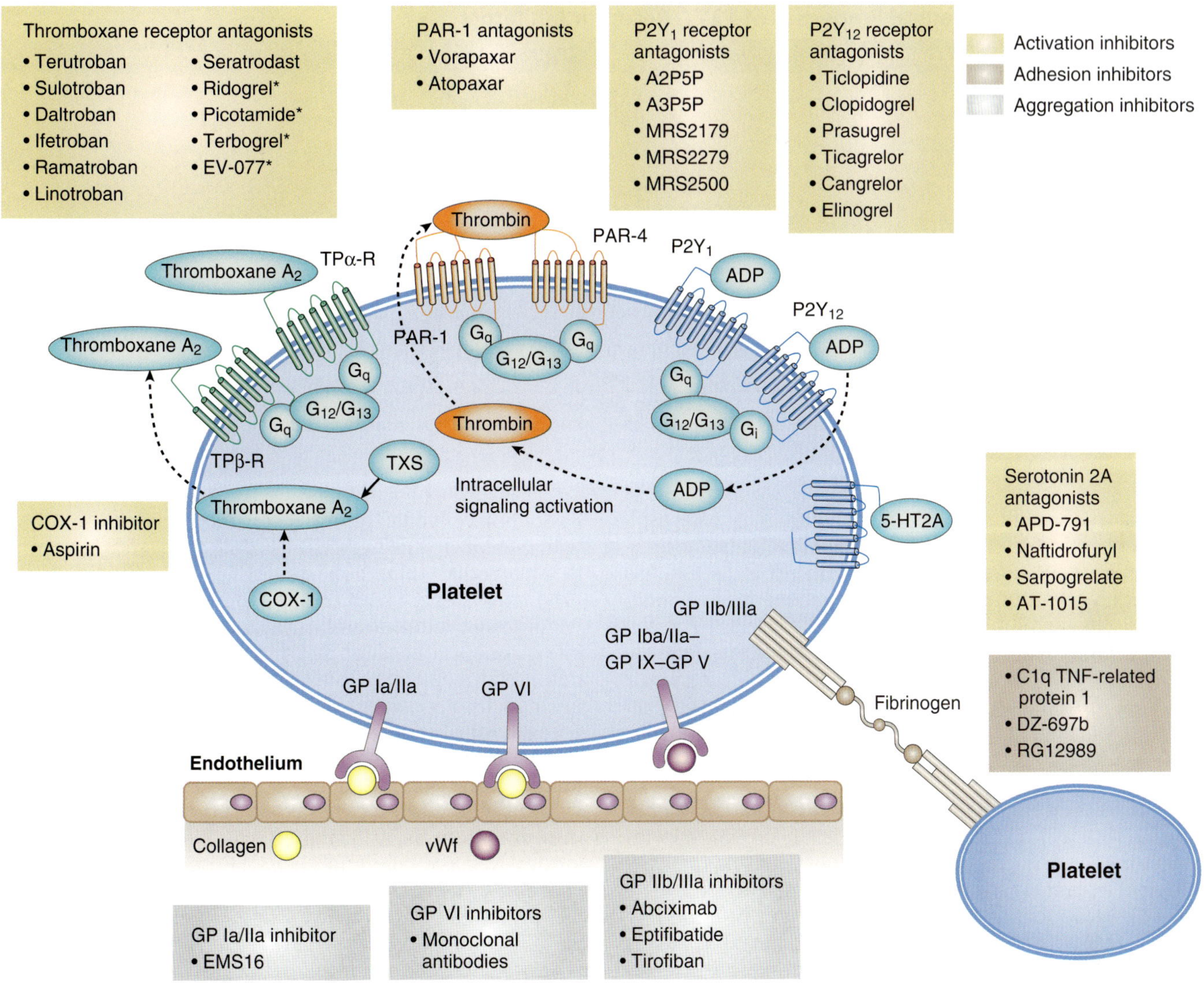

FIGURE 19-2 Platelet activation pathways and sites of action of current and emerging antiplatelet agents. Platelet adherence to the endothelium occurs at sites of vascular injury through the binding of glycoprotein (GP) receptors to exposed extracellular matrix proteins (collagen and von Willebrand factor [vWf]). Platelet activation occurs via complex intracellular signaling processes, and causes the production and release of multiple agonists, including thromboxane A_2 (TXA_2) and adenosine diphosphate (ADP), and local production of thrombin. These factors bind to their respective G-protein–coupled receptors, mediating paracrine and autocrine platelet activation. Further, they potentiate each other's actions ($P2Y_{12}$ signaling modulates thrombin generation). The major platelet integrin GP IIb/IIIa mediates the final common step of platelet activation by undergoing a conformational shape change and binding fibrinogen and vWf, which leads to platelet aggregation. The net result of these interactions is thrombus formation mediated by platelet–platelet interactions with fibrin. Current and emerging therapies inhibiting platelet receptors, integrins, and proteins involved in platelet activation include the TXA_2 synthase inhibitors, thromboxane receptor (TP) receptor inhibitors, the ADP receptor antagonists, the GP IIb/IIIa inhibitors, and the novel protease-activated receptor (PAR) antagonists and adhesion antagonists. *Combined thromboxane-receptor antagonists and thromboxane A2 synthase inhibitors. *5-HT2A*, 5-hydroxy tryptamine 2A receptor. *(Adapted from Franchi F, Angiolillo DJ: Novel antiplatelet agents in acute coronary syndrome.* Nat Rev Cardiol *12:30, 2015.)*

variability in response to aspirin and cardiovascular events has led to inconsistent findings.[13,14,16] This is likely attributable to the type of tests being used for pharmacodynamic evaluation of aspirin effects. When tests specific for COX-1 activity are used, aspirin resistance is extremely rare and is likely caused by noncompliance; drug–drug interactions (i.e., ibuprofen) and enteric coating may also represent contributing causes.[13,14,17] The residual ischemic risk is thus mainly because of the fact that aspirin specifically targets the TXA_2 pathway, and it is not effective in reducing platelet activation stimulated by other pathways involved in arterial thrombosis.[3,4,18]

$P2Y_{12}$ Receptor Antagonists

The agonist ADP exerts its effects on platelets through the purinergic G-protein–coupled $P2Y_1$ and $P2Y_{12}$ receptors (see Figure 19-2).[3,4,13,14] Although both receptors are involved in aggregation, ADP-stimulated effects on platelets are mediated mainly by G_i-coupled $P2Y_{12}$ receptor activation, which leads to sustained platelet aggregation and stabilization of platelet aggregates, whereas $P2Y_1$ is responsible for an initial weak and transient phase of aggregation and change in platelet shape.[3] The addition of a $P2Y_{12}$ receptor inhibitor to aspirin is able to reduce platelet aggregation more than what each single drug is able to achieve,[4] and this synergism has been shown to be beneficial in clinical trials that have assessed the optimal antithrombotic regimen in patients undergoing coronary stent implantation.[12,14]

Several oral $P2Y_{12}$ receptor inhibitors (ticlopidine, clopidogrel, prasugrel, and ticagrelor) have been developed to be used in addition to aspirin for the prevention of ischemic events during the acute management and secondary prevention after an MI (Table 19-1). The first available $P2Y_{12}$ receptor inhibitor was the first-generation thienopyridine ticlopidine.[14] Although ticlopidine in combination with aspirin was shown to be superior compared with either

TABLE 19-1 Pharmacological Properties of $P2Y_{12}$ Receptor Inhibitors

	CLOPIDOGREL	PRASUGREL	TICAGRELOR	CANGRELOR
Pharmacological class	Thienopyridine	Thienopyridine	CPTP	ATP analogue
Receptor blockade	Irreversible	Irreversible	Reversible	Reversible
Administration route	Oral	Oral	Oral	IV
Frequency	Once daily	Once daily	Twice daily	Bolus plus infusion
Prodrug	Yes	Yes	No*	No
Onset of action	2–8 hrs	30 min–4 hrs†	30 min–4 hrs†	2 min
Offset of action	7–10 days	7–10 days	3–5 days	30–60 min
CYP drug interaction	CYP2C19	No	CYP3A	No
Approved settings	ACS and stable CAD PCI	ACS undergoing PCI	ACS (full spectrum)	$P2Y_{12}$ receptor inhibitors naïve patients undergoing PCI

ACS, Acute coronary syndrome; *CAD*, coronary artery disease; *CYP*, cytochrome P450; *CPTP*, cyclopentyltriazolopyrimidine; *IV*, intravenous; *PCI*, percutaneous coronary intervention.
*Although most ticagrelor-mediated antiplatelet effects are direct, approximately 30% to 40% are attributed to an active metabolite (AR-C124910XX).
†Depending on the clinical setting.

aspirin alone or anticoagulation in combination with aspirin for prevention of thrombotic events in patients undergoing percutaneous coronary intervention (PCI), its use has been largely abandoned because of its frequent side effects, including life-threatening hematologic disorders.[14] The following sections will provide an overview on the pharmacology and clinical trial development of $P2Y_{12}$ receptor inhibitors currently approved for clinical use, focusing on studies performed in the acute phase of ACS.

Clopidogrel

Clopidogrel (see Figure 19-2) is a second-generation thienopyridine with a more favorable safety profile compared with ticlopidine.[4,12,14] Furthermore, clopidogrel has a pharmacological advantage over ticlopidine, because it achieves a faster onset of action through administration of a loading dose (LD).[4,12,14] Clopidogrel is orally administrated and is a prodrug that requires metabolic transformation to exert its antiplatelet effects (Table 19-1; see also Figure 20-1).[4,12,14] After intestinal absorption, approximately 85% of clopidogrel is hydrolyzed by carboxylase to an inactive metabolite. The remaining approximately 15% is rapidly metabolized by hepatic cytochrome P450 (CYP) isoenzymes, in particular CYP2C19, in a two-step oxidation process with the generation of a highly unstable active metabolite that irreversibly binds to the $P2Y_{12}$ receptor (Figure 19-3).[4,12,14]

Several clinical trials have shown the benefit of dual antiplatelet therapy (DAPT) with a combination of aspirin and clopidogrel in patients with ACS or who are undergoing PCI (Table 19-2).[12,14] In the CURE (Clopidogrel in Unstable Angina to Prevent Recurrent Events) trial, the administration of clopidogrel (300 mg LD followed by 75 mg once daily), in addition to aspirin, significantly reduced a composite of death from cardiovascular causes, nonfatal MI, or stroke by 20%, compared with aspirin alone in patients with NSTE-ACS (n = 12,562) who were medically managed or underwent revascularization (PCI or coronary artery bypass graft [CABG]).[14] However, this occurred at the expense of an increased risk of major bleeding complications.[14] A post hoc analysis of aspirin dose showed that bleeding events were less likely to occur with lower doses of aspirin (≤100 mg) without any trade-off in efficacy. The clinical benefit of DAPT with aspirin and clopidogrel was also shown in a lower risk population of patients who underwent elective PCI (including patients with ACS) in the CREDO (Clopidogrel for the Reduction of Events During Observation) trial and in patients with STEMI in the COMMIT (Clopidogrel and Metoprolol in Myocardial Infarction) and CLARITY (Clopidogrel as Adjunctive Reperfusion Therapy) trials.[14]

Although clopidogrel is still the most widely used $P2Y_{12}$ receptor antagonist,[19,20] a considerable number of patients still continue to experience recurrent thrombotic events while receiving clopidogrel.[4,14] This risk has been partially attributed to the high interindividual variability that characterizes the response to clopidogrel.[21] Several factors have been associated with clopidogrel response variability, including clinical (i.e., poor absorption, drug–drug interactions, ACS, diabetes mellitus, obesity, chronic kidney disease), genetic (i.e., CYP polymorphisms), and cellular (i.e., accelerated platelet turnover, reduced CYP3A4 metabolic activity, or up-regulation of $P2Y_{12}$ pathway) factors (see Chapter 20).[21] Pharmacodynamic studies have shown that approximately 30% to 40% of patients have high platelet reactivity while on clopidogrel treatment, which translates into worse outcomes.[21–23] Overall, these observations underscore the need for more potent and less variable antiplatelet agents for the treatment of MI patients.

Prasugrel

Prasugrel is an irreversible, orally administered third-generation thienopyridine. It is a prodrug, which after intestinal absorption, requires a single-step oxidation process through hepatic CYP to generate its active metabolite (see Table 19-1 and Figure 19-3).[4,13] Although prasugrel's active metabolite has the same in vitro affinity for the $P2Y_{12}$ receptor as clopidogrel's active metabolite, the metabolic conversion of prasugrel is more efficient, leading to higher in vivo availability.[4,13] These pharmacological properties translate into a more prompt (faster onset of action), potent (enhanced platelet inhibition), and predictable (lower interindividual variability in effects) antiplatelet effect compared with clopidogrel.[4,13] In particular, a 60-mg LD of prasugrel achieves 50% platelet inhibition by 30 minutes and 80% to 90% inhibition by 2 hours.[4,13]

In the TRITON-TIMI 38 (Trial to Assess Improvement in Therapeutic Outcomes by Optimizing Platelet Inhibition with Prasugrel-Thrombolysis in Myocardial Infarction 38) trial, patients (n = 13,608) with moderate- to high-risk ACS scheduled for PCI were randomized to receive either

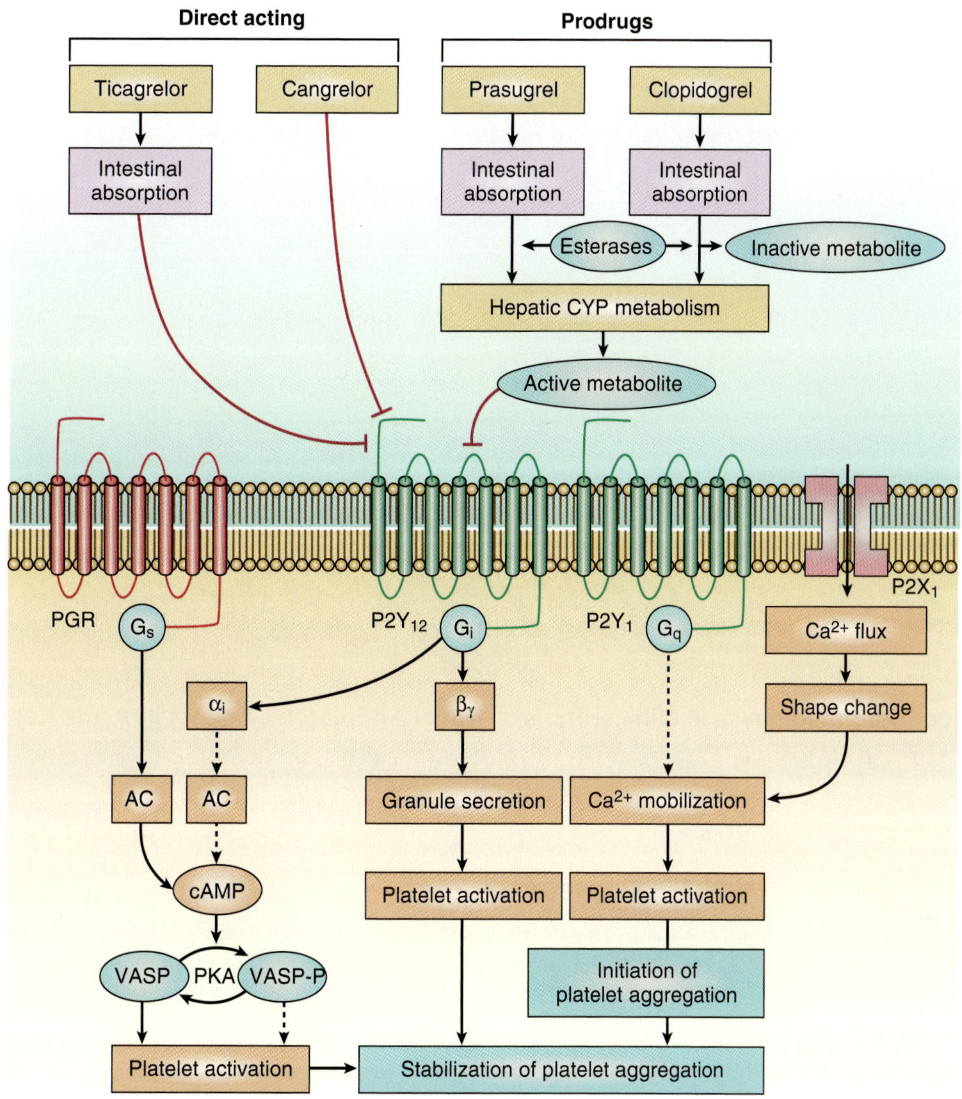

FIGURE 19-3 **$P2Y_{12}$ metabolism inhibitors and mechanism of action.** Clopidogrel is an oral prodrug, and after intestinal absorption, approximately 85% of clopidogrel is hydrolyzed by carboxylase to an inactive metabolite. The remaining approximately 15% is rapidly metabolized by hepatic cytochrome (CYP) P450 isoenzymes in a two-step oxidation process, with the generation of a highly unstable active metabolite. Prasugrel is also an oral prodrug with a similar intestinal absorption process. However, in contrast to clopidogrel, esterases are part of prasugrel's activation pathway, and prasugrel is oxidized more efficiently to its active metabolite via a single CYP-dependent step. Direct-acting antiplatelet agents (cangrelor and ticagrelor) have reversible effects and do not require hepatic metabolism for achieving pharmacodynamic activity. Ticagrelor is orally administered, and after intestinal absorption, it directly inhibits platelet activation by allosteric modulation of the $P2Y_{12}$ receptor, binding to a site on the receptor distinct from the adenosine diphosphate (ADP)-binding site. Cangrelor is intravenously administered, and directly inhibits the $P2Y_{12}$ receptor, bypassing intestinal absorption. P2Y receptors are a family of purinergic G-protein–coupled receptors and are activated by extracellular nucleotides such as ADP. Platelets express at least two ADP receptors, $P2Y_1$ and $P2Y_{12}$, which couple to Gq and Gi, respectively. The activation of $P2Y_{12}$ inhibits adenylyl cyclase (AC), causing a decrease in the cyclic adenosine monophosphate (cAMP) level, and the activation of $P2Y_1$ causes an increase in the intracellular calcium (Ca^{2+}) level, leading to platelet aggregation through the change in the ligand-binding properties of the glycoprotein IIb/IIIa receptor. Clopidogrel, prasugrel, ticagrelor, and cangrelor bind to the $P2Y_{12}$ receptor and ultimately inhibit platelet activation and aggregation processes by modulating intraplatelet levels of cAMP and phosphorylation of vasodilator-stimulated phosphoprotein. *Solid black arrows* indicate activation. *Dotted black arrows* indicate inhibition. *PDE*, Phosphodiesterase; *PKA*, protein kinases. *(Adapted from Franchi F, Angiolillo DJ: Novel antiplatelet agents in acute coronary syndrome.* Nat Rev Cardiol *12:30, 2015.)*

prasugrel 60 mg LD followed by a 10 mg/day maintenance dose (MD) or clopidogrel 300 mg LD and 75 mg/day MD, in addition to aspirin (Table 19-3) (Table 19-e1).[4] Prasugrel significantly reduced the primary efficacy endpoint (a composite of cardiovascular death, nonfatal MI, or nonfatal stroke) compared with clopidogrel over a median follow-up of 14.5 months (9.9% vs. 12.1%; hazard ratio [HR], 0.81; 95% confidence interval [CI], 0.73 to 0.90; P <.001), which was mainly driven by a reduction in nonfatal MI. A significant 52% reduction in the rate of stent thrombosis, irrespective of stent type, and a 34% decrease in need for urgent target vessel revascularization were also seen when prasugrel was used.

This effect was hampered by significantly increased rates of non-CABG–related Thrombolysis In Myocardial Infarction (TIMI) major bleeding; CABG-related TIMI major bleeding, life-threatening bleeding, and fatal bleeding were also increased. However, the net clinical benefit was still in favor of prasugrel-treated patients.[4] The benefit achieved by prasugrel over clopidogrel was consistent in patients with STEMI and was particularly notable in patients with DM and in those who experienced recurrent events.[4,24,25] Clinical outcomes with prasugrel treatment were not affected by CYP polymorphisms or drug interference with CYP2C19 enzymes.[26,27] The results were also consistent, irrespective of aspirin dose.[28] In contrast, a neutral effect was found in low body weight

TABLE 19-2 Major Clinical Trials of Clopidogrel in Patients with Acute Myocardial Infarction

TRIAL	PATIENTS (NO.)	SETTING	TREATMENT ARMS	PRIMARY ENDPOINT	RESULTS
CURE[14]	12,562	NSTE-ACS	Aspirin+clopidogrel vs. aspirin	CV death, nonfatal MI, or stroke at 1 yr	9.3% vs. 11.4%; HR, 0.80; 95% CI, 0.72–0.90; *P* <.001
PCI-CURE[76]	2658	NSTE-ACS treated with PCI	Aspirin+clopidogrel vs. aspirin	CV death, MI, or revascularization within 30 days	4.5% vs. 6.4%; RR, 0.70; 95% CI, 0.50–0.97; *P* = .03
CREDO[14]	2116	Patients undergoing PCI (including ACS)	Aspirin+clopidogrel vs. aspirin	CV death, MI, or stroke at 1 yr	8.5% vs. 11.5%; RRR, 26.9%; 95% CI, 3.9%–44.4%; *P* = .02
COMMIT[14]	45,852	STEMI	Aspirin+clopidogrel vs. aspirin	Death, reinfarction, or stroke at 28 days	9.2% vs. 10.1%; OR, 0.91; 95% CI, 0.86–0.97; *P* = .002
CLARITY[14]	3491	STEMI	Aspirin+clopidogrel+FA vs. aspirin+FA	Occluded infarct-related artery, death, or recurrent MI before angiography	15.0% vs. 21.7%; OR, 0.64; 95% CI, 0.53–0.76; *P* <.001
CURRENT-OASIS 7[15]	25,087	ACS referred for an early invasive strategy	Aspirin+double-dose clopidogrel vs. aspirin+standard dose clopidogrel	CV death, MI, or stroke at 30 days	4.2% vs. 4.4%; HR, 0.94; 95% CI, 0.83–1.06; *P* = .30

ACS, Acute coronary syndrome; *CV*, cardiovascular; *FA*, fibrinolytic agent; *HR*, hazard ratio; *MI*, myocardial infarction; *NSTE-ACS*, non–ST-elevation acute coronary syndrome; *OR*, odds ratio; *PCI*, percutaneous coronary intervention; *RR*, relative risk; *RRR*, relative risk reduction; *STEMI*, ST-elevation myocardial infarction.
Clopidogrel was given as a 300-mg loading dose and then 75 mg/day in CURE, PCI-CURE, CREDO, COMMIT, and CLARITY. In CURRENT-OASIS 7, a double dose of clopidogrel was defined as a 600-mg loading dose and 150 mg once daily for 7 days, followed by 75 mg once daily; standard-dose clopidogrel was defined as a 300-mg loading dose, followed by 75 mg once daily. Patients were also randomized to receive low-dose (75–100 mg/day) or high-dose (300–325 mg/day) aspirin.

TABLE 19-3 Major Completed Phase III Clinical Trials of Novel Antiplatelet Agents in Acute Coronary Syndrome

TRIAL	PATIENTS (NO.)	SETTING	TREATMENT ARMS	PRIMARY ENDPOINT	RESULTS
TRITON-TIMI 38[4]	13,608	ACS patients undergoing PCI	Aspirin+prasugrel vs. aspirin+clopidogrel	CV death, nonfatal MI or nonfatal stroke	9.9% vs. 12.1% (15 mos); HR, 0.81; 95% CI, 0.73–0.90; *P* <.001
TRILOGY-ACS[30]	9326	Medically managed NSTE-ACS	Aspirin+prasugrel vs. aspirin+clopidogrel	CV death, MI, or stroke at 17 mos in patients with age <75 yrs	13.9% vs. 16.0%; HR, 0.91; 95% CI, 0.79–1.05; *P* = .21
ACCOAST[82]	4033	NSTEMI scheduled for angiography	Pretreatment with prasugrel 30 mg vs. placebo	CV death, MI, stroke, GPI bailout, or urgent revascularization at 7 days	10.0% vs. 9.8%; HR, 1.02; 95% CI, 0.84–1.25; *P* = .81
PLATO[34]	18,624	ACS	Aspirin+ticagrelor vs. aspirin+clopidogrel	Death from vascular causes, MI. or stroke	9.8% vs. 11.7% (12 mos); HR, 0.84; 95% CI, 0.77–0.92; *P* <.001
CHAMPION PHOENIX[58]	11,145	Patients undergoing PCI	Aspirin+clopidogrel+ cangrelor vs. aspirin+clopidogrel	Death from any cause, MI, IDR, and stent thrombosis at 48 hr	4.7% vs. 5.9%; OR, 0.78; 95% CI, 0.66–0.93; *P* = .005
TRACER[65]	12,944	NSTE-ACS	Standard APT+vorapaxar vs. standard APT+placebo	CV death, MI, stroke, recurrent ischemia with rehospitalization, or urgent coronary revascularization	18.5% vs. 19.9% (2 yrs); HR, 0.92; 95% CI, 0.85–1.01; *P* = .07
TRA 2P-TIMI 50[66]	26,449	Patients with history of MI, ischemic stroke, or PAD	Standard APT+vorapaxar vs. standard APT+placebo	CV death, MI, or stroke	9.3% vs. 10.5% (36 mos); HR, 0.87; 95% CI, 0.80–0.94; *P* <.001

ACS, Acute coronary syndrome; *APT*, antiplatelet therapy; *CI*, confidence interval; *CV*, cardiovascular; *GPI*, glycoprotein IIb/IIIa inhibitor; *HR*, hazard ratio; *IDR*: ischemia-driven revascularization; *MI*: myocardial infarction; *NSTE*, non–ST-elevation; *OR*, odds ratio; *PAD*, peripheral artery disease; *PCI*, percutaneous coronary intervention.
Adapted from Franchi F, Angiolillo DJ: Novel antiplatelet agents in acute coronary syndrome. Nat Rev Cardiol *12:30, 2015.*

patients (<60 kg) and older adults (≥75 years), and a net harm was shown in patients with a history of stroke or transient ischemic attack.[4] Among patients (n = 346) who underwent isolated CABG and who received the study drug before the procedure, there was a reduction in all-cause and cardiovascular mortality with prasugrel compared with clopidogrel, although there was a higher 12-hour chest tube blood loss.[29]

The efficacy of prasugrel compared with clopidogrel in medically managed ACS was tested in the TRILOGY-ACS (Targeted Platelet Inhibition to Clarify the Optimal Strategy to Medically Manage Acute Coronary Syndromes) trial (see Table 19-3).[30] Aspirin-treated patients (n = 9326) with an NSTE-ACS who underwent medical management were randomized to receive either prasugrel (30 mg LD followed by 10 mg MD) or clopidogrel (300 mg LD and 75 mg MD). Prasugrel MD was adjusted to 5 mg for patients who were aged 75 years or older or who weighed less than 60 kg. Clopidogrel pretreatment before randomization occurred in approximately 96% of patients. The primary endpoint was a composite of cardiac death, MI, or stroke among patients aged younger than 75 years (n = 7243). After a median follow-up of 17 months, there were no differences between prasugrel and clopidogrel in the primary ischemic endpoint (13.9% vs. 16%; HR, 0.91; 95% CI, 0.79 to 1.05; P = .21). Importantly, the rates of non-CABG–related severe or life-threatening bleeding according to the GUSTO (Global Use of Strategies to Open Occluded Coronary Arteries) criteria, TIMI major bleeding, and intracranial bleeding were low and similar between groups.[30] Moreover, in the secondary analysis on patients (n = 2083) aged 75 years or older, prasugrel 5 mg was not associated with an ischemic benefit compared with standard clopidogrel, although there was no increase in bleeding.[31] Importantly, in the prespecified substudy on patients aged younger than 75 years who underwent angiography before randomization (n = 3085), prasugrel led to a significant reduction in the risks of the composite primary endpoint compared with clopidogrel, with a trend toward an increased risk of major bleeding. These data suggest that when angiography is performed for ACS and anatomic coronary disease is confirmed, the benefits and risks of a more intense antiplatelet therapy exist whether the patient is treated with drugs or PCI.[32]

Ticagrelor

Ticagrelor is an orally administered cyclopentyltriazolopyrimidine that directly and reversibly inhibits the platelet $P2Y_{12}$ receptor (Table 19-1 and Figure 19-3).[4,13] Ticagrelor is not a prodrug and does not require metabolic activation, although approximately 30% to 40% of its antiplatelet effects are attributed to an active metabolite (AR-C124910XX) generated through the hepatic CYP3A system (CYP3A4 and CYP3A5).[4,13] Ticagrelor does not bind directly to the platelet ADP-binding site on the $P2Y_{12}$ receptor; it reversibly binds to a distinct site on the receptor and prevents ADP from causing activation of the $P2Y_{12}$ pathway in a noncompetitive fashion through allosteric modulation.[4,13] Ticagrelor is rapidly absorbed after oral administration and has a half-life of 7 to 12 hours, thus requiring twice daily dosing. Compared with clopidogrel, ticagrelor achieves a faster, more potent and more predictable antiplatelet effect, with a faster offset of action.[33]

The efficacy and safety of ticagrelor in patients with ACS were evaluated in the Phase III PLATO (Platelet Inhibition and Patient Outcomes) trial (see Table 19-3).[34] There are key differences between the PLATO and TRITON-TIMI 38 trial designs, as summarized in Table 19-e1. In the PLATO trial, ACS patients (n = 18,624) were randomized to receive either ticagrelor (180 mg LD followed by 90 mg twice daily MD) or clopidogrel (300 to 600 mg LD followed by 75 mg/day MD) in addition to aspirin for 12 months. The trial embraced the whole spectrum of patients with ACS, including those intended to undergo invasive as well as noninvasive management. Patients pretreated with clopidogrel were eligible for study entry, and study drug LD administration occurred before or after angiography, but before PCI. Compared with clopidogrel, ticagrelor significantly reduced the primary endpoint (a composite of death from vascular causes, MI, or stroke) at 12 months (9.8% vs. 11.7%; HR, 0.84; 95% CI, 0.77 to 0.92; P <.001), including a significant 21% reduction in cardiovascular death and a 16% reduction of MI. Ticagrelor treatment also significantly reduced the rates of definite or probable stent thrombosis.

Although protocol-defined major bleeding was similar between groups (11.6% vs. 11.2%; P = .43), ticagrelor led to a significantly increased hazard of non-CABG–related PLATO and TIMI major bleeding, as well as fatal intracranial hemorrhage.[34] Importantly, the benefit of ticagrelor over clopidogrel was consistent across multiple prespecified subgroups, including patients who were treated initially with a noninvasive or invasive (followed by PCI or CABG) strategy.[35–38] Accordingly, patients with STEMI, diabetes mellitus, who were older than 75 years of age, weighed less than 60 kg, who had a previous stroke or transient ischemic attack, with recurrent cardiovascular events, chronic kidney disease, and with or without CYP2C19 loss-of function polymorphisms, also benefitted from ticagrelor therapy.[34,39–45] Bleeding outcomes were also consistent across subgroups, with no groups experiencing harm with ticagrelor.[46]

Importantly, a geographic interaction was found in the trial, with patients enrolled in North America not experiencing a reduction in the primary endpoint by ticagrelor treatment. Although these findings can be attributed to play of chance, a post hoc assessment found this to be possibly explained by the use of high-dose (≥300 mg/day) aspirin, which was more common in North America.[47] Although subsequent studies failed to demonstrate any effect of aspirin dosing on the pharmacokinetic and pharmacodynamic profile of ticagrelor,[48] the use of low-dose aspirin (≤100 mg) is currently recommended in ticagrelor-treated patients.[5–10]

Non-$P2Y_{12}$–mediated effects of ticagrelor related to increased plasma levels of adenosine have been described.[49] Under normal conditions, adenosine has a short half-life and is rapidly up-taken by red blood cells and metabolized.[49] Ticagrelor has been shown to significantly inhibit cellular uptake of adenosine by blocking the sodium-dependent equilabrative nucleoside transporters (ENT-1), and thus, increasing adenosine plasma concentrations.[50,51] Adenosine has multiple cardiac and extracardiac properties that include inhibition of platelet aggregation (mainly through the activation of A_{2A} G-coupled receptors), arterial vasodilation, reduction in inflammatory response, negative chronotropic and dromotropic effects, stimulation of pulmonary vagal C fibers that mediate the sensation of dyspnea, and a role in the regulation of kidney glomerular filtration.[49] Although ticagrelor does not directly act on adenosine receptors, it enhances the biological effects of adenosine, which may contribute to the overall benefits of ticagrelor, including a reduction in cardiovascular mortality, and to the nonbleeding side effects of ticagrelor, such as a higher incidence of dyspnea (15% to 22% of ticagrelor-treated patients) and ventricular pauses and increased levels of creatinine and uric acid during treatment compared with clopidogrel (Figure 19-4).[49] These side effects are usually self-limiting and have no impact on clinical outcomes, but were responsible for the higher discontinuation rate of ticagrelor compared with clopidogrel in the PLATO trial.[34] Importantly, no effect of ticagrelor on specific pulmonary function parameters, such as spirometry, lung volumes, diffusion capacity, and pulse oximetry, have been shown.[52]

Cangrelor

Although prasugrel and ticagrelor are characterized by more prompt, potent, and predictable antiplatelet effects, leading to greater clinical efficacy over clopidogrel, these drugs still present limitations inherent to orally administered antiplatelet agents, including delayed pharmacodynamic effects in patients with STEMI, slow offset of action, and an inability to exert reliable and predictable platelet inhibition in patients who are hemodynamically unstable or sedated, intubated, in shock, under therapeutic hypothermia, or who have nausea or vomiting.[4,53] Cangrelor is an analogue of adenosine triphosphate (ATP) and is the first reversible intravenous $P2Y_{12}$ inhibitor. It directly binds to the $P2Y_{12}$ receptor in a predominantly competitive manner without the need for being metabolized (see Table 19-1 and Figure 19-3).[4,54] Cangrelor achieves very potent (>80%) antiplatelet effects, reaching steady-state concentrations within a few minutes, and is characterized by a linear dose-dependent pharmacokinetic profile that leads to very stable pharmacodynamic effects.[54,55] Because of its very short half-life (3 to 5 minutes), cangrelor has a fast offset of action, with platelet aggregation returning to baseline levels within 30 to 60 minutes.[54,55]

The role of cangrelor as adjunctive antiplatelet therapy in patients who require PCI has been tested in three large-scale phase III clinical trials.[56-58] Although the first two trials, namely the CHAMPION (Cangrelor versus Standard Therapy to Achieve Optimal Management of Platelet Inhibition)-PCI and the CHAMPION-PLATFORM trials, were interrupted for futility and failed to document any ischemic benefit of cangrelor over DAPT with aspirin and clopidogrel,[56,57] pitfalls in study endpoint definitions (i.e., the definition of MI) may have contributed to these results.[54] A pooled analysis of the CHAMPION-PCI and CHAMPION-PLATFORM trials, which used the Universal Definition of MI

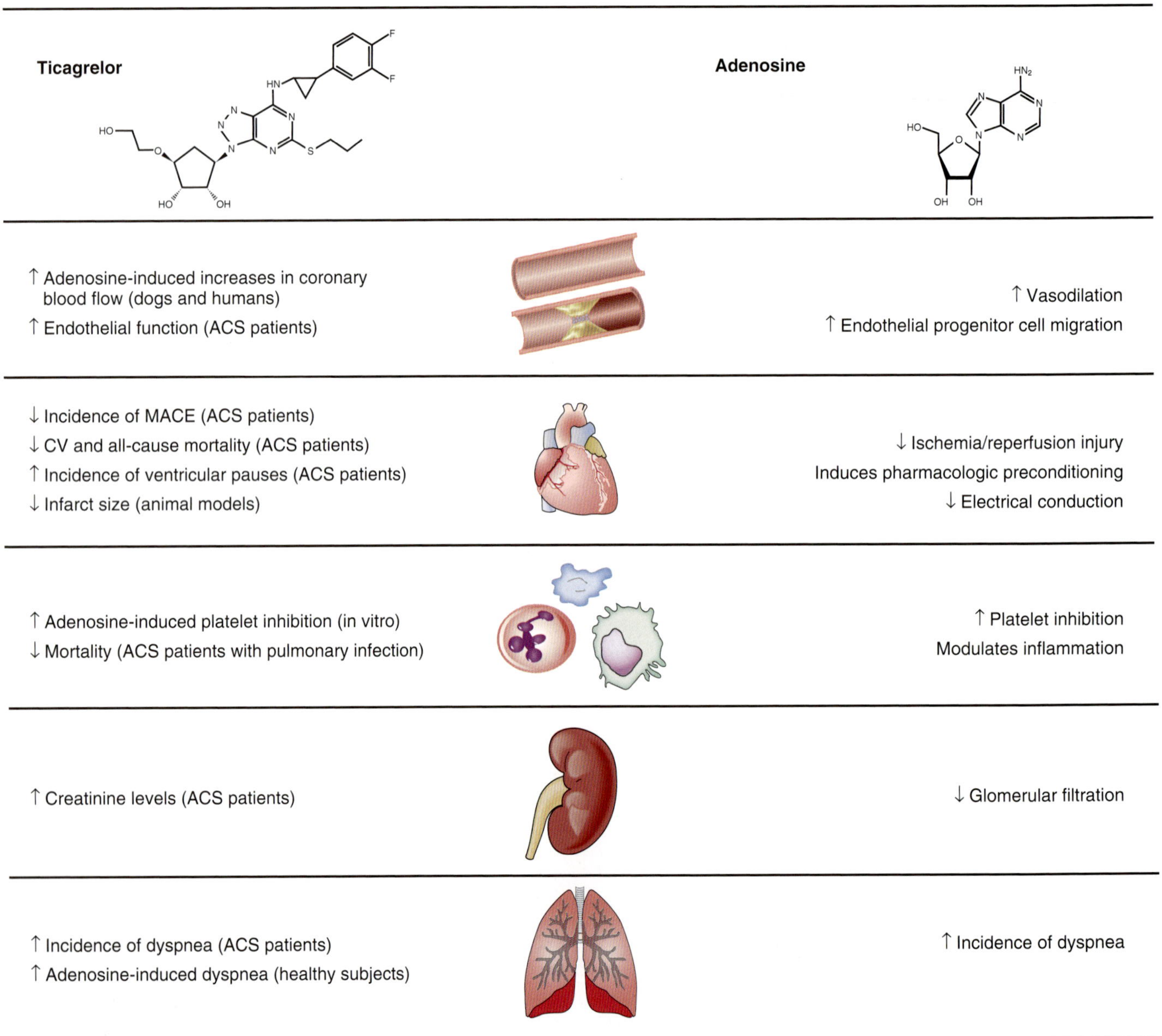

FIGURE 19-4 Major biological effects mediated by ticagrelor and adenosine. There are similarities between the biological effects of adenosine (*right*) and the pharmacological effects of ticagrelor (*left*), which suggests that at least some of the non-$P2Y_{12}$–mediated effects of ticagrelor may be mediated by the drug-induced inhibition of the cellular sodium-independent equilibrative nucleoside transporter type 1 (ENT-1). Because adenosine degradation is primarily restricted to the intracellular space, inhibition of cellular uptake of adenosine via ENT-1 results in prolonging the half-life of adenosine, thereby increasing its extracellular (plasma) concentration. Hence, ENT-1 inhibition by ticagrelor results in enhanced responses to adenosine, mediated by interaction with the adenosine receptor subtypes A_1R, $A_{2A}R$, $A_{2B}R$, and A_3R, which are coupled to G_s or G_i proteins. *ACS*, Acute coronary syndrome; *CV*, cardiovascular; *MACE*, major adverse cardiovascular events. *(Adapted from Cattaneo M, Schulz R, Nylander S: Adenosine-mediated effects of ticagrelor: evidence and potential clinical relevance.* J Am Coll Cardiol *63:2503, 2014.)*

(see Chapter 1 and Chapter 7) to define MI events, showed a significant reduction in the primary endpoint with the use of cangrelor.[59]

The hypothesis-generating data from this analysis led to the design of the CHAMPION PHOENIX trial, which evaluated if addition of cangrelor on top of DAPT with aspirin and clopidogrel in patients undergoing PCI could reduce the occurrence of acute ischemic complications (see Table 19-3).[58] The study included $P2Y_{12}$ receptor inhibitor–naïve patients across the spectrum of coronary artery disease (CAD) manifestations (stable angina, NSTE-ACS, and STEMI). After angiography, patients (n = 11,145) were randomized to receive either a cangrelor bolus (30 μg/kg) followed by infusion (4 μg/kg per minute for 2 to 4 hours) or a clopidogrel LD (300 or 600 mg before or immediately after the PCI, as per institutional standard). In the cangrelor arm, patients received 600 mg of clopidogrel at the end of the infusion. Adjunctive cangrelor therapy significantly reduced the primary efficacy endpoint (a composite of death from any cause, MI, ischemia-driven revascularization, and stent thrombosis) at 48 hours (4.7% vs. 5.9%; adjusted odds ratio [OR] with cangrelor, 0.78; 95% CI, 0.66 to 0.93; $P = .005$), which was primarily driven by a reduction in the hazard of MI (3.8% vs. 4.7%; $P = .02$). The use of cangrelor led to a significant reduction in the rate of stent thrombosis at 48 hours (0.8% vs 1.4%; OR, 0.62; 95% CI, 0.43 to 0.90; $P = .01$).[58] Intraprocedural stent thrombosis, which was shown to be associated with an increase in adverse outcomes at 48 hours and 30 days, was also significantly reduced.[60]

The rate of severe bleeding at 48 hours was not significantly increased by cangrelor using the GUSTO criteria and other definitions of bleeding. However, the rate of major bleeding according to the more sensitive ACUITY criteria was significantly higher in patients treated with cangrelor, which was primarily driven by a higher incidence of hematomas at the vascular access sites. Overall, the net rate of adverse clinical events (ischemic plus bleeding events) was significantly reduced by the use of cangrelor.[58] The clinical benefit of adjunctive cangrelor therapy was consistent at 30 days and across multiple prespecified subgroups, such as those defined by different clinical presentations (stable angina, NSTE-ACS, or STEMI), dose and timing of clopidogrel loading, stent type, and duration of study drug infusion.[58]

These results were further confirmed by a pooled analysis on approximately 25,000 patients enrolled in the three CHAMPION trials, which showed consistent results using the PHOENIX definition of MI.[61] Cangrelor was also tested as a bridging strategy in patients (n = 210) on thienopyridine treatment (including patients with a recent MI) and who required CABG; it showed high and stable levels of platelet inhibition up to 7 days of infusion, with a rapid offset after discontinuation before surgery. This strategy was not associated with an increased risk of major bleeding or side effects before or during CABG, although these findings need to be interpreted with caution because the study was not powered for clinical outcomes.[62]

Glycoprotein IIb/IIIa Inhibitors

GP IIb/IIIa inhibitors (GPIs) are only available for intravenous use, and include abciximab, eptifibatide, and tirofiban.[63] GPIs are classified into two groups: small (eptifibatide, tirofiban) and nonsmall (abciximab) molecules. GPIs are characterized by different pharmacological properties, as summarized in Table 19-4. They target the final pathway of platelet aggregation, competing with fibrinogen and vWf for GP IIb/IIIa receptor binding and provide fast and potent antiplatelet effects.[63] GPIs have been shown to improve ischemic outcomes in patients with STEMI and NSTEMI who are undergoing PCI, although most of these studies did not include the use of novel generation $P2Y_{12}$ receptor inhibitors.[63] The administration of GPIs is an accepted treatment option in high-risk ACS patients undergoing PCI. However,

TABLE 19-4 Pharmacology of Glycoprotein IIb/IIIa Inhibitors

	ABCIXIMAB	EPTIFIBATIDE	TIROFIBAN
Trade name	ReoPro	Integrilin	Aggrastat
Molecule	Fragment antigen binding (Fab)[7E3]	Synthetic peptide	Nonpeptide mimetic
Molecular weight	~50,000	~800	~500
Stoichiometry (drug to GP IIb/IIIa)	~1.5:1	>>100:1	>>100:1
Binding	Noncompetitive	Competitive	Competitive
Half-life	Plasma: 10–15 hrs Biologic: 12–24 hrs	Plasma: 2–2.5 hrs Biologic = plasma	Plasma: 2–2.5 hrs Biologic = plasma
PCI dosing	Bolus: 0.25 mg/kg (10–60 min) Infusion: 0.125 μg/kg/min (12h)	Bolus: 180 μg/kg* + 180 μg/kg (after 10 min) Infusion: 2 μg/kg/min (24–48 hrs) †	Bolus: 25 μg/kg (30 min) Infusion: 0.10 μg/kg/min (48 hrs)
Renal adjustment	No	Bolus: 180 μg/kg Infusion: 1 μg/kg/min (24–48 hrs)	Bolus: 12.5 μg/kg (30 min) Infusion: 0.10 μg/kg/min (48 hrs)

GP, Glycoprotein; *PCI*, percutaneous coronary intervention.
*Started immediately before PCI.
†Started immediately after the first bolus..
Adapted from Muñiz-Lozano A, Rollini F, Franchi F, Angiolillo DJ: Update on platelet glycoprotein IIb/IIIa inhibitors: recommendations for clinical practice. Ther Adv Cardiovasc Dis *7:197, 2013.*

their role is currently reduced because of their high rates of bleeding complications and because of the development of alternative treatment strategies with a more favorable safety profile. Available data support a selective (i.e., bailout in cases of large residual thrombus) rather than a routine use of GPIs for patients with ACS treated with PCI.[63] Intracoronary administration of GPIs has been tested in several small studies and associated with some benefits compared with intravenous administration, but these have not been confirmed in large-scale clinical trials.[63]

Protease-Activated Receptor-1 Antagonists

DAPT with a combination of aspirin and a $P2Y_{12}$ receptor inhibitor primarily targets pathways associated with TXA_2 and ADP-mediated platelet activation.[3,4] Thus, other pathways, such as thrombin-mediated platelet activation remain unaffected and may in part account for the residual risk of ischemic events (see Figure 19-2).[11] Because thrombin is a key mediator of platelet activation, and levels of thrombin are known to be elevated after an ACS, targeting thrombin-mediated effects has been an important area of clinical investigation.[4,11] Two different strategies can be pursued to block thrombin effects: indirect modulation by blockade of the platelet PAR receptor and direct inhibition of either thrombin or other upstream coagulation factors (i.e., factor X).[4,11,12] Leveraging this latter strategy, several trials have tested the use of nonvitamin K antagonist oral anticoagulants in patients with MI. These therapies are described in Chapter 21.

The serine protease thrombin is one of the most potent platelet activators, and the surface of activated platelets is the main source of circulating thrombin.[4,11] PARs are a family of G-protein–coupled receptors, and four types of PARs have been described in humans; PAR-1 and PAR-4 are expressed on human platelets, and PAR-1 has the principal role of mediating platelet activation at low concentrations of thrombin, whereas PAR-4 reacts only at high concentrations.[4,64] Several PAR-1 antagonists have been developed so far[11]; only vorapaxar has completed phase III clinical investigations and is available for clinical use. Vorapaxar was tested in two large-scale phase III clinical trials: the TRACER (Thrombin Receptor Antagonist for Clinical Event Reduction in Acute Coronary Syndrome) and TRA 2°P-TIMI 50 (Thrombin Receptor Antagonist in Secondary Prevention of Atherothrombotic Ischemic Events - TIMI 50) trials (see Table 19-3).[65,66] Although vorapaxar did not have a favorable balance of efficacy and bleeding in the acute management of ACS in the TRACER trial, this PAR-1 antagonist was effective for long-term secondary prevention after MI in the TRA 2°P-TIMI 50 trial. The use of PAR-1 antagonists in patients with MI is detailed in Chapter 35.

PRACTICAL RECOMMENDATIONS AND GUIDELINES

Guideline recommendations from the American College of Cardiology (ACC)/American Heart Association (AHA) and the European Society of Cardiology (ESC) for the use of antiplatelet therapy in patients with MI are summarized in Tables 19-5 and 19-6. The following sections will provide practical considerations for the initial management of antiplatelet strategies in patients with NSTEMI and STEMI.

Indications and Dosing of Antiplatelet Therapies

Oral Antiplatelet Therapies

Aspirin

Aspirin is the established first-line therapy in patients with MI.[5–10] Nonenteric-coated aspirin (150 to 325 mg) should be administered promptly after presentation in patients with both NSTEMI and STEMI, and then continued indefinitely irrespective of the treatment strategy. An aspirin LD should preferably be given orally, including chewing, to ensure complete inhibition of TXA_2-dependent platelet aggregation. However, an intravenous formulation is available in certain countries and can be used as a 300- to 500-mg dose in patients who are unable to swallow. Even if the optimal dosing regimen for prevention of cardiovascular

TABLE 19-5 Summary of ACC/AHA and ESC Guidelines for the Initial Management of Oral and Intravenous Antiplatelet Therapy in Patients with Non–ST-Elevation Myocardial Infarction

RECOMMENDATIONS	ACC/AHA		ESC	
	COR	LOE	COR	LOE
Oral Therapy				
Nonenteric coated oral aspirin (150–325 mg) promptly after presentation (or 80–150 mg IV). Aspirin MD (preferably ≤100 mg/day) continued indefinitely.	I	A	I	A
A $P2Y_{12}$ inhibitor is recommended in addition to aspirin, and maintained over 12 mos unless there are contraindications, such as excessive risk of bleeding:	I	B	I	A
• Prasugrel (60 mg LD, 10 mg/daily MD) in patients in whom coronary anatomy is known and who are proceeding to PCI.	IIa	B	I	B
• Ticagrelor (180 mg LD, 90 mg bid MD) regardless of initial treatment strategy, including those pretreated with clopidogrel.	IIa	B	I	B
• Clopidogrel (600 mg LD, 75 mg/day MD), only when prasugrel or ticagrelor are not available, or are contraindicated			I	B
Pretreatment with prasugrel in patients in whom coronary anatomy is not known is not recommended.			III	B
Intravenous Therapy				
GPIs should be considered for bailout situation or thrombotic complications.			IIa	C
GPIs added to aspirin should be considered before angiography in high-risk patients not preloaded with $P2Y_{12}$ inhibitors.	I	A	IIa	C
In high-risk patients, eptifibatide or tirofiban may be considered before early angiography in addition to DAPT.	IIa	B	IIb	C
In patients undergoing PCI, routine upstream use of GPIs is not recommended.			III	A

bid, Twice a day; *COR*, class of recommendation; *DAPT*, dual antiplatelet therapy; *GPI*, glycoprotein IIb/IIIa inhibitor; *IV*, intravenously; *LD*: loading dose; *LOE*, level of evidence; *MD*, maintenance dose; *PCI*, percutaneous coronary intervention.

events has been subject of controversy, current evidence suggest the use of low-dose aspirin (≤100 mg) following the initial LD administration of aspirin. In aspirin-treated patients, nonsteroidal anti-inflammatory drugs should be avoided because of their competition for the COX-1 active site.[13,14]

Clopidogrel

Clopidogrel (300 to 600 mg LD and 75 mg/day MD) is currently approved for the treatment of patients with MI, irrespective of the clinical presentation or the treatment strategy, and in patients undergoing PCI.[5–10] Although the LD regimen varies according to different guidelines, available data suggest that a 600 mg LD should be preferred in MI patients who are undergoing PCI.[5–10,14] In patients with STEMI treated with fibrinolytics, clopidogrel is also the only $P2Y_{12}$ receptor inhibitor currently recommended, and should be administered as a 300 mg LD followed by 75 mg/day in patients who are aged 75 years or younger, and 75 mg/day without an LD in patients who are aged older than 75 years.[7–10] Clopidogrel is contraindicated in patients with active pathological bleeding, such as peptic ulcer or intracranial hemorrhage. Alternative treatments should be considered in patients identified as CYP2C19 poor metabolizers (see Chapter 20). In patients taking clopidogrel, the use of drugs that are strong or moderate CYP2C19 inhibitors should be avoided; in particular, the concomitant use of omeprazole and clopidogrel should be avoided because of the effect on clopidogrel's active metabolite levels and antiplatelet activity. Pantoprazole and esomeprazole have less effect on the pharmacological activity of clopidogrel than omeprazole, whereas dexlansoprazole and lansoprazole have marginal effects on clopidogrel metabolism. If interruption is needed before surgery, clopidogrel should be stopped for at least 5 days.[67]

Prasugrel

Prasugrel (60 mg LD and 10 mg/day MD) is currently approved for patients with ACS who are undergoing PCI, and should be administered only after the coronary anatomy has been established, with the exception of STEMI patients who are undergoing primary PCI. Prasugrel is not recommended in noninvasively managed ACS patients and in stable non-ACS patients undergoing PCI. It is contraindicated in patients with previous stroke and/or transient ischemic attack and patients who have a high risk of bleeding.[5–10,68,69] In older adult patients, prasugrel is generally not recommended, except for those with a high-risk ACS and in those with a history of diabetes mellitus or previous MI. In this scenario, the Food and Drug Administration (FDA) recommends the standard 10-mg dose, whereas the European Medicines Agency (EMA) recommends a 5-mg dose. Both agencies recommend dose adjustment to 5 mg in low-body-weight patients (<60 kg).[68,69] The rationale for the 5-mg dose is primarily derived from pharmacodynamic and pharmacokinetic studies, which showed that prasugrel 5 mg achieved similar platelet inhibitory effects in low-weight and older adult patients as the 10-mg dose in non–low-weight patients and the nonelderly.[4] Because of its irreversible binding to the $P2Y_{12}$ receptor and the potent platelet inhibition, prasugrel administration should be stopped for at least 7 days before surgery to reduce the risk of bleeding.[68,69]

Ticagrelor

Ticagrelor (180 mg LD and 90 mg MD twice daily) is currently approved for the treatment and prevention of secondary atherothrombotic events across the entire spectrum of patients with ACS, irrespective of the treatment strategy (invasive or noninvasive).[5–10,70,71] It can be administered before the coronary anatomy is known and to patients pretreated with clopidogrel. Ticagrelor has not been tested in patients with stable CAD, and thus, it is not indicated for this condition. Ticagrelor is contraindicated in patients with hypersensitivity, high risk of bleeding, in those with a previous hemorrhagic stroke or intracranial bleeding, and those with severe hepatic dysfunction. Ticagrelor should not be used in patients with a high-degree atrioventricular block or sick sinus syndrome without pacemaker protection. No dose adjustment is required according to age or body weight. Despite the more rapid speed of offset of antiplatelet effects compared with thienopyridines, the high levels of platelet inhibition achieved with ticagrelor warrant a 5-day washout period for patients requiring surgery. Because ticagrelor is also metabolized by CYP3A4/5 enzymes, which leads to the generation of an active metabolite (AR-C124910XX)

TABLE 19-6 Summary of ACC/AHA and ESC Guidelines for the Initial Management of Oral and Intravenous Antiplatelet Therapy in Patients with ST-Elevation Myocardial Infarction

RECOMMENDATIONS	ACC/AHA		ESC	
	COR	LOE	COR	LOE
Oral Therapy				
Oral aspirin (150–325 mg) promptly after presentation (or 80–150 mg IV). Aspirin MD (preferably ≤100 mg/day) continued indefinitely.	I	A	I	A
A $P2Y_{12}$ inhibitor is recommended in addition to aspirin early as possible or at time of primary PCI, and maintained over 12 mos unless there are contraindications:	I	B	I	A
• Prasugrel (60 mg LD, 10 mg/day MD) if no contraindications.	I	B	I	B
• Ticagrelor (180 mg LD, 90 mg bid MD) if no contraindications.	I	B	I	B
• Clopidogrel (600 mg LD, 75 mg/day MD), only when prasugrel or ticagrelor are not available or are contraindicated.	I	B	I	B
In patients receiving fibrinolytic therapy, clopidogrel is indicated in addition to aspirin (300 mg LD for patients ≤75 yrs of age, 75-mg dose for patients >75 yrs of age) followed by an MD of 75 mg/day.	I	A	I	A
Intravenous Therapy				
GPIs should be considered for bailout or evidence of no-reflow or a thrombotic complication.			IIa	C
Upstream use of a GPIs may be considered in high-risk patients	IIb	B	IIb	B

bid, Twice a day; *COR*, class of recommendation; *GPI*, glycoprotein IIb/IIIa inhibitor; *IV*, intravenously; *LD*, loading dose; *LOE*, level of evidence; *MD*, maintenance dose; *PCI*, percutaneous coronary intervention.

responsible for 30% to 40% of its platelet inhibitory effects, patients taking ticagrelor should avoid the use of strong inhibitors (i.e., ketoconazole, itraconazole, voriconazole, clarithromycin, nefazodone, ritonavir, saquinavir, nelfinavir, indinavir, atazanavir, and telithromycin) or inducers (i.e., rifampin, dexamethasone, phenytoin, carbamazepine, and phenobarbital) of CYP3A. In addition, with initiation of, or any change in, ticagrelor therapy, the use of simvastatin and lovastatin doses more than 40 mg should be avoided, and monitoring of digoxin levels is recommended.[70,71]

Vorapaxar

Vorapaxar is not recommended for the acute management of MI.[72,73]

Intravenous Antiplatelet Therapies

Glycoprotein IIb/IIIa Receptor Inhibitors

GPIs use should be considered for patients with NSTEMI who are undergoing PCI, because limited benefit has been shown in medically managed patients; their dosing is summarized in Table 19-4. GPIs use is a reasonable treatment in high-risk patients with ACS, such as those with elevated cardiac biomarkers who are not pretreated with a $P2Y_{12}$ receptor antagonist.[5–10] GPIs can also be used in patients receiving the more potent $P2Y_{12}$ receptor inhibitors prasugrel and ticagrelor, because these agents have different pharmacodynamic profiles, and trial data have shown them to be of additive benefit, irrespective of the use of GPIs. Clinical data do not support routine upstream use of GPIs, which therefore should be started in the catheterization laboratory if considered clinically indicated.[5–10] In patients with STEMI who are undergoing primary PCI, GPI use has been shown to be beneficial. If a GPI is deemed necessary, this should be administered in the catheterization laboratory, because most trial data have not shown any benefit with upstream use. Intracoronary administration with standard infusion does not offer any benefit over systemic infusion.[7–10]

Cangrelor

Cangrelor (30 µg/kg bolus plus 4 µg/kg/min infusion initiated before PCI and continued for at least 2 hours or for the duration of PCI, whichever is longer) was recently approved for clinical use by the FDA as an adjunct to PCI for reducing the risk of periprocedural MI, repeat coronary revascularization, and stent thrombosis in patients who have not been treated with a $P2Y_{12}$ platelet inhibitor and are not being given a GPI. Cangrelor was also approved for clinical use by the EMA for patients undergoing PCI who have not received an oral $P2Y_{12}$ inhibitor before the PCI procedure and in whom oral therapy with $P2Y_{12}$ inhibitors is not feasible or desirable.[74,75] Cangrelor has yet to be tested as a bridging strategy in surgeries other than CABG.

Timing of Administration of Antiplatelet Therapies

General Considerations

In patients presenting with an MI, timely use of antiplatelet therapy is critical. At time of presentation, all patients should be treated with aspirin. Timing of administration of the oral $P2Y_{12}$ receptor inhibitors has been a subject of controversy in patients with both NSTEMI and STEMI.[76] In the past, particularly before the introduction of novel $P2Y_{12}$ inhibiting therapies, when time from clinical presentation to the catheterization laboratory was more delayed than currently, upstream treatment with GPIs was commonly used. However, in the setting of current practice patterns, the evidence for upstream treatment with GPIs in patients with NSTEMI and STEMI is weak. At least one large randomized clinical trial did not show any additional benefit of routine upstream use of GPIs compared with a delayed provisional administration.[63] However, in selected high-risk cases, upstream GPI use may still be considered. There are no studies with upstream treatment with cangrelor, which is reserved for use in the catheterization laboratory in patients with defined coronary anatomy who are undergoing PCI.

Timing of Administration of Oral $P2Y_{12}$ Receptor Antagonists

The term pretreatment embraces a variety of different clinical scenarios, where the antiplatelet drug is given in the ambulance, in the medical emergency department, at the referral hospital, in the cardiac intensive care unit, or in the catheterization laboratory after coronary angiography and before PCI. Pretreatment can be defined as any treatment given before the coronary anatomy has been defined and a decision about revascularization is undertaken.[76] Although the need for early adequate platelet inhibition is emphasized among invasively managed patients with MI, the evidence supporting pretreatment with $P2Y_{12}$ receptor inhibitors is mixed and controversial.[76–78] Furthermore, changes in practice patterns in patients who require an invasive strategy and who are currently undergoing cardiac catheterization in a more expedited fashion, particularly in the United States, have amplified the debate on the benefits of pretreatment (Figure 19-5).[76] On one hand, early administration of antiplatelet therapy may protect the patient from thrombotic events in the vulnerable period before and immediately after PCI. On the other hand, pretreatment may result in an unnecessary excess of platelet inhibition and related bleeding risk when patients do not undergo PCI, such as those patients without CAD or patients who require CABG (~10% to 15% of patients hospitalized for NSTE-ACS).[76] Although pretreatment with $P2Y_{12}$ receptor inhibitors seems to be a highly prevalent practice (from 57% to 90% of patients with MI), particularly in some countries,[79,80] evidence and guideline recommendations vary according to the clinical presentation.

Non–ST-Elevation Myocardial Infarction

For years, the ACC/AHA and ESC guidelines provided a class I recommendation for preloading with $P2Y_{12}$ receptor inhibitors as soon as possible after admission in patients with NSTEMI.[76] Although the level of evidence for pretreatment was high in these documents, the supporting references did not relate to any randomized trial of upstream versus downstream use of $P2Y_{12}$ inhibitors. Notably, in the more recent 2014 ESC guidelines for myocardial revascularization and ACC/AHA guidelines for NSTE-ACS, there is no longer a specific recommendation for early initiation of $P2Y_{12}$ inhibitors in this setting, and pretreatment with prasugrel is now not recommended (class III).[5,10]

The data to support pretreatment with clopidogrel are limited and inconsistent.[76–78] Results of the PCI-CURE study support the hypothesis that an effective antiplatelet regimen with clopidogrel started before PCI could reduce long-term adverse ischemic events. However, this reflects a practice pattern that is now outdated because of the long pretreatment period (median of 10 days) in this setting and the use

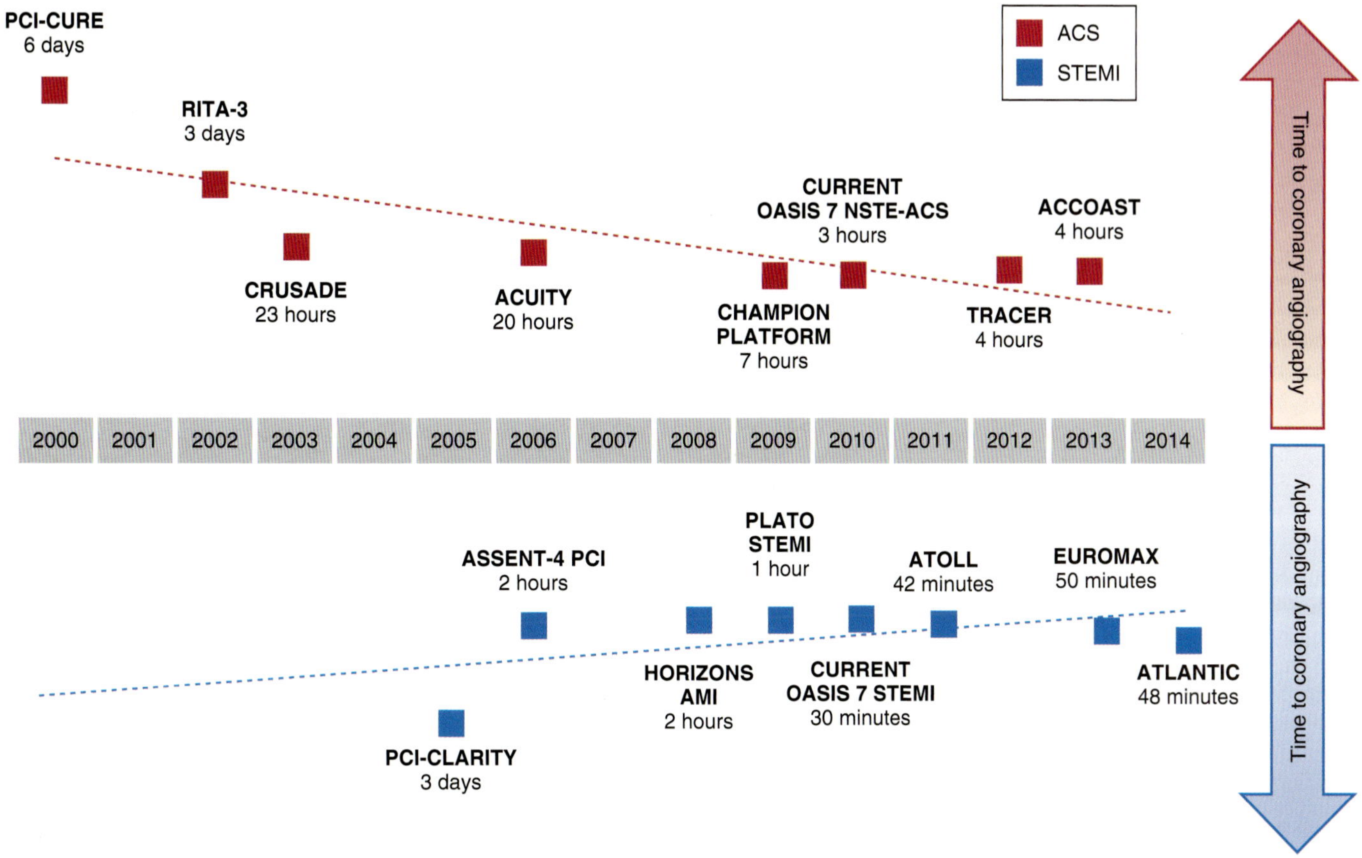

FIGURE 19-5 **Time from hospital admission or first medical contact to coronary angiography in studies of non–ST-elevation acute coronary syndrome (NSTE-ACS) and ST-elevation myocardial infarction (STEMI).** *(Adapted from Capodanno D, Angiolillo DJ: Pretreatment with antiplatelet drugs in invasively managed patients with coronary artery disease in the contemporary era: review of the evidence and practice guidelines.* Circ Cardiovasc Interv *8:e002301, 2015.)*

of a 300 mg LD.[76] Importantly, a meta-analysis in patients with NSTE-ACS from randomized clinical trials and from observational analyses of randomized clinical trials found no differences in mortality with clopidogrel pretreatment versus no pretreatment.[81]

The benefits of pretreatment with ticagrelor in patients with NSTEMI have not been tested in any randomized clinical trial, because all patients in the PLATO trial were pretreated. The study design of PLATO, as well as the lack of a significant statistical interaction with antiplatelet pretreatment, supports the current practice of administering ticagrelor before the coronary anatomy is defined.[34,76]

In the TRITON-TIMI 38 trial, administration of prasugrel before coronary angiography was not allowed in enrolled patients with NSTE-ACS.[4] Because of this gap, the impact of prasugrel pretreatment in patients with NSTE ACS was tested in the ACCOAST [Comparison of Prasugrel at the Time of Percutaneous Coronary Intervention (PCI) or as Pretreatment at the Time of Diagnosis in Patients with Non-ST Elevation Myocardial Infarction] trial (see Table 19-3).[82] In this trial, $P2Y_{12}$ receptor inhibitor–naïve patients with NSTEMI were randomly assigned to receive either pretreatment with a prasugrel 30 mg LD or matching placebo as soon as possible after diagnosis. After angiography (performed after a median time of 4.3 hours), patients (n = 4033) who underwent PCI received an additional prasugrel 30 mg LD if in the pretreatment arm or a 60 mg LD if in the control arm. Prasugrel pretreatment failed to improve the primary efficacy endpoint (a composite of death from cardiovascular causes, MI, stroke, urgent revascularization, or GP IIb/IIIa inhibitor bailout) at 7 days compared with standard delayed administration (10.0% vs. 9.8%; HR, 1.02; 95% CI, 0.84 to 1.25; *P* = .81), but it was associated with a significant threefold increase in non-CABG–related TIMI major bleeding and a sixfold increase in life-threatening bleeding. Importantly, results were consistent across the cohort that underwent PCI (68.7% of the patients), the cohort that underwent CABG (6.2%), and the cohort that received medical treatment only (25.1%).[82] Therefore, the results of the ACCOAST trial do not support the use of prasugrel before angiography in patients with NSTEMI. Accordingly, in a recent meta-analysis of patients who presented with NSTE-ACS, pretreatment with thienopyridines (clopidogrel or prasugrel) was associated with no significant reduction in mortality, but did have a significant excess of major bleeding regardless of the strategy adopted (invasive or conservative).[83] It is currently unknown if these data could be also applied to pretreatment with ticagrelor.

ST-Elevation Myocardial Infarction

In the 2014 ESC guidelines for myocardial revascularization, administration of a $P2Y_{12}$ inhibitor, including clopidogrel, prasugrel, and ticagrelor, is recommended at first medical contact in patients with STEMI who are undergoing primary PCI.[10] The ACC/AHA guidelines for STEMI give a class I recommendation for the administration of an LD of a $P2Y_{12}$ receptor inhibitor as early as possible or at time of primary PCI.[7] Because pharmacodynamic studies have shown a delayed onset of the antiplatelet effects of $P2Y_{12}$ inhibitors in patients with STEMI,[53] pretreatment seems an appealing strategy to provide a stronger platelet inhibition at the time of primary PCI, even if there are insufficient available supporting data. Although evidence supporting clopidogrel pretreatment in patients undergoing primary PCI is conflicting,[76] in the STEMI subgroup of a large meta-analysis on patients who underwent PCI, pretreatment with clopidogrel was associated with an approximately 50% reduction in mortality.[81] In the TRITON-TIMI 38, only 32% of patients with STEMI who underwent primary PCI (≤12 hours after symptom onset) and 20% of those who underwent secondary PCI (>12 hours) received the loading dose before PCI; therefore, the value of pretreatment with prasugrel in STEMI has not been specifically demonstrated.[4,24]

The role of ticagrelor pretreatment in STEMI was tested in the ATLANTIC (Administration of Ticagrelor in the Cath-Laboratory or in the Ambulance for New ST-Segment-Elevation Myocardial Infarction to Open the Coronary Artery) trial, in which patients (n = 1862) who underwent emergency angiography were randomly assigned to receive either prehospital (in the ambulance) or in-hospital (in the cardiac catheterization laboratory) treatment with a 180-mg loading dose of ticagrelor, in addition to aspirin.[84] The median time difference in the administration of the LD between the two strategies was only 31 minutes. Prehospital ticagrelor did not reduce the co-primary endpoints (the proportion of patients without a 70% or greater resolution of ST-segment elevation before PCI and the proportion of patients without TIMI flow grade 3 in the infarct-related artery at initial angiography). Although the trial was not powered for clinical endpoints, rates of major bleeding were low and similar between the two groups, which suggested the safety of prehospital ticagrelor administration. Because of the extremely low number of events, the finding of a significant reduction in the rate of definite acute (≤24 hours) stent thrombosis (0% in the prehospital group vs. 0.8% in the in-hospital group) should be considered as exploratory only.[84]

These results, along with the study design of the PLATO trial, provide evidence that pretreatment with ticagrelor is safe in STEMI. Notably, the small platelet function substudy of the ATLANTIC study showed no significant differences in platelet inhibition between the two strategies at any time point.[84] Overall, available data suggest that if primary PCI is performed with a short medical contact-to-balloon time, residual platelet reactivity before PCI is also considerably high in patients treated or pretreated with prasugrel or ticagrelor.[53,84] In-catheterization laboratory use of intravenous agents, such as GPIs or cangrelor, has the potential to provide immediate platelet inhibition until the full antiplatelet effect of oral $P2Y_{12}$ inhibitors is achieved.[54,63]

Selection of Oral $P2Y_{12}$ Receptor Antagonist

For more than a decade, DAPT with aspirin and clopidogrel has been the cornerstone of antiplatelet treatment in patients with MI.[14] Despite the efficacy of this combination, trials of newer agents have consistently shown that the more prompt, potent, and predictable platelet inhibition achieved with the novel $P2Y_{12}$ receptor antagonists leads to significantly better clinical outcomes, albeit at the expense of an increase in the rates of major bleeding.[4,14] Therefore, prasugrel and ticagrelor are preferred for the initial treatment of patients with MI, irrespective of the clinical presentation (STEMI/NSTEMI) in patients undergoing invasive management. Ticagrelor is preferred over clopidogrel in patients undergoing non-invasive management of NSTEMI. Algorithms for consideration of $P2Y_{12}$ receptor antagonists at each stage of management in patients with NSTEMI or STEMI are shown in Figures 19-6 and 19-7.

Clopidogrel should only be used when both prasugrel and ticagrelor are contraindicated. Clopidogrel is still the treatment of choice in patients with STEMI undergoing fibrinolysis and patients with MI who require a triple antithrombotic therapy (see Chapter 21), such as patients with atrial fibrillation, in whom the use of prasugrel and ticagrelor is not recommended because of the increased bleeding risk.[5–10] In the absence of head-to-head clinical comparisons between these two agents, the selection of one drug over the other should take into account the specific contraindications of each drug and the patient characteristics.[4] The ongoing ISAR-REACT (Prospective, Randomized Trial of Ticagrelor Versus Prasugrel in Patients With Acute Coronary Syndrome - Intracoronary Stenting and Antithrombotic Regimen: Rapid Early Action for Coronary Treatment) 5 trial (NCT01944800) will provide a head-to-head clinical comparison between prasugrel and ticagrelor in approximately 4000 patients with ACS, with a planned invasive strategy.[85] Moreover, although platelet function and genetic testing have been proposed to help identify patients who may benefit from treatment with the novel $P2Y_{12}$ receptor inhibitors (see Chapter 20), these agents are generally preferred based on clinical grounds.

Because of its reversible binding to the $P2Y_{12}$ receptor and its plasma half-life of 8 to 12 hours, ticagrelor requires twice daily administration.[4] Therefore, patients with poor compliance may not be optimal candidates for ticagrelor, and the use of an irreversible inhibitor, which only requires a once daily administration with $P2Y_{12}$ receptors blocked for the lifetime of a platelet (7 to 10 days), could be the preferred choice. However, the reversible binding property of ticagrelor also translates into a faster offset of action, leading to a shorter washout period before surgery and potentially to reduced periprocedural-related bleeding.[4] It may also be hypothesized that reversible agents with twice daily dosing such as ticagrelor, which provide stable plasma concentrations, may enable more effective antiplatelet effects in patients with high platelet turnover rates, such as those with MI or diabetes mellitus, which are characterized by higher levels of reticulated platelets, which are hyperreactive and associated with worse outcomes.[4]

The type of management strategy should also be considered in the choice of the $P2Y_{12}$ receptor inhibitor. In patients with MI who are treated with PCI, all three agents, clopidogrel, prasugrel and ticagrelor, can be used.[5–10] Although in patients with STEMI, the probability of performing PCI is usually high, thus allowing to choose among all drugs, in patients with NSTEMI, either the choice to pretreat or uncertainties about the following management strategy can limit the choice between clopidogrel and ticagrelor. These agents, but not prasugrel, are approved for pretreatment and for treatment of NSTEMI patients who are medically managed.[5,6,9,10] In this latter scenario, ticagrelor represents the first-line treatment, because of the benefit shown over clopidogrel in the medically managed subgroup of the PLATO trial.[35]

Switching $P2Y_{12}$ Receptor Antagonists

Switching $P2Y_{12}$ inhibiting therapies occurs commonly in clinical practice, particularly in the acute setting of patients who present with an MI.[80,86,87] Several circumstances may lead clinicians to switch antiplatelet agents in the acute phase of an MI. Switching from clopidogrel to a newer agent usually occurs in patients who are pretreated with clopidogrel, because of the better clinical profile of prasugrel and ticagrelor.[80,86,87] Switching from clopidogrel to ticagrelor

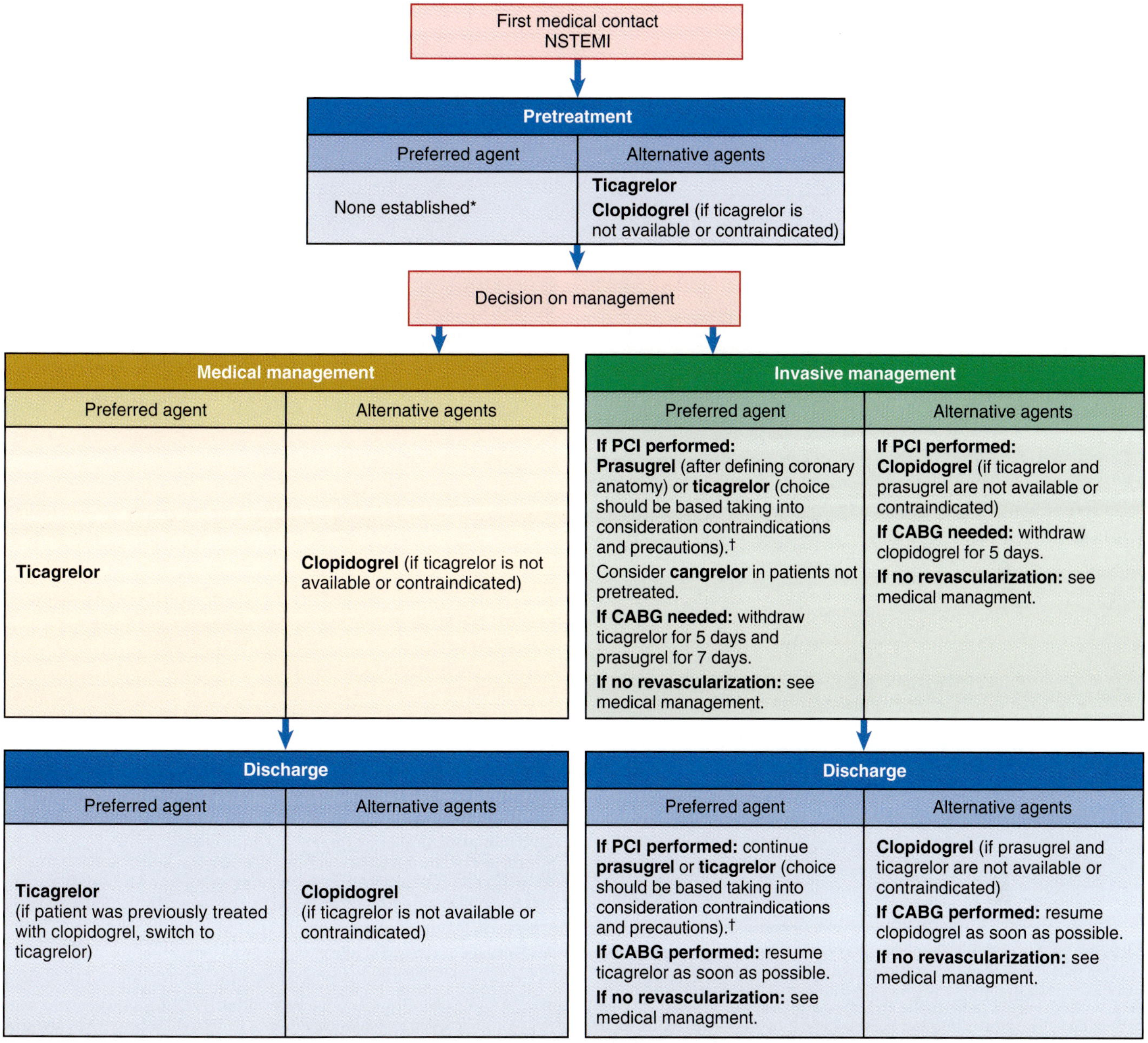

FIGURE 19-6 **Algorithm for choice of $P2Y_{12}$ receptor antagonists in patients with non–ST-elevation myocardial infarction (NSTEMI).** *The choice to pretreat with a $P2Y_{12}$ receptor antagonist should be based on the risk/benefit ratio of such an approach, taking into consideration the thrombotic and bleeding risk. Early administration of antiplatelet therapy may protect the patient from thrombotic events in the vulnerable period before and immediately after percutaneous coronary intervention (PCI). However, pretreatment may result in an unnecessary excess of platelet inhibition and related bleeding risks when patients do not undergo PCI, such as patients without coronary artery disease or patients who require coronary artery bypass graft (CABG) surgery. †If the patient was previously treated with clopidogrel, switching to prasugrel or ticagrelor should be considered.

occurred in nearly half of the patients enrolled in the PLATO trial, which showed consistent safety and efficacy results, irrespective of previous exposure to clopidogrel. In the trial, patients randomized to ticagrelor therapy were treated with a 180 mg LD, irrespective of timing of the last dose of clopidogrel.[34] Accordingly, a similar approach should be applied in clinical practice whenever switching from clopidogrel to ticagrelor in the acute phase of MI.

Switching from clopidogrel to prasugrel was not explored in the TRITON TIMI 38 trial.[4] Data from registries have not shown any major safety concerns (i.e., bleeding) related to switching.[80,86,87] Surrogate data from dedicated pharmacodynamic studies showed that patients pretreated with clopidogrel can switch to prasugrel, which leads to enhanced levels of platelet inhibition. These are achieved more promptly when switching to a 60 mg LD rather than a 10 mg MD, and without any drug interactions, irrespective of whether a patient was on maintenance 75 mg/day therapy or recently received a 600 mg LD of clopidogrel.[88,89] Therefore, administering a 60 mg LD should be the strategy to use when switching from clopidogrel to prasugrel in patients with acute MI.[87]

Switching from a novel $P2Y_{12}$ receptor inhibitor to clopidogrel occurs commonly in clinical practice, but with limited data to support this approach.[80,86,87] Reduced costs associated with a generic formulation of clopidogrel, as well as concerns about bleeding with prasugrel and ticagrelor, remain key reasons for switching to clopidogrel. In the absence of clinical studies investigating the effects of such a strategy, based on pharmacodynamic considerations,

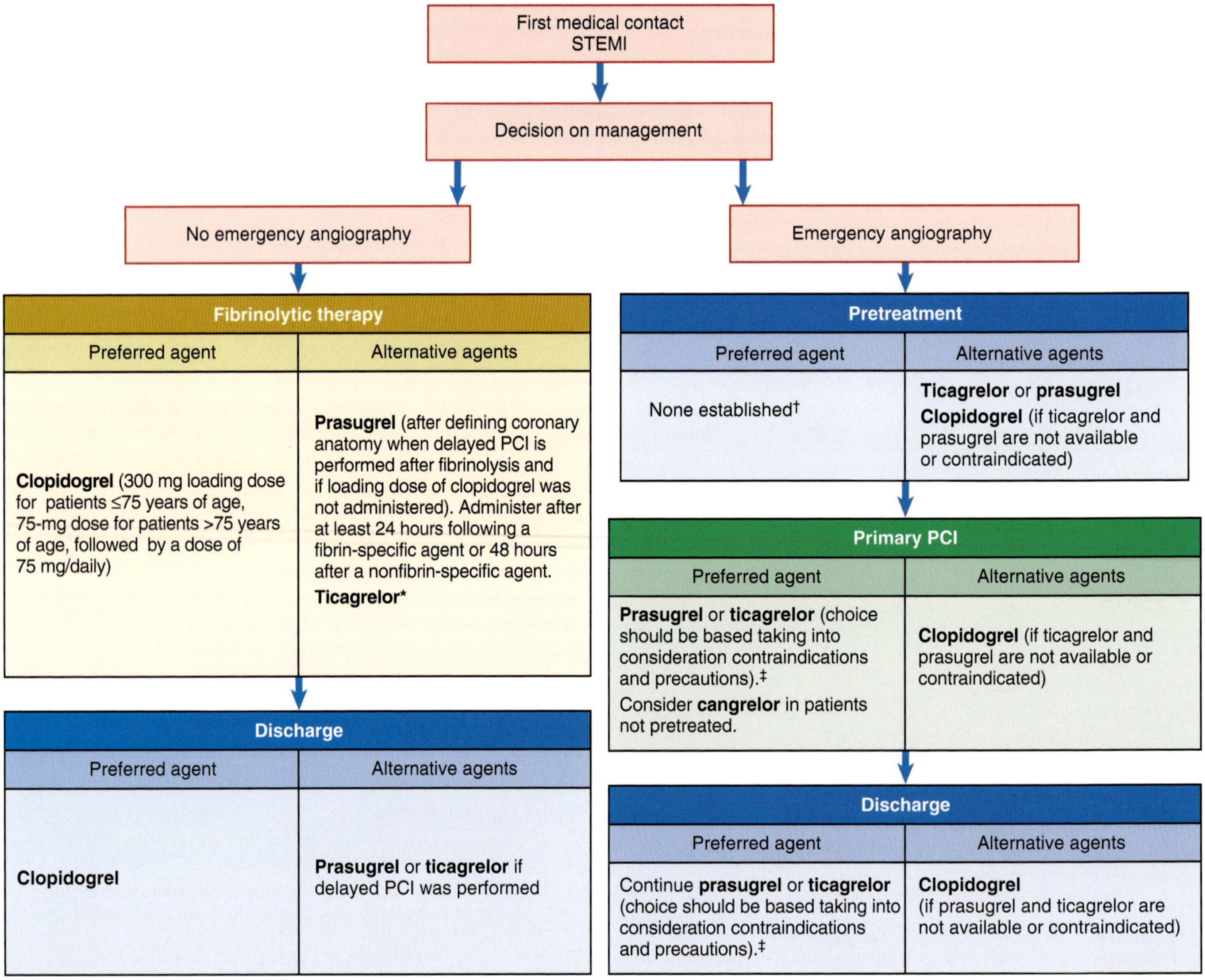

FIGURE 19-7 Algorithm for choice of $P2Y_{12}$ receptor antagonists in patients with ST-elevation myocardial infarction (STEMI). *Tested only in few small nonrandomized studies of patients undergoing delayed percutaneous coronary intervention (PCI). †The choice to pretreat with a $P2Y_{12}$ receptor antagonist should be based on the risk/benefit ratio of such an approach, taking into consideration the thrombotic and bleeding risk. Early administration of antiplatelet therapy may protect the patient from thrombotic events in the vulnerable period before and immediately after PCI. However, pretreatment may result in an unnecessary excess of platelet inhibition and related bleeding risk when patients do not undergo PCI, such as patients without coronary artery disease or patients requiring coronary artery bypass graft (CABG) surgery. ‡If the patient was previously treated with clopidogrel, switching to prasugrel or ticagrelor should be considered.

whenever switching from prasugrel or ticagrelor is required, clopidogrel should be administered with a 600 mg LD, because of its unpredictable platelet inhibitory profile.[87]

Registry data indicate that switches between novel $P2Y_{12}$ receptor inhibitors occur rarely, ranging from 2% to 4% of patients.[80,86,87] In this setting, clinical data are lacking, and pharmacodynamic studies are also limited. However, switching from ticagrelor to prasugrel has been shown to be associated with an acute (24 to 48 hours) increase in platelet reactivity, potentially because of a drug interaction, which is reduced with the administration of a 60 mg LD.[90] Conversely, small pharmacodynamic investigations showed that platelet inhibition was enhanced when switching from prasugrel to ticagrelor.[91] Based on the best available evidence, the administration of an LD is preferred when switching between new $P2Y_{12}$ receptor inhibitors.

Switching from the intravenous cangrelor to clopidogrel has been tested in large-scale clinical trials, whereas data on switching to the new agents have been derived from small pharmacodynamic studies. Overall, available data suggest that clopidogrel and prasugrel should be administered immediately after discontinuation of cangrelor infusion to avoid a pharmacodynamic interaction, because these agents compete for the same ADP binding site.[87,92] In contrast, ticagrelor is a noncompetitive ADP antagonist and thus can be administered before, during, or after cangrelor infusion.[93] No drug interaction has been described when transitioning from any oral $P2Y_{12}$ receptor inhibitor to cangrelor, which can thus be started at any time.[87,92,93]

SUMMARY

Antiplatelet therapy has a pivotal role in the treatment of patients with MI. Currently, DAPT with a combination of aspirin and either prasugrel or ticagrelor should be considered the treatment of choice in the setting of acute MI, because these agents achieve a faster and more potent platelet inhibition compared with clopidogrel and improve outcomes with an overall satisfactory safety profile. Clopidogrel should be considered for patients with contraindications to prasugrel and ticagrelor and for those who require adjunctive oral anticoagulant therapy. The findings that patients still continue to experience ischemic events despite COX-1 and $P2Y_{12}$ receptor blockade has raised interest toward alternative antithrombotic strategies, such as agents that target the different pathways involved in thrombosis, or intravenous drugs, which are particularly attractive to achieve an immediate antiplatelet effect in the early phase of an ACS.

Classic References

Chen ZM, et al.: Addition of clopidogrel to aspirin in 45,852 patients with acute myocardial infarction: randomised placebo-controlled trial, *Lancet* 366:1607, 2005.

ISIS-2 (Second International Study of Infarct Survival) Collaborative Group: Randomised trial of intravenous streptokinase, oral aspirin, both, or neither among 17,187 cases of suspected acute myocardial infarction: ISIS-2. ISIS-2 (Second International Study of Infarct Survival) Collaborative Group, *Lancet* 1988(2):349, 1988.

Mehta SR, et al.: Effects of pretreatment with clopidogrel and aspirin followed by long-term therapy in patients undergoing percutaneous coronary intervention: the PCI-CURE study, *Lancet* 358:527, 2001.

Sabatine MS, et al.: Addition of clopidogrel to aspirin and fibrinolytic therapy for myocardial infarction with ST-segment elevation, *N Engl J Med* 352:1179, 2005.

Steinhubl SR, et al.: Early and sustained dual oral antiplatelet therapy following percutaneous coronary intervention: a randomized controlled trial, *JAMA* 288:2411, 2002.

Wiviott SD, et al.: Prasugrel versus clopidogrel in patients with acute coronary syndromes, *N Engl J Med* 357:2007, 2001.

Yusuf S, et al.: Effects of clopidogrel in addition to aspirin in patients with acute coronary syndromes without ST-segment elevation, *N Engl J Med* 345:494, 2001.

References

1. Falk E, et al.: Update on acute coronary syndromes: the pathologists' view, *Eur Heart J* 34:719, 2013.
2. Libby P: Mechanisms of acute coronary syndromes and their implications for therapy, *N Engl J Med* 368:2013, 2004.
3. Angiolillo DJ, Ueno M, Goto S: Basic principles of platelet biology and clinical implications, *Circ J* 74:597, 2010.
4. Franchi F, Angiolillo DJ: Novel antiplatelet agents in acute coronary syndrome, *Nat Rev Cardiol* 12:30, 2015.
5. Amsterdam EA, et al.: 2014 AHA/ACC Guideline for the management of patients with non-ST-elevation acute coronary syndromes: a report of the American College of Cardiology/American Heart Association Task Force on Practice Guidelines, *Circulation* 130:e344, 2014.
6. Roffi M, et al.: 2015 ESC guidelines for the management of acute coronary syndromes in patients presenting without persistent ST-segment elevation: Task Force for the Management of Acute Coronary Syndromes in Patients Presenting without Persistent ST-Segment Elevation of the European Society of Cardiology (ESC), *Eur Heart J* 37:267, 2016.
7. O'Gara PT, et al.: 2013 ACCF/AHA guideline for the management of ST-elevation myocardial infarction: a report of the American College of Cardiology Foundation/American Heart Association Task Force on Practice Guidelines, *J Am Coll Cardiol* 61:e78, 2013.
8. Steg PG, et al.: ESC guidelines for the management of acute myocardial infarction in patients presenting with ST-segment elevation, *Eur Heart J* 33:2569, 2012.
9. Levine GN, et al.: 2011 ACCF/AHA/SCAI guideline for percutaneous coronary intervention. A report of the American College of Cardiology Foundation/American Heart Association Task Force on Practice Guidelines and the Society for Cardiovascular Angiography and Interventions, *J Am Coll Cardiol* 58:e44, 2011.
10. Windecker S, et al.: 2014 ESC/EACTS guidelines on myocardial revascularization: the Task Force on Myocardial Revascularization of the European Society of Cardiology (ESC) and the European Association for Cardio-Thoracic Surgery (EACTS) Developed with the special contribution of the European Association of Percutaneous Cardiovascular Interventions (EAPCI), *Eur Heart J* 35:2541, 2014.
11. Angiolillo DJ, Capodanno D, Goto S: Platelet thrombin receptor antagonism and atherothrombosis, *Eur Heart J* 31:17, 2010.
12. Angiolillo DJ, Ferreiro JL: Antiplatelet and anticoagulant therapy for atherothrombotic disease: the role of current and emerging agents, *Am J Cardiovasc Drugs* 13:233, 2013.
13. Mega JL, Simon T: Pharmacology of antithrombotic drugs: an assessment of oral antiplatelet and anticoagulant treatments, *Lancet* 386:281, 2015.
14. Angiolillo DJ: The evolution of antiplatelet therapy in the treatment of acute coronary syndromes: from aspirin to the present day, *Drugs* 72:2087, 2012.
15. Mehta SR, et al.: Dose comparisons of clopidogrel and aspirin in acute coronary syndromes, *N Engl J Med* 363:930, 2010.
16. Pettersen AÅ, et al.: High on-aspirin platelet reactivity and clinical outcome in patients with stable coronary artery disease: results from ASCET (Aspirin Nonresponsiveness and Clopidogrel Endpoint Trial), *J Am Heart Assoc* 1:e000703, 2012.
17. Grosser T, et al.: Drug resistance and pseudoresistance: an unintended consequence of enteric coating aspirin, *Circulation* 127:377, 2013.
18. Capodanno D, et al.: Pharmacodynamic effects of different aspirin dosing regimens in type 2 diabetes mellitus patients with coronary artery disease, *Circ Cardiovasc Interv* 4:180, 2011.
19. Karve AM, et al.: Contemporary use of ticagrelor in interventional practice (from Blue Cross Blue Shield of Michigan Cardiovascular Consortium), *Am J Cardiol* 115:1502, 2015.
20. Bueno H, et al.: Opportunities for improvement in anti-thrombotic therapy and other strategies for the management of acute coronary syndromes: insights from EPICOR, an international study of current practice patterns, *Eur Heart J Acute Cardiovasc Care* 5:3, 2016.
21. Tantry US, et al.: Consensus and update on the definition of on-treatment platelet reactivity to adenosine diphosphate associated with ischemia and bleeding, *J Am Coll Cardiol* 62:2261, 2013.
22. Stone GW, et al.: Platelet reactivity and clinical outcomes after coronary artery implantation of drug-eluting stents (ADAPT-DES): a prospective multicentre registry study, *Lancet* 382:614, 2013.
23. Aradi D, et al.: Bleeding and stent thrombosis on P2Y12-inhibitors: collaborative analysis on the role of platelet reactivity for risk stratification after percutaneous coronary intervention, *Eur Heart J* 36:1762, 2015.
24. Montalescot G, et al.: Prasugrel compared with clopidogrel in patients undergoing percutaneous coronary intervention for ST-elevation myocardial infarction (TRITON-TIMI 38): double-blind, randomised controlled trial, *Lancet* 373:723, 2009.
25. Wiviott SD, et al.: Greater clinical benefit of more intensive oral antiplatelet therapy with prasugrel in patients with diabetes mellitus in the trial to assess improvement in therapeutic outcomes by optimizing platelet inhibition with prasugrel-Thrombolysis in Myocardial Infarction 38, *Circulation* 118:1626, 2008.
26. Mega JL, et al.: Cytochrome P450 genetic polymorphisms and the response to prasugrel: relationship to pharmacokinetic, pharmacodynamic, and clinical outcomes, *Circulation* 119:2553, 2009.
27. O'Donoghue ML, et al.: Pharmacodynamic effect and clinical efficacy of clopidogrel and prasugrel with or without a proton-pump inhibitor: an analysis of two randomised trials, *Lancet* 374:989, 2009.
28. Kohli P, et al.: Discharge aspirin dose and clinical outcomes in patients with acute coronary syndromes treated with prasugrel versus clopidogrel: an analysis from the TRITON-TIMI 38 study (Trial to Assess Improvement in Therapeutic Outcomes by Optimizing Platelet Inhibition with Prasugrel-Thrombolysis In Myocardial Infarction 38), *J Am Coll Cardiol* 63:225, 2014.
29. Smith PK, et al.: Mortality benefit with prasugrel in the TRITON-TIMI 38 coronary artery bypass grafting cohort: risk-adjusted retrospective data analysis, *J Am Coll Cardiol* 60:388, 2012.
30. Roe MT, et al.: Prasugrel versus clopidogrel for acute coronary syndromes without revascularization, *N Engl J Med* 367:1297, 2012.
31. Roe MT, et al.: Elderly patients with acute coronary syndromes managed without revascularization: insights into the safety of long-term dual antiplatelet therapy with reduced-dose prasugrel versus standard-dose clopidogrel, *Circulation* 128:823, 2013.
32. Wiviott SD, et al.: Prasugrel versus clopidogrel for patients with unstable angina or non-ST-segment elevation myocardial infarction with or without angiography: a secondary, prespecified analysis of the TRILOGY ACS trial, *Lancet* 382:605, 2013.
33. Gurbel PA, et al.: Randomized double-blind assessment of the ONSET and OFFSET of the antiplatelet effects of ticagrelor versus clopidogrel in patients with stable coronary artery disease: the ONSET/OFFSET study, *Circulation* 120:2577, 2009.
34. Wallentin L, et al.: Ticagrelor versus clopidogrel in patients with acute coronary syndromes, *N Engl J Med* 361:1045, 2009.
35. James SK, et al.: Ticagrelor versus clopidogrel in patients with acute coronary syndromes intended for non-invasive management: substudy from prospective randomised PLATelet inhibition and patient Outcomes (PLATO) trial, *BMJ* 342:d3527, 2011.
36. Cannon CP, et al.: Comparison of ticagrelor with clopidogrel in patients with a planned invasive strategy for acute coronary syndromes (PLATO): a randomised double-blind study, *Lancet* 375:283, 2010.
37. Held C, et al.: Ticagrelor versus clopidogrel in patients with acute coronary syndromes undergoing coronary artery bypass surgery: results from the PLATO (Platelet Inhibition and Patient Outcomes) trial, *J Am Coll Cardiol* 57:672, 2011.
38. Lindholm D, et al.: Ticagrelor vs. clopidogrel in patients with non-ST-elevation acute coronary syndrome with or without revascularization: results from the PLATO trial, *Eur Heart J* 35:2083, 2014.
39. Steg PG, et al.: Ticagrelor versus clopidogrel in patients with ST-elevation acute coronary syndromes intended for reperfusion with primary percutaneous coronary intervention: a Platelet Inhibition and Patient Outcomes (PLATO) trial subgroup analysis, *Circulation* 122:2131, 2010.
40. James S, et al.: Ticagrelor vs. clopidogrel in patients with acute coronary syndromes and diabetes: a substudy from the PLATelet inhibition and patient Outcomes (PLATO) trial, *Eur Heart J* 31:3006, 2010.
41. Husted S, et al.: Ticagrelor versus clopidogrel in elderly patients with acute coronary syndromes: a substudy from the prospective randomized PLATelet inhibition and patient Outcomes (PLATO) trial, *Circ Cardiovasc Qual Outcomes* 5:680, 2012.
42. James SK, et al.: Ticagrelor versus clopidogrel in patients with acute coronary syndromes and a history of stroke or transient ischemic attack, *Circulation* 125:2914, 2012.
43. Kohli P, et al.: Reduction in first and recurrent cardiovascular events with ticagrelor compared with clopidogrel in the PLATO Study, *Circulation* 127:673, 2013.
44. James S, et al.: Ticagrelor versus clopidogrel in acute coronary syndromes in relation to renal function: results from the Platelet Inhibition and Patient Outcomes (PLATO) trial, *Circulation* 122:1056, 2010.
45. Wallentin L, et al.: Effect of CYP2C19 and ABCB1 single nucleotide polymorphisms on outcomes of treatment with ticagrelor versus clopidogrel for acute coronary syndromes: a genetic substudy of the PLATO trial, *Lancet* 376:1320, 2010.
46. Becker RC, et al.: Bleeding complications with the P2Y12 receptor antagonists clopidogrel and ticagrelor in the PLATelet inhibition and patient Outcomes (PLATO) trial, *Eur Heart J* 32:2933, 2011.
47. Mahaffey KW, et al.: Ticagrelor compared with clopidogrel by geographic region in the Platelet Inhibition and Patient Outcomes (PLATO) trial, *Circulation* 124:544, 2011.
48. Teng R, Maya J, Butler K: Evaluation of the pharmacokinetics and pharmacodynamics of ticagrelor co-administered with aspirin in healthy volunteers, *Platelets* 24:615, 2013.
49. Cattaneo M, Schulz, Nylander S: Adenosine-mediated effects of ticagrelor: evidence and potential clinical relevance, *J Am Coll Cardiol* 63:2503, 2014.
50. Armstrong D, et al.: Characterization of the adenosine pharmacology of ticagrelor reveals therapeutically relevant inhibition of equilibrative nucleoside transporter 1, *J Cardiovasc Pharmacol Ther* 19:209, 2014.
51. Bonello L, et al.: Ticagrelor increases adenosine plasma concentration in patients with an acute coronary syndrome, *J Am Coll Cardiol* 63:872, 2014.
52. Storey RF, et al.: Pulmonary function in patients with acute coronary syndrome treated with ticagrelor or clopidogrel (from the Platelet Inhibition and Patient Outcomes [PLATO] pulmonary function substudy), *Am J Cardiol* 108:1542, 2011.
53. Alexopoulos D, Xanthopoulou I, Goudevenos J: Effects of P2Y12 receptor inhibition in patients with ST-segment elevation myocardial infarction, *Am J Cardiol* 113:2064, 2014.
54. Franchi F, Rollini F, Muñiz-Lozano A, et al.: Cangrelor: a review on pharmacology and clinical trial development, *Expert Rev Cardiovasc Ther* 11:1279, 2013.
55. Angiolillo DJ, Schneider DJ, Bhatt DL, et al.: Pharmacodynamic effects of cangrelor and clopidogrel: the platelet function substudy from the Cangrelor versus Standard Therapy to Achieve Optimal Management of Platelet Inhibition (CHAMPION) trials, *J Thromb Thrombolysis* 34:44, 2012.
56. Harrington RA, et al.: Platelet inhibition with cangrelor in patients undergoing PCI, *N Engl J Med* 361:2318, 2009.
57. Bhatt DL, et al.: Intravenous platelet blockade with cangrelor during PCI, *N Engl J Med* 361:2330, 2009.
58. Bhatt DL, et al.: Effect of platelet inhibition with cangrelor during PCI on ischemic events, *N Engl J Med* 368:1303, 2013.
59. White HD, et al.: Reduced immediate ischemic events with cangrelor in PCI: a pooled analysis of the CHAMPION trials using the universal definition of myocardial infarction, *Am Heart J* 163:182.e4, 2012.
60. Généreux P, et al.: Impact of intraprocedural stent thrombosis during percutaneous coronary intervention: insights from the CHAMPION PHOENIX Trial (Clinical Trial Comparing Cangrelor to Clopidogrel Standard of Care Therapy in Subjects Who Require Percutaneous Coronary Intervention), *J Am Coll Cardiol* 63:619, 2014.
61. Steg PG, et al.: Effect of cangrelor on periprocedural outcomes in percutaneous coronary interventions: a pooled analysis of patient-level data, *Lancet* 382:2013, 1981.
62. Angiolillo DJ, et al.: Bridging antiplatelet therapy with cangrelor in patients undergoing cardiac surgery: a randomized controlled trial, *JAMA* 307:265, 2012.
63. Muñiz-Lozano A, et al.: Update on platelet glycoprotein IIb/IIIa inhibitors: recommendations for clinical practice, *Ther Adv Cardiovasc Dis* 7:197, 2013.
64. Franchi F, et al.: Platelet thrombin receptor antagonism with vorapaxar: a review on pharmacology and clinical trial development, *Future Cardiol* 11:547, 2015.
65. Tricoci P, et al.: Thrombin-receptor antagonist vorapaxar in acute coronary syndromes, *N Engl J Med* 366:20, 2012.

66. Morrow DA, et al.: Vorapaxar in the secondary prevention of atherothrombotic events, *N Engl J Med* 366:1404, 2012.
67. FDA Clopidogrel Full Prescribing Information. http://www.accessdata.fda.gov/drugsatfda_docs/label/2010/020839s048lbl.pdf. Accessed May 1, 2015.
68. FDA Prasugrel Full Prescribing Information. http://www.accessdata.fda.gov/drugsatfda_docs/label/2010/022307s002lbl.pdf. Accessed May 1, 2015.
69. EMA: Assessment Report for Efient. http://www.ema.europa.eu/docs/en_GB/document_library/EPAR_-_Public_assessment_report/human/000984/WC500021975.pdf. Accessed May 1, 2015.
70. FDA: Ticagrelor Full Prescribing Information. www.accessdata.fda.gov/drugsatfda_docs/label/2013/022433s010lbl.pdf. Accessed May 1, 2015.
71. EMA: Assessment Report for Brilique. http://www.ema.europa.eu/docs/en_GB/document_library/EPAR_-_Public_assessment_report/human/001241/WC500100492.pdf. Accessed May 1, 2015.
72. FDA: Vorapaxar Prescribing Information. http://www.accessdata.fda.gov/drugsatfda_docs/label/2014/204886s000lbl.pdf. Accessed May 1, 2015.
73. EMA: Vorapaxar Assessment Report. http://www.ema.europa.eu/ema/index.jsp?curl=pages/medicines/human/medicines/002814/human_med_001839.jsp&mid=WC0b01ac058001d124. Accessed May 1, 2015.
74. Cangrelor United States full prescribing information [online]. www.kengreal.com/pdfs/kengreal-us-prescribing-information.pdf. Accessed July 1, 2015.
75. Cangrelor EMA prescribing information [online]. www.ema.europa.eu/docs/en_GB/document_library/EPAR_-_Product_Information/human/003773/WC500188098.pdf. Accessed July 1, 2015.
76. Capodanno D, Angiolillo DJ: Pretreatment with antiplatelet drugs in invasively managed patients with coronary artery disease in the contemporary era: review of the evidence and practice guidelines, *Circ Cardiovasc Interv* 8:e002301, 2015.
77. Valgimigli M: Pretreatment with P2Y12 inhibitors in non-ST-segment-elevation acute coronary syndrome is clinically justified, *Circulation* 130:1891, 2014.
78. Collet JP, et al.: Pretreatment with P2Y12 inhibitors in non-ST-segment-elevation acute coronary syndrome: an outdated and harmful strategy, *Circulation* 130:1904, 2014.
79. Sherwood MW, et al.: Early clopidogrel versus prasugrel use among contemporary STEMI and NSTEMI patients in the US: insights from the National Cardiovascular Data Registry, *J Am Heart Assoc* 3:e000849, 2014.
80. De Luca L, et al.: Contemporary antithrombotic strategies in patients with acute coronary syndrome admitted to cardiac care units in Italy: The EYESHOT Study, *Eur Heart J Acute Cardiovasc Care* 4:441–445, 2015.
81. Bellemain-Appaix A, et al.: Association of clopidogrel pretreatment with mortality, cardiovascular events, and major bleeding among patients undergoing percutaneous coronary intervention: a systematic review and meta-analysis, *JAMA* 308:2507, 2012.
82. Montalescot G, et al.: Pretreatment with prasugrel in non-ST-segment elevation acute coronary syndromes, *N Engl J Med* 369:999, 2013.
83. Bellemain-Appaix A, et al.: Reappraisal of thienopyridine pretreatment in patients with non-ST elevation acute coronary syndrome: a systematic review and meta-analysis, *BMJ* 349:g6269, 2014.
84. Montalescot G, et al.: Prehospital ticagrelor in ST-segment elevation myocardial infarction, *N Engl J Med* 371:1016, 2014.
85. Schulz S, et al.: Randomized comparison of ticagrelor versus prasugrel in patients with acute coronary syndrome and planned invasive strategy–design and rationale of the Intracoronary Stenting and Antithrombotic Regimen: Rapid Early Action for Coronary Treatment (ISAR-REACT) 5 trial, *J Cardiovasc Transl Res* 7:91, 2014.
86. Bagai A, et al.: In-hospital switching between adenosine diphosphate receptor inhibitors in patients with acute myocardial infarction treated with percutaneous coronary intervention: insights into contemporary practice from the TRANSLATE-ACS study, *Eur Heart J Acute Cardiovasc Care* 4:499–508, 2014.
87. Rollini F, Franchi F, Angiolillo DJ: Switching P2Y12 receptor inhibitors in patients with coronary artery disease, *Nat Rev Cardiol* 13:11–27, 2016.
88. Angiolillo DJ, et al.: Increased platelet inhibition after switching from maintenance clopidogrel to prasugrel in patients with acute coronary syndromes: results of the SWAP (SWitching Anti Platelet) study, *J Am Coll Cardiol* 56:1017, 2010.
89. Diodati JG, et al.: Effect on platelet reactivity from a prasugrel loading dose after a clopidogrel loading dose compared with a prasugrel loading dose alone: Transferring From Clopidogrel Loading Dose to Prasugrel Loading Dose in Acute Coronary Syndrome Patients (TRIPLET): a randomized controlled trial, *Circ Cardiovasc Interv* 6:567, 2013.
90. Angiolillo DJ, et al.: Pharmacodynamic evaluation of switching from ticagrelor to prasugrel in patients with stable coronary artery disease: results of the SWAP-2 Study (Switching Anti Platelet-2), *J Am Coll Cardiol* 63:1500, 2014.
91. Bassez C, et al.: Effectiveness of switching 'low responders' to prasugrel to ticagrelor after acute coronary syndrome, *Int J Cardiol* 176:1184, 2014.
92. Schneider DJ, et al.: Pharmacodynamic effects during the transition between cangrelor and prasugrel, *Coron Artery Dis* 26:42, 2015.
93. Schneider DJ, et al.: Pharmacodynamic effects during the transition between cangrelor and ticagrelor, *JACC Cardiovasc Intv* 7:435, 2014.

20 Clinical Practice/Controversy

Individualization of Antiplatelet Therapy for Patients with Acute Coronary Syndromes

Jean Philippe Collet and Guillaume Cayla

INTRODUCTION

The combination of aspirin with $P2Y_{12}$ inhibitors, which is also known as dual antiplatelet therapy, is the standard of care for oral antiplatelet treatment in patients presenting with an acute coronary syndrome (ACS) and/or who are undergoing percutaneous coronary intervention (PCI).[1] The widely variable pharmacological effects of clopidogrel and the heterogeneous relationship between the extreme value of adenosine diphosphate (ADP)–induced platelet aggregation and the occurrence of ischemic and bleeding events are limitations of this prodrug. In contrast, second-generation oral $P2Y_{12}$ inhibitors (i.e., prasugrel and ticagrelor) display a more consistent, rapid, and profound inhibition of the $P2Y_{12}$ receptor and produce further reductions in the risk of ischemic events, albeit with more bleeding complications (see Chapter 19).[2] Clopidogrel is the second-leading drug sold worldwide, and its nonselective administration is counterintuitive when it is possible to assess for a measurable drug effect and when there is the possibility of identifying patients at risk of developing adverse outcomes. Individualized treatment based on point-of-care assays is now technically possible with the potential to improve the risk and/or benefit of oral $P2Y_{12}$ therapy by identifying extreme responses and adjusting treatment.[3] There is a consensus that high on-treatment platelet reactivity (HPR) or inhibition to ADP is a major risk factor for post-PCI ischemic and/or bleeding events, respectively. However, guidelines have given a class IIb recommendation for platelet function testing or genotyping if the results of testing may alter management.[1] In this chapter, we develop the concept that individualization of oral antiplatelet therapy reflects multifaceted influences with a variety of potential clinical implications.

CLOPIDOGREL METABOLISM AND BIOLOGICAL RESPONSE

Clopidogrel is a second-generation thienopyridine derivative that binds specifically and irreversibly to the platelet $P2Y_{12}$ purinergic receptor, inhibiting ADP-mediated platelet activation and aggregation (see Chapter 19). It is an inactive prodrug that requires oxidation by the hepatic cytochrome P450 (CYP) system to generate clopidogrel H4-thiol, the putative-only active metabolite that selectively binds the $P2Y_{12}$ receptor. Platelet aggregation is affected not only when triggered by ADP, but also by other substances that require released ADP as an amplifier (Figure 20-1).

The wide interindividual variability of the biological response to clopidogrel is an established limitation of clopidogrel, and it has multiple determinants, including environmental, cellular, clinical, and genetic factors (Figure 20-2).[3] HPR and low-on treatment platelet reactivity (LPR) have been associated with recurrent ischemic and bleeding events.[4,5] The aim of platelet function testing is to measure individual responses to the drug to avoid HPR and LPR. Multiple methods exist, without consensus with regard to the best method to use.[6]

METHODS FOR PLATELET FUNCTION TESTING

There are currently four ADP-stimulated assays (vasodilator-stimulated phosphoprotein [VASP] phosphorylation:VASP-P assay, [Diagnostica Stago, Biocytex, Asnières, France]; Multiplate impedance aggregometry, [Dynabyte Medical, Munich, Germany]; VerifyNow [Accumetrics, San Diego, California]; and light transmission aggregometry [LTA]) that are validated for the prediction of stent thrombosis and bleeding in patients with ACS. There are substantial methodological differences that explain the imperfect agreement among ADP-stimulated assays

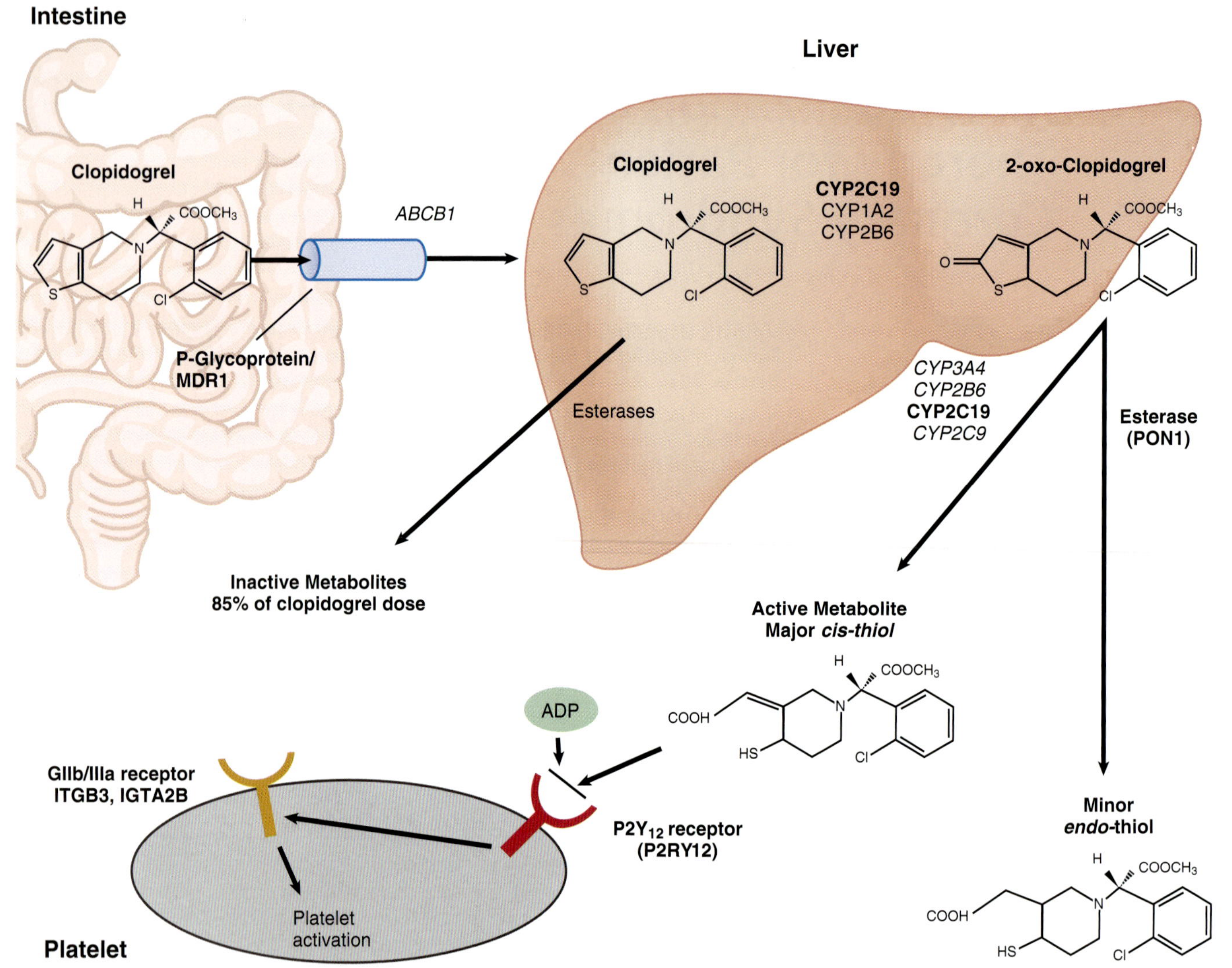

FIGURE 20-1 Metabolite activation of clopidogrel. Bioavailability of the prodrug is determined by intestinal absorption, which might be limited by the efflux pump MDR1 (encoded by ABCB1). Subsequently, 85% of the prodrug is converted into inactive metabolites by esterases. The remaining 15% is converted into an active metabolite through two-step oxidations. The first oxidative step (CYP2C19) produces the intermediate 2-oxo-clopidogrel. The second step (CYP2C19) produces the bioactive metabolite, which irreversibly binds to $P2Y_{12}$ receptors. *ADP*, Adenosine diphosphate; *PON1*, paraoxonase-1.

and the heterogeneity in classification of subjects at risk for thrombotic events. The global aggregation measure approach (platelet aggregation) is usually less specific to the drug action, whereas analysis of the drug effect with high specificity at subcellular levels (such as VASP phosphorylation) provides less information with regard to the overall state of the activation–aggregation cascade. LTA with ADP stimulation is only recommended when no standardized assays are available. Based on the currently available evidence, the best preliminary cutoffs for risk stratification include 95 and 208 $P2Y_{12}$ reaction units (PRUs) for VerifyNow, 19 and 46 U for Multiplate, and 10% and 50% platelet reactivity index (PRI) for VASP-P for bleeding and stent thrombosis, respectively (Table 20-1). These suggested cutoffs might be different according to clinical presentation, timing from PCI, procedural success, and ethnicity and therefore need further validation.

Vasodilator-Stimulated Phosphoprotein Phosphorylation

Measuring the phosphorylation state of VASP using flow cytometry is a completely $P2Y_{12}$ receptor–specific method for the evaluation of ADP-receptor inhibition. VASP is a second messenger in the signaling pathway of the $P2Y_{12}$ receptor. The ratio of dephosphorylated and phosphorylated VASP is a selective measure of $P2Y_{12}$ inhibition. The measurement is not influenced by the presence of glycoprotein IIb/IIIa receptor inhibitors (GPIs), and it is the only assay that is able to evaluate the extent of $P2Y_{12}$ receptor inhibition without the influence of the $P2Y_1$ receptor. It requires a special laboratory environment and staff experienced in flow cytometric analysis, making the method inappropriate for routine clinical purposes, but ideal for platelet function research.

Multiplate Impedance Aggregometry

Muliplate impedance aggregometry is a semi-automated, standardized aggregometry that evaluates the efficacy of platelet inhibition in whole blood. The assessment is significantly faster and more reliable than conventional aggregometry. It uses an impedance aggregometer that detects changes in electric impedance over time between two electrodes immersed in hirudin-anticoagulated whole blood diluted with saline. Changes in impedance are plotted over time, resulting in an aggregation curve that is similar to LTA. This technique requires sample preparation and pipetting throughout the assessment. The cost of testing is between the costs of LTA and VerifyNow.

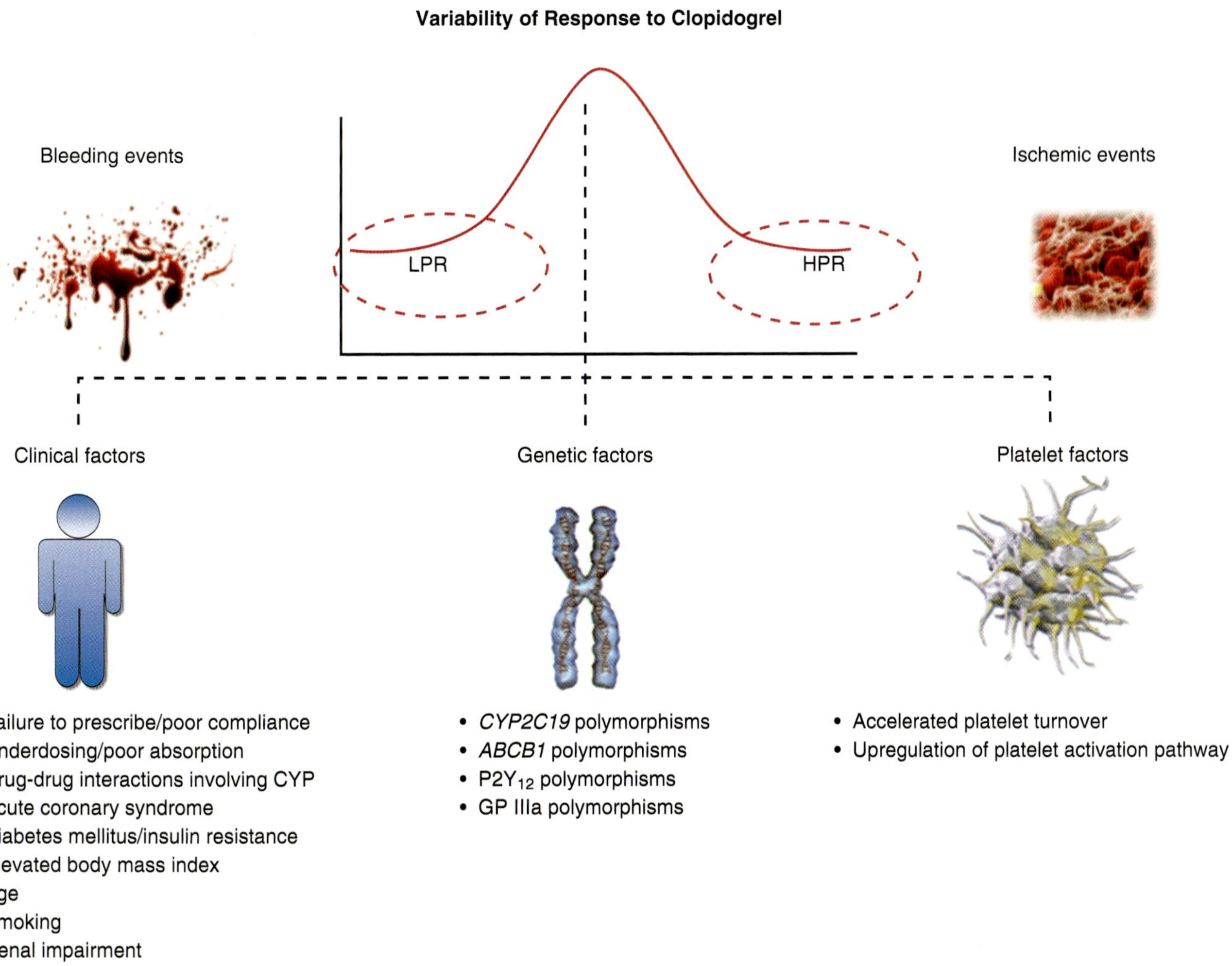

FIGURE 20-2 **Factors associated with variability of response to clopidogrel.** *GP*, Glycoprotein; *HPR*, high platelet reactivity; *LPR*, low platelet reactivity.

TABLE 20-1 Best Validated Cutoffs of Platelet Reactivity to Predict Stent Thrombosis and Bleeding.[3,4]

ASSAYS	STENT THROMBOSIS		BLEEDING	
	Cutoff	n	Cutoff	n
VerifyNow	>208 PRU	11,245	<95 PRU	8449
Multiplate	>46 U	1608	<19 U	2533
VASP-P	>50% PRI	640	<10% PRI	1542

PRI, Platelet reactivity index; *PRU*, platelet reactivity unit; *U*, aggregation unit; *VASP-P*, vasodilator stimulated phosphoprotein phosphorylation.

VerifyNow

The VerifyNow System is a point-of-care assay that measures agonist-induced platelet aggregation by turbidimetric-based optical detection. Platelets are activated by the presence of agonists and bind to fibrinogen-coated beads, causing agglutinates to drop out of solution. Results are reported as PRUs, with a lower PRU value corresponding to a higher degree of $P2Y_{12}$ receptor inhibition. Advantages of the VerifyNow system include simplicity, sensitivity, speed, and user-friendliness.

Light Transmission Aggregometry

Infrared light transmittance passing through platelet-poor plasma is used to represent 100% aggregation, and the optical changes from 0%, set by the unstimulated platelet-rich plasma, is evaluated in response to inductors. As activated platelets aggregate after the inductors, optical density decreases in the absence of antiplatelet medication. It is inexpensive and the historical gold standard tool for platelet function studies, with widespread use and with significant clinical experience in both pharmacodynamic and clinical studies. However, LTA is time-consuming and requires trained laboratory personnel, which precludes testing 24-hour/7-day service at the bedside. The lack of standardization caused by the diversity in the concentration of agonist used (5, 10, 20 μM), the preferred estimate for evaluation (peak aggregation, late aggregation), the choice of anticoagulants (citrate, hirudin, or phenylalanyl-prolyl-arginyl chloromethyl ketone [PPACK] anticoagulation), and the different specifications in sample preparation techniques (centrifuging time and speed) are other important limitations.

RATIONALE FOR PLATELET FUNCTION TESTING

Prognostic Usefulness of Platelet Function Testing for Thrombotic Events

Platelet function testing has confirmed that $P2Y_{12}$-receptor signaling is a major component of pathophysiological thrombus formation in patients with ACS treated with PCI. In particular, HPR has emerged as an independent predictor for stent thrombosis. In the ADAPT-DES (Assessment of Dual AntiPlatelet Therapy with Drug-Eluting Stents) trial, the largest observational platelet function study conducted to date, approximately 50% of 30-day post-PCI stent thrombosis was attributable to high platelet reactivity (propensity-adjusted hazard ratio [HR], 3.0; 95% confidence interval [CI], 1.39 to 6.49; *P* = .005), defined as a PRU value of more than 208 when using the bedside test VerifyNow.[5] HPR was also independently correlated with a 1-year definite and/or probable stent thrombosis (adjusted HR, 2.49; 95% CI, 1.43 to 4.31; *P* = .001) and myocardial infarction (MI) (adjusted HR, 1.42; 95% CI, 1.09 to 1.86; *P* = .01). However, the risk associated with HPR is modulated by the clinical characteristics and procedural results of the studied individual. For example, the predictive accuracy of HPR to ADP was higher in patients with ACS (adjusted HR, 3.91; 95% CI, 1.51 to 10.11; *P* = .005) than in patients with stable coronary artery disease (adjusted HR, 1.49; 95% CI, 0.35 to 6.36; *P* = .59). In the TRILOGY-ACS (Targeted Platelet Inhibition to Clarify the Optimal Strategy to Medically Manage Acute Coronary Syndromes) trial, HPR in patients treated by clopidogrel or prasugrel was not an independent predictor of adverse events.[7] Finally, HPR is much less prevalent in prasugrel- or ticagrelor-treated patients than in patients treated with clopidogrel, and its correlation with outcome in patients treated with these third-generation ADP antagonists has still not been established.[6]

Prognostic Usefulness of Platelet Function Testing for Bleeding Events

Among patients treated with $P2Y_{12}$ inhibitors, LPR, defined in Table 20-1, is associated with an increased risk of major bleeding complications compared with optimal platelet reactivity (relative risk [RR] 1.74; 95% CI, 1.47 to 2.06; *P* <.00001).[4] Of interest, the increase in the risk of bleeding using current generation potent $P2Y_{12}$ inhibitors is becoming closer to the magnitude of reduction in stent thrombosis or MI. The lack of standardization in the definition of bleeding events, duration of follow-up, adjudication of bleeding events in many studies, and predefined cutoff value of LPR are recognized limitations. In addition, evidence with the current generation $P2Y_{12}$ inhibitors is much less compared with clopidogrel, and the relevance of clopidogrel thresholds to define LPR with prasugrel and ticagrelor needs to be verified.[8] A therapeutic window for $P2Y_{12}$ inhibition has been suggested and has raised the possibility of tailoring antiplatelet therapy for optimization of the benefit-to-risk ratio in clinical practice (Figure 20-3).

PLATELET FUNCTION TEST-GUIDED TREATMENT STRATEGY

Even if on-treatment platelet reactivity appears to be a reliable and independent measure of the risk of future events, the concept of selective intensive antiplatelet therapy based on a measured drug effect has never been successfully proven. Randomized trials that have examined the platelet function testing hypothesis have been limited by low event rates, insufficient pharmacological interventions, bias toward low-risk patient recruitment, and intervention in patients who are considered to be nonresponders after stent placement.

The GRAVITAS (Gauging Responsiveness with A VerifyNow assay-Impact on Thrombosis And Safety) trial[9] tested a strategy of a fixed regimen of high-dose clopidogrel (600 mg followed by 150 mg/day for 6 months) in patients with high on-treatment reactivity (defined as 230 PRUs according to the VerifyNow $P2Y_{12}$ test). This strategy of a fixed higher dose, regardless of the achieved level of platelet inhibition, did not reduce cardiovascular death, MI, and stent thrombosis after PCI compared with a standard dose of clopidogrel (75 mg/day). Interpretation of these results should take into account the following limitations: a stringent definition of clopidogrel poor response (PRU >230); a low-intensity intervention to overcome poor response; a small proportion of ACS patients (15.5% with positive biomarkers); and a low event rate (observed event rate was 2.3% compared with the expected 5%) because of randomization after coronary intervention. A post hoc analysis of the study showed that PRU values less than 208 were independently associated with the 60-day primary endpoint, which was a composite of death, MI, and stent thrombosis (HR, 1.68; 95% CI, 0.76 to 1.32).[10]

In Testing Platelet Reactivity in Patients Undergoing Elective Stent Placement on Clopidogrel to Guide Alternative Therapy with Prasugrel (TRIGGER-PCI), 2150 low-risk stable coronary artery disease patients with successfully implanted drug-eluting stents and more than 208 PRUs on VerifyNow were planned to be randomized to receive either prasugrel administered as a 60-mg loading dose, followed by 10-mg/day clopidogrel administered with a 600-mg loading dose and followed by 75 mg/day.[11] Although TRIGGER-PCI was terminated early because of futility, the active strategy was effectively reduced HPR, which was 6% on prasugrel. Only 1 occurrence of the primary endpoint was reported among 236 patients who

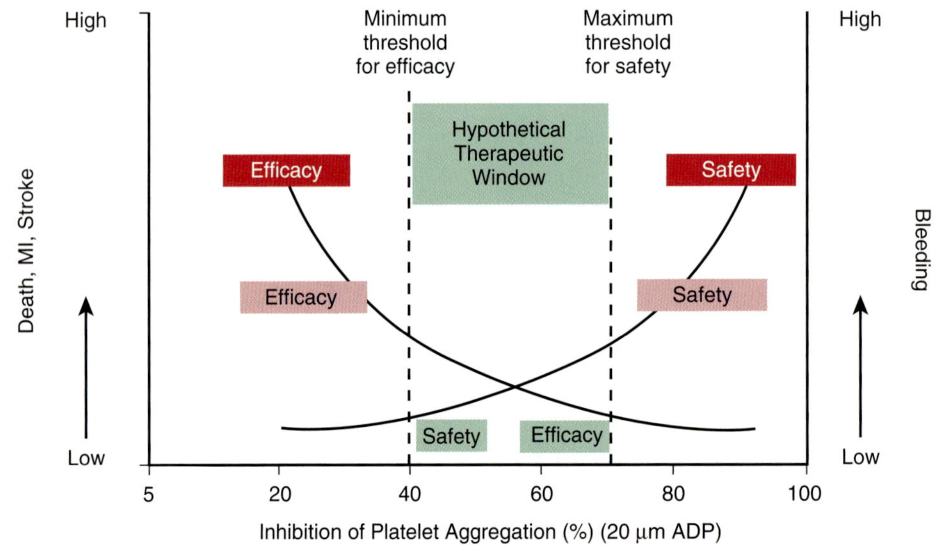

FIGURE 20-3 Therapeutic window of $P2Y_{12}$ inhibition and outcomes. *ADP*, Adenosine diphosphate; *MI*, myocardial infarction. *(Modified from Becker RC: Pharmacogenetics and safety parameters for platelet P2Y12 receptor antagonists.* J Thromb Thrombolysis *28:513–514, 2009.)*

completed 6 months of follow-up. Of importance, 30% of the enrolled patients declined randomization after being identified as having HPR, which underscored the limitation of a trial strategy based on identification of deemed nonresponders instead of randomizing the use of platelet function testing and adjusting treatment.

In the ARCTIC (Assessment by a Double Randomization of a Conventional Antiplatelet Strategy Versus a Monitoring Guided Strategy for Drug-Eluting Stent Implantation and of Treatment Interruption Versus Continuation One year After Stenting) trial (n = 2440),[12] HPR was identified in patients allocated by randomization to the strategy of platelet function monitoring, and treatments were adjusted to control this risk factor as much as possible both before and after hospital discharge (Figure 20-4). However, this strategy failed to show a benefit on ischemic events that occurred during the first year after hospitalization for revascularization with coronary drug-eluting stents (Figure 20-5). High-platelet reactivity during treatment with aspirin was defined as ≥550 aspirin reaction units. High-platelet reactivity during treatment with thienopyridine was defined as ≥235 PRU and 15% or less inhibition compared with a baseline measurement of aggregation, or both. Drug adjustment consisted of a new loading dose of clopidogrel or use of prasugrel, infusion of GPI, and an increased maintenance dose of clopidogrel or use of prasugrel. The low ACS rate (30%) and the inability of the intervention to overcome HPR in 15% of patients were the major drawbacks of the ARCTIC study. The same results were confirmed after excluding all in-hospital events,[13] refuting the hypothesis that HPR is not only a marker of risk, but is also a risk factor that can possibly be modified with the antiplatelet drugs available. This study was appropriately powered with a significant more aggressive pharmacological intervention in nonresponders, leading to a twofold reduction in the rate of nonresponders. Of interest, patients with major bleeding were more likely to have HPR than those who did not bleed (34.4% vs. 15.2%; $P = .001$).[14] This demonstrates that HPR is a complex trait that solely integrates treatment response, and it furthermore explains why it was not an independent predictor of death in the ADAPT-DES registry.

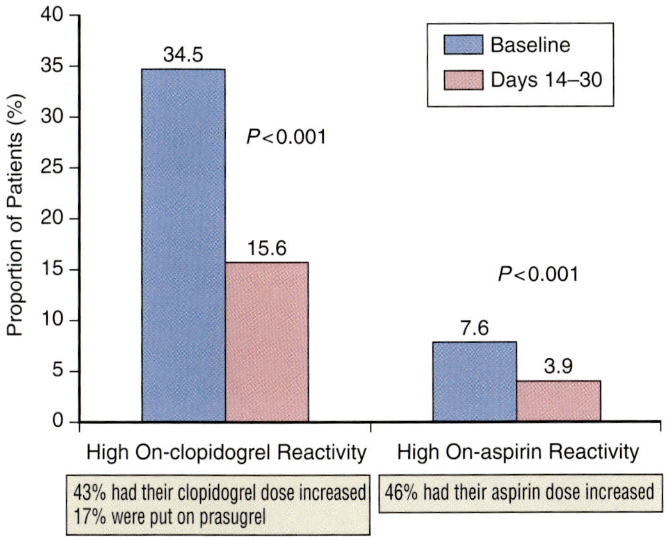

FIGURE 20-4 Treatment adjustment during follow-up in the ARCTIC trial.[12] High-on platelet reactivity was halved at the time of PCI and during the maintenance phase as a result of treatment adjustment.

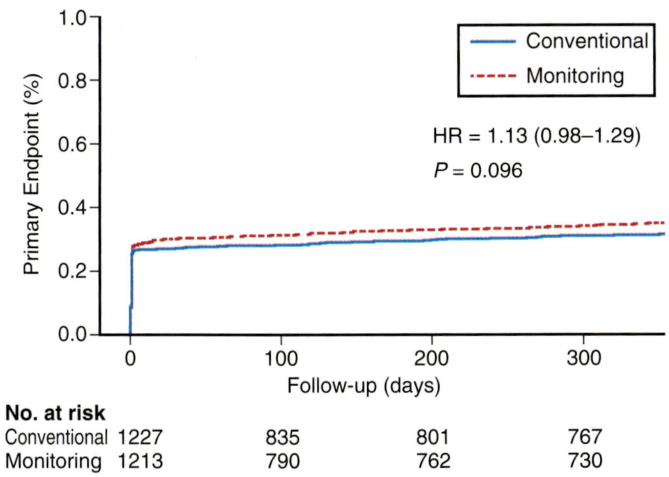

FIGURE 20-5 Proportion of patients with primary outcome events (composite of death, myocardial infarction, stent thrombosis, stroke, or urgent revascularization 1 year after stent implantation) in the ARCTIC trial.[12] *HR*, Hazard ratio.

Limitations of Platelet Function Testing

Altogether, the risk level of the population, the cutoff value used to define HPR to ADP, and the heterogeneity in treatment adjustment in those who are deemed nonresponders are potential explanations for the lack of benefit of platelet function testing to guide antiplatelet therapy. The lack of impact of treatment adjustment on other major determinants of platelet reactivity, including treatment compliance, should also to be considered.

The low predictive performance of platelet function tests also remains a major limitation. This poor performance first reflects the low prevalence of stent thrombosis in stable patients. However, the lack of a strong association between platelet reactivity and stent thrombosis remains a concern and accounts for the poor discrimination of this parameter,[15] which should be viewed as a risk predictor rather than a "diagnostic" tool.[16] According to the ARCTIC study, it seems likely that the reclassification of the performance of platelet function tests appears limited, further supporting platelet reactivity as a marker of risk rather than a risk factor.

Seeking a Therapeutic Window of $P2Y_{12}$ Inhibition

Taken together, these data suggest that measuring treatment response by platelet function assays should be limited to research or unexpected situations, and as stated in current professional guidelines, should not be routinely used clinically. Studies of treatment individualization that target different populations and types of events are ongoing and have the potential to change the guidelines (Table 20-2). However, there are specific situations in which platelet function assays may guide therapy, especially in cases of unexpected events such as stent thrombosis, treatment compliance issues, or a high likelihood of treatment poor response, if the results could change the treatment strategy.

The ANTARCTIC study (Assessment of a Normal versus Tailored Dose of Prasugrel after Stenting in Patients Aged >75 Years to Reduce the Composite of Bleeding, Stent Thrombosis and Ischemic Complications; ClinicalTrials.gov number, NCT01538446) trial is designed to demonstrate the superiority of a strategy of platelet function monitoring with dose and drug adjustment in patients who are initially treated with prasugrel 5 mg compared with a conventional

TABLE 20-2 Summary of the Randomized Studies Testing the Hypothesis of Individualized Antiplatelet Therapy

	GRAVITAS	TRIGGER	ARCTIC	ANTARCTIC	TROPICAL ACS
No. of Patients	2214	423	2440	852	2600
	CAD PCI	CAD PCI	CAD PCI	Older Adults ACS PCI	ACS PCI
ACS (%)	40	0	27	100	100
PFT assay	VerifyNow	VerifyNow	VerifyNow	VerifyNow	Multiplate
Intervention if HPR	High-dose clopidogrel	Prasugrel 10 mg	High-dose clopidogrel/prasugrel	Prasugrel 10 mg	Prasugrel
Intervention if LPR	NA	NA	NA	Downgrade to clopidogrel	NA
Primary endpoint	CV death, MI, ST at 6 mos	Cardiac death or MI	CV death, MI, urgent revascularization, stroke	CV death, MI, stroke, urgent revascularization, ST, BARC 2,3,5	CV death, MI, stroke, urgent revascularization, ST, BARC ≥2
Follow-up	6 mos	6 mos	1 yr	1 yr	1 yr
Results	2.3% vs. 2.3%; *P* = .97	0% vs. 0.004%	34.6% (monitoring) vs. 31.1 (conventional *P* = .1)	Ongoing	Ongoing
Event reduction	No	No	No	Ongoing	Ongoing

ACS, Acute coronary syndrome; *BARC*, Bleeding Academic Research Consortium; *CAD*, coronary artery disease; *CV*, cardiovascular; *HPR*, high platelet reactivity; *LPR*, low platelet reactivity; *MI*, myocardial infarction; *PCI*, percutaneous coronary intervention; *PFT*, platelet function test.

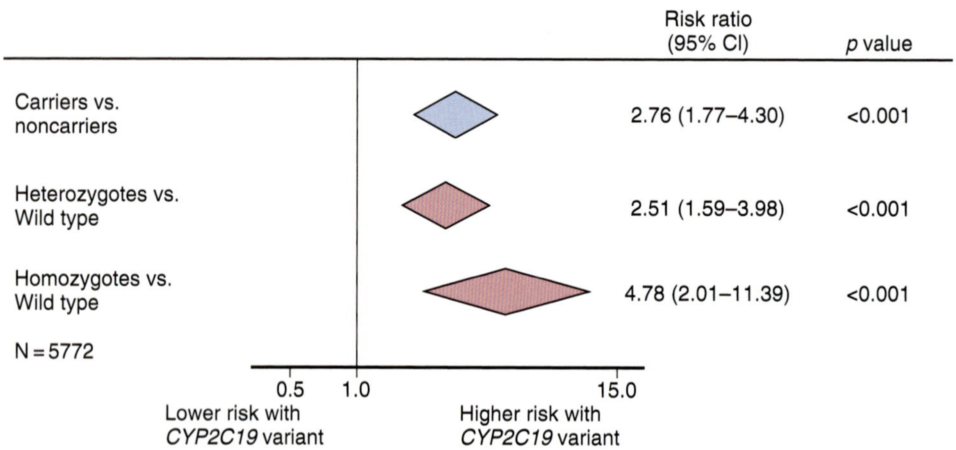

FIGURE 20-6 Effects of *CYP2C19* variants on stent thrombosis in acute coronary syndrome.[20] Carriers of the loss-of-function allele CYP219*2 had an increased risk of stent thrombosis with a gene–dose effect. *CI*, Confidence interval.

strategy using prasugrel 5 mg without monitoring and drug adjustment (Fig. 20-e1).[17] The study population includes ACS patients aged 75 years or older who are treated by PCI with stent implantation. Patients in the monitoring arm will be tested with the VerifyNow $P2Y_{12}$ 2 weeks after initiation of 5 mg of prasugrel. For the first time, the ANTARCTIC study will test the concept of a therapeutic window, with a reduction of intensity of $P2Y_{12}$ inhibition switching from prasugrel to clopidogrel in patients with LPR. In contrast, the prasugrel dose will be increased in HPR patients. In contrast to previous randomized studies, the primary endpoint is investigating the net clinical benefit, a combination of Bleeding Academic Research Consortium (BARC) 2, 3, and 5 bleeding, and ischemic endpoints.

The TROPICAL ACS (Testing Responsiveness to Platelet Inhibition on Chronic Antiplatelet Treatment for Acute Coronary Syndromes Trial; ClinicalTrials.gov number, NCT01959451) study is testing the noninferiority of multiplate-guided $P2Y_{12}$ inhibition compared with 1-year use of prasugrel in high-risk ACS patients after PCI. As in the ANTARCTIC study, the primary endpoint is a composite endpoint of ischemic and bleeding events.

GENETIC TESTS FOR CLOPIDOGREL RESPONSE

Genetic variability in clopidogrel absorption and metabolism has a direct impact on generation of the active drug metabolite. The two-step hepatic cytochrome P450 (CYP)–dependent oxidative metabolism of the prodrug appears to be of particular importance. Carriage of the loss-of-function allele *CYP2C19*2* observed in 15% of whites and up to 30% of Asians alters the pharmacodynamic response to clopidogrel, leading to an increased rate in cardiovascular events.[18–20] In particular, the risk of stent thrombosis is augmented in both carriers of one (HR, 2.67; 95% CI, 1.69 to 4.22; *P* <.0001) and two (HR, 3.97; 95% CI, 1.75 to 9.02; *P* = .001) reduced function alleles (Figure 20-6). This risk appears to be independent of the clinical and procedural factors and platelet reactivity. However, none of the studies used in this metanalysis was randomized, and there is some uncertainty with respect to the impact of a clopidogrel loading dose. There is evidence that demonstrates that a higher dose of clopidogrel is effective in improving platelet aggregation responses in *CYP2C19*2* carriers with a gene–dose effect,[21,22] but that prasugrel and ticagrelor are much better alternatives in homozygous carriers.[23] In brief, prognostic performance of genetic testing

TABLE 20-3 Clopidogrel-Predicted Metabolizers Phenotype According to Genetic Polymorphism Carriage Genetic Factors

METABOLIZER TYPE	GENETIC VARIANT	CLINICAL PHENOTYPE
Ultra	*17/*17, *1/*17	Rapid metabolizers
Extensive	*1/*1	
Intermediate	*1/*2, *1/*3	Slow metabolizers
Poor	*2/*2, *2/*3, *3/*3	
Unknown	*2/*17, *3/*17	

appears to be weak mainly because of the low prevalence of adverse events and little discrimination.[15]

The *CYP2C19*17* allele (c.-806C>T; rs12248560) is a regulatory, gain-of-function variant that has been associated with increased CYP2C19 transcription that results in a modest gain of function. The *17 allele is common, with an average multiethnic allele frequency of approximately 3% to 21%. Carriage of the gain-of-function polymorphism *2C19*17* is associated with LPR and a higher risk of bleeding. The two polymorphisms (*17 and *2) are in complete linkage disequilibrium, and the combination of both *17 and *2 variant is rare. On the basis of combinations of alleles, patients can be classified into one of five categories of metabolizer phenotypes (Table 20-3).

The *ABCB1* gene encodes a glycoprotein called MDR1 or P-glycoprotein (P-GP), which is located in the intestinal cell membrane that is involved in the efflux of different drugs, including clopidogrel. The common C3435T polymorphism results in overexpression of the ABCB1 protein and has been associated with a lower concentration of clopidogrel active metabolite, a higher rate of high on-clopidogrel platelet reactivity, and an increase in cardiovascular events.

Paraoxonase-1 (PON1) is a hepatic esterase that binds circulating high-density lipoproteins to prevent oxidative modification of low-density lipoproteins and has been proposed as an important factor in the transformation of the intermediate metabolite of clopidogrel. The PON 1Q192 variant gene polymorphism has been suggested to play a major role on both pharmacokinetic and pharmacodynamic responses.[24] However, none of the further studies published after this one were able to replicate these findings, which suggested that PON1 likely had no major role in clopidogrel response.[25]

Genotype Test-Guided Treatment Strategy

The consistent prognostic value of *CYP2C19*2* carriage in stented patients and the warning of the Food and Drug Administration (FDA) stating that there can be a diminished effect of standard doses of clopidogrel in CYP2C19 slow metabolizers[26] has led to the rationale for genotype test–guided treatment strategies. Bedside genetic testing has been used to select poor responders to clopidogrel and altering therapy toward more potent $P2Y_{12}$ inhibitors, but the safety and the efficacy of such a strategy remains unknown.

The ReAssessment of Anti-Platelet Therapy Using an InDividualized Strategy Based on GENetic Evaluation (RAPID GENE) trial was the first proof of concept study in which 200 patients who underwent PCI for ACS or stable coronary artery disease (SCAD) were randomly assigned to rapid point-of-care genotyping for the *CYP2C19*2* allele or to standard treatment.[27] Carriers in the genotyping arm were treated with

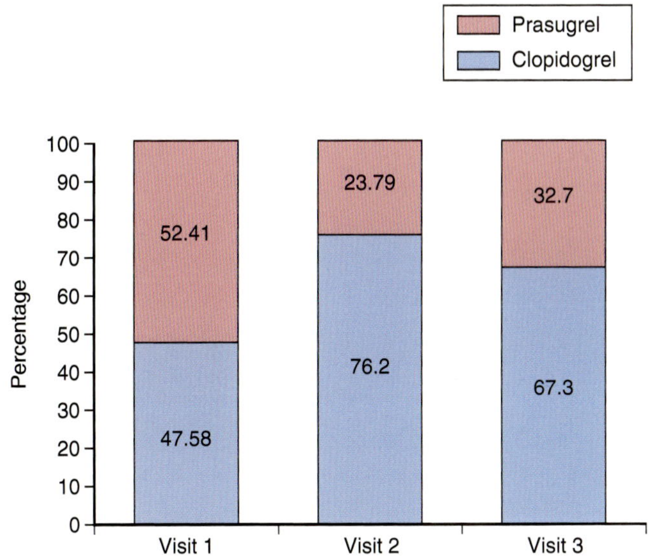

FIGURE 20-7 The GAMMA study. Proportional representation of antiplatelet therapy at the time of inclusion in the study (visit 1), after genetic profiling (visit 2), and after genetic profiling and platelet function testing (visit 3).

10 mg/day of prasugrel, and noncarriers in the control arm were given 75 mg/day of clopidogrel. At day 7, none of the 23 carriers in the rapid genotyping group had a PRU value of more than 234 compared with 7 (30%) carriers who received standard treatment (P = .0092). There were nonsignificant differences in the proportion of patients above this PRU value between the genotype group and the standard group in patients who were homozygous for the wild-type *CYP2C19*1*. However, a strategy tailoring anti-$P2Y_{12}$ therapy to CYP2C19 status ignored the HPR to ADP in up to one-third of the "rapid" metabolizers treated with clopidogrel,[19,28] leaving them exposed to a three-fold higher risk of stent thrombosis.[29]

Genotype and Platelet Function Test-Guided Strategy

The GAMMA (Point of care Genetic profiling Approach for a fast identification of clopidogrel Metabolizer phenotype to optimize Maintenance treatment after an Acute Coronary Syndrome; ClinicalTrials.gov Identifier NCT01390974) trial further tested the hypothesis that the sequential use of the Verigene rapid CYP2C19 test for genetic profiling and the VerifyNow bedside test for platelet function measurement in 269 ACS patients might improve $P2Y_{12}$ inhibition. Patients who were slow metabolizers were switched to prasugrel and rapid metabolizers were switched to clopidogrel. This study demonstrated that point-of-care genotyping and platelet function testing were complementary in selecting prasugrel or clopidogrel maintenance doses in ACS patients. In particular, by using genetic information only, 50% of patients still remained outside the optimal window of platelet reactivity, thus demonstrating a loose relationship between genotype and platelet function phenotype. Interestingly, more than one-third of clopidogrel-treated patients with HPR had previous LPR on prasugrel.[30] The combination of genetic and pharmacodynamics information led to a drastic reduction in the need for more potent $P2Y_{12}$ inhibitors (Figure 20-7).

Although such approaches are attractive, none of these studies were outcome-driven, and platelet reactivity has to be considered as a surrogate endpoint. The GIANT (Genotyping Infarct Patients to Adjust and Normalize Thienopyridine

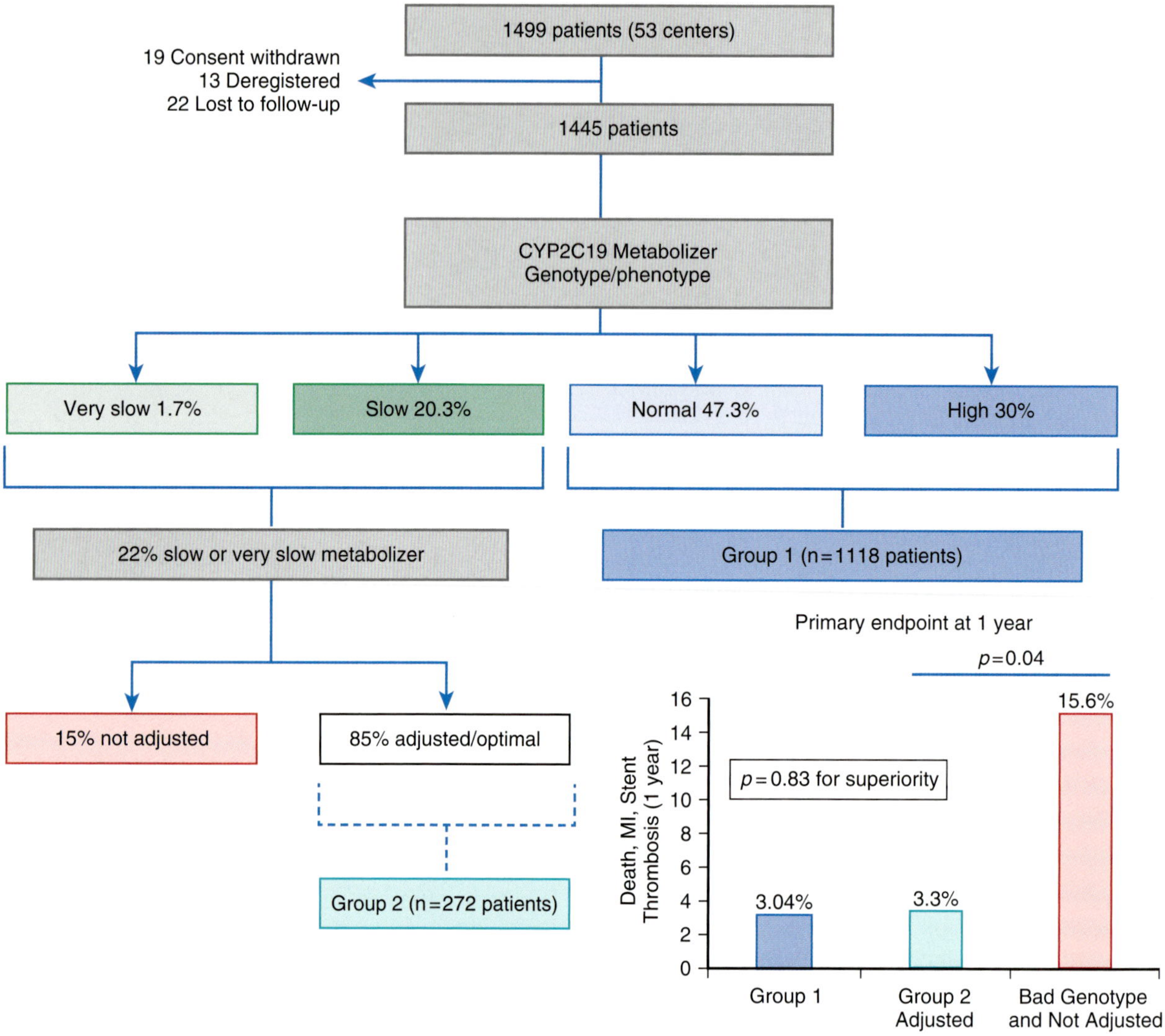

FIGURE 20-8 The GIANT study. Genotype-guided $P2Y_{12}$ inhibition following primary percutaneous coronary intervention. Carriers of the loss-of-function allele *CYP2C19*2* who underwent treatment adjustment had similar clinical outcomes as no-carriers without treatment adjustment. *MI*, Myocardial infarction.

Treatment; ClinicalTrials.gov Identifier: NCT01134380) trial was one of the first clinical studies with a genotype-guided antiplatelet therapy in patients who received a stent for an acute MI. A total of 1445 patients were included in this study (Figure 20-8).[31] Genotype information regarding CYP2C19 polymorphisms was available within 48 hours after stenting. A drug adjustment was strongly recommended for patients who carried the CYP2C19 clopidogrel loss of function. Among the 272 patients with the loss-of-function genotype and antiplatelet adjustment (prasugrel), the 1-year composite risk of ischemic events was similar compared with patients with a normal genotype (n = 1118). Although the results of GIANT are interesting, the use of the genotyping was not randomized. The ongoing Patient Outcome after Primary PCI (POPULAR) genetics study is randomizing 2700 ST-elevation myocardial infarction (STEMI) patients to a CYP2C19-guided genotype therapy or a conventional therapy to improve net clinical benefit.[32]

Genotype Test and Clinically Guided Approach

A clinically-guided approach integrating genotyping has been evaluated in the ONline ASSIstance for Stent Thrombosis (ONASSIST) study, in which 123 patients who survived an early stent thrombosis were matched for age and gender with 246 control subjects.[33] Six nongenetic factors (type C lesion, proton pump inhibitor use, diabetes mellitus, left ventricular dysfunction <40%, PCI in an acute setting, and clopidogrel loading dose) and three genetic factors (CYP2C19 metabolic status, ABCB1 3435 TT genotype, and ITGB3 PLA2 polymorphism) were independently associated with early stent thrombosis. Risk models to identify at-risk patients were created, and it was demonstrated that the combination of clinical and genetic features provided the greatest power to discriminate stent thrombosis cases compared with the clinical-only model (Figures 20-9 and 20-10). Further prospective evaluation of such an approach is now needed.

SUMMARY

The use of platelet function information to stratify risk and to inform treatment decisions as a routine approach remains to be demonstrated, and therefore, cannot be recommended as a routine approach. However, the evidence is strong enough now to recommend genotyping and phenotyping in high-risk PCI patients and especially when

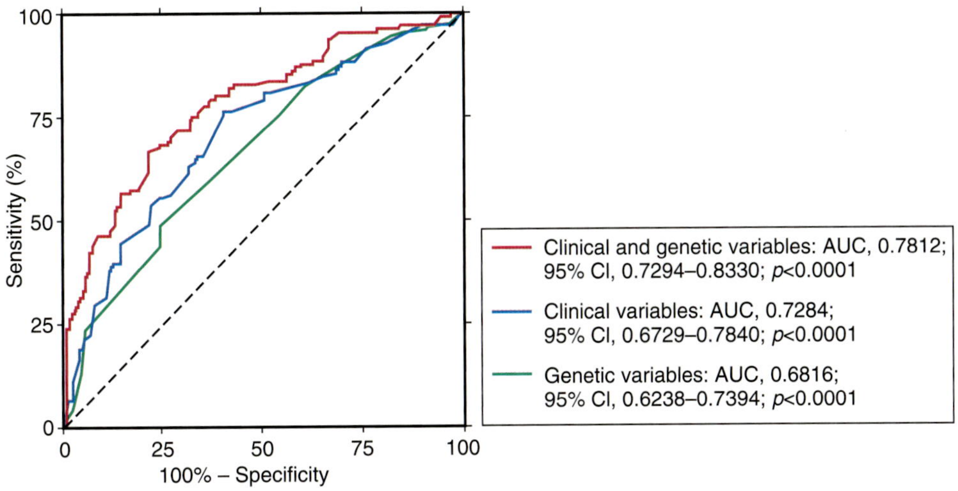

FIGURE 20-9 Receiver-operator character curve for association with early stent thrombosis in the ONASSIST registry. The clinical model is based on nongenetic factors (type C lesion, proton pump inhibitor use, diabetes mellitus, left ventricular dysfunction <40%, percutaneous coronary intervention in acute setting, and clopidogrel loading dose), with a sensitivity of 60% and a specificity of 70%, for a positive likelihood ratio of 2.1 (area under the curve [AUC], 0.73; 95% confidence interval [CI], 0.67 to 0.78; *P* <.001).The genetic model contains CYP2C19 metabolic status, an ABCB1 3435 TT genotype, and an ITGB3 PLA2 polymorphism, with a sensitivity of 48% and a specificity of 78%, for a positive likelihood ratio of 2.0 (AUC, 0.68; 95% CI, 0.62 to 0.74; *P* <.001). The combined model contains all clinical, angiographic, and genetic predictors, with a sensitivity of 67% and a specificity of 79%, for a positive likelihood ratio of 3.4 (AUC, 0.78; 95% CI, 0.73 to 0.83; *P* <.001). The *diagonal dotted line* is the expected receiver-operating characteristic curve for a totally random classifier.

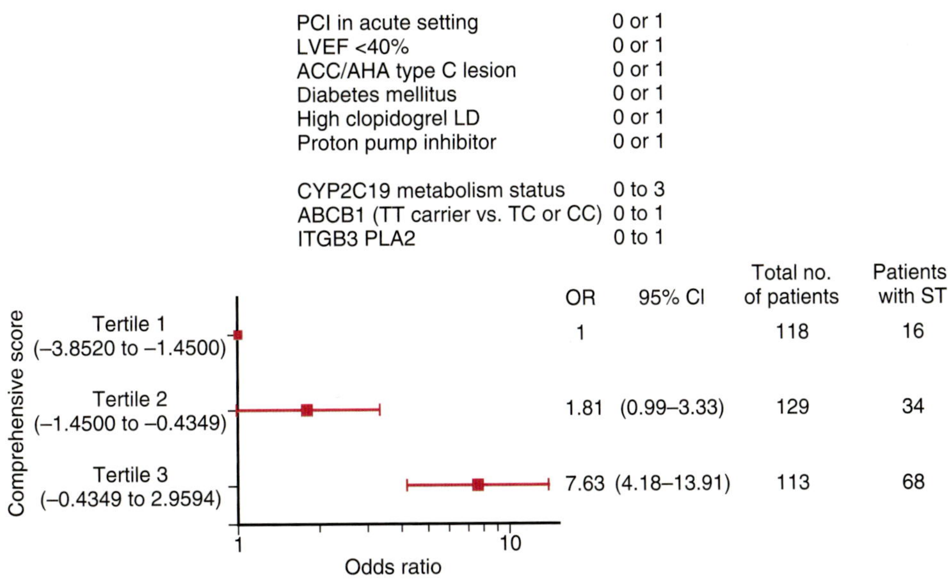

FIGURE 20-10 ONASSIST scoring system. Estimation of the risk of early stent thrombosis according to a comprehensive model based on clinical factors (n = 6) and genetic factors. Patients in the highest tertile have a seven-fold increased risk of stent thrombosis. *ACC/AHA*, American College of Cardiology/American Heart Association; *CI*, confidence interval; *LD*, loading dose; *LVEF*, left ventricular ejection fraction; *OR*, odds ratio; *PCI*, percutaneous coronary intervention.

an unexpected event occurs after an ACS (Figure 20-11). Whether high-risk selected patients, such as older adults who present with ACS, would have a better benefit-to-risk profile with tailored therapy is the next step of clinical investigation. Cardiogenic shock complicating acute MI with and without left ventricular assist devices is another area of potential investigation. The benefit of revascularization is sometimes questionable in patients with multiorgan failure in whom the use of intense platelet inhibition may add risk. Finally, post–transcatheter aortic valve replacement (TAVR) is another potential situation of interest. The benefit of antiplatelet therapy is unknown in an older adult population in whom bleeding complications are frequent and treatment compliance is a concerning issue. Platelet reactivity is a complex trait that integrates many effects of comorbidities, and the question arises as to whether clinical characteristics are sufficient to tailor treatment. This becomes an even more relevant issue because the debates of prolongation of dual antiplatelet therapy duration after an ACS is ongoing.

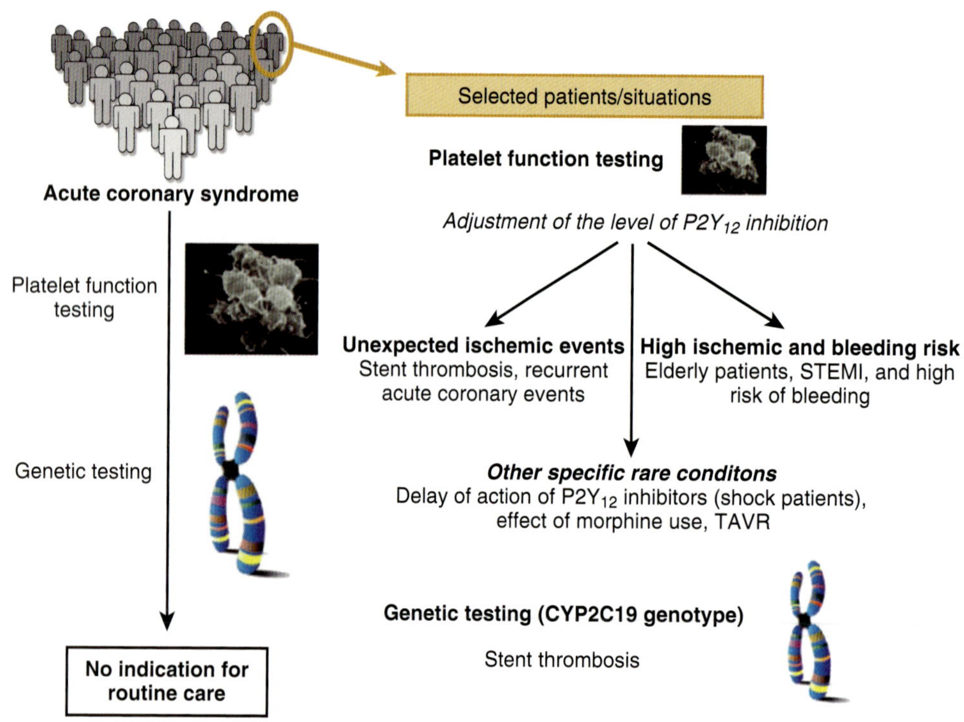

FIGURE 20-11 **Overview of current role for assessment of platelet responsiveness in clinical care.** *STEMI*, ST-elevation myocardial infarction.

References

1. Windecker S, et al.: Authors/Task Force Members. 2014 ESC/EACTS Guidelines on myocardial revascularization: The Task Force on Myocardial Revascularization of the ESC/EACTS, developed with the special contribution of the EAPCI, *Eur Heart J* 35:2541–2619, 2014.
2. Bellemain-Appaix A, et al.: New P2Y12 inhibitors versus clopidogrel in percutaneous coronary intervention: a meta-analysis, *J Am Coll Cardiol* 56:1542–1551, 2010.
3. Aradi D, et al.: on behalf of the Working Group on Thrombosis of the European Society of Cardiology. Expert position paper on the role of platelet function testing in patients undergoing percutaneous coronary intervention, *Eur Heart J* 35:209–215, 2014.
4. Aradi D, et al.: Bleeding and stent thrombosis on P2Y12-inhibitors: collaborative analysis on the role of platelet reactivity for risk stratification after percutaneous coronary intervention, *Eur Heart J* 36:1762–1771, 2015.
5. Stone GW, et al.: Platelet reactivity and clinical outcomes after coronary artery implantation of drug-eluting stents (ADAPT-DES): a prospective multicentre registry study, *Lancet* 382:614–623, 2013.
6. Kerneis M, et al.: Switching acute coronary syndrome patients from prasugrel to clopidogrel, *JACC Cardiovasc Interv* 6:158–165, 2013.
7. Gurbel PA, et al.: TRILOGY ACS Platelet Function Substudy Investigators. Platelet function during extended prasugrel and clopidogrel therapy for patients with ACS treated without revascularization: the TRILOGY ACS platelet function substudy, *JAMA* 308:1785–1794, 2012.
8. Cayla G, et al.: Prasugrel monitoring and bleeding in real world patients, *Am J Cardiol* 111:38–44, 2013.
9. Price MJ, et al.: for GRAVITAS Investigators. Standard- vs high-dose clopidogrel based on platelet function testing after percutaneous coronary intervention: the GRAVITAS randomized trial, *JAMA* 305:1097–1105, 2011.
10. Price MJ, et al.: Platelet reactivity and cardiovascular outcomes after percutaneous coronary intervention: a time-dependent analysis of the Gauging Responsiveness with a VerifyNow P2Y12 assay: impact on Thrombosis and Safety (GRAVITAS) trial, *Circulation* 124:1132–1137, 2011.
11. Trenk D, et al.: A randomized trial of prasugrel versus clopidogrel in patients with high platelet reactivity on clopidogrel after elective percutaneous coronary intervention with implantation of drug-eluting stents: Results of the TRIGGER-PCI (Testing Platelet Reactivity In Patients Undergoing Elective Stent Placement on Clopidogrel to Guide Alternative Therapy With Prasugrel) Study, *J Am Coll Cardiol* 59:2159–2164, 2012.
12. Collet J-P, et al.: Bedside monitoring to adjust antiplatelet therapy for coronary stenting, *N Engl J Med* 367:2100–2109, 2012.
13. Montalescot G, et al.: ARCTIC Investigators. High on-treatment platelet reactivity as a risk factor for secondary prevention after coronary stent revascularization: a landmark analysis of the ARCTIC study, *Circulation* 129:2136–2143, 2014.
14. Collet J, et al.: High on-treatment platelet reactivity, a marker of bleeding risk? An analysis of the ARCTIC. Presented at ESC: European Society of Cardiology, August 31–September 4, 2013. Abstract 86472. Amsterdam.
15. Krishna V, Diamond GA, Kaul S: The role of platelet reactivity and genotype testing in the prevention of atherothrombotic cardiovascular events remains unproven, *Circulation* 125:1288–1303, 2012.
16. Aradi D, et al.: on behalf of the Working Group on Thrombosis of the European Society of Cardiology. Expert position paper on the role of platelet function testing in patients undergoing percutaneous coronary intervention, *Eur Heart J* 62:2261–2273, 2013.
17. Cayla G, et al.: ANTARCTIC Investigators. Platelet function monitoring in elderly patients on prasugrel after stenting for an acute coronary syndrome: design of the randomized ANTARCTIC study, *Am Heart J* 168:674–681, 2014.
18. Collet J-P, et al.: Cytochrome P450 2C19 polymorphism in young patients treated with clopidogrel after myocardial infarction: a cohort study, *Lancet* 373:309–317, 2009.
19. Hulot JS, et al.: Cardiovascular risk in clopidogrel-treated patients according to cytochrome P450 2C19*2 loss-of-funtion allele or proton pump inhibitor co-administration: a systematic meta-analysis, *J Am Coll Cardiol* 56:134–143, 2010.
20. Mega JL, et al.: Reduced-function CYP2C19 genotype and risk of adverse clinical outcomes among patients treated with clopidogrel predominantly for PCI: a meta-analysis, *JAMA* 304: 1821–1830, 2010.
21. Collet JP, et al.: High doses of clopidogrel to overcome genetic resistance (The CLOVIS-2 study), *J Am Coll Cardiol Intv* 4:392–402, 2011.
22. Mega JL, et al.: Dosing clopidogrel based on CYP2C19 genotype and the effect on platelet reactivity in patients with stable cardiovascular disease, *JAMA* 306:2221–2228, 2011.
23. Pena A, et al.: Can we override clopidogrel resistance? *Circulation* 119:2854–2858, 2009.
24. Bouman HJ, et al.: Paraoxonase-1 is a major determinant of clopidogrel efficacy, *Nat Med* 17: 110–116, 2010.
25. Hulot J-S, et al.: CYP2C19 but not PON1 genetic variants influence clopidogrel pharmacokinetics, pharmacodynamics, and clinical efficacy in post-myocardial infarction patients, *Circ Cardiovasc Interv* 4:422–428, 2011.
26. FDA Drug Safety Communication: Reduced effectiveness of Plavix (clopidogrel) in patients who are poor metabolizers of the drug. www.fda.gov/Drugs/DrugSafety/Postmarket rs/ucm203888.htm. Accessed April 28, 2010.
27. Roberts JD, et al.: Point-of-care genetic testing for personalisation of antiplatelet treatment (RAPID GENE): a prospective, randomised, proof-of-concept trial, *Lancet* 379:1705–1711, 2012.
28. Mega JL, et al.: Genetic variants in ABCB1 and CYP2C19 and cardiovascular outcomes after treatment with clopidogrel and prasugrel in the TRITON-TIMI 38 trial: a pharmacogenetic analysis, *Lancet* 376:1312–1319, 2010.
29. Parodi G, et al.: High residual platelet reactivity after clopidogrel loading and long-term cardiovascular events among patients with acute coronary syndromes undergoing PCI, *JAMA* 306:1215–1223, 2011.
30. Collet J, et al.: Point-of-care genetic profiling and/or platelet function testing in acute coronary syndrome, *Thromb Haemost* 115:382–391, 2016.
31. Chevalier B: Genotyping infarct patients to adjust and normalize thienopyridine treatment, Presented at TCT, October 27–November 1, 2013. Transcatheter Cardiovascular Therapeutics 25th Annual Scientific Symposium.
32. Bergmeijer TO, et al.: CYP2C19 genotype-guided antiplatelet therapy in ST-segment elevation myocardial infarction patients—rationale and design of the Patient Outcome after Primary PCI (POPular) genetics study, *Am Heart J* 168:16–22.e1, 2014.
33. Cayla G, et al.: Clinical, angiographic, and genetic factors associated with early coronary stent thrombosis, *JAMA* 306:1765–1774, 2011.

21 Old and New Oral Anticoagulant Therapy After Myocardial Infarction

Jessica L. Mega and Edward T. Carreras

INTRODUCTION

Despite improvements in secondary preventive care and risk factor modification, there is a persistently elevated risk of recurrent cardiovascular (CV) events after experiencing a myocardial infarction (MI), with more than 10% of patients developing recurrent MI, refractory angina, hospitalization, or death within the subsequent 6 months.[1] Therapies to minimize atherothrombotic complications in patients with MI have evolved over the past several decades. The current standard of care for antithrombotic therapy during the initial presentation of acute coronary syndrome (ACS) focuses on dual antiplatelet therapy (DAPT) in addition to parenteral anticoagulation (see Chapter 18 and Chapter 19).[2,3] However, once ACS is stabilized, long-term secondary prevention of recurrent thromboembolic events focuses on antiplatelet therapy only. Despite the development of more potent and effective antiplatelet medications, patients with stabilized ACS continue to experience recurrent adverse CV events after their index event.[4,5]

During the acute management of ACS, parenteral anticoagulants are administered to inhibit the generation of thrombin, the levels of which remain elevated long after ACS.[6] Because of the persistently elevated risk of recurrent adverse CV events after ACS, oral anticoagulants have been studied for the long-term care of patients following ACS. Initial studies that investigated warfarin in this setting showed promising results with regard to reducing ischemic events; however, because of an associated increased bleeding risk, in addition to the inherent difficulties with the prescription and administration of warfarin, routine adoption of vitamin K antagonists (VKAs) for secondary prevention into standard clinical practice did not occur.[1]

With the advent of nonvitamin K oral anticoagulants (NOACs), in addition to the emerging pathobiological evidence that emphasizes the role of thrombin in thrombus formation and thromboembolic events after ACS, there has been renewed interest in the use of long-term anticoagulation in patients who are stable after ACS. The results have been mixed, with the most promising data coming from the addition of low-dose oral direct factor Xa inhibitors to standard therapy for stabilized ACS.[7] Importantly, using optimal dosing strategies and applying therapies to the appropriate populations provides the ability to maximize benefit and minimize risk.

ROLE OF THROMBIN IN ACUTE CORONARY SYNDROME

In ACS, disruption of an atherosclerotic plaque exposes the underlying thrombogenic contents to circulating blood (see Chapter 3).[8] Platelets adhere to exposed collagen and von Willebrand factor, resulting in platelet activation and release of thromboxane A_2 and adenosine diphosphate, which triggers further platelet activation. Plaque rupture also prompts the subendothelial release of tissue factor, which activates coagulation factors. Coagulation factors assemble on activated platelets, which results in the formation of factor Xa and leads to the conversion of prothromin into thrombin (factor IIa). Thrombin triggers further coagulation and platelet activation, and prevents the degradation of fibrin (see Chapter 18).

Thrombin induces further platelet activation by binding to transmembrane proteins with extracellular thrombin-binding sites known as protease-activated receptors (PARs).[1] There are two human PARs: PAR-1, which is the most important source of platelet activation, and PAR-4. Thrombin binds to the extracellular PAR domain, cleaves the receptor, and triggers a cellular process that ultimately induces platelet activation. Thrombin is also responsible for triggering its own generation and expansion, with approximately 95% of thrombin generation occurring after initial thrombus formation.

The formation of a thrombus after ACS occurs via two pathways: one driven by platelets and one driven by thrombin (Figure 21-1). High-shear conditions, such as those in the coronary arteries, tend to form platelet-rich thrombi. However, because thrombin generation leads to further thrombin production and platelet aggregation, a reduction in blood flow creates a setting for a more thrombin- and fibrin-rich thrombus.

Importantly, although thrombin generation is enhanced immediately after the onset of ACS, it does not return to normal after clinical stabilization.[6] Biomarkers of thrombin generation, such as D-dimer, prothrombin fragments, and thrombin–antithrombin complexes, remain elevated for at least 6 months to 1 year after ACS.[1,6] Nonetheless, the contribution of thrombin to thrombus formation is not routinely targeted by medical therapy once ACS is stabilized. During this period, patients continue to experience an appreciable risk of adverse CV events, which may be partially caused by the elevated thrombin levels that continue to enhance thrombus formation.

CURRENT THERAPY AND OUTCOMES FOLLOWING ACUTE CORONARY SYNDROME

The current standard of care for antithrombotic therapy during the acute management of MI includes DAPT, which consists of aspirin in addition to a $P2Y_{12}$ inhibitor and parenteral anticoagulation, usually with either intravenous unfractionated heparin or low-molecular-weight heparin (see Chapter 13).[2,3] These therapies target multiple components of the coagulation cascade to maximally inhibit thrombus growth and minimize atherothrombotic complications (Figure 21-2).

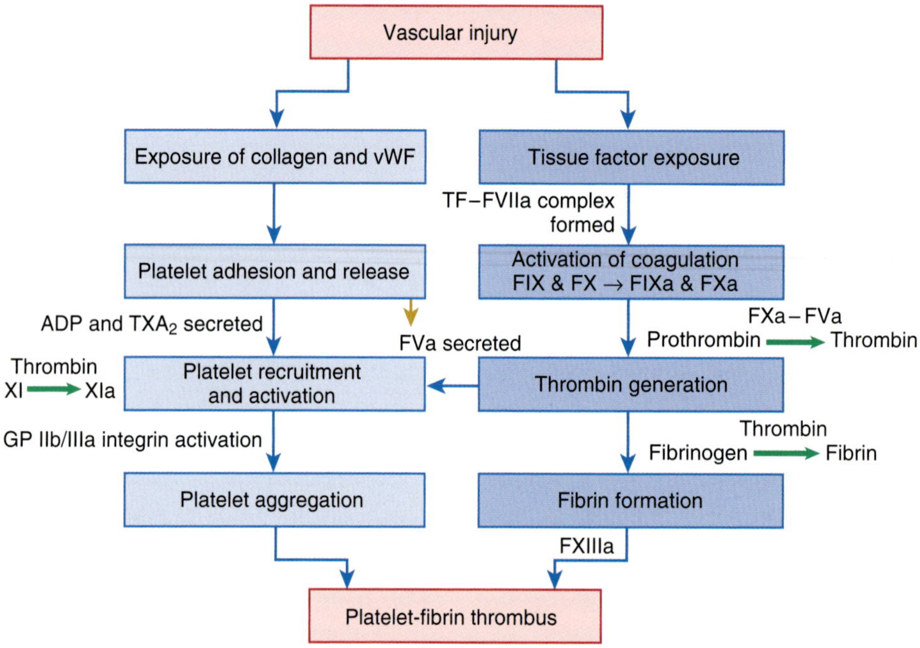

FIGURE 21-1 Thrombus formation in acute coronary syndrome. Thrombus formation in acute coronary syndrome is driven by platelet aggregation and fibrin formation. Thrombin plays a central role, because it is generated after vascular injury and leads to fibrin formation while also activating and recruiting platelets, which promotes platelet aggregation. *ADP*, Adenosine diphosphate; *F*, factor; *GP*, glycoprotein, *TF*, tissue factor; TXA_2, thromboxane A_2; *vWF*, von Willebrand factor. *(Adapted from Weitz JI: Insights into the role of thrombin in the pathogenesis of recurrent ischaemia after acute coronary syndrome.* Thromb Haemost *112:924–931, 2014; Fig. 1.)*

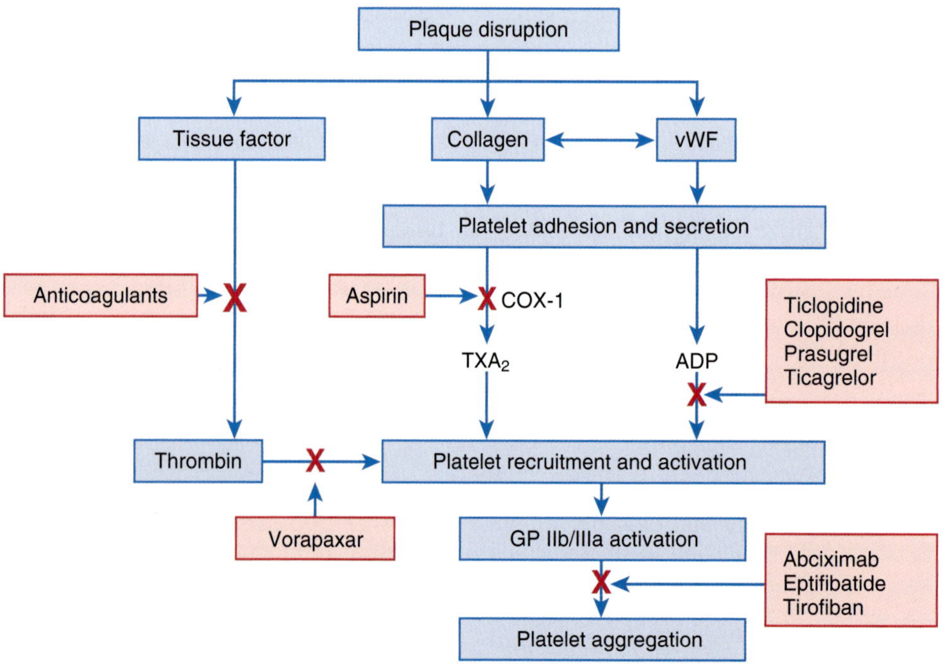

FIGURE 21-2 Pathophysiology and treatment targets in atherothrombosis. Therapies for atherothrombosis target multiple components of the coagulation cascade to maximally inhibit thrombus generation and expansion. *ADP*, Adenosine diphosphate; *COX*, cyclooxygenase; *GP*, glycoprotein, TXA_2, thromboxane A_2; *vWF*, von Willebrand factor. *(From Weitz JI: Taking a closer look at thrombin and its role in ACS. Medscape Education Cardiology, 2012, WebMD, LLC. www.medscape.org/viewarticle/769566_transcript. Accessed April 25, 2015.)*

After the acute period, therapy for stabilized ACS shifts away from the early emphasis on reducing elevated thrombin levels to focus solely on targeting the contribution of platelets to thrombus formation.

Despite medical therapy for stabilized ACS with DAPT, mortality risk persists for at least 6 months after admission for MI (Figure 21-3).[9] Furthermore, the risks of hospital readmissions, recurrent adverse CV events, and mortality persist for up to 5 years after MI, with greater morbidity and mortality in high-risk patients.[9] The persistently elevated risk of recurrent ischemic events after MI has prompted research into alternative and more potent antithrombotic strategies. One approach has been the investigation of prolonged administration of more potent antiplatelet therapies (see Chapter 35). Clopidogrel, prasugrel, and ticagrelor are each platelet $P2Y_{12}$ inhibitors; the latter two achieve higher degrees of platelet inhibition than clopidogrel and have an associated reduction in recurrent major CV events. Moreover, the addition of the PAR-1 antagonist vorapaxar has also been shown to improve efficacy for secondary prevention.[10] Each of these alternatives for enhanced antiplatelet therapy comes with a cost of an increased rate of moderate or severe bleeding.

These studies all support the concept that platelets contribute to the pathogenesis of thromboembolic events in patients stabilized after an MI and that more potent platelet inhibition reduces the recurrence of adverse CV events. However, their results also show a persistent appreciable risk of major CV events even in patients treated with potent antiplatelet strategies. For these reasons, investigators have studied the use of long-term anticoagulation for the secondary prevention of adverse CV events in patients stabilized after an MI.

VITAMIN K ANTAGONIST THERAPY AFTER MYOCARDIAL INFARCTION

The use of oral anticoagulants to treat MI dates back to the 1940s, when oral VKAs were found to reduce mortality in this setting.[1] Subsequently, numerous studies in the 1990s and early 2000s investigated the usefulness of warfarin after MI. In the WARIS II trial, patients with recent MI were randomized to either aspirin 160 mg, warfarin with an international normalized ratio (INR) target of 2.8 to 4.2, or aspirin 75 mg in

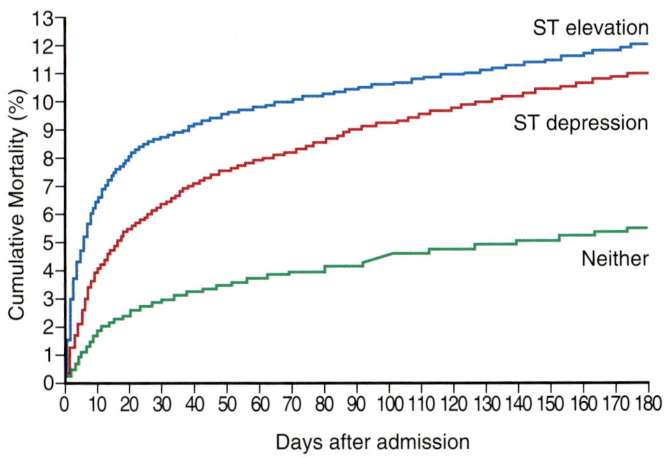

FIGURE 21-3 Cumulative mortality after acute coronary syndrome. Patients with acute coronary syndrome experience a rise in mortality rates for at least 6 months after admission. *(From Fox KA, Anderson FA, Jr., Goodman SG, et al: Time course of events in acute coronary syndromes: implications for clinical practice from the GRACE registry.* Nat Clin Pract Cardiovasc Med *5:580–589, 2008; Fig. 1B.)*

combination with warfarin with an INR target of 2.0 to 2.5.[11] Warfarin (relative risk [RR], 0.81; 95% confidence interval [CI], 0.69 to 0.95; P = .03) and warfarin plus aspirin (RR, 0.71; 95% CI, 0.60 to 0.83; P = 0.001) significantly reduced death, nonfatal MI, or thromboembolic stroke compared with aspirin 160 mg, at the cost of significant increases in major nonfatal bleeding (P <.001). There were no significant differences in efficacy between the two anticoagulation arms. In the ASPECT-2 trial, patients were randomized to three similar arms and had similar results to that in the WARIS II study.[11] High-intensity anticoagulation (hazard ratio [HR], 0.55; 95% CI, 0.30 to 1.00; P = .0479) and moderate-intensity anticoagulation, in addition to aspirin (HR, 0.50; 95% CI, 0.27 to 0.92; P = .03), significantly reduced death, MI, or stroke compared with aspirin alone. There were no significant differences in efficacy between the two anticoagulation arms.

A meta-analysis of 10 trials of warfarin after ACS was conducted, including the WARIS II and ASPECT-2 trials (Figure 21-4).[11] The results, which were driven strongly by the results in the WARIS II and ASPECT-2 trials, demonstrated that warfarin plus aspirin reduced the annual rate of MI (2.2% vs. 4.1%; RR, 0.56; 95% CI, 0.46 to 0.69), ischemic stroke (0.4% vs. 0.8%; RR, 0.46; 95% CI, 0.27 to 0.77), and revascularization (11.5% vs. 13.5%; RR, 0.80; 95% CI, 0.67 to 0.95) compared with aspirin alone, at the cost of an increase in major bleeding (1.5% vs. 0.6%; RR, 2.5; 95% CI, 1.7 to 3.7). There was no observed differences in mortality between aspirin plus warfarin versus aspirin alone.

Despite warfarin's promising ability to reduce recurrent adverse CV events in patients with stabilized ACS, its use in this setting has ultimately not been favored. The reasons behind the lack of adoption of warfarin for routine secondary prevention after MI are multifactorial; they are driven mostly by concerns with regard to bleeding, the practical challenges of administering warfarin, and the advent of more potent antiplatelet strategies.

NEW ORAL ANTICOAGULANT THERAPY IN STABILIZED ACUTE CORONARY SYNDROME

Warfarin has multiple limitations, including drug and food interactions, variability in dosing based on genetics, delayed onset and offset, and the need for frequent monitoring and dose adjustments. NOACs that avoid many of these issues have been studied in several disease states, such as atrial fibrillation (AF) and venous thromboembolism (VTE). Because of the previously promising results of warfarin in MI, several studies were conducted to determine whether NOACs might have a role after ACS (Table 21-1).

Initial Phase II Trials

The direct thrombin inhibitor, ximelagatran, was the first NOAC to be studied in patients with stabilized ACS. In the ESTEEM trial, 1883 patients with a recent MI were randomized to ximelagatran, at one of four doses or placebo. Standard medical therapy in these patients otherwise consisted of single antiplatelet therapy with aspirin 160 mg/day, and few patients underwent PCI.[1] Ximelagatran reduced the risk of death, nonfatal MI, or severe recurrent ischemia (HR, 0.76; 95% CI, 0.59 to 0.98; P = .036) for the combined ximelagatran groups versus placebo, but had a dose-dependent increase in bleeding. Ultimately, ximelagatran was deemed unsafe because of an associated risk of hepatotoxicity.

Study, year	Rate ratio (95% CI)	Weight (%)	Events/patient-years Warfarin	Events/patient-years ASA
ATACS, pilot, 1990	0.22 (0.01–4.66)	0.5	0/9	1/7
ATACS main, 1994	0.69 (0.29–1.65)	5.7	6/24	9/25
Williams et al., 1997	0.19 (0.03–1.16)	1.3	1/6	5/5
APRICOT-2, 2002	0.28 (0.09–0.92)	3.1	3/34	11/35
OASIS main, 2001	0.58 (0.38-0.98)	23.9	30/373	52/375
OASIS pilot, 1998	0.51 (0.20–1.26)	5.2	5/25	10/25
Huynh et al., 2001	2.07 (0.20–21.85)	0.8	2/38	1/39
ASPECT-2, 2002	0.69 (0.31–1.53	6.8	10/298	14/289
Zibaeenezhad et al., 2004	0.87 (0.20–2.28)	2.9	4/70	6/70
WARIS II, 2002	0.56 (0.42–0.75)	49.8	69/4927	117/4669
Overall	0.56 (0.48–0.69)	100.0	130/5834	228/5539

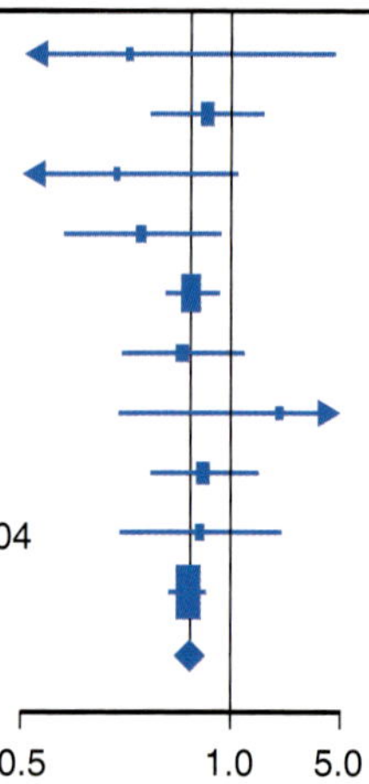

FIGURE 21-4 Rate ratios of recurrent myocardial infarction (MI) for warfarin plus aspirin (ASA) compared with ASA alone. The results of a meta-analysis of studies that evaluated patients with MI managed with warfarin plus ASA versus ASA alone, which showed a trend toward a reduction in the rate of recurrent MI in patients treated with warfarin plus ASA. *CI*, Confidence interval. *(Adapted from Rothberg MB, Celestin C, Fiore LD, et al: Warfarin plus aspirin after myocardial infarction or the acute coronary syndrome: meta-analysis with estimates of risk and benefit.* Ann Intern Med *143:241–250, 2005; Fig 1.)*

Dabigatran, another direct thrombin inhibitor, was studied in stabilized ACS in the phase 2 RE-DEEM trial. Patients with recent ACS were randomized to dabigatran, at one of three doses (50, 100, or 150 mg twice daily), or placebo, in addition to standard medical therapy, including DAPT.[12] At 6 months, dabigatran was associated with a dose-dependent increase in major and nonmajor bleeding (50-mg dose: HR, 1.77; 95% CI, 0.70 to 4.50; 150-mg dose: HR, 4.27; 95% CI, 1.86 to 9.81). Although this phase II trial was not powered for efficacy, there was no observed differences in death, MI, or stroke between dabigatran or placebo. However, all dabigatran doses were associated with a 45% reduction in D-dimer concentrations at 4 weeks compared with placebo ($P < .001$). Further investigation of dabigatran in stabilized ACS has not been pursued.

Darexaban tested the oral direct factor Xa inhibitor in stabilized ACS. In the phase II RUBY-1 trial, patients with recent ACS were randomized to receive darexaban, at doses ranging from 10 to 60 mg/day, or placebo, in addition to standard medical therapy with DAPT.[13] At 6 months, darexaban was associated with a significant dose-dependent increase in bleeding (overall HR, 2.28; 95% CI, 1.13 to 4.60; $P = .022$), without any corresponding observed efficacy benefit. There were no further studies of darexaban in stabilized ACS. Another oral direct factor Xa inhibitor, TAK-442, was studied in patients with recent ACS.[14] A wide range of doses was tested, and the investigators observed a significant dose-dependent increase in bleeding, without any clear efficacy benefit. As with dabigatran and darexaban, further investigation of TAK-442 was halted based on the phase II trial results.

Large Outcome Trials

Apixaban and rivaroxaban, which are oral direct factor Xa inhibitors, are the two most extensively studied NOACs in patients following an ACS (see Table 21-1).

Apixaban

In the phase II APPRAISE-1 trial, apixaban was tested versus placebo, in addition to standard therapy, in 1751 patients with recent ACS.[15] Apixaban showed a dose-dependent reduction in ischemic events at the cost of increased bleeding. In the phase III APPRAISE-2 trial, 7392 patients with recent ACS who received standard medical therapy, including DAPT with aspirin and clopidogrel for most patients, were randomized to placebo or apixaban 5 mg twice daily (which is equivalent to the full anticoagulant dose tested for stroke prevention in patients with AF).[16,17] The study population was high risk, and included patients with previous strokes and/or transient ischemic attacks (TIAs). Apixaban increased TIMI major bleeding compared with placebo (1.3% vs. 0.5%; HR, 2.59; 95% CI, 1.50 to 4.46; $P = .001$) without a significant reduction in ischemic events (7.5% vs. 7.9%; HR, 0.95; 95% CI, 0.20 to 1.11; $P = .51$).

Because of the increase in major bleeding without a corresponding reduction in ischemic events, the APPRAISE-2 trial was terminated early. Notably, if patients with previous strokes or TIAs were excluded, apixaban was associated with nonsignificant reductions in CV death, MI, or ischemic stroke (HR, 0.89; 95% CI, 0.74 to 1.06). In addition, there was a trend toward a reduction in stent thrombosis (HR 0.73; 95% CI, 0.47 to 1.12; $P = .15$) compared with placebo, despite the premature termination of the trial.

Rivaroxaban

In terms of rivaroxaban, the phase II dose-ranging ATLAS ACS-TIMI 46 trial studied rivaroxaban versus placebo in 3491 patients with recent ACS, most of whom were also taking aspirin and clopidogrel.[18] Patients received one of four doses of rivaroxaban: 5, 10, 15, or 20 mg, given either once daily or the same total daily dose divided twice daily. Rivaroxaban resulted in a dose-dependent increase

TABLE 21-1 Nonvitamin K Oral Anticoagulants in Patients Following Acute Coronary Syndrome

TRIAL	STUDY DRUG AND DOSES	DURATION	MECHANISM OF ACTION	PRIMARY ENDPOINT	SECONDARY ENDPOINT
RE-DEEM[23] (2011): 1861 patients (phase II)	Dabigatran 50 mg bid; 75 mg bid; 110 mg bid; 150 mg bid vs. placebo	6 mos	Oral direct thrombin inhibitor	Major and nonmajor clinically relevant bleeding; vs. placebo: dabigatran 50 mg: HR, 1.77; 95% CI, 0.70–4.50 dabigatran 75 mg: HR, 2.17; 95% CI, 0.88–5.31 dabigatran 110 mg: HR, 3.92; 95% CI, 1.72–8.95 Dabigatran 150 mg: HR, 4.27; 95% CI, 1.86–9.81	Reduction in D-dimer concentration; dabigatran analysis: 45% reduction compared with placebo (P <.001)
RUBY-1[24] (2011): 1279 patients (phase II)	Darexaban 5 mg bid; 10 mg qd; 15 mg bid; 30 mg qd; 30 mg bid; 60 mg qd vs. placebo	26 wks	Oral direct factor Xa inhibitor	Major and nonmajor clinically relevant bleeding; vs. placebo: darexaban: HR, 2.28; 95% CI, 1.13–4.60; P = .022	All-cause mortality, nonfatal MI, nonfatal stroke, and severe recurrent ischemia: no significant difference for darexaban vs. placebo
AXIOM-ACS[25] (2011): 2753 patients (phase II)	TAK-442 Stage 1: 10 mg bid; 20 mg bid; 40 mg qd Stage 2: 40 mg bid; 80 mg qd; 80 mg bid Stage 3: 160 mg qd; 120 mg bid vs placebo	24 wks	Oral direct factor Xa inhibitor	Incidence of TIMI major bleeding; no significant difference for TAK-442 vs. placebo	No efficacy outcomes
APPRAISE[26] (2009): 1715 patients (phase II)	Apixaban 2.5 mg bid; 10 mg od; 10 mg bid; 20 mg qd	6 mos	Oral direct factor Xa inhibitor	Major and nonmajor clinically relevant bleeding; vs. placebo: apixaban 2.5 mg bid: HR, 1.78; 95% CI, 0.91–3.48; P = .09 apixaban 10 mg qd: HR, 2.45; 95% CI, 1.31–4.61; P = .005 apixaban 10 mg bid and 20 mg qd discontinued because of excess total bleeding	CV death, MI, or ischemic stroke; vs. placebo: apixaban: HR, 0.95; 95% CI, 0.80–1.11; P = .51
APPRAISE-2[27] (2011): 7392 patients (phase III)	Apixaban 5 mg bid vs. placebo	Maximum follow-up of 241 days (early termination)	Oral direct factor Xa inhibitor	CV death, MI or ischemic stroke; vs. placebo: HR, 0.95; 95% CI, 0.80–1.11; P = .51	Major bleeding: HR, 2.59; 95% CI, 1.50–4.46; P = .001
ATLAS ACS-TIMI 46[28] (2009): 3491 patients (phase II)	Rivaroxaban Range of od and bid doses (5–20 mg) vs. placebo	6 mos	Oral direct factor Xa inhibitor	Major bleeding; significantly increased with rivaroxaban in a dose-dependent manner	Death, MI, stroke, or severe recurrent ischemia; vs. placebo: HR, 0.79; 95% CI, 0.60–1.05; P = .10
ATLAS ACS 2-TIMI 51[29,30] (2012): 15,526 patients (phase III)	Rivaroxaban 2.5 mg bid; 5 mg bid vs. placebo	Maximum follow-up of 31 mos (mean, 13)	Oral direct factor Xa inhibitor	CV death, MI, or stroke; vs. placebo: HR, 0.84; 95% CI, 0.74–0.96; P = .008	Non-CABG major bleeding; incidence compared with placebo: rivaroxaban (2.1% vs 0.6%; P <.001)

ACS, Acute coronary syndrome; *bid*, twice daily; *CABG*, coronary artery bypass graft; *CI*, confidence interval; *CV*, cardiovascular; *HR*, hazard ratio; *MI*, myocardial infarction; *od*, once daily; *qd*, every day; *TIMI*, Thrombolysis in Myocardial Infarction.
From Weitz JI: Insights into the role of thrombin in the pathogenesis of recurrent ischaemia after acute coronary syndrome. Thromb Haemost *112:924–931, 2014; p 928, Table 2.*

in clinically significant bleeding (Figure 21-5). In addition, rivaroxaban reduced CV death, MI, or stroke (3.9% vs. 5.5%; HR, 0.69; 95% CI, 0.50 to 0.96; P = .027), with the numerically lowest HRs seen with the lowest twice daily doses.

Based on the phase II results, in the phase III ATLAS ACS 2-TIMI 51 trial, doses of rivaroxaban 2.5 and 5 mg twice daily (which are just one-quarter and one-half, respectively, of the total daily doses tested for stroke prevention in patients with AF) were compared with placebo. The study included 15,526 patients with recent ACS on a background of standard post-ACS therapy, which included DAPT with aspirin and clopidogrel in most patients.[7,19] Notably, patients with previous stroke or TIA on background DAPT were excluded from this trial. Patients were followed for a mean of 13 months and up to 31 months. Rivaroxaban reduced the primary endpoint of CV death, MI, or stroke (8.9% vs. 10.7%; HR, 0.84; 95% CI, 0.74 to 0.96; P = .008). There was an overall increase in non–coronary artery bypass graft (CABG)-related TIMI major bleeding (2.1% vs. 0.6%; HR, 3.96; 95% CI, 2.46 to 6.38; P <.001). However, there was no significant difference between rivaroxaban and placebo with respect to fatal bleeding (0.3% vs. 0.2%; HR 1.19; 95% CI, 0.54 to 2.59; P = .66).

With respect to the individual doses, both the 2.5 and 5 mg twice daily doses reduced the primary endpoint of CV death, MI, or stroke, as well as the secondary endpoint of stent thrombosis compared with placebo. In addition, the 2.5 mg twice daily dose significantly reduced CV mortality (2.7% vs. 4.1%; HR 0.66; 95% CI, 0.51 to 0.86; P = .002) and all-cause mortality (2.9% vs. 4.5%; HR 0.68; 95% CI, 0.53 to 0.87; *P* = .002) compared with placebo (Figure 21-6). The 5 mg twice daily dose did not demonstrate differences in CV or all-cause mortality compared with placebo. In a direct comparison of the 2.5 and 5 mg twice daily doses, the 2.5-mg dose demonstrated significantly less TIMI bleeding that required medical attention (12.9% vs. 16.2%; *P* <.001) and less fatal bleeding (0.1% vs. 0.4%; *P* = .04) (Figure 21-7).[20] In aggregate, the results demonstrate that the 2.5 mg twice daily dose offers the more favorable balance of efficacy and safety. Based on these results, the European Medicines Agency has approved rivaroxaban 2.5 mg twice daily for patients with recent ACS with elevated markers of cardiac necrosis. Rivaroxaban has not been approved in the United States for secondary prevention after ACS.

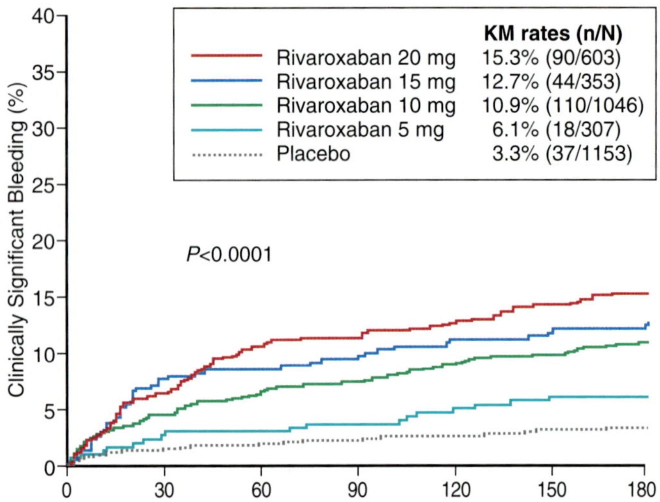

FIGURE 21-5 Clinically significant bleeding across rivaroxaban doses. In the ATLAS ACS-TIMI 46 trial, rivaroxaban showed a dose-dependent increase in clinically significant bleeding (Thrombolysis In Myocardial Infarction [TIMI] major, TIMI minor, or requiring medical attention). *KM*, Kaplan-Meier. *(From Mega JL, Braunwald E, Mohanavelu S, et al: Rivaroxaban versus placebo in patients with acute coronary syndromes [ATLAS ACS-TIMI 46]: a randomised, double-blind, phase II trial.* Lancet *374:29–38, 2009; Fig. 3.)*

Specific Patient Populations

Regarding particular populations, among the patients in ATLAS ACS 2-TIMI 51 trial who presented with an ST-elevation myocardial infarction (STEMI), there was a 19% relative reduction in CV death, MI, or stroke, with rivaroxaban compared with placebo (HR, 0.81; 95% CI, 0.67 to 0.97; *P* = .019).[21] In patients in the ATLAS-ACS 2-TIMI 51 trial who underwent PCI, rivaroxaban led to a significant reduction in stent thrombosis (HR 0.65; *P* = .017).[22] An additional analysis characterized the specific effects of rivaroxban on the size and type of MI. It determined that in patients with ACS, most of the MI events were spontaneous in nature, and rivaroxaban significantly reduced these events by 20%. Notably, rivaroxaban compared with placebo reduced MIs with extensive biomarker release and STEMI events.[23]

Synthesis Across Divergent Clinical Trials

Overall, the studies that have examined the addition of oral anticoagulants to antiplatelet therapies post-ACS suggest that there is a dose-dependent increased risk of bleeding. This concept is supported by all of the available studies. Regarding efficacy, in the phase II studies, the reductions in ischemic events were directionally consistent in the APPRAISE 1 and ATLAS ACS-TIMI 46 trials, but these reductions were not seen in the other studies. Notably, the phase II studies of dabigatran, darexaban, and TAK-442 were designed and powered to assess safety, so the lack of observed efficacy benefit was likely a result of small and underpowered studies. In terms of the large phase III studies and efficacy, the findings in the ATLAS ACS 2-TIMI 51 and APPRAISE-2 trials were divergent, and the two main issues that likely accounted for the results were dosing and the patient population.

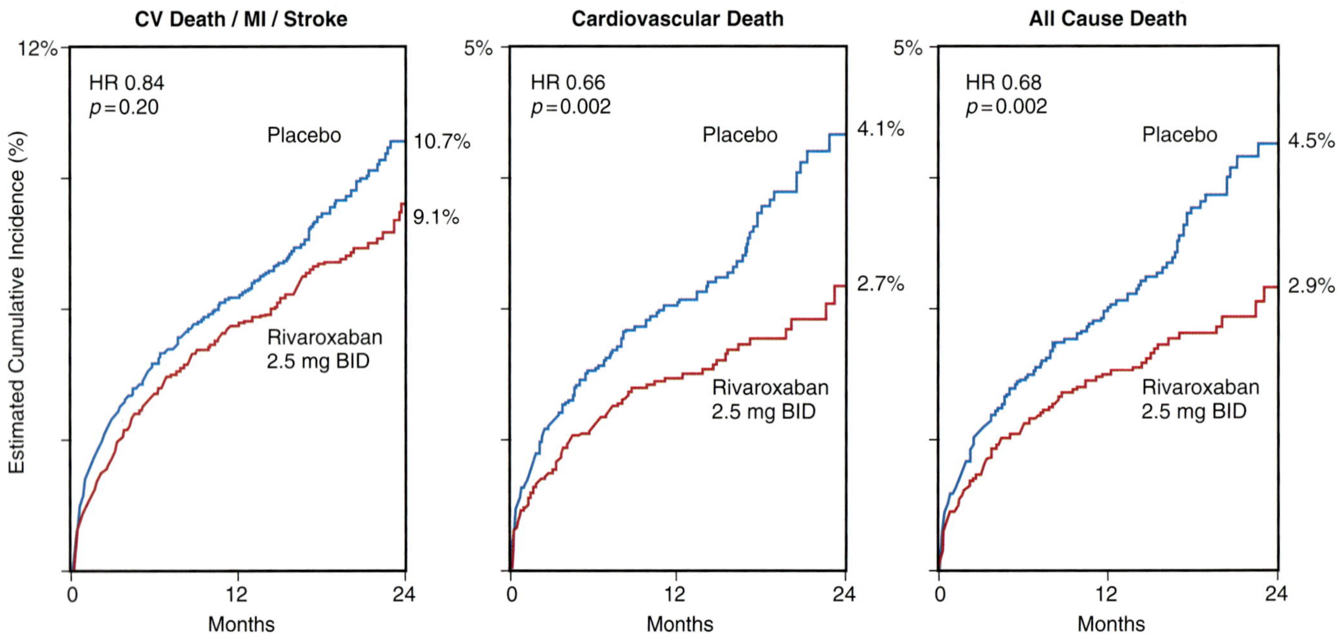

FIGURE 21-6 Outcomes with rivaroxaban 2.5 mg twice daily (BID) versus placebo. In the ATLAS ACS-TIMI 51 trial, rivaroxaban 2.5 mg BID was associated with significant reductions in cardiovascular (CV) death, myocardial infarction (MI) or stroke, CV death alone, and mortality alone, compared with placebo in patients with stabilized acute coronary syndrome. *HR*, Hazard ratio. *(Adapted from Mega JL, Braunwald E, Wiviott SD, et al: Rivaroxaban in patients with a recent acute coronary syndrome.* N Engl J Med *366:9–19, 2012; Fig. 3.)*

There appears to be a dose of an antithrombotic agent at which the overall risk versus benefit ratio is optimized and the reduction in CV and all-cause mortality is maximized. This observation has been apparent with several medications in this class of drugs, including warfarin, heparin, and aspirin. In APPRAISE-2, apixaban was tested at the full anticoagulant dose used for stroke prevention in patients with AF, which resulted in an unacceptable increase in bleeding when layered on top of antiplatelet therapy.[17] In the ATLAS ACS 2-TIMI 51 trial, the 2.5 and 5 mg twice daily doses of rivaroxaban were tested at one-quarter and one-half, respectively, of the 20 mg/day dose tested for stroke prevention in patients with AF.[19] The 2.5 mg twice daily dose is also only one-half of the 10 mg/day dose tested for the prevention of VTE after elective hip and knee replacement.[24] At these low doses, although there was an overall increase in non-CABG–related TIMI, there was no significant increase in fatal bleeding. In addition, with the 2.5 mg twice daily dose of rivaroxaban, there was an overall reduction in CV and all-cause mortality.

In addition to precise dosing, patient selection is critically important when using anticoagulation after ACS. The APPRAISE-2 and ATLAS ACS 2-TIMI 51 trials have shown that different populations and disease states respond differently to anticoagulant therapy for stabilized ACS. Specifically, patients with previous stroke or TIA do not appear to benefit from the addition of anticoagulation to DAPT after ACS; this is a finding that has also been seen with layering antiplatelet therapies.[25] When excluding these subjects from the APPRAISE-2 trial, there was a trend toward a reduction in CV death, MI, or stroke, although further conclusions are limited because the trial was terminated early. Other patient populations, such as those individuals who presented with STEMI or those with elevated cardiac biomarkers, appear to experience particular benefit. Future investigation will hopefully identify other populations and disease states that are more or less likely to benefit from long-term anticoagulant therapy after stabilized MI.

CURRENT ROLE FOR ORAL ANTICOAGULATION FOR SECONDARY PREVENTION AFTER MYOCARDIAL INFARCTION

Upon the initial presentation of MI, treatment with aspirin and a $P2Y_{12}$ receptor antagonist, as recommended by current guidelines, should be initiated (see Chapter 19). In many patients in whom more potent platelet inhibition is desired, prasugrel or ticagrelor are reasonable choices for $P2Y_{12}$ receptor antagonism. In these patients, DAPT with ticagrelor or prasugrel in addition to aspirin once the ACS is stabilized is frequently continued, and there is no current role for adding oral anticoagulation to improve secondary prevention. In some countries outside of the United States, in patients managed with aspirin and clopidogrel in whom a more potent antithrombotic strategy is desired, the addition of low-dose rivaroxaban is one option to further reduce the risk of adverse CV events. Further understanding of the pathobiology of ACS, combined with ongoing clinical investigations, will hopefully identify the unique characteristics of patient populations and disease states that maximize the benefit of either antiplatelet or anticoagulant therapy in stabilized ACS.

Patients with Another Indication for Oral Anticoagulant Therapy

The patients discussed thus far were treated with anticoagulation for the purpose of secondary prevention after MI. Patients with stabilized MI who have a preexisting or newly developed independent indication for long-term oral anticoagulation, such as AF or VTE, are a separate and particularly challenging group to treat. For example, the optimal antithrombotic treatment for a patient with AF who

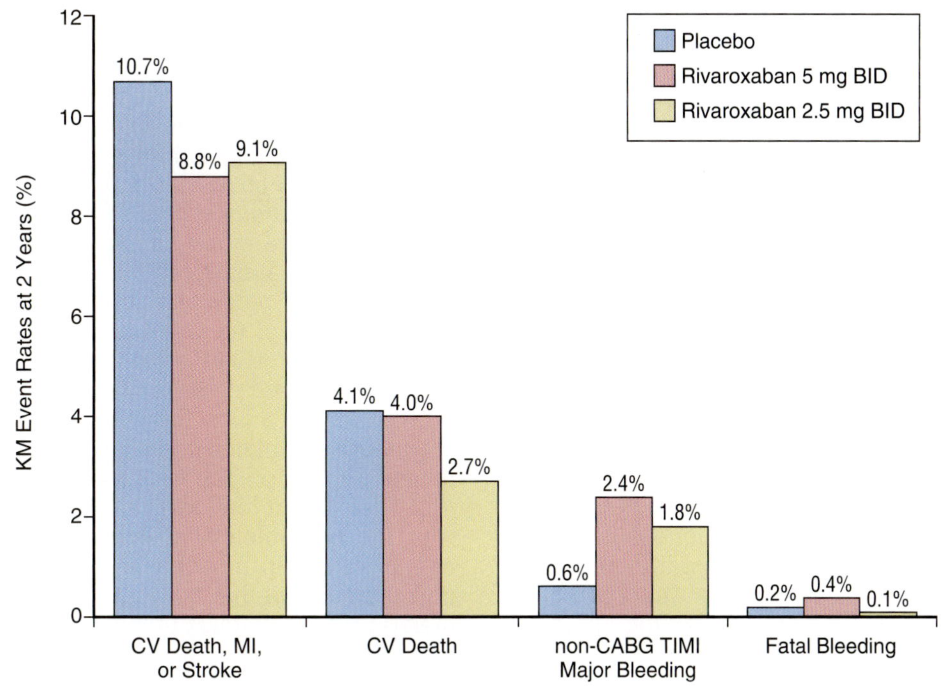

FIGURE 21-7 Outcomes with rivaroxaban 5 mg twice daily (BID), 2.5 mg BID, and placebo. In a comparison of the 2.5 and 5 mg BID doses in the ATLAS ACS-TIMI 51 trial, the 2.5-mg dose was associated with a significant reduction in cardiovascular (CV) death, as well as significantly less non–coronary artery bypass graft (CABG) Thrombolysis In Myocardial Infarction (TIMI) major bleeding and fatal bleeding. *KM,* Kaplan-Meier. *(Adapted from Mega JL, Braunwald E, Wiviott SD, et al: Comparison of the efficacy and safety of two rivaroxaban doses in acute coronary syndrome [from ATLAS ACS 2-TIMI 51].* Am J Cardiol *112:472–478, 2013.)*

experiences ACS and who undergoes PCI depends on a number of factors, including atherothrombotic and bleeding risk. Although there is evidence to suggest that patients with ACS may benefit from the addition of low-dose anticoagulation to DAPT, it is unclear what the optimal antithrombotic strategy is for patients who require full-dose anticoagulation.

Triple Oral Antithrombotic Therapy

These patients are often treated with DAPT in addition to full-dose oral anticoagulation, which is also known as triple oral antithrombotic therapy (TOAT). However, studies have suggested that the balance of efficacy and safety with TOAT is tipped toward an excess of bleeding. Initial observational data found TOAT to be associated with an approximately threefold higher risk of major bleeding compared with DAPT alone.[26] A recent large Denmark registry study found that TOAT versus VKAs plus single antiplatelet therapy was associated with significantly more bleeding at 90 days (HR, 1.47; 95% CI, 1.04 to 2.08) and 1 year (HR, 1.36; 95% CI, 0.95 to 1.95), with statistically similar efficacy results (HR, 1.15; 95% CI, 0.95 to 1.40).[27]

The WOEST trial was an open-label trial that randomized 573 patients who underwent PCI and who had a preexisting indication for oral anticoagulation to receive either double therapy (warfarin and clopidogrel 75 mg) or TOAT (warfarin, clopidogrel 75 mg, and aspirin 80 mg). At 1 year, patients who received double therapy compared with TOAT experienced a significantly lower cumulative incidence of all TIMI bleeding (44.9% vs. 19.5%; HR, 0.36; 95% CI, 0.26 to 0.50; $P < .001$), which was driven mostly by differences in TIMI minor and minimal bleeding without a difference in intracranial bleeding. There were no changes in the primary endpoint when controlling for age, gender, indication for oral anticoagulation (OAC), stent type, or ACS presentation. Interestingly, double therapy also resulted in a significantly lower rate of death, MI, stroke, systemic embolism, target vessel revascularization, or stent thrombosis compared with double therapy (17.7% vs. 11.3%; HR, 0.60; 95% CI, 0.38 to 0.94; $P = .025$); this was driven mostly by a reduction in all-cause mortality at 1 year (6.4% vs. 2.6%; HR, 0.39; 95% CI, 0.16 to 0.93; $P = .027$).

In the WOEST trial, the double therapy group did not receive aspirin rather than clopidogrel because of concerns that stent thrombosis might be unacceptably increased without clopidogrel. In the Denmark registry study, although VKA plus single antiplatelet therapy was associated with an overall decrease in bleeding compared with TOAT, the subset of patients who received clopidogrel as the single antiplatelet agent experienced an incidence of bleeding similar to that seen with triple therapy. In addition, the safety results in the WOEST trial were driven largely by reductions in TIMI minor and minimal bleeding, without any significant differences in major or fatal bleeding. Furthermore, none of the available studies included patients treated with either prasugrel or ticagrelor. As such, although oral anticoagulation plus single antiplatelet therapy may be the preferred strategy in patients who would otherwise be treated with TOAT, the optimal antiplatelet agent is unclear, and further investigation is ongoing. Moreover, it is important to interpret the available data with caution. The WOEST trial was relatively small and designed to evaluate safety. Although the secondary efficacy composite endpoint of death, MI, stroke, systemic embolism, target vessel revascularization, or stent thrombosis did meet statistical significance, confirmation in additional studies will be helpful to further guide clinical practice.

Consensus Practice Guidelines

Several consensus guidelines have been drafted to address the management of patients with atrial fibrillation and ACS and/or PCI.[26,28–30] Guidelines such as those from the joint consensus statements of the European Society of Cardiology Working Group on Thrombosis, the European Heart Rhythm Association, the European Association of Percutaneous Cardiovascular Interventions, and the European Association of Acute Cardiac Care, suggest that the stroke and bleeding risk be assessed using the CHA_2DS_2-VASc and HAS-BLED scores, respectively (Figure 21-8).[30] It is also important to evaluate whether patients present with stable disease versus ACS and whether PCI is performed. Based on this information, the appropriate antiplatelet and anticoagulant strategies can be recommended. Considering the WOEST results, in patients at high risk of stroke and bleeding and low risk of stent thrombosis, a VKA plus clopidogrel may be a reasonable alternative to an initial brief period of TOAT. However, in patients at high risk of stent thrombosis atherothrombotic disease, a period of TOAT is reasonable.

Regarding the type of anticoagulant, the guidance document indicates that in patients with MI who develop AF and are at high risk of stroke, anticoagulation with a VKA or a NOAC should be initiated. The usefulness of NOACs in TOAT is unknown, although several studies are ongoing.[31–33] Because of the evidence for improved safety and efficacy with NOACs versus warfarin in other populations, there is great interest in these studies, particularly in terms of safety.[34]

SUMMARY

Patients with an MI have a persistently increased long-term risk of adverse CV events despite current therapies. Thrombin plays a major role in platelet activation and thrombus formation, and thrombin levels remain elevated for months after an ACS. Although anticoagulants are commonly used to address the downstream effects of thrombin in the acute management of MI, antiplatelet therapy is the focus of antithrombotic regimens for stabilized MI. Because of the persistently elevated thrombin levels and continued risk of recurrent adverse CV events, long-term anticoagulation is an appealing option to consider in patients stabilized after an MI. Studies of anticoagulation for stabilized ACS have shown mixed results, which is likely secondary to anticoagulant dosing and selection of the patient population. The results of the ATLAS ACS 2–TIMI 51 trial, which used low doses of rivaroxaban, are congruent with the pathobiological evidence for the fundamental role of thrombin in ischemic events after ACS, and support the concept that both antiplatelet and anticoagulant therapies can minimize the risk of recurrent thromboembolic events after ACS. Moving forward, it will be important to continue to explore patient characteristics that predict better or worse responses to anticoagulation for secondary prevention after MI.

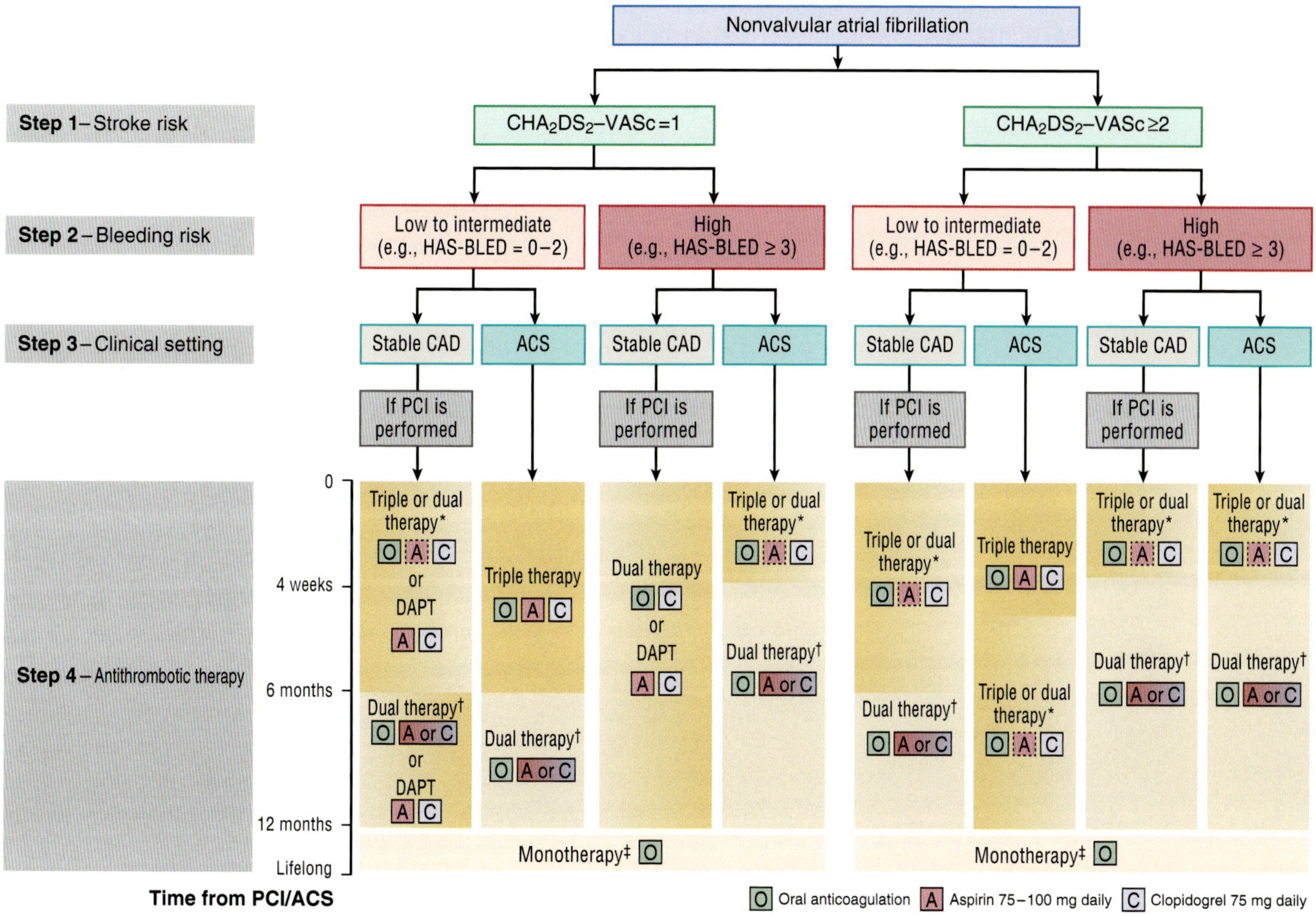

FIGURE 21-8 Antithrombotic therapy in patients with atrial fibrillation after acute coronary syndrome (ACS) or percutaneous coronary intervention (PCI). Choice of antithrombotic therapy, including combination strategies of oral anticoagulation, aspirin, and/or clopidogrel (OAC) is illustrated. *Solid boxes* represent recommended drugs. *Dashed boxes* represent optional drugs depending on clinical judgment. *Dual therapy with OAC may be considered in selected patients. †Aspirin as an alternative to clopidogrel may be considered in patients on dual therapy (i.e., oral anticoagulation plus single antiplatelet). ‡Dual therapy with oral anticoagulation and an antiplatelet agent (aspirin or clopidogrel) may be considered in patients at high risk of coronary events. *CAD,* Coronary artery disease; *DAPT,* dual antiplatelet therapy. *(Adapted from Lip GY, Windecker S, Huber K, et al: Management of antithrombotic therapy in atrial fibrillation patients presenting with acute coronary syndrome and/or undergoing percutaneous coronary or valve interventions: a joint consensus document of the European Society of Cardiology Working Group on Thrombosis, European Heart Rhythm Association [EHRA], European Association of Percutaneous Cardiovascular Interventions [EAPCI] and European Association of Acute Cardiac Care [ACCA] endorsed by the Heart Rhythm Society [HRS] and Asia-Pacific Heart Rhythm Society [APHRS].* Eur Heart J *35:3155–3179, 2014; Fig 1.)*

References

1. Weitz JI: Insights into the role of thrombin in the pathogenesis of recurrent ischaemia after acute coronary syndrome, *Thromb Haemost* 112:924–931, 2014.
2. Amsterdam EA, et al.: 2014 AHA/ACC guideline for the management of patients with non-ST-elevation acute coronary syndromes: a report of the American College of Cardiology/American Heart Association Task Force on Practice Guidelines, *J Am Coll Cardiol* 64:e139–228, 2014.
3. O'Gara PT, et al.: 2013 ACCF/AHA guideline for the management of ST-elevation myocardial infarction: a report of the American College of Cardiology Foundation/American Heart Association Task Force on Practice Guidelines, *Circulation* 127:e362–425, 2013.
4. Montalescot G, et al.: Prasugrel compared with clopidogrel in patients undergoing percutaneous coronary intervention for ST-elevation myocardial infarction (TRITON-TIMI 38): double-blind, randomised controlled trial, *Lancet* 373:723–731, 2009.
5. Wallentin L, et al.: Ticagrelor versus clopidogrel in patients with acute coronary syndromes, *N Engl J Med* 361:1045–1057, 2009.
6. Skeppholm M, et al.: Is fibrin formation and thrombin generation increased during and after an acute coronary syndrome? *Thromb Res* 128:483–489, 2011.
7. Mega JL, et al.: Rivaroxaban in patients with a recent acute coronary syndrome, *N Engl J Med* 366:9–19, 2012.
8. Libby P: Mechanisms of acute coronary syndromes, *N Engl J Med* 369:883–884, 2013.
9. Fox KA, et al.: Underestimated and under-recognized: the late consequences of acute coronary syndrome (GRACE UK-Belgian Study), *Eur Heart J* 31:2755–2764, 2010.
10. Scirica BM, et al.: Vorapaxar for secondary prevention of thrombotic events for patients with previous myocardial infarction: a prespecified subgroup analysis of the TRA 2 degrees P-TIMI 50 trial, *Lancet* 380:1317–1324, 2012.
11. Carreras ET, Mega JL: Balancing antiplatelet and anticoagulant therapies in patients with cardiovascular disease, *Cardiol Ther* 2:85–96, 2013.
12. Oldgren J, et al.: Dabigatran vs. placebo in patients with acute coronary syndromes on dual antiplatelet therapy: a randomized, double-blind, phase II trial, *Eur Heart J* 32:2781–2789, 2011.
13. Steg PG, et al.: RUBY-1: a randomized, double-blind, placebo-controlled trial of the safety and tolerability of the novel oral factor Xa inhibitor darexaban (YM150) following acute coronary syndrome, *Eur Heart J* 32:2541–2554, 2011.
14. Goldstein S, et al.: Phase 2 study of TAK-442, an oral factor Xa inhibitor, in patients following acute coronary syndrome, *Thromb Haemost* 111:1141–1152, 2014.
15. Alexander JH, et al.: Apixaban, an oral, direct, selective factor Xa inhibitor, in combination with antiplatelet therapy after acute coronary syndrome: results of the Apixaban for Prevention of Acute Ischemic and Safety Events (APPRAISE) trial, *Circulation* 119:2877–2885, 2009.
16. Alexander JH, et al.: Apixaban with antiplatelet therapy after acute coronary syndrome, *N Engl J Med* 365:699–708, 2011.
17. Granger CB, et al.: Apixaban versus warfarin in patients with atrial fibrillation, *N Engl J Med* 365:981–992, 2011.
18. Mega JL, et al.: Rivaroxaban versus placebo in patients with acute coronary syndromes (ATLAS ACS-TIMI 46): a randomised, double-blind, phase II trial, *Lancet* 374:29–38, 2009.
19. Patel MR, et al.: Rivaroxaban versus warfarin in nonvalvular atrial fibrillation, *N Engl J Med* 365:883–891, 2011.
20. Mega JL, et al.: Comparison of the efficacy and safety of two rivaroxaban doses in acute coronary syndrome (from ATLAS ACS 2-TIMI 51), *Am J Cardiol* 112:472–478, 2013.
21. Mega JL, et al.: Rivaroxaban in patients stabilized after a ST-segment elevation myocardial infarction: results from the ATLAS ACS-2-TIMI-51 trial (Anti-Xa Therapy to Lower Cardiovascular Events in Addition to Standard Therapy in Subjects with Acute Coronary Syndrome-Thrombolysis In Myocardial Infarction-51), *J Am Coll Cardiol* 61:1853–1859, 2013.
22. Gibson CM, et al.: Reduction of stent thrombosis in patients with acute coronary syndromes treated with rivaroxaban in ATLAS-ACS 2 TIMI 51, *J Am Coll Cardiol* 62:286–290, 2013.
23. Cavender MA, et al.: The effect of rivaroxaban on myocardial infarction in the ATLAS ACS 2-TIMI 51 trial, *Eur Heart J Acute Cardiovasc Care* 4:468–474, 2015.
24. Eriksson BI, et al.: Oral rivaroxaban for the prevention of symptomatic venous thromboembolism after elective hip and knee replacement, *J Bone Joint Surg Br* 91:636–644, 2009.
25. Lee M, et al.: Risk-benefit profile of long-term dual- versus single-antiplatelet therapy among patients with ischemic stroke: a systematic review and meta-analysis, *Ann Intern Med* 159:463–470, 2013.
26. You JJ, et al.: Antithrombotic therapy for atrial fibrillation: antithrombotic therapy and prevention of thrombosis, 9th ed: American College of Chest Physicians Evidence-Based Clinical Practice Guidelines, *Chest* 141:e531S–575S, 2012.
27. Lamberts M, et al.: Bleeding after initiation of multiple antithrombotic drugs, including triple therapy, in atrial fibrillation patients following myocardial infarction and coronary intervention: a nationwide cohort study, *Circulation* 126:1185–1193, 2012.

28. Lip GY, et al.: Antithrombotic management of atrial fibrillation patients presenting with acute coronary syndrome and/or undergoing coronary stenting: executive summary–a Consensus Document of the European Society of Cardiology Working Group on Thrombosis, endorsed by the European Heart Rhythm Association (EHRA) and the European Association of Percutaneous Cardiovascular Interventions (EAPCI), *Eur Heart J* 31:1311–1318, 2010.
29. Faxon DP, et al.: Antithrombotic therapy in patients with atrial fibrillation undergoing coronary stenting: a North American perspective: executive summary, *Circ Cardiovasc Interv* 4:522–534, 2011.
30. Lip GY, et al.: Management of antithrombotic therapy in atrial fibrillation patients presenting with acute coronary syndrome and/or undergoing percutaneous coronary or valve interventions: a joint consensus document of the European Society of Cardiology Working Group on Thrombosis, European Heart Rhythm Association (EHRA), European Association of Percutaneous Cardiovascular Interventions (EAPCI) and European Association of Acute Cardiac Care (ACCA) endorsed by the Heart Rhythm Society (HRS) and Asia-Pacific Heart Rhythm Society (APHRS), *Eur Heart J* 35:3155–3179, 2014.
31. Gibson CM, et al.: An open-label, randomized, controlled, multicenter study exploring two treatment strategies of rivaroxaban and a dose-adjusted oral vitamin k antagonist treatment strategy in subjects with atrial fibrillation who undergo percutaneous coronary intervention (PIONEER AF-PCI), *Am Heart J* 169:472–478 e5, 2015.
32. Evaluation of Dual Therapy With Dabigatran vs. Triple Therapy With Warfarin in Patients With AF That Undergo a PCI With Stenting (REDUAL-PCI). https://clinicaltrials.gov/ct2/show/NCT02164864?term=redual+pci&rank=1. Accessed April 17, 2015.
33. Study Apixaban to Vitamin K Antagonist for the Prevention of Stroke or Systemic Embolism and Bleeding in Patients With Non-valvular Atrial Fibrillation and Acute Coronary Syndrome/Percutaneous Coronary Intervention. https://www.clinicaltrials.gov/ct2/show/NCT02415400?term=apixaban&rank=8. Accessed April 17, 2015.
34. Ruff CT, et al.: Comparison of the efficacy and safety of new oral anticoagulants with warfarin in patients with atrial fibrillation: a meta-analysis of randomised trials, *Lancet* 383:955–962, 2014.

22 Stem Cell Therapy in Patients with Myocardial Infarction

Roberto Bolli and Shahab Ghafghazi

INTRODUCTION

Cell-based therapy is an exciting new treatment modality that has the potential to revolutionize cardiovascular (CV) medicine. Research on the application of cell therapy for ischemic heart disease emerged in the late 1990s, when conventional wisdom regarded the heart as an organ devoid of capacity for endogenous repair. The dogma that the mammalian heart was a terminally differentiated organ incapable of regeneration and repair was predicated on the lack of significant tissue repair seen after acute myocardial infarction (MI) and during the ensuing period of left ventricular (LV) remodeling and heart failure (HF). However, this paradigm changed dramatically at the dawn of the new millennium, when evidence began to accumulate that formation of new myocytes in the adult heart is possible, and that cell therapy enhances cardiac function after MI.[1] Over the past 15 years, the field of regenerative cardiology has grown exponentially, to the point that it is now generally accepted that cardiac myocytes can be regenerated. We believe that we are witnessing a veritable conceptual and therapeutic revolution that is likely to change CV medicine profoundly.

Various types of stem and/or progenitor cells have been tested in preclinical and clinical studies of cardiac repair or regeneration, mostly in the settings of MI and ischemic cardiomyopathy (ICM), but also in that of nonischemic cardiomyopathy (NICM).[2,3] These cells include skeletal myoblasts, bone marrow mononuclear cells (BMMNCs), mesenchymal stromal cells (MSCs), proangiogenic progenitor cells, and cardiac progenitor cells (CPCs) (Figure 22-1). Experimental and clinical work has advanced in parallel, leading to rapid translation of basic discoveries into clinical trials. Considering that the first preclinical study of cell therapy was published in 1998[4] and the first clinical application was used in 2001,[5] the rapidity in which basic and clinical research has progressed in a relatively short time is truly remarkable. In the clinical arena, almost 100 trials of cell therapy for CV disease have been published, some of which have reported promising results. A large number of ongoing clinical trials have been registered with the National Institutes of Health (NIH); in April 2015, a search in the NIH-sponsored clinicaltrials.gov website for cell therapy trials in the context of MI or HF revealed 36 actively recruiting studies in adult populations, including phase III trials.[3]

As mentioned previously, the two major clinical settings in which cell therapy has been studied are acute MI and chronic HF. In this chapter, we specifically review the application of stem and/or progenitor cells for the treatment of acute MI. Treatment of HF with stem and/or progenitor cells has been reviewed recently,[3] and is beyond the scope of the present chapter.

RATIONALE FOR CELL THERAPY IN ACUTE MYOCARDIAL INFARCTION

The worldwide incidence of acute MI continues to increase at an accelerated pace (see Chapter 2). Acute MI leads to adverse LV remodeling (see Chapter 36), which causes further cardiomyocyte attrition, ventricular dilation, and HF (see Chapter 25), thereby initiating a downward spiral that can eventually culminate in death. Although it is now appreciated that the adult heart has some capacity for renewal,[6,7] this capacity is limited and is overwhelmed by the ischemic insult and subsequent remodeling. The loss of cardiomyocytes associated with acute MI cannot be reversed with contemporary treatment modalities. Current therapies for LV remodeling and HF are predominantly palliative (see Chapter 36); they can improve symptoms and prolong life, but they do not address the underlying loss of contractile tissue. Consequently, the prognosis of patients with ischemic heart disease and HF remains bleak.[8,9] Cell therapy offers a novel strategy that has the potential to reconstitute dead myocardium, and for the first time, reverse the fundamental cause of HF rather than merely delay its progression.

CELL TYPES USED FOR CELL THERAPY IN MYOCARDIAL INFARCTION

Embryonic Stem Cells

Pluripotent stem cells, that is, cells that have the ability to differentiate into tissues derived from all three germ layers (ectoderm, endoderm, and mesoderm), include

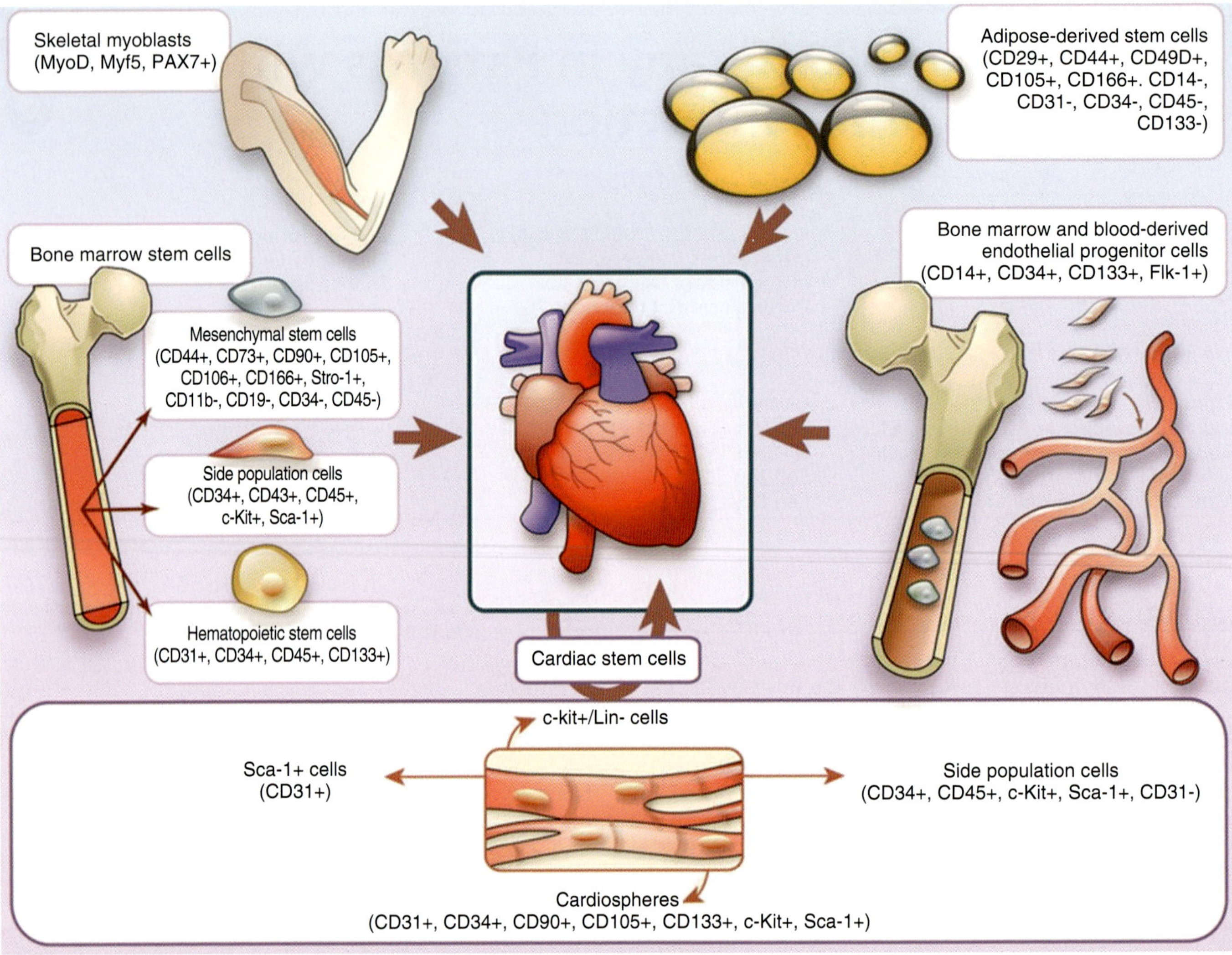

FIGURE 22-1 Sources of stem cells used for cardiac repair. Bone marrow–derived stem cells include a broad range of cells, from mesenchymal stem cells to endothelial progenitor cells, hematopoietic stem cells, and unfractionated mononuclear cells. *(From Sanganalmath SK, Bolli R: Cell therapy for heart failure: a comprehensive overview of experimental and clinical studies, current challenges, and future directions.* Circ Res *113:810–34, 2013; Figure 2.)*

embryonic stem cells (ESCs), which are harvested from the inner cell mass of preimplantation-stage blastocysts, and induced pluripotent stem cells (iPSCs), which are embryonic-like stem cells derived from adult cells. The functional components of the human heart (cardiomyocytes, endothelial cells, and smooth muscle cells) are of mesodermal origin.

Preclinical Studies

ESC-derived cardiomyocytes (hESC-CMs) display adult cardiomyocyte morphology with properly organized sarcomeric proteins, spontaneous beating activity, and characteristic atrial, ventricular, and nodal action potentials.[10] The ability of ESCs to generate bona fide cardiomyocytes has spurred interest in the use of ESCs or hESC-CMs for cardiac regeneration after MI. A number of preclinical reports have described engraftment of hESC-CMs and/or differentiation of ESCs into adult cardiomyocytes with subsequent attenuation of LV remodeling and improvement in left ventricular ejection fraction (LVEF) in rodent models. In one study, investigators transplanted murine cardiac-committed ESCs into the infarcted myocardium of sheep 2 weeks after MI. One month after transplantation, the ESCs had differentiated into cardiomyocytes, engrafted to the host heart, and improved LV function.[3] Shiba and colleagues demonstrated, in a guinea pig model of MI, that implanted hESC-CMs partially integrated into the host myocardium and contracted synchronously with the host muscle.[11] The engrafted hearts showed improved mechanical function and a reduced incidence of both spontaneous and induced ventricular tachycardia. Chong and colleagues transplanted one billion hESC-CMs into a nonhuman primate model of reperfused MI under intense immunosuppression.[12] They reported extensive remuscularization of the infarcted area, which averaged 2.1% of the LV and 40% of the infarct volume, as well as formation of electromechanical junctions between the graft and host cardiomyocytes. Study of calcium transients indicated electrical activation of the cardiomyocyte grafts and electromechanical coupling. However, this study raised significant concerns in the scientific community,[13] primarily because the observations were anecdotal (1 to 2 monkeys were assessed at each time point), the infarcts were small (7% to 10% of the LV), the infarct size was not reduced, the evidence for remuscularization of the infarcted tissue was inadequate, cardiac function was not assessed, and importantly, malignant ventricular arrhythmias were observed in all monkeys that received the transplants.

Barriers to Clinical Development

Despite the obvious promise of hESCs and hESC-CMs, the use of these cells faces formidable hurdles[10,14] and is unlikely to become a therapy for CV disease.[3] The allogeneic nature of ESCs necessitates lifelong use of immunosuppressive therapy, with its attendant risks and morbidity, which could be worse than the disease being treated. The recent finding that hESC-CMs are arrhythmogenic constitutes another problem.[12] Even more concerning is the risk of teratoma formation, which is inherent in the embryonic nature of the cells; despite attempts to minimize it, the occurrence of this serious consequence cannot be completely eliminated. These risks and problems are all the more unacceptable because potentially safer alternatives are available, including iPSCs and adult stem cells; the latter have already been tested in numerous clinical trials, with an excellent safety profile (vide infra). In view of these considerations, it is difficult to rationalize using ESCs for therapeutic purposes in patients with CV disease.[3] Not surprisingly, no clinical trial of ESC-based therapy for CV disease has been published despite the fact that these cells have been studied for two decades; meanwhile, over this time period, thousands of patients have been safely treated with adult stem and/or progenitor cells with results that have been sufficiently encouraging to warrant phase III trials.

Induced Pluripotent Stem Cells

Preclinical Studies

In 2006, Takahashi and Yamanaka reported generation of iPSCs by transducing adult mouse fibroblasts with a cocktail of transcription factors, including Oct3/4, Sox2, c-Myc, and Klf4, which are the so-called Yamanaka factors.[15] The embryonic-like cells expressed ESC marker genes and exhibited morphology and growth properties similar to those of ESCs. It was subsequently demonstrated that iPSCs possess a cardiogenic potential comparable to that of ESCs, and more importantly, functional properties typical of cardiac cells, such as cardiac ion channel expression, spontaneous beating, and contractility.[16] iPSCs have a capacity equivalent to ESCs to differentiate into nodal-, atrial-, and ventricular-like cardiomyocyte phenotypes, based on action potential characteristics. iPSC-derived cardiomyocytes (iPSC-CMs) exhibit typical sarcomeric organization and respond to β-adrenergic stimulation, with an increase in the spontaneous rate and a decrease in action potential duration.[17] Initial studies in small animal models have reported improvement in cardiac function as a result of iPSC administration.[18] In a porcine model of MI, intramyocardial transplantation of human iPSC-CMs, endothelial cells, and smooth muscle cells, in combination with a three-dimensional fibrin patch loaded with insulin growth factor–encapsulated microspheres, resulted in human iPSC-CMs being integrated into the host myocardium and generating organized sarcomeric structures[19]; moreover, endothelial and smooth muscle cells were also incorporated into the host vasculature, although their contribution was minimal. At 4 weeks, LV function was significantly improved compared with untreated animals, along with a trend toward a reduction in infarct size. In this study, cell treatment was delivered after reperfusion, and the animals were immunosuppressed.

Barriers to Clinical Development

Despite these promising results, the iPSC technology is associated with a number of safety concerns, including the potential for genetic and epigenetic abnormalities related to the origin and manipulation of the cells and for tumorigenicity related to retroviral transgene activation, insertional mutagenesis, and contamination with undifferentiated pluripotent stem cells and/or differentiation-resistant cells.[20] Despite the initial hope that these autologous cells would not require immunosuppression, issues of immunogenicity of transplanted cells have emerged.[20] Some of these safety concerns have been addressed (e.g., virus-free induction of iPSCs[14]), but other concerns persist. Furthermore, clinical translation is hindered by major practical hurdles related to cell procurement, including efficient induction of cardiomyocyte lineages from iPSCs, selective expansion and/or survival of iPSC-CM lineages, and purification of differentiated iPSC-CMs by elimination of residual undifferentiated iPSCs.[20] Although major progress has been made in differentiation protocols,[21] significant problems remain to be resolved. Additional limiting factors are the cost and effort required to generate autologous iPSCs in every patient who is treated. Although iPSC technology is evolving rapidly, and these challenges may be overcome, at present it seems unlikely that these cells will be used in clinical trials in the near future.

A new strategy that has recently emerged for cardiac regeneration is in vivo direct reprogramming of nonmyocyte cardiac cells, which make up more than 50% of the cells in the heart.[22] This direct reprogramming strategy entails direct transdifferentation of one cell type (i.e., cardiac fibroblast) to another (i.e., cardiomyocyte), bypassing the need for dedifferentiation to an earlier embryonic state before redifferentiation toward a cardiomyocyte fate. This approach is still in its nascent phase, and it is unclear whether clinical translation will ever be feasible.

Bone Marrow Mononuclear Cells

Most clinical trials of cell therapy in the setting of acute MI have been performed using BMMNCs (Table 22-1). An advantage of these cells includes not needing to be cultured, and thus, they can be delivered quickly and relatively inexpensively. In acute MI, BMMNCs have usually been infused intracoronarily because of the concern that transendocardial injection into freshly infarcted myocardium might result in complications (e.g., arrhythmias or perforation of the LV wall). However, subsequent experience with transendocardial injection of BMMNCs at an average of 10 days after MI has not corroborated these concerns. The safety of this delivery modality has not been tested in the first week after MI.

Clinical Trials

Since the initial report of cell therapy in patients with acute MI,[24] many phase I and some phase II clinical trials have been performed using BM cells in patients with ST-elevation MI (STEMI). The preponderance of these investigations have tested unfractionated BMMNCs, with only a small number of studies using selected BM populations, such as $CD34^+$ cells, $CD133^+$ cells, and MSCs. The results have been inconsistent (see Table 22-1).

In the BOOST trial, 60 patients with STEMI were randomized 4 to 6 days after MI to receive intracoronary BM cells (which included, but were not limited to, BMMNCs that were depleted of erythrocytes and platelets) or no treatment.[25] At 6 months, there was a statistically significant improvement in global and regional LVEF and border zone wall

TABLE 22-1 Key Clinical Trials of Cell-Based Therapy after Acute Myocardial Infarction

STUDY NAME/FIRST AUTHOR (YEAR)	DESIGN	PATIENT NUMBER	CELL TYPE/DOSE	ROUTE OF INJECTION	IMAGING MODALITIES	TIMING FROM MI TO CELL DELIVERY	FOLLOW-UP/RESULTS
BOOST Wollert[25] (2004) Meyer[26] (2006, 2009)	RCT	Treated: 30 Control: 30	Nucleated BM cells $24.6 \pm 0.94 \times 10^8$	IC	CMR Echo	4–6 days	6 mos: Improvement in EF 18 mos: No improvement in EF, LV volumes, and RWM 5 yrs: No improvement in EF, LV volumes, infarct size, and RWM
Janssens (2006)	RDBCT	Treated: 33 Placebo: 34	Nucleated BM cells $3 \pm 1.28 \times 10^8$ containing $1.72 \pm 0.72 \times 10^8$ BMMNCs	IC	CMR	1–2 days	4 mos: No improvement in EF; ↓infarct size, ↑RWM 12 mos: No improvement in EF, LV volumes, and infarct size; ↑ RWM
ASTAMI Lunde (2006, 2008) Beitnes[31] (2009)	RCT	Treated: 47 Controls: 50	BMMNCs 0.7×10^8 (0.54×10^8 to 1.3×10^8)	IC	SPECT Echo CMR	4–8 days	6 mos: No improvement in EF, infarct size, and LV volumes 12 mos: No improvement in EF, LV volumes, and RWM 3 yrs: No improvement in EF, LV volumes, LV mass, infarct size, and RWM
REPAIR-AMI Schächinger[27] (2006) Assmus[28,29] (2010, 2014)	RDBCT	Treated: 101 Placebo: 98	BMMNCs $2.36 \pm 1.74 \times 10^8$	IC	LV angiography	3–6 days	4 mos: Improvement in EF, ESV and RWM 1 yr: ↓MACE, ↑RWM, 2 yrs: ↓MACE, ↑RWM, ↓infarct size, no improvement in EF and LV volumes 5 yrs: ↓MACE
FINCELL Huikiri (2008)	RDBCT	Treated: 40 Placebo: 40	BMMNCs $4.02 \pm 1.96 \times 10^6$	IC	Echo LV angiography	2–6 days	6 mos: No improvement in EF; improved ΔEF
REGENT Tendera[49] (2009)	RCT	Treated: 160 Controls: 40	BMMNCs 1.78×10^8 $CD34^+/CXCR4^+$ 1.9×10^6	IC	CMR LV angiography	3–12 days	6 mos: No improvement in EF and LV volumes
Hare[54] (2009)	RDBCT	Treated: 34 Placebo: 19	Allogeneic BM MSCs 0.5, 1.6, 5×10^6/kg	IV	Echo CMR	1–10 days	6 mos: No improvement EF
TIME Traverse[34] (2012)	RDBCT	Treated: 80 Placebo: 40	BMMNCs 1.5×10^8	IC	CMR	3–7 days	6 mos: No improvement in EF, LV volumes, RWM, and infarct size
LateTIME Traverse[35] (2011)	RDBCT	Treated: 58 Placebo: 29	BMMNCs 1.5×10^8	IC	CMR	15–20 days	6 mos: No improvement in EF, LV volumes, RWM, and infarct size
SWISS-AMI Surder[37] (2013)	RCT	Treated early: 60 Treated late: 58 Controls: 49	BMMNCs $1.4–1.6 \times 10^8$	IC	CMR	5–7 days 3–4 wks	4 mos: No improvement in EF, LV volumes, and scar mass

↑, Increased; ↓, decreased, *BM*, bone marrow; *BMMNCs*, bone marrow mononuclear cells; *CMR*, cardiac magnetic resonance imaging; *Echo*, echocardiography; *EF*, ejection fraction; *ESV*, end-systolic volume; *IC*, intracoronary; *IV*, intravenous; *LV*, left ventricular; *MACE*, major adverse cardiovascular events; *MSCs*, mesenchymal stromal/stem cells; *RCT*, randomized controlled trial; *RDBCT*, randomized double-blind controlled trial; *RWM*, regional wall motion; *SPECT*, single-photon emission computed tomography.

motion (measured by cardiac magnetic resonance imaging [CMR]) in the treated group compared with the control group, although there was no improvement in LV volumes. However, despite this early benefit, the difference between the control and treated groups was no longer significant at 18 months and 5 years, primarily because of an improvement in the control group.[26]

REPAIR-AMI

REPAIR-AMI, a double-blind, randomized controlled trial (RCT), is the largest study of cell therapy in acute MI performed so far.[27] Two hundred four patients with STEMI were assigned to intracoronary infusion of BMMNCs or placebo 3 to 6 days after successful percutaneous coronary intervention (PCI). At 4 months, there was a statistically significant improvement in LVEF, as measured by contrast ventriculography, in the patients in the cell group compared with those in the placebo group. Furthermore, at 1 year, the number of major adverse cardiac events (MACE) (death and recurrent MI) was significantly reduced by cell treatment. However, the CMR substudy, which included 54 of the 204 patients, did not show any difference between the treated and placebo groups with regard to LVEF at 4 or 12 months. In another substudy of 58 patients, coronary flow reserve in the infarct-related artery became normal in the treated group at 4 months, suggesting that intracoronary BMMNC therapy may restore microvascular function.

All of the composite clinical endpoints remained significantly improved in the treated cohort at 2 years[28]; at the 5-year follow-up, only the composite of death, recurrent MI, and any revascularization remained significantly different between the treated and placebo groups, which was driven mainly by revascularization.[29] Further analysis by CMR suggested that BMMNC therapy attenuated adverse LV remodeling, as demonstrated by a decrease in end-diastolic wall thickness in the infarcted and remote regions, and an increase in regional contractility.[30] However, LV volumes were not significantly affected by cell therapy.

REPAIR-AMI was a landmark trial in cell therapy not only because of its size and design (randomized, double-blinded, and placebo-controlled with BM aspiration and sham cell infusion in control subjects), but also because it provided important insights that have had a profound influence on clinical research in this field. The REPAIR-AMI investigators made observations that were adopted in the design of most subsequent trials. In a prespecified subgroup analysis, they noted that the benefits of BMMNC therapy were confined to patients with LVEF at or below the median value of 48.9%. At 4 months, in the subset of patients with LVEF ≤48.9%, the increase in LVEF affected by BMMNC therapy was approximately 5 EF units (95% confidence interval [CI], 2.0 to 8.1) greater than that in the placebo group, whereas in the subset of patients with LVEF greater than 48.9%, the increase relative to placebo was only 0.3 unit (95% CI, −2.2 to 2.8). This dichotomy is not difficult to rationalize; if LV function is normal or near normal, it seems unlikely that cell therapy (or any therapy) could effect a significant improvement. The inverse relation between baseline LV function and magnitude of therapeutic effect reported in REPAIR-AMI formed the basis for the design of subsequent trials of cell therapy in acute MI, which have almost invariably excluded patients with normal or near-normal LV function. In these subjects, not only is the therapeutic effect likely to be small, but the need for cell therapy is less obvious. Conversely, in patients with large MIs (particularly those with anterior MIs), there is a clearer rationale for cell therapy, and the benefits are likely to be greater. Thus, in general, clinical trials performed after REPAIR-AMI have enrolled patients with baseline LVEF of ≤45%.

The other important insight garnered in REPAIR-AMI was the interaction between improvement in LVEF and time of cell infusion. Specifically, the beneficial effects of BMMNC infusion on the recovery of contractile function were observed only in patients who were treated ≥5 days after PCI, suggesting that early (within 4 days) administration of cell therapy may be ineffective, possibly because of the intense inflammatory response and the hostile environment that it creates for transplanted cells. However, this concept has not been supported by later studies, as detailed in the following.

Other Randomized Trials of Bone Marrow Mononuclear Cells

In contrast to REPAIR-AMI, two other contemporaneous RCTs reported no benefit from BMMNCs in acute MI. In the open-label ASTAMI trial, 100 patients with STEMI were randomized to BMMNCs or control (no treatment) at 4 to 8 days after MI. The two groups did not differ with respect to LVEF, LV end-diastolic volume, or infarct size at 6 months (as measured by single-photon emission computed tomography, echocardiography, and CMR) and 1 year (as measured by echocardiography). Long-term follow-up at 3 years also failed to demonstrate any benefit with respect to LVEF, LV volumes, infarct size, and wall motion, as evaluated both by CMR and echocardiography.[31] Janssens and colleagues randomized 67 patients with STEMI to BMMNCs or placebo early (1 day) after PCI and measured outcome 4 months later using CMR. There was no improvement in LVEF, although infarct size and regional LV function improved in the cell therapy group. Similarly, at 1 year, LVEF and LV volumes did not differ between the two groups, although the favorable effects of cell therapy on selected LV remodeling parameters remained, such as wall motion in the infarct border zone and regional contraction in segments with transmural hyperenhancement (the early difference in infarct size was no longer significant at 1 year).

In addition, four other phase II RCTs examined the effect of BMMNCs in the context of acute MI and yielded negative results (see Table 22-1). In the multicenter open-label HEBE trial, 200 patients with a first large MI, baseline EF ≤45%, and successful PCI were assigned to intracoronary BMMNCs, peripheral blood mononuclear cells, or no treatment (control subjects) in addition to standard therapy 3 to 8 days after successful reperfusion.[32] At 4 months, there was no difference among the groups with respect to LVEF (assessed by CMR), LV volumes, LV mass, infarct size, or clinical events. Long-term follow-up at 2 years showed no difference among the groups with regard to LVEF (evaluated by CMR); interestingly, the authors reported that the composite endpoint of death or recurrent MI was significantly more frequent in the peripheral blood mononuclear cell group at 5 years.[33] In the National Heart, Lung, and Blood Institute Cardiovascular Cell Therapy Research Network (CCTRN) TIME trial, 120 patients with STEMI, LVEF ≤45%, and successful reperfusion, were randomized 2:1 to early intracoronary BMMNCs or placebo at either 3 or 7 days after acute MI.[34] The purpose of this design was to verify the observation made earlier in REPAIR-AMI that BMMNC therapy was only helpful if delivered 5 days or more after MI. At the 6-month follow-up, there was no significant effect of cell therapy on recovery of global or regional LV function or LV volumes, as measured by CMR. Furthermore, no difference was observed between the patients treated at 3 and 7 days after MI. The CCTRN Late-TIME trial was designed to investigate the effects of BMMNCs administered 2 to 3 weeks after AMI; in this study, 87 patients with STEMI and LVEF ≤45% were assigned, in a 2:1 fashion, to intracoronary BMMNCs or placebo.[35] The hypothesis was that the inflammation associated with acutely infarcted myocardium produces a hostile environment that is toxic to the cells, and that allowing the inflammation to subside may lead to greater cell survival and larger therapeutic effects. Again, the investigators found no improvement in global or regional LV function or LV volumes measured by CMR at 6 months. A combined analysis of all patients enrolled in TIME and Late-TIME was also neutral[36]; when this combined data set was examined for the effects of age, baseline LVEF, and time from PCI to infusion, only baseline LVEF was found to be significantly associated with changes in the LVEF (patients with lower LVEF exhibited greater increases in LVEF and vice versa). This relationship was observed regardless of treatment. Finally, in the SWISS-AMI trial, 200 patients with successfully reperfused STEMI were randomized 1:1:1 to an open-label control (no treatment) or two intracoronary BMMNC treatment groups (early, 5 to 7 days, and late, 3 to 4 weeks after MI).[37] This trial was also designed to investigate the effects of early versus late administration of BMMNCs. Again, the treatment did not produce any improvement in LVEF, scar mass, or LV volumes at 4 months, as measured by CMR.

Reconciling Discordant Results from Clinical Trials

Multiple potential reasons have been proposed to explain the conflicting results of BMMNC trials in acute MI. A major problem with cell therapy is that the properties of the cell product may vary enormously from one study to another, and from one laboratory to another, depending on the specific protocol used to isolate and expand the cells. Even seemingly meaningless (and thus unrecognized) details can have a profound effect on the viability and potency of the cell product. For example, although all trials used density gradient centrifugation to separate mononuclear cells from the BM aspirate, there were significant differences in the protocols that could have resulted in differences in the composition and quality of the cell product (e.g., the percent of progenitor cells such as $CD34^+$ and $CD133^+$ cells or the functional competence of the cells). A recent retrospective analysis of TIME suggested that the content of $CD31^+$ cells in the BM injectate was an important determinant of LV functional recovery.[38] Along these lines, the discrepancy between REPAIR-AMI and ASTAMI has been attributed to the efficiency of the cell isolation protocol, which resulted in different degrees of cell viability. By comparing the two protocols, the REPAIR-AMI investigators concluded that the protocol used in ASTAMI resulted in lower cell recovery, a lower number of hematopoietic, endothelial, and mesenchymal colony-forming units (CFUs), significantly reduced migration capacity of the cells in response to the chemotactic stromal-derived factor-1 (SDF-1), and abolished capacity of the cells to promote neovascularization in an experimental hind limb ischemia model. However, the investigators in the negative HEBE trial validated the cell isolation protocol against the one used in REPAIR-AMI before enrolling the first patient and demonstrated that the quantity and quality of the cells were similar in both studies. Similarly, the CCTRN investigators argued that such concerns were not warranted.[39] Going forward, it is crucial that trials of cell therapy incorporate appropriate assays to verify the viability and functional competence of the cell product under investigation.

Another potential explanation for the discrepancies is erythrocyte contamination of the BM cell product. In an exploratory analysis of the injectate in the REPAIR-AMI cohort, the number of red blood cells (RBCs) contaminating the final cell product was significantly correlated with reduced recovery of LVEF 4 months after BMMNC therapy.[40] Higher numbers of RBCs in the BMMNC preparation were associated with reduced cell viability, CFU capacity, and migratory capacity in vitro; furthermore, neovascularization capacity was significantly impaired in vivo in a murine model of hind limb ischemia after infusion of BMMNCs contaminated with RBCs compared with BMMNCs alone. An additional variable that has been proposed to contribute to the discrepancies is the use of heparin. The REPAIR-AMI investigators found that heparin profoundly and dose-dependently inhibits SDF-1–induced BMMNC migration in vitro, and that pretreatment of BMMNCs with heparin significantly reduces the homing of the injected cells in a murine ear-wound model.[41] However, it is doubtful that the RBC and heparin issues account for the inconsistent results of clinical trials. For example, in the CCTRN TIME trial, the cell product was devoid of significant RBC contamination and contained only minuscule amounts of heparin, and in the SWISS-AMI trial, no heparin was used in the final product. Nonetheless, both trials were null.

A factor that may have contributed to the negative results of the CCTRN TIME and Late-TIME trials is that the enrollment of patients was based upon the LVEF measured in the qualifying echocardiograms, which were obtained earlier after PCI than the baseline CMRs. In the TIME trial, LVEF averaged approximately 37% in the qualifying echocardiograms, but they increased to approximately 45% in the baseline CMR; in the Late-TIME trial, these values were approximately 36% and approximately 48%, respectively.[36] In patients with baseline LVEF of approximately 45% to 48%, the benefits of cell therapy would be expected to be attenuated. However, SWISS-AMI did not experience this limitation (the baseline LVEF averaged 37.4% at an average of 6 days after MI) and was still negative. Finally, the possibility that the preceding trials had insufficient statistical power cannot be excluded. For example, the HEBE and SWISS-AMI trials were powered to detect a 6.0- and 3.5-unit improvement in LVEF, respectively[32,37]; a smaller effect would likely have been missed.

Meta-Analyses of Bone Marrow Cell Therapy

Many of the individual trials in acute MI were limited by their size and/or design. Therefore, in the absence of phase III trials, no definitive conclusions can be made regarding the effects of cell therapy in this setting. At present, the best available evidence comes from meta-analyses. In a collaborative meta-analysis, Delewi and colleagues pooled the data from 16 RCTs that had enrolled more than 30 patients in the BM arm, reaching a total of 1494 patients.[42] At 3 to 6 months, LVEF improved by 2.55 units among BM cell–treated patients compared with control subjects (P <.001)

(Figure 22-2). Moreover, cell therapy significantly reduced end-systolic and end-diastolic LV volumes. In subgroup analyses, the benefit of treatment on LVEF was more pronounced in younger patients compared with older ones, and in patients with baseline LVEF of less than 40% compared with those with LVEF ≥40%. There was also a trend in favor of patients treated ≥7 days after primary PCI compared with patients treated at less than 7 days and in patients who received more than 10^8 BMMNCs compared with ≥10^8 cells (see Figure 22-2).

Another meta-analysis that combined the results of 22 RCTs involving 1513 patients arrived at similar conclusions; the overall improvement in LVEF at 6 months and at 6 to 18 months after cell therapy was 2.10 and 3.04 units, respectively (P = .004 and P = .0008, respectively) (Fig. 22-e1).[43] In addition, this study pooled the clinical endpoints and reported no beneficial effects after a median follow-up of 6 months. Contrary to the meta-analysis by Delewi and colleagues,[42] however, the subsets of patients who were treated less than 8 days after PCI benefited more than the patients treated at ≥8 days (P = .009). However, both of these studies failed to detect a beneficial effect of cell therapy on LVEF when the analysis was restricted to trials that used CMR for outcome assessment, an important finding that has been echoed by other meta-analyses.[44,45] Of note, all of the major trials that used CMR as the method for LVEF quantification have been negative.[36]

In contrast to these group-based meta-analyses, an individual patient data (IPD)–based meta-analysis provided sobering conclusions. ACCRUE is an ongoing collaborative database that includes IPDs from randomized and cohort studies of cell therapy in patients with ischemic heart disease.[46] The investigators compiled 12 studies involving 1085 patients, including 2 studies that used cell types other than BMMNCs, although most patients received BMMNCs. Importantly, the availability of IPDs enabled them to perform an intention-to-treat analysis. Using this approach, at a median of 6 months after MI (range, 3 to12 months), no effect of cell therapy was identified with the combined endpoint of all-cause death, recurrent MI, stroke, and target vessel revascularization (14.0% in cell-treated patients vs. 16.3% in control subjects; hazard ratio, 0.86; 95% CI, 0.63 to 1.18), on death (1.4% vs. 2.1%), or on the composite endpoint of death, recurrent MI, and stroke (2.9% vs. 4.7%), nor were any difference in LVEF observed in comparison with control subjects (mean difference between treated and control subjects: 0.96%, 95% CI, −0.2 to 2.1) (Figure 22-3). Subgroup analyses did not reveal any interaction between improvement in EF on one hand and baseline LVEF, use of CMR for EF quantification, and time from reperfusion to cell therapy on the other hand.

Thus far, ACCRUE is the only meta-analysis that used patient-level data to assess the effects of cell therapy in acute MI. Despite the advantages of using IPD, this study

Characteristics	N	Treatment effect (95%CI)	*p*-value*
Overall†	1494	2.55 (1.83, 3.26)	
Age (years)			
<55	676	3.38 (2.36, 4.39)	0.03
≥55	809	1.77 (0.80, 2.74)	
Diabetes			
Yes	229	2.87 (1.32, 4.41)	0.39
No	1263	2.10 (1.29, 2.90)	
Symptoms to PCI (hours)			
<6	764	1.79 (0.81, 2.77)	0.13
≥6	509	2.98 (1.79, 4. 16)	
IRA			
LAD	1239	1.98 (1.16, 2.80)	0.11
RCA/LCX	235	3.53 (1.82, 5.23)	
LVEDVI (mL/m²)			
<100	988	1.79 (0.84, 2.73)	0.11
≥100	326	3.00 (1.85, 4. 15)	
LVEF (%)			
<40	503	5.30 (4.27, 6.33)	<0.001
≥40	991	1.45 (0.60, 2.31)	
Infarct size (g)			
<20	169	1.50 (−0.69, 3.69)	0.84
≥20	355	1.54 (−1.46, 4.54)	
MVO			
Presence	350	1.41 (−0.79, 3.61)	0.67
Absence	196	1.80 (−0.21, 3.80)	

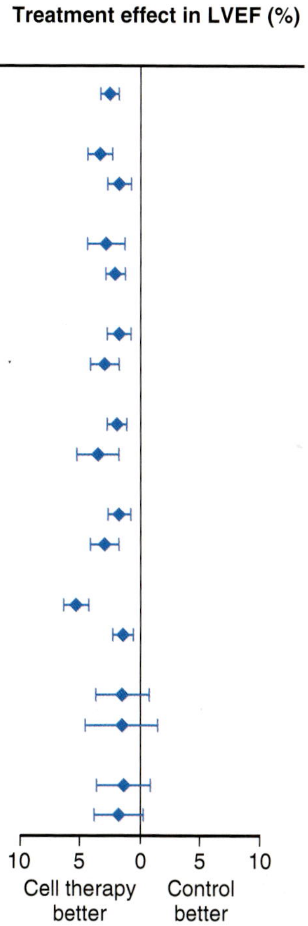

FIGURE 22-2 Forest plot of change in left ventricular ejection fraction (LVEF) with cell therapy among trials that assessed specific subgroups. *CI*, Confidence interval; *IRA*, infarct-related artery; *LAD*, left anterior descending artery; *LCX*, left circumflex artery; *LVEDVI*, left ventricular end-diastolic volume index; *MVO*, microvascular obstruction; *PCI*, percutaneous coronary intervention; *RCA*, right coronary artery. **P* value for subgroup differences. †Frequencies can vary across subgroups because of missing baseline characteristics values. *(From Delewi R, et al: Impact of intracoronary bone marrow cell therapy on left ventricular function in the setting of ST-segment elevation myocardial infarction: a collaborative meta-analysis.* Eur Heart J *35:989–98, 2014; Figure 2.)*

Study or subgroup	Cell therapy Mean (%)	SD (%)	Total	Control Mean (%)	SD (%)	Total	Weight (%)	Mean difference 95% CI (%)
Aalst	5.2	11.8	19	4.32	13.15	14	2.7	0.88 (−7.81, 9.57)
ASTAMI	8.06	11.16	50	6.84	9.5	50	8.3	1.22 (−2.84, 5.28)
BONAMI	1.19	5.21	47	1.71	6.65	47	13.2	−0.52 (−2.94, 1.90)
BOOST	6.66	6.47	30	0.69	8.12	30	9.1	5.97 (2.25, 9.69)
CADUCEUS	5.03	9.64	17	6.48	4.41	8	5.6	−1.45 (−6.96, 4.06)
FINCELL	7.18	12.64	34	2.39	10.13	36	5.8	4.79 (−0.60, 10.18)
LATE-TIME	0.51	8.19	55	3.56	9.34	26	8.0	−3.05 (−7.24, 1.14)
REGENT	2.96	11.61	90	−0.27	10.93	32	7.3	3.23 (−1.25, 7.71)
REPAIR-AMI	5.51	7.28	95	3.01	6.51	92	14.8	2.50 (0.52, 4.48)
SCAMI	−0.69	7.74	22	4.12	10.04	12	4.3	−4.81(−11.35, 1.73)
SWISS-AMI	1.34	8.04	107	−0.38	8.78	60	12.2	1.72 (−0.97, 4.41)
TIME	3.16	10.34	75	3.27	9.69	37	8.7	−0.11(−4.01, 3.79)
Total (95% CI)			**641**			**444**	**100.0%**	**1.15 (−0.38,2.69)**

Heterogeneity $Tau^2 = 3.13$; $Chi^2 = 21.04$, df = 11 ($P = 0.03$); $I^2 = 48\%$
Test for overall effect: $Z = 1.47$ ($P = 0.14$)

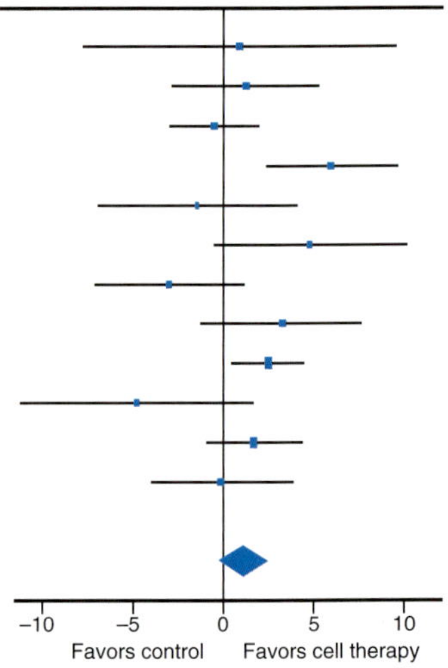

FIGURE 22-3 Forest plot of changes in left ventricular ejection fraction (LVEF) in the ACCRUE patient-level meta-analysis. *CI*, Confidence interval; *df*, degree of freedom. *(From Gyöngyösi M, et al: Meta-Analysis of Cell-based CaRdiac stUdiEs [ACCRUE] in patients with acute myocardial infarction based on individual patient data.* Circ Res *116:1346–1360, 2015; Fig 4A.)*

had limitations, including the fact that there was a significant baseline difference in LVEF, end-systolic volumes, and end-diastolic volumes between the treated and control groups, and that only approximately 60% of all patients with acute MI enrolled in cell therapy trials were included (because of refusal of several investigators to participate in ACCRUE), which increased the risk of bias in this meta-analysis. Another limitation was that ACCRUE included CADUCEUS, which was a study of cardiosphere-derived cells administered 62 ± 11 days after MI. Combining studies of BM cells and cardiosphere-derived cells and patients with acute MI and subacute MI may not be justified.

These conflicting data highlight the need for a large phase III RCT. The BAMI trial (NCT01569178) is an ongoing multinational, multicenter, randomized, open-label, controlled, parallel-group phase III study funded by the European Union. Its aim is to demonstrate that intracoronary infusion of autologous BMMNCs is safe and reduces all-cause mortality in patients with reduced LVEF (≤45%) after successful reperfusion for acute MI compared with a control group of patients treated with standard medical care. A sample size of 3000 patients was calculated on the basis of the results of REPAIR-AMI, and the protocol is derived from that study.

Selected Bone Marrow Cells

Because the efficacy of BMMNCs has been increasingly questioned by the results of "negative" trials, attention has turned to selected BM cell populations, including $CD34^+$, $CD133^+$, and MSCs. $CD34^+$ and $CD133^+$ cells are present among BMMNCs in small proportions (approximately 1% to 2%)[34] and are selected out of the BMMNCs by immunomagnetic sorting. $CD34^+$ and $CD133^+$ cells (sometimes loosely termed endothelial progenitor cells [EPCs] or proangiogenic progenitor cells) are both vasculogenic and hematopoietic. CD34 is a surface marker of both hematopoietic stem cells and EPCs, and $CD34^+$ cells are found both in the BM and in the peripheral blood. There is currently no consensus regarding the definition of EPCs, which have been identified as cells that express CD34, CD133, KDR, or any combination thereof.[47] It has been suggested in observational studies that EPCs, including $CD34^+$ and $CD133^+$ cells, are mobilized in patients with acute MI, and that this phenomenon is correlated with improved LVEF and attenuation of adverse LV remodeling.[48] In preclinical models, the administration of $CD34^+$ and $CD133^+$ cells has been found to enhance cardiac perfusion and function by stimulating neovascularization.

Autologous proangiogenic progenitors have been investigated in the context of acute MI, ICM, and NICM. In the open-label REGENT trial, 200 patients with LVEF of less than 40% after MI were randomized to BMMNCs, BM $CD34^+$/$CXCR4^+$ cells, and to control (no treatment) in a 2:2:1 fashion.[49] Overall, there was no significant difference among the groups with regard to LVEF, LV volumes (assessed by CMR), and clinical endpoints at the 6-month follow-up. This trial was limited by imbalances in baseline LVEF and incomplete follow-up, with paired CMR analysis available only in 117 of 200 patients. Importantly, the median number of cells injected in the $CD34^+$/$CXCR4^+$ group was 1.9×10^6. This is not dissimilar from the content of $CD34^+$/$CD133^+$ cells in the cell product administered in trials that used unselected BMMNCs. The question naturally arises as to whether higher numbers of proangiogenic cells would be beneficial. This was investigated in a small study in which 31 patients who presented with STEMI were randomized to $CD34^+$ cell therapy or control (no treatment).[50] In the cell therapy group, patients received three escalating doses of 5, 10, and 15×10^6 cells (5 or 6 patients per cohort). Although at the 6-month follow-up there was no difference among the groups in terms of LV function, a positive trend was noted in favor of the ≥10 million cohorts; in addition, improved perfusion was correlated with the quantity and mobility of the infused $CD34^+$ cells. The phase II ENACT-AMI double-blind trial (NCT00936819) is recruiting 100 patients with moderate to large STEMIs and assigning them to 3 groups, including intracoronary administration of placebo, autologous blood-derived EPCs (20×10^6), or autologous EPCs transfected with human endothelial nitric oxide synthase (20×10^6), to investigate the effects of cell therapy alone or in combination with gene therapy on myocardial function in patients with MI.

In summary, as is the case for BMMNCs, the effects of CD34+ cells and CD133+ cells in patients with acute MI are unclear; additional studies will be needed to assess this issue.

Mesenchymal Stromal Cells

MSCs are a population of cells of mesodermal origin that exist in almost all postnatal organs and connective tissues, including BM, adipose tissue, and the heart.[51] They give rise to stromal cells such as fibroblasts and to other cells of mesodermal origin, such as those found in bone, cartilage, and adipose tissue. They have been studied most thoroughly in the BM, where they constitute a rare nonhematopoietic population.

MSCs are being increasingly used in clinical trials of stem cell therapy because of their favorable characteristics, including in vitro stemness features, ease of isolation and ex vivo expansion, and a favorable immunoprivileged profile[52]; the latter characteristic has been exploited particularly in studies of stem cells in patients with acute MI. Purportedly, MSCs are hypoimmunogenic and immunomodulatory, and therefore, capable of evading or even suppressing the immune system. They have been used in allogeneic fashion in preclinical models and clinical studies without appreciable immune response.[53] This behavior is partly because they lack expression of the surface structures involved in immunogenicity, including MHC class II molecules and co-stimulatory molecules for T-cell induction, such as CD40, CD40 ligand, and the B7 molecules CD80 and CD86. In addition, MSCs are capable of suppressing the immune response by direct cell–cell interactions and release of soluble factors that inhibit proliferation, maturation, and function of various immune cells. As a consequence of these properties, the use of allogeneic MSCs does not necessitate concurrent immunosuppression,[53] and the cells can be used "off-the-shelf," which is particularly suitable for acute MI. In addition, because of the adverse effects of co-morbidities on stem cell function, procurement of cells from a young healthy donor may translate into a more efficacious product.

A number of promising preclinical studies have paved the way for the use of MSCs in cardiac cell therapy trials.[52] Clinically, MSCs have been used mainly in chronic cardiomyopathy, but a few studies have also investigated them in acute MI. In a phase I randomized, double-blind, placebo-controlled, dose-escalation, multicenter trial, a total of 53 patients with first acute MI were randomized in a 2:1 fashion to different doses of allogeneic hMSCs or placebo.[54] Both the treatment and placebo groups exhibited a statistically significant improvement in LVEF (measured by echocardiography) at 6 months compared with baseline, with no difference between the two groups. However, the CMR substudy of 34 patients showed that MSC treatment led to a significant improvement in LVEF and reverse remodeling compared with placebo.[54] A phase II trial of allogeneic BM-derived MSCs is planned in patients who present with non–ST-elevation MI (NSTEMI) (NCT02277613).

Although the BM is the most common source of MSCs, these cells are also procured from other tissues, most notably, adipose tissue. In the adipose tissue, MSCs are located in perivascular niches; the adipose-derived stromal vascular fraction is enriched in MSCs 2500-fold compared with freshly isolated BMMNCs from the BM. Because of the abundance and availability of adipose tissue through liposuction, MSCs can be readily harvested in large enough numbers for acute administration after STEMI without the need for ex vivo expansion; an average of 20 to 40 million MSCs can be isolated and prepared within 2 hours after liposuction from as little as 200 g of lipoaspirate.[55] These properties make adipose-derived MSCs attractive for use in STEMI patients. The APOLLO trial was a double-blind, placebo-controlled study that investigated the safety and feasibility of intracoronary adipose-derived MSCs in STEMI. Fourteen patients with anterior STEMI were randomized 3:1 to receive either 20 million cells ($n = 10$) or placebo. There was a trend toward improved LVEF according to CMR analysis, with a 4.6% increase in the treated group from baseline to 6 months (P = NS), whereas in the placebo group, LVEF deteriorated by 1.7% ($P = .114$ for the comparison of changes in LVEF in the two groups). In the treated group, there was also a 52% reduction in infarct size versus baseline ($P = .002$), whereas in the placebo group, infarct size did not differ from baseline. A phase II trial using these cells is currently underway (NCT01216995). MSCs from other tissues, including bone and placenta, have also been studied in the preclinical setting.

Finally, the method for isolating MSCs from the BM aspirate continues to evolve. The traditional method results in a somewhat heterogeneous population of immature and mature cells, with mixed potential.[53,51] To overcome this limitation, attempts have been made to isolate a more homogenous and primitive population of cells. It has been shown that immunomagnetic isolation of cells based on cell surface markers, such as stromal precursor antigen-1 (STRO-1) and nontissue specific alkaline phosphatase (STRO-3), results in a subset of MSCs that exhibit enhanced stemness characteristics, such as clonogenicity, proliferative capacity, and trilineage differentiation capacity, as well as a superior proangiogenic and cardioprotective paracrine profile compared with plastic adherent MSCs.[56,57] After encouraging preclinical studies in large animal models,[58] STRO-3–selected MSCs are being tested in a phase II, placebo-controlled RCT, the ongoing AMICI trial (NCT01781390), which is randomizing 225 patients with anterior STEMI. Another approach to arrive at a more potent cell population is to treat cells with a cocktail of growth factors and cytokines to "prime" them toward cardiopoiesis, a process termed lineage guidance.[59] So far, these cardiogenically oriented MSCs have been investigated clinically in the context of ICM, but not acute MI; phase II studies are underway.[59]

In summary, MSCs are a promising cell population for cardiovascular therapy. Advantages include ease of procurement and expansion, possibility of allogeneic treatment, and encouraging preclinical and clinical results. Their use in the setting of acute MI is being investigated in ongoing trials, which, along with studies performed in the context of ischemic cardiomyopathy, should shed further light on the therapeutic potential of these cells.

ROUTES OF CELL DELIVERY

The methods used for cell delivery are of immense importance for any successful clinical cell therapy. Important considerations in choosing a cell delivery method include safety of cell administration, cell retention, uniformity of cell distribution, and efficiency of engraftment in the scarred myocardium (Table 22-2). Cells can be administered systematically through the intravenous route or locally. Local administration can be done via intracoronary infusion, percutaneous transendocardial injection, or transepicardial injection at the time of bypass surgery (Figure 22-4). Another less common method of delivery includes the surgical placement of in vitro manufactured cell sheets, some of which are impregnated with cytokines and growth factors to improve survival and/or differentiation. Thus far, all delivery routes have proven to be safe, but these delivery routes have also been plagued with poor cell retention and survival. Identifying the optimal cell delivery method that can ensure acceptable cell retention and survival is one of the major current challenges in cell-based therapy. This problem has been the focus of much attention in the bioengineering community. Multiple types of injectable scaffolds have been tested to improve cell retention, survival, and functional integration[60]; however, these scaffolds are not yet ready for clinical testing and will require additional research.

Intravenous Delivery

Intravenous delivery of stem cells is particularly appealing because of the ease of administration. The major problem is that cells become trapped in the pulmonary microcirculation, and a negligible fraction of cells homes to the heart. Preclinical studies have shown that the cardiac homing of intravenously injected stem cells is close to zero. So far, only one clinical trial has delivered cells (MSCs) intravenously[54] (the rationale was that MSCs, by virtue of their size, may

TABLE 22-2 Advantages and Disadvantages of the Intracoronary and Transendocardial Delivery Modes of Stem Cells

CHARACTERISTICS	INTRACORONARY INFUSION	TRANSENDOCARDIAL INJECTION
Duration of the procedure	Shorter	Longer
Cost	No additional cost beyond standard cardiac catheterization	Expensive, secondary to the use of the intramyocardial diagnostic and injection catheters
Required skills	Not beyond routine cardiac catheterization	Steep learning curve for the use of the intramyocardial catheter and injection system
Safety profile	Minimally invasive. Standard cardiac catheterization risk profile. May need multiple balloon inflations in stop-flow technique	Minimally invasive. Standard cardiac catheterization risk and risk of myocardial perforation, hemopericardium, and cardiac tamponade
Selectivity to the infarct region	Relatively selective by injecting cells down the infarct-related artery. Dependent on homing signal for accumulation of cells in the infarct territory.	Selective by injecting cells around the scar
Distribution of cells	Homogenous within the infused bed	Not homogeneous; cells are clustered around the injection site
Feasibility	Not feasible with chronic total occlusion	Feasible in all patients
No. of administered cells	Practically unlimited for BMMNCs; limited for MSCs and CPCs	Practically unlimited for all cell types
Cell retention	Poor	Poor; higher initial retention than intracoronary infusion
Time point for cell administration after MI	Can be done within hours after reperfusion therapy	Earliest time used so far after acute MI is 10 days

BMMNCs, Bone marrow mononuclear cells; *CPCs*, cardiac progenitor cells; *MI*, myocardial infarction; *MSCs*, mesenchymal stromal cells.

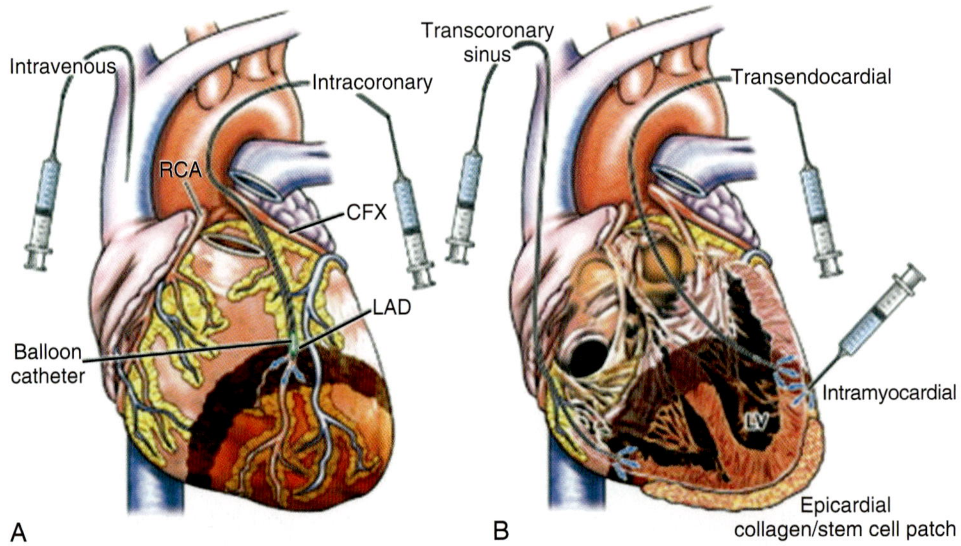

FIGURE 22-4 **(A)** Intracoronary and **(B)** intramyocardial transplantation methods in heart disease. The clinically used methods for vascular and myocardial cell delivery in cardiac intervention and cardiac surgery. *CFX*, Circumflex artery; *LAD*, left anterior descending artery; *LV*, left ventricle; *RCA*, right coronary artery. *(From Strauer BE, Steinhoff G: 10 Years of intracoronary and intramyocardial bone marrow stem cell therapy of the heart: from the methodological origin to clinical practice.* J Am Coll Cardiol *58:1095–1104, 2011; Figure 1.)*

cause microcirculatory obstruction if given intracoronarily). Surprisingly, the results of this study were encouraging, and a phase II trial (NCT00877903) of intravenously delivered MSCs is underway.

As mentioned previously, observational studies have indicated that mobilization of EPCs and $CD34^+$ cells after acute MI is correlated with improved LV function and remodeling, supporting the hypothesis that systemic induction of circulating progenitor cells after acute MI may be associated with favorable outcomes.[48] In the STEM-AMI trial, 60 patients with a first anterior STEMI and an echocardiographic LVEF of ≤45% after successful revascularization were randomized to granulocyte-colony stimulating factor (G-CSF) or placebo.[61] There was no difference between the two groups in terms of LVEF either at 6 months or at 3 years. In a head-to-head comparison of systemic (intravenous) G-CSF versus placebo in 86 patients with LVEF less than 45% after anterior STEMI,[62] G-CSF therapy was associated with a significantly lower LVEF relative to placebo at 6 months. However, in a meta-analysis of 14 randomized trials of G-CSF versus placebo (N = 566), there was no difference with respect to LVEF or clinical outcomes, even in the subset of patients with baseline LVEF of less than 45%. In summary, current evidence suggests that mobilization of stem and/or progenitor cells with G-CSF is not an effective modality for cell therapy.

Intracoronary Delivery

The most common delivery route for cell therapy in preclinical and clinical studies of acute MI is the intracoronary route. This is particularly true for BM cells; in almost all trials, these cells have been administered intracoronarily. Conversely, MSCs have been delivered mostly by transendocardial injection, although some studies are ongoing with intracoronary administration of MSCs (e.g., RELIEF, NCT01652209). Advantages of the intracoronary route include selectivity relative to the infarct region, more uniform distribution of cells in the target region, simplicity of the procedure, availability in virtually every hospital, relatively short procedure time, minimal invasiveness, and low cost (see Table 22-2). The safety of intracoronary infusion of BM cells (up to 300 million) and cardiac-derived cells (up to 25 million) has been demonstrated repeatedly. In contrast, there still exist important safety concerns with intracoronary injection of MSCs. Using an ovine model, Grieve and colleagues demonstrated that intracoronary administration of 25 million MSCs was safe, but that administration of 75 million cells was associated with biochemical and histological evidence of MI.[63] Similarly, dose-dependent ST-segment elevation has been shown in a canine model with intracoronary administration of MSCs.[64] The average size of MSCs and BMMNCs is approximately 21.0 ± 3.3 μm and 8.6 ± 1.8 μm, respectively. At 7 to 10 μm, the typical capillary luminal diameter is smaller than the average-sized MSCs, likely expounding the findings in the aforementioned studies.

Another important issue pertaining to the intracoronary route is whether to use the stop-flow technique (balloon inflation) at the time of infusion. The rationale for balloon inflation is that stopping coronary flow may facilitate marginalization of the injected cells and their migration through the endothelium into the adjacent tissue. Typically, a catheter balloon is inflated for 2 to 3 minutes while the cells are infused via the central lumen of the catheter; this process is usually repeated multiple times. Although most clinical trials performed to date have used the stop-flow technique, this method entails the risk of coronary dissection. The seriousness of this complication (particularly in nonstented coronary segments) warrants studies aimed at determining the need for balloon inflation. We have recently addressed this question in a swine model of chronic infarction, and found that there was no difference between balloon inflation and no balloon inflation in terms of cell retention at 24 hours. This finding has important implications in terms of lowering the risk of complications in clinical trials in which cell therapy is administered by intracoronary infusion.

Intramyocardial Injection

Direct intramyocardial injection can be performed either by the transepicardial approach during thoracotomy, or by the transendocardial route through left heart catheterization. To perform transendocardial injection, a special LV mapping catheter is used to generate a three-dimensional electromechanical map of the LV by recording electrical signals from the endocardial surface (Figure 22-e2); the goal is to discern viable myocardium from scar tissue based on unipolar surface voltages. Cell injection to the scar border is then performed using the injection catheter, which is equipped with a protruding retractable needle at the tip. The advantage of intramyocardial injection is that it obviates the need for homing signals, because cells are delivered directly to the target myocardium where they are required. Although early cell attrition is still considerable, preclinical studies have shown that direct injection is superior to intravenous and intracoronary delivery with regard to cell retention. The disadvantages include longer duration of the procedure, higher cost, a steep learning curve of the operator, lack of familiarity on the part of interventional cardiologists (in cases of percutaneous injection), and risk of myocardial perforation, especially in the setting of freshly infarcted, friable tissue in patients with acute MI (see Table 22-2). Consequently, intramyocardial injection has mostly been used in the context of cardiomyopathy, although injection in the peri-infarct myocardium has been performed in both preclinical and clinical studies of MI.[23,65]

There has never been a head-to-head clinical comparison of intracoronary versus intramyocardial injection in the setting of acute MI. Two trials compared these delivery methods in HF patients, but reported dissimilar results.[66,67]

In summary, the experimental data regarding myocardial cell retention with different routes of delivery are not entirely consistent and may vary depending on the cell type used. The preponderance of the evidence indicates that short-term cell retention is higher after transendocardial injection rather than after intracoronary infusion. In the previously conducted clinical trials, BM and peripheral blood–derived cells (except for MSCs) have been administered mostly by the intracoronary route. In the setting of acute MI, BM cells have been usually injected into the infarct-related coronary artery. In contrast, MSCs have been delivered mostly through transendocardial injection.

MECHANISM OF ACTION OF CELL THERAPY

The mechanism(s) responsible for the salutary effects of adult stem and/or progenitor cells in preclinical and clinical studies remain unclear, and have been a matter of much debate and controversy. Three main mechanisms have been proposed: (1) differentiation of transplanted cells into new cardiomyocytes; (2) differentiation of transplanted cells into new vessels; and (3) the paracrine effect (Figure 22-5). The first two mechanisms were initially believed to account for the therapeutic actions of cell therapy, but it is now clear that the contribution of stem cell differentiation to the improvement in cardiac function seen in preclinical and clinical studies is negligible. Earlier reports of (trans)differentiation of BM cells and MSCs into mature cardiomyocytes have not been corroborated.[3] Most studies that claimed formation of new cardiomyocytes from transplanted cells only reported immature phenotypes. In the case of BM cells, some studies suggested that fusion of these cells with resident cardiomyocytes might explain their beneficial effects, but this, too, has not been corroborated. An overarching argument against differentiation of transplanted cells as a mechanism of improvement is that the retention of transplanted cells (regardless of their nature) in the recipient heart is extremely poor, such that the number of remaining cells, even if all of them (trans) differentiated into cardiomyocytes, would not be sufficient to account for the beneficial effects observed.[68] Regarding vasculogenesis, differentiation of transplanted cells into new blood vessels has been reported with various cells, including MSCs and EPCs,[69] and it has been proposed that new vessel formation may lead to salvage of cardiomyocytes in the region at risk. Although it is possible that this phenomenon accounts for some of the beneficial effects of cell-based therapy, it is difficult to envision how it could be a major mechanism in patients with ischemic heart disease who have undergone successful coronary revascularization and have little or no hibernating myocardium.

Because of these facts, the paradigm has shifted from the aforementioned mechanisms to the paracrine theory, which postulates that most of the improvement following cell delivery is attained through signals (cytokines, chemokines, growth factors, exosomes, microparticles, and so on) that are released in a paracrine fashion by the transplanted cells and modify the adjacent cells and matrix of the recipient heart. These paracrine signals may promote a number of restorative processes, including activation of endogenous CPCs (resulting in myocyte regeneration), neovascularization, inhibition of apoptosis, inhibition of hypertrophy, and favorable alterations of the extracellular matrix.[3]

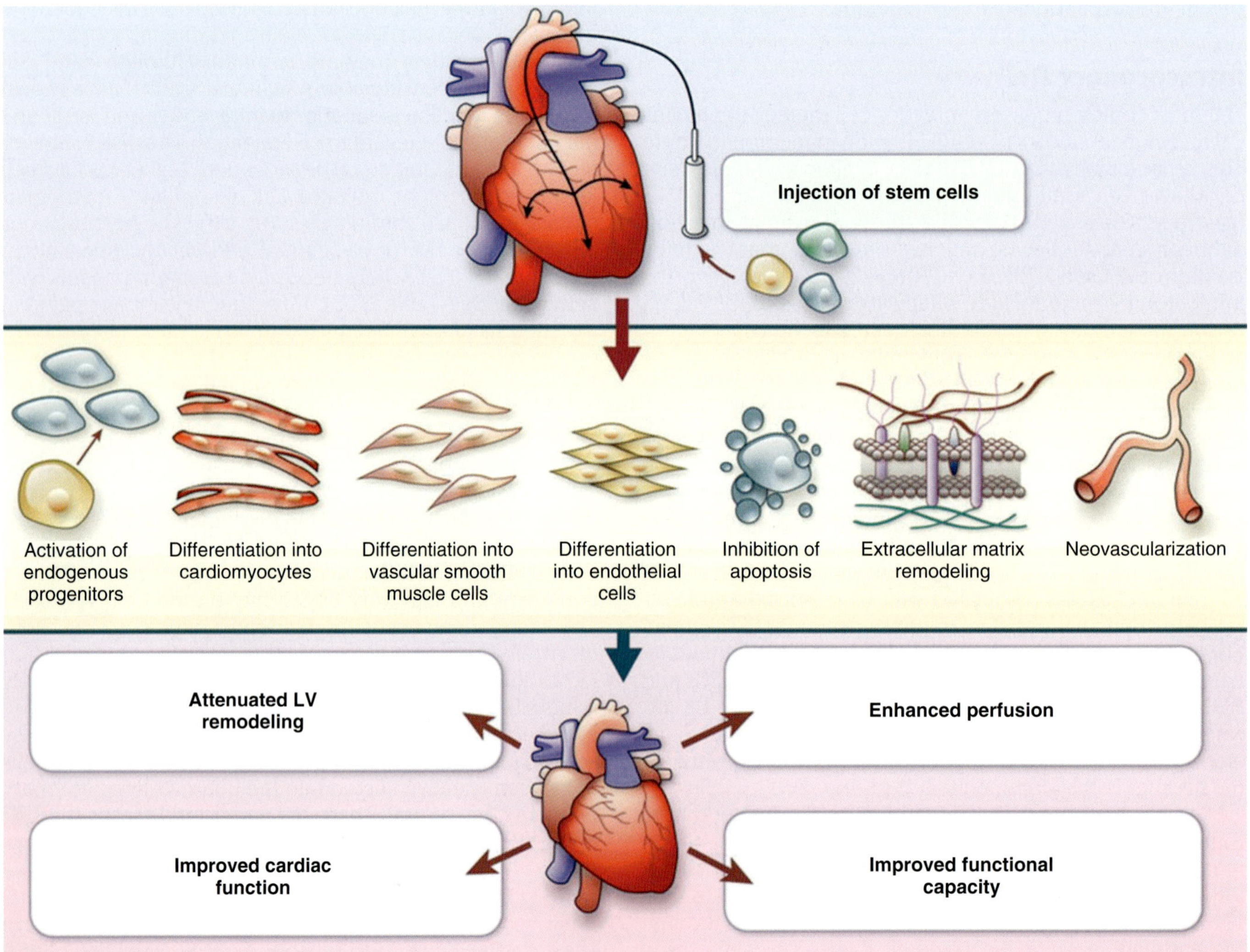

FIGURE 22-5 Potential mechanisms of action of stem cells. Implantation of stem cells in the injured heart initiates myocardial repair via several direct and indirect mechanisms: activation of endogenous precursors, differentiation into cardiac and vascular cells, promotion of neovascularization, favorable modulation of the extracellular matrix, and inhibition of apoptosis. Together, these events reduce adverse cardiac remodeling and hypertrophy, increase perfusion, and improve cardiac function, leading to improvement in clinical status. *LV*, Left ventricular. *(From Sanganalmath SK, Bolli R: Cell therapy for heart failure: a comprehensive overview of experimental and clinical studies, current challenges, and future directions.* Circ Res *113:810–834, 2013; Figure 3.)*

In support of the paracrine theory, a study by Tang and colleagues found that exogenous CPCs increased viable myocardium in the risk region, reduced infarct size, and improved LV performance in a rat model of ICM despite the fact that the transplanted cells had almost disappeared from the recipient heart.[70] The salubrious effects of exogenous CSCs were associated with activation of endogenous CPCs in both the infarcted and noninfarcted regions.[70] Activation of endogenous CPCs has also been demonstrated after adoptive transfer of MSCs in a swine model of acute MI, in which intramyocardial injection of MSCs resulted in a 20-fold increase in endogenous c-kit$^+$ CPCs in MSC-treated animals versus controls.[71] Reduction of apoptosis may also be part of the paracrine actions of transplanted cells. For example, MSCs have been shown to reduce apoptosis in models of acute MI.[72] Finally, paracrine factors released by transplanted stem cells may alter the extracellular matrix and influence postinfarction LV remodeling in a favorable manner. As mentioned previously, MSCs have been shown to reduce fibrosis and scar mass, in addition to increasing viable mass, in a number of clinical trials. A similar effect has also been shown with BMMNCs, albeit inconsistently. The mechanism underlying this effect is likely complex, and may include diminished expression of proinflammatory cytokines (e.g., tumor necrosis factor-α and interleukins-1α and -6) and modification of matrix metalloproteinases that are intimately involved in regulating LV remodeling.[72]

UNMET CHALLENGES IN SUCCESSFUL TRANSLATION OF CELL THERAPY AND FUTURE DIRECTIONS

An enormous amount of basic, preclinical, and clinical work related to cell therapy has been performed in the last 15 years, including more than 100 clinical trials. Phase III RCTs are already underway using BMMNCs in acute MI and MSCs in cardiomyopathy. By now, the safety of cell therapy has been well established across different cell types, doses, and routes of administration. Nevertheless, many unresolved issues remain that need to be answered before cell therapy can be applied in clinical practice. Among the most important unresolved issues are the following (Table 22-3). What is the most efficacious cell type? What is the optimal dose or range of doses? In the case of acute MI, when is the optimal time to administer cells? Is combined cell therapy superior to single cell therapy? Are repeated administrations of cells superior to single administration? What is the most appropriate route of administration?

Cell Type

Few studies have attempted to compare different cell types.[3] Such experiments are complicated even at the preclinical level, because before attempting a comparison between two different cell types, the optimal cell dose for each cell type first has to be defined through a dose-escalation study; merely comparing an arbitrary dose of one cell type against another would not be sufficient. At the preclinical level, there is evidence that the combination of two cell types may be superior to single cell therapy. In a proof-of-concept study that combined human MSCs and c-kit$^+$ CPCs in a swine model of MI, the combination therapy resulted in greater scar size reduction and a seven-fold greater engraftment of stem cells compared with either of these cell types alone.[73]

Cell Dose

Dose-escalation studies should be done for every cell type that is being tested for clinical translation. Few studies have attempted to address this question, and this has mostly been done at the preclinical level. The results have often been incongruent between different studies or between preclinical and clinical studies.[3] In one clinical study of allogeneic MSCs in the context of acute MI, no difference was reported between different doses[54]; a larger study is planned (NCT00877903). As for BMMNCs in acute MI, there is a conspicuous lack of data, although, realistically, further clinical work on BMMNCs will depend on the result of the BAMI trial (that is, a negative result of the BAMI trial would likely render BMMNCs obsolete in cardiac regeneration studies). Another unexplored issue is whether administering multiple doses of cells could be advantageous as opposed to one dose of cells. The ongoing RELIEF trial (NCT01652209) is attempting to

TABLE 22-3 Ongoing Challenges and Future Opportunities for Cell Therapy after Acute Myocardial Infarction

CHALLENGES	OPPORTUNITIES AND FUTURE DIRECTIONS
Low cell retention	Improvement in delivery systems: a. New injection catheters b. Bioscaffolds, patches, and tissue engineering c. Use of magnetic fields and magnetically labeled cells
Suboptimal cell viability and function in vivo	Optimization of cell product: a. Purity of isolation (e.g., immunoselection) b. In vitro modifications • Preconditioning with drugs, cytokines • Functional modification/enhancement by gene therapy • Lineage commitment Allogeneic therapy Combination cell therapy
Uncertain mechanism of action	Mechanistic studies with molecular biology techniques, cell imaging, and so on
Key unresolved questions: • Optimal cell type • Single vs. combined cell types • Optimal dose • Optimal timing • Single vs. repeat administration • Optimal delivery route	In vivo and in vitro comparison studies
Lack of standardization of trials	Rigorous trial design: • Multicenter • Randomized, double blind (placebo-controlled) • Conservative sample size calculation/large sample size • Meaningful, uniformly defined, reproducible clinical endpoints with core laboratory analysis Standardization of techniques for cell isolation and processing

assess the effect of single versus double doses of autologous MSCs in patients with acute MI and LVEF of less than 45%.

Cell Retention

Poor cell retention has plagued cell-based therapy regardless of the type of cell used and likely limits the benefits of therapy.[74,75] Therefore, to optimize therapeutic benefits, it is imperative to implement strategies that improve cell homing, survival, and engraftment in the hostile infarcted and/or ischemic environment. Several approaches are under investigation, including ex vivo pretreatment of cells (genetic modifications; physical or pharmacological preconditioning), tissue engineering approaches, such as cardiac patches (i.e., in vitro–engineered sheets of myocardial tissue), and injectable scaffolds, which limit adverse remodeling or act as vehicles to support the delivery of cells and other therapeutics.[60] These scaffolds can also be impregnated with cytokines and growth factors to promote cell survival, engraftment, and differentiation and activate the endogenous progenitor pool.

Timing of Cell Therapy

An important, yet unanswered question in cell therapy for ischemic heart disease is the timing of treatment; that is, whether patients should be treated in the setting of acute MI (and how soon after MI) or chronic ischemic cardiomyopathy. There are theoretical considerations in support of different approaches. It has been suggested that the stronger homing signals present after acute MI facilitate cell engraftment and attract the injected cells to the injured myocardium. Acute MI produces a global inflammatory reaction associated with increased local production of chemoattractants, including SDF-1 and G-CSF, in the ischemic myocardium, and neural and humoral signals that promote the egress of stem and/or progenitor cells from the BM.[48] It is now appreciated that hematopoietic stem cells, EPCs, MSCs, proangiogenic progenitor cells, and pluripotent very small embryonic-like cells are rapidly mobilized in the blood in the setting of acute MI,[76] although the contribution of these cells to myocardial repair is unclear. In this context, administration of exogenous cells may be efficacious by leveraging the chemoattractants and cytokines and/or growth factors associated with acute MI. In contrast, it has been argued that the acutely infarcted myocardium constitutes a hostile environment for the transplanted cells and adversely affects their survival. As mentioned previously, a subset analysis in the REPAIR-AMI study suggested that treatment should be delayed until 5 days from the onset of acute MI for the cells to be effective[27]; however, subsequent trials in which cells were given 5 days or later have found no effect (see Table 22-3).

Trial Endpoints

In addition to the preceding fundamental questions, there are other issues in need of attention. For example, thus far, LVEF has been the surrogate endpoint of choice in phase I and II trials of cell-based therapy. Although a study powered to detect improvement in hard clinical outcomes will eventually be required for clinical translation of any cell-based therapy, the suitability of LVEF as the surrogate outcome of choice in phase I and II studies has been questioned. A significant amount of reverse LV remodeling has been observed in clinical and preclinical studies of cell therapy that, although clinically significant, may not be large enough to be reflected in LVEF.[77] Thus, it seems appropriate to use indexes of regional function and LV remodeling (including LV volume, scar size and mass, and strain analysis) in addition to parameters of global function such as LVEF. CMR, with its unique capabilities to quantify all of the previous parameters, is best suited for this purpose and has become the standard technique used in clinical trials of cell-based therapy that are not powered for clinical endpoints (see Chapter 33).

SUMMARY

Only a few years ago, the mere suggestion that a therapy may regenerate myocardial tissue would have been considered science fiction. Notwithstanding the many unresolved mechanistic, pathophysiological, and practical issues, it is important to keep a historical perspective and remember that tremendous progress has been made in a relatively short time. What we know after 15 years of research on cell therapy in acute MI is the following: (1) at the preclinical level, several cell types have been consistently effective in improving LV function and remodeling in a variety of experimental models of post-MI cardiomyopathy; (2) all clinical trials in patients with acute MI have found cell therapy to be safe; and (3) some trials have suggested that cell therapy is beneficial, whereas other trials have not. The reason(s) for this discrepancy is unknown; however, the discrepancy is not surprising considering the following: (1) many clinical trials performed so far have been small and underpowered, and some have not been well designed; (2) cell therapy is a novel treatment, and we still do not know how best to use it; specifically, we do not know the optimal cell type(s), dose, route, timing, and frequency of administration; and (3) unlike pharmacologic therapies, the quality of the cell product is highly variable from one laboratory to another, because they are affected by a myriad of conditions (known and unknown) used during cell isolation and expansion. In view of our lack of knowledge regarding the use of cell therapy, it is remarkable that beneficial effects have been observed in some clinical trials. It seems reasonable to assume that a better understanding of the preceding issues may enhance the efficacy of cell therapy. The current uncertainty will not be resolved by surrendering to therapeutic nihilism; it will only be resolved by conducting rigorous, large-scale, rationally designed, RCTs to conclusively determine whether cell therapy is efficacious in patients with acute MI.

ACKNOWLEDGMENTS

This work was supported in part by NIH grants P01 HL-78825 and UM1 HL-113530 (CCTRN).

Classic References

Beltrami AP, et al.: Adult cardiac stem cells are multipotent and support myocardial regeneration, *Cell* 114:763–776, 2003.

Menasche P, et al.: Myoblast transplantation for heart failure, *Lancet* 357:279–280, 2001.

Perin EC, et al.: Transendocardial, autologous bone marrow cell transplantation for severe, chronic ischemic heart failure, *Circulation* 107:2294–2302, 2003.

Quaini F, et al.: Chimerism of the transplanted heart, *N Engl J Med* 346:5–15, 2002.

Taylor DA, et al.: Regenerating functional myocardium: improved performance after skeletal myoblast transplantation, *Nature Medicine* 4:333–929, 1998.

References

1. Loughran JH, et al.: Cardiac stem cells in patients with ischemic cardiomyopathy: discovery, translation, and clinical investigation, *Current Atherosclerosis Reports* 14:491–503, 2012.
2. Psaltis PJ, et al.: An update on stem cell therapies for acute coronary syndrome, *Current Cardiology Reports* 16:526, 2014.

3. Sanganalmath SK, Bolli R: Cell therapy for heart failure: a comprehensive overview of experimental and clinical studies, current challenges, and future directions, *Circulation Research* 113: 810–834, 2013.
4. Taylor DA, et al.: Regenerating functional myocardium: improved performance after skeletal myoblast transplantation, *Nature Medicine* 4:929–933, 1998.
5. Menasche P, et al.: Myoblast transplantation for heart failure, *Lancet* 357:279–280, 2001.
6. Senyo SE, et al.: Mammalian heart renewal by pre-existing cardiomyocytes, *Nature* 493:433–436, 2013.
7. Bergmann O, et al.: Evidence for cardiomyocyte renewal in humans, *Science (New York, NY)* 324:98–102, 2009.
8. Mozaffarian D, et al.: Heart disease and stroke statistics-2015 update: a report from the American Heart Association, *Circulation* 131:e29–e322, 2015.
9. Heidenreich PA, et al.: Forecasting the future of cardiovascular disease in the United States: a policy statement from the American Heart Association, *Circulation* 123:933–944, 2011.
10. Burridge PW, et al.: Production of de novo cardiomyocytes: human pluripotent stem cell differentiation and direct reprogramming, *Cell Stem Cell* 10:16–28, 2012.
11. Shiba Y, et al.: Human ES-cell-derived cardiomyocytes electrically couple and suppress arrhythmias in injured hearts, *Nature* 489:322–325, 2012.
12. Chong JJ, et al.: Human embryonic-stem-cell-derived cardiomyocytes regenerate non-human primate hearts, *Nature* 510:273–277, 2014.
13. Anderson ME, et al.: Embryonic stem cell-derived cardiac myocytes are not ready for human trials, *Circulation Research* 115:335–338, 2014.
14. Barad L, et al.: Human embryonic stem cells vs human induced pluripotent stem cells for cardiac repair, *Canadian Journal of Cardiology* 30:1279–1287, 2014.
15. Takahashi K, Yamanaka S: Induction of pluripotent stem cells from mouse embryonic and adult fibroblast cultures by defined factors, *Cell* 126:663–676, 2006.
16. Liang P, et al.: Drug screening using a library of human induced pluripotent stem cell-derived cardiomyocytes reveals disease-specific patterns of cardiotoxicity, *Circulation* 127:1677–1691, 2013.
17. Zhang J, et al.: Functional cardiomyocytes derived from human induced pluripotent stem cells, *Circulation Research* 104:e30–e41, 2009.
18. Mauritz C, et al.: Induced pluripotent stem cell (iPSC)-derived Flk-1 progenitor cells engraft, differentiate, and improve heart function in a mouse model of acute myocardial infarction, *European Heart Journal* 32:2634–2641, 2011.
19. Ye L, et al.: Cardiac repair in a porcine model of acute myocardial infarction with human induced pluripotent stem cell-derived cardiovascular cells, *Cell Stem Cell* 15:750–761, 2014.
20. Okano H, et al.: Steps toward safe cell therapy using induced pluripotent stem cells, *Circulation Research* 112:523–533, 2013.
21. Burridge PW, et al.: Chemically defined generation of human cardiomyocytes, *Nature Methods* 11:855–860, 2014.
22. Qian L, Srivastava D: Direct cardiac reprogramming: from developmental biology to cardiac regeneration, *Circulation Research* 113:915–921, 2013.
23. Krause K, Jaquet K, Schneider C, et al.: Percutaneous intramyocardial stem cell injection in patients with acute myocardial infarction: first-in-man study, *Heart* 95:1145–1152, 2009.
24. Assmus B, et al.: Transplantation of Progenitor Cells and Regeneration Enhancement in Acute Myocardial Infarction (TOPCARE-AMI), *Circulation* 106:3009–3017, 2002.
25. Wollert KC, et al. Intracoronary autologous bone-marrow cell transfer after myocardial infarction: the BOOST randomised controlled clinical trial. *Lancet* 364:141–148, 2004.
26. Meyer GP, et al.: Intracoronary bone marrow cell transfer after myocardial infarction: 5-year follow-up from the randomized-controlled BOOST trial, *European Heart Journal* 30:2978–2984, 2009.
27. Schachinger V, et al.: Intracoronary bone marrow-derived progenitor cells in acute myocardial infarction, *New England Journal of Medicine* 355:1210–1221, 2006.
28. Assmus B, et al.: Clinical outcome 2 years after intracoronary administration of bone marrow-derived progenitor cells in acute myocardial infarction, *Circulation Heart Failure* 3:89–96, 2010.
29. Assmus B, et al.: Long-term clinical outcome after intracoronary application of bone marrow-derived mononuclear cells for acute myocardial infarction: migratory capacity of administered cells determines event-free survival, *European Heart Journal* 35:1275–1283, 2014.
30. Rolf A, et al.: Maladaptive hypertrophy after acute myocardial infarction positive effect of bone marrow-derived stem cell therapy on regional remodeling measured by cardiac MRI, *Clinical Research Cardiology* 100:983–992, 2011.
31. Beitnes JO, et al.: Long-term results after intracoronary injection of autologous mononuclear bone marrow cells in acute myocardial infarction: the ASTAMI randomised, controlled study, *Heart* 95:1983–1989, 2009.
32. Hirsch A, et al.: Intracoronary infusion of mononuclear cells from bone marrow or peripheral blood compared with standard therapy in patients after acute myocardial infarction treated by primary percutaneous coronary intervention: results of the randomized controlled HEBE trial, *European Heart Journal* 32:1736–1747, 2011.
33. Delewi R, et al.: Long term outcome after mononuclear bone marrow or peripheral blood cells infusion after myocardial infarction, *Heart* 101:363–368, 2015.
34. Traverse JH, et al.: Effect of the use and timing of bone marrow mononuclear cell delivery on left ventricular function after acute myocardial infarction: The TIME randomized trial, *Journal of the American Medical Association* 308:2380–2389, 2012.
35. Traverse JH, et al.: Effect of intracoronary delivery of autologous bone marrow mononuclear cells 2 to 3 weeks following acute myocardial infarction on left ventricular function: The LateTIME randomized trial, *Journal of the American Medical Association* 306:2110–2119, 2011.
36. Simari RD, et al.: Bone marrow mononuclear cell therapy for acute myocardial infarction: a perspective from the cardiovascular cell therapy research network, *Circulation Research* 114: 1548–1564, 2014.
37. Surder D, et al.: Intracoronary injection of bone marrow-derived mononuclear cells early or late after acute myocardial infarction: effects on global left ventricular function, *Circulation* 127: 1968–1979, 2013.
38. Schutt RC, et al.: Bone marrow characteristics associated with changes in infarct size after STEMI: a biorepository evaluation from the CCTRN TIME trial, *Circulation Research* 116:99–107, 2015.
39. Gee AP, et al.: Multicenter cell processing for cardiovascular regenerative medicine applications: the Cardiovascular Cell Therapy Research Network (CCTRN) experience, *Cytotherapy* 12: 684–691, 2010.
40. Assmus B, et al.: Red blood cell contamination of the final cell product impairs the efficacy of autologous bone marrow mononuclear cell therapy, *Journal of the American College of Cardiology* 55:1385–1394, 2010.
41. Seeger FH, et al.: Heparin disrupts the CXCR4/SDF-1 axis and impairs the functional capacity of bone marrow-derived mononuclear cells used for cardiovascular repair, *Circulation Research* 111:854–862, 2012.
42. Delewi R, et al.: Impact of intracoronary bone marrow cell therapy on left ventricular function in the setting of ST-segment elevation myocardial infarction: a collaborative meta-analysis, *European Heart Journal* 35:989–998, 2014.
43. de Jong R, et al.: Intracoronary stem cell infusion after acute myocardial infarction: a meta-analysis and update on clinical trials, *Circulation Cardiovascular Interventions* 7:156–167, 2014.
44. Traverse JH, Henry TD, Moye LA: Is the measurement of left ventricular ejection fraction the proper end point for cell therapy trials? An analysis of the effect of bone marrow mononuclear stem cell administration on left ventricular ejection fraction after ST-segment elevation myocardial infarction when evaluated by cardiac magnetic resonance imaging, *American Heart Journal* 162:671–677, 2011.
45. Clifford DM, et al.: Stem cell treatment for acute myocardial infarction, *Cochrane Database Systematic Reviews* 2:Cd006536, 2012.
46. Gyongyosi M, et al.: Meta-Analysis of Cell-based CaRdiac stUdiEs (ACCRUE) in patients with acute myocardial infarction based on individual patient data, *Circulation Research* 116:1346–1360, 2015.
47. Yoder MC: Defining human endothelial progenitor cells, *Journal of Thrombosis and Haemostasis* 7(Suppl 1):49–52, 2009.
48. Wojakowski W, et al.: Mobilization of stem and progenitor cells in cardiovascular diseases, *Leukemia* 26:23–33, 2012.
49. Tendera M, et al.: Intracoronary infusion of bone marrow-derived selected CD34+CXCR4+ cells and non-selected mononuclear cells in patients with acute STEMI and reduced left ventricular ejection fraction: results of randomized, multicentre Myocardial Regeneration by Intracoronary Infusion of Selected Population of Stem Cells in Acute Myocardial Infarction (REGENT) Trial, *European Heart Journal* 30:1313–1321, 2009.
50. Quyyumi AA, et al.: CD34(+) cell infusion after ST elevation myocardial infarction is associated with improved perfusion and is dose dependent, *American Heart Journal* 161:98–105, 2011.
51. Williams AR, Hare JM: Mesenchymal stem cells: biology, pathophysiology, translational findings, and therapeutic implications for cardiac disease, *Circulation Research* 109:923–940, 2011.
52. Karantalis V, et al.: Allogeneic cell therapy: a new paradigm in therapeutics, *Circulation Research* 116:12–15, 2015.
53. Psaltis PJ, Spoon DB, Wong DT: Utility of mesenchymal stromal cells for myocardial infarction. Transitioning from bench to bedside, *Minerva Cardioangiologica* 61:639–663, 2013.
54. Hare JM, et al.: A randomized, double-blind, placebo-controlled, dose-escalation study of intravenous adult human mesenchymal stem cells (prochymal) after acute myocardial infarction, *Journal of the American College of Cardiology* 54:2277–2286, 2009.
55. Houtgraaf JH, et al.: First experience in humans using adipose tissue-derived regenerative cells in the treatment of patients with ST-segment elevation myocardial infarction, *Journal of the American College of Cardiology* 59:539–540, 2012.
56. See F, et al.: Therapeutic effects of human STRO-3-selected mesenchymal precursor cells and their soluble factors in experimental myocardial ischemia, *Journal of Cellular and Molecular Medicine* 15:2117–2129, 2011.
57. Psaltis PJ, et al.: Enrichment for STRO-1 expression enhances the cardiovascular paracrine activity of human bone marrow-derived mesenchymal cell populations, *Journal of Cellular Physiology* 223:530–540, 2010.
58. Houtgraaf JH, et al.: Intracoronary infusion of allogeneic mesenchymal precursor cells directly after experimental acute myocardial infarction reduces infarct size, abrogates adverse remodeling, and improves cardiac function, *Circulation Research* 113:153–166, 2013.
59. Bartunek J, et al.: Cardiopoietic stem cell therapy in heart failure: the C-CURE (Cardiopoietic stem Cell therapy in heart failURE) multicenter randomized trial with lineage-specified biologics, *Journal of the American College of Cardiology* 61:2329–2338, 2013.
60. Radisic M, Christman KL: Materials science and tissue engineering: repairing the heart, *Mayo Clinic Proceedings* 88:884–898, 2013.
61. Achilli F, et al.: G-CSF treatment for STEMI: final 3-year follow-up of the randomised placebo-controlled STEM-AMI trial, *Heart* 100:574–581, 2014.
62. Hibbert B, et al.: Granulocyte colony-stimulating factor therapy for stem cell mobilization following anterior wall myocardial infarction: the CAPITAL STEM MI randomized trial. *Canadian Medical Association Journal* 186:E427–E434, 2014.
63. Grieve SM, et al.: Microvascular obstruction by intracoronary delivery of mesenchymal stem cells and quantification of resulting myocardial infarction by cardiac magnetic resonance, *Circulation Heart Failure* 3:e5–e6, 2010.
64. Vulliet PR, et al.: Intra-coronary arterial injection of mesenchymal stromal cells and microinfarction in dogs, *Lancet* 363:783–784, 2004.
65. Gyongyosi M, et al.: Combined delivery approach of bone marrow mononuclear stem cells early and late after myocardial infarction: the MYSTAR prospective, randomized study, *Nature Clinical Practice Cardiovascular Medicine* 6:70–81, 2009.
66. Mozid A, et al.: Safety and feasibility of intramyocardial versus intracoronary delivery of autologous cell therapy in advanced heart failure: the REGENERATE-IHD pilot study, *Regenerative Medicine* 9:269–278, 2014.
67. Vrtovec B, et al.: Comparison of transendocardial and intracoronary CD34+ cell transplantation in patients with nonischemic dilated cardiomyopathy, *Circulation* 128:S42–S49, 2013.
68. Hong KU, et al.: c-kit+ Cardiac stem cells alleviate post-myocardial infarction left ventricular dysfunction despite poor engraftment and negligible retention in the recipient heart, *PloS One* 9:e96725, 2014.
69. Cai L, et al.: IFATS collection: Human adipose tissue-derived stem cells induce angiogenesis and nerve sprouting following myocardial infarction, in conjunction with potent preservation of cardiac function, *Stem Cells* 27:230–237, 2009.
70. Tang XL, et al.: Intracoronary administration of cardiac progenitor cells alleviates left ventricular dysfunction in rats with a 30-day old infarction, *Circulation* 121:293–305, 2010.
71. Hatzistergos KE, et al.: Bone marrow mesenchymal stem cells stimulate cardiac stem cell proliferation and differentiation, *Circulation Research* 107:913–922, 2010.
72. Mirotsou M, et al.: Paracrine mechanisms of stem cell reparative and regenerative actions in the heart, *Journal of Molecular and Cellular Cardiology* 50:280–289, 2011.
73. Williams AR, et al.: Enhanced effect of combining human cardiac stem cells and bone marrow mesenchymal stem cells to reduce infarct size and to restore cardiac function after myocardial infarction, *Circulation* 127:213–223, 2013.
74. Alestalo K, et al.: High number of transplanted stem cells improves myocardial recovery after AMI in a porcine model, *Scandinavian Cardiovascular Journal* 49:82–94, 2015.
75. Cheng K, et al.: Magnetic enhancement of cell retention, engraftment, and functional benefit after intracoronary delivery of cardiac-derived stem cells in a rat model of ischemia/reperfusion, *Cell Transplantation* 21:1121–1135, 2012.
76. Wojakowski W, et al.: Mobilization of bone marrow-derived Oct-4+ SSEA-4+ very small embryonic-like stem cells in patients with acute myocardial infarction, *Journal of the American College of Cardiology* 53:1–9, 2009.
77. Kramer DG, et al.: Quantitative evaluation of drug or device effects on ventricular remodeling as predictors of therapeutic effects on mortality in patients with heart failure and reduced ejection fraction: a meta-analytic approach, *Journal of the American College of Cardiology* 56:392–406, 2010.

SECTION IV

In-Hospital Complications and Assessment

23 Recurrent Ischemia and Recurrent Myocardial Infarction: Detection, Diagnosis, and Outcomes

Harvey D. White

INTRODUCTION

There has been a major decline in the incidence of myocardial infarction (MI) in the developed world, with the proportion of ST-elevation MI (STEMI) decreasing and the proportion of non–ST-elevation MI (NSTEMI) increasing (see Chapter 2).[1] As survival following MI improves, more survivors are candidates for recurrent events, including recurrent MI. However, the incidence of recurrent MI in the community has fallen, with a similar magnitude as the decline in incident MI.[2] In addition to improvements in secondary preventive pharmacotherapy, the shift toward invasive evaluation and management of the initial MI has contributed to this reduction in subsequent recurrent ischemic events. For example, in patients with STEMI, recurrent MI is less frequent after primary percutaneous coronary intervention (pPCI) (see Chapter 17) than after fibrinolysis, with in-hospital rates being approximately 2.0% versus 4.0%; readmission rates with recurrent MI at 1 year are approximately 4.8% and 9.6%, respectively.[3]

Other changes in clinical practice have also affected the epidemiology of recurrent MI, with competing directions. MI event rates are sensitive to changes in MI definitions, and after the introduction of the Universal Definition of MI in 2000,[4] the epidemiology of MI has continued to evolve (see Chapter 1). Moreover, the use of biomarkers with increased sensitivity (e.g., high-sensitivity troponin assays)[5] have greatly increased the detection of MI (see Chapter 7). Increased use of revascularization will increase the incidence of periprocedural MIs. At the same time, the frequency of recurrent MI may be underestimated because patients dying from recurrent MI may be classified as experiencing sudden death.

DETECTION OF RECURRENT ISCHEMIA AND INFARCTION

Recurrent Ischemia Without Infarction

Recurrent ischemia after presentation with an acute coronary syndrome (ACS) portends an unfavorable outcome and has major implications for use of health care resources. Ischemic symptoms at rest carry a worse prognosis than ischemia with exercise. In the thrombolytic era, in the GUSTO (Global Utilization of Streptokinase and Tissue Plasminogen Activator for Occluded Coronary Arteries) IIb fibrinolytic trial, recurrent ischemia occurred in approximately 23% of patients with STEMI and 35% of patients with NSTEMI.[6]

Refractory ischemia, which was defined as symptoms of ischemia for 10 minutes with ST-segment deviation or definite T-wave inversion, and/or new hypotension, pulmonary edema, or cardiac murmur believed to represent myocardial ischemia (despite the use of nitrates and either β-blocker or calcium channel blockers), occurred in approximately 20% of patients with ischemia. Refractory ischemia was associated with an approximate doubling of 30-day mortality among patients with ST-segment elevation (11.8 % vs. 5.4%; $P < .001$) and an even greater mortality risk among patients without ST-segment elevation (12.0% vs. 2.7%; $P < .001$).

Most ischemia is silent, and can be detected on 24-hour continuous electrocardiographic (ECG) monitoring. The frequency and duration of silent ischemia has a direct relationship to prognosis.[7] Several studies that used continuous ST-segment monitoring showed that 15% to 30% patients with NSTE-ACS had transient episodes of

ST-segment changes.[8] These patients had an increased risk of subsequent cardiac events, including cardiovascular death. ST monitoring has been shown to add independent prognostic information to the ECG, troponins, and other clinical variables.[8,9]

In the MERLIN–TIMI 36 (Metabolic Efficiency With Ranolazine for Less Ischemia in Non–ST-Elevation Acute Coronary Syndrome–TIMI 36) trial, continuous ECG recording was performed for 7 days in 6355 patients with NSTE-ACS; 42% of the patients underwent revascularization during the index hospitalization.[8] Patients with ≥1 episode of ischemia (20%) during the first 7 days were at increased risk of cardiovascular death (7.7% vs. 2.7%; $P < .001$), MI (9.4% vs. 5.0%; $P < .001$), and clinically manifested ischemia (17.5% vs. 12.3%; $P < .001$) over the following year.

With early invasive evaluation and management of MI, the incidence of early recurrent ischemia has decreased substantially. Among patients with STEMI in the PAMI (Primary Angioplasty in Acute Myocardial Infarction) study,[10] recurrent ischemia was significantly less frequent in patients who had reperfusion with pPCI (10.3%) than in those who received fibrinolytic therapy (28.0%). Similarly, a major effect of early invasive management for NSTEMI is the reduction in recurrent ischemic events (see Chapter 16).

Because of the adverse prognosis of recurrent ischemia, clinical practice incorporates the performance of serial ECGs, monitoring for recurrent ischemic symptoms, and in some centers, continuous ST-segment monitoring. Many STEMI and NSTEMI patients are discharged 3 to 4 days after they have undergone an invasive strategy with pPCI or a pharmacoinvasive strategy with stenting of the culprit and often nonculprit lesions, either at initial angiography or subsequently. In patients who have typical ischemic pain at rest, a stress test is not necessary to define the need for additional therapy. A test for inducible ischemia may be considered in patients who are not fully revascularized before hospital discharge to help determine whether coronary angiography should be performed and revascularization, as appropriate, should be undertaken (see Chapter 30).

Diagnosis of Recurrent Myocardial Infarction

Classification of Recurrent Myocardial Infarction

The criteria for the diagnosis of MI according to the Third Universal Definition of MI are discussed in Chapter 1 and shown in Table 1-2. MIs are a heterogeneous group of events and are classified by the Universal Definition of MI into five types that differ according to pathophysiology, prognosis, and treatment (Table 1-4).[11,12] The diagnosis of the initial MI is discussed in Chapter 1, Chapter 6, and Chapter 7. This section focuses on the diagnosis of recurrent MI as a complication in patients who have presented with an initial MI event.

Spontaneous Myocardial Infarction

Spontaneous MIs (type 1) are the most commonly observed MIs in clinical practice,[13–15] and they are also the most common type of recurrent MI during the long-term. Clinical judgment is required to distinguish type 2 (supply–demand imbalance) MIs from type 1 MIs by taking into account the contribution of increased myocardial demand and decreased supply and the likely absence of acute plaque rupture based on all of the clinical information available (see Figure 1-3).[16]

Myocardial Infarction Related to Percutaneous Coronary Intervention (Type 4a)

Myocardial necrosis associated with PCI is a frequent cause of early recurrent MI and may be caused by several mechanisms, including distal embolization of plaque and/or thrombus with resultant microvascular plugging, occlusion of a side branch or a major coronary artery, coronary dissection, spasm, or endothelial dysfunction.[17] The association between type 4a MI and mortality is controversial and less important than spontaneous MI.[13–15]

Myocardial Infarction Caused by Stent Thrombosis (Type 4b)

Stent thrombosis after PCI for STEMI and NSTEMI is an infrequent but medically important event because of its adverse prognosis. This risk is higher with drug-eluting stents (DES) than with bare metal stents, and is associated with MI and death. MI may also occur that is unrelated to the stent.[18] The risk of stent thrombosis is less with the new generation DES,[19] and the risk is approximately 50% lower than with the first-generation DES.

Myocardial Infarction with Coronary Artery Bypass Grafting (Myocardial Infarction Type 5)

During coronary artery bypass grafting (CABG), numerous factors can lead to periprocedural myocardial injury with necrosis. These include direct myocardial injury from (1) suture placement or manipulation of the heart, (2) coronary dissection, (3) global or regional ischemia related to inadequate intraoperative cardiac protection, (4) microvascular events related to reperfusion, (5) myocardial injury induced by oxygen free radical generation, or (6) failure to reperfuse areas of the myocardium that are not subtended by graftable vessels. Magnetic resonance imaging studies suggest that most necrosis in this setting is not focal, but diffuse and localized in the subendocardium.[20]

Recurrent Myocardial Infarction and the Electrocardiogram

The ECG diagnosis of suspected recurrent MI following the initial MI may be confounded by the initial evolutionary ECG changes. Recurrent MI should be considered when ST-segment elevation of more than 0.1 mV recurs, or new pathologic Q waves appear, in at least two contiguous leads, particularly when associated with ischemic symptoms for 20 minutes or longer. In the presence of persistent ST-segment elevation (failed resolution of ST-segment elevation because of impaired microvascular flow) early after reperfusion, detection of reinfarction by ECG alone is difficult and requires consideration whether there has been a proportional increase since the preceding ECG, together with clinical symptoms of ischemia. Coronary angiography to detect reocclusion is sometimes necessary in such cases to resolve uncertainty. However, reelevation of the ST-segment can also be seen in threatened myocardial rupture and the presence of a left ventricular aneurysm, and should lead to consideration of these alternatives.

Biomarkers and Recurrent Myocardial Infarction

Because of persistent elevation of biomarkers of necrosis in the first days to weeks after a large initial MI, the diagnosis of recurrent MI can be challenging and is dependent on identifying a dynamic pattern of biomarker values separate from the initial MI, rather than simply elevation above the 99th percentile alone. In patients in whom recurrent MI is suspected from clinical signs or symptoms following the initial MI, an immediate measurement of troponin is recommended. A second sample should be obtained 3 to 6 hours later if the troponin level is elevated, but stable or decreasing at the time of suspected recurrent MI. Recurrent MI can be diagnosed if there is a more than 20% increase of the contemporary troponin value in the second sample. Two troponin values are considered to be analytically different if they are separated by more than 3 SDs of the variance (see Chapter 7).[11] For most contemporary non–high-sensitivity troponin assays, the SD is 5% to 7% at the levels involved with recurrent MI. Therefore, a 20% change should be considered significant (i.e., more than 3 SDs than expected from the analytical variability itself). This value should also exceed the 99th percentile upper reference limit (URL). If the initial troponin concentration is normal, the criteria for diagnosing a new acute MI apply (see Chapter 7).

Comparison of Different Definitions of Myocardial Infarction

In the OAT (Occluded Artery Trial) study, the OAT definition for the diagnosis of recurrent MI required two of three criteria: symptoms, the ECG, and an elevation of biomarkers. The ECG requirements were new Q waves >0.03 s and/or Q-wave voltage >⅓ QRS in >2 related leads on ECG.[21] The biomarker criteria included a ≥2-fold elevation for type 1 MI, a ≥3-fold elevation for type 4a, and a ≥5-fold elevation for type 5 infarction. The 2007 Universal Definition had similar criteria for type 4a and type 5 MI, but this definition had a lower threshold for type 1 MI based on any biomarker elevation above the upper limit of normal (ULN).[11] Consequently, more MIs were detected by the Universal Definition (Table 23-1).[21]

In a pooled analysis of two large negative phase III trials with the $P2Y_{12}$ antagonist, cangrelor, which used the Universal Definition of MI instead of the protocol definition of MI, there was a significant reduction in the primary endpoint, which included MI as opposed to a null result.[22] This result contributed to further development of cangrelor with a further large phase III trial, the CHAMPION PHOENIX (Cangrelor versus Standard Therapy to Achieve Optimal Management of Platelet Inhibition PHOENIX) trial, which used the Universal Definition of MI in the primary endpoint. The trial showed a significant 20% reduction in MI and a significant reduction in the primary endpoint.[23]

TABLE 23-1 Comparison of Recurrent Myocardial Infarctions Using Universal and OAT Definitions[21]

TYPE OF RE-MIs BY UNIVERSAL DEFINITION	NO. OF RE-MIs BY UNIVERSAL DEFINITION	NO. OF ADDITIONAL RE-MIs PICKED UP BY UNIVERSAL DEFINITION
Type 1: spontaneous	106	9
Type 2: secondary	7	4
Type 3: sudden death	12	10
Type 4a: PCI related	10	4
Type 4b: stent related	33	1
Type 5: CABG related	1	1
Total	169	29

CABG, Coronary artery bypass grafting; *PCI*, percutaneous coronary intervention; *Re-MI*, recurrent myocardial infarction.

Adapted from White HD, et al: Reinfarction after percutaneous coronary intervention or medical management using the universal definition in patients with total occlusion after myocardial infarction: results from long-term follow-up of the Occluded Artery Trial (OAT) cohort. Am Heart J 163:563–571, 2012.

CAUSES AND PREDICTORS OF RECURRENT MYOCARDIAL INFARCTION

Causes of Recurrent Myocardial Infarction

There are a number of causes of recurrent MI related to features of the plaque, features of the blood (thrombogenesis), and features of the patient. Activation of the coagulation system continues for at least 6 months[24] and plays a major role in the occurrence of recurrent MI related to the culprit lesion and at other sites in the coronary tree (Table 23-2). Recurrent MI may also be procedurally related, as described in the preceding section on Classification of Recurrent Myocardial Infarction.

Predictors of Recurrent Myocardial Infarction

Factors that have been shown to be predictors of recurrent MI are shown in the Table 23-3. Some are contradictory (e.g., smoking). Other traditional risk factors for coronary artery disease (CAD) (e.g., hypertension, diabetes, dyslipidemia) are also likely to increase the risk for recurrent MI.

TABLE 23-2 Causes of Recurrent Myocardial Infarction

- Ongoing thrombogenesis
- New plaque rupture or fissuring
- Recurrent or new dissection
- Recurrent or new embolism
- Decreased supply and/or increased demand
- Periprocedural MI (associated with PCI or CABG)
- Stent thrombosis
- Restenosis
- Withdrawal of antiplatelet therapy

CABG, Coronary artery bypass grafting; *MI*, myocardial infarction; *PCI*, percutaneous coronary intervention.

TABLE 23-3 Factors Shown to Be Predictors of Recurrent Myocardial Infarction

- Advanced age
- Shorter time to fibrinolysis
- Nonsmoking/smoking
- Female sex
- Anterior MI
- Lower systolic blood pressure
- Diabetes
- Hypertension
- Increasing baseline creatinine levels
- Killip class >1/Killip class <2
- Ejection fraction <50%
- Previous PCI
- No new Q waves
- Shorter time from MI
- Presence of thrombus
- Final coronary stenosis >30%
- Coronary dissection
- Complex type C lesion:
  - Diffuse (>2 cm length)
  - Total occlusion >3 mos old
  - Excessive tortuosity of proximal segment
  - Inability to protect major side branches
  - Extremely angulated segments >90°
  - Degenerated vein grafts with friable lesions
- Not on β-blockers
- Thrombocytosis
- Multivessel disease
- Longer symptom onset-to-balloon time
- Total stent length

MI, Myocardial infarction; *PCI*, percutaneous coronary intervention.

In patients with STEMI enrolled in the GUSTO I and GUSTO III fibrinolytic trials, recurrent MI occurred in 4.3% of patients at a median of 3.8 days after administration of fibrinolytic therapy. Advanced age, shorter time to fibrinolysis, non-U.S. enrollment, nonsmoking status, previous MI or angina, female sex, anterior MI, and lower systolic blood pressure were associated significantly with the occurrence of recurrent MI.[25] In the pooled PAMI trials, predictors of recurrent MI at 30-days were Killip class higher than 1, ejection fraction less than 50%, final coronary stenosis more than 30%, coronary dissection, and presence of thrombus.[26]

Among patients with NSTEMI, in the TRILOGY ACS (Targeted Platelet Inhibition to Clarify the Optimal Strategy to Medically Manage Acute Coronary Syndromes) trial,[27] which evaluated patients with NSTEMI and/or unstable angina who were managed medically without planned revascularization, MI was the most common endpoint, representing 45.3% of all first events, which included cardiovascular (CV) death and stroke. A prediction model for a first spontaneous MI event included 17 variables. The strongest predictors of spontaneous MI were older age, NSTEMI versus unstable angina as the index event, diabetes mellitus, no pre-randomization angiography, and higher baseline creatinine values. The prediction model performed well in terms of predictive capabilities (c index = 0.732) and had good calibration, especially in patients with a low-to-moderate risk of spontaneous MI (Figure 23-1).

Characteristics of the culprit lesion on angiography, and in particular, the American College of Cardiology/American Heart Association type C lesions (Table 23-3)[28] have been associated with worse prognosis.[29] Among the 3661 patients who underwent PCI in the ACUITY (Acute Catheterization and Urgent Intervention Triage Strategy) study, patients with type C lesions had higher 30-day rates of mortality (1.2% vs. 0.6%; P = .049), MI (9.2% vs. 6.3%; P = .0006), and unplanned revascularization (4.3% vs. 3.1%; P = .04) compared with those without type C lesions. In multivariable analysis, type C lesions were independently associated with MI (odds ratio [OR], 1.37; 95% confidence interval [CI], 1.04 to 1.80; P = .02) and composite ischemia (OR, 1.49; 95% CI, 1.17 to 1.88; P = .001) at 30 days (Figure 23-2).

In the OAT trial, recurrent MI tended to occur at a higher rate in patients randomized to PCI. Most recurrent MIs were spontaneous (type 1), which occurred at a similar frequency in both randomized treatment groups. However, in the PCI group, there were more type 4a (both protocol PCI-related and other PCI-related infarctions) and type 4b (stent thrombosis) infarctions. The recurrent MIs were clinically significant, with approximately 10% being rapidly fatal. A number of nonmodifiable predictors of recurrent MI were identified (Table 23-4). No single angiographic predictive factor was identified in the HORIZONS-AMI (Harmonizing Outcomes with Revascularization and Stents in Acute Myocardial Infarction) trial.[30] The independent predictors of reinfarction were current smoking, Killip class ≥2, baseline thrombocytosis, multivessel disease, longer symptom onset-to-balloon time, and total stent length.

Several genetic mutations are associated with increased risk of MI.[31–33] Patients with severe coronary artery stenoses have an increased risk of MI not only because of the stenoses, but because the stenoses are markers for widespread atherosclerosis.

Recurrent Myocardial Infarction in the Culprit or Nonculprit Arteries

Recurrent MI may occur in the territory of the culprit artery or in different arteries than the culprit artery.[18] If recurrent MI occurs in the culprit artery territory after administration of fibrinolytic therapy, it is likely caused by reocclusion or spasm, and after PCI, it may be the result of stent thrombosis, restenosis, or spasm. Plaque rupture can also occur proximally or distally to the previous culprit stenosis or in a nonculprit artery. In patients with ACS, multiple plaque ruptures are frequently found apart from the culprit lesion, indicating that plaque vulnerability is present throughout the coronary tree.[34]

Efforts to identify patients who are at a high risk of having an MI have focused on using advanced imaging methods to detect "vulnerable" atherosclerotic plaques with thin fibrous caps and lipid-rich cores (see also Chapter 10).[35] In the PROSPECT (Providing Regional Observations to Study Predictors of Events in the Coronary Tree) study, which was conducted in patients with ACS over 3.4 years, there was a 20.4% rate in the composite of cardiac death, cardiac arrest, MI, or rehospitalization for unstable or progressive angina. Events related to culprit lesions occurred in 12.9% of patients and to nonculprit lesions in 11.6% of patients.[18] Nonculprit MI occurred related to stenoses of less than 50% in 67% of cases. Intravascular ultrasound imaging showed that high-risk features of vulnerable plaques, including thin-cap fibroatheromas, were related to recurrent events in nonculprit lesions. However the presence of vulnerable plaques may be markers of more extensive and/or active atherosclerotic disease rather than independent risk predictors. The most powerful predictors of the risk of a new MI are the magnitude and activity of the coronary atherosclerotic plaque burden and the number of risk factors for a prothrombotic milieu.[36]

The guidelines for treating nonculprit arteries are evolving based on recent trials that showed that complete revascularization of all significantly stenosed arteries lead to better outcomes. In the recently reported PRAMI (Preventive Angioplasty in Acute Myocardial Infarction) trial, a preventive stenting strategy for stenoses of more than 50% was associated with a clinically significant reduction in cardiac death, MI, or refractory angina of 65% (see Chapter 17).[37]

INCIDENCE OF RECURRENT MYOCARDIAL INFARCTION

Although 6-month mortality rates have decreased in clinical trials of NSTEMI, from 6.7% (1994 to 1998) to 5.1% (2004 to 2008), 30-day MI rates have remained stable (9.2% [1994 to 1998] to 10% [2004 to 2008]) (Figure 23-3A).[38] As mortality has declined, the contribution of MI to the composite of death and/or MI has increased, reflecting a change in competing risk in which more patients are at risk of recurrent MI. Over that same period, the incidence of periprocedural MIs increased, whereas that for spontaneous MIs decreased (Figure 23-3B).

Table 23-5 shows the frequency of MI types in contemporary trials. The incidence of type 2 MIs has ranged from 3.5% to 9.8%. Spontaneous MIs have been shown to be the most common MI in cardiovascular trials with long-term follow-up, with proportions ranging from 32% to 94% of all MIs. Figure 23-4 shows the distribution of new or recurrent MIs (n = 1218) according to the Universal Definition of MI clinical classification in the TRITON-TIMI 38 (Trial to Assess Improvement

Spontaneous MI Risk Prediction Calculator

*Only for use in patients who present with unstable angina or an MI without ST-segment elevation and are not indicated for revascularization

	Risk Factors	Units	Valid Values	Patient Values (enter new values here)
Baseline Lab Values and Concomitant Medication Usage	Creatinine	Milligrams per deciliter (mg/dL)	(0.07/1.73)	1.50
	Proton pump inhibitor usage	N = no PPI usage; Y = PPI usage	(N, Y)	Y
	Statin usage	N = no statin usage; Y = statin usage	(N, Y)	Y
Demographics and Presentation Characteristics	Disease classification (NSTEMI vs unstable angina)	N = unstable angina; Y= NSTEMI	(N, Y)	N
	Killip class (I vs. II-IV)	N = Killip class II-IV; Y = Killip class I	(N, Y)	Y
	Age	Years (yrs.)	(26, 101)	76
Cardiovascular Risk Factors	Diabetes mellitus	N = not diabetic; Y = diabetic	(N, Y)	Y
	Hypertension	N = no hypertension; Y = hypertension	(N, Y)	Y
	Family history of CAD	N = no family history of CAD; Y= family history of CAD	(N, Y)	N
	Angiography at presentation	N = no angiography; Y = angiography	(N, Y)	N
	Current smoker (cigarettes)	N = not current cigarette smoker; Y = smokes cigarettes	(N, Y)	Y
	Hyperlipidemia	N = no hyperlipidemia; Y = hyperlipidemia	(N, Y)	Y
Cardiovascular Disease History	Peripheral artery disease	N = no PAD; Y = PAD	(N, Y)	N
	Prior MI	N = no previous MI; Y = previous MI occurred	(N, Y)	Y
	Chronic heart failure	N = no chronic heart failure; Y= chronic heart failure	(N, Y)	N
	Prior PCI	N = no prior PCI; Y= prior PCI	(N, Y)	N
	Prior CABG	N = no prior CABG; Y = prior CABG	(N, Y)	N

†Predicted risk at time (please choose between 1 and 1200 days): 900	days	17.33%
	95% CI of the predicted risk:	(12.17%, 24.36%)

†The risk prediction given above is an estimate of the probability that a patient with the given risk profile will have a spontaneous MI at the given time point. The 95% confidence interval given below the risk estimate provides an estimate of the uncertainty in the estimate (i.e., how variable it is).

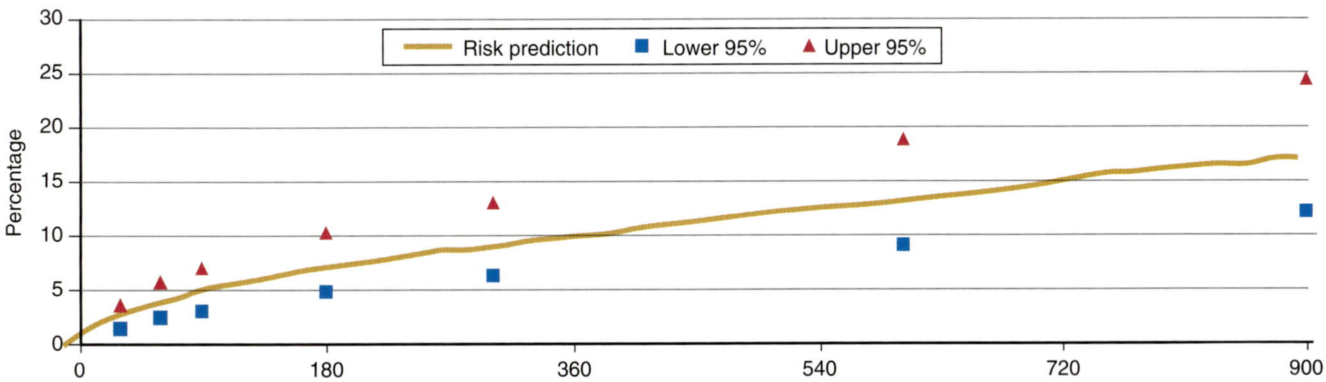

FIGURE 23-1 A patient with a relatively low risk of spontaneous myocardial infarction (MI). A 58-year-old male admitted for unstable angina with normal creatinine (0.7 mg/dL) has a 2-year risk of spontaneous MI of 8.7% (95% confidence interval [CI], 5.7% to 13.1%). *(Adapted from Lopes RD, et al: Spontaneous MI after non–ST-segment elevation acute coronary syndrome managed without revascularization: The TRILOGY ACS trial.* J Am Coll Cardiol *67[11]:1289-97,2016.)*

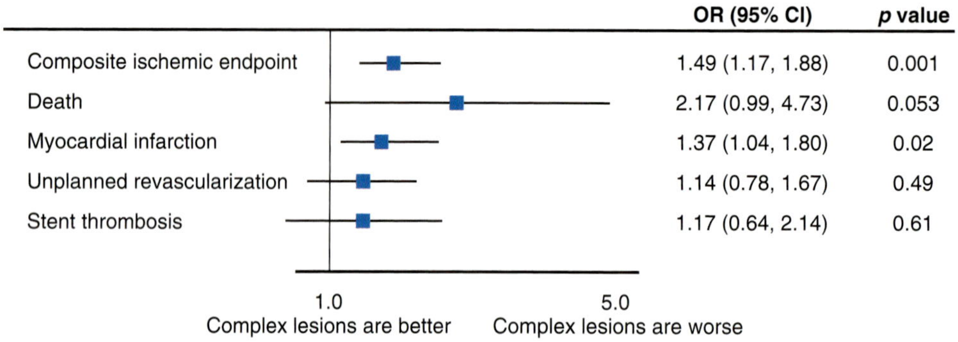

FIGURE 23-2 Multivariate analysis demonstrating the association of type C lesions with 30-day outcomes. *CI*, confidence interval; *OR*, odds ratio. Stent thrombosis was defined as definite and/or probable stent thrombosis according to the Academic Research Consortium definitions. *(Adapted from Goto K, Lansky AJ, Ng VG, et al: Prognostic value of angiographic lesion complexity in patients with acute coronary syndromes undergoing percutaneous coronary intervention [from the Acute Catheterization and Urgent Intervention Triage Strategy Trial].* Am J Cardiol *114:1638–1645, 2014; Fig. 3.)*

TABLE 23-4 Multivariable Predictors of Recurrent Infarction in the OAT Study[21]

PARAMETER	HR	95% CI	*P* VALUE
Randomized to PCI	1.33	0.98–1.81	0.07
Previous MI	1.57	1.04–2.39	0.03
Previous PCI	2.28	1.38–3.77	0.001
Diabetes	1.63	1.16–2.28	0.005
Lower age*	1.16	1.01–1.34	0.03
No new Q waves	1.51	1.10–2.06	0.01
Shorter time from MI†	1.03	1.01–1.05	0.02
Lower ejection fraction‡	1.17	1.02–1.34	0.03

CI, Confidence intervals; *HR*, hazard ratio; *MI*, myocardial infarction; *PCI*, percutaneous coronary intervention.
*By 10-year intervals.
†Time from MI to randomization.
‡By 10% intervals.
Adapted from White HD, et al: Reinfarction after percutaneous coronary intervention or medical management using the universal definition in patients with total occlusion after myocardial infarction: results from long-term follow-up of the Occluded Artery Trial (OAT) cohort. Am Heart J *163:563–571,2012.*

in Therapeutic Outcomes by Optimizing Platelet Inhibition with Prasugrel–Thrombolysis in Myocardial Infarction 38) trial.[39] The TRA·CER (Thrombin Receptor Antagonist for Clinical Event Reduction in Acute Coronary Syndrome) trial compared vorapaxar, a novel platelet protease-activated receptor-1 antagonist, with placebo in 12,944 patients with high-risk NSTE-ACS.[40] During a median follow-up of 502 days, 1580 MIs, as defined by the Universal Definition of MI, occurred in 1319 patients. Most were type 1 (spontaneous) MI, followed by type 4a (PCI)-related MI (Table 23-5). The lesion types were also defined in TRA·CER and are shown in Table 23-6. Restenosis was more common than stent thrombosis, and de novo lesions were three times as common as stent thrombosis. In the TRILOGY trial, after a median follow-up of 16 months, 695 spontaneous MI events occurred, representing 94% of all 737 adjudicated MI events. The Kaplan-Meier event rate of spontaneous MI through 30 months was 10.7%.

In the TRA 2ºP-TIMI 50 (Thrombin Receptor Antagonist in Secondary Prevention of Atherothrombotic Ischemic Events) trial, if the pre-PCI biomarkers were higher than the ULN, an increase by at least 50% over the previous value and documentation that the biomarker was decreasing before the suspected recurrent MI were required.[41] Troponins were available in 94% of patients, and most of the MIs (84%) were in patients who qualified for the trial with a history of MI. Among patients with an MI after randomization, 159 patients had multiple events accounting for 245 (22%) of the 1095 MIs. The annualized rate of any new or recurrent MI after trial enrollment was 2% per year. Type 1 MI was the most common type of MI, and most MIs (81%) were NSTEMIs. Most were associated with a more than 10-fold elevation of cardiac biomarkers. Type 2 MI accounted for 9.8% of MIs.

In the HORIZONS-AMI trial, recurrent MIs following insertion of first-generation DES and bivalirudin anticoagulation in the contemporary era occurred in 1.8% at 30 days, 4.0% at 1 year, and 6.9% at 3 years.[30] Definite stent thrombosis was responsible for 76.3% of recurrent MIs within 30 days and 52% of all recurrent MIs within 3 years. Bivalirudin, compared with heparin plus glycoprotein IIb/IIIa inhibitors, did not reduce recurrent MI.

Time Course of Recurrent Myocardial Infarction

Recurrent MI is more common in the first 30 days than subsequently. In the TRITON-TIMI 38 trial, an analysis of the timing of procedural versus spontaneous recurrent MI demonstrated a substantially higher early hazard of procedurally related MI and a consistent risk of spontaneous MI. In the HORIZONS-AMI trial, the highest risk period was the first 30 days for both stent thrombosis and recurrent MI, with an ongoing risk over time.[30]

OUTCOMES WITH RECURRENT MYOCARDIAL INFARCTION

Outcomes with recurrent MI are related to the size of the infarction and the cumulative effect on left ventricular function. Other factors such as the severity of CAD and diabetes, modification of risk factors, and adherence with evidence-based therapies are also important. Patients with recurrent MI in the GUSTO I and III fibrinolytic trials had higher mortality at 30 days (11.3% vs. 3.5% without recurrent MI; OR, 3.5; $P < .001$) and from 30 days to 1 year (4.7% vs. 3.2%; hazard ratio [HR], 1.5; $P < .001$).[25] In the PAMI studies, recurrent MI was independently related to mortality at 6 months (OR, 7.14; 95% CI, 3.28 to 15.5).[26]

In the TRITON-TIMI 38 trial, patients who experienced an MI during follow-up had a higher risk of CV death at 6 months than patients without an MI (6.5% vs. 1.3%; $P < .001$).[14] This higher risk was present across all subtypes

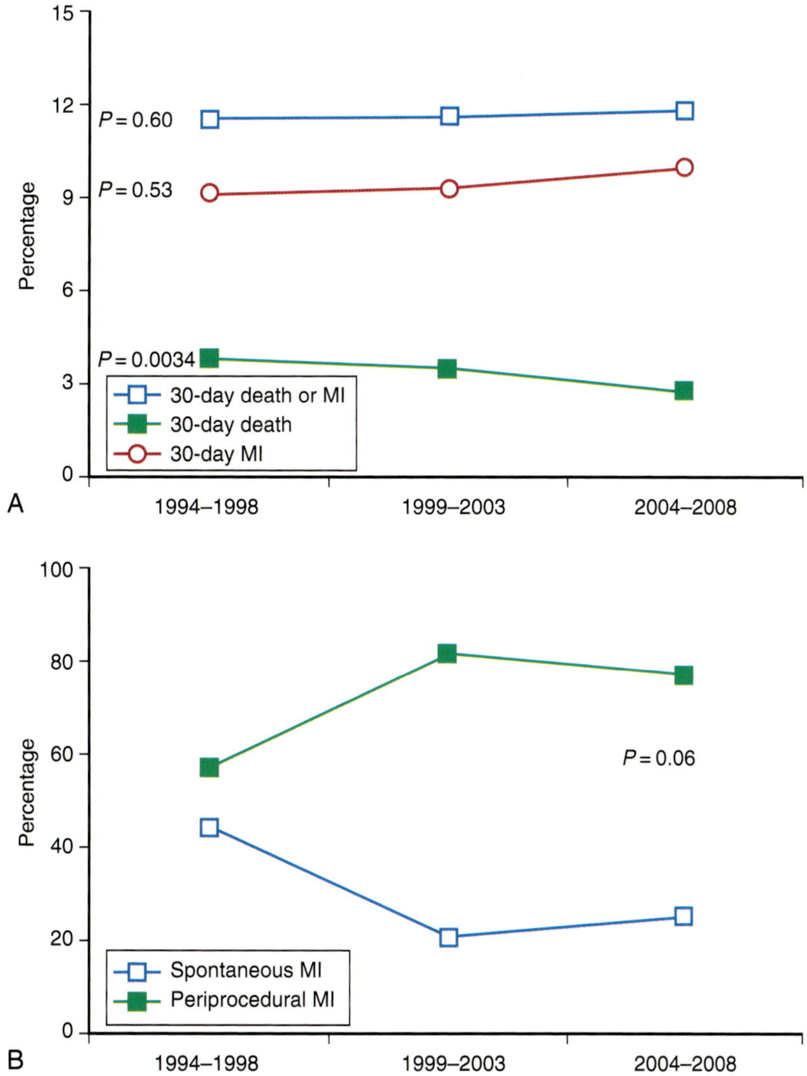

FIGURE 23-3 **(A)** Temporal trends in the rates of clinical outcomes of 30-day death or myocardial infarction (MI) and **(B)** the proportion of myocardial infarctions that are spontaneous versus periprocedural. *(Adapted from Chan MY, Sun JL, Newby LK, et al: Trends in clinical trials of non-ST-segment elevation acute coronary syndromes over 15 years.* Int J Cardiol *167:548–554, 2013; Fig 2.)*

TABLE 23-5 Universal Definition of Myocardial Infarction and Proportion of Recurrent Myocardial Infarction by Type in Clinical Trials of Patients with Acute or Previous Myocardial Infarction[14]

	TYPE I	TYPE 2	TYPE 3	TYPE 4A	TYPE 4B	TYPE 5
TRA 2°P-TIMI 50[39,45] Stable CAD	77%	9.8%	<1%	13% (Types 4A and 4B combined)		<1%
TRITON–TIMI 38 (ACS)[14]	32%	3.7%	0%	53%	13.8%	0.6%
TRACER (ACS)[38]	64.9%	5.2%	0.1%	22.3%	5.4%	2.1%
ATLAS ACS 2 TIMI 51 (ACS)[46]	80.5%	3.5%	0.2%	2.7%	12.8%	0.5%
TRILOGY (ACS)[27] Medical Treatment	94%			6% (Types 4A to 5 combined)		

ACS, Acute coronary syndromes; *CAD*, coronary artery disease.

of MI, including type 4a (peri-PCI, 3.2%; $P < .001$) and type 4b (stent thrombosis, 15.4%; $P < .001$) (Figure 23-5). After adjustment for important clinical covariates, the occurrence of any MI was associated with a fivefold higher risk of death at 6 months (95% CI, 3.8 to 7.1), with a similar increased risk across subtypes. Also, all subtypes of MI were associated with an increased risk of CV death. There was a fourfold increased risk in patients who experienced type 1 MI (spontaneous; adjusted HR, 4.1; 95% CI, 2.7 to 6.3; $P < .001$) and an approximately threefold increased risk (adjusted HR, 2.8; 95%

TABLE 23-6 Nonprocedural Myocardial Infarction Rates and Associated Type of Coronary Lesion in the TRA·CER Trial[38]

TYPE OF LESION	NO. (%)
Lesion type with PCI	438
De novo	267 (61)
Restenosis	119 (27)
Stent thrombosis	89 (20)

MI, Myocardial infarction; *PCI*, percutaneous coronary intervention.
Among 12,944 randomized subjects, 1194 nonprocedural MIs occurred, and 441 had a PCI performed within 7 days. Because there could be multiple lesions treated during a PCI, the percentages of type of lesions (de novo, restenosis, and stent thrombosis) add up more than 100%.
Adapted from Leonardi S, et al: Effect of vorapaxar on myocardial infarction in the thrombin receptor antagonist for clinical event reduction in acute coronary syndrome (TRA·CER) trial. Eur Heart J *34:1723–1731, 2013.*

CI, 0.9 to 8.8; $P = .085$) in patients who experienced type 2 MI (supply-demand imbalance). The risk of CV death was increased more than twofold (adjusted HR, 2.4; 95% CI, 1.6 to 3.7; $P < .001$) in patients who experienced type 4a MI (peri-PCI) and more than 10-fold (adjusted HR, 10.5; 95% CI, 1.18 to 93.6; $P = .035$) in those who experienced type 5 MI (CABG-related). When examined relative to the timing of the recurrent MI, there was a qualitatively similar risk associated with type 1 MI that occurred early and late after the initial ACS presentation and a particularly high risk of early type 4b MI (Table 23-7).

The OAT compared PCI with medical therapy in patients with occluded infarct-related arteries (IRAs). After adjustment for baseline characteristics, the patients who developed recurrent MI according to the Universal Definition had a 4.15-fold (95% CI, 3.03 to 5.69; $P < .001$) increased risk of death compared with patients without recurrent MI.[21] This risk was similar for both treatment groups (interaction $P = 0.26$). Recurrent MIs that occurred within 6 months of randomization had a similar relationship with mortality as recurrent MI that occurred later, and the impact of recurrent MI because of the same IRA and a different epicardial vessel was similar. The independent association of recurrent MI with mortality was not affected by the timing of recurrent MI, definition of MI by more or less stringent criteria, or management of the index MI with PCI or medical therapy alone. Recurrent MI was also a strong independent predictor of subsequent class III or IV heart failure.

In the ACUITY trial, both MI and major bleeding had a similar overall strength of association with mortality in the first year after ACS.[42] The occurrence of an MI was associated with an OR of 3.1 compared with patients who did not have an MI, after adjustment for baseline predictors. MI within 30 days markedly increased the mortality risk for the first 2 days after the events (adjusted HR, 17.6), but this risk declined rapidly postinfarction (HR, 1.4 beyond 1 month after the MI event). In contrast, major bleeding had a prolonged association with mortality risk (HR, 3.5), which remained fairly steady over time throughout 1 year (Figure 23-6).[42]

Recurrent MI in the HORIZONS-AMI trial was also associated with stroke, ischemia-driven target vessel revascularization, and non-CABG surgery–related major bleeding. The occurrence of recurrent MI conferred an approximate eightfold and an approximate threefold increase in the risk of cardiac mortality (HR, 7.65; 95% CI, 4.47 to 13.09; $P < .0001$) and all-cause mortality (HR, 2.88; 95% CI, 1.74 to 4.78; $P < .0001$).[30]

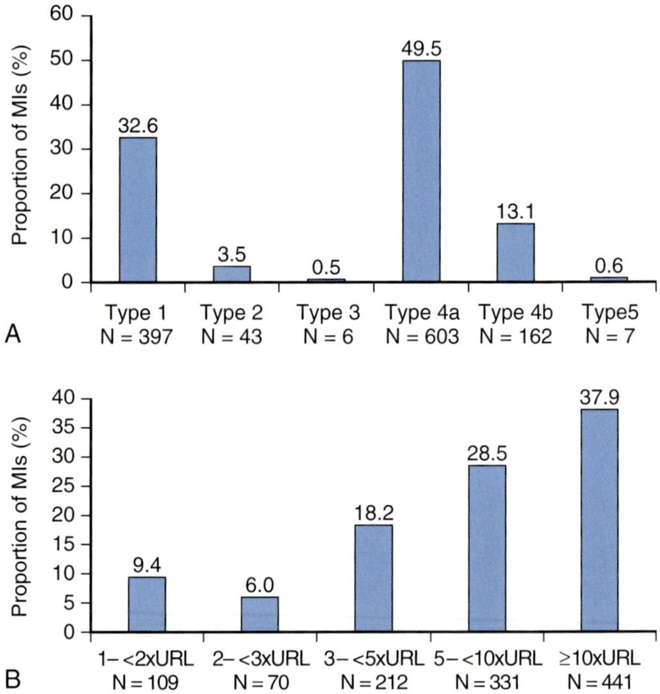

FIGURE 23-4 **(A)** Distribution of new or recurrent myocardial infarctions (MIs) (n = 1218) by the Universal Definition of MI clinical classification. **(B)** Distribution of new or recurrent MIs with available biomarker and reference limit data (n = 1163) by the Universal Definition of MI categories of biomarker of necrosis elevation. *URL*, Upper reference limit. *(Adapted from Morrow DA, Wiviott SD, White HD, et al: Effect of the novel thienopyridine prasugrel compared with clopidogrel on spontaneous and procedural myocardial infarction in the TRial to Assess Improvement in Therapeutic Outcomes by Optimizing Platelet InhibitioN with Prasugrel–Thrombolysis In Myocardial Infarction 38: An application of the classification system from the Universal Definition of Myocardial Infarction.* Circulation *119:2758–2764, 2009; Fig. 1.).*

Prognosis with Type 4a Myocardial Infarction

The prognostic implication of type 4a MI is controversial. A collaborative analysis of individual patient data from the FRISC II (Framingham and Fast Revascularization During Instability in Coronary Artery Disease) trial, the ICTUS (Invasive Versus Conservative Treatment in Unstable Coronary Syndromes), and the RITA-3 (Intervention Versus Conservative Treatment Strategy in Patients With Unstable Angina or Non-ST Elevation Myocardial Infarction [the Third Randomised Intervention Treatment of Angina]) (FRISC II, ICTUS, and RITA-3 [FIR]) trials showed there was no association between type 4a MI and mortality.[43]

In contrast, in the TRITON-TIMI 38 trial, type 4a MI was associated with an adjusted 2.4-fold higher (95% CI, 1.6 to 3.7) risk of CV death at 6 months.[14] This risk was statistically significant, but qualitatively less, than that related to type 1 MI. The most important differentiating factor between these two studies was the definition used for type 4a MI. In the FIR analysis, multiple trials with differing definitions of periprocedural MI were entered into a combined analysis with a variable threshold (1, 1.5, or 2) relative to the URL for the biomarker of necrosis. In TRITON-TIMI 38, to identify periprocedural MI more definitively, creatine kinase-myocardial band (CK-MB) was used preferentially for the diagnosis of type 4a MI and required a CK-MB more than three times the URL on two samples after PCI. In addition, and most importantly, the definition required that the MI was distinct from

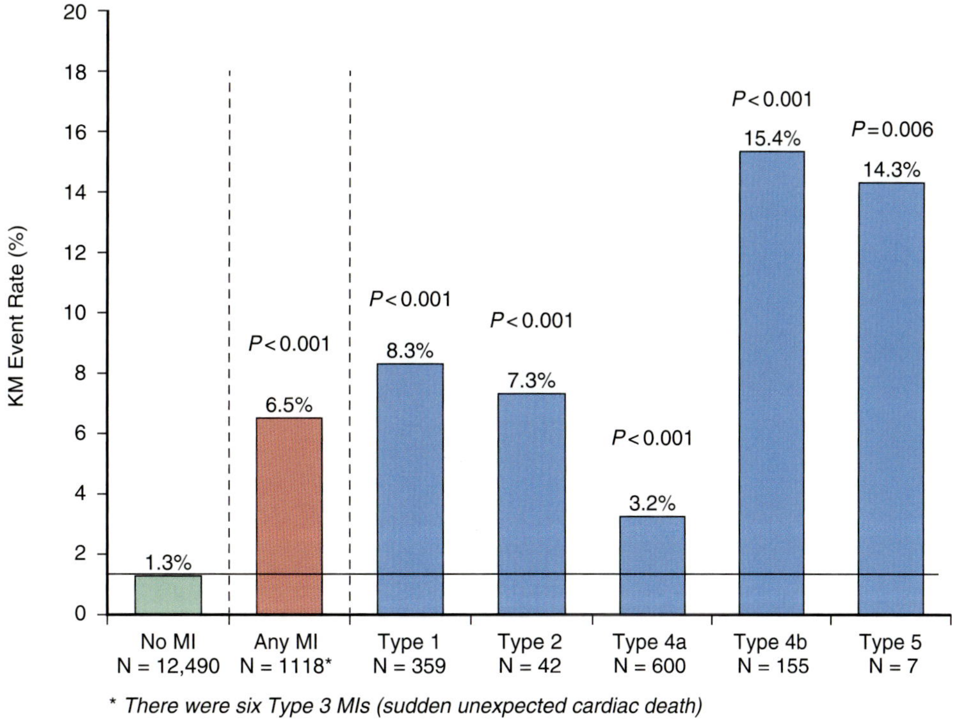

FIGURE 23-5 Cardiovascular death at 180 days by myocardial infarction (MI) subtype. Cumulative incidence of cardiovascular death at 180 days stratified by the occurrence of new or recurrent MI during study follow-up (*red bar*) and by the universal definition of MI subtypes (*green bar*; no MI; *red bar*, any MI; *blue bars*; type 1: spontaneous, type 2: demand related, type 3: sudden unexpected cardiac death, type 4a: percutaneous coronary intervention related, type 4b: stent thrombosis, type 5: related to coronary artery bypass grafting). *KM*, Kaplan-Meier. *(Adapted from Bonaca MP, Wiviott SD, Braunwald E, et al: American College of Cardiology/American Heart Association/European Society of Cardiology/World Heart Federation universal definition of myocardial infarction classification system and the risk of cardiovascular death: observations from the TRITON-TIMI 38 trial [Trial to Assess Improvement in Therapeutic Outcomes by Optimizing Platelet Inhibition With Prasugrel–Thrombolysis in Myocardial Infarction 38].* Circulation *125:577–583, 2012; Fig 1.)*

TABLE 23-7 Cardiovascular Death at 180 Days after a New Myocardial Infarction, Stratified by Time from Index Event[14]

	MI ≤30 DAYS FROM INDEX EVENT		MI >30 DAYS FROM INDEX EVENT	
FOLLOW-UP	**NO MI**	**ANY MI**	**NO MI***	**ANY MI**
Cardiovascular death KM%	1.26%	6.41% (n = 756)†	0.49%	6.94% (n = 362)†
Adjusted HR (95% CI)		5.1 (3.6–7.3)†		11.7 (7.0–19.5)†
Type 1 MI		10.6% (n = 67)		7.9% (n = 292)
Adjusted HR (95% CI)		4.0 (1.6–9.8)		10.2 (6.1–17.2)
Type 2 MI		12.5% (n = 8)		6.2% (n = 34)
Adjusted HR (95% CI)		6.9 (0.95–50.1)		5.4 (1.3–22.9)
Type 4a MI		3.3% (n = 592)		NS‡
Adjusted HR (95% CI)		2.4 (1.6–3.7)		NS‡
Type 4b MI		22.0% (n = 96)		3.7% (n = 59)
Adjusted HR (95% CI)		16.7 (10.1–27.6)		5.8 (1.4–24.0)
Type 5 MI		33.3% (n = 3)		NS‡
Adjusted HR (95% CI)		36.6 (5.0–270.0)		NS‡

CI, Confidence interval; *HR*, hazard ratio; *KM%*, Kaplan-Meier percentage; *MI*, myocardial infarction.
*Landmark analysis at 30 days.
†$P < .001$.
‡Insufficient number of events.
Adapted from Bonaca MP, et al: American College of Cardiology/American Heart Association/European Society of Cardiology/World Heart Federation universal definition of myocardial infarction classification system and the risk of cardiovascular death: observations from the TRITON-TIMI 38 trial (Trial to Assess Improvement in Therapeutic Outcomes by Optimizing Platelet Inhibition With Prasugrel–Thrombolysis in Myocardial Infarction 38). Circulation *125:577–583,2012.*

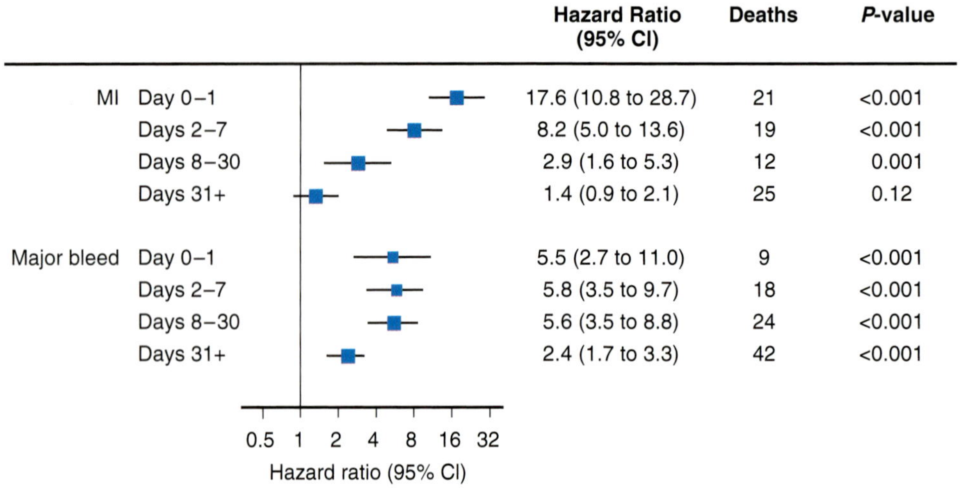

FIGURE 23-6 **Association of recurrent myocardial infarction (MI) and major bleeding with mortality, adjusted for baseline predictors (age, white blood cell count, diabetes, ST-deviation, left bundle branch block, gender, planned treatment, cerebrovascular event, creatinine clearance, hemoglobin, elevated creatine kinase-MB/troponin, current smoker, treatment).** *(Adapted from Mehran R, Pocock SJ, Stone GW, et al: Associations of major bleeding and myocardial infarction with the incidence and timing of mortality in patients presenting with non-ST-elevation acute coronary syndromes: a risk model from the ACUITY trial.* Eur Heart J *30:1457–1466, 2009; Fig. 4.)*

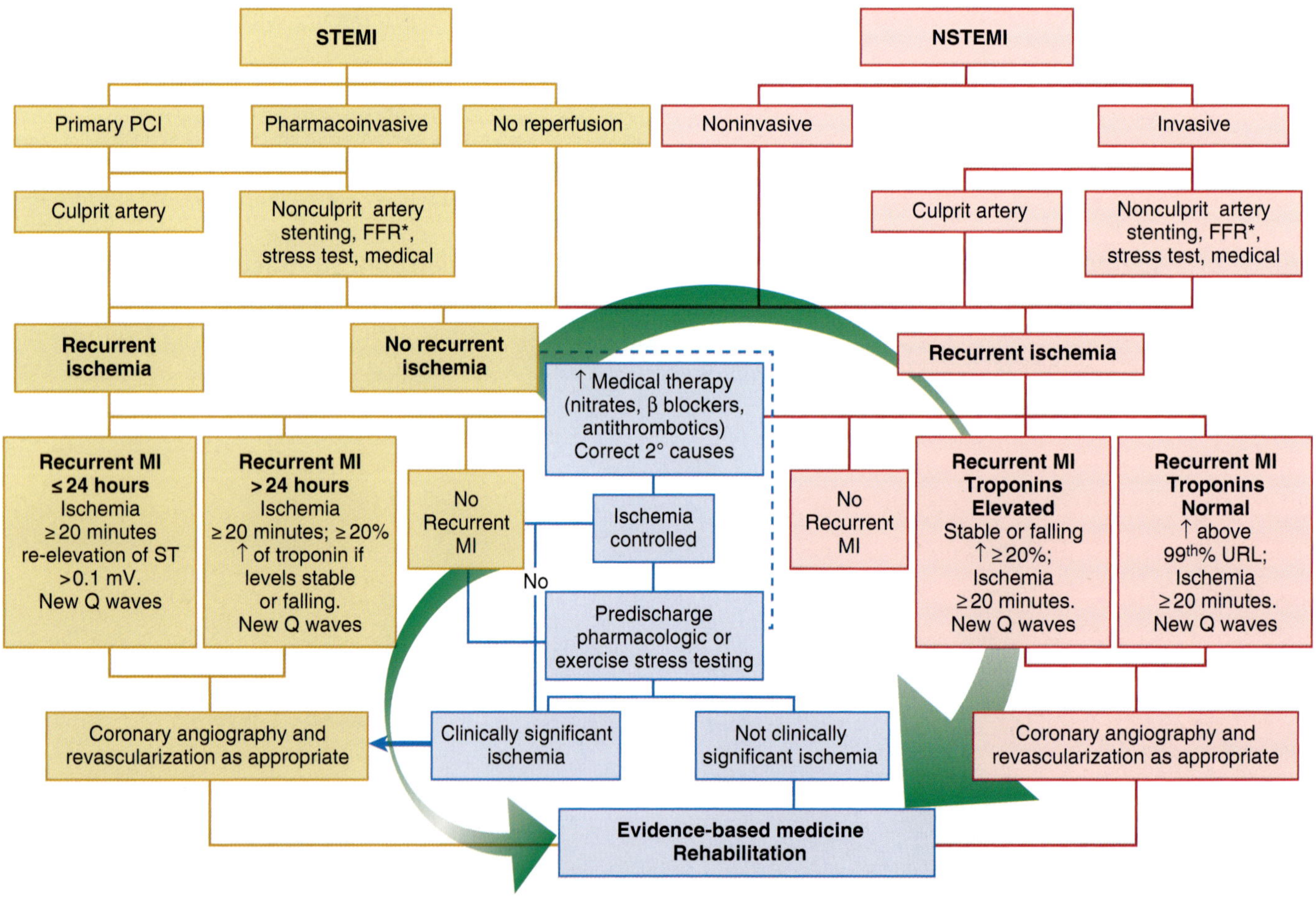

FIGURE 23-7 **Algorithm for managing of patients with ST-elevation myocardial infarction (STEMI) or non–ST-elevation MI (NSTEMI) and recurrent ischemia and/or recurrent MI.** For patients undergoing primary percutaneous coronary intervention (PCI) of only the culprit artery without recurrent ischemia or recurrent MI, the *large arrow* shows bypass tracts. There is a direct pathway to the use of evidence-based medicine without undergoing pharmacological or exercise stress testing if a new culprit artery was treated predischarge, and there is no recurrent ischemia. Medically, it is recommended that stress testing should be undertaken. *FFR*, Fractional flow reserve (*can be performed acutely or delayed); *PCI*, percutaneous coronary intervention; *URL*, upper reference limit.

the index event; in the setting of biomarker elevation from a preceding event, a diagnosis of type 4a MI required both that the concentration decreased before the new event and that there was a subsequent increase of at least 50%. Using this approach, it is plausible that a new MI was more accurately discriminated from biomarker elevation related to the ACS that led to the PCI being performed.

Several other studies have also shown that patients with type 1 MIs have a worse prognosis than type 4a MIs. In a combination of the EARLY ACS (Early Glycoprotein IIb/

IIIa Inhibition in Non–ST-Segment Elevation Acute Coronary Syndrome) and the SYNERGY (Superior Yield of the New Strategy of Enoxaparin, Revascularisation and Glycoprotein IIb/IIIa Inhibitors Datasets) trials, type 1 MIs had an approximate four times higher 1-year mortality than type 4a MIs.[47]

PREVENTION OF RECURRENT MYOCARDIAL INFARCTION

Figure 23-7 shows an algorithm for the diagnosis and management of recurrent ischemia and/or recurrent MI. Lifestyle modifications such as quitting smoking, body weight control with prevention of diabetes, and adherence to secondary evidence-based medications could help reduce the incidence of recurrent MI. Secondary preventive therapy is discussed in Chapter 34 and considerations regarding the use of long-term antithrombotic therapies are reviewed in Chapter 21 and Chapter 35.

SUMMARY

Recurrent MI is important because it is not uncommon and is associated with increased hospital complications, including heart failure, arrhythmias, increased rates of stroke, increased ischemia-driven revascularization, bleeding, and increased in-hospital and long-term mortality.[44] There may also be decreased quality of life, increased hospital stay, and increased costs. Further studies are required to define predictors and to identify better treatments, including pharmacotherapy, better stents, and evolution of implantation techniques to reduce the occurrence of recurrent MI and its complications.

References

1. Yeh RW, et al.: Population trends in the incidence and outcomes of acute myocardial infarction, *N Engl J Med.* 362:2155–2165, 2010.
2. Jokhadar M, et al.: Sudden death and recurrent ischemic events after myocardial infarction in the community, *Am J Epidemiol.* 159:1040–1046, 2004.
3. Stenestrand U, Lindback J, Wallentin L: Long-term outcome of primary percutaneous coronary intervention vs prehospital and in-hospital thrombolysis for patients with ST-elevation myocardial infarction, *JAMA.* 296:1749–1756, 2006.
4. The Joint European Society of Cardiology/American College of Cardiology Committee: Myocardial infarction redefined – a consensus document of the Joint European Society of Cardiology/American College of Cardiology Committee for the Redefinition of Myocardial Infarction, *J Am Coll Cardiol.* 36:959–969, 2000.
5. Keller T, et al.: Sensitive troponin I assay in early diagnosis of acute myocardial infarction, *N Engl J Med.* 361:868–877, 2009.
6. Armstrong PW, et al.: Acute coronary syndromes in the GUSTO-IIb trial: prognostic insights and impact of recurrent ischemia, *Circulation.* 98:1860–1868, 1998.
7. Langer A, et al.: Prognostic significance of ST segment shift early after resolution of ST elevation in patients with myocardial infarction treated with thrombolytic therapy: the GUSTO-I ST Segment Monitoring Substudy, *J Am Coll Cardiol.* 31:783–789, 1998.
8. Scirica BM, et al.: Ischemia detected on continuous electrocardiography after acute coronary syndrome: observations from the MERLIN-TIMI 36 (Metabolic Efficiency With Ranolazine for Less Ischemia in Non-ST-Elevation Acute Coronary Syndrome-Thrombolysis In Myocardial Infarction 36) trial, *J Am Coll Cardiol.* 53:1411–1421, 2009.
9. Akkerhuis KM, et al.: Recurrent ischaemia during continuous multilead ST-segment monitoring identifies patients with acute coronary syndromes at high risk of adverse cardiac events: meta-analysis of three studies involving 995 patients, *Eur Heart J.* 22:1997–2006, 2001.
10. Stone GW, et al.: Implications of recurrent ischemia after reperfusion therapy in acute myocardial infarction: a comparison of thrombolytic therapy and primary angioplasty, *J Am Coll Cardiol.* 26:66–72, 1995.
11. Thygesen K, et al.: Universal definition of myocardial infarction, *Circulation.* 116:2634–2653, 2007.
12. Thygesen K, et al.: Third universal definition of myocardial infarction, *Circulation.* 126:2020–2035, 2012.
13. Prasad A, et al.: Prognostic significance of periprocedural versus spontaneously occurring myocardial infarction after percutaneous coronary intervention in patients with acute coronary syndromes: an analysis from the ACUITY (Acute Catheterization and Urgent Intervention Triage Strategy) trial, *J Am Coll Cardiol.* 54:477–486, 2009.
14. Bonaca MP, et al.: American College of Cardiology/American Heart Association/European Society of Cardiology/World Heart Federation universal definition of myocardial infarction classification system and the risk of cardiovascular death: observations from the TRITON-TIMI 38 trial (Trial to Assess Improvement in Therapeutic Outcomes by Optimizing Platelet Inhibition With Prasugrel–Thrombolysis in Myocardial Infarction 38), *Circulation.* 125:577–583, 2012.
15. Damman P, et al.: Long-term cardiovascular mortality after procedure-related or spontaneous myocardial infarction in patients with non-ST-segment elevation acute coronary syndrome: a collaborative analysis of individual patient data from the FRISC II, ICTUS, and RITA-3 trials (FIR), *Circulation.* 125:568–576, 2012.
16. Alpert JS, et al.: Diagnostic and therapeutic implications of type 2 myocardial infarction: review and commentary, *Am J Med.* 127:105–108, 2014.
17. White HD: Torrent of troponin, *Circ Cardiovasc Interv.* 7:435–438, 2014.
18. Stone GW, et al.: A prospective natural-history study of coronary atherosclerosis, *N Engl J Med.* 364:226–235, 2011.
19. Palmerini T, et al.: Stent thrombosis with drug-eluting and bare-metal stents: evidence from a comprehensive network meta-analysis, *Lancet.* 379:1393–1402, 2012.
20. Selvanayagam JB, et al.: Relationship of irreversible myocardial injury to troponin I and creatine kinase-MB elevation after coronary artery bypass surgery: insights from cardiovascular magnetic resonance imaging, *J Am Coll Cardiol.* 45:629–631, 2005.
21. White HD, et al.: Reinfarction after percutaneous coronary intervention or medical management using the universal definition in patients with total occlusion after myocardial infarction: results from long-term follow-up of the Occluded Artery Trial (OAT) cohort, *Am Heart J.* 163:563–571, 2012.
22. White HD, et al.: Reduced immediate ischemic events with cangrelor in PCI: a pooled analysis of the CHAMPION trials using the universal definition of myocardial infarction, *Am Heart J.* 163:182–190, 2012. e184.
23. Bhatt DL, et al.: Effect of platelet inhibition with cangrelor during PCI on ischemic events, *N Engl J Med.* 368:1303–1313, 2013.
24. Merlini PA, et al.: Persistent activation of coagulation mechanism in unstable angina and myocardial infarction, *Circulation.* 90:61–68, 1994.
25. Hudson MP, et al.: Early reinfarction after fibrinolysis: experience from the global utilization of streptokinase and tissue plasminogen activator (alteplase) for occluded coronary arteries (GUSTO I) and global use of strategies to open occluded coronary arteries (GUSTO III) trials, *Circulation* 104:1229–1235, 2001.
26. Kernis SJ, et al.: The incidence, predictors, and outcomes of early reinfarction after primary angioplasty for acute myocardial infarction, *J Am Coll.Cardiol.* 42:1173–1177, 2003.
27. Lopes RD, et al.: Spontaneous MI after non–ST-segment elevation acute coronary syndrome managed without revascularization: The TRILOGY ACS trial, *J Am Coll Cardiol.* 67(11): 1289–1297, 2016.
28. Ellis SG, et al.: Coronary morphologic and clinical determinants of procedural outcome with angioplasty for multivessel coronary disease: implications for patient selection, *Circulation.* 82:1193–1202, 1990.
29. Goto K, et al.: Prognostic value of angiographic lesion complexity in patients with acute coronary syndromes undergoing percutaneous coronary intervention (from the Acute Catheterization and Urgent Intervention Triage Strategy Trial), *Am J Cardiol.* 114:1638–1645, 2014.
30. Stone SG, et al.: Incidence, predictors, and implications of reinfarction after primary percutaneous coronary intervention in ST-segment-elevation myocardial infarction: the Harmonizing Outcomes with Revascularization and Stents in Acute Myocardial Infarction Trial, *Circ Cardiovasc Interv.* 7:543–551, 2014.
31. Damani SB, Topol EJ: Emerging genomic applications in coronary artery disease, *JACC Cardiovascular Interventions.* 4:473–482, 2011.
32. Makinen VP, et al.: Integrative genomics reveals novel molecular pathways and gene networks for coronary artery disease, *PLoS Genet.* 10:e1004502, 2014.
33. Traylor M, et al.: Genetic risk factors for ischaemic stroke and its subtypes (the METASTROKE collaboration): a meta-analysis of genome-wide association studies, *Lancet Neurol.* 11:951–962, 2012.
34. Arbab-Zadeh A, Fuster V: The myth of the "vulnerable plaque": transitioning from a focus on individual lesions to atherosclerotic disease burden for coronary artery disease risk assessment, *J Am Coll Cardiol.* 65:846–855, 2015.
35. Fleg JL, et al.: Detection of high-risk atherosclerotic plaque: report of the NHLBI Working Group on current status and future directions, *JACC Cardiovasc Imaging.* 5:941–955, 2012.
36. Budoff MJ, et al.: Progression of coronary artery calcium predicts all-cause mortality, *JACC Cardiovasc Imaging.* 3:1229–1236, 2010.
37. Wald DS, et al.: Randomized trial of preventive angioplasty in myocardial infarction, *N Engl J Med.* 369:1115–1123, 2013.
38. Chan MY, et al.: Trends in clinical trials of non-ST-segment elevation acute coronary syndromes over 15 years, *Int J Cardiol.* 167:548–554, 2013.
39. Morrow DA, et al.: Effect of the novel thienopyridine prasugrel compared with clopidogrel on spontaneous and procedural myocardial infarction in the TRial to Assess Improvement in Therapeutic Outcomes by Optimizing Platelet InhibitioN with Prasugrel–Thrombolysis In Myocardial Infarction 38: an application of the classification system from the Universal Definition of Myocardial Infarction, *Circulation.* 119:2758–2764, 2009.
40. Leonardi S, et al.: Effect of vorapaxar on myocardial infarction in the thrombin receptor antagonist for clinical event reduction in acute coronary syndrome (TRA·CER) trial, *Eur Heart J.* 34:1723–1731, 2013.
41. Kidd S, et al.: Universal classification system type of incident myocardial infarction in patients with stable atherosclerosis: observations from TRA 2°P-TIMI 50, *J Am Coll Cardiol.* 63:A1568, 2014.
42. Mehran R, et al.: Associations of major bleeding and myocardial infarction with the incidence and timing of mortality in patients presenting with non-ST-elevation acute coronary syndromes: a risk model from the ACUITY trial, *Eur Heart J.* 30:1457–1466, 2009.
43. Damman P, et al.: Timing of angiography with a routine invasive strategy and long-term outcomes in non-ST-segment elevation acute coronary syndrome: a collaborative analysis of individual patient data from the FRISC II (Fragmin and Fast Revascularization During Instability in Coronary Artery Disease), ICTUS (Invasive Versus Conservative Treatment in Unstable Coronary Syndromes), and RITA-3 (Intervention Versus Conservative Treatment Strategy in Patients With Unstable Angina or Non-ST Elevation Myocardial Infarction) trials, *JACC Cardiovasc.Interv.* 5:191–199, 2012.
44. Fokkema ML, et al.: Incidence, predictors, and outcome of reinfarction and stent thrombosis within one year after primary percutaneous coronary intervention for ST-elevation myocardial infarction, *Catheter Cardiovasc Interv.* 73:627–634, 2009.
45. Bonaca MP, et al.: Coronary stent thrombosis with vorapaxar versus placebo: results from the TRA 2º P-TIMI 50 trial, *J Am Coll Cardiol.* 64:2309–2317, 2014.
46. Cavender MA, et al.: The effect of rivaroxaban on myocardial infarction in the ATLAS ACS 2-TIMI 51 trial, *Eur Heart J Acute Cardiovasc Care* 4:468–474, 2015.
47. Leonardi S, et al.: Comparison of the prognosis of spontaneous and percutaneous coronary intervention-related myocardial infarction, *J Am Coll Cardiol.* 60:2296–2304, 2012.

24 Reperfusion Injury: Prevention and Management

Robert A. Kloner and Sharon L. Hale

INTRODUCTION

The term "reperfusion injury" refers to cellular damage that occurs during the reperfusion phase after an episode of ischemia.[1] If reperfusion occurs after a short period of ischemia, all cells are salvaged (Figure 24-1A). However, as the duration of ischemia increases, cells become irreversibly injured, and the territory of cell death increases in size over time (Figure 24-1B). Sorting out damage that occurs primarily because of reperfusion rather than during the preceding ischemic phase can be difficult, because it is impossible to have reperfusion without ischemia. For this reason, the resulting myocardial damage is often referred to as an ischemia/reperfusion injury. Evidence that reperfusion itself is harmful to the heart comes from studies that showed that certain phenomena first manifest during the reperfusion phase (no-reflow, ventricular arrhythmias) and then worsen as the phase of reperfusion progresses. In addition, studies of therapies administered only at the time of or solely during the reperfusion phase that result in some benefit also provide evidence that reperfusion itself has detrimental effects. Examples include the administration of oxygen radical scavengers at reperfusion, which results in improved function of stunned myocardium; the initiation of hypothermia at 30 minutes after reperfusion that results in a reduction of the zone of no-reflow[2]; and administering a pharmacologic agent to the patient undergoing postconditioning at reperfusion, which results in a reduction of myocardial infarct size. In this chapter, we describe the pathobiology and clinical manifestations of reperfusion injury, as well as therapeutic strategies for which studies are completed or ongoing. The pathobiology of infarct healing is described in Chapter 4. Adverse remodeling of the myocardium after myocardial infarction (MI) is addressed in Chapter 36.

PATHOLOGICAL AND CLINICAL COMPONENTS OF REPERFUSION INJURY

There are four basic components of "reperfusion injury": (1) stunned myocardium; (2) reperfusion arrhythmias; (3) the no-reflow phenomenon, which is also known as microvascular obstruction; and (4) lethal myocardial cell injury caused by reperfusion. In our opinion, there is little doubt that the first three phenomena are caused by reperfusion itself. However, we still question the significance and importance of lethal myocardial cell injury caused by reperfusion and address this uncertainty later in this chapter (see the section on Lethal Myocardial Cell Injury Caused by Reperfusion).

Stunned Myocardium

Stunned myocardium refers to myocardium that has been subjected to a period of ischemia that results in reversible injury (i.e., the cells become ischemic, but are not necrotic) in which there is prolonged but transient contractile dysfunction after reperfusion.[3] In early studies in canine models of proximal coronary artery occlusion followed by reperfusion, 5- to 15-minute episodes of ischemia resulted in regional wall motion abnormalities that persisted for several hours to days, despite the absence of cell death. Hence, in such experiments, the myocardium behaved as if it were "stunned" by a brief episode of ischemia followed by reperfusion. The entire hypoperfused area of myocardium is described as the area at risk (Figure 24-1A). However, when occlusion of the coronary artery is prolonged, irreversible cellular injury occurs, which results in infarction (Figure 24-1B).

The mechanism of stunning is believed to involve damage from the release of reactive oxygen species and from calcium overload that occurs in the early stages of reperfusion, which results in reduced responsiveness of the contractile apparatus to calcium. Calcium uptake by the sarcoplasmic reticulum appears to be impaired in stunned myocardium and might contribute to contractile dysfunction.[4] The observation that therapy with oxygen radical scavengers at reperfusion improves function supports the concept that stunning is a form of functional reperfusion injury. Clinical examples of stunned myocardium include: (1) slow recovery of salvaged myocardium in the outer wall of the ventricle after thrombolytic therapy or percutaneous coronary intervention (PCI) therapy for ST-elevation MI (STEMI); (2) slow recovery of ventricular function after cardiopulmonary bypass procedures; (3) persistent regional wall motion abnormalities after exercise-induced ischemia or prolonged angioplasty balloon inflation during PCI; and (4) slow recovery of function in those with Takotsubo cardiomyopathy.[5]

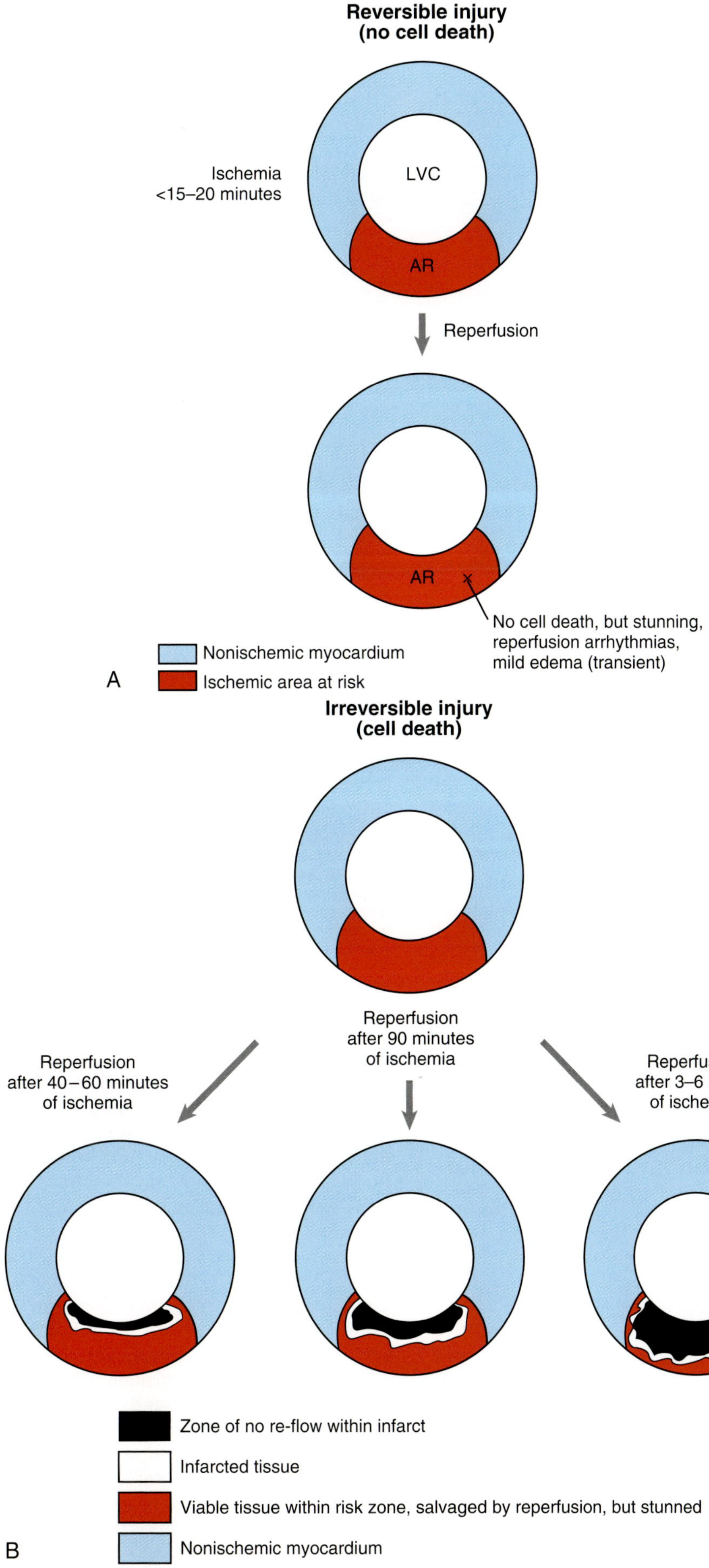

FIGURE 24-1 **(A)** Schematic of a transmural section of the heart after a short period of ischemia (≤20 minutes). Cell death does not occur (reversible injury), but tissue is stunned and reperfusion arrhythmias might ensue. **(B)** Schematic of a transmural section of the left ventricle derived from studies in the anesthetized canine model of proximal coronary occlusion and reperfusion. After 40 to 60 minutes of ischemia, irreversible cell damage is confined to the subendocardium. A smaller area of no-reflow is present within the necrotic region. If reperfusion is delayed to 90 minutes, the necrotic region expands from the subendocardium to the mid-myocardium within the ischemic risk zone, accompanied by an expansion of the no-reflow region. After 3 to 6 hours of ischemia, necrosis becomes nearly transmural, and the no-reflow region, although contained within the necrotic area, becomes larger. *AR*, Area at risk; *LVC*, left ventricular cavity.

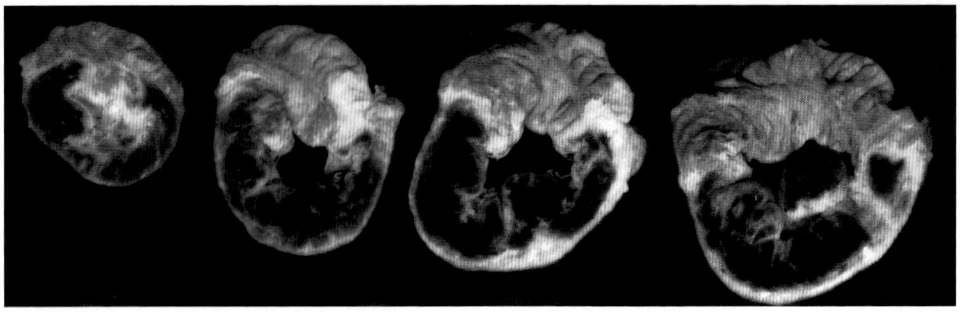

FIGURE 24-2 Thioflavin S–stained sections of rabbit heart subjected to 30 minutes of ischemia plus reperfusion viewed under ultraviolet light. The *fluorescent white* areas are within the risk zone that received blood flow during reperfusion. *Black areas* in the subendocardium did not receive blood flow containing the fluorescent thioflavin S, even after reperfusion of the epicardial coronary artery and represent the anatomic zone of no-reflow. *Gray areas* at the top contain an overlap of blue dye used to delineate the nonischemic risk zone during coronary artery occlusion plus thioflavin S.

Reperfusion Arrhythmias

Our laboratory and others have observed that reperfusion, after a brief period of ischemia (only 5 minutes in the anesthetized rat model), results in a barrage of ventricular arrhythmias, including polymorphic ventricular tachycardia and ventricular fibrillation. The release of toxic oxygen radicals at the time of reperfusion, as well as electrolyte disturbances (including sodium and calcium overload of cardiomyocytes) may contribute to the onset of these arrhythmias. In addition, during the first seconds of reperfusion, inhomogeneity of action potential amplitude and duration in the previously ischemic zone and border zone might contribute to reentry-related arrhythmias. Certain therapies introduced at the time of reperfusion, such as postconditioning (transient episodes of brief coronary reocclusion and reperfusion) markedly diminish reperfusion-induced arrhythmias. Reperfusion arrhythmias, including accelerated idioventricular rhythms, ventricular tachycardia, and ventricular premature beats, have been observed in patients after reperfusion therapy for STEMI (see Chapter 28). Bursts of reperfusion-induced ventricular arrhythmias may be associated with larger infarcts and might represent a biomarker of reperfusion injury.[6] Reperfusion arrhythmias may also pose a potentially unrecognized problem in the setting of reversal of coronary vasospasm (such as in Prinzmetal angina), which is, on rare occasion, followed by sudden death.[7]

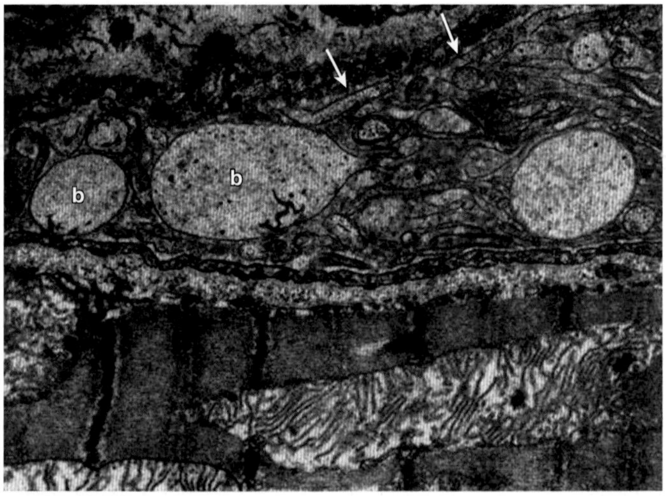

FIGURE 24-3 Posterior papillary region of the heart from a canine model made temporarily ischemic for 90 minutes with 10 to 12 seconds of coronary blood reperfusion (from area of no-reflow). Endothelial pinocytotic vesicles are sparse. The capillary lumen is full of endothelial protrusions (*arrows*) and membrane-bound bodies (*b*), some of which might represent degranulated platelets. Mitochondria are swollen with amorphous matrix dense bodies. I bands and intermyofibrillar edema are present (magnification 22,640×). *(From Kloner RA, et al: The "no-reflow" phenomenon after temporary coronary occlusion in the dog.* J Clin Invest *56:1496, 1974; Fig 8a.)*

No-Reflow Phenomenon and Microvascular Obstruction

Pathobiology

The no-reflow phenomenon refers to the inability to perfuse portions of the myocardium because of microvascular obstruction after successful reopening of a closed proximal epicardial coronary artery.[8] The fluorescent dye, thioflavin S, is used in animal models to show the anatomic no-reflow zone (Figure 24-2). In a study performed in anesthetized canines in the mid-1970s, we observed that when the proximal circumflex coronary artery was occluded for 90 minutes, followed by reperfusion, that thioflavin S, when injected into the vasculature, failed to penetrate the subendocardium of the posterior left ventricular wall.[8] An electron microscopic examination (Figure 24-3) of these nonfluorescent zones of no-reflow revealed capillaries with focal endothelial swelling, or "blebs" that appeared to be obstructing blood flow. Areas of microvascular hemorrhage with extrusion of red blood cells into the interstitial space adjacent to endothelial gaps were also observed. Occasionally, capillaries appeared to be compressed by adjacent swollen cardiomyocytes, and damaged vessels appeared to be plugged by fibrin tactoids, platelets, and neutrophils. It is likely that the cause of no-reflow is structural damage to the microvasculature within the MI zone (Figure 24-4). The size of the zone of no-reflow within the infarct is correlated with the duration of coronary occlusion (Figure 24-1B). We showed that streptokinase, tissue plasminogen activator, or dabigatran[9] could not prevent no-reflow. The size of the no-reflow zone expanded over several hours after reperfusion of the proximal, patent coronary artery.[8] The growth of the anatomic no-reflow zone, which was assessed by injecting fluorescent dye into the vasculature, was accompanied by a deterioration of regional myocardial blood flow within this zone.[8] These findings suggest that whatever damage occurs to the microvasculature happens partially during the reperfusion phase, and therefore, no-reflow is a form of reperfusion injury.

An influx of electrolytes, fluid, calcium, and reactive oxygen species during the early minutes of reperfusion might result in damage to endothelial cells, including

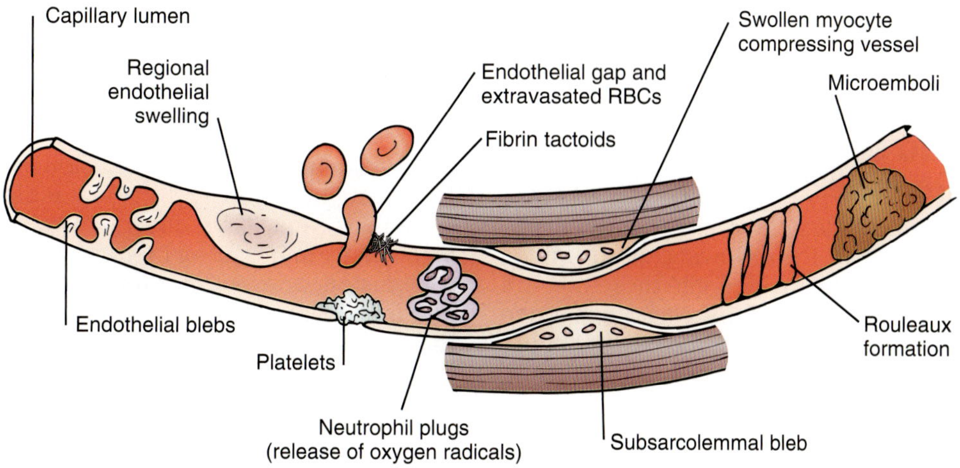

FIGURE 24-4 **Different mechanisms involved in the development of no-reflow, and accompanying ultrastructural alterations of the microvascular bed.** *RBC*, Red blood cell. *(From Reffelmann T, Kloner RA: The "no-reflow" phenomenon: basic science and clinical correlates.* Heart *87:162, 2002; Figure 2.)*

focal and diffuse edema, and eventual rupture of endothelial cells that then blocks flow. The zone of no-reflow rapidly expands outward within the infarcted region, finally leveling off at approximately 2 to 8 hours. In general, we observed that the zone of no-reflow is contained within the MI zone (myocyte cell death). We do not believe that no-reflow contributes directly to myocyte cell death. However, experimental and clinical studies increasingly suggest that the no-reflow phenomenon is an important marker of prognosis. The larger the extent of no-reflow, the more myocardial infarct expansion and left ventricular remodeling was likely to occur.[8] This observation makes intrinsic sense; if blood elements cannot access the zone of necrotic debris, healing of the scar is impaired.

Clinical Manifestations

No-reflow is now well documented in patients and is clinically manifest in up to 30% of those undergoing reperfusion therapy for acute MI.[8] Several imaging techniques, including nuclear imaging (see Chapter 32), echo-contrast (see Chapter 31), and magnetic resonance imaging (see Chapter 33) have visualized anatomic zones of no-reflow or microvascular obstruction in patients. Similar to the findings in experimental animal studies, the zones of no-reflow observed in humans are typically subendocardial to mid-myocardial and appear to be confined to the necrotic zone. As in animal studies, the presence of no-reflow in patients is associated with greater left ventricular dilation and adverse left ventricular remodeling, as well as a worse clinical outcome, including higher mortality rates and more congestive heart failure.[10–14] Some studies have shown that the size of the no-reflow zone is a marker of poor clinical outcome, independent of the size of the MI.[12–14]

No-reflow in humans is complicated by the fact that during PCI, atherosclerotic fragments and thrombi can break off and cause distal embolization, which contributes to additional distal microvascular obstruction. No-reflow may be observed in the catheterization laboratory even during routine nonemergent coronary angioplasties or stenting procedures. In the catheterization laboratory, sluggish flow in an otherwise patent epicardial coronary artery and reduced myocardial blush grade are signs of low or no-reflow and predict a poor outcome.

TABLE 24-1 Potential Mechanisms of Lethal Myocyte Injury because of Reperfusion

1. An influx of sodium, calcium, or water into myocytes with leaky sarcolemmal membranes, resulting in volume and calcium overload of the cells and cellular organelles, such as mitochondria
2. Damage to cellular membranes and structures because of the generation of reactive oxygen species at the time of reperfusion
3. Opening of the mitochondrial permeability transition pore during reperfusion
4. Hypercontracture of myocytes because of calcium overload with the formation of contraction bands
5. Changes in pH that occur with reperfusion
6. Damage caused by the presence of inflammatory cytokines and neutrophil infiltration into the previously ischemic reperfused zone

Lethal Myocardial Cell Injury Caused by Reperfusion

The fourth, most important, but still controversial component of reperfusion injury, is lethal myocardial cell injury caused by reperfusion itself. In this construct, cardiomyocytes are injured, but still alive at the end of ischemia. However, once reperfusion occurs, the cardiomyocytes become irreversibly injured and die because of the act of reperfusion. Potential mechanisms in which reperfusion could cause a reversibly injured cardiomyocyte to become irreversibly injured (dead) are listed in Table 24-1. In particular, the generation of oxygen-free radicals and the opening of the mitochondrial permeability transition pore during reperfusion are believed to be important contributors to ischemia/reperfusion injury and have become targets for therapy (see the section on Prevention and Management of Reperfusion Injury). The mitochondrial permeability transition pore is a large-conductance megachannel that is closed under physiological conditions, but it opens in response to changes in the mitochondrial membrane potential, reactive oxygen species, and increased calcium concentration. Opening of the pore is believed to be a key event in the initiation of apoptotic cell death.

Support for the concept that lethal cardiomyocyte reperfusion injury is a real phenomenon comes largely from studies in which therapies given right at or shortly before reperfusion further reduce MI size above and beyond reperfusion alone.[1,15] However, few clinical trials have shown such benefit. Worsening of chest pain or reelevation of ST segments on the electrocardiogram at reperfusion are sometimes interpreted as a clinical manifestation of reperfusion injury.

PREVENTION AND MANAGEMENT OF REPERFUSION INJURY

The prevention and management of ischemia/reperfusion injury are discussed in the following. Interventions to achieve these goals may be divided into those that are directed at managing the clinical manifestations of reperfusion injury, such as supporting contractility in the setting of myocardial stunning, treating reperfusion arrhythmias or limiting infarct size, and those interventions that are aimed at the prevention of the reperfusion injury itself. At present, all therapies in this latter category are investigational only.

General Interventions to Manage Complications of Ischemia/ Reperfusion Injury

Stunned Myocardium

Stunned myocardium can be prevented by avoiding the initial episode of ischemia. Stunning has been successfully treated by administering oxygen radical scavenging agents at the time of reperfusion. In addition, stunned myocardium can be overcome by using inotropic drugs. Because stunned myocardium is a transient phenomenon and responds to inotropic drugs, it can usually be managed in the clinical setting with appropriate titration of such drugs.

Reperfusion Arrhythmias

In general, reperfusion arrhythmias that occur in the setting of MI are amenable to therapy, and in most instances, are not a major clinical problem. Studies in our laboratory have shown that reperfusion-induced ventricular arrhythmias are responsive to treatment with lidocaine, sotalol, ranolazine, and postconditioning.[16,17]

Interventions Aimed at Reducing Microvascular Obstruction

In general, we have observed that most agents that reduce MI size also reduce the size of the no-reflow zone within the ischemic risk zone. A few therapies have been notable for their ability to reduce no-reflow, even when administered relatively late during the occlusion or even after reperfusion has begun.

Hypothermia

When hypothermia was introduced early during a coronary artery occlusion/reperfusion protocol in the rabbit, it reduced both MI size and the extent of the anatomic zone of no-reflow. When hypothermia was introduced 5 minutes before or 5 minutes after reperfusion, it failed to reduce MI size, but still reduced no-reflow. In one study, we introduced hypothermia as late as 30 minutes after reperfusion. Again, it had no effect on MI size, but it still reduced the area of no-reflow.[2,18]

Agents Influencing Free Radicals

Bendavia (Stealth Biotherapeutics, Newton, Mass.), a mitochondrial targeting peptide given at reperfusion, resulted in a nonsignificant trend toward reducing infarct size, but it also reduced the anatomic zone of no-reflow for any ischemic risk zone size.[19] The oxygen radical scavenging agents, superoxide dismutase plus catalase, which were given at reperfusion in our canine model of 2 hours of proximal coronary artery occlusion and 4 hours of reperfusion, did not reduce MI size, but it did reduce microvascular injury and also reduced low reflow. These studies all show that administering therapy at or close to the time of reperfusion, or even after reperfusion reduces no-reflow and microvascular injury, provides additional support for the concept that no-reflow is a true form of reperfusion injury.

Various therapies that have shown some success in improving low or no-reflow after cardiac catheterization include vasodilators (e.g., nitroprusside, adenosine, and calcium channel blockers) such as verapamil, diltiazem, and others.[14]

Interventions Aimed at Preventing Reperfusion Injury That Causes Cellular Necrosis

The primary treatment of acute STEMI should be early and complete reperfusion of the occluded culprit epicardial coronary artery (see Chapter 13). Reperfusion salvages tissue, has a substantial impact on infarct size, and improves clinical outcome. However, if the act of reperfusion also kills some population of cardiomyocytes that are hovering between life and death, then efforts to reduce this reperfusion injury might further improve outcome (Figure 24-5). Numerous clinical trials have attempted to further reduce MI size by administering adjunctive therapies near the time of reperfusion to mitigate reperfusion injury.[20–25] There is a long list of the agents that showed promise in preclinical trials but that failed in clinical trials. We have previously described these trials, and discussed reasons why these trials may have failed.[21–25]

Therapies that have been used clinically in an attempt to reduced MI size by inhibiting reperfusion injury have included oxygen radical scavengers, calcium blockers, and anti-inflammatory agents. Early studies with these and other agents primarily yielded negative results. One reason for the failure of early studies is likely that therapy was administered too late after reperfusion. In general, we have observed that most therapies aimed at reducing MI size work only when they are present early enough to protect the myocardium during at least a portion of the ischemic phase and are present at the moment of reperfusion. Because oxygen radical generation, sodium and calcium overload, and myocardial edema occur within seconds of the release of a coronary artery occlusion, therapies aimed at these adverse reperfusion phenomena must be present in the early phase of reperfusion to confer a benefit. Despite the substantial number of clinical trials that failed to show a benefit of strategies to reduce reperfusion injury, some studies have had more promising results.

Table 24-2[26–52] shows selected clinical trials that suggest that some, but not all, adjunctive agents and maneuvers administered near the time of reperfusion reduced MI size above and beyond reperfusion alone. In particular, administration of mitochondrial permeability transition pore closers (e.g., cyclosporine or postconditioning protocols, with brief

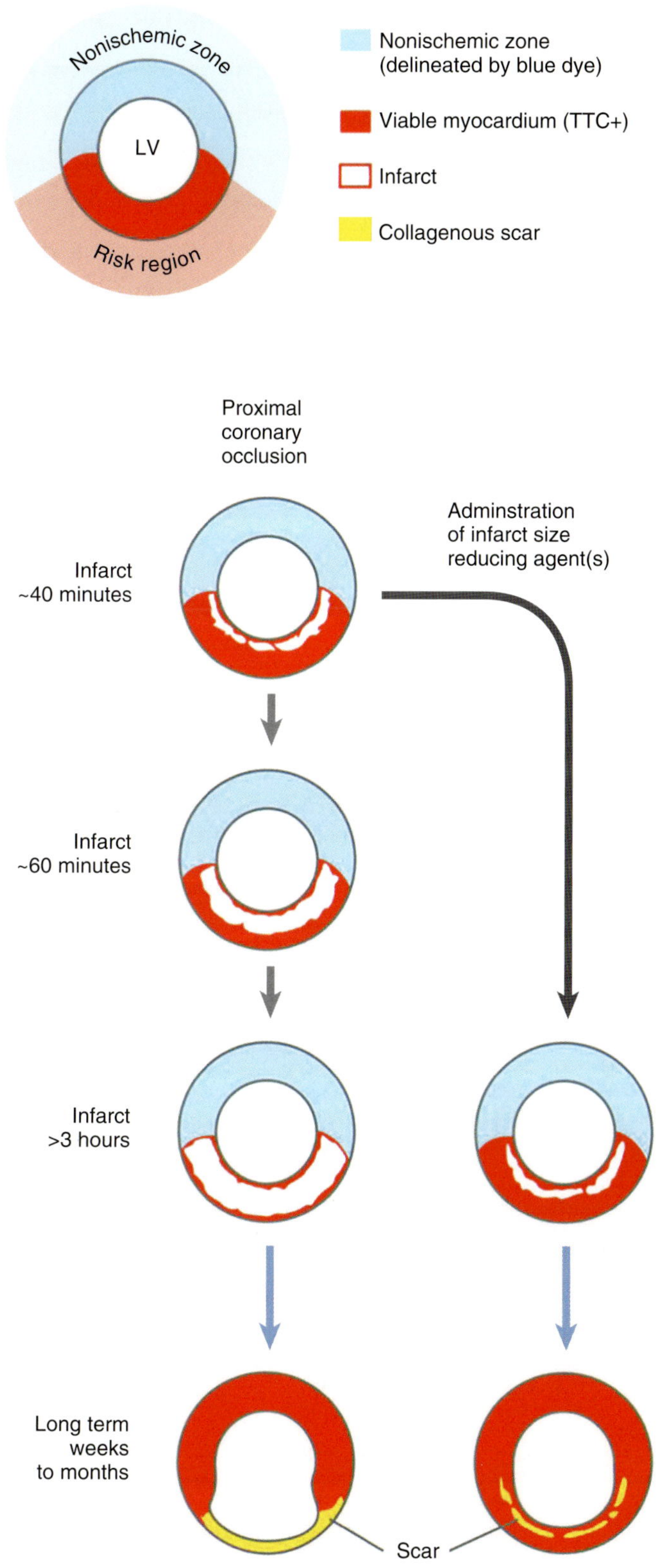

FIGURE 24-5 Schematic showing how reducing myocardial infarct size early could have a benefit on the long-term structure of the heart. *Top panel*, The wavefront concept of Reimer and Jennings. After proximal coronary occlusion, a portion of the left ventricle (LV) becomes ischemic, defined as the ischemic risk region. When a blue dye is injected into the vasculature, the blue dye circulates to areas receiving blood flow and fails to penetrate the ischemic zone. If reperfusion occurs after approximately 40 minutes of ischemia, irreversible myocardial damage (i.e., necrosis; *pale white areas*) is confined to the subendocardial myocardium. Viable myocardium within the risk zone is stained red by triphenyltretazolium chloride (TTC). If reperfusion is delayed (after 60 minutes) or after 3 to 6 hours, the extent of necrosis expands from the subendocardium to the mid-myocardium to the subepicardium within the ischemic risk zone. This development of necrosis becomes transmural or nearly transmural if reperfusion is not instituted within approximately 3 to 6 hours or if reperfusion does not occur. Large transmural infarcts may then go on to result in severe LV remodeling with infarct expansion, LV cavity dilation, LV aneurysm formation, and eccentric hypertrophy of the noninfarcted tissue (*bottom left*). If agents are administered to reduce infarct size or if early reperfusion is instituted, the size of the infarct can be limited (first transverse LV slice shown in the *right column*). During the long term, this smaller infarct will shrink in size with a minimum of subendocardial scar tissue and substantial viable tissue remaining in the mid-myocardial wall. LV remodeling will be minimized with less infarct wall thinning, less LV dilation, and less eccentric hypertrophy. In addition, LV function will be better preserved. *(From Kloner RA: Current state of clinical translation of cardioprotective agents for acute myocardial infarction.* Circ Res *113:451, 2013.)*

episodes of coronary artery reocclusion and reperfusion) or pharmacologic agents related to the Reperfusion Injury Salvage Kinase (RISK) pathway, given right at or shortly before reperfusion) have each markedly reduced MI size.[1] Some of these agents also appeared to improve clinical outcome. Because of these results, some experts have attributed up to 50% of all cell death associated with MI in the setting of ischemia/reperfusion as being caused by reperfusion, rather than ischemic damage.[1]

However, it is important to point out that in most studies, it is not possible to determine whether the benefits observed were because of a reduction in the initial ischemic damage, a reduction in reperfusion injury, or some combination of the two. In many of these studies, therapies were started before reperfusion (see Table 24-2); thus, therapies given during the later phase of an episode of ischemia might have conferred benefit by protecting the heart during critical phases of the ischemic insult, rather than by protecting the heart during the reperfusion phase alone. There are a few exceptions in which therapy did not commence until after reperfusion had begun. Selected interventions of particular interest in the evolution of this field are discussed in the following paragraphs.

Postconditioning

Postconditioning reduced MI size in at least three prospective trials.[26–28] Because of the timing of the intervention, postconditioning plausibly works only during the reperfusion phase. However, in other trials, postconditioning was ineffective.[29,30] In our own laboratory, although postconditioning was very effective at reducing reperfusion-induced ventricular arrhythmias, it was ineffective at reducing MI size.

Cyclosporin A

Both postconditioning and cyclosporine A are believed to prevent opening of the mitochondrial permeability transition pore during the early phase of reperfusion (see the section on Lethal Myocardial Cell Injury Caused by Reperfusion). The opening of this pore has been linked to mitochondrial damage and reperfusion injury (see Table 24-1). Early small studies with cyclosporine A suggested that administration of cyclosporine A at reperfusion reduced MI size, as assessed both by serial cardiac biomarkers of necrosis and by magnetic resonance imaging. However, in a study by Ghaffari and colleagues[31] in which cyclosporine A was administered just before fibrinolytic therapy in 101 patients with STEMI, no benefit was observed (see Table 24-2). A large randomized trial of cyclosporin A (n = ~975) in patients with STEMI called CIRCUS (Cyclosporin and Prognosis in Acute Myocardial Infarction Patients; NCT01502774) was recently reported as negative, with no clinical benefit of cyclosporin A.

TABLE 24-2 Examples of Major Clinical Studies of Pharmacological Interventions Aimed at Reducing Myocardial Infarct Size

INTERVENTION	TIME TREATMENT INITIATED	OUTCOME	TOTAL PATIENTS	REFERENCE
Cyclosporine-A	Immediately before thrombolytic therapy	Failed to reduce arrhythmias or myocardial enzyme release. In-hospital and 6-mo mortality rates similar.	101	Ghaffari S et al. 2013[31]
Exenatide	15 min before PCI	Infarct size normalized to risk area, assessed by imaging at 90 ± 21 days, 23% smaller than in placebo; 0.30 vs. 0.39; $P = 0.003$	172	Lonborg J et al. 2012[39]
Exenatide	Before PCI	Treatment increased salvage index in both hyperglycemic and normoglycemic patients.	210	Lonborg J et al. 2014[40]
Exenatide	Peri-PCI	Release of CK-MB and troponin I over 72 hrs were significantly reduced in treated group.	58	Woo JS et al. 2013[41]
Metoprolol	Before PCI	IS measured by imaging at 7 days 20% smaller in treated group ($P = .012$), as was IS assessed by CK-AUC release.	270	Ibanez B et al. 2013[34]
Atorvastatin	Before PCI	Treatment failed to decrease IS or improve cardiac function or microvascular perfusion	42	Post S et al. 2012[42]
Rosuvastatin (high vs. conventional dose)	Peri-PCI	Early high dose (40 mg + maintenance of 10 mg/day) did not reduce infarct volume vs. conventional dose (placebo + maintenance of 10 mg/day).	185	Ko YG et al. 2014[43]
Clopidogrel (600- vs. 300-mg loading doses)	Peri-PCI	IS assessed by CK release was significantly lower in the high-dose group (32%; $P = .0001$). Both microvascular perfusion and ejection fraction were better in the high-dose group.	201	Patti G et al. 2011[44]
Streptokinase as adjunct to PCI	Immediately after PCI	Coronary flow reserve at 2 days significantly better in streptokinase group ($P < .001$). At 6 months, IS (imaging) was smaller (22.7% vs. 32.9%; $P = .003$) and ejection fraction better in treated group.	95	Sezer M et al. 2009[45]
Erythropoietin	Before PCI	30% reduction in IS assessed by CK-MB release ($P = .025$)	30	Ferrario M et al. 2011[46]
Erythropoietin	Within 4 hrs reperfusion	Treatment did not reduce IS but was associated with a higher incidence of adverse cardiac events.	222	Najjar S et al. 2011[47]
Darbepoetin-α	Onset of reflow after PCI	Release of CK similar in treated and placebo groups	56	Roubille F et al. 2013[48]
Endothelin receptor blockade	Onset of PCI	Treatment with BQ-123 resulted in smaller enzymatic infarct sizes ($P = .014$)	57	Adlbrecht C et al. 2012[49]
FX06	At reperfusion after PCI	Necrotic core zone assessed at 5 days by imaging was reduced by 58% in the treated group, but no significant difference in troponin I levels	234	Atar D et al. 2009[50]
Intracoronary delivery of supersaturated oxygen	At PCI Pts within 6 hrs of onset of symptoms	Infarct size (imaging) was 20% in the treated group vs. 26.5% in controls ($P = .02$)	301	Stone GW et al. 2009[32]
Hypothermia	Core body temperature <35°C before reperfusion by PCI	38% reduction in IS (imaging) normalized to myocardium at risk in group treated by cold saline and endovascular cooling (29.8% vs. 48% in control; $P = .041$). Cumulative release of troponin T also lower in hypothermia group ($P = .03$)	20	Götberg M et al. 2010[51]
Hypothermia	Core body temperature 34.7°C before reperfusion by PCI	Pts in hypothermia group treated by cold saline and endovascular cooling. Mean IS (imaging) as percent of myocardium at risk was similar in both groups (40.5% in hypothermic group vs. 46.6% in control; $P = .15$). Post hoc analysis showed 33% IS reduction in early (<4 hr) anterior infarctions in hypothermia group.	120	Erlinge D et al. 2014[52]

AUC, Area under the curve; *CK*, creatine kinase; *IS*, infarct size; *MI*, myocardial infarction; *pts*, patients; *PCI*, percutaneous coronary intervention.

Bendavia

Bendavia is an agent that targets the inner mitochondrial membrane; it stabilizes the configuration of the election transport chain and reduces formation of reactive oxygen species during ischemia/reperfusion. When given before reperfusion, it resulted in a modest trend toward reduction of infarct size (~11%) in our rabbit model.[19] It resulted in an approximately18% reduction in infarct size in animals with ischemic risk zones of more than 20% ($P = .09$). Bendavia resulted in greater reductions in infarct size when administered at reperfusion in other models and in other laboratories (in guinea pig, sheep, rats, rabbits).[19] However, in a recent clinical trial, Bendavia did not significantly reduce infarct size.[53]

Other Pharmacotherapeutic Approaches

Therapeutic hyperoxemia in the Acute Myocardial Infarction with Hyperoxemic Therapy (AMIHOT) trial[32,33] and atrial natriuretic peptide[25] have been studied, with initiation commencing after reperfusion; both therapies demonstrated favorable effects. Therefore, the reported benefits of these agents would have to represent a reduction in lethal myocardial cell injury. We observed a signal that suggested that some salvaging of tissue occurred when olmesartan[54] was administered shortly before reperfusion. Because olmesartan was given 5 minutes before reperfusion, we could not rule out that some degree of salvage occurred because of cardioprotection during the last few minutes of ischemia. Similarly, therapies, such as remote preconditioning, hypothermia, adenosine, exenetide, glucose-insulin-potassium (GIK), intravenous cyclosporine, and metoprolol,[34–53] reduced infarct size and/or had beneficial clinical effects (see Table 24-2). However, because these agents were all initiated before reperfusion, at least some component of any benefit might have been caused by therapy during ischemia rather than during reperfusion alone.[25]

Hypothermia

Therapeutic hypothermia has consistently reduced MI size in our laboratory. However, it must be present during the ischemic phase, and an adequate degree of temperature reduction must be achieved before reperfusion for the intervention to be effective.[18] Studies in humans (see Table 24-2) also suggest that reducing core temperature to less than 35°C in anterior infarcts, coupled with timely reperfusion, may reduce MI size. The issue has been how to achieve rapid hypothermia. A technique called the Thermosuit (Life Recovery Systems, Kinnelon, N.J.) (already approved by the Food and Drug Administration to treat hyperthermia) uses immersion-convection cooling and is able to reduce core temperature to desired levels in humans in approximately 20 minutes. Therapeutic hypothermia attained using the Thermosuit technique remains the single most effective therapy for reducing infarct size in our laboratory.[18]

Importance of Timing of Administration

Despite the few apparent successes described previously, our group has observed less evidence for the ability of agents to reduce MI size when administered only at the time of reperfusion. Most cardioprotective agents that we have tested have required that the agent be present for at least a portion of the ischemic phase.[2,55] We have been unable to verify that postconditioning or oxygen radical scavengers given at reperfusion reduce MI size. Hypothermia reduced infarct size when present during at least the last one-third of the ischemic time, but when initiated after reperfusion had commenced, it failed to reduce infarct size, although it did reduce the zone of no-reflow.[2] Preliminary reports from the Consortium for Preclinical Assessment of Cardioprotective Therapies (CEASAR) group, which included a randomized, blinded, multicenter study, showed that sodium nitrite and the phosphodiesterase-5 inhibitor, sildenafil, failed to reduce MI size when administered shortly before reperfusion.[56,57]

Lessons Learned from Previous Studies

Whether adjunctive agents work only during ischemia, during reperfusion, or during both may not be such a crucial question. Therapies can be started either in the catheterization laboratory or emergency department before the infarct-related coronary artery is opened, ensuring that a portion of the ischemic period is treated. Some studies, such as those that evaluated remote ischemic preconditioning[37] and glucose-insulin-potassium,[38] have shown the feasibility of starting therapy even before a patient with acute MI is admitted to the hospital. Hence, adjunctive therapies could be instituted during the ischemic phase, the reperfusion phase, or both, protecting the patient from ischemia/reperfusion injury. In addition, it might be naive to think that only one adjunctive agent needs to be given to further protect against ischemia/reperfusion injury. For example, perhaps an intervention such as hypothermia or metropolol, which can reduce oxygen demand during ischemia, should be administered during the ischemic phase, and then a mitochondrial permeability transition pore closing agent, such as cyclosporine, or a mitochondrial protective agent that reduces generation of reactive oxygen species (e.g., Bendavia), should be given during the reperfusion phase. In other words, a cocktail of compounds might be needed to optimally reduce MI size. We observed that a combination of hypothermia, preconditioning, and sodium–hydrogen exchange inhibition profoundly reduced MI size to levels greater than what would have been expected with any of these agents given alone.

SUMMARY

Reperfusion injury in the setting of acute MI consists of four main components: (1) stunned myocardium; (2) reperfusion-induced arrhythmias; (3) no-reflow phenomenon (microvascular obstruction); and (4) lethal myocardial cell injury. Data supporting stunned myocardium, reperfusion-induced arrhythmias, and no-reflow as a form of reperfusion injury are solid. The importance of lethal myocardial cell injury caused by reperfusion remains controversial. However, despite improvements in reperfusion therapy, morbidity and mortality from MI are still unacceptable. There is still a need to further reduce MI size and no-reflow, which are both determinants of poor outcome following MI (see Chapter 13). The search for agents and therapies that reduce ischemic damage, reperfusion injury, or some combination of the two should continue to be of high priority to optimize outcome following MI.

References

1. Fröhlich GM, et al.: Myocardial reperfusion injury: looking beyond primary PCI, *Eur Heart J* 34:1714, 2013.
2. Hale SL, Herring MJ, Kloner RA: Delayed treatment with hypothermia protects against the no-reflow phenomenon despite failure to reduce infarct size, *J Am Heart Assoc* 2:e004234, 2013.
3. Pomblum VJ, et al.: Cardiac stunning in the clinic: the full picture, *Interact Cardiovasc Thorac Surg* 10:86, 2010.
4. Kumar S, et al.: Myocardial stunning is associated with impaired calcium uptake by sarcoplasmic reticulum, *Biochem Biophys Res Commun* 387:77–82, 2009.
5. Wittstein IS: Stress cardiomyopathy: a syndrome of catecholamine-mediated myocardial stunning? *Cell Mol Neurobiol* 32:847, 2012.
6. Majidi M, et al.: Reperfusion ventricular arrhythmia 'bursts' predict larger infarct size despite TIMI 3 flow restoration with primary angioplasty for anterior ST-elevation myocardial infarction, *Eur Heart J* 30:757, 2009.
7. Matsue Y, et al.: Clinical implications of an implantable cardioverter-defibrillator in patients with vasospastic angina and lethal ventricular arrhythmia, *J Am Coll Cardiol* 60:908, 2012.
8. Kloner RA: No-reflow phenomenon: maintaining vascular integrity, *J Cardiovasc Pharmacol Ther* 16:244, 2011.
9. Hale SL, Kloner RA: Dabigatran treatment: effects on infarct size and the no-reflow phenomenon in a model of acute myocardial ischemia/reperfusion, *J Thromb Thrombolysis* 39:50, 2015.
10. Kranenburg MV, et al.: Prognostic value of microvascular obstruction and infarct size, as measured by CMR in STEMI patients, *JACC Cardiovasc Imaging* 7:930, 2014.
11. Hamirani YS, et al.: Effect of microvascular obstruction and intramyocardial hemorrhage by CMR on LV remodeling and outcomes after myocardial infarction: a systematic review and meta-analysis, *JACC Cardiovasc Imaging* 7:940, 2014.
12. Niccoli G, et al.: Myocardial no-reflow in humans, *J Am Coll Cardiol* 54:281, 2009.
13. Ndrepepa G, et al.: 5-year prognostic value of no-reflow phenomenon after percutaneous coronary intervention in patients with acute myocardial infarction, *J Am Coll Cardiol* 55:2383, 2010.
14. Rezkalla SH, et al.: No-reflow phenomenon following percutaneous coronary intervention for acute myocardial infarction: incidence, outcome, and effect of pharmacologic therapy, *J Interv Cardiol* 23:429, 2010.
15. Jennings RB: Historical perspective on the pathology of myocardial ischemia/reperfusion injury, *Circ Res* 113:428, 2013.
16. Dhalla AK, et al.: Ranolazine, an antianginal agent, markedly reduces ventricular arrhythmias induced by ischemia and ischemia - reperfusion, *Am J Physiol Heart Circ Physiol* 297:H1923, 2009.
17. Kloner RA, Dow JS, Bhandari A: First direct comparison of the late sodium current blocker ranolazine to established antiarrhythmic agents in an ischemia/reperfusion model, *J Cardiovasc Pharmacol Ther* 16:192, 2011.

18. Herring MJ, et al.: Hypothermia in the setting of experimental acute myocardial infarction: A comprehensive review, *Ther Hypothermia Temp Manag* 4:159, 2014.
19. Kloner RA, et al.: Reduction of ischemia/reperfusion injury with Bendavia, a mitochondrial-targeting cytoprotective peptide, *J Am Heart Assoc* 1:e001644, 2012.
20. Ibáñez B, et al.: Evolving therapies for myocardial ischemia/reperfusion injury, *J Am Coll Cardiol* 65:1454, 2015.
21. Gerczuk PZ, Kloner RA: An update on cardioprotection: a review of the latest adjunctive therapies to limit myocardial infarction size in clinical trials, *J Am Coll Cardiol* 59:969, 2012.
22. Gerczuk PZ, Kloner RA: Protecting the heart from ischemia: an update on ischemic and pharmacologic conditioning, *Hosp Pract* 39(35):2011, 1995.
23. Kloner RA, Schwartz Longacre L: State of the science of cardio-protection: challenges and opportunities. Proceedings of the 2010 NHLBI Workshop on Cardio-protection, *J Cardiovasc Pharmacol Ther* 16:223, 2011.
24. Schwartz Longacre L, et al.: New horizons in cardioprotection. Recommendations from the 2010 National Heart, Lung, and Blood Institute Workshop, *Circulation* 124:1172, 2011.
25. Kloner RA: Current state of clinical translation of cardioprotective agents for acute myocardial infarction, *Circulation Research* 113:451, 2013.
26. Lønborg J, et al.: Cardioprotective effects of ischemic postconditioning in patients treated with primary percutaneous coronary intervention, evaluated by magnetic resonance, *Circ Cardiovasc Interv* 3:34, 2010.
27. Garcia S, et al.: Long-term follow-up of patients undergoing postconditioning during ST-elevation myocardial infarction, *J Cardiovasc Transl Res* 4:92, 2011.
28. Thuny F, et al.: Post-conditioning reduces infarct size and edema in patients with ST-segment elevation myocardial infarction, *J Am Coll Cardiol* 59:2175, 2012.
29. Khalili H, et al.: Surrogate and clinical outcomes following ischemic postconditioning during primary percutaneous coronary intervention of ST-segment elevation myocardial infarction: a meta-analysis of 15 randomized trials, *Catheter Cardiovasc Interv* 15(84):978, 2014.
30. Favaretto E, et al.: Meta-analysis of randomized trials of postconditioning in ST-elevation myocardial infarction, *Am J Cardiol* 114:946, 2014.
31. Ghaffari S, et al.: The effect of prethrombolytic cyclosporine-A injection on clinical outcome of acute anterior ST-elevation myocardial infarction, *Cardiovasc Ther* 31:e34, 2013.
32. Stone GW, et al.: AMIHOT-II Trial Investigators. Effect of supersaturated oxygen delivery on infarct size after percutaneous coronary intervention in acute myocardial infarction, *Circ Cardiovasc Interv* 2:366, 2009.
33. Sattur S, Brener SJ, Stone GW: Pharmacologic therapy for reducing myocardial infarct size in clinical trials: failed and promising approaches, *J Cardiovasc Pharmacol Ther* 20:21, 2015.
34. Ibanez B, et al.: Effect of early metoprolol on infarct size in ST-segment-elevation myocardial infarction patients undergoing primary percutaneous coronary intervention: the Effect of Metoprolol in Cardioprotection During an Acute Myocardial Infarction (METOCARD-CNIC) trial, *Circulation* 128:1495, 2013.
35. Pizarro G, et al.: Long-term benefit of early pre-reperfusion metoprolol administration in patients with acute myocardial infarction: results from the METOCARD-CNIC trial (Effect of Metoprolol in Cardioprotection During an Acute Myocardial Infarction), *J Am Coll Cardiol* 63:2356, 2014.
36. Mateos A, et al.: METOCARD-CNIC Investigators. Efficacy and safety of out-of-hospital intravenous metoprolol administration in anterior ST-segment elevation acute myocardial infarction: insights from the METOCARD-CNIC Trial, *Ann Emerg Med* 65:318, 2015.
37. Bøtker HE, et al.: Remote ischaemic conditioning before hospital admission, as a complement to angioplasty, and effect on myocardial salvage in patients with acute myocardial infarction: a randomised trial, *Lancet* 375:727, 2010.
38. Selker HP, et al.: Out-of-hospital administration of intravenous glucose-insulin-potassium in patients with suspected acute coronary syndromes: the IMMEDIATE randomized controlled trial, *JAMA* 307:1925, 2012.
39. Lonborg J, et al.: Exenatide reduces reperfusion injury in patients with ST-segment elevation myocardial infarction, *Eur Heart J* 33:149, 2012.
40. Lonborg J, et al.: Impact of acute hyperglycemia on myocardial infarct size, area at risk, and salvage in patients with STEMI and the association with exenatide treatment: results from a randomized study, *Diabetes* 63:2474, 2014.
41. Woo JS, et al.: Cardioprotective effects of exenatide in patients with ST-segment-elevation myocardial infarction undergoing primary percutaneous coronary intervention: results of exenatide myocardial protection in revascularization study, *Arterioscler Thromb Vasc Biol* 33:2252, 2013.
42. Post S, et al.: Early statin treatment prior to primary PCI for acute myocardial infarction: REPERATOR, a randomized placebo-controlled pilot trial, *Catheter Cardiovasc Interv* 80:756, 2012.
43. Ko YG, et al.: Efficacy of early intensive rosuvastatin therapy in patients with ST-segment elevation myocardial infarction undergoing primary percutaneous coronary intervention (ROSEMARY Study). *Am J Cardiol* 114:29, 2014.
44. Patti G, et al.: Outcome comparison of 600- and 300-mg loading doses of clopidogrel in patients undergoing primary percutaneous coronary intervention for ST-segment elevation myocardial infarction: results from the ARMYDA-6 MI (Antiplatelet therapy for Reduction of MYocardial Damage during Angioplasty-Myocardial Infarction) randomized study, *J Am Coll Cardiol* 58:1592, 2011.
45. Sezer M, et al.: Effect of intracoronary streptokinase administered immediately after primary percutaneous coronary intervention on long-term left ventricular infarct size, volumes, and function, *J Am Coll Cardiol* 54:1065, 2009.
46. Ferrario M, et al.: High-dose erythropoietin in patients with acute myocardial infarction: a pilot, randomised, placebo-controlled study, *Int J Cardiol* 147:124, 2011.
47. Najjar SS, et al.: Intravenous erythropoietin in patients with ST-segment elevation myocardial infarction: REVEAL: a randomized controlled trial, *JAMA* 305:1863, 2011.
48. Roubille F, et al.: Intracoronary administration of darbepoetin-alpha at onset of reperfusion in acute myocardial infarction: results of the randomized Intra-Co-EpoMI trial, *Arch Cardiovasc Dis* 106:135, 2013.
49. Adlbrecht C, et al.: Systemic endothelin receptor blockade in ST-segment elevation acute coronary syndrome protects the microvasculature: a randomised pilot study, *EuroIntervention* 7:1386, 2012.
50. Atar D, et al.: Effect of intravenous FX06 as an adjunct to primary percutaneous coronary intervention for acute ST-segment elevation myocardial infarction results of the F.I.R.E. (Efficacy of FX06 in the Prevention of Myocardial Reperfusion Injury) trial, *J Am Coll Cardiol* 53:720, 2009.
51. Götberg M, et al.: A pilot study of rapid cooling by cold saline and endovascular cooling before reperfusion in patients with ST-elevation myocardial infarction, *Circ Cardiovasc Interv* 3:400, 2010.
52. Erlinge D, et al.: Rapid endovascular catheter core cooling combined with cold saline as an adjunct to percutaneous coronary intervention for the treatment of acute myocardial infarction The CHILL-MI trial: a randomized controlled study of the use of central venous catheter core cooling combined with cold saline as an adjunct to percutaneous coronary intervention for the treatment of acute myocardial infarction, *J Am Coll Cardiol* 63:1857, 2014.
53. Gibson CM, et al.: EMBRACE STEMI study: a phase 2a trial to evaluate the safety, tolerability, and efficacy of intravenous MTP-131 on reperfusion injury in patients undergoing primary percutaneous coronary intervention, *Eur Heart J* 37:1296-1303, 2016.
54. Dai W, et al.: Cardioprotective effects of angiotensin II type 1 receptor blockade with olmesartan on reperfusion injury in a rat myocardial ischemia reperfusion model, *Cardiovasc Ther* 28:30, 2010.
55. Herring MJ, et al.: Rapid induction of hypothermia by the Thermosuit system profoundly reduces infarct size and anatomic zone of no-reflow following ischemia/reperfusion in rabbit and rat hearts, *J Cardiovasc Pharmacol Ther* 20:193, 2015.
56. Lefer D, et al.: Sodium nitrite fails to limit myocardial infarct size: results from the CAESAR Cardioprotection Consortium, *FASEB J* 28(Supplement, LB645), 2014.
57. Kukreja R, et al.: Administration of sildenafil at reperfusion fails to reduce infarct size: results from the CAESAR Cardioprotection Consortium, *FASEB J* 28(Supplement, LB650), 2014.

25 Heart Failure and Cardiogenic Shock After Myocardial Infarction

David A. Morrow and Erin A. Bohula

INTRODUCTION

Myocardial infarction (MI) is defined by myocyte necrosis. If large in its territory or critical in its location, this injury can lead to loss of contractile function or other structural complications (see Chapter 26) that result in insufficient cardiac output and consequent heart failure or cardiogenic shock. Despite significant advancements in the acute management of MI, incident heart failure still occurs in 10% to 30% of patients during the initial hospitalization for acute MI and is associated with at least a two-fold higher adjusted risk of in-hospital death compared to patients without heart failure.[1,2] Cardiogenic shock occurs in aproximately 5% to 7% of patients presenting with an acute MI and carries a substantial 40% to 60% mortality rate.[3,4]

This chapter reviews the current understanding of the epidemiology, pathophysiology, evaluation, and management of heart failure and cardiogenic shock after MI. The mechanical complications of MI are detailed in Chapter 26. The implementation of mechanically assisted circulatory support for cardiogenic shock after MI is discussed in Chapter 27.

Defining and Classifying Heart Failure and Cardiogenic Shock

Heart failure after MI is a clinical syndrome typically defined by evidence of pulmonary venous or central venous congestion. Cardiogenic shock is characterized by congestion and inadequate tissue or end-organ perfusion secondary to cardiac insufficiency. This reduction in perfusion results in decreased oxygen and nutrient delivery to tissues, which, if severe or protracted, can lead to multiorgan dysfunction and death. Generally accepted criteria for shock include (1) frank or relative hypotension defined by a systolic blood pressure below 80 or 90 mm Hg or by a reduction in mean arterial pressure of 30 mm Hg; (2) inadequate cardiac index defined as below 1.8 L/min/m^2 without mechanical or pharmacologic support or less than 2.2 L/min/m^2 with support; (3) elevated end-diastolic pressures on the right (greater than 10 to 15 mm Hg) and/or left (greater than 18 mm Hg) side of the heart; and (4) evidence of end-organ hypoperfusion.[5] End-organ hypoperfusion may manifest as altered mental status, decreased urine output, acute kidney injury, cool or mottled extremities, acute liver injury, or lactic acidosis.

Heart failure and cardiogenic shock can be categorized by severity using one of several classification systems (Table 25-1). The Killip classification system, derived specifically in patients with acute MI, is defined by physical examination findings consistent with heart failure.[6] Killip class I is characterized by an absence of heart failure; class II is consistent with mild to moderate heart failure (S_3 gallop, pulmonary rales, or jugular venous distention); class III heart failure includes overt pulmonary edema; and class IV is defined as cardiogenic shock. The Killip classification has a strong graded relationship with mortality after acute MI, in that patients with class II or III heart failure have a 4-fold increased risk of in-hospital death, and those with cardiogenic shock, a 10-fold increased risk.[2] The New York Heart Association (NYHA) system describes a functional or symptomatic status, whereby classes I to IV are defined by the spectrum of no symptomatic limitation of physical activity (NYHA class I), slight limitation (NYHA class II), marked limitation without symptoms at rest (NYHA class III) and symptoms with minimal exertion or symptoms at rest (NYHA class IV), respectively. NYHA class also is a marker of heart failure severity and therefore is associated with survival.[6] Finally, investigators with the Interagency Registry of Mechanically Assisted Circulatory Support (*INTERMACS*) developed a classification system based on combination of signs, symptoms and level of therapeutic support, with the goal of refining the description of NYHA class III-IV and shock patients to best define populations that would benefit from advanced therapies such as pacing, cardiac transplantation, and mechanical circulatory support (MCS).[7] The INTERMACS profiles (Table 25-1) range from NYHA class III (INTERMACS 7), exertion-limited, exertion-intolerant, symptoms at rest, stable but inotrope-dependent, progressive decline on inotropes, to critical cardiogenic shock (INTERMACS 1).

TABLE 25-1 Heart Failure and Cardiogenic Shock Classification Systems

CLASSIFICATION SYSTEM	DEFINITION
Killip	
Class I	No evidence of heart failure
Class II	Mild to moderate heart failure, including S_3 gallop, rales auscultated over less than one half of the posterior lung fields, or jugular venous distention
Class III	Overt pulmonary edema
Class IV	Cardiogenic shock
NYHA	
Class I	No limitation of physical activity
Class II	Slight limitation of physical activity; comfortable at rest, but ordinary physical activity results in symptoms of heart failure
Class III	Marked limitation of physical activity; comfortable at rest, but less than ordinary activity causes symptoms of heart failure
Class IV	Unable to carry on any physical activity without symptoms of heart failure or symptoms of heart failure at rest
INTERMACS	
Profile 1	Critical cardiogenic shock ("crash and burn"); life-threatening hypotension despite rapidly escalating inotropic support
Profile 2	Progressive decline ("sliding on inotropes"); declining function despite intravenous inotropic support
Profile 3	Stable but inotrope-dependent ("dependent stability"); stable blood pressure, organ function, and symptoms on continuous intravenous inotropic support or temporary circulatory support or both with repeated failure to wean
Profile 4	Resting symptoms; stabilized close to normal volume status but experiences daily symptoms at rest or during activities of daily living (ADLs)
Profile 5	Exertion intolerant ("housebound"); comfortable at rest or with ADLs, symptoms with any further activity
Profile 6	Exertion limited ("walking wounded"); fatigues after first few minutes of anything beyond minor activity
Profile 7	Advanced NYHA III

INTERMACS, Interagency Registry of Mechanically Assisted Circulatory Support; *NYHA,* New York Heart Association.

EPIDEMIOLOGY AND OUTCOMES

Left ventricular failure is the predominant mechanism of cardiac insufficiency in approximately 75% of patients in whom shock develops after MI (Figure 25-1).[8] Mechanical causes of heart failure and shock (see Chapter 26), including ventricular septal rupture, severe mitral regurgitation, and free wall rupture with tamponade, account for 12% of cases, and predominant right ventricular failure, another 3%.

Incidence and Risk Factors

Depending on the characteristics of the study population and heart failure definitions applied, the incidence of new-onset heart failure after acute MI is estimated at 10% to 30%.[1] For example, in four major trials of fibrinolysis, 13% of the 61,041 patients presenting with ST-elevation MI (STEMI) had heart failure without shock on admission, and 29% had heart failure that emerged some time during admission. Of 13,707 patients in the Global Registry of Acute Coronary Events (GRACE) registry without previous heart failure or cardiogenic shock, 13% of patients presenting with an acute coronary syndrome had Killip class II or III heart failure, and heart failure developed in an additional 5% during the initial hospitalization.[9]

The available data are conflicting regarding the trends in incident heart failure without shock after acute MI, with some evidence to support a decrease in early heart failure due to improved reperfusion strategies, but an increase in chronic heart failure rates due to increased survival of patients with substantial left ventricular damage.[1] For example, investigators with the GRACE registry found that with increasing rates of percutaneous coronary intervention (PCI) and evidence-based pharmacotherapies, rates of incident heart failure decreased by 9% in patients with STEMI and by 6.9% in patients with non–ST-elevation MI (NSTEMI) between 1999 and 2006. In this registry, predictors of incident heart failure in the setting of acute coronary syndromes included older age, prior MI, atherosclerotic disease in non-coronary vascular beds, presentation with an MI (versus unstable angina), diabetes, and increased heart rate.[9] Other studies have identified left ventricular systolic dysfunction and infarct size as predictors of new-onset heart failure after MI.[10,11]

The incidence of cardiogenic shock complicating acute MI has been declining, a trend that also may relate to increased use of more efficacious reperfusion strategies (see Chapter 13). For example, in a registry of 13,663 residents of Worcester, Massachusetts, hospitalized with acute MI, the incidence of cardiogenic shock decreased from 7.3% in 1975 to approximately 5% in 2005[4] (Figure 25-2). Similarly, an analysis of data for 7,531 patients from three French registries reported that the incidence decreased from 6.9% in 1995 to 5.7% in 2005; a period over which the rate of PCI increased dramatically.[3]

Cardiogenic shock occurs more frequently in the setting of STEMI than NSTEMI, with estimated rates of 5% to 8% and 2% to 3%, respectively.[5] Other risk factors for the development of cardiogenic shock, identified in French and Danish registries, include older age, female sex, hypertension, diabetes, previous MI, heart failure, anterior MI, left bundle branch block, and reduced left ventricular systolic function.[3,5]

Outcomes with Heart Failure and Cardiogenic Shock

As noted, heart failure without cardiogenic shock continues to be a common complication of acute MI and portends a worse prognosis. In the previously described GRACE registry of 13,707 patients with ACS without shock or previous heart failure, presentation with heart failure or development of heart failure after admission identified patients with markedly higher in-hospital mortality than that for patients without heart failure (12.0% versus 17.8% versus 2.8%; $P < .0001$), representing a greater than two-fold increased risk after adjustment for other predictors of mortality.[9] Analysis of data for 3,343 patients with STEMI in the Harmonizing Outcomes with Revascularization and Stents in Acute Myocardial Infarction (HORIZONS-AMI) trial revealed that development of new-onset heart failure was associated not only with higher mortality but also with increased risk for recurrent MI, stent thrombosis, and need for coronary revascularization.[11]

Cardiogenic shock is a relatively infrequent complication of acute MI, but the mortality rate associated with the

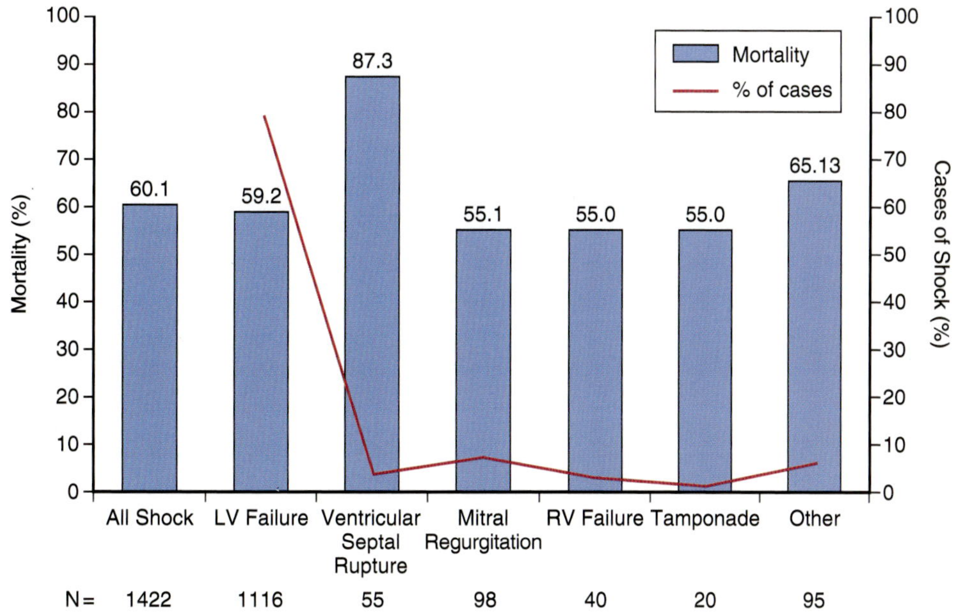

FIGURE 25-1 Mortality by etiology of cardiogenic shock following acute myocardial infarction (AMI). In-hospital mortality rates *(bars, left axis)* are shown for various primary etiologic conditions associated with death due to cardiogenic shock after AMI: left ventricular (LV) failure, ventricular septal rupture (VSR), acute severe mitral regurgitation (MR), isolated right ventricular (RV) failure, cardiac tamponade/rupture (tamp), and "other" (includes previous severe valvular heart disease and excessive beta or calcium channel blockade). The proportion of patients in each category is shown *(line graph, right axis). (Adapted from Hochman JS, Buller CE, Sleeper LA, et al: Cardiogenic shock complicating acute myocardial infarction—etiologies, management and outcome: a report from the SHOCK Trial Registry. SHould we emergently revascularize Occluded Coronaries for cardiogenic shocK?* J Am Coll Cardiol *36(3 Suppl A):1063-1070, 2000.)*

condition is staggeringly high. Although in-hospital mortality rates have decreased, from 70% to 80% in the 1970s to approximately 40% to 60% currently, cardiogenic shock remains the major cause of death among patients hospitalized with acute MI (see Figure 25-2).[3,4] The improvement in mortality over time is certainly multifactorial. During this period, multiple medical therapies that reduce the rate of recurrent cardiovascular events have been incorporated into standard practice, including lipid-lowering therapies, β-adrenergic blockade (beta-blockade), inhibition of the renin-angiotensin-aldosterone system (RAAS), and use of potent antiplatelet agents (see Chapter 13).[12,13] In addition, the options for and prioritization of reperfusion strategies for acute coronary syndromes have advanced significantly.

Mortality Risk Prediction

Clinical predictors of higher mortality rates among patients with shock include delayed or inadequate revascularization, older age, anoxic brain injury, lower left ventricular ejection fraction, low systolic blood pressure, vasopressor requirements, renal dysfunction, elevated lactate levels, and complicated coronary disease, such as left main artery or three-vessel disease.[5,14-16] Of interest, outcomes are relatively similar in patients with cardiogenic shock after STEMI and in those after NSTEMI, and also for cardiogenic shock due to predominant left ventricular failure and that due to right ventricular failure.[5] A depressed cardiac power output, defined as the product of mean arterial pressure and cardiac output, was found to be the strongest, most independent hemodynamic predictor of in-hospital mortality in the Should We Emergently Revascularize Occluded Coronaries for Cardiogenic Shock? (SHOCK) trial.[5] Biomarkers of inflammation, such as interleukin-6 (IL-6), and of microcirculatory dysfunction or vascular leakage (angiopoietins) also have been associated with poorer prognosis and higher mortality in these patients but are not currently used for clinical risk stratification.[17,18]

PATHOPHYSIOLOGY

The pathophysiology of cardiogenic shock is complex and dynamic, involving adaptive and maladaptive compensatory mechanisms coordinated by multiple organ systems.

Hemodynamic Considerations

The multiple myocardial and vascular parameters that determine stroke volume and work are represented in the left ventricular pressure-volume loops (Figure 25-3A).[19] The left ventricular end-diastolic pressure is a function of the end-diastolic volume and myocardial compliance, represented by the end-diastolic pressure-volume relationship (EDPVR). The difference between the end-diastolic and end-systolic volume represents the stroke volume and area contained in the pressure-volume loop, the stroke work. The timing of the events in the cycle is determined by both myocardial and vascular characteristics. For example, the load-independent left ventricular contractility (E_{max}), described by the end-systolic pressure-volume relationship (ESPVR) across the range of loading conditions, and the effective arterial elastance (E_a) define the timing of aortic valve closure and thus of end systole. E_a is a measure of arterial loading, approximated as the ratio of end-systolic pressure and stroke volume and is influenced by peripheral resistance, vascular compliance and impedance, and systolic and diastolic time intervals. Stroke work or left ventricular pump efficiency is maximal when the ratio of effective arterial elastance and left ventricular contractility (E_a/E_{max}) approaches 1.

In the setting of an acute MI, left ventricular contractility is reduced through myocardial necrosis and stunning, thereby shifting the ESPVR down, and reducing stroke volume (see Figure 25-3B). In many cases, myocardial compliance decreases as well, shifting the EDPVR up, leading to an increase in left ventricular end-diastolic pressure for

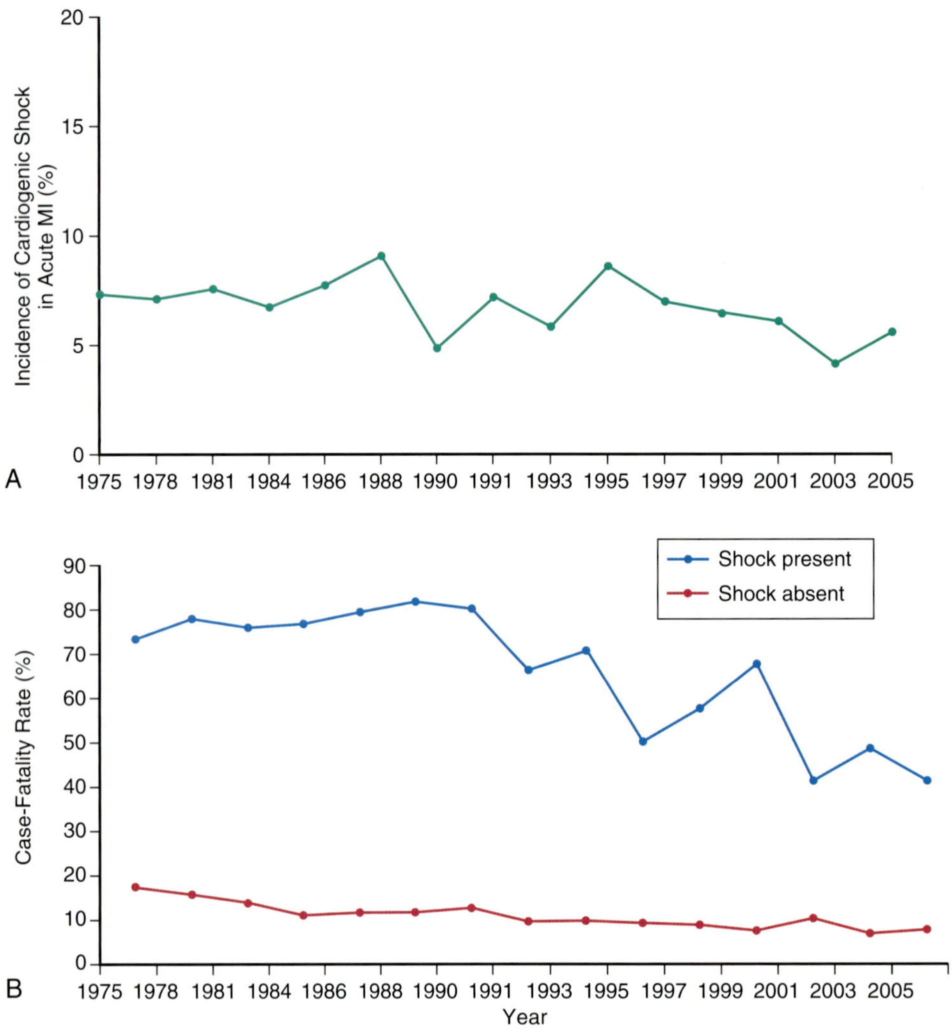

FIGURE 25-2 Trends in the incidence and case fatality rates of cardiogenic shock complicating acute myocardial infarction (MI). Registry data for 13,663 patients hospitalized with acute MI in Worcester, Massachusetts, from 1975 to 2005 demonstrated a small but significant decline in the incidence of cardiogenic shock complicating acute MI over time (**A**), as well as a decrease in the case-fatality rate in patients in whom cardiogenic shock develops (**B**). *(From Goldberg RJ, Spencer FA, Gore JM, et al: Thirty-year trends (1975 to 2005) in the magnitude of, management of, and hospital death rates associated with cardiogenic shock in patients with acute myocardial infarction: a population-based perspective.* Circulation *119:1211-1219, 2009.)*

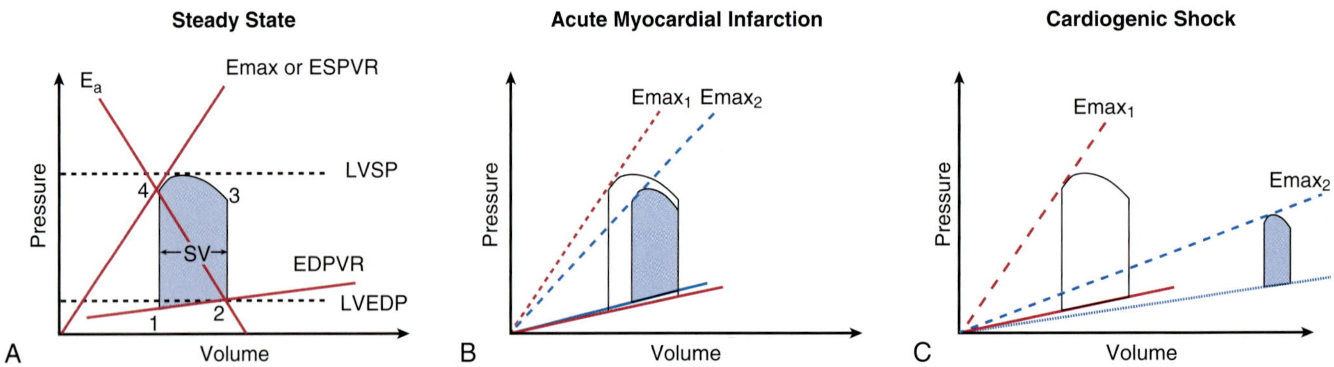

FIGURE 25-3 Normal and pathologic pressure-volume loops. Each pressure-volume loop represents one cardiac cycle. **(A)** In the normal steady state, left ventricular filling occurs at the end of isovolumic relaxation (period between points 4 and 1) on opening of the mitral valve (point 1 on the diagram). The left ventricular end-diastolic pressure (LVEDP) is a function of the end-diastolic volume and myocardial compliance, represented by the end-diastolic pressure-volume relationship (EDPVR). Once left ventricular volume is maximal at end-diastole (point 2), isovolumic contraction (period between points 2 and 3) begins. Systolic ejection occurs when left ventricular pressure exceeds aortic pressure, leading to aortic valve opening (point 3), and continues until the point at which aortic pressure exceeds the left ventricular pressure, the end-systolic pressure-volume point (point 4). The difference between the end-diastolic and end-systolic volumes represents the stroke volume (SV) and area contained in the pressure-volume loop, the stroke work. *LVSP,* left ventricular systolic pressure. **(B)** In the setting of an acute myocardial infarction, left ventricular contractility is reduced, shifting the ESPVR down and reducing SV. In addition, a decrease in myocardial compliance may lead to an increase in LVEDP. **(C)** In cardiogenic shock, left ventricular contractility and SV are severely reduced, and LVEDP is increased. *(Adapted from Rihal CS, Naidu SS, Givertz MM, et al: 2015 SCAI/AC/HFSA/STS Clinical Expert Consensus Statement.* J Am Coll Cardiol *65(19):e7-e26, 2015.)*

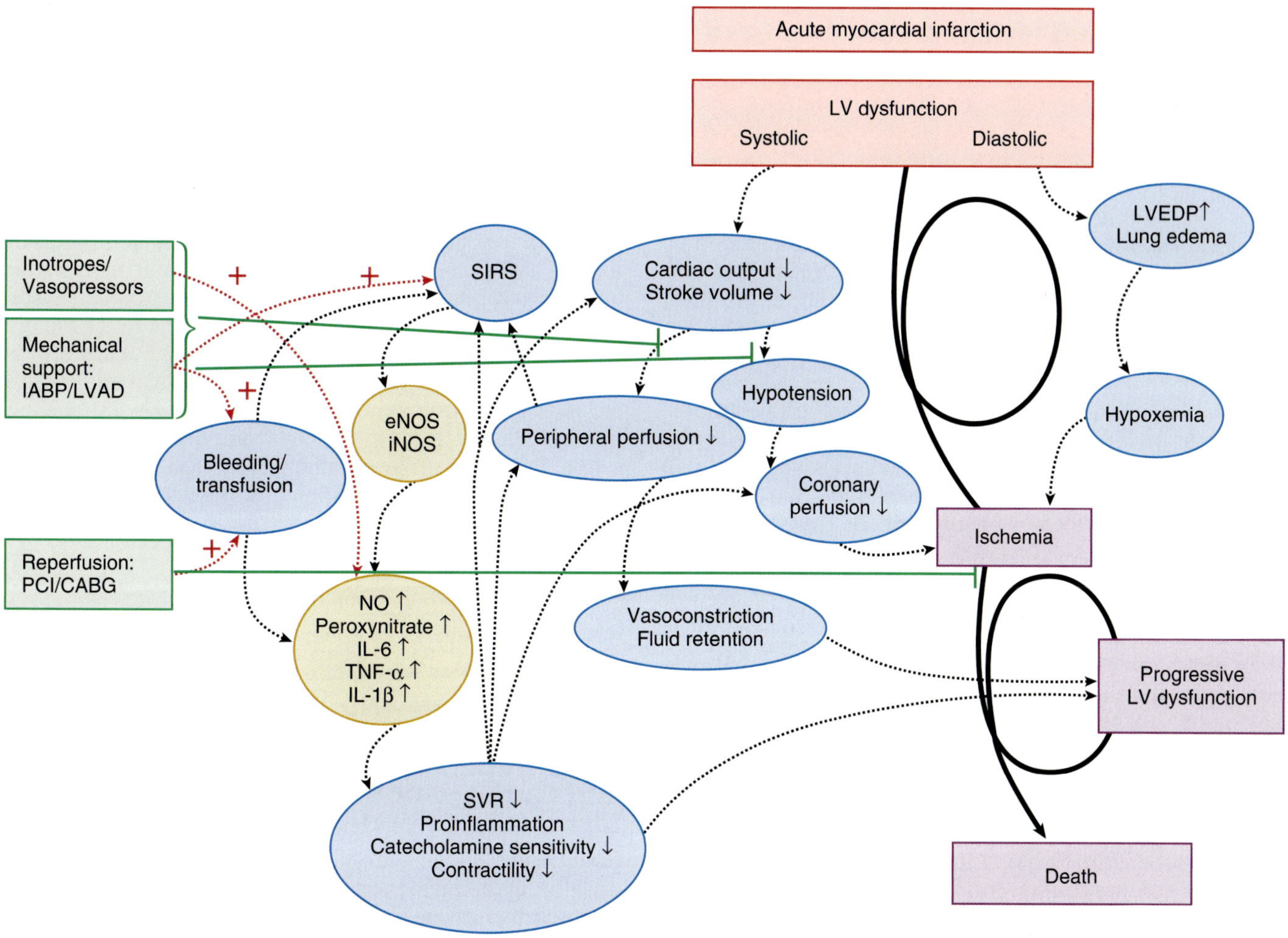

FIGURE 25-4 **Pathophysiology of cardiogenic shock.** The classic shock spiral following acute myocardial infarction involves left ventricular dysfunction, leading to further ischemia, progressive ventricular dysfunction and death. Systolic dysfunction results in insufficient cardiac output, hypotension, and peripheral and coronary hypoperfusion, with subsequent ischemia. Diastolic dyfunction results in pulmonary congestion, hypoxemia, and additional ischemia. Finally, a systemic inflammatory response leads to inappropriate vasodilation with further hypotension, hypoperfusion, and ischemia, as well as direct myocardial suppression, leading to worsened ventricular dysfunction. Several therapeutic strategies aim to abort this spiral through improvement in coronary perfusion (revascularization), myocardial contractility (inotropes), and peripheral perfusion (vasopressors and mechanical circulatory support). These therapeutic interventions also may contribute to bleeding, infection, and exacerbation of the systemic inflammatory response syndrome (SIRS). *eNOS,* Endothelial nitric oxide synthase; *IABP/LVAD,* intra-aortic ballooon pump/left ventricular assist device; *IL-6,* interleukin-6; *iNOS,* inducible nitric oxide synthase; *LV,* left ventricular; *LVEDP,* LV end-diastolic pressure; *NO,* nitric oxide; *PCI/CABG,* percutaneous coronary intervention/coronary artery bypass grafting; *SVR,* systemic vascular resistance; *TNF-α,* tumor necrosis factor-alpha. *(Adapted from Reynolds HR, Hochman JS: Cardiogenic shock: current concepts and improving outcomes.* Circulation *117(5):686-697, 2008.)*

a given volume. If severe, these acute alterations in systolic and diastolic function can lead to decreased cardiac output and stroke work and increased pulmonary congestion, resulting in clinical heart failure.

In the extreme case of these perturbations (Figure 25-3C), left ventricular contractile function is severely reduced and left ventricular end-diastolic volume and pressures are significantly increased, culminating in cardiogenic shock. Without appropriate interventions, cardiogenic shock begets worsened cardiogenic shock and death (Figure 25-4). That is, the shock state, defined by inadequate cardiac output and congestion, results in a cascade of events that reinforce and exacerbate the underlying pathology of ischemia and progressive left ventricular dysfunction (see also Figure 27-1).

Impact of Altered Hemodynamics

The primary insult, myocyte necrosis in the setting of an acute MI, results in reduced myocardial contractility and systolic dysfunction. The resultant reduction in cardiac output leads to hypotension and peripheral hypoperfusion. Hypotension can promote further ischemia and myocardial depression through decreased coronary perfusion, which can be exacerbated by atherosclerotic lesions in non-culprit coronary vessels (Figure 25-4). In an attempt to maintain perfusion to vital organs, the body releases endogenous catecholamines (e.g., norepinephrine) and other vasopressors (e.g., angiotensin II). These catecholamines and vasoconstrictors may mediate improved blood pressure through increased systemic vascular resistance (SVR) as well as myocardial contractility; however, this increase in blood pressure may come at the cost of increased myocardial oxygen demand resulting from increased afterload and heart rate, promoting further ischemia. Hypoperfusion also activates the neurohormonal cascade, resulting in sodium and fluid retention, thereby increasing perfusion through increased intravascular volume. In the setting of diastolic dysfunction, however, this compensatory response can lead to a greater elevation of left ventricular end-diastolic pressures, translating to more pulmonary edema and hypoxemia with further ischemia and progressive left ventricular dysfunction.

Vasodilatory and Inflammatory Response in Cardiogenic Shock

In addition to the critical myocardial hemodynamic changes, cardiogenic shock can be complicated by development of a systemic inflammatory response syndrome (SIRS). The development of SIRS is more common with a longer duration of shock and often is not associated with superimposed infection.[5] For example, approximately 20% of patients enrolled in the SHOCK trial had suspected sepsis. Only three quarters of those patients ultimately had positive blood cultures, however, and the vasodilatory state generally preceded bacteremia by several days, suggesting an earlier noninfectious inflammatory process.

Several mechanisms may be contributors to this vasodilatory state, including (1) the development of a vasopressin deficiency, (2) activation of ATP-sensitive potassium (K_{ATP}) channels on vascular smooth muscle, and (3) release of inflammatory cytokines.[5,20] Vasopressin, or antidiuretic hormone, promotes vasoconstriction, free water absorption, decreased plasma osmolality, and increased blood volume. It is secreted in response to increased plasma osmolality, angiotensin II, cardiac wall stress, and adrenergic stimuli.[21] Vasopressin levels are notably lower in vasodilatory shock after cardiopulmonary bypass or ventricular assist device placement, possibly as a result of depletion of neurohypophyseal stores. Patients in this setting tend to respond with brisk increases in arterial pressure with vasopressin administration, even when refractory to catecholamines.[20]

K_{ATP} channels on vascular smooth muscle allow for efflux of potassium, resulting in cellular hyperpolarization, decreased calcium influx, and vasodilation.[20] A number of factors present during shock contribute to K_{ATP} channel activation, including acidosis (e.g., hydrogen ion and lactate), decreased energy stores, reduced vasopressin levels, and increased atrial natriuretic peptide and nitric oxide levels.

Inflammatory cytokines are elevated in the setting of cardiogenic shock complicating acute MI—a phenomenon that is even more pronounced in the subset of patients with SIRS.[17,22] These cytokines, particularly IL-6 and tumor necrosis factor-alpha (TNF-α), are believed to promote progressive shock through a number of mechanisms. IL-6 and TNF-α stimulate expression of inducible nitric oxide synthase (iNOS). Increased iNOS results in higher levels of nitric oxide, which in turn cause inappropriate vasodilation through induction of soluble guanylate cyclase and increased cyclic guanosine monophosphate (cGMP), as well as activation of K_{ATP} channels in vascular smooth muscle. This cascade of inflammatory activation drives progressive hypotension with worsened peripheral and coronary hypoperfusion and, as a result, further myocardial depression and worsened shock. Nitric oxide exerts additional negative effects by promoting further release of inflammatory cytokines, induction of DNA damage through generation of peroxynitrite, suppression of mitochondrial respiration, and reduced contractility as a result of decreased calcium release from the sarcoplasmic reticulum.[22,23] IL-6 also may contribute to myocardial depression through downregulation of sarcoplasmic reticulum calcium ATPase (SERCA2) and myosin expression, upregulation of the IL-6 receptor, and generation of oxygen free radicals secondary to increased xanthine oxidase activity.[23]

The inflammatory cascade in cardiogenic shock is thought to be driven by myocyte necrosis, as well as hypoxemia and hypoperfusion of other tissues, most notably the gut.[5,24] Intestinal ischemia–reperfusion is believed to lead to increased intestinal permeability, bacterial translocation and endotoxin release, and, in a subset, development of bacteremia and sepsis. Endotoxin, a lipopolysaccharide (LPS) found in the cell walls of gram-negative bacteria, binds to Toll-like receptors on macrophages, resulting in production of inflammatory cytokines, including TNF and the interleukins IL-1β and IL-6. The link between intestinal hypoperfusion and endotoxin is supported by a study demonstrating a correlation between biomarkers of intestinal injury, including urinary intestinal fatty acid–binding protein (IFABP) and plasma citrulline, and endotoxin levels in 21 patients with out-of-hospital cardiac arrest (OHCA).[25] Furthermore, those patients with post-arrest shock demonstrated increasing levels of endotoxin over time, and those without shock had decreasing levels in the days after the arrest. In this setting, high endotoxin levels after OHCA were associated with increased severity and duration of shock, as indicated by the mean dose of vasopressor and days requiring vasopressor therapy.[26]

Studies attempting to target systemic inflammation and inappropriate vasodilation in cardiogenic shock are described later in the chapter.

PRESENTATION AND INITIAL EVALUATION

Presentation of Heart Failure and Cardiogenic Shock After Myocardial Infarction

Cardiogenic shock secondary to acute MI typically develops during the initial hospitalization, with only 15% of cases documented as present at the time of hospital arrival.[13] For patients who develop shock after hospitalization, the onset tends to occur early, usually within 24 hours, of STEMI and later, on the order of 3 to 4 days, for NSTEMI.

Nohria and colleagues described a classification system for heart failure states based on the presence or absence of congestion, described as "wet" or "dry," and on the presence or absence of hypoperfusion, described as "cold" or "warm."[6] The physical examination in patients with heart failure without cardiogenic shock reveals congestion with preserved perfusion ("warm and wet") and the examination in cardiogenic shock indicates both hypoperfusion and congestion ("cold and wet"). On physical examination, congestion is identified by the presence of jugular venous distention, hepatojugular reflux or a square-wave blood pressure response to the Valsalva maneuver, orthopnea, peripheral edema, or a third heart sound (S_3 gallop). Hypoperfusion is identified by hypotension, a narrow pulse pressure, cool extremities (except in patients who develop a low-SVR state), or altered mental status. A narrow pulse pressure, defined by a ratio of the pulse pressure (systolic minus diastolic pressure) to systolic pressure of 25% or less, has been shown to have a 91% sensitivity and 83% specificity for a cardiac index below 2.2 L/min/m^2.[6]

Differential Diagnosis

Findings on the history and physical examination assist in the differentiation among types of shock, including cardiogenic, hypovolemic, distributive, and mixed (e.g., cardiogenic and distributive). Once a cardiogenic component is suspected, it is prudent to consider a broad group of possible etiologic

TABLE 25-2 Differential Diagnosis of Cardiogenic Shock

Acute myocardial infarction or ischemia, including right ventricular infarction
Mechanical complications of acute myocardial infarction
Acute mitral regurgitation/papillary muscle rupture
Ventricular septal rupture
Free wall rupture and tamponade
Stress cardiomyopathy
Myocarditis
Myocardial contusion
Pericarditis and tamponade
Type A dissection with acute aortic insufficiency or tamponade
Native valvular dysfunction
Complication of prosthetic valves
Acute thrombosis
Valve dehiscence
Dysrhythmia
Pulmonary embolism

disorders. Multiple causes of cardiogenic shock may coexist, and the treatment may vary accordingly. For example, in a patient hospitalized after an anterior STEMI, cardiogenic shock may develop secondary to left ventricular dysfunction, as well as from mechanical complications, such as ventricular septal rupture. Potential causes of cardiogenic shock, including those possible after MI, are listed in Table 25-2. These etiologic factors include complications of MI, such as left, right, and biventricular pump dysfunction in the setting of the initial ischemic event, as well as mechanical complications (see Chapter 26), including acute mitral regurgitation, ventricular septal rupture, free wall rupture, and cardiac dysrhythmia (see Chapter 28). The differential diagnosis also includes entities not related to epicardial coronary disease, such as stress cardiomyopathy, inflammatory myocarditis, pericarditis with tamponade, native or prosthetic valvular dysfunction, and massive pulmonary embolism (see Chapter 6).

Approach to Evaluation of a Patient with Shock

Evaluating a patient with shock requires integration of data from multiple sources, including the clinical history, physical examination, laboratory data, electrocardiography, imaging, and invasive hemodynamic assessments.

Clinical History and Physical Examination

The clinical history and physical examination are critical elements in the evaluation of patients with shock. The history can provide important information regarding etiology, duration, and progression. The physical examination is invaluable for rapidly assessing the likely type of shock. For example, in patients with hypovolemic shock, the physical examination will expose manifestations of decreased preload, including low jugular venous pressure, dry mucous membranes, decreased skin turgor, and possibly cool, mottled extremities (reflective of high SVR). Distributive shock is characterized by an inappropriate decrease in SVR, which typically results in an augmentation of heart rate and compensatory increase in cardiac output. Preload may be low or normal in the case of distributive shock. Although many of the physical examination findings may be similar to those in hypovolemic shock (e.g., tachycardia, low jugular venous pressure), a distinguishing feature of distributive shock is warm or hyperemic extremities, reflecting a low-SVR state. Finally, as described previously, the physical examination in cardiogenic shock often reveals congestion, as manifested by pulmonary or peripheral edema, ascites, an S_3 gallop, and jugular venous distention, as well as hypoperfusion with cool extremities (elevated SVR), altered mental status, or oliguria.

Laboratory Assessments

Depending on the severity of shock, laboratory evaluation may demonstrate evidence of anaerobic metabolism with a lactic acidosis and organ hypoperfusion, including acute kidney and liver injury. Biomarkers of myonecrosis, including troponin, are important in the diagnosis and prognostication in patients with acute MI (see Chapter 6 and Chapter 7), and also may be elevated in patients with shock outside of the setting of acute MI.[27] Additionally, troponin has been associated with worse clinical outcomes and higher mortality in patients with acute decompensated heart failure.[28] B-type natriuretic peptide (BNP) and the amino-terminal cleavage product (NT-proBNP) are released by cardiomyocytes in the setting of increased myocardial wall stress. These biomarkers are useful to support clinical judgment for diagnosis or exclusion of acute decompensated heart failure, as well as for risk stratification.[6] Natriuretic peptides can be elevated in other cardiac and noncardiac conditions and may be falsely decreased in the setting of obesity.

Several investigational biomarkers have shown promise for risk stratification in cardiogenic shock. Consistent with the inflammatory response to myocardial necrosis and prolonged cardiogenic shock, investigators found that higher levels of interleukins, including IL-6, predicted occurrence of death in 40 patients with acute MI and cardiogenic shock in the IABP-SHOCK trial.[17] Similarly, markers of vascular integrity, the angiopoietins, were independently associated with mortality in cardiogenic shock.[18] As described earlier, the presence of endotoxin probably reflects end-organ (intestinal) hypoperfusion, with higher levels indicating more severe shock.[26] Endotoxin is known to drive production of procalcitonin, a precursor to the hormone calcitonin, which is used as a relatively specific biomarker of systemic bacterial infections and sepsis. Of interest, in a study of 29 patients with acute cardiogenic shock without bacteremia, Brunkhorst and colleagues found that in 18 of 20 patients who survived for more than 12 hours, pyrexia and an increase in procalcitonin level developed in the absence of positive cultures, supporting the hypothesis that the development of SIRS in cardiogenic shock may be related to exposure to bacterial endotoxin.[5] Further studies are needed to determine the optimal combination of biomarkers for risk stratification and, possibly, to monitor response to therapy in cardiogenic shock.

Electrocardiogram, Imaging, and Other Assessments

Electrocardiogram

An electrocardiogram (ECG) should be obtained immediately at the time of presentation, to assist with diagnosis, prognosis, and therapeutic decision making (see Chapter 6). The extent of ST-segment deviation on the ECG, location of infarction, and QRS duration correlate with risk of adverse outcomes, including the risk for onset of severe heart failure or shock.

Echocardiography

Noninvasive imaging with echocardiography is recommended in patients with acute MI and should be performed urgently in such patients with cardiogenic shock.[12,13,29] Echocardiography is a widely available and rapidly applied modality that can identify left and right ventricular dysfunction, myocardial wall motion abnormalities, pericardial tamponade, severe valvular disease, papillary muscle rupture, and ventricular septal rupture (see Chapter 31). In addition, echocardiography can be used to estimate left ventricular filling pressures using several different techniques.[30] For example, the ratio of the peak transmitral pulsed Doppler inflow velocity (E), a marker of early diastolic flow, to the tissue Doppler-derived mitral annular velocity (e′), a marker of myocardial relaxation, is well correlated with invasively measured pulmonary capillary wedge pressure (r = 0.87; P < .001)[30] (Figure 25-5). Specifically, an E/e′ ratio of 12 or higher using the lateral annulus, or an E/e′ ratio of 15 or higher using the septal annulus, are correlated with a wedge pressure of 15 mm Hg or more, and an E/e′ less than 8 at either annular location is correlated with normal left ventricular filling pressures. Doppler echocardiography also has been studied as a method to estimate cardiac output in critically ill or perioperative patients, using small probes placed in the esophagus after appropriate sedation and mechanical ventilation have been instituted. With this technique, the cardiac output is based on the diameter and velocity of flow in the aorta and an estimation of the proportion of output delivered to the descending aorta.[31]

Cardiovascular Magnetic Resonance

Cardiovascular magnetic resonance (CMR) combines an excellent spatial and temporal resolution to allow for the simultaneous assessment of cardiac function, anatomy (including coronary and valvular), stress and rest myocardial perfusion, and viability during the same test (see Chapter 33). Despite the diagnostic potential of CMR, its clinical usefulness in patients with shock often is limited by availability and by the ability of hemodynamically unstable patients to tolerate this time-intensive testing.

Invasive Coronary Angiography

Invasive coronary angiography is the optimal strategy for identification of epicardial coronary disease in the setting of cardiogenic shock, because it allows for simultaneous revascularization of culprit lesions. On the basis of the benefit of early revascularization observed in the SHOCK trial, an immediate invasive strategy is recommended for all patients with cardiogenic shock and acute MI.[12,13,29,32] The role of revascularization is discussed later under Coronary Reperfusion and Revascularization.

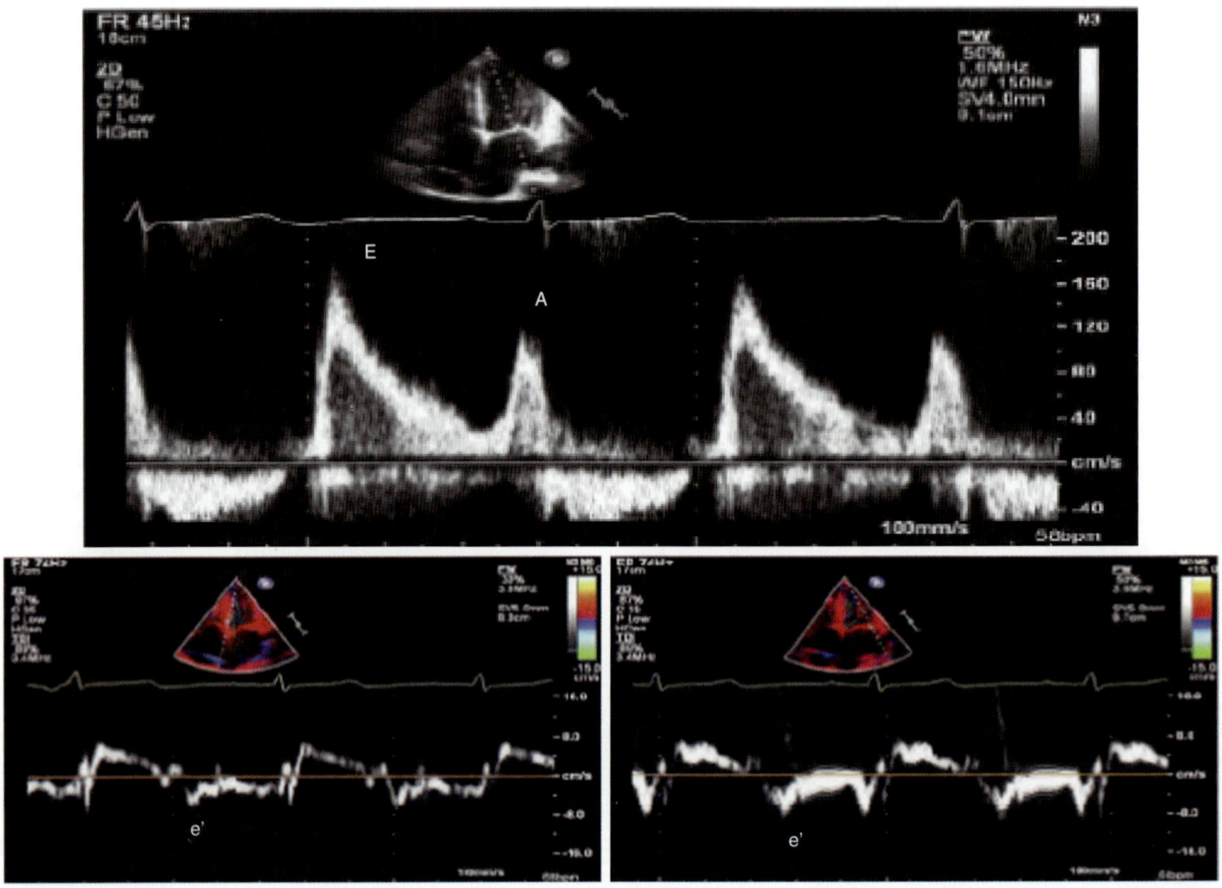

Septal E/e' = 160/8 = 20 Lateral E/e' =160/8 = 20

FIGURE 25-5 Echocardiographic estimation of left ventricular filling pressures. Echocardiographic measurements in a patient with impaired left ventricular relaxation and elevated left ventricular filling pressures. A ratio of the peak transmitral pulsed Doppler inflow velocity (*E* in cm/s, shown in *top panel*) to the Doppler tissue imaging at the septal (e′ in cm/s, *bottom left panel*) or lateral (e′ in cm/s, *bottom right panel*) mitral annulus of 12 or greater is correlated with an elevated pulmonary capillary wedge pressure. *(Adapted from Mor-Avi V, Lang RM, Badano LP, et al: Current and evolving echocardiographic techniques for the quantitative evaluation of cardiac mechanics: ASE/EAE consensus statement on methodology and indications endorsed by the Japanese Society of Echocardiography.* J Am Soc Echocardiogr *24:277-313, 2011.)*

Hemodynamic Monitoring

Invasive assessment of hemodynamics by means of right heart catheterization allows for identification of hypervolemia or hypovolemia, assessment of cardiac output and SVR, and detection and quantification of shunting, such as in the setting of ventricular septal rupture, and may be useful to guide the titration of inotropes, vasopressors, and vasodilators. To date, no randomized trials have been conducted to evaluate right heart catheterization in patients with cardiogenic shock after MI, and data on use of a pulmonary artery catheter to guide management in heart failure without shock in this setting are limited. Specific hemodynamic goals of therapy measured with a pulmonary artery catheter are described briefly later in the Pharmacotherapy section.

Consideration of data outside the setting of cardiogenic shock and acute MI may or may not be helpful to understanding the role of right heart catheterization in this setting. The Evaluation Study of Congestive Heart Failure and Pulmonary Artery Catheterization Effectiveness (ESCAPE) trial demonstrated no difference in death or hospitalization at 6 months, but increased rates of adverse events (21.9% versus 11.5%; $P = .04$) in 433 patients with heart failure not accompanied by shock randomly assigned to placement of a pulmonary artery catheter or to noninvasive standard care.[6] A meta-analysis by Shah and colleagues of data for 5051 patients from 13 randomized control trials of pulmonary artery catheterization in patients undergoing surgery admitted to the intensive care unit with advanced heart failure or diagnosed with acute respiratory distress syndrome or sepsis did not demonstrate a difference in mortality.[6] Based on these limited data and expert consensus, placement of a pulmonary artery catheter is recommended in only a subset of patients, including those with presumed cardiogenic shock and need for escalating vasopressor therapy or mechanical support; those exhibiting clinical decompensation with equivocal findings on assessment of filling pressures, perfusion, and vascular tone; and patients with ongoing significant symptoms or dependence on inotropes despite attempts at noninvasive optimization of recommended therapies.[6]

In light of the risks of invasive monitoring and the desire to intermittently or continuously monitor cardiac output and tissue perfusion, several minimally invasive monitoring techniques have been developed. However, to date, none have been adopted as a complete replacement for placement of a pulmonary artery catheter. These strategies include employing Doppler ultrasound (e.g., transesophageal echocardiography), bioimpedance, pulse pressure analysis, and applied Fick principle.[31] Pulse pressure or pulse contour analysis is based on the principle that stroke volume can be estimated from the pressure waveform obtained using an arterial line, and consequently cardiac output can be estimated using the product of stroke volume and heart rate. Devices utilizing this technique are commercially available (e.g., Vigileo, Edwards Lifesciences, Irvine, California). Devices based on this principle are of limited usefulness in the presence of artifact on arterial waveforms, peripheral atherosclerosis limiting pulse pressure, or significant arrhythmias (e.g., atrial fibrillation). Bioimpedance uses electric current stimulation, often delivered to skin or endotracheal tube electrodes, to estimate hemodynamic parameters such as stroke volume, heart rate, and cardiac output using changes in impedance throughout the cardiac cycle.

Other noninvasive strategies involve assessment of the microcirculation as a surrogate marker of splanchnic perfusion. For example, a darkfield imaging technique that estimates sublingual microcirculatory flow by means of red blood cell absorption of device-emitted green light, was found to be predictive of multiorgan dysfunction and death in patients with cardiogenic shock after acute MI.[33] Another technique, near-infrared spectroscopy (NIRS), takes advantage of the differential absorption of near-infrared light (wavelengths between 700 and 1000 nm) by oxygenated and deoxygenated hemoglobin to determine postcapillary oxygenation, reflecting a combination of oxygen delivery, consumption, and extraction as a measure of adequacy of local tissue oxygen delivery.[34] Although this easily applied technique has shown promise in the setting of traumatic, hemorrhagic shock, its usefulness in the setting of cardiogenic shock remains to be determined.

MANAGEMENT OF HEART FAILURE AND SHOCK DUE TO IMPAIRED VENTRICULAR CONTRACTILITY

General Principles of Management

The general principles of management of heart failure without shock in the setting of acute MI include reversal of ischemia by means of reperfusion, anti-ischemic pharmacotherapy, treatment of volume overload, afterload reduction, and initiation of therapy to minimize adverse left ventricular remodeling (see Chapter 36).[6] The therapeutic priorities for cardiogenic shock due to acute MI include early coronary revascularization, assessment for and treatment of mechanical complications of MI, maintenance of perfusion with pharmacologic (i.e., vasopressors and inotropes) and non-pharmacologic (i.e., MCS) methods, and correction of metabolic disturbances, such as acidosis or hyperglycemia, which may exacerbate cardiac dysfunction and limit the efficacy of pharmacologic support (Figure 25-6). Unfortunately, current treatments for cardiogenic shock are based largely on extrapolation from pathophysiologic principles in the absence of data from randomized controlled trials of adequate size evaluating their efficacy and safety. Moreover, most evidence-based therapies applied in patients with acute MI have been studied in clinical trials that excluded subjects with hemodynamic instability or shock. To date, on the order of only 2000 patients with cardiogenic shock have been included in randomized clinical trials of therapies targeted at the management of this condition (Figure 25-7). Additional investigation in patients with cardiogenic shock is needed to provide guideposts for evidence-based therapy, with a goal of improving survival in this high-mortality condition.

Coronary Reperfusion and Revascularization

Early invasive coronary revascularization is recommended for patients with acute MI complicated by heart failure without shock based on recognition of heart failure as a potent independent indicator of increased risk for poor outcomes (see Chapter 11, Chapter 16, and Chapter 17).[12,13]

Of note, coronary revascularization is the single therapy that is recommended (class I) in professional guidelines for the management of cardiogenic shock after

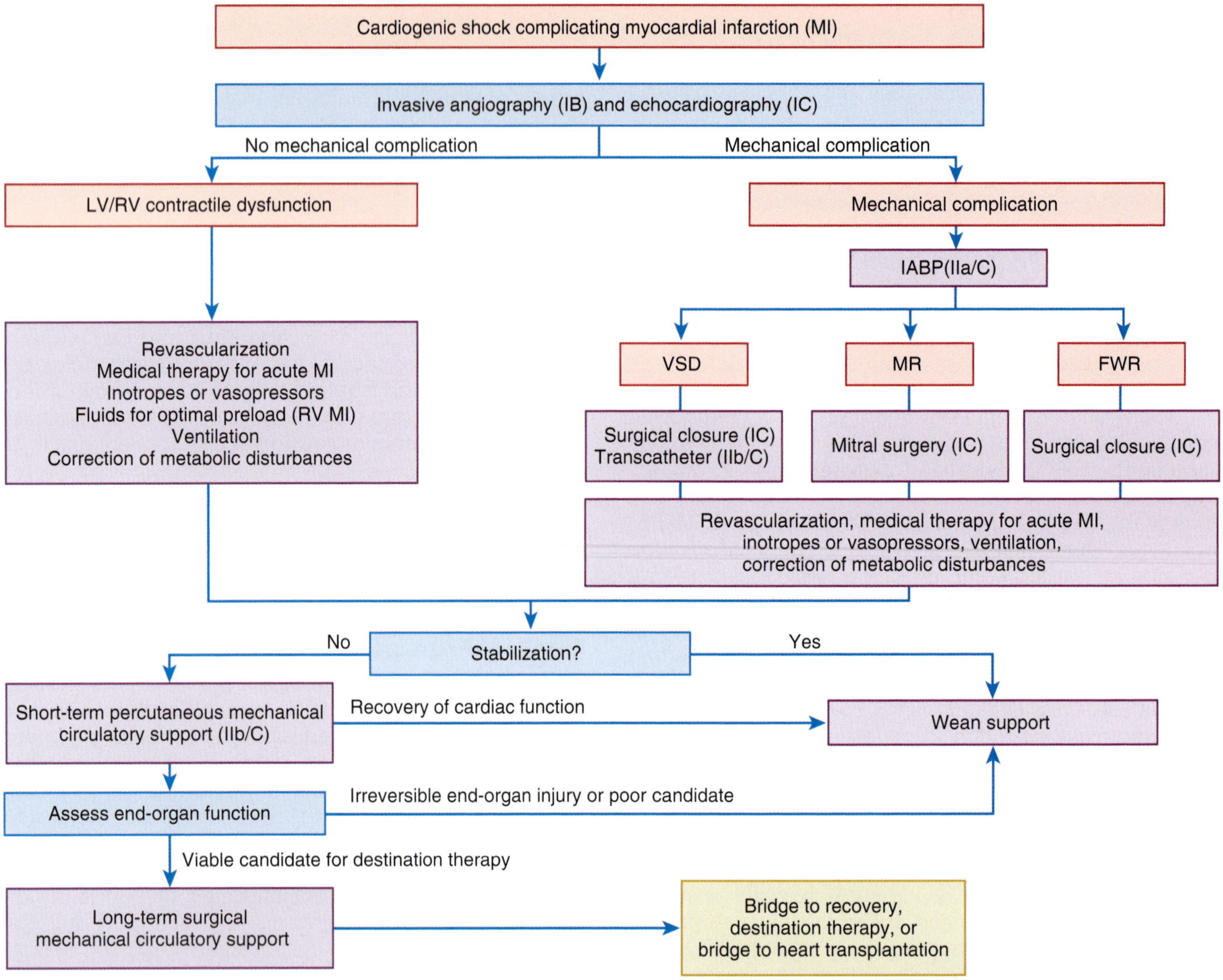

FIGURE 25-6 **Treatment algorithm for patients with cardiogenic shock and acute myocardial infarction.** *FWR,* Free wall rupture; *IABP,* intraaortic balloon pump; *LV/RV,* left ventricular/right ventricular; *MR,* mitral regurgitation; *VSD,* ventricular septal defect. *(Adapted from Thiele H, Ohman EM, Desch S, et al. Management of cardiogenic shock.* Eur Heart J *36:1223-1230, 2015.)*

MI. This recommendation is based on the results from two randomized trials; however, the strength of this evidence, when viewed critically, is modest. The SHOCK trial included 302 patients with STEMI and cardiogenic shock due to left ventricular failure who were randomly assigned to either early revascularization (within 6 hours) or initial medical therapy, including fibrinolysis, with delayed revascularization more than 54 hours after institution of treatment, if appropriate.[5] The study did not meet the primary endpoint of all-cause mortality at 30 days, with mortality rates of 46.7% and 56.0% in the early revascularization and control groups, respectively (hazard ratio [HR], 0.83; 95% confidence interval [CI], 0.67 to 1.04). In supplementary analyses during subsequent longer-term follow-up, however, mortality was significantly reduced at 6 months (50.3% versus 63.1%; HR, 0.80; $P = .027$), 1 year (53.3% versus 66.4%; HR, 0.72; $P < .03$), and 6 years (67.2% versus 80.4%; HR, 0.59; $P = .03$) (Figure 25-8).[35]

The underpowered Swiss Multicenter Study of Angioplasty for Shock (SMASH) study included 55 patients with acute MI and shock and demonstrated a trend toward a reduction in mortality with early revascularization (HR, 0.88; 95% CI, 0.6 to 1.2).[5]

Timing of Revascularization in Shock

Patients with a shorter time from symptom onset to revascularization (less than 6 hours) in the SHOCK trial had superior outcomes to those in late presenters (up to 48 hours after MI and 18 hours after onset of shock); however, even this late-presentation group showed a pattern of benefit from revascularization (Figure 25-9). Observational data from registries similarly provide support for more favorable outcomes among patients with cardiogenic shock undergoing early rather than late revascularization. In the Arbeitsgemeinschaft Leitende Kardiologische Krankenhausarzte (ALKK) registry of patients with cardiogenic shock due to MI undergoing PCI, early revascularization (less than 6 hours from symptom onset) and the success of reperfusion as defined by the post-PCI Thrombolysis in Myocardial Infarction (TIMI) flow grade were predictors of improved survival.[16]

On the basis of these data, early invasive evaluation is recommended in all patients with acute MI and cardiogenic shock, with a view toward immediate culprit vessel revascularization (see Figure 25-6). In view of the persistent benefit of revascularization over medical therapy irrespective of time delay from MI, revascularization should be pursued as

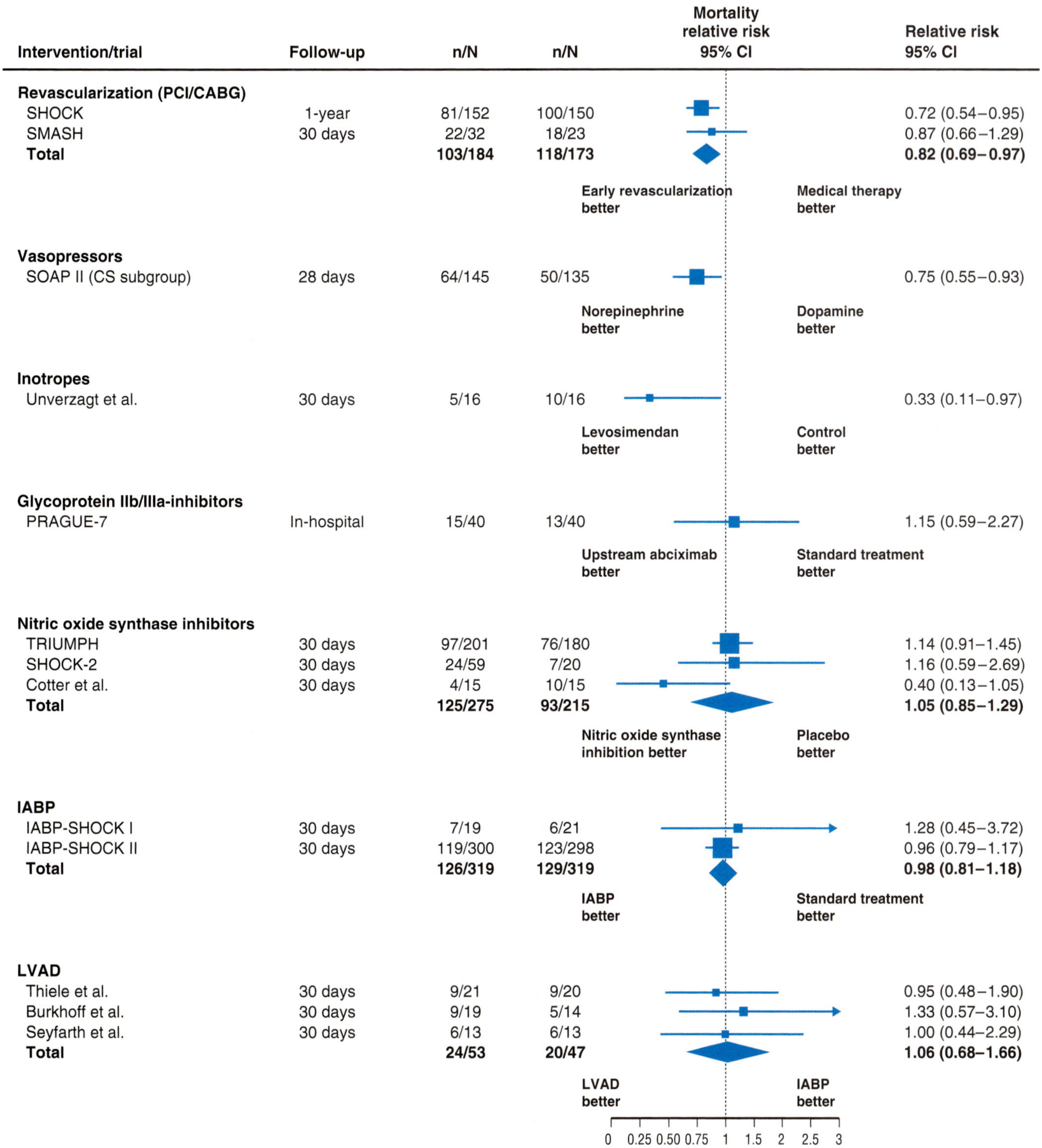

FIGURE 25-7 Randomized clinical trial data of cardiogenic shock (CS). Randomized trial data for reperfusion therapy, vasoactive medications, including vasopressors, inotropes, and nitric oxide synthase (NOS) inhibitors, antiplatelet therapy, and mechanical circulatory support in patients with cardiogenic shock. *IABP,* Intraaortic balloon pump; *LVAD,* left ventricular assist device; *PCI/CABG,* percutaneous coronary intervention/coronary artery bypass grafting. *(From Thiele H, Ohman EM, Desch S, et al: Management of cardiogenic shock.* Eur Heart J *36:1223-1230, 2015.)*

soon as possible, and generally even among patients with late presentation.[12,13,29]

Method of Reperfusion

PCI or, in some cases, coronary artery bypass grafting (CABG) is the recommended approach to reperfusion therapy in patients with STEMI complicated by cardiogenic shock.[12,13,29] Fibrinolysis is recommended only for patients presenting with STEMI who have no contraindication to fibrinolytic therapy but are unsuitable candidates for percutaneous and surgical revascularization owing to technical, anatomic, or patient-specific reasons. As a result, immediate transfer to a PCI-capable facility is recommended for all patients with cardiogenic shock and acute MI, irrespective of time from symptom onset (see Chapter 5 and Chapter 17). Moreover, in patients who undergo initial fibrinolytic therapy,

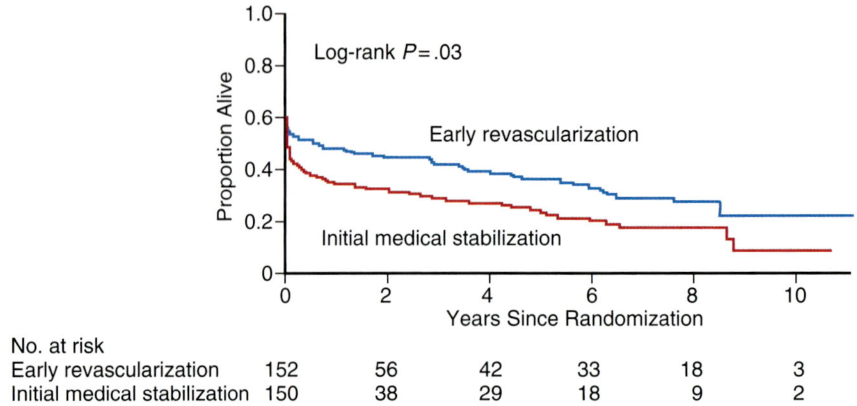

FIGURE 25-8 Mortality benefit of early revascularization in patients with cardiogenic shock after acute myocardial infarction. The SHOCK trial randomly assigned 302 patients with STEMI and cardiogenic shock due to left ventricular failure to undergo early revascularization within 6 hours or initial medical stabilization with delayed revascularization more than 54 hours after initiation of treatment, if appropriate. Survival rates in these two groups were 53.3% versus 44.0% (P = .11) at 30 days, 49.7% versus 36.9% (P = .027) at 6 months, 46.7% versus 33.6% (P < .03) at 1 year, and 32.8% versus 19.6% (P = .03) at 6 years, respectively. *(Data from Hochman JS, Sleeper LA, Webb JG, et al: Early revascularization and long-term survival in cardiogenic shock complicating acute myocardial infarction.* JAMA *295(21):2511, 2006.)*

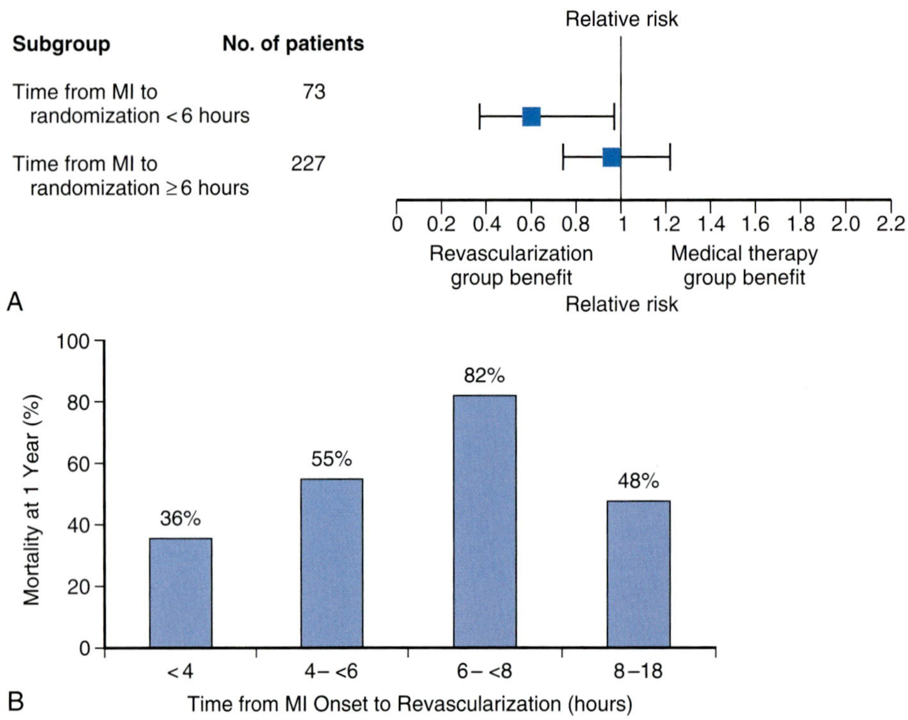

FIGURE 25-9 Timing of revascularization in the SHOCK trial. (A) Subgroup analysis for 30-day mortality rate found no significant difference in benefit for early revascularization (ERV), either earlier (less than 6 hours from MI onset) or later (6 hours or longer from MI onset), compared with initial medical stabilization (IMS) (P-interaction = nonsignificant). **(B)** Within the ERV group, mortality increased with increasing time from MI until after 8 hours, which was thought to represent survivor bias. *MI,* Myocardial infarction. *(Data from Hochman JS, Sleeper LA, Webb JG, et al: Early revascularization in acute myocardial infarction complicated by cardiogenic shock. SHOCK Investigators. Should We Emergently Revascularize Occluded Coronaries for Cardiogenic Shock.* N Engl J Med *341(9):625, 1999; and from Hochman JS, Sleeper LA, Webb JG, et al: Early revascularization and long-term survival in cardiogenic shock complicating acute myocardial infarction.* JAMA *295(21):2511, 2006.)*

the development of severe heart failure or shock are considered indications for urgent angiography (class I).

These recommendations are based on findings from the SHOCK trial, in which 49% (n = 152) of patients assigned to the early revascularization group and 63% (n = 150) of those assigned to initial medical stabilization received fibrinolytic therapy for STEMI.[13] Among patients receiving initial medical therapy, administration of fibrinolytic therapy at the discretion of the treating physician was associated with a lower mortality rate at 1 year (unadjusted HR of 0.59; P = .01). However, among patients randomly assigned to undergo early revascularization, no association was found between administration of a fibrinolytic and subsequent mortality (unadjusted HR = 0.93; P = .76).

Although PCI is the preferred approach to revascularization when the coronary anatomy is suitable, favorable outcomes also can be achieved with early CABG. Of patients who underwent revascularization in the SHOCK trial, 63% had PCI and 37% CABG.[5] Despite higher rates of diabetes, three-vessel and left main coronary artery disease in the CABG cohort, survival was similar at 1 year between patients who were revascularized with PCI compared with CABG (51.9% versus 46.8%; P = 0.71). In patients with papillary muscle rupture, or acute severe mitral regurgitation related to MI, emergent surgical revascularization and valvular replacement may be preferable to a staged approach of percutaneous revascularization followed by surgical valve repair (see Chapter 26).

Study	Multi-vessel PCI Mortality n/N	%	Culprit-lesion-only PCI n/N	%	Adjusted OR or HR (95% CI)	P value
Mylotte et al.	37/66	56.1	82/103	79.6	0.57	0.005
Yang et al.	21/60	35.0	85/278	30.6	1.06	0.83
Cavender et al.	158/433	36.5	737/265	27.8	1.54	<0.01
Zeymer et al.	81/173	46.8	201/562	35.8	1.5	<0.05
Bauer et al.	40/82	48.8	95/254	37.4	1.28	NS
Webb et al.	6/11	54.5	14/71	20	2.75	0.040

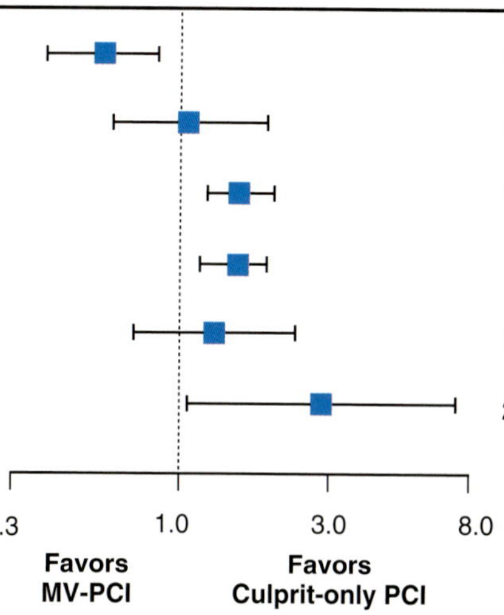

FIGURE 25-10 **Mortality for multivessel versus culprit vessel–only percutaneous coronary intervention (PCI) in several registries of patients with cardiogenic shock.** *HR,* Hazard ratio; *OR,* odds ratio. *(Data from Thiele H, Ohman EM, Desch S, et al: Management of cardiogenic shock.* Eur Heart J *36:1223-1230, 2015.)*

Non–Culprit Artery Revascularization in Shock

Multivessel disease is identified in 70% to 90% of patients with cardiogenic shock and acute MI; however, the optimal extent of the initial revascularization is not yet known.[5,36] Although multiple small studies, including PRAMI (Preventive Angioplasty in Acute Myocardial Infarction) (*n* = 465), DANAMI-3 PRIMULTI (*n* = 627), and CvLPRIT (Complete Versus Lesion-Only Primary PCI trial) (*n* = 296), have demonstrated robust reductions in recurrent cardiovascular events with multivessel or complete revascularization compared with infarct artery–only revascularization in patients with STEMI, all of these studies excluded subjects with cardiogenic shock.[37-39] In a prospective observational study of 266 subjects with resuscitated cardiac arrest and cardiogenic shock, multivessel PCI was associated with decreased mortality compared with culprit vessel–only PCI (Figure 25-10).[40] In contrast, all other observational studies suggest equivalent or worse outcomes with multivessel as compared with culprit lesion–only PCI (see Figure 25-10).[16] The role of multivessel PCI is being addressed in the ongoing CULPRIT-SHOCK trial (NCT0127549), in which approximately 700 patients with onset of cardiogenic shock within 12 hours of acute MI (both ST-elevation and non–ST-elevation MI) will be randomly assigned to infarct artery–only or acute multivessel revascularization. Current guidelines suggest that in patients with cardiogenic shock due to pump failure, PCI to open a severely stenotic large noninfarct artery might improve hemodynamic stability and should be considered during the primary procedure.[13]

Pharmacotherapy

In general, the acute antithrombotic therapy and secondary preventive treatments for patients with acute MI and heart failure or shock should mirror that recommended for patients with an acute coronary event without heart failure or shock (see Chapter 13). Of note, however, patients with hemodynamic instability were rarely included in the clinical trials supporting these guideline-based therapies. Furthermore, certain agents routinely used during treatment of an acute MI will exacerbate shock and are therefore contraindicated, including negative inotropic agents and antihypertensives. In addition, gastric and intestinal absorption of oral agents may be impaired in patients with shock. The role of anticoagulant and antiplatelet agents are discussed in Chapter 18 and Chapter 19, respectively. Long-term secondary preventive therapies are discussed in Chapter 34. The focus of this section is on pharmacotherapy relevant to the acute management of heart failure and shock.

Agents with negative inotropic properties are contraindicated in cardiogenic shock. Specifically, these agents include beta-blockade; nondihydropyridine calcium channel blockers, such as verapamil and diltiazem; and specific classes of antiarrhythmics, notably class I sodium channel blockers (e.g., procainamide and quinidine) and certain class III agents (e.g., sotalol). If needed, amiodarone is the recommended antiarrhythmic of choice. Angiotensin-converting enzyme (ACE) inhibitors should not be administered in the hypotensive patient with shock.

Vasoactive Medications

In addition to early coronary reperfusion, preservation of cardiac output, blood pressure, and end-organ perfusion is paramount in patients with acute MI complicated by cardiogenic shock. These parameters can often be improved with a combination of pharmacologic and nonpharmacologic (e.g., advanced MCS) measures.

General Considerations

Inotropes and vasopressors may be administered with the goal of maintaining perfusion so as to preserve end-organ function. To achieve this goal, therapy is generally targeted at supporting the mean arterial pressure. Once the blood pressure is stabilized with resuscitation and/or vasopressor therapy, therapies can be tailored to address the underlying pathophysiology (e.g., addition of further inotropic support or vasodilator therapy).

In general, the dose of vasopressor and inotropic therapy should be maintained at the minimal dose and duration of therapy necessary to achieve these aims, as these agents can have adverse consequences. Catecholamines increase

TABLE 25-4 Inotropic and Vasopressor Dose Range, Receptor Binding, Indications, and Major Clinical Side Effects

DRUG	CLINICAL INDICATION(S)	DOSE RANGE	RECEPTOR BINDING α1	β1	β2	DA	MAJOR SIDE EFFECTS
Catecholamines							

the concern that the adverse effects of epinephrine may outweigh the benefits.

Phenylephrine

Phenylephrine is a synthetic, selective α_1-agonist that results in systemic vasoconstriction and often, reflex bradycardia. Based on its potent vasoconstrictor properties, its use is primarily reserved for vasodilatory shock. As with other vasoconstrictors, phenylephrine can cause significant peripheral ischemia at high doses.

Vasopressin

Vasopressin, or antidiuretic hormone (ADH), is a peptide hormone that is synthesized in the hypothalamus and secreted from the pituitary gland in response to decreased intravascular volume or plasma hyperosmolality. Its vasopressor activity is thought to result from arterial smooth muscle contraction mediated through V_1 receptor agonism on the systemic vasculature (see Table 25-4). Vasopressin typically is used for refractory vasodilatory shock, particularly septic shock. Vasopressin often is used as an adjunct in septic shock, allowing for lower doses of norepinephrine—a strategy that has been shown to carry mortality rates equivalent to those for high-dose norepinephrine.[47] In our own practice, we also occasionally use this "adrenergic-sparing" approach in patients with severe heart failure, particularly in the setting of mixed cardiogenic and vasodilatory shock. This strategy is based on the hypothesis that endogenous vasopressin may fall over time owing to depletion of neurohypophyseal stores and norepinephrine-induced inhibition of vasopressin, and that vasopressin may counter the mechanisms underlying inflammatory vasodilation, including K_{ATP} channel activation and nitric oxide production.[21] Although clinical trial data on outcomes are limited with vasopressin use in cardiogenic shock, a single retrospective study of 36 patients with cardiogenic shock after MI reported that vasopressin use significantly improved mean arterial pressure without changing cardiac index or pulmonary capillary wedge pressure.[48]

Inotropes

Inotropes augment cardiac output through an increase in contractility. Those agents used most commonly for this effect (dobutamine and milrinone) also increase heart rate and reduce SVR (see Table 25-4). Dobutamine is a synthetic sympathomimetic amine, and milrinone is a phosphodiesterase-3 enzyme (PDE) inhibitor; thus, with both agents, intracellular cyclic adenosine monophosphate (cAMP) is increased. Milrinone has a longer half-life than dobutamine (approximately 2.5 hours versus 2 minutes with normal renal function) and also tends to be associated with a greater degree of pulmonary vasodilation and fewer arrhythmic events. Of note, in a randomized trial of this drug for acute heart failure (Outcomes of a Prospective Trial of Intravenous Milrinone for Exacerbations of Chronic Heart Failure), milrinone did not reduce mortality, and in a retrospective analysis of the Acute Decompensated Heart Failure National Registry (ADHERE), dobutamine was associated with higher mortality.[2,48] Consequently, inotropic therapy typically is restricted to patients who cannot be managed with vasodilator and diuretic therapy alone.

Levosimendan is a "calcium sensitizer" that increases myofilament response to calcium at lower concentrations, thereby improving myocardial contractility without increasing oxygen demand or intracellular calcium overload. In addition, levosimendan has systemic and coronary vasodilatory effects through action on the K_{ATP} channels in vascular smooth muscle. Despite the theoretical benefits of increased contractility and vasodilation in heart failure, improved survival has not been observed in the larger-scale clinical trials.[8] Although an apparent benefit has been noted in patients with cardiogenic shock, particularly when levosimendan is combined with catecholamines to maintain adequate perfusion pressures, the small number of patients with cardiogenic shock studied limits interpretation.[8,48,49]

Vasodilators

Nitrates are endothelium-independent vasodilators of the peripheral and coronary vasculature. Venodilation decreases cardiac preload, and more modest arterial dilation may result in decreased afterload. Additionally, nitrates can improve coronary flow, including that from collaterals. Despite a lack of data showing a reduction in recurrent major adverse cardiovascular events, because of these favorable physiologic effects as determined by expert consensus, intravenous nitroglycerin carries a class I indication in patients with acute MI and heart failure and/or persistent ischemia.[12,13] Sodium nitroprusside is an intravenous vasodilator with a more balanced effect on venodilation and arteriodilation that is easily titrated and may be particularly useful in the setting of heart failure with hypertension or acute ischemic mitral regurgitation. Of note, nitroprusside can produce significant hypotension and, in the setting of prolonged use or renal dysfunction, thiocyanate toxicity. Nitroprusside can also precipitate "coronary steal" in setting of epicardial coronary stenoses. Owing to the arterial vasodilation and associated drop in blood pressure, neither agent should be used early in the setting of cardiogenic shock. However, vasodilators (particularly intravenous nitroglycerin) can be cautiously added in patients after stabilization of blood pressure, to decrease preload and congestion.

Volume Management

Diuretics are the mainstay of therapy to reduce preload in patients with heart failure without shock. Intravenous loop diuretics are the recommended first-line therapeutic agents, with bolus dosing and continuous infusions producing similar results in terms of symptoms, effective diuresis, and clinical outcomes.[6,50] Thiazide diuretics can be added to improve diuretic responsiveness. Ultrafiltration (UF) generally is reserved for patients with persistent congestion that is refractory to maximally escalated medical therapy. This limited use is based on findings from Cardiorenal Rescue Study in Acute Decompensated Heart Failure (CARRESS-HF), in which 188 patients with acute decompensated heart failure, progressive renal dysfunction, and ongoing congestion were randomly assigned to stepped medical therapy, including loop and thiazide diuretics and selective use of vasodilators and inotropes, or to UF.[51] The UF modality was inferior to medical therapy as assessed by worsening renal function in the UF group, compared with improved renal function in the medical therapy group.

Additional Therapies for Heart Failure without Shock

Renin-Angiotensin-Aldosterone System Inhibition

Inhibition of the RAAS is recommended in post-MI patients with heart failure or left ventricular dysfunction on the basis of improved survival. The rationale for RAAS inhibition includes experimental and clinical evidence of a favorable impact on ventricular remodeling, improvement in hemodynamics, and reductions in congestive heart failure. Unequivocal evidence from randomized, placebo-controlled trials shows that ACE inhibitors reduce the mortality rate in patients with reduced ejection fraction or clinical signs of heart failure after acute MI. In all but one trial in such patients, ACE inhibitor therapy was initiated between 3 and 16 days after MI and maintained for 1 to 4 years.

In unselected patients with acute MI, ACE inhibitors administered for a short duration of therapy saves 5 lives per 1000 patients treated. In patients at higher risk of adverse remodeling, such as patients with anterior infarction, ACE inhibitors offer a greater benefit from early administration (11 lives saved/1000). In patients with ventricular dysfunction or heart failure among whom ACE inhibitors were administered for longer duration (years), this benefit is greater with 42 to 76 lives saved per 1000 patients treated. In patients with acute MI at risk for heart failure, the mortality reduction with ACE inhibitors is accompanied by significant reductions in the development of heart failure, supporting the underlying pathophysiologic rationale for administering this class of drugs in patients with acute MI. Patients with acute MI and anterior infarction, previous infarction, Killip class II or worse, or evidence of depressed global ventricular function on an imaging study should receive lifelong treatment with ACE inhibitors.

An alternative method of pharmacologic inhibition of the RAAS is by administration of angiotensin II receptor blockers (ARBs). The VALIANT trial compared the effects of the ARB valsartan versus captopril alone and in combination with captopril on mortality in patients with acute MI complicated by left ventricular systolic dysfunction and/or heart failure, randomly assigned to the three drug regimens within 10 days of MI.[52] Mortality rates were similar in the three treatment groups: 19.9% in the valsartan group, 19.3% in the valsartan plus captopril group, and 19.5% in the captopril alone group. The choice between ACE inhibition and an ARB after acute MI should be based on physician experience with the agents, patient tolerability, safety, convenience, and cost.

Aldosterone blockade is another pharmacologic strategy for inhibition of the RAAS. The EPHESUS trial randomly assigned 6642 patients with acute MI complicated by left ventricular dysfunction and heart failure to a regimen of the selective aldosterone blocker eplerenone or placebo in conjunction with contemporary postinfarction pharmacotherapy.[53,54] During a mean follow-up period of 16 months, a 15% reduction occurred in the relative risk of mortality in the eplerenone treatment group. Cardiovascular mortality or hospitalization for cardiovascular events also was reduced by eplerenone. Serious hyperkalemia (serum potassium concentration above 6 mmol/L) occurred in 5.5% of patients in the eplerenone group compared with 3.9% of patients in the placebo group ($P < .002$). We favor long-term administration of aldosterone blockade for high-risk patients after STEMI (ejection fraction less than 40%, clinical heart failure, diabetes mellitus) who are already receiving an ACE inhibitor and beta-blocker and do not have contraindications. In view of the small but definite increase in the risk of serious hyperkalemia associated with aldosterone blockade, particularly with concurrent use of other measures for inhibition of the RAAS, periodic monitoring of the serum potassium level is recommended.

β-Adrenergic Blockers

Although beta-blockade is recommended in the setting of uncomplicated acute MI (class I), it is contraindicated for patients with shock, and caution is advised regarding use in patients at risk for cardiogenic shock.[12,13] The recommendations for at-risk patients are based on findings from the Clopidogrel and Metoprolol in Myocardial Infarction Trial (COMMIT) in 45,852 patients randomly assigned to a regimen of early intravenous and subsequent high-dose oral metoprolol or placebo within 24 hours of MI, most of whom presented with STEMI and were treated with fibrinolysis or medical therapy alone.[13] Lower rates of recurrent MI and ventricular fibrillation were counterbalanced by higher rates of cardiogenic shock, particularly in association with older age (older than 70 years), lower systolic blood pressure (below 120 mm Hg), elevated heart rate (above 110 beats/min), and late presentation. An observational study in the NCDR registry of 34,661 patients with NSTEMI or STEMI treated with more contemporary therapies, including PCI, found that in addition to older age, increased heart rate, and lower blood pressure, a history of heart failure and left ventricular dysfunction (ejection fraction below 40%) were risk factors for cardiogenic shock or death with beta-blocker use.[55]

By contrast, other studies have demonstrated improved long-term outcomes with subacute initiation of chronic beta-blockade after MI in patients with left ventricular dysfunction or heart failure. For example, the Carvedilol Post-Infarct Survival Control in Left Ventricular Dysfunction (CAPRICORN) study, which randomly assigned 1959 patients with reduced left ventricular systolic dysfunction after MI to receive carvedilol or placebo an average of 10 days after MI, observed lower rates of death, recurrent MI, and atrial and ventricular arrhythmias with beta-blockade.[6] As a result, the professional society guidelines recommend that beta-blocker therapy be withheld in the first 24 hours for patients with heart failure or other risk factors for the development of shock. However, in-hospital eligibility for beta-blocker therapy should be reassessed after 24 hours. Furthermore, patients with heart failure or left ventricular function should receive chronic beta-blocker therapy for long-term secondary prevention.[12,13]

Investigational Agents

Randomized studies of therapies that target systemic inflammation or vasodilation in MI, heart failure, or shock are limited and generally have not proved successful to date. For example, the anti-inflammatory agent pexelizumab, a monoclonal antibody against complement, did not reduce mortality in acute STEMI.[5] Owing to the putative role of nitric oxide in causing inappropriately low SVR and myocardial depression in cardiogenic shock, tilarginine acetate, an inhibitor of nitric oxide synthase, was studied in patients with acute MI and cardiogenic shock (see Figure 25-3). The Tilarginine Acetate Injection in a Randomized International Study in Unstable MI Patients with Cardiogenic Shock (TRIUMPH) trial in 398 patients was stopped for futility with no difference in all-cause mortality at 30 days, despite an increase in blood pressure.[8,48]

In view of the link between inflammation, increased xanthine oxidase (XO) activity, and free radical production, XO has been identified as a potential target in heart failure. An observational study of continuous allopurinol therapy was associated with reduced heart failure readmissions or deaths in more than 25,000 patients with heart failure.[56] The Xanthine Oxidase Inhibition for Hyperuricemic Heart Failure Patients (EXACT-HF) trial, which randomly assigned 253 patients with symptomatic heart failure, left ventricular dysfunction, and hyperuricemia to receive allopurinol versus placebo, did not identify a difference in clinical status, function, or ejection fraction after 24 weeks of therapy.[57] To date, allopurinol has not been studied in the setting of cardiogenic shock.

Methylene blue is an inhibitor of guanylate cycle that decreases cGMP in vascular smooth muscle, resulting in vasoconstriction. Methylene blue increased mean arterial pressure and SVR, as well as reducing mortality, in a small study of patients with vasoplegia following cardiopulmonary bypass ($n = 58$).[48] Its use is contraindicated in patients with cardiogenic shock with normal or high SVR, owing to a resultant decrease in cardiac output.

Mechanical Circulatory Support

In severe cases of cardiogenic shock, pharmacologic therapy may not provide sufficient hemodynamic support. It is hypothesized that early and appropriate use of MCS will interrupt the spiral of shock through improvement in cardiac output, blood pressure, and perfusion and thereby help to correct or limit ongoing ischemia, progressive ventricular dysfunction, development of multiorgan dysfunction, and risk of death (see Figure 25-4; see also Figure 27-1). However, demonstration of an improvement in long-term survival in randomized trials is lacking. The options for temporary MCS, which include use of the intra-aortic balloon pump (IABP), TandemHeart percutaneous ventricular assist device, Impella Recover System, extracorporeal membrane oxygenation (ECMO), and CentriMag blood pump, are discussed in detail in Chapter 27. Presented here is a brief review of considerations in the selection of patients for initiation of MCS and in the timing of this intervention.

In general, the choice of temporary mechanical support should be guided by patient characteristics in the context of institutional expertise/experience and consultation with a multidisciplinary team, including the critical care staff, interventional cardiology, cardiac surgery, and advanced heart failure. Not infrequently, temporary MCS is employed in acutely ill patients as a "bridge to decision," allowing time to assess the likelihood of recovery and/or appropriateness for destination therapy with placement of a ventricular assist device (VAD) or transplantation (see Figure 25-6). The 2015 ACAI/ACC/HFSA/STS statement, based primarily on expert consensus, recommends that in light of the superior hemodynamic support provided by MCS compared with pharmacologic therapy, early institution of MCS may be considered in patients with cardiogenic shock who fail to stabilize quickly after initial interventions (e.g., reperfusion) and may even be considered for those undergoing high-risk PCI (e.g., multivessel or unprotected left main coronary artery) with severe heart failure or left ventricular dysfunction.[19] On account of the lack of data for MCS after MI, prospective, randomized studies comparing different strategies are necessary to determine the benefit of initiating MCS after MI, as well as to determine the optimal timing and choice of device.

In clinical practice, a rational approach is to initiate a preliminary discussion of the options for temporary percutaneous MCS in patients who have had an inadequate response to initial pharmacotherapy, so that if they fail to respond to additional titration of the pharmacotherapeutic regimen, MCS can be instituted before severe end-organ dysfunction ensues. In our own experience, once shock has progressed, with consequent severe hepatic injury, overt bowel ischemia, or the development of SIRS, outcomes with MCS are extremely poor. We therefore strive to initiate MCS once there is reasonable evidence that pharmacological support is likely to fail and before these severe consequences of end-organ hypoperfusion emerge

Device selection should be based on the amount of hemodynamic support required, whether biventricular support is necessary (favoring ECMO or TandemHeart), whether oxygenation is needed (requiring ECMO), and on the temporal urgency of initiation, with acknowledgment that placement of some devices (e.g., TandemHeart) is more time-consuming. Institutional experience and operator expertise tend to play heavily in the options available for MCS.

SUMMARY

Heart failure, characterized by pulmonary or central venous congestion, and cardiogenic shock, defined by heart failure with inadequate end-organ perfusion, are complications of acute MI that portend poor short- and long-term outcomes. The primary goal of therapy in both cases is reversal of ischemia via reperfusion. Heart failure management in the absence of shock should focus on treatment of volume overload, afterload reduction, and prevention of adverse left ventricular remodeling. Additional therapy for cardiogenic shock should prioritize maintenance of blood pressure and end-organ perfusion through pharmacologic or mechanical means. In light of the persistently high mortality associated with cardiogenic shock after acute MI, additional investigations are critically needed to support evidence-based practices in this little-studied population.

References

1. Jhund PS, McMurray JJ: Heart failure after acute myocardial infarction: a lost battle in the war on heart failure? *Circulation* 118(20):2019–2021, 2008.
2. Flaherty JD, Bax JJ, De Luca L, et al.: Acute heart failure syndromes in patients with coronary artery disease: early assessment and treatment, *J Am Coll Cardiol* 53(3):254–263, 2009.
3. Aissaoui N, Puymirat E, Tabone X, et al.: Improved outcome of cardiogenic shock at the acute stage of myocardial infarction: a report from the USIK 1995, USIC 2000, and FAST-MI French nationwide registries, *Eur Heart J* 33(20):2535–2543, 2012.
4. Goldberg RJ, Spencer FA, Gore JM, et al.: Thirty-year trends (1975 to 2005) in the magnitude of, management of, and hospital death rates associated with cardiogenic shock in patients with acute myocardial infarction: a population-based perspective, *Circulation* 119(9):1211–1219, 2009.
5. Reynolds HR, Hochman JS: Cardiogenic shock: current concepts and improving outcomes, *Circulation* 117(5):686–697, 2008.
6. Yancy CW, Jessup M, Bozkurt B, et al.: 2013 ACCF/AHA guideline for the management of heart failure: a report of the American College of Cardiology Foundation/American Heart Association Task Force on practice guidelines, *Circulation* 128(16):e240–e327, 2013.
7. Stevenson LW, Pagani FD, Young JB, et al.: INTERMACS profiles of advanced heart failure: the current picture, *J Heart Lung Transplant* 28(6):535–541, 2009.
8. Thiele H, Allam B, Chatellier G, et al.: Shock in acute myocardial infarction: the Cape Horn for trials? *Eur Heart J* 31(15):1828–1835, 2010.
9. Steg PG, Dabbous OH, Feldman LJ, et al.: Determinants and prognostic impact of heart failure complicating acute coronary syndromes: observations from the Global Registry of Acute Coronary Events (GRACE), *Circulation* 109(4):494–499, 2004.
10. McAlindon E, Bucciarelli-Ducci C, Suleiman MS, Baumbach A: Infarct size reduction in acute myocardial infarction, *Heart* 101(2):155–160, 2015.
11. Kelly DJ, Gershlick T, Witzenbichler B, et al.: Incidence and predictors of heart failure following percutaneous coronary intervention in ST-segment elevation myocardial infarction: the HORIZONS-AMI trial, *Am Heart J* 162(4):663–670, 2011.
12. Amsterdam EA, Wenger NK, Brindis RG, et al.: 2014 AHA/ACC guideline for the management of patients with non-ST-elevation acute coronary syndromes: executive summary: a report of the American College of Cardiology/American Heart Association Task Force on Practice Guidelines, *Circulation* 130(25):2354–2394, 2014.
13. O'Gara PT, Kushner FG, Ascheim DD, et al.: 2013 ACCF/AHA guideline for the management of ST-elevation myocardial infarction: a report of the American College of Cardiology Foundation/American Heart Association Task Force on Practice Guidelines, *Circulation* 127(4):e362–e425, 2013.
14. Katz JN, Stebbins AL, Alexander JH, et al.: Predictors of 30-day mortality in patients with refractory cardiogenic shock following acute myocardial infarction despite a patent infarct artery, *Am Heart J* 158(4):680–687, 2009.
15. Thiele H, Zeymer U, Neumann FJ, et al.: Intra-aortic balloon counterpulsation in acute myocardial infarction complicated by cardiogenic shock (IABP-SHOCK II): final 12 month results of a randomised, open-label trial, *Lancet* 382(9905):1638–1645, 2013.
16. Thiele H, Ohman EM, Desch S, Eitel I, de Waha S: Management of cardiogenic shock, *Eur Heart J* 36(20):1223–1230, 2015.
17. Prondzinsky R, Unverzagt S, Lemm H, et al.: Interleukin-6, -7, -8 and -10 predict outcome in acute myocardial infarction complicated by cardiogenic shock, *Clin Res Cardiol* 101(5):375–384, 2012.
18. Link A, Pöss J, Rbah R, et al.: Circulating angiopoietins and cardiovascular mortality in cardiogenic shock, *Eur Heart J* 34(22):1651–1662, 2013.
19. Rihal CS, Naidu SS, Givertz MM, et al.: 2015 SCAI/ACC/HFSA/STS Clinical Expert Consensus Statement on the Use of Percutaneous Mechanical Circulatory Support Devices in Cardiovascular Care: Endorsed by the American Heart Assocation, the Cardiological Society of India, and Sociedad

Latino Americana de Cardiologia Intervencion; Affirmation of Value by the Canadian Association of Interventional Cardiology–Association Canadienne de Cardiologie d'Intervention, *J Am Coll Cardiol* 65(19):e7–e26, 2015.

20. Landry DW, Oliver JA: The pathogenesis of vasodilatory shock, *N Engl J Med* 345(8):588–5895, 2001.
21. Overgaard CB, Dzavik V: Inotropes and vasopressors: review of physiology and clinical use in cardiovascular disease, *Circulation* 118(10):1047–1056, 2008.
22. Shpektor A: Cardiogenic shock: the role of inflammation, *Acute Card Care* 12(4):115–118, 2010.
23. Tamariz L, Hare JM: Inflammatory cytokines in heart failure: roles in aetiology and utility as biomarkers, *Eur Heart J* 31(7):768–770, 2010.
24. Frangogiannis NG: The inflammatory response in myocardial injury, repair, and remodelling, *Nat Rev Cardiol* 11(5):255–265, 2014.
25. Grimaldi D, Guivarch E, Neveux N, et al.: Markers of intestinal injury are associated with endotoxemia in successfully resuscitated patients, *Resuscitation* 84(1):60–65, 2013.
26. Grimaldi D, Sauneuf B, Guivarch E, et al.: High level of endotoxemia following out-of-hospital cardiac arrest is associated with severity and duration of postcardiac arrest shock, *Crit Care Med* 43(12):2597–2604, 2015.
27. Thygesen K, Alpert JS, Jaffe AS, et al.: Third universal definition of myocardial infarction, *Circulation* 126(16):2020–2035, 2012.
28. Januzzi Jr JL, Filippatos G, Nieminen M, Gheorghiade M: Troponin elevation in patients with heart failure: on behalf of the third Universal Definition of Myocardial Infarction Global Task Force: Heart Failure Section, *Eur Heart J* 33(18):2265–2271, 2012.
29. Authors/Task Force members, Windecker S, Kolh P, et al.: 2014 ESC/EACTS Guidelines on myocardial revascularization: the Task Force on Myocardial Revascularization of the European Society of Cardiology (ESC) and the European Association for Cardio-Thoracic Surgery (EACTS). Developed with the special contribution of the European Association of Percutaneous Cardiovascular Interventions (EAPCI), *Eur Heart J* 35(37):2541–2619, 2014.
30. Mor-Avi V, Lang RM, Badano LP, et al.: Current and evolving echocardiographic techniques for the quantitative evaluation of cardiac mechanics: ASE/EAE consensus statement on methodology and indications endorsed by the Japanese Society of Echocardiography, *J Am Soc Echocardiogr* 24(3):277–313, 2011.
31. Alhashemi JA, Cecconi M, Hofer CK: Cardiac output monitoring: an integrative perspective, *Crit Care* 15(2):214, 2011.
32. Task Force on the Management Of ST-Segment Elevation Acute Myocardial Infarction of the European Society of Cardiology (ESC), Steg PG, James SK, et al.: ESC guidelines for the management of acute myocardial infarction in patients presenting with ST-segment elevation, *Eur Heart J* 33(20):2569–2619, 2012.
33. den Uil CA, Lagrand WK, van der Ent M, et al.: Impaired microcirculation predicts poor outcome of patients with acute myocardial infarction complicated by cardiogenic shock, *Eur Heart J* 31(24):3032–3039, 2010.
34. Scheeren TW, Schober P, Schwarte LA: Monitoring tissue oxygenation by near infrared spectroscopy (NIRS): background and current applications, *J Clin Monit Comput* 26(4):279–287, 2012.
35. Hochman JS, Sleeper LA, Webb JG, et al.: Early revascularization and long-term survival in cardiogenic shock complicating acute myocardial infarction, *JAMA* 295(21):2511–2515, 2006.
36. Thiele H, Zeymer U, Neumann FJ, et al.: Intraaortic balloon support for myocardial infarction with cardiogenic shock, *N Engl J Med* 367(14):1287–1296, 2012.
37. Engstrom T, Kelbæk H, Helqvist S, et al.: Complete revascularisation versus treatment of the culprit lesion only in patients with ST-segment elevation myocardial infarction and multivessel disease (DANAMI-3-PRIMULTI): an open-label, randomised controlled trial, *Lancet* 386(9994): 665–671, 2015.
38. Wald DS, Morris JK, Wald NJ: Preventive angioplasty in myocardial infarction, *N Engl J Med* 370(3):283, 2014.
39. Gershlick AH, Khan JN, Kelly DJ, et al.: Randomized trial of complete versus lesion-only revascularization in patients undergoing primary percutaneous coronary intervention for STEMI and multivessel disease: the CvLPRIT trial, *J Am Coll Cardiol* 65(10):963–972, 2015.
40. Mylotte D, Morice MC, Eltchaninoff H, et al.: Primary percutaneous coronary intervention in patients with acute myocardial infarction, resuscitated cardiac arrest, and cardiogenic shock: the role of primary multivessel revascularization, *JACC Cardiovasc Interv* 6(2):115–125, 2013.
41. Asfar P, Teboul JL, Radermacher P: High versus low blood-pressure target in septic shock, *N Engl J Med* 371(3):283–284, 2014.
42. Chen HH, Anstrom KJ, Givertz MM, et al.: Low-dose dopamine or low-dose nesiritide in acute heart failure with renal dysfunction: the ROSE acute heart failure randomized trial, *JAMA* 310(23):2533–2543, 2013.
43. De Backer D, Biston P, Devriendt J, et al.: Comparison of dopamine and norepinephrine in the treatment of shock, *N Engl J Med* 362(9):779–789, 2010.
44. Dellinger RP, Levy MM, Rhodes A, et al.: Surviving sepsis campaign: international guidelines for management of severe sepsis and septic shock, *Crit Care Med* 41(2):580–637, 2013.
45. Hagihara A, Hasegawa M, Abe T, et al.: Prehospital epinephrine use and survival among patients with out-of-hospital cardiac arrest, *JAMA* 307(11):1161–1168, 2012.
46. Dumas F, Bougouin W, Geri G, et al.: Is epinephrine during cardiac arrest associated with worse outcomes in resuscitated patients? *J Am Coll Cardiol* 64(22):2360–2367, 2014.
47. Russell JA: Bench-to-bedside review: vasopressin in the management of septic shock, *Crit Care* 15(4):226, 2011.
48. Nativi-Nicolau J, Selzman CH, Fang JC, Stehlik J: Pharmacologic therapies for acute cardiogenic shock, *Curr Opin Cardiol* 29(3):250–257, 2014.
49. Unverzagt S, Wachsmuth L, Hirsch K, et al.: Inotropic agents and vasodilator strategies for acute myocardial infarction complicated by cardiogenic shock or low cardiac output syndrome, *Cochrane Database Syst Rev*(1)CD009669, 2014.
50. Felker GM, Lee KL, Bull DA, et al.: Diuretic strategies in patients with acute decompensated heart failure, *N Engl J Med* 364(9):797–805, 2011.
51. Bart BA, Goldsmith SR, Lee KL, et al.: Ultrafiltration in decompensated heart failure with cardiorenal syndrome, *N Engl J Med* 367(24):2296–2304, 2012.
52. Welch TD, Yang EH, Reeder GS, Gersh BJ: Modern management of acute myocardial infarction, *Curr Probl Cardiol* 37(7):237–310, 2012.
53. Lang CC, Struthers AD: Targeting the renin-angiotensin-aldosterone system in heart failure, *Nat Rev Cardiol* 10(3):125–134, 2013.
54. Rassi AN, Cavender MA, Fonarow GC, et al.: Temporal trends and predictors in the use of aldosterone antagonists post-acute myocardial infarction, *J Am Coll Cardiol* 61(1):35–40, 2013.
55. Kontos MC, Diercks DB, Ho PM, et al.: Treatment and outcomes in patients with myocardial infarction treated with acute β-blocker therapy: results from the American College of Cardiology's NCDR(R), *Am Heart J* 161(5):864–870, 2011.
56. Thanassoulis G, Brophy JM, Richard H, Pilote L: Gout, allopurinol use, and heart failure outcomes, *Arch Intern Med* 170(15):1358–1364, 2010.
57. Givertz MM, Anstrom KJ, Redfield MM, et al.: Effects of xanthine oxidase inhibition in hyperuricemic heart failure patients: the Xanthine Oxidase Inhibition for Hyperuricemic Heart Failure Patients (EXACT-HF) study, *Circulation* 131(20):1763–1771, 2015.

26 Mechanical Complications of Myocardial Infarction

James C. Fang and Jack H. Morshedzadeh

INTRODUCTION

Myocardial infarction (MI) caused by coronary artery disease remains the leading cause of death in the United States (see Chapter 2).[1] Although the advent of coronary care units and early reperfusion therapy has decreased in-hospital mortality rates for acute MI by one-third, acute MI remains an important cause of death.[1] Along with cardiogenic shock (see Chapter 25), complications from severe myocardial injury are a major contributor to the in-hospital mortality of MI. Among these complications are right ventricular (RV) infarction, mechanical complications (left ventricular [LV] free-wall rupture, pseudoaneurysm, ventricular septal rupture, or acute mitral regurgitation), ventricular aneurysm, and LV thrombus with or without embolization. Rapid diagnosis of MI and rapid reperfusion therapy have decreased the incidence of these complications; however, when they do occur, survival remains dependent upon timely diagnosis and emergent or urgent treatment.

RIGHT VENTRICULAR INFARCTION

RV infarction rarely occurs in isolation. Fifty percent of patients with inferior MI and ≤10% of patients with anterior infarction have some degree of RV involvement.[2] Significant RV infarction almost always results from a proximal occlusion of the right coronary artery, which compromises flow to major RV branches. Infarction of the ventricular septum from a proximal left anterior descending (LAD) artery occlusion can also affect RV performance because of the important impact of septal systolic function on RV ejection. The RV is more resistant to infarction than the LV because it has less myocardial oxygen consumption, which is caused by its smaller muscle mass and some oxygen delivery from the endocardium into the thin free wall. Because RV function often recovers after infarction, some investigators have preferred the concept of RV "stunning" rather than permanent infarction.[3]

RV infarction may lead to decreased cardiac output as a result of acute RV distension, a reduction in RV contractility, and the inability to fill the LV through the pulmonary circulation. Acute RV diastolic dysfunction and enlargement produces an impediment to RV filling and leads to venous congestion. The decreased RV forward stroke volume from decreased RV contractility is further compromised by significant functional tricuspid regurgitation as a consequence of acute RV dilation. Moreover, RV systolic performance may be further impeded by passive pulmonary hypertension as a consequence of increased LV end-diastolic pressure (EDP) from concomitant LV infarction. The decrease in RV forward stroke volume ultimately leads to an inability to fill the LV.

Increased RV volume and RVEDP also displaces the interventricular septum toward the volume-compromised LV, further impairing LV filling and compliance. Ischemia of the interventricular septum, with loss of contribution to global RV systolic function, will further reduce RV stroke volume. Finally, RV dilation within the noncompliant pericardium results in elevated intrapericardial pressures, causing a further decrease in LV filling and equalization of diastolic pressures (Figure 26-1).[4]

Diagnosis of Right Ventricular Infarction

Physical Examination in Right Ventricular Infarction

The clinical triad of hypotension, clear lung fields, and an elevated jugular venous pressure has been traditionally considered a marker of RV infarction in patients with inferior MI. However, this triad has a low sensitivity (25%) and high specificity (96%). Kussmaul sign (distention of the jugular vein with inspiration), which is indicative of poor RV compliance, and pulsus paradoxus (a decrease in systolic blood pressure >10 mm Hg with inspiration), which is indicative of increased interventricular dependence when the RV suddenly distends in the fixed pericardial space, may also occur with RV infarction. The primary differential diagnostic consideration is cardiac tamponade from free-wall rupture, which is characterized by the presence of pulsus paradoxus but a lack of Kussmaul sign. Auscultation may reveal a right-sided S3 and S4 gallop and a tricuspid regurgitation murmur. An RV heave may be present from the acutely dilated RV. Occasionally, a harsh systolic murmur may signify the coexistence of an inferobasal ventricular septal defect complicating the concomitant inferoposterior MI. Cannon a-waves in the jugular pulse and bradycardia may suggest concomitant heart block as

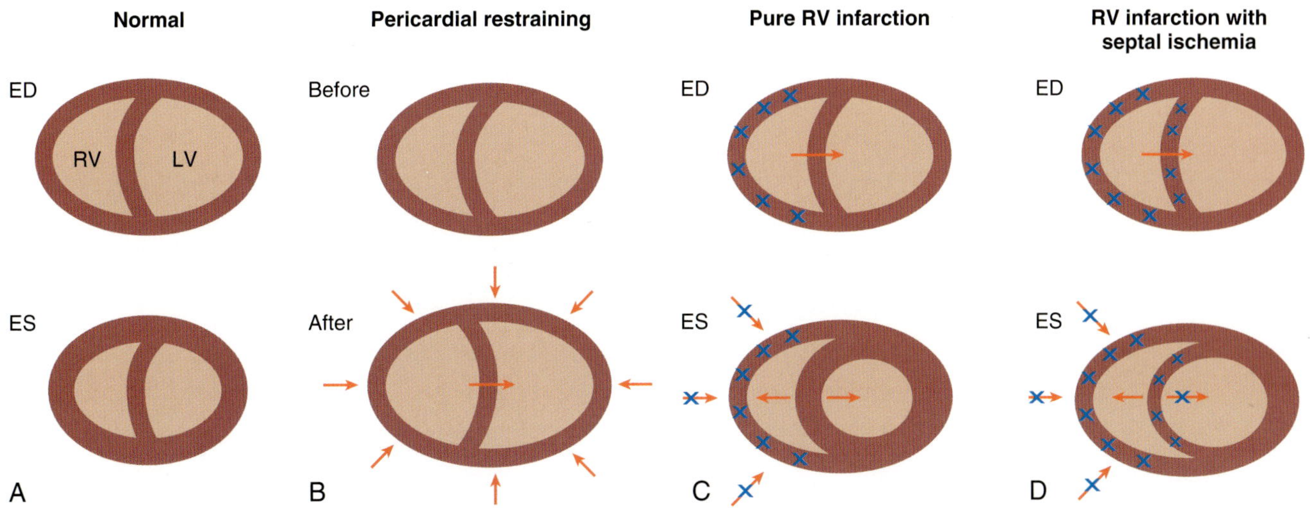

FIGURE 26-1 Two physiological concepts explaining the detrimental effects of excessive volume loading. (**A**) Normal ventricle: at end-systole (ES), the right ventricular (RV) free wall moves toward the septum compared with end-diastole (ED). (**B**) Pericardial restraining effects (*top*, before volume loading; *bottom*, after excessive volume loading); RV dilation, as a result of excessive volume loading, can lead to the elevation of intrapericardial pressure, an increase in pericardial constraint (*red arrow*), and change geometry because of interventricular septum shift. These changes contribute to the low-output state by decreasing left ventricular (LV) distensibility, preload, and ventricular elastance. (**C** and **D**) Role of the interventricular septum (**C**, pure RV infarction; **D**, RV infarction with septal ischemia). (**C**) At ES, the RV free wall moves toward the septum. At ED, the RV dilates during diastole, and the septum reverse curves toward the volume-reduced LV. At ES, the septum thickens, but moves paradoxically into the RV, displacing the RV volume despite RV free wall dyskinesis. (**D**) Septal ischemia depresses septal contraction and global LV function, resulting in LV dilation. The septum stops thickening, and there is increased systolic septal displacement into the RV. Pansystolic septal thinning and more extensive paradoxical displacement are associated with further depression of RV performance. *(From Inohara T, et al: The challenges in the management of right ventricular infarction.* Eur Heart J: Acute Cardiovasc Care *2:231, 2013.)*

well. Hepatojugular reflux may also be present. Hypoxemia that does not correct using high-flow oxygen may be indicative of an in atrial shunt through a patent foramen ovale if right atrial pressure exceeds left atrial pressure. However, electrocardiography and noninvasive imaging are the cornerstones of the diagnosis of RV infarction because of their high specificity and the low sensitivity associated with physical examination.

Electrocardiography of Right Ventricular Infarction

RV infarction is frequently diagnosed with the electrocardiogram (ECG) and is best accomplished with the right precordial leads. Because of the association of RV infarction with inferior MI, ST-segment elevation in the inferior leads (II, III, avF) should always be accompanied by assessment of the right precordial leads. Suspicion for RV infarction is heightened further when there is disproportionate ST-segment elevation of lead III greater than lead II. On a right-sided ECG, ST-segment elevation of more than 1 mm in lead V_4R is considered significant, and it is also a strong independent predictor of major complications and in-hospital mortality. This ST-segment elevation is believed to represent an ischemic injury to the posterobasal septum. Several other ECG criteria have been proposed in the evaluation of patients with suspected RV infarction (Figure 26-2).

Hemodynamics in Right Ventricular Infarction

The use of invasive hemodynamics at the time of revascularization or during the initial management of an inferior MI can provide insight into the degree of right heart dysfunction (Figure 26-e1). If right atrial function is not compromised, the a-wave and x descent of the right atrial pressure are enhanced, but the y descent may be blunted because of pandiastolic RV dysfunction. In patients with associated right atrial dysfunction, the right atrial pressures are often higher, but the a-wave will be depressed, and the x and y descents will form an "M or W" pattern. A rapid y descent in RV infarction should also prompt consideration of concomitant tricuspid regurgitation (TR). If the TR is severe, the right atrial waveform will approximate the RV waveform. A "square root" sign may be present in the RV tracing, and it reflects poorly compliant RV filling exclusively in early diastole before the filling is suddenly truncated. Criteria for hemodynamically significant RV infarction include: (1) elevated right atrial pressure (RAP) more than 10 mm Hg; (2) an elevated RAP to pulmonary capillary wedge pressure (PCWP) ratio of more than 0.86; (3) a narrow pulmonary artery pulse pressure; (4) an increased ratio of RVEDP to LVEDP; and (5) a decreased pulmonary artery pulsatility index of less than 1 (PAPi = PA pulse pressure/RAP).[5]

Echocardiography of Right Ventricular Infarction

Echocardiography is a widely available and inexpensive tool for the comprehensive evaluation of the structure, function, and hemodynamics of the RV (see also Chapter 31). Echocardiography of the RV has many technical challenges, including the complex shape of the RV, incomplete visualization in any single echocardiographic view, and the afterload dependence of the RV, which can lead to inaccurate interpretation of RV performance.[6] Several traditional and novel parameters have been used to assess the degree of RV dysfunction in the setting of inferior MI (Table 26-1 and Figure 26-3). It is important to note that echocardiographic findings of RV dysfunction may be temporary and can resolve within a few hours. Cardiac magnetic resonance (CMR) imaging (see Chapter 33) has become the gold standard for noninvasive assessment of RV function, and it is the most accurate method for determining the extent of infarction and RV mass, volume, and ejection fraction (Figure 26-e2).

Prognosis with Right Ventricular Infarction

Although RV infarction may result in profound acute hemodynamic effects, arrhythmias, and higher in-hospital

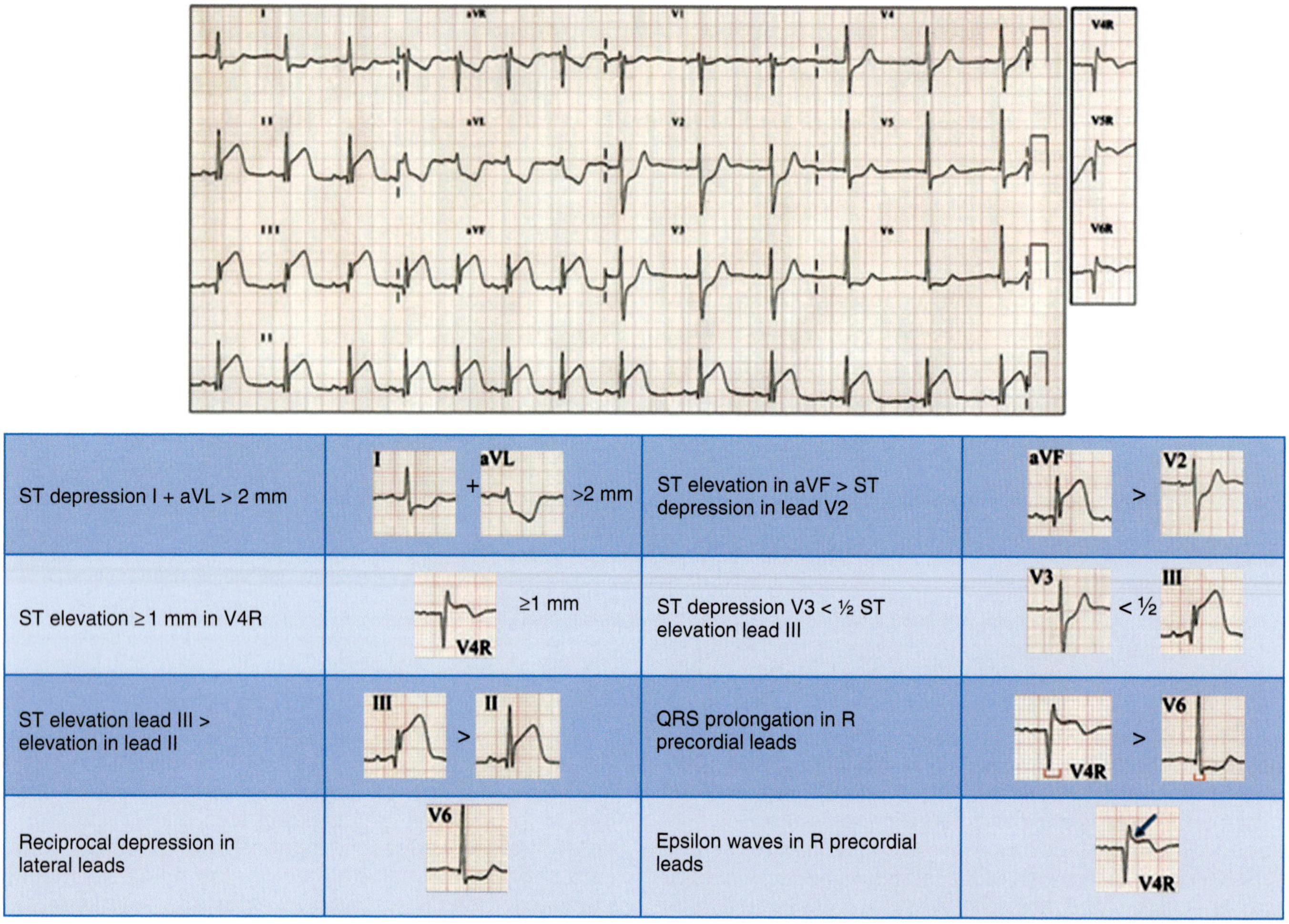

FIGURE 26-2 **Summary of electrocardiography features of right ventricular myocardial infarction (MI) complicating inferior MI.** Coronary angiography confirmed proximal occlusion of the right coronary artery with minor left anterior descending artery disease. *(From Kakouros N, Cokkinos D: Right ventricular myocardial infarction: pathophysiology, diagnosis, and management.* Postgrad Med J *86:722, 2010.)*

mortality, chronic right heart failure secondary to RV infarction is rare. Patients with inferior MI have a substantially increased risk of short-term death during hospitalization if RV involvement is present, but those who survive hospitalization have a relatively good long-term prognosis. This paradox is attributed to the favorable supply–demand characteristics of the RV. Other unique anatomic and physiologic characteristics of the RV also contribute to recovery from RV infarction. First, the pulmonary circulation poses a significantly lower afterload compared with the systemic circulation, thus a minimal perfusion gradient is sufficient to maintain pulmonary blood flow. Second, the thin RV free wall allows for coronary perfusion in both systole and diastole. Third, the RV has a rich collateral arterial supply from the LAD artery, which also provides most of the blood flow to the ventricular septum.

TABLE 26-1 Echocardiographic Parameters Used to Evaluate Right Ventricular Dysfunction in the Setting of Myocardial Infarction

Parameter
Increased ratio of RV to LV end-diastolic dimension
RV free wall motion abnormalities
Paradoxical interventricular septal motion
Fractional area change
Tricuspid annular plane systolic excursion
Doppler tissue imaging of the peak systolic tricuspid lateral annulus velocity (S′)
RV myocardial performance index or Tei index
RV peak systolic longitudinal strain
RV ejection fraction as assessed by 3D echocardiography

3D, Three-dimensional; *LV*, left ventricular; *RV*, right ventricular.

Treatment of Right Ventricular Infarction

A concise summary of the assessment and treatment of inferior MI complicated by RV dysfunction is provided in Figure 26-4. The mainstay of management of RV infarction is immediate revascularization. Once coronary flow has been established, attention is then directed toward hemodynamic and electrical stabilization. In patients with RV infarction, the dilated noncompliant RV is preload dependent, which will exacerbate a stiff LV that may be preload-deprived. Any measure that further reduces LV preload will be detrimental; therefore, vasodilators and diuretics are contraindicated. Although most patients (75%) with RV infarction are clinically silent without significant hemodynamic compromise, RV infarction may be subsequently "unmasked" with standard treatment for LV infarction (e.g., β-blockade, morphine, and nitroglycerin) that exacerbates the preload sensitive state.

Adequate plasma volume expansion, ideally with the aid of invasive monitoring, is essential in the treatment of RV infarction when a low cardiac output and shock are present

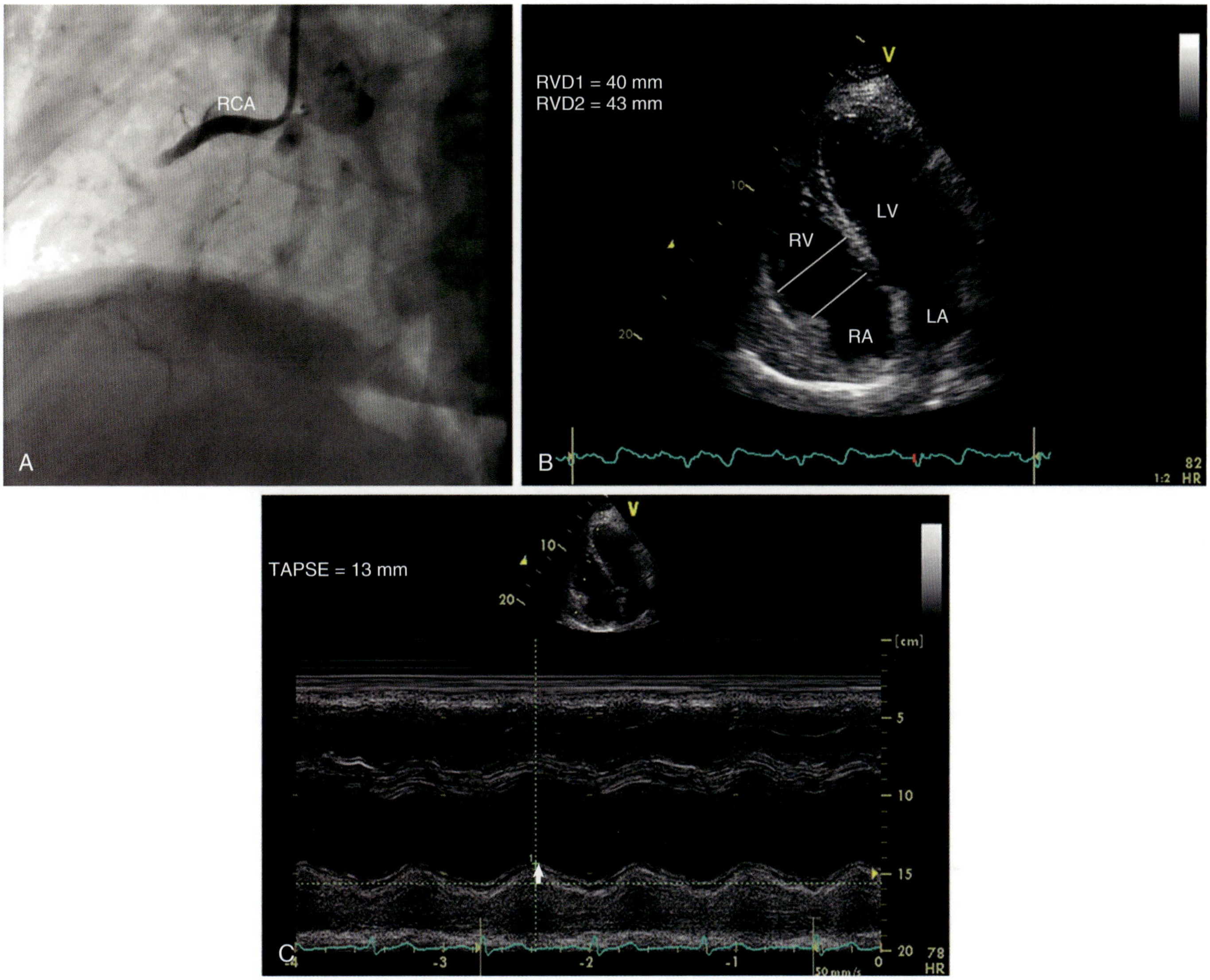

FIGURE 26-3 (**A**) A patient with acute proximal right coronary artery (RCA) occlusion, resulting in (**B**) right ventricular dilation and (**C**) depressed right ventricular performance as indicated by reduced tricuspid annular plane systolic excursion (TAPSE). The apical four-chamber view is focused on the right ventricle (RV) to optimize the imaging of the lateral wall and to measure basal (RVD1) and midcavity (RVD2) right ventricular diameters. *LA*, Left atrium; *LV*, left ventricle; *RA*, right atrium. *(From Rallidis L, Makavos G, Nihoyannopoulos P: From right ventricular involvement in coronary artery disease: role of echocardiography for diagnosis and prognosis.* J Am Soc Echocardiogr *27:227, 2014.)*

1. Coronary revascularization
2. Assessment of RV function and/or hemodynamics

Echocardiogram	Hemodynamics
Abnormal RV wall motion	RAP >10 mm Hg
RV enlargement	RAP/PCWP > 0.86
Paradoxical septal motion	Narrow pulmonary artery pulse pressure
TAPSE <10 mm	Increase ratio of RVEDP/LVEDP
S' <12 cm/sec	PAPi <1

3. Avoid beta-blockers, diuretics, vasodilators, and morphine.
4. Plasma volume expansion (ideally RAP <16 mm Hg)
5. For continued hypotension, begin inotropic therapy (dobutamine).
6. Optimize AV synchrony and chronotropic competence with temporary AV pacing.
7. For refractory hypotension consider mechanical support with pRVAD or IABP.
8. For continued compromise consider ECMO.

FIGURE 26-4 Treatment algorithm for patients with suspected right ventricular (RV) infarction. *ECMO*, Extracorporeal membrane oxygenation; *IABP*, intra-aortic balloon pump; *LVEDP*, left ventricular end-diastolic pressure; *PAPi*, pulmonary artery pulsatility index; *PCWP*, pulmonary capillary wedge pressure; *pRVAD*, percutaneous right ventricular assist device; *RAP*, right atrial pressure; *RVEDP*, right ventricular end-diastolic pressure; S′, pulse-wave Doppler tissue imaging of the lateral tricuspid annulus; *TAPSE*, tricuspid annular plane systolic excursion.

(see Chapter 25). Fluid replacement can be challenging in patients with severe RV dysfunction, but it is recommended to passively "drive" filling of the LV (e.g., a Fontan-like circulation). An overly aggressive approach to volume expansion can result in further clinical deterioration because of the detrimental effects of excess volume loading. Consequent excessive RV dilation can compromise LV output because of pericardial restraint and exaggeration of biventricular interdependence. By compromising LV filling, this situation will decrease LV stroke volume and precipitate a low-output state, particularly if concomitant bradycardia is present. The optimal RV filling pressure in RV infarction is not known; studies that used standard volume loading protocols have not demonstrated improvements in cardiac output, but may have been limited by the variable initial volume status of patients.

Interventricular septal contraction contributes to 30% to 50% of RV stroke work. Patients with intact LV septal contraction (manifest as paradoxical septal motion with preserved thickening on echocardiography) have a better prognosis. In RV infarction associated with significant septal dysfunction, hypotension and low cardiac output may be refractory to initial fluid optimization. Under these circumstances, the use of inotropic stimulation (commonly with dobutamine) will improve RV performance by enhancing global LV contraction and increasing septal displacement into the RV.

Electrical stabilization, including an adequate heart rate and atrioventricular (AV) synchrony, are essential in preserving cardiac output in RV infarction. High-grade AV block and bradycardia-related hypotension without AV block commonly complicate inferior MI. These arrhythmias are attributed to the effects of AV nodal ischemia and cardioinhibitory (Bezold-Jarisch) reflexes arising from stimulation of vagal afferents in the ischemic LV inferoposterior wall. The ischemic RV has a relatively fixed stroke volume as does the preload-deprived LV. Therefore, biventricular output is heart rate–dependent. In some hypotensive bradycardic patients, atropine may restore physiologic rhythm. If temporary pacing is required, right atrial rather than RV pacing is favored to maintain AV synchrony. Acute transvenous pacing can be technically difficult with placing and securing a transvenous lead in the right atrial appendage. In the case of emergency ventricular pacing, both sensing and pacing may be inadequate in an acutely infarcted RV, which is also prone to perforation and ventricular arrhythmias.

Mechanical circulatory support (see Chapter 27) may also be necessary for those with refractory hypotension unresponsive to volume resuscitation, inotropic therapy, and treatment of bradyarrhythmias. The use of an intra-aortic balloon pump may be beneficial in patients with RV infarction, although the exact mechanism of benefit is unclear. Balloon pump counterpulsation does not directly improve RV performance; however, the increase in coronary perfusion pressure and effects on LV systolic and diastolic function (e.g., improved contraction of the interventricular septum) may be critical. When RV failure is unresponsive to medical therapy and balloon pump support, an RV assist device may be appropriate. These devices are discussed in Chapter 27.

MECHANICAL COMPLICATIONS OF MYOCARDIAL INFARCTION

The most dramatic complication of acute MI involves tearing or rupture of acutely infarcted tissue. Such a diagnosis should be considered in MI whenever there is severe hemodynamic instability or a sudden change in clinical condition. The clinical presentation of myocardial rupture depends upon the extent and site of rupture, which includes the interventricular septum, papillary muscles, or the free wall of either ventricle (Figure 26-5). Most ruptures occur in the first 2 to 5 days after MI, when the necrotic myocardium is most vulnerable to rupture from the systolic pressures arising within the LV. Before the reperfusion era, the reported incidence of rupture was up to 6%. In the current era, with advances in timely revascularization and adjunctive pharmacologic therapies, the reported incidence is less than 2% (Figure 26-e3).[7] Definitive management requires surgical intervention but is limited in practice by different thresholds for surgical risk by cardiac surgeons. Figure 26-6 provides an overview of the clinical findings, diagnosis, and treatment of these mechanical complications encountered after an MI.

Left Ventricular Free-Wall Rupture

Rupture of the ventricular free wall usually presents catastrophically with hemodynamic collapse, electromechanical dissociation, tamponade, shock, and death. Free-wall rupture has been described in the anterior, posterior, and lateral walls of the LV. Pathologically, three types of rupture have been identified (Figure 26-7). Type 1 rupture is characterized as an abrupt slit-like tear that occurs during the acute phase of a MI (<24 hours).

Type 2 rupture results from a subacute process with localized necrosis of the myocardium, resulting in a slow progressive tear, often at the border zone between necrotic and viable myocardium. Type 3 rupture is preceded by the development of myocardial thinning, with rupture in the center of the thinned area, which typically occurs during the late phase of MI (>7 days). Intramyocardial hemorrhage is also commonly noted at autopsy, and paradoxically, is associated with reperfusion therapy.[7]

Free-wall rupture is more commonly seen in patients who present with their first MI, with anterior infarction, who are older adults (>70 years), and in women. Other possible risk factors for rupture include hypertension during the acute phase of MI, lack of antecedent angina or previous MI, lack of collateral blood supply, use of corticosteroids or nonsteroidal anti-inflammatory drugs, and the administration of fibrinolytics more than 14 hours after symptom onset.

The clinical diagnosis of free-wall rupture should be considered whenever there is severe and/or sudden hemodynamic instability and is suggested by the physical examination findings of cardiac tamponade and electromechanical dissociation (Figure 26-6). Rarely, patients can present with a subacute ventricular rupture, which is manifested by pericardial pain, ECG evidence of pericarditis, and a pericardial rub. Because of the usual abrupt and catastrophic nature of rupture, confirmatory diagnostic evaluation is not always feasible. However, if time allows, echocardiography can be diagnostic (see Chapter 31). If available, pulmonary arterial catheterization will reveal equalization of right atrial, RV diastolic, and pulmonary capillary wedge pressures consistent with cardiac tamponade, and should be distinguished from RV infarction. The presence of a moderately sized (>1 cm) pericardial effusion is associated with high mortality after acute MI and should always prompt consideration of free-wall rupture.[8] If clinical stability can be achieved, cardiac computed tomography or CMR should be considered

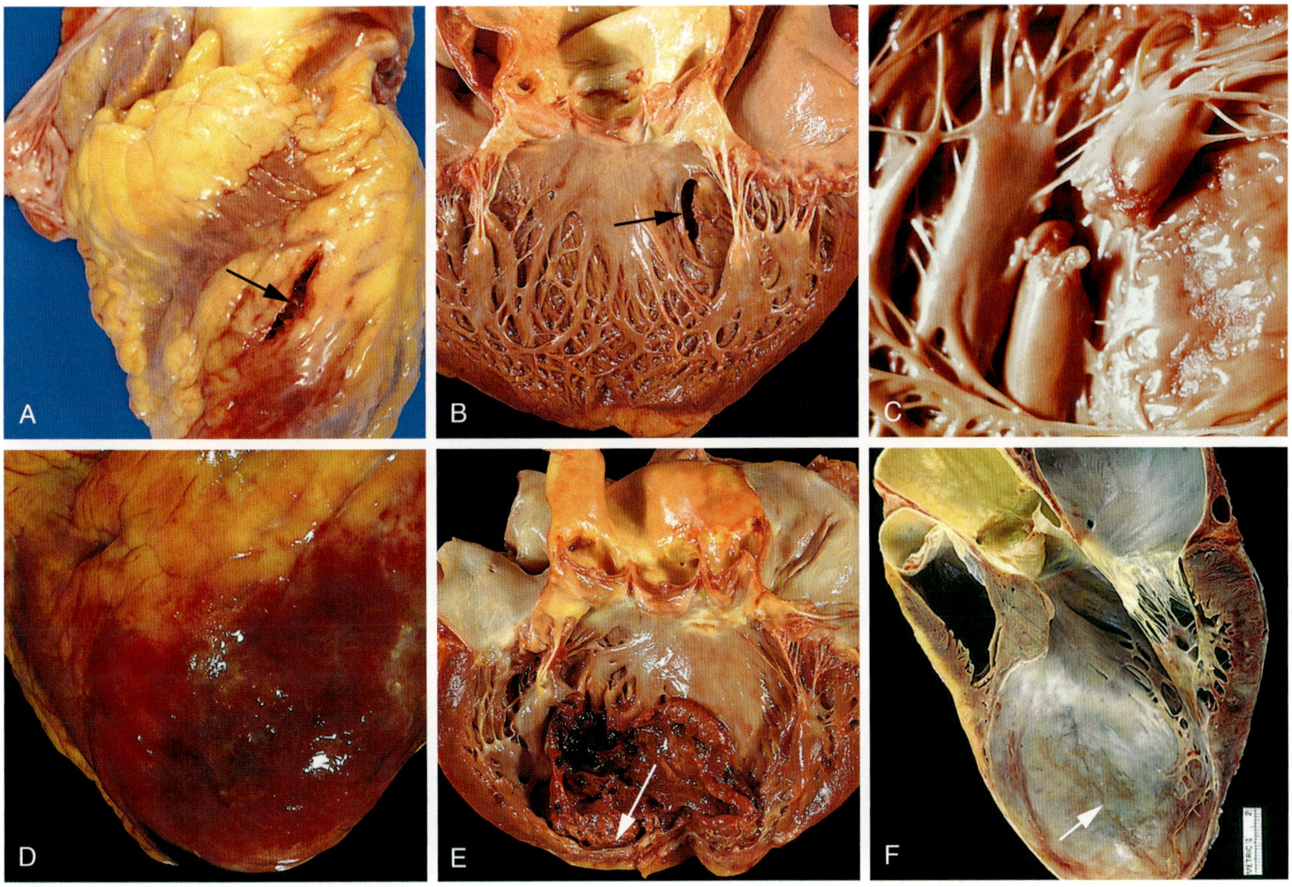

FIGURE 26-5 Complications of myocardial infarction. (**A**) Anterior myocardial rupture in an acute infarct (*arrow*). (**B**) Rupture of the ventricular septum (*arrow*). (**C**) Complete rupture of a necrotic papillary muscle. (**D**) Fibrinous pericarditis, showing a dark, roughened epicardial surface overlying an acute infarct. (**E**) Early expansion of anteroapical infarct with wall thinning (*arrow*) and mural thrombus. (**F**) Large apical left ventricular aneurysm. The left ventricle is on the right in this apical four-chamber view of the heart. *(From Schoen FJ, Mitchell RN: The heart. In Kumar V, et al, editors:* Robbins and Cotran pathologic basis of disease, *9th ed. Saunders, Philadelphia, 2015.)*

to confirm and localize the perforation in such cases (see Chapter 33). If such secondary imaging is not available or feasible to perform, pericardiocentesis with measurement of fluid hematocrit can be confirmatory for free-wall rupture.

Survival for patients with free-wall rupture depends upon prompt diagnosis, hemodynamic stabilization, and immediate surgical intervention. In-hospital mortality for cardiac rupture may be declining because the rate and success of emergent surgery for this condition has increased (Figure 26-8).[7] The use of pericardial drainage should be considered cautiously, if at all; drainage may provide short-term hemodynamic improvement, but extension of the rupture can occur with loss of the "pressure" tamponade. In patients who have the diagnosis recognized and undergo surgical repair, the operative mortality ranges from 18% to 54%, depending on late (>7 days) or early surgical repair.[9]

Pseudoaneurysm

Incomplete rupture of the myocardium may occur when thrombus is organized in concert with the pericardium, sealing a rupture of the ventricle, which thus prevents the development of hemopericardium. Over time, this combination of thrombus and pericardium will result in a pseudoaneurysm that maintains communication with the cavity of the LV (Figure 26-9 and Figure 26-10; see Figure 31-19, Video 31-20, and Video 31-21), and this most commonly occurs in the inferior and inferolateral locations. Pseudoaneurysms may present with systemic embolization, heart failure, chest pain, ventricular tachycardia, and incidentally on imaging (e.g., cardiomegaly on a chest x-ray). Diagnosis is confirmed by noninvasive imaging (see Chapter 31) and should be suspected when the mouth of an aneurysm is narrow, in contrast to the wide neck of true myocardial aneurysms. When a rupture is subacute and the diagnosis of pseudoaneurysm is made, emergency surgery should be considered. The natural history of surgically treated and untreated pseudoaneurysms is not clearly defined and is largely based on retrospective single-center case series. Historically, pseudoaneurysms are considered to confer a high risk of rupture of up to 45%.[10] Surgical management should also be considered even if the pseudoaneurysm is asymptomatic because of the unpredictable risk of rupture.

Ventricular Septal Rupture

Ventricular septal rupture (VSR) is similar in many ways to free-wall rupture. There is a bimodal temporal distribution of presentation, depending on the pathologic characteristics of the rupture. Typically, septal ruptures are classified as simple or complex. A simple VSR is a single defect or tear with openings to both ventricles at approximately the same level (Figure 26-e4). However, most VSRs are complex with serpinginous channels through the myocardium that enter and exit at different levels of the right and left ventricular septal walls and approximate a "tearing" of the septum (Figure 26-e4) (Figure 26-11). The risk factors for developing VSR are also similar to that of free-wall rupture.

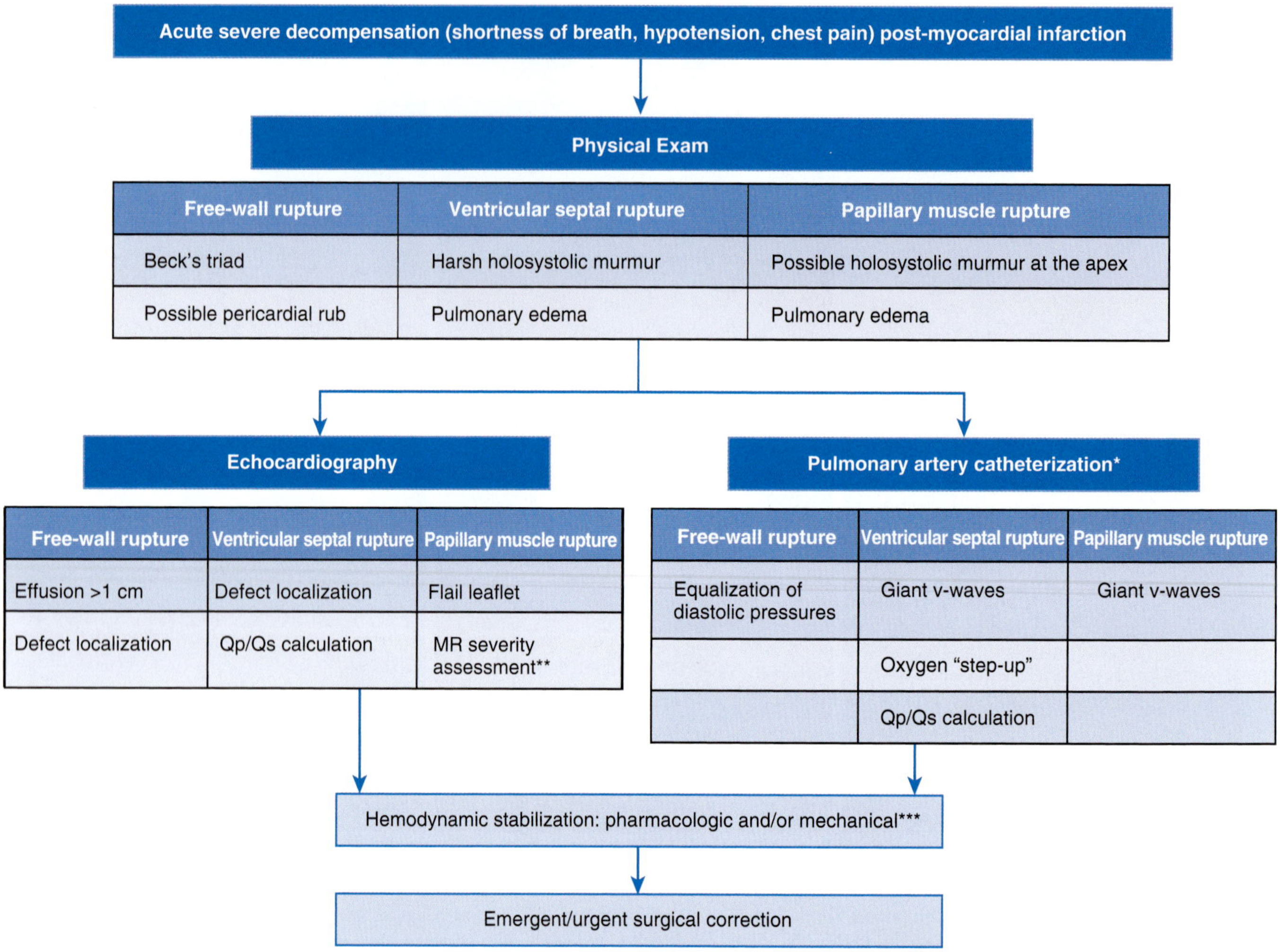

FIGURE 26-6 Assessment of acute severe decompensation after myocardial infarction. *Pulmonary artery catheterization is not required to confirm diagnosis. If already in place, findings can be supportive and/or suggestive. To be performed if echocardiographic findings are unclear. **Using standard color, continuous-wave and pulse-wave Doppler evaluation, pulmonary venous flow assessment, regurgitant volume, and fraction calculation. ***Pharmacologic therapy (vasodilators, inotropes, or vasopressors) and mechanical support uses are dependent on systemic blood pressure and should not delay surgical intervention. *MR*, Mitral regurgitation.

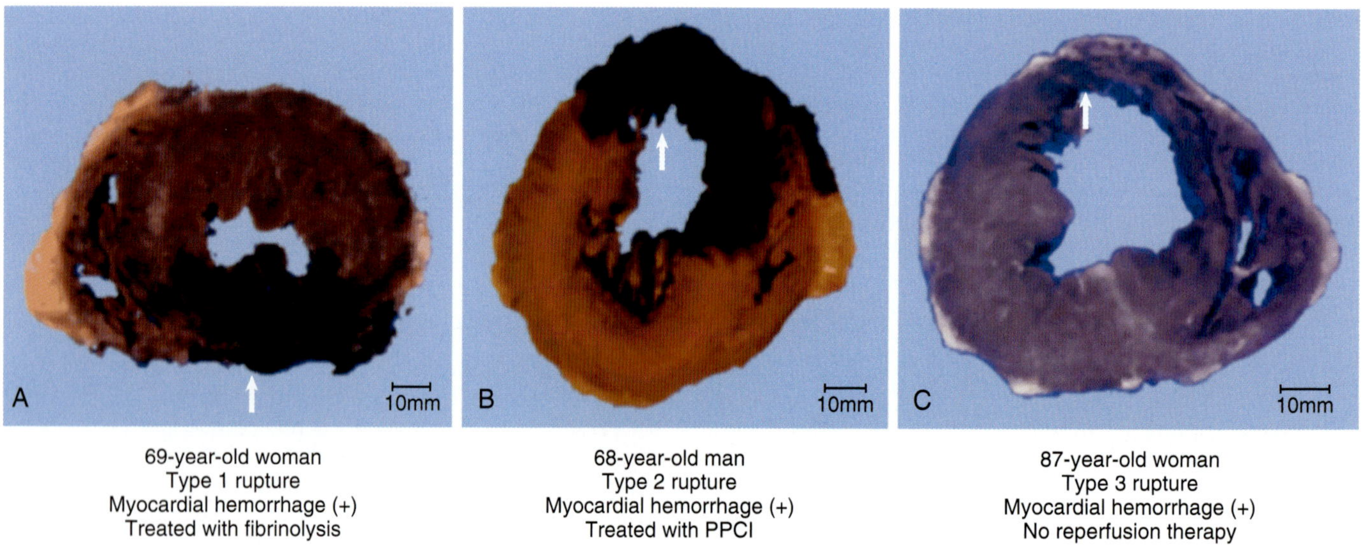

FIGURE 26-7 Representative autopsy cases of cardiac rupture (CR). (**A**) A 69–year–old woman with inferior acute myocardial infarction (AMI) and Becker type 1 rupture. She underwent fibrinolysis 4 hours after the onset of AMI, and developed CR 8 hours after the onset of AMI. *Arrow*, the inferior free–wall rupture with massive myocardial hemorrhage. There is no wall thinning in the infarcted area. (**B**) A 68–year–old man with anterior AMI and Becker type 2 rupture. He underwent primary percutaneous coronary intervention (PPCI) 5 hours after the onset of AMI, and developed CR 11 hours after the onset of AMI. *Arrow*, the anterior free–wall rupture with massive myocardial hemorrhage and erosion. Myocardial erosion at the site of rupture can be observed. (**C**) An 87–year–old woman with anterior AMI and Becker type 3 rupture; reperfusion therapy was not performed. She developed CR 12 days after the onset of AMI. *Arrow*, the anterior free–wall rupture with marked thinning of the infarcted myocardium. *(Adapted from Honda S, et al: Trends in the clinical and pathological characteristics of cardiac rupture in patients with acute myocardial infarction over 35 years.* J Am Heart Assoc *3:e000984, 2014.)*

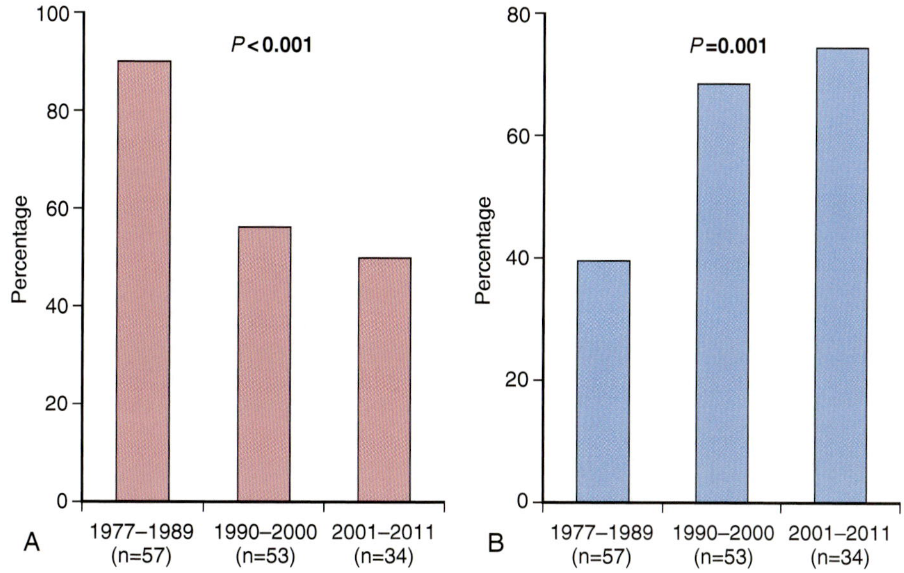

FIGURE 26-8 **Decreased in-hospital mortality is associated with an increased rate of emergent surgery in 144 patients with cardiac rupture (CR).** (**A**) The in-hospital mortality rate in patients with CR. (**B**) The rate of emergent surgery for CR. *(From Honda S, et al: Trends in the clinical and pathological characteristics of cardiac rupture in patients with acute myocardial infarction over 35 years.* J Am Heart Assoc *3:e000984, 2014.)*

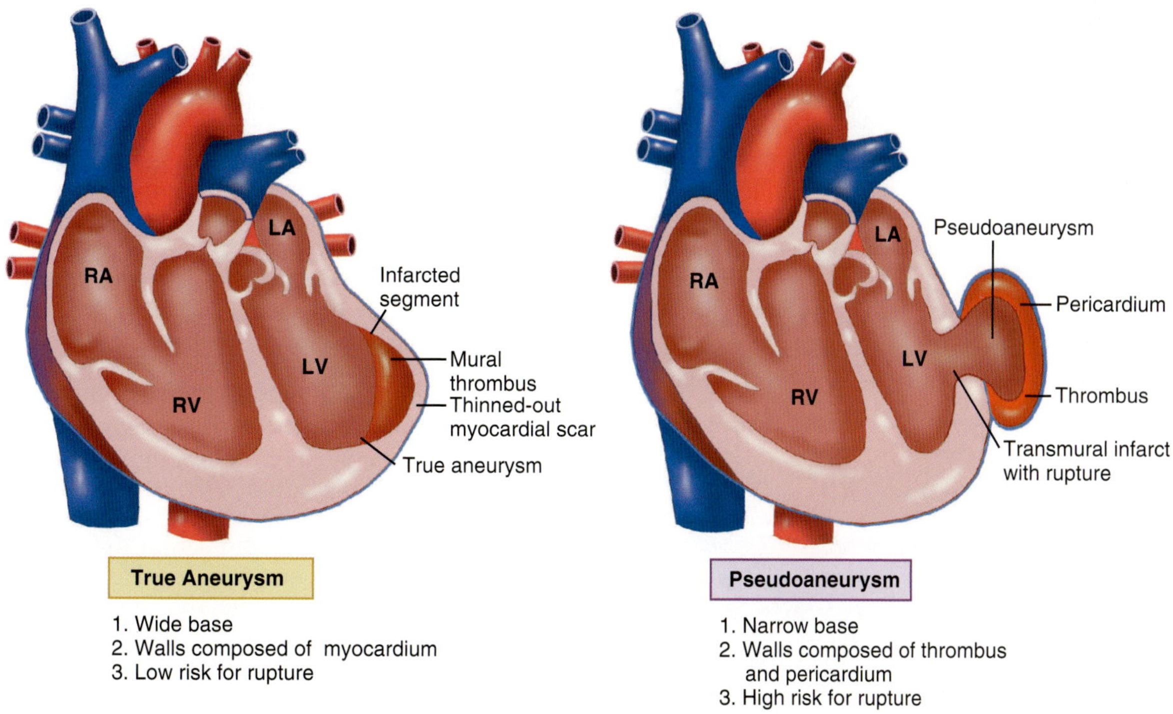

FIGURE 26-9 **Differences between a pseudoaneurysm and a true aneurysm.** *LA*, Left atrium; *LV*, left ventricle; *RA*, right atrium; *RV*, right ventricle. *(From Shah PK: Complications of acute myocardial infarction. In Parmley W, Chatterjee K, editors:* Cardiology. *Philadelphia, JB Lippincott, 1987.)*

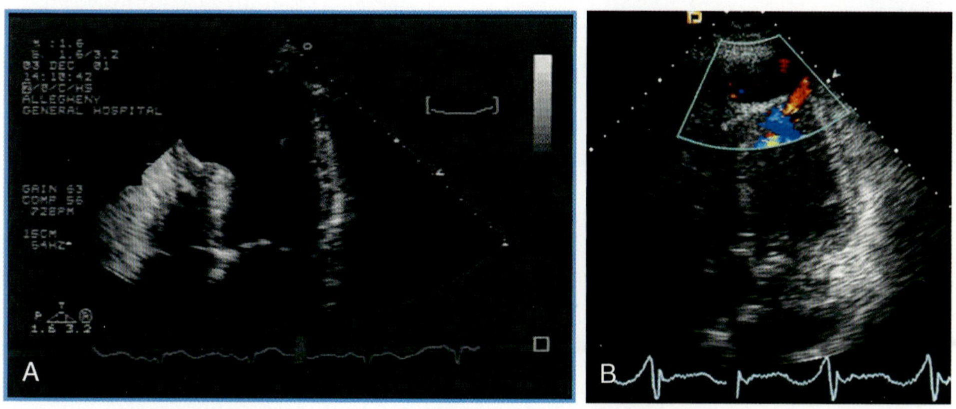

FIGURE 26-10 Echocardiography is useful at differentiating (**A**) left ventricular (LV) aneurysm (wide entry neck) from (**B**) an LV pseudoaneurysm (narrow entry neck). *(From Tsang MG, et al: Echocardiography in acute myocardial infarction. In Lang RM ,et al, editors:* ASE's comprehensive echocardiography, *3rd ed. Philadelphia, Saunders, 2016.)*

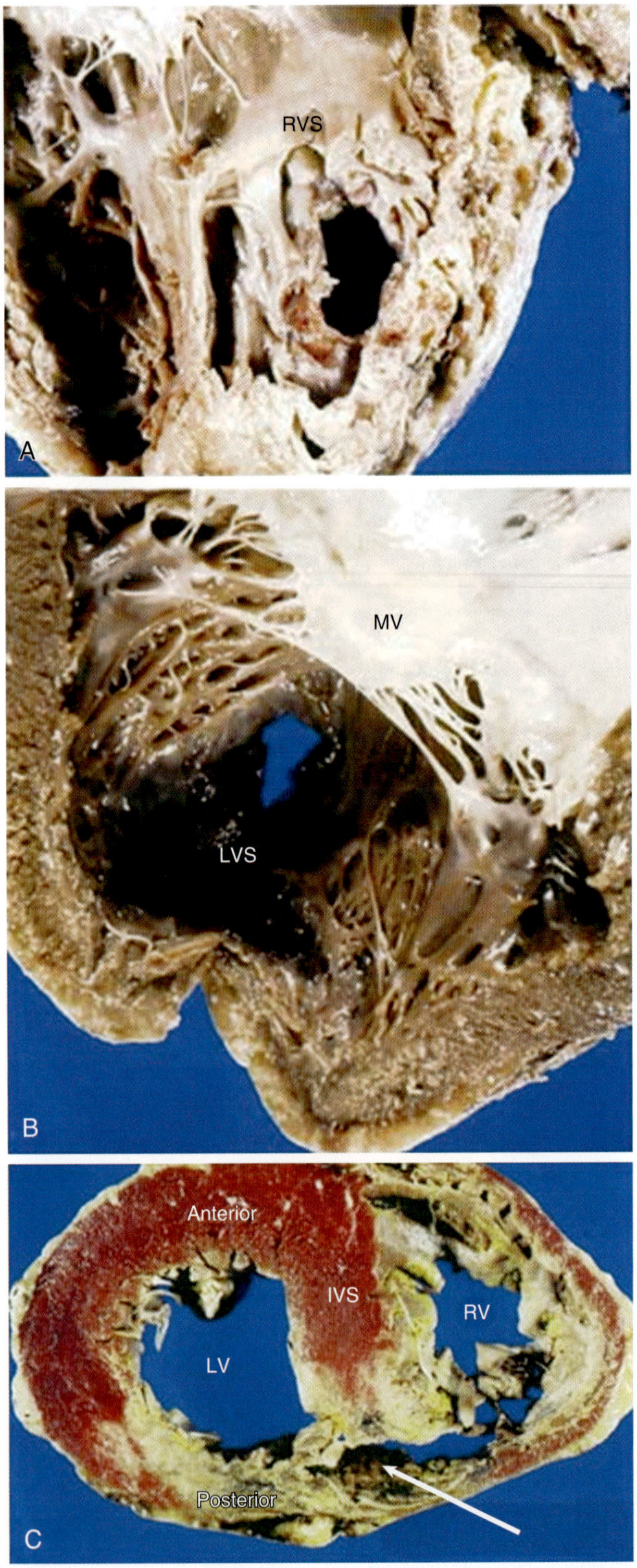

FIGURE 26-11 (**A** and **B**) Findings at autopsy in a patient with a simple ventricular septal rupture. There is a discrete defect with a direct through-and-through communication across the septum. The perforation is at the same level on both sides of the septum: the left ventricular aspect of the interventricular septum (LVS), and the right ventricular aspect of the interventricular septum (IVS). (**C**) Gross findings in a patient with a posterior ventricular septal rupture. There is an infarction involving the basal inferior septum, the basal posteroinferior wall, and the right ventricle (RV). The ventricular septal rupture (*arrow*) is complex, with an irregular, serpiginous tract at the junction of the inferior wall and the interventricular septum (IVS). *LV*, Left ventricle; *MV*, mitral valve. *(From Birnbaum Y, et al: Ventricular septal rupture after acute myocardial infarction.* N Engl J Med *347:1427, 2002.)*

The clinical manifestations of VSR are directly related to the size of the defect and magnitude of left-to-right shunting. A harsh pansystolic murmur with findings of right or left ventricular heart failure, or sudden and/or severe hemodynamic instability should alert the clinician to the presence of VSR. Pulmonary edema and hypotension are common. Echocardiography (see Chapter 31) is essential at confirming the diagnosis, and distinguishing between papillary muscle rupture and VSR (Figure 26-12) (Figure 26-e5) (see Figure 31-20A and Videos 31-22, 31-23, 32-24, 31-25, and 31-26). Echocardiography can also characterize the site, size, and degree of left-to-right shunting. Calculation of shunt magnitude can be assessed using the relative flows across the pulmonic and aortic valves; a ratio greater than two suggests a large shunt and indicates greater urgency for its repair. Although right heart catheterization has been largely replaced by echocardiography, it can help to confirm a diagnosis if the echocardiographic data are unclear. The demonstration of an oxygen saturation "step-up" between right atrial and pulmonary artery samples confirms the presence of a ventricular shunt, but is limited to detection of shunts of at least 1.5:1. A large v-wave is also common because the large recirculated volume overwhelms the compliance of the left atrium and can be confused with the giant v-waves of acute severe mitral regurgitation (MR) from papillary muscle rupture.

The mortality rate with septal rupture is as high as 50% for surgically treated patients, and 90% for those treated medically but biased by surgical risk (Figure 26-13).[11] VSR from inferior wall MI generally occurs in the inferobasal septum, is difficult to repair, and is associated with a worse prognosis than anterior MI-related VSR, which often occurs in the apical septum. Hemodynamic optimization with inotropic, vasodilatory, and mechanical support should not delay definitive surgical treatment (Figure 26-e6).

Repair of Ventricular Septal Rupture: Timing and Approaches

Controversy remains as to the optimal timing of surgery in hemodynamically stable patients or patients with modest degree shunts (e.g., Qp/Qs <1.5–2.0). Delay in surgery allows for maturing and fibrosis of the infarcted tissue, which allows easier surgical repair. Unfortunately, few patients (<5%) allow for a delayed repair. However, deferring surgery carries the risk of rupture extension, heart failure, arrhythmia, and sudden death. Early surgery is technically more difficult, has a higher risk of recurrent ventricular rupture or residual shunt, and is associated with significant surgical mortality (Figure 26-14).

Assessing operative candidacy is the first priority in clinical decision making for VSR repair and integrates evaluation of surgical risk with consideration with the consulting surgeon as to whether there is a prohibitive risk (Figure 26-15).[12] If the patient is an operative candidate, the timing, and method of VSR repair will be predicated by hemodynamic status, the location and size of VSR, and the availability of operative and percutaneous expertise. Most experts recommend urgent surgical intervention (e.g., within 24–48 hours of diagnosis).[13] Emergent repair (e.g., <6 hours) has been associated with high mortality, but is most likely a reflection of underlying patient illness rather than the surgical intervention itself. There is little evidence to support extended delays in operative repair despite the theoretical advantages of allowing for tissue healing to overcome surgical technical

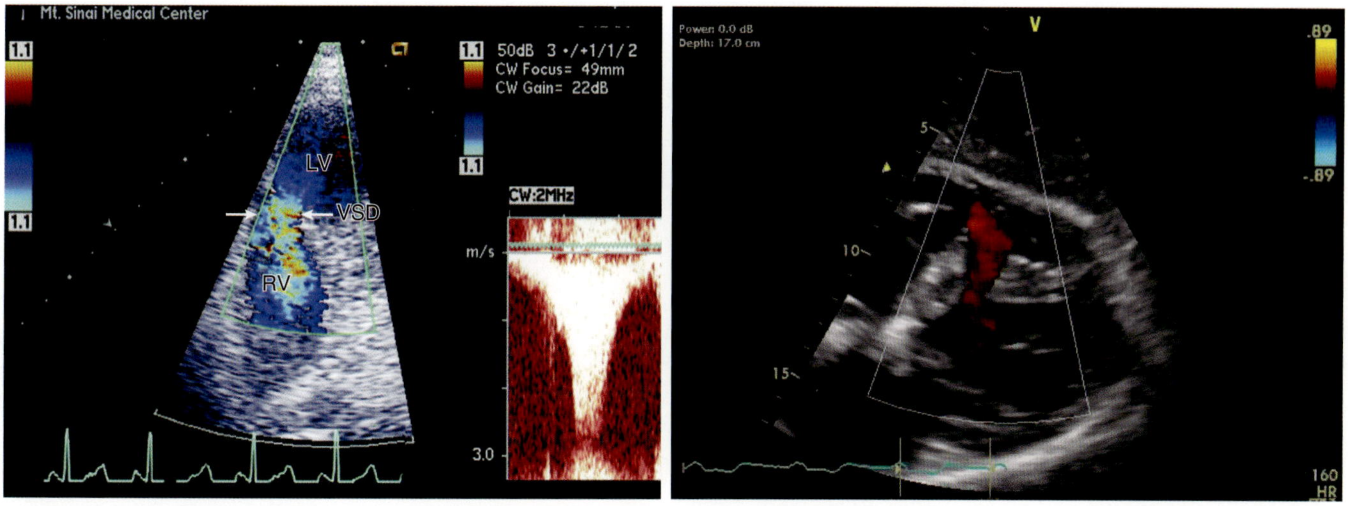

FIGURE 26-12 Echocardiography of two ventricular septal defects (VSDs) that developed after ST-elevation myocardial infarction (STEMI). A close-up of the ventricular septum in an apical four-chamber view demonstrates turbulent systolic color flow Doppler across a VSD and continuous-wave Doppler demonstrates systolic flow across a VSD (*left*). A subcoastal view demonstrates color flow Doppler across a VSD (*right*). *LV*, Left ventricular; *RV*, right ventricular. *(From Kamran M, et al: Images in cardiovascular medicine. Ventricular septal defect complicating an acute myocardial infarction.* Circulation *112:e337, 2005; and Brigham and Women's Hospital, 2013.)*

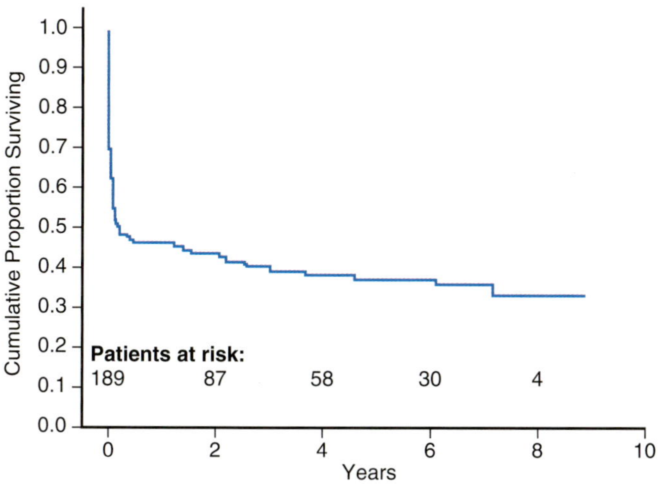

FIGURE 26-13 Cumulative survival in all postinfarction ventricular septal defect patients (n = 189). *(From Jeppsson A, et al: Surgical repair of post infarction ventricular septal defects: a national experience.* Eur J Cardiothorac Surg *27:216, 2005.)*

challenges. For select nonoperative candidates, percutaneous repair can be considered if available.

Percutaneous closure is a less invasive option, but limited to patients with simple discrete defects that are less than 15 mm in diameter. Percutaneous closure has been attempted in the acute setting with variable results. The procedural success rate of any device closure varies from 74% to 91%; however, these procedures are ultimately associated with a high mortality (18% to 65%) and complication rate (41%).[14] In a series of 29 consecutive patients who underwent primary transcatheter VSR closure (median 1 day after recognition), the initial procedural success rate was 86%. Procedure-related complications, such as major residual shunting, LV rupture, and device embolization, occurred in 41%. The 30-day survival rate was 88% for patients in shock before the procedure versus 38% in patients without shock. As such, outcomes appear to be dominated by the clinical status of the patient preceding the procedure more than the technical aspects or immediate procedural success of the intervention.[15] Markers of multisystem organ dysfunction have been proposed as a tool for selection of appropriate candidates for intervention.[16] Further technical developments and prospective studies are required to identify the patients best suited for a percutaneous approach.

Acute Mitral Regurgitation

MR after MI occurs via two mechanisms: (1) partial or total rupture of a papillary muscle, and (2) postinfarction LV remodeling with lateral and apical displacement of the papillary muscles, leaflet tethering, and annular dilation (e.g., ischemic or functional MR). Acute rupture more commonly affects the posteromedial papillary muscle (often in association with inferior MI) than the anterolateral papillary muscle because of the singular blood supply of the former. Complete transection of the papillary muscle body is usually fatal because of the sudden massive magnitude of the MR. Rupture of the tip or partial head of the papillary muscle also results in severe MR and is more likely to be encountered than transection of the papillary muscle body, and it may not be immediately fatal (Figure 26-e7). Unlike ruptures of the septum and free wall, papillary muscle rupture can occur with small infarctions (e.g., those involving the branches of the circumflex artery).

Patients with papillary muscle rupture usually present within 1 week after MI with acute pulmonary edema with or without shock. The classic holosystolic murmur of MR may not always be appreciated because of the rapid rise of left atrial pressure. Echocardiography is often diagnostic (see Figure 31-21, Figure 31-22, and Video 31-27). Right heart catheterization is of limited use, but can help to differentiate VSR from acute MR when there is a detectable oximetric "step-up." The pulmonary capillary wedge pressure tracing may show giant v-waves, but may be also seen in VSR or severe LV failure.

Acute MR is associated with an in-hospital mortality of up to 80% with medical treatment alone but again, it is biased by perceived surgical risk. Surgical mortality is approximately 20%.[13] Medical treatment with afterload reduction, diuretics, and mechanical support may allow for stabilization in preparation for surgery (Figure 26-16). Intravenous nitroprusside is an ideal acute vasodilator when hypotension is absent. Intra-aortic balloon counterpulsation should

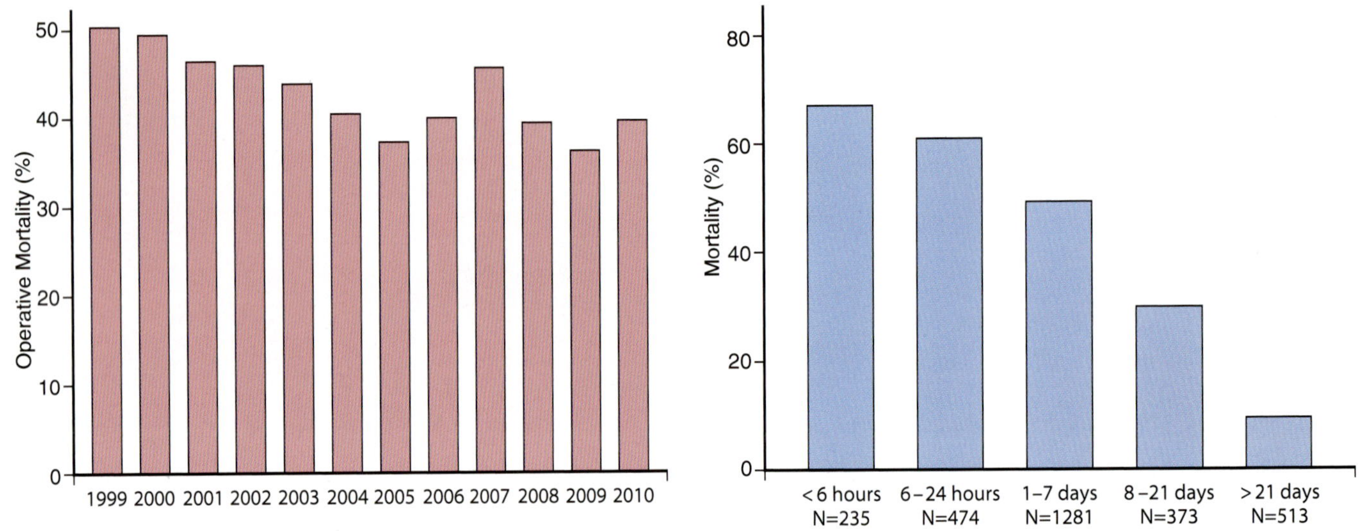

FIGURE 26-14 Ventricular septal rupture surgical repair. Society of Thoracic Surgery National Database: ventricular septal defect repair in 2876 patients, 1999 to 2010. *(From Arnaoutakis GJ, et al: Surgical repair of ventricular septal defect after myocardial infarction: outcomes from the Society of Thoracic Surgeons National Database.* Ann Thorac Surg *94:436, 2012.)*

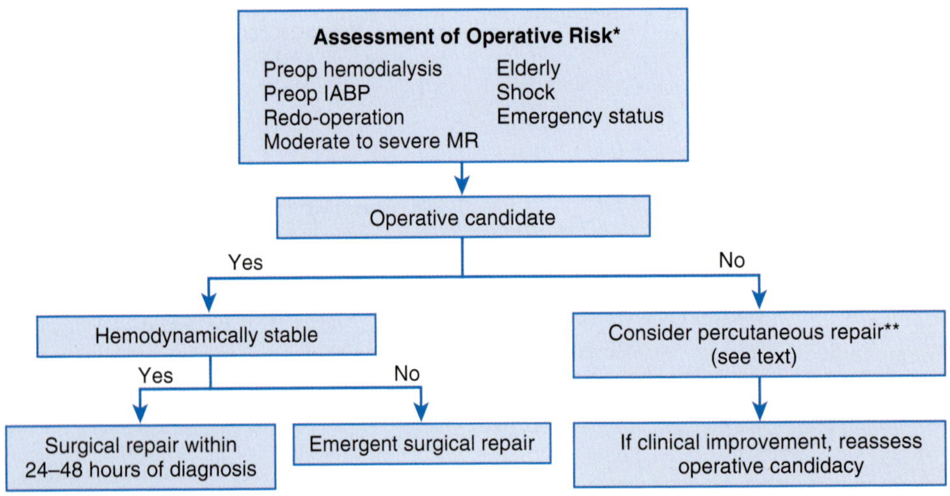

FIGURE 26-15 Approach to ventricular septal rupture management. *Final risk assessment must be made in conjunction with the surgical team. **Should be considered if expertise is available. Should be followed by a definitive surgical repair if a satisfactory result is not achieved. *IABP*, Intra-aortic balloon pump; *MR*, mitral regurgitation.

be strongly considered in almost all cases, but particularly if hypotension is present. Surgical mitral valve replacement, rather than repair, is usually performed in conjunction with revascularization. Although there is no difference in early mortality between patients undergoing concomitant coronary artery bypass grafting (CABG) and those who are not revascularized at the time of emergent mitral surgery (CABG 27% vs. no CABG 26%), the long-term survival is improved by concomitant revascularization at 15 years (CABG 64% vs. no CABG 23%).[17]

Left Ventricular Aneurysm

True aneurysms of the ventricular wall describe a discrete thin-walled area of dyskinesis with a broad neck involving all three layers of myocardium. True aneurysms occur in less than 5% of patients with MI. It is more commonly associated with large anteroapical infarctions with delayed reperfusion and poorly collateralized blood flow. Rupture of true aneurysms is rare. However, the rate of mortality in patients with LV aneurysm is up to six times higher than that in patients without aneurysms, even in patients with comparable LV ejection fractions. Death in these patients is most likely related to ventricular tachyarrhythmias. Heart failure is also common and is a consequence of LV stroke volume being partially ejected into the "dead space" of the aneurysm, decreasing forward stroke volume. Furthermore, the poorly compliant aneurysm impairs diastolic performance and exacerbates diastolic dysfunction. The physical examination may demonstrate a palpable dyskinetic apex that is laterally displaced. Diagnosis is often suspected in patients with persistent ST-segment elevation on ECG. However, the diagnosis is generally made with surveillance echocardiography after MI (see Chapter 30 and Chapter 31).

Surgical correction of LV aneurysm is considered when there are refractory ventricular arrhythmias that are not amendable to medications or radiofrequency ablation, heart failure, or recurrent thromboembolism despite appropriate anticoagulant therapy. A randomized clinical trial failed to demonstrate a benefit of routine surgical reconstruction of akinetic or dyskinetic anteroapical segments, but this study may have been limited by the modest surgical reduction in

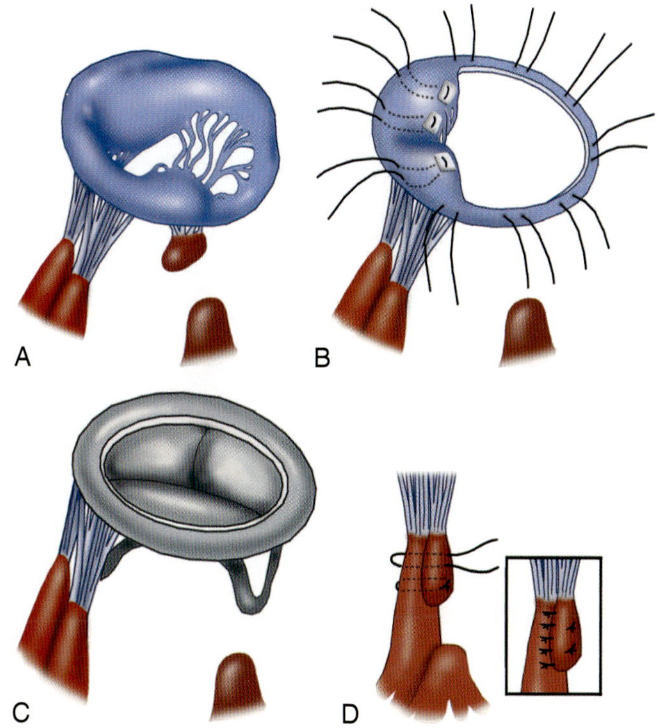

FIGURE 26-16 Surgical management of mitral regurgitation caused by ruptured papillary muscle. (**A**) An acute papillary muscle rupture results in severe mitral regurgitation as a result of leaflet and commissural prolapse. Mitral valve replacement is usually necessary. (**B**) Mitral debridement with retention of the unruptured commissural and leaflet segment is performed to preserve partial continuity of the annular papillary muscle. (**C**) Mitral valve replacement is then performed. (**D**) Occasionally, mitral valve repair can be performed by transfer of a papillary head to a nonruptured segment. *(Courtesy of Dr. David Adams, Mt. Sinai Hospital, New York.)*

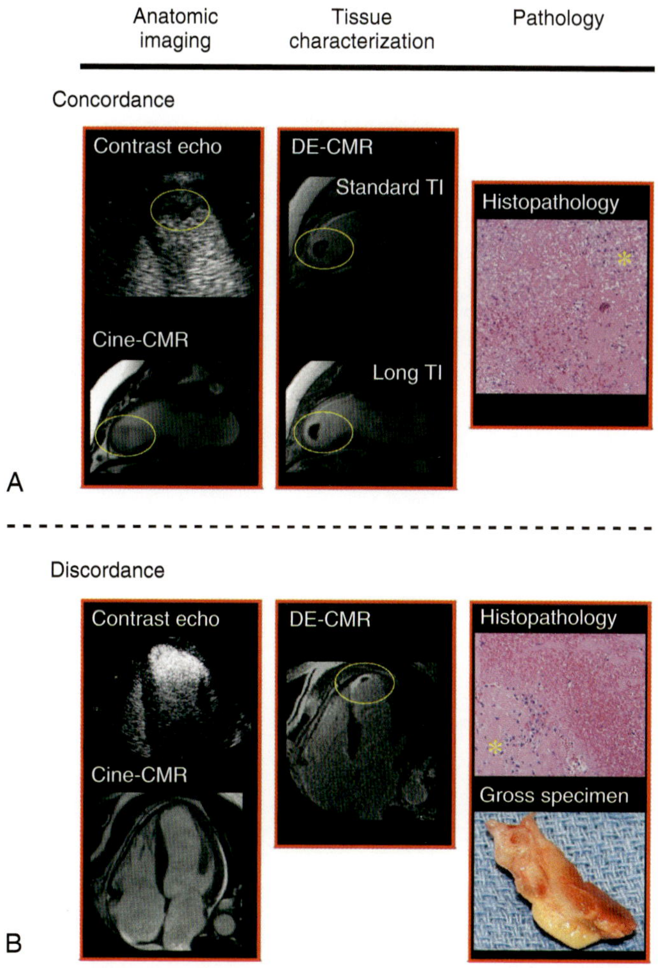

FIGURE 26-17 Apical thrombus by anatomic and tissue characterization imaging. (**A**) Representative example of apical thrombus (*circle*) concordantly detected by anatomic imaging (*left*, contrast echocardiography four-chamber, cine-cardiac magnetic resonance [CMR] two-chamber) and delayed enhancement (DE)-CMR (*center*). (**B**) Representative example of discordance between anatomic imaging and DE-CMR. DE-CMR identified a small mural thrombus (*circle*) within the apex. Cine-CMR and contrast echocardiography were interpreted as negative. For both examples, surgical resection enabled thrombus verification based on histopathology (*right*, hematoxylin and eosin stain, low power), which showed thrombus with associated fibroblasts (*asterisk*). *(From Weinsaft JW, et al: Contrast-enhanced anatomic imaging as compared to contrast-enhanced tissue characterization for detection of left ventricular thrombus.* JACC Cardiovasc Imaging *2:972, 2009.)*

end-diastolic volume compared with revascularization alone (see Chapter 25).[18] Percutaneous exclusion of large anteroapical segments may be possible with newer devices such as the PARACHUTE device (Cardiokinetix, Menlo Park, Calif.).

Anticoagulation to either treat or prevent intra-aneurysm thrombus formation is often recommended. In one contemporary series of 648 patients with post-MI LV aneurysms, anticoagulation did not predict improved outcomes (death, nonfatal MI, stroke, embolization) (hazard ratio [HR], 1.05; 95% confidence interval [CI], 0.67 to 1.64; $P = .84$), even in the presence of LV thrombus (HR, 1.38; 95% CI, 0.32 to 5.97; $P = .66$).[19] Moreover, no specific subgroup (e.g., older age, dual antiplatelet therapy, LV ejection fraction <40%) appeared to either to be benefited or harmed. Randomized trials have not been conducted to date.

LEFT VENTRICULAR THROMBUS

During the acute phase of MI, endocardial inflammation, stasis of blood, and hypercoaguability can lead to mural thrombus formation; this largely depends upon MI size and location. Thrombus is most often seen in patients with large infarctions and associated aneurysms. The reported incidence of LV thrombus varies depending on the imaging modality used (e.g., echocardiography with or without contrast vs. CMR), as well as the frequency and timing of cardiac imaging after MI (Figure 26-17) (Figure 26-e8) (see Figure 31-23 and Video 31-32). In the prereperfusion era, mural thrombus was associated with up to 40% of acute MIs, but is now likely less than 20%[20] because of the limitation of infarct size with rapid reperfusion. The predominant use of echocardiography as the diagnostic imaging modality may underestimate the true incidence. CMR has superior sensitivity and specificity in the detection of mural thrombus, and is the current gold standard for its diagnosis.[21]

Clinical suspicion for LV thrombus should be considered for patients presenting with stroke or systemic embolism in the context of a recent (<3 months) MI, LV aneurysm, or decreased LV ejection fraction. The risk of thromboembolism caused by mural thrombus has been reported to be as high as 10%,[22] and an increased risk is associated with thrombus mobility and its protrusion into the LV. Most thromboembolic events occur within the first 3 months of diagnosis.

There are no randomized trials that have evaluated the efficacy of extended duration of anticoagulation to prevent embolization in patients with LV thrombus after MI. However, in studies of low-molecular-weight heparin during the initial hospitalization for acute MI, anticoagulation with the more effective anticoagulant also reduced the short-term risk of ischemic stroke. Current recommendations are based upon observational studies in patients with documented LV thrombus who had a reduced risk of embolization with anticoagulation and extrapolation from experiences when atrial fibrillation or heart failure complicated MI. Individual assessment regarding the risk of thromboembolization should be balanced against the risk of bleeding. It is reasonable to consider 3 months of anticoagulation in patients at high risk of thromboembolism, absent any data from prospective randomized data.[23] There are currently no data on the use of specific oral anticoagulants in the setting of LV thrombus associated with MI. Dual antiplatelet therapy does not appear to prevent mural thrombus formation in observational studies,[24,25] but prospective randomized data are not available.

References

1. Mozaffarian D, et al.: Heart disease and stroke statistics – 2015. A report from the American Heart Association, *Circulation* 131:e29–e322, 2015.
2. Kakouros N, Cokkinos D: Right ventricular myocardial infarction: pathophysiology, diagnosis, and management, *Postgrad Med J* 86:719–728, 2010.
3. Goldstein JA: Acute right ventricular infarction, *Cardiol Clin* 30:219–232, 2012.
4. Inohra T, et al.: The challenges in the management in right ventricular infarction. *Eur Heart J: Acute Cardiovasc Care* 2:226–234, 2013.
5. Korabathina R, et al.: The pulmonary artery pulsatility index identifies severe right ventricular dysfunction in acute inferior myocardial infarction, *Catheter Cardiovasc Interv* 80:593–600, 2012.
6. Rallidis LS, Makavos G: Nihoyannopoulos. Right ventricular involvement in coronary artery disease: role of echocardiography for diagnosis and prognosis, *J Am Soc Echocardiogr* 27:223–229, 2014.
7. Honda S, et al.: Trends in the clinical and pathological characteristics of cardiac rupture in patients with acute myocardial infarction over 35 years, *J Am Heart Assoc* 3:e000984, 2014.
8. Figuera J, et al.: Hospital outcome of moderate to severe pericardial effusion complicating ST-elevation acute myocardial infarction, *Circulation* 122:1902–1909, 2010.
9. Arnaoutakis GJ, et al.: Surgical repair of ventricular septal defect after myocardial infarction: outcomes from the Society of Thoracic Surgeons National Database, *Ann Thorac Surg* 92:436–444, 2012.
10. Hulten EA, Blankstein R: Pseudoaneurysms of the heart, *Circulation* 125:920–1925, 2012.
11. Nozoe M, et al.: Clinical manifestation of early phase left ventricular rupture complicating acute myocardial infarction in the primary PCI era, *J Cardiol* 63:14–18, 2014.
12. Arnaoutakis GJ, et al.: Surgical repair of ventricular septal defect after myocardial infarction: outcomes from the Society of Thoracic Surgeons National Database, *Ann Thorac Surg* 94: 436–444, 2012.
13. Agnihotri AK, Madsen JC, Daggett WM: Surgical treatment of complications of acute myocardial infarction: postinfarction ventricular septal defect and free wall rupture. In Cohn LH, editor: *Cardiac surgery in the adult*, 4th Ed., New York, 2012, McGraw Hill, pp 602–628.
14. Isoda S, et al.: Surgical repair of postinfarction ventricular septal defects – 2013 update, *Ann Thorac Cardiovasc Surg* 19:95–102, 2013.
15. Thiele H, et al.: Immediate primary transcatheter closure of postinfarction ventricular septal defects, *Eur Heart J* 30:81–88, 2009.
16. Jones BM, et al.: Ventricular septal rupture complicating acute myocardial infarction: a contemporary review, *Eur Heart J* 35:2060–2068, 2014.
17. Kutty RS, Jones N, Moorjani N: Mechanical complications of acute myocardial infarction, *Cardiol Clin* 31:519–531, 2013.
18. Jones RH, et al.: Coronary bypass surgery with or without surgical ventricular reconstruction, *N Engl J Med* 360:1705–1717, 2009.
19. Lee GY, et al.: Anticoagulation in ischemic left ventricular aneurysm, *Mayo Clin Proc* 90:441–449, 2015.
20. Delewi R, Zijlsttra F, Piek JJ: Left ventricular thrombus formation after acute myocardial infarction, *Heart* 98:1743–1749, 2012.
21. Weinsaft JW, et al.: Left ventricular thrombus detection by routine echocardiography—insights into performance characteristics using delayed enhancement CMR, *JACC Cardiovasc Imaging* 4:702–712, 2011.
22. Lee JM, et al.: Left ventricular thrombus and subsequent thromboembolism, comparison of anticoagulation, surgical removal and antiplatelet agents, *J Atheroscler Thromb* 20:73–93, 2013.
23. O'Gara PT, et al.: 2013 ACCF/AHA guideline for the management of ST-Elevation myocardial infarction: a report of the American College of Cardiology Foundation/American Heart Association Task Force on Practice Guidelines, *J Am Coll Cardiol* 61:e78–140, 2013.
24. Osherov AB, et al.: Incidence of early left ventricular thrombus after acute anterior wall myocardial infarction in the primary coronary intervention era, *Am Heart J* 157:1074–1080, 2009.
25. Solheim S, et al.: Frequency of left ventricular thrombus in patients with anterior wall acute myocardial infarction treated with percutaneous coronary intervention and dual antiplatelet therapy, *Am J Cardiol* 106:1197–1200, 2010.

27

Clinical Practice/Controversy

Mechanical Circulatory Support for Complications of Myocardial Infarction: Role of Currently Available Devices

E. Magnus Ohman and Jacob A. Doll

INTRODUCTION

Mortality for patients with myocardial infarction (MI) remains unacceptably high despite improvements in medical therapy and revascularization. Death, when it occurs, is often caused by cardiac dysfunction, which leads to low cardiac output, hypotension, and end-organ failure (Figure 27-1). This syndrome is broadly referred to as cardiogenic shock, and can be considered a continuum of severity from pre-shock to refractory shock (see Chapter 25). Cardiogenic shock can result from a variety of complications of MI, including left ventricular (LV) dysfunction, mitral regurgitation (MR), ventricular septal rupture, right ventricular failure, or cardiac tamponade (see Chapter 26).

Temporary mechanical circulatory support (MCS) devices improve hemodynamic parameters of patients with cardiogenic shock. In theory, timely and appropriate use of MCS will interrupt the shock cascade and prevent multiorgan dysfunction and death (see Figure 27-1). Devices such as the intra-aortic balloon pump (IABP), Impella (Abiomed, Danvers, Massachusetts), TandemHeart (Cardiac Assist, Pittsburgh, Pennsylvania), and extra-corporeal membrane oxygenation (ECMO) can be deployed rapidly and can provide clinically significant hemodynamic support. To date, these hemodynamic benefits have not been translated into improved outcomes in randomized trials, and the role of MCS remains uncertain despite decades of clinical use. A recent position paper from the American Heart Association and Society of Cardiac Angiography and Intervention highlights this uncertainty, noting definitive clinical evidence is unavailable or controversial in many cases.[1] Nonetheless, use of MCS is increasing in the United States.[2,3]

We provide a review of currently available technologies with a detailed look at the advantages and disadvantages of each, a summary of available trial evidence, and guidance for clinical situations in which each device may be helpful. Clinicians should carefully weigh the putative benefit of circulatory support with an increased risk of complications for each patient when persuasive evidence of improved clinical outcomes with MCS is not available.

MECHANICAL CIRCULATORY SUPPORT DEVICES

The ideal MCS device is able to be placed quickly at the bedside, corrects the hemodynamic deficits resulting from MI, causes few serious complications, and may be removed easily when it is no longer needed. MCS should (1) restore systemic circulation to normalize end-organ function and prevent multisystem shock, (2) increase myocardial blood flow to normal and ischemic coronary territories, and (3) decrease myocardial oxygen demand and limit the extent of ischemia and/or infarct. No current devices fully meet these criteria. Thoughtful use of MCS devices requires an understanding of the hemodynamic effects of each device, the ease of use and frequency of complications, and available clinical trial evidence (Figure 27-2).

Studies of MCS devices have focused on cardiogenic shock caused by LV dysfunction, which is the dominant cause of shock after ST-elevation MI (STEMI) (see Chapter 25). Evidence of use for patients with acute MR, right ventricular failure, or ventricular septal defects (VSDs) is explicitly noted, when available.

Intra-Aortic Balloon Pump

Hemodynamic Effects

Aortic counterpulsation is the most widely used and mature technology for hemodynamic support. This support modality uses a balloon positioned in the descending aorta that inflates during diastole and deflates immediately before systole. With inflation, the balloon displaces blood from the descending aorta and increases diastolic pressure. This leads to improved peripheral and coronary artery perfusion. With deflation, early systolic blood pressure falls and results in reduced LV afterload. Overall, mean arterial pressure is increased, mostly because of diastolic augmentation by balloon inflation (Figure 27-2).

The benefits of aortic counterpulsation include (1) increased mean arterial pressure and cardiac output, (2) increased coronary blood flow, and (3) decreased myocardial oxygen demand (Figure 27-e1). As such, IABP fits the hemodynamic criteria for an ideal MCS device. However, the

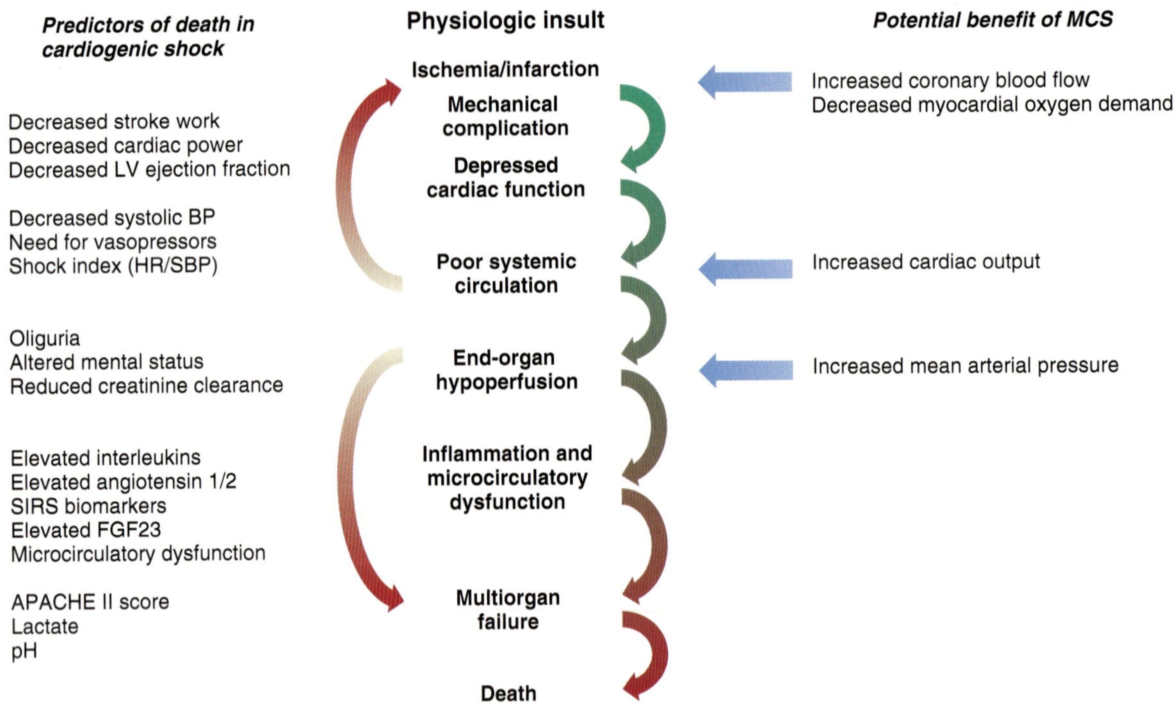

FIGURE 27-1 Clinical deterioration following myocardial infarction and potential hemodynamic benefits of mechanical circulatory support (MCS). *BP*, Blood pressure; *FGF*, fibroblast growth factor; *HR*, heart rate; *LV*, left ventricular; *SBP*, systolic blood pressure. *(Adapted from Werdan K, et al: Mechanical circulatory support in cardiogenic shock.* Eur Heart J *35:156–167, 2014; and Shah NR, et al: Serum biomarkers in severe refractory cardiogenic shock.* JACC Heart Fail *1:200-206, 2013.)*

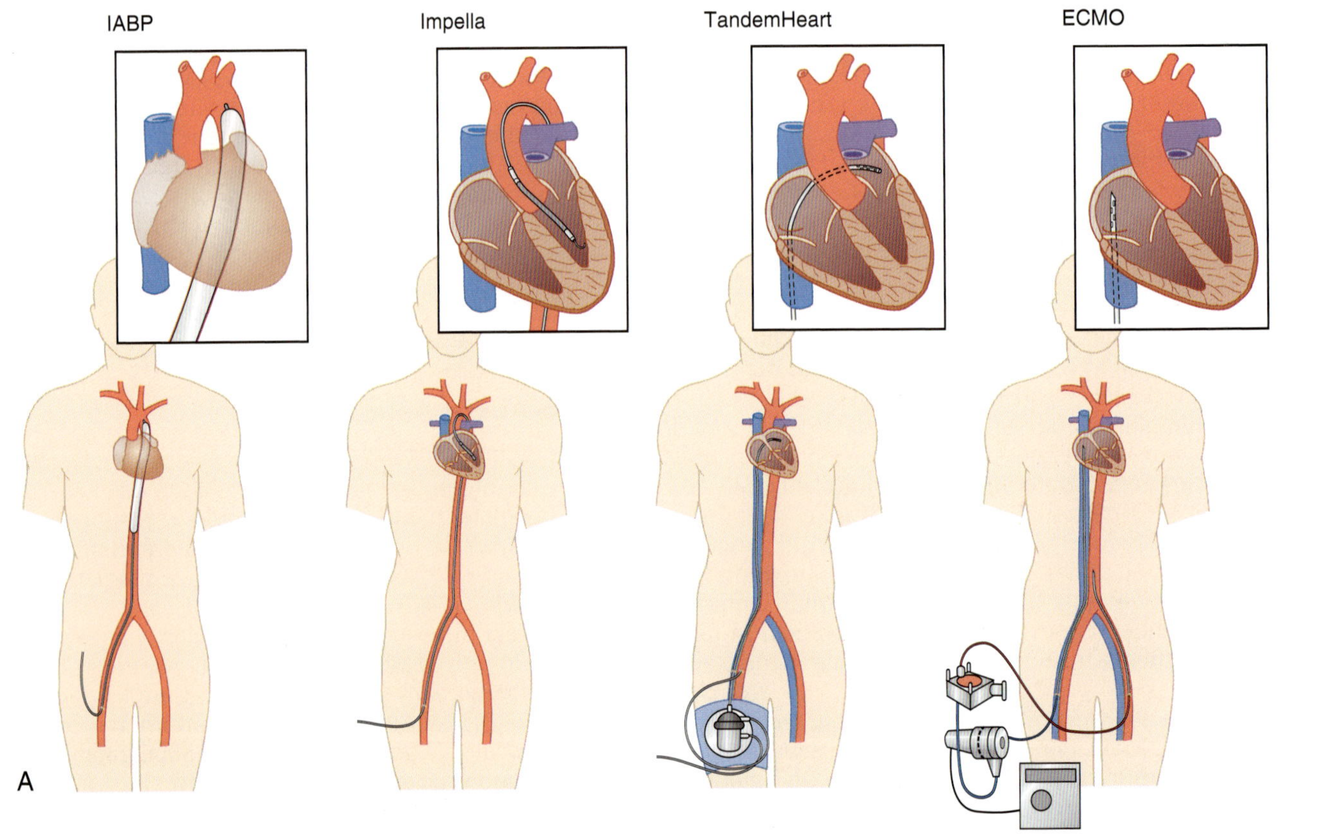

FIGURE 27-2 Comparison of percutaneous mechanical circulatory support devices. (**A**) Four major types of devices. (**B**) Details on the mechanism and hemodynamic and clinical effects of each device. *ECMO*, Extra-corporeal membrane oxygenation; *IABP*, intra-aortic balloon pump; *MAP*, mean arterial pressure; *PCWP*, pulmonary capillary wedge pressure. *(Adapted from Werdan K, et al: Mechanical circulatory support in cardiogenic shock.* Eur Heart J *35:156–167, 2014.)*

	IABP	Impella 2.5	Impella CP	TandemHeart	ECMO
Mechanism	Pneumatic	Axial	Axial	Centrifugal	Centrifugal
Hemodynamic					
Flow augmentation	Dependent on LV function	2.5 L/min	2.5-3.5 L/min	4-5 L/min	Variable, up to full physiologic support
Cardiac index	↑	↑	↑↑	↑↑	↑↑
MAP	↑	↑	↑↑	↑↑	↑↑
Coronary perfusion	↑	↑	↑	?	?
PCWP	↓	↓	↓	↓↓	Variable
Myocardial work	↓	↓	↓↓	↓↓	↔/↑
LV afterload	↓	↔	↔	↑	↑
Clinical					
Arterial femoral access	7-8 F	13 F	14 F	15-19 F or 12-15 F x 2	15-17 F
Venous access	None	None	None	21 F femoral with transeptal puncture	19-25 F
Systemic anticoagulation	Recommended	Required	Required	Required	Required

B

FIGURE 27-2, cont'd

impact of IABP on cardiac output is generally small and is dependent on the loading conditions and function of the LV. No more than a 0.5 to 1.0 L/min increase in cardiac output should be expected. Similarly, improvement of coronary perfusion is likely modest and dependent on patient factors. IABP delivers an increase in blood flow to the aortic root (6.4% of balloon volume on 1:1 assistance)[4] and improves flow in open coronary arteries, but the effect on blood flow past coronary stenosis or in patients with acute coronary syndromes is unclear.[5] IABP improves coronary blood flow after thrombolysis and can increase the rate of clot lysis in canine models. Independent of coronary blood flow effects, IABP reduces myocardial ischemia by decreasing oxygen demand. Decreased demand results from a decrease in LV afterload and wall stress, and may be the dominant hemodynamic effect of IABP in the setting of active ischemia.[6]

Clinical Use

IABP is commonly placed percutaneously via the femoral artery, although axillary artery or subclavian artery access is also possible using a surgical cutdown. The IABP is placed over a guidewire and positioned in the descending aorta just distal to the origin of the left subclavian artery (2 to 4 cm below the aortic arch). Modern devices provide automatic balloon inflation based on electrocardiographic or hemodynamic triggers. Timing can be adjusted manually. Inflation should occur at the dicrotic notch and fully deflate before the onset of systole. Inappropriate device timing will limit hemodynamic benefits of the device (Figure 27-3). One inflation per cardiac cycle (1:1) provides maximum hemodynamic support. A reduced assist ratio (1:2 or 1:3) may be more appropriate for patients with tachycardia, arrhythmia, or for weaning before device removal. Systemic anticoagulation is commonly used when using IABP with an assist ratio of less than 1:1. However, systematic evaluations of the effects of anticoagulation versus placebo are lacking. Device use at 1:1 for limited periods (<24 hours) without anticoagulation is probably safe and is often used to allow anticoagulation to dissipate before IABP removal.[7] Moderate or severe aortic insufficiency may worsen with IABP use and is an absolute contraindication, as is the presence of aortic dissection. Relative contraindications include severe peripheral arterial disease, aortic aneurysm, bleeding, or inability to safely administer a systemic anticoagulant.[8] The IABP exists in several sizes, from 34 to 50 mL. The most commonly used size is 40 mL. Recently, the 50-mL IABP has been evaluated, and it may be associated with slightly better hemodynamic augmentation compared with the 40-mL device.[9]

An IABP is relatively easy to insert and has a low complication rate. The Benchmark Counterpulsation Outcomes Registry prospectively registered 5495 patients who received an IABP in the setting of MI from 1996 to 2001. Balloon insertion was successful in 97.7% of patients, and in-hospital mortality was 20%. Only 2.7% of patients experienced major complications (severe bleeding [1.4%], major limb ischemia [0.5%], balloon leak [0.8%], or death related to IABP [0.05%]). Prolonged use of IABP is also associated with thrombocytopenia, hemolysis, and infection.[7]

In real-world practice, MI complications account for only a minority of IABP insertions. In the Benchmark Registry, 27.3% of patients received an IABP because of cardiogenic

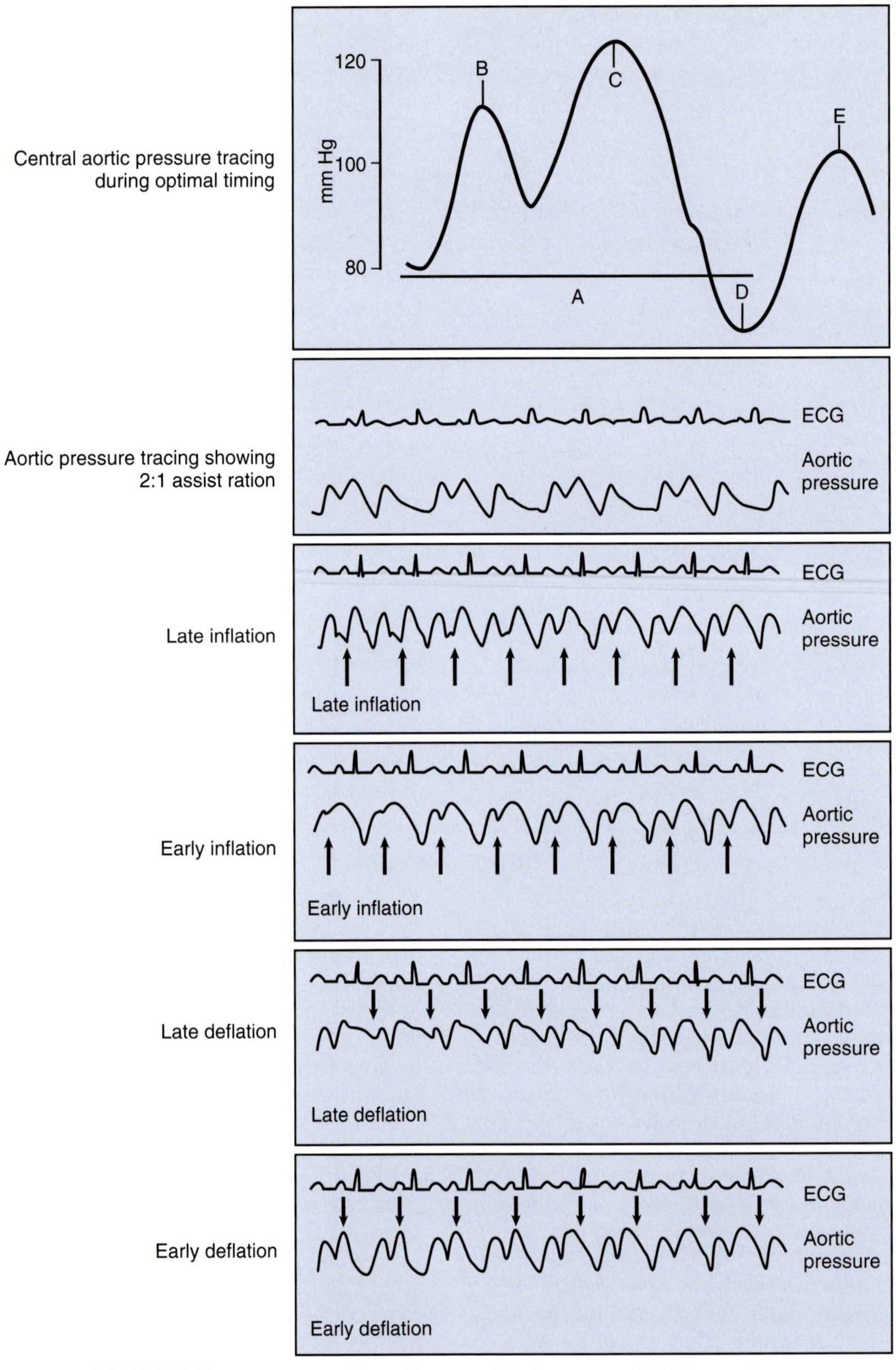

FIGURE 27-3 **Hemodynamic effects of intra-aortic balloon pump.** *ECG*, Electrocardiogram.

shock, and 11.7% received it for mechanical complications of MI. Although use of MCS is increasing overall in the United States, there has been a slight decline in IABP use since 2008.[3]

Observational Evidence

Kantrowitz and Kantrowitz suggested the concept of balloon counterpulsation in 1953, and the first clinical use occurred in 1967. The IABP gained popularity in subsequent decades, supported by promising observational evidence. The GUSTO-I trial included 2972 patients with STEMI complicated by cardiogenic shock. Of these, the 25% of patients treated with early IABP demonstrated a trend toward lower 30-day mortality compared with patients not treated with IABP or treated later in the clinical course (47% vs. 60%; $P = .06$).[10,11] Use of an IABP was 86% in both arms of the SHOCK trial, which showed benefit of early revascularization compared with medical management for patients with STEMI and cardiogenic shock.[12] In the SHOCK trial registry, 51% of patients were treated with IABP, and IABP use was associated with lower mortality (50% vs. 72%; $P < .0001$). Among 23,180 patients with acute MI and cardiogenic shock in the NRMI-2 cohort, 31% were treated with IABP. IABP use was associated with reduced mortality in patients who

TABLE 27-1 Randomized Clinical Trials Assessing Use of Temporary Mechanical Circulatory Support for Treatment of Acute Myocardial Infarction with Cardiogenic Shock

STUDY	PERIOD	SAMPLE SIZE	SETTING	REVASCULARIZATION TYPE	HEMODYNAMIC OUTCOMES	CLINICAL OUTCOMES
IABP vs. Medical Therapy						
Ohman, 2005 (TACTICS)	1996–1999	57	Multicenter	Thrombolysis (100%), PCI (23%), CABG (18%)	Not reported	Mortality at 6 mos similar for IABP and control (34% vs. 43%; *P* = .23) Trend toward benefit for IABP among patients with Killip III/IV classification
Prondzinsky, 2010 (IABP SHOCK I)	2003–2004	40	Single-center	PCI (100%)	No significant difference in cardiac output, SVR, PCWP	No difference in APACHE II score
Thiele, 2012[16] (IABP SHOCK II)	2009–2012	598	Multicenter	PCI (96%), CABG (4%), None (3%)	No difference in HR, BP, or serum lactate	Mortality at 30 days similar for IABP and control (39.7% vs. 41.3%)
TandemHeart vs. IABP						
Thiele, 2005	2000–2003	41	Single-center	PCI (95%), CABG (5%)	Patients treated with TandemHeart had greater improvements in cardiac power index, PCWP, CVP, and serum lactate	Mortality at 30 days was similar for patients treated with TandemHeart and IABP (43% vs. 45%; *P* = .86)
Burkhoff, 2006	2002–2004	33	Multicenter	Among AMI patients: PCI (85%), CABG (12%)	Patients treated with TandemHeart had greater improvements in CI, MAP, and PCWP	No difference in 30-day mortality.
Impella vs. IABP						
Seyfarth, 2008	2004–2007	26	Two centers	PCI (94%), CABG (4%)	Patients treated with Impella had significantly improved CI	No difference in 30-day mortality (46% in both arms)

AMI, Acute myocardial infarction; *APACHE*, Acute Physiology and Chronic Health Evaluation; *CABG*, coronary artery bypass graft; *CI*, cardiac index; *CVP*, central venous pressure; *IABP*, intra-aortic balloon pump; *MAP*, mean arterial pressure; *PCI*, percutaneous coronary intervention; *PCWP*, pulmonary capillary wedge pressure; SVR, systemic vascular resistance.

received thrombolytic therapy, but who did not undergo primary angioplasty.[10,13]

In 2004, IABP use for patients with MI complicated by shock became a class I recommendation despite a lack of randomized data. A later meta-analysis of observational data showed no association of IABP therapy with survival for patients treated with percutaneous coronary intervention (PCI) in the setting of STEMI with cardiogenic shock, although IABP was associated with survival among patients treated with thrombolysis.[10]

Randomized Trials

Subsequently, several randomized trials have addressed this question (Table 27-1). The IABP SHOCK I trial randomized patients with MI and shock to IABP or no IABP. This small trial assessed hemodynamic endpoints only. Temporal improvements in cardiac output and systemic vascular resistance were seen in patients managed both with and without IABP, with no significant difference between groups, which is in contrast to other physiological studies.[14] The IABP-SHOCK II study then randomized 600 patients with cardiogenic shock that complicated STEMI to IABP or medical therapy at the time of PCI. There was no significant difference between groups in any clinical endpoints at 30 days or 1 year.[15,16] These neutral results were consistent across all of the major subgroups in which a benefit of IABP would have been plausibly more likely. The CRISP-AMI trial randomized 337 patients with anterior STEMI to elective versus provisional insertion of IABP. Although performed in patients with stable hemodynamics, this study tested the hypothesis that IABP might reduce the area of MI in patients at risk of cardiogenic shock. The mean infarct size, as assessed by cardiac magnetic resonance imaging, was not significantly different between groups. Clinical endpoints were similar at hospital discharge and 30 days. A nonsignificant trend toward a mortality benefit with IABP was seen at 6 months.[17]

In summary, current observational evidence supports use of IABP for patients with post-MI shock who are receiving thrombolytics. Routine use of IABP for MI patients who are undergoing PCI is not supported by current observational or randomized trial data (Table 27-2; see also the section on Suggested Approach). A provisional strategy of selective use for refractory shock has not been tested. Use of IABP has been described for patients with acute VSDs and MR with cardiogenic shock (see Chapter 26). In one series, IABP support was associated with lower preoperative mortality.[18] IABP may have a role in stabilization of shock to permit definitive surgical correction.

TandemHeart

Hemodynamic Effects

TandemHeart is a percutaneous ventricular assist device (VAD) that can provide up to 4 L/min of circulatory support, making it attractive for patients with poor intrinsic systolic function and/or prolonged anticipated periods of shock. TandemHeart draws blood from the left atrium and injects

TABLE 27-2 Guideline Recommendations for Mechanical Circulatory Support for Patients with Acute Myocardial Infarction

	GERMAN-AUSTRIAN S3: CARDIOGENIC SHOCK (2012)	ACCF/AHA: STEMI (2013)	ESC/EACTS: REVASCULARIZATION (2014)
IABP: Shock	In the setting of lytic therapy: IABP should be carried out adjunctively. In the setting of PCI: May be considered, but the available evidence is unclear.	IIa, B IABP can be useful for patients with cardiogenic shock after STEMI who do not quickly stabilize with pharmacological therapy.	III, A Routine use of IABP in patients with cardiogenic shock is not recommended.
IABP: Mechanical complications of MI	No recommendation	No formal recommendation. "IABP can provide temporary circulatory support."	IIa, C IABP insertion should be considered in patients with hemodynamic instability due to mechanical complications.
TandemHeart, Impella: Shock	No recommendation	IIb, C Alternative LV assist devices for circulatory support may be considered in patients with refractory cardiogenic shock.	IIb, C Short-term mechanical circulatory support in ACS patients with cardiogenic shock may be considered.

ACCF/AHA, American College of Cardiology Foundation/American Heart Association; *ACS*, acute coronary syndrome; *ESC/EACTS*, European Society of Cardiology/European Association of Cardiothoracic Surgery; *IABP*, intra-aortic balloon pump; *LV*, left ventricular; *MI*, myocardial infarction; *PCI*, percutaneous coronary intervention; *STEMI*, ST-elevation myocardial infarction.

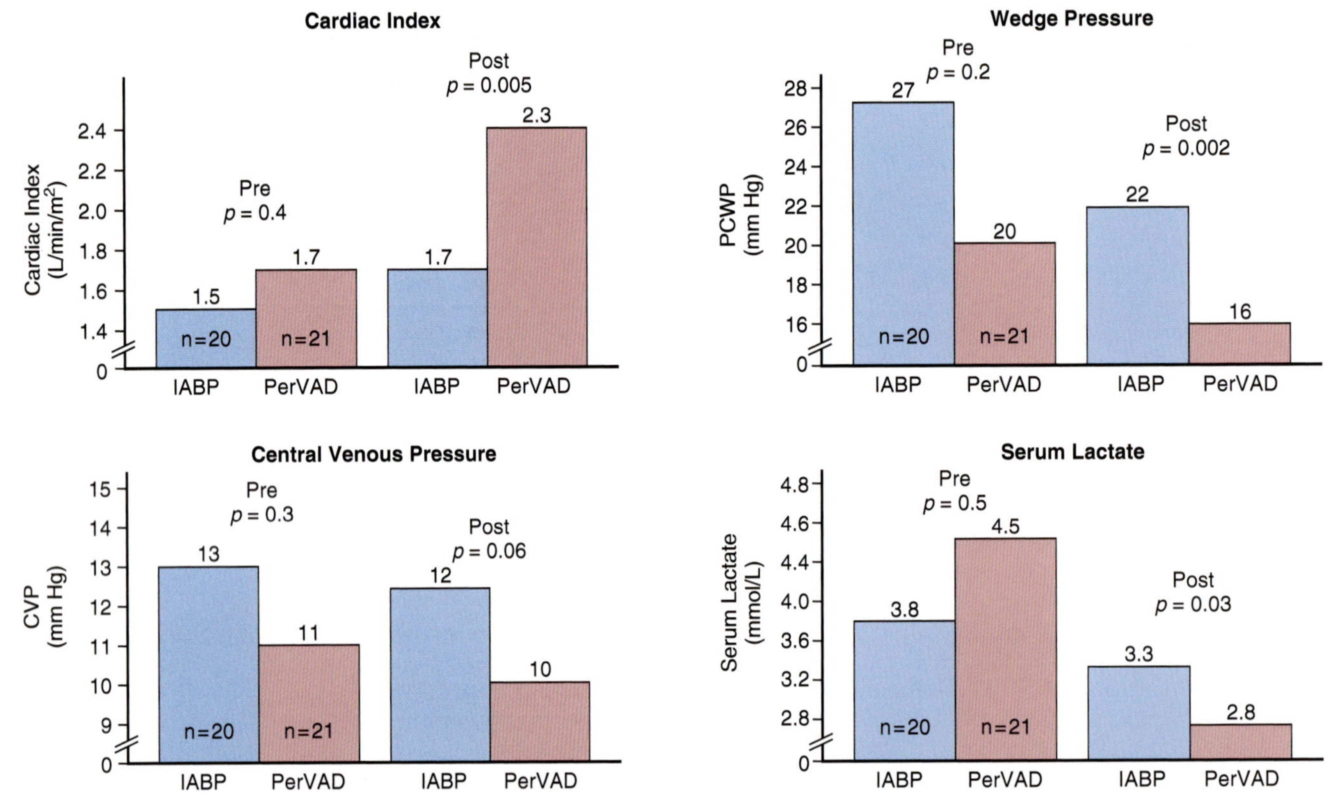

FIGURE 27-4 Hemodynamic and metabolic changes with initiation of TandemHeart support. *CVP*, Central venous pressure; *IABP*, intra-aortic balloon pump; *PCWP*, pulmonary capillary wedge pressure; *VAD*, ventricular assist device. *(Data from Thiele H, et al. Randomized comparison of intraaortic balloon support with a percutaneous left ventricular assist device in patients with revascularized acute myocardial infarction complicated by cardiogenic shock.* Eur Hear J *1276–1283, 2005.)*

it into the iliac artery or abdominal aorta. It consists of a left atrial drainage catheter, an extracorporeal centrifugal pump, and a femoral artery inflow catheter (Figure 27-2).[5]

For patients with cardiogenic shock, TandemHeart results in a reduction in pulmonary capillary wedge pressure (PCWP) and pulmonary artery pressure, augmented systolic blood pressure, and an improved cardiac index (Figure 27-4; also see Figure 27-2).[19] Compared with IABP, TandemHeart provides superior left heart preload reduction because of direct aspiration of blood from the left atrium, significantly reducing LV volume and pressure (see Figure 27-e1), which results in greater reduction in the PCWP. The cardiac index was also improved more effectively with TandemHeart.[20] The effect of TandemHeart on coronary perfusion is unknown.

Clinical Use

TandemHeart was first described in 2001 and received US Food and Drug Administration (FDA) 510(k) approval in 2006. Use is less common than IABP because of its greater complexity of deployment and a higher complication rate. A 21F venous catheter is advanced via the right femoral vein to the right atrium (Animation 27-1). A transseptal puncture under fluoroscopic and/or echocardiographic guidance introduces this inflow cannula into the left atrium. A 15F to 17F catheter is placed via percutaneous puncture of the common femoral artery and positioned in the iliac artery or distal aorta. The extracorporeal pump then provides up to 4 L/min of cardiac output at speeds of up to 7500 rpm.[5] Bilateral 12F femoral artery cannulae may be used instead of the 17F cannula, but this will limit overall flow to 3 L/min. Device placement, even in experienced hands, can take between 15 minutes and 1 hour.[19] Complications are common. In a series of 117 patients with refractory cardiogenic shock, the most frequent complications included sepsis (29.9%), bleeding around the cannula site (29.1%), gastrointestinal bleeding (19.7%), coagulopathy (11.0%), stroke (6.8%), groin hematoma (5.1%), and limb ischemia (3.4%). Overall, 59.8% of patients received blood transfusions.[19] In a population of patients who received short-term support for elective high-risk PCI, major vascular complications occurred in 13% of patients, and thrombocytopenia in 10%.[21] In addition, the inflow cannula can migrate back into the right atrium, which requires repositioning to avoid delivery of unoxygenated blood from the right atrium to the systemic circulation. Cardiac tamponade and perforation can also occur. Anticoagulation is mandatory, with a target partial thromboplastin time of 60 to 80 seconds.[5]

Clinical Trial Evidence

Two randomized studies have compared TandemHeart to IABP in patients with cardiogenic shock (Table 27-1). Thiele and colleagues randomized 41 patients with shock following MI to either TandemHeart or IABP. The TandemHeart group demonstrated greater improvement in the cardiac power index, cardiac output, PCWP, pulmonary artery pressure, and serum lactate. There was no significant difference in mortality, and the TandemHeart group had a higher incidence of limb ischemia (33% vs. 0%), bleeding requiring transfusion (91% vs. 40%), and disseminated intravascular coagulation (62% vs. 15%). In a similar study by Burkhoff and colleagues, 33 patients with shock, 70% presenting with MI, were randomized to TandemHeart or IABP. Again, patients randomized to TandemHeart had a significantly improved cardiac index and PCWP, with no change in clinical outcomes. Adverse events were balanced between the two groups. There are no studies that have compared TandemHeart to medical therapy or MCS other than IABP.[20] Evidence of successful treatment of patients with mechanical complications is lacking. Use of TandemHeart for right ventricular support via right atrium and pulmonary artery cannulation has been described.[22]

In summary, this device provides a high level of cardiac output, but with high complication rates. TandemHeart might be considered in centers where there is substantial experience with its use.

Impella

Hemodynamic Effects

The Impella devices are microaxial flow rotary pumps that are deployed across the aortic valve, drawing blood from the LV and depositing it in the ascending aorta. The Impella device is available in several sizes for support of the left heart (2.5, CP, LD, and 5.0) and the right heart (RP). The Impella 2.5 provides up to 2.5 L/min of augmented cardiac output. In the limited published data with the larger device, the Impella CP, cardiac output augmentation of up to 3.5 L/min has been reported. The Impella 5.0 and Impella LD (placed directly into the aorta) provide up to 5 L/min of support, but require surgical placement. Like other MCS devices, the Impella devices increase cardiac output and mean arterial pressure and decrease PCWP (Figure 27-5).[6] The Impella unloads the LV directly, which results in an immediate reduction in end-diastolic wall stress (see Figure 27-e1).[23] Coronary perfusion pressure is increased, potentially because of an elevation of aortic pressure and decreased LV intramyocardial pressure.[24,25] Unlike the IABP, augmentation of cardiac output is independent of native cardiac function, making it a useful device for patients with moderate to

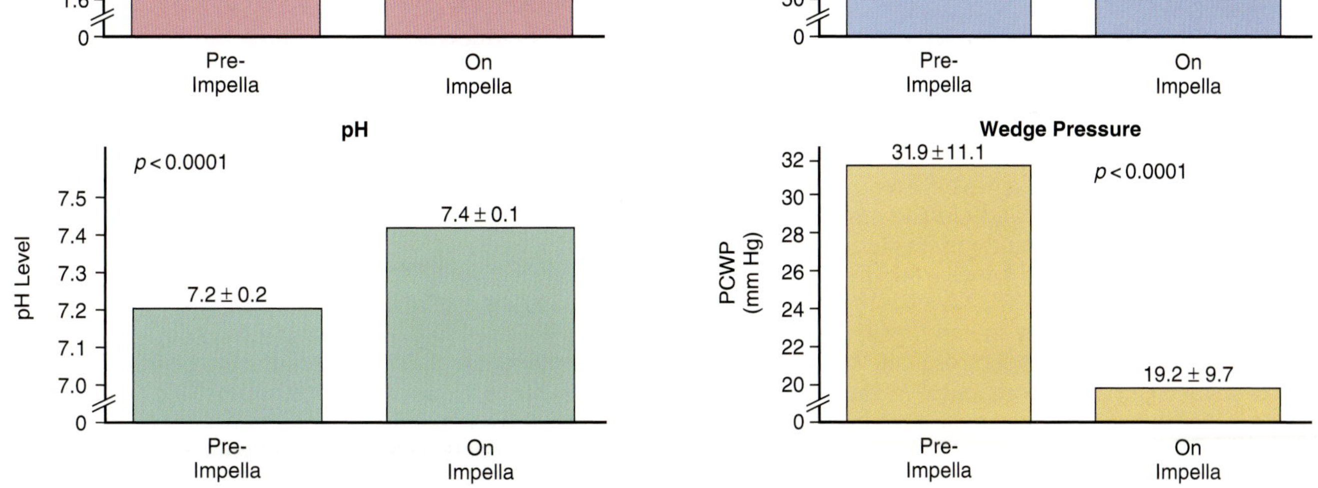

FIGURE 27-5 **Hemodynamic and metabolic changes with initiation of Impella support in the USPella Registry.** *PWCP*, Pulmonary capillary wedge pressure.

severe reduction in cardiac performance. In the USpella registry of 154 patients with MI and cardiogenic shock across 38 US hospitals, hemodynamic parameters improved after deployment of Impella, including mean arterial pressure (94 mm Hg vs. 63 mm Hg), PCWP (19 mm Hg vs. 32 mm Hg), and cardiac index (2.7 L/min/m^2 vs. 1.9 L/min/m^2).[26] The Impella RP is placed via femoral venous access and provides up to 5 L/min of support.

Clinical Use

The Impella 2.5 is a 12F device mounted on a 9F catheter that is inserted percutaneously in the femoral artery via a 13F sheath. The Impella CP uses a 14F device inserted via a 14F sheath. The Impella 5.0 is inserted via cutdown of the femoral or axillary artery, and the Impella LD is placed directly into the ascending aorta.[27] Both have 21F pumps mounted on 9F catheters. In the USpella registry, common complications included acute renal dysfunction (18.1%), bleeding requiring transfusion (17.5%), infection (12.9%), hemolysis (10.3%), and vascular injury that required surgical repair (9.7%). Anticoagulation is recommended to maintain an activated clotting time (ACT) of 160 to 180 seconds during use. A mechanical aortic valve or presence of LV thrombus are absolute contraindications. The Impella devices are approved in the United States for partial circulatory support for up to 6 hours, whereas they are approved in Europe for up to 5 days. The Impella RP is currently available for clinical use in the United States and Europe. This device, which is designed to support patients with right ventricular failure, draws blood from the inferior vena cava and injects it into the pulmonary artery.[28]

Clinical Trial Evidence

The ISAR-SHOCK trial randomized 26 patients to Impella 2.5 or IABP (Table 27-1). Impella 2.5 provided relative improvements in the cardiac index (0.49 ± 0.46 L/min/m^2) and mean arterial pressures (9.0 ± 14 mm Hg) at 30 minutes. Mortality at 30 days was 46% in both groups.[20] Subsequently, a European registry of Impella 2.5 use in cardiogenic shock (Impella-EUROSHOCK) reported results from 120 patients from 2005 to 2010.[29] This high-risk cohort (mean ejection fraction of 27%, 85% use of inotropes, 69% mechanically ventilated) had predictably poor outcomes, with 42% mortality during Impella support and 64.2% mortality at 30 days. However, Impella use in this population was technically feasible and improved hemodynamics. Implantation of the device was considered "easy or suitable" in 95% of patients, and explantation was easy or suitable in 95.7% of the surviving patients. The device was used for prolonged support (mean duration 43.5 hours), not just for periprocedural assistance. In the USpella registry, use of Impella before PCI, compared with post-PCI, was associated with improved survival to discharge (65.1% vs. 40.7%; $P = .003$).[26] Other case series have reported the feasibility of Impella use in STEMI and cardiac arrest patients.[30,31] Unfortunately, there are no randomized studies of sufficient size to assess the impact of Impella on clinical endpoints. Two larger studies (IMPRESS, RECOVER II) have been terminated because of an inability to enroll patients.[32] Treatment of mechanical complications such as acute MR and VSD has been described in case reports only.[33,34] Patients with right heart failure may benefit from a right-sided Impella device.

In summary, the family of Impella devices offers reasonable balance between stronger hemodynamic support and ease of use. There is a limited published experience of its use in cardiogenic shock, but it suggests that this device may be a reasonable choice in the more severe forms of shock.

Percutaneous Extra-Corporeal Membrane Oxygenation

Hemodynamic Effects

ECMO, which is a form of cardiopulmonary bypass, can be deployed rapidly at the bedside for treatment of cardiogenic shock or cardiac arrest. Although approved for pediatric use, ECMO has never undergone an FDA approval process for adults, because its current use is achieved by combining several individual components that all have independent 510k approval. Deoxygenated blood is aspirated from the right atrium or the vena cava, pumped through an oxygenator, and injected into the arterial circulation, thus bypassing the heart and lungs.[35] Full cardiopulmonary support of greater than 6 L/min can be provided over extended periods of time. The hemodynamic effects of ECMO in the setting of cardiogenic shock are poorly understood and may be deleterious for some patients. Veno-arterial (VA) ECMO is appropriate for patients with cardiac failure, and is distinct from the veno-venous (VV) ECMO used for patients with advanced respiratory failure.

VA ECMO maintains mean arterial pressure and end-organ perfusion independent of cardiac function, although this is potentially at the cost of increased LV afterload, myocardial oxygen demand, and worsening myocardial ischemia (see Figure 27-e1).[36] Coronary oxygen delivery may also be impaired. When using VA ECMO, coronary flow is composed of the oxygenated blood returning retrograde from the peripheral cannula and the blood expelled anterograde by native cardiac function. If the patient has respiratory failure, anterograde blood flow may be relatively deoxygenated, further exacerbating ischemia. ECMO flow rates can be increased to provide more retrograde oxygenated blood flow to the coronary and cerebral circulations.[37] Finally, a VA circuit will not directly decompress the LV. LV ballooning, pulmonary edema, and respiratory failure can result (see Figure 27-e1). A transseptal or transapical "vent" can be surgically placed in the LV to provide decompression, or combined use of ECMO with Impella may be considered.

Clinical Use

A venous outflow cannula is placed in the right atrium or inferior vena cava via the femoral or internal jugular vein (see Figure 27-2). The outflow cannula is connected to an external pump and oxygenator. Blood is returned to the systemic circulation via a femoral or axillary artery cannula. Venous and arterial cannulae can be matched to patient size and peripheral vasculature. For adults, venous drainage cannulae are typically 23F to 25F, and arterial return cannulae are 17F to 21F.[38] Multiple pumps and oxygenators are commercially available, including integrated, self-contained systems.

Maintenance of ECMO circuits may be challenging, and in most cases, requires full-time supervision by a perfusionist. Arterial oxyhemoglobin saturation should be maintained at ≥90%. Patients must be therapeutically anticoagulated, with a target ACT of 180 to 210 seconds or a plasma partial thromboplastin time of at least 1.5 times normal.[38] Sedation is not mandatory, and some patients with stable central cannula can be awake and ambulatory. However, sedation and mechanical ventilation are strongly advised for patients with peripheral cannulation in the setting of acute cardiogenic shock. Weaning of ECMO can be attempted after recovery of cardiac function.

Observational Evidence

No randomized trials have investigated the use of ECMO for cardiogenic shock. The literature is currently limited to case series and registries. A systematic review of 84 reports with a total of 1494 patients with cardiogenic shock of various causes or cardiac arrest reported that ECMO was successfully weaned in 65% of patients, and median survival to discharge was 40%. Among cardiogenic shock patients, survival to discharge was 52%. This review found evidence of publication bias that might have overestimated survival rates with ECMO therapy.[39] Two studies with historical controls reported improved survival of MI-related cardiogenic shock after availability of ECMO.[40,41] A cohort of 81 patients with MI and cardiac arrest refractory to cardiopulmonary resuscitation received ECMO to facilitate PCI. A 30-day survival rate of 29% in this extreme-risk population demonstrated the promise of ECMO as a salvage therapy.[42]

Reports of complication rates vary, although bleeding (5% to 79%), infection (17% to 49%), renal failure (30% to 58%), and limb ischemia (13% to 25%) are most common.[38] Vascular complication rates vary between 10% and 70%, and are related to the type of access and cannulae size. These may include acute embolism, peripheral arterial dissection, pseudoaneurysm, and compartment syndrome.[43] Finally, device failure is relatively common, potentially because of blood clots (0.13% to 22%), pump failure (4.7% to 30%), and oxygenator failure (21% to 27%).[38] Review by the United Kingdom National Institute for Health and Care Excellence identified major safety concerns and uncertainty about which patients are likely to benefit. This committee recommended that ECMO be used only by experienced teams for patients whose condition is refractory to other treatments. Patients and caregivers should receive detailed information explaining the uncertainty about safety and efficacy of ECMO.[44] Ongoing randomized trials of ECMO for cardiac arrest could provide some guidance. At least two trials are testing a hyperinvasive approach of early ECMO deployment in the emergency department for survivors of cardiac arrest (CT.gov ID NCT01605409 and NCT01511666). However, a large randomized efficacy trial for ECMO in cardiogenic shock is also needed.

In summary, ECMO is complex to use, with limited published information available to assess its safety and efficacy in adults with cardiogenic shock. It may be most well indicated for the cardiac arrest situation only, and the ongoing trials will provide important information on this device.

Surgically Implanted Devices

Patients may also undergo emergency surgery via sternotomy for MCS. Options include ECMO via central cannulation or temporary VADs. Central cannulation for ECMO can provide more stable access and improved patient comfort compared with ECMO via percutaneous cannulation. Temporary VADs such as the Centrimag (Thoratec, Pleasanton, California), the Thoratec Paracorporeal VAD, and the BVS 5000 and AB5000 (Abiomed) may be used for LV support (LVAD), right ventricular support, or biventricular support, depending on the clinical scenario. The temporary VAD systems can be used as a bridge to ventricular recovery, as a bridge to a durable VAD, or as a bridge to transplantation. There are no randomized controlled trials to compare the temporary surgical VADs to medical therapy or alternative MCS devices, although numerous case series have described successful prolonged support.[45] Although some centers report use of these devices as a "Bridge to Decision" to permit assessment of end-organ function and planning for possible durable VAD or transplantation, this strategy remains untested. At present, surgical MCS is not ideal for initial treatment of MI complications. However, MCS may have a role in the transition of care for patients who remain unstable despite use of a percutaneous device and have a well-defined long-term strategy, such as a listing for heart transplantation.

Improved patient mobility is a potential advantage of surgically implanted devices. Ambulatory VV ECMO can bridge critically ill patients to lung transplantation, and has been associated with improved long-term survival, potentially because of avoidance of critical illness myopathy and improved fitness before transplantation.[46] Similarly, central or upper extremity placement of ECMO or temporary VAD cannulae can allow ambulation while patients receive full cardiopulmonary support. This may be useful when bridging a patient to heart transplantation, or if myocardial recovery is anticipated. Axillary placement of an IABP and Impella are also technically feasible and allows patients to sit up and walk.

IMPORTANCE OF CLINICAL JUDGMENT IN THE ABSENCE OF ADEQUATE CLINICAL TRIALS

Recent negative randomized trials and meta-analyses have led some to abandon use of MCS for cardiogenic shock after MI. However, because of the high mortality of these patients and the absence of effective alternative therapies, many other clinicians continue to use MCS devices for their sickest patients. Optimal use of MCS remains unclear in the face of insufficient data. Although definitive evidence of efficacy is lacking, many potential uses of MCS have been poorly studied or completely untested.

Randomized trials of MCS have been underpowered and may not represent real-world populations. The IABP SHOCK II trial is the only randomized study that has been adequately powered to assess mortality.[16] Although a well-performed trial, the overall negative results of this study have been challenged for several reasons: (1) most patients received IABP after completion of PCI (86.6%); (2) 17.4% of the control group crossed over to receive IABP; and (3) the enrolled population was incompletely defined.[47] Randomized trials in this high-risk population may be limited by selection bias. Many physicians may not believe there is sufficient equipoise to randomize all patients with cardiogenic shock. MCS may be used preferentially for patients most likely to benefit, with clinical trial enrollment reserved for patients who are perceived to have unclear benefit from hemodynamic support. In addition, lack of long-term follow-up may hide benefit. Assessment of mortality after MCS use has generally been limited to the period of hospitalization or 30 days. Longer term follow-up of the CRISP-AMI study and the PROTECT II study of hemodynamic support for high-risk PCI showed potential benefits for MCS.[17,48]

Observational studies may also be confounded by selection bias. Clinicians may be more likely to use MCS devices in patients with greater likelihood to benefit, potentially because they have a greater likelihood of survival. This would bias observational studies to show a benefit for MCS. Alternatively, some MCS devices such as ECMO may be used predominantly as a salvage therapy. High mortality rates would be expected in this population.

In addition, devices with greater hemodynamic impact have not been adequately studied in randomized trials. There are no randomized studies of TandemHeart, Impella, or ECMO powered to assess mortality in the MI population. Circulatory support provided by IABP may be insufficient to produce a mortality benefit, and the greater hemodynamic effects of alternative MCS devices could result in greater likelihood of clinical recovery. Larger studies are clearly needed, but are challenging to conduct in the setting of more severe forms of cardiogenic shock, as evidenced by several aborted trials because of slow enrollment. It may be that these devices should all be evaluated against historical outcomes, as was done for surgically implanted LVADs. Although not ideal, it would allow a better safety and efficacy evaluation than is currently done.

Finally, appropriate use of MCS for patients with mechanical complications of MI is unclear. Studies of MCS for cardiogenic shock have primarily enrolled patients with shock caused by LV dysfunction, because this is the most common etiology of cardiogenic shock. Studies that address treatment of mechanical complications such as acute MR and VSD are lacking. Further research is needed to better clarify the role of existing MCS devices, develop new devices, and identify subgroups of patients that may benefit. In the meantime, clinicians who choose to use MCS devices should do so judiciously, with consideration of the risk/benefit ratio of each device and in consultation with the patient and family when possible.

Suggested Approach

Routine use of IABP for patients with cardiogenic shock in the setting of STEMI was previously recommended (class I) in the American College of Cardiology Foundation/American Heart Association and European Society of Cardiology guidelines, but this recommendation has subsequently been revised to a class IIa (reasonable to use) on the basis of the IABP-SHOCK II trial results (Table 27-2).[24] Current recommendations in the US professional society guidelines are that the use of MCS devices is reasonable (IABP) or may be considered (class IIb, for advanced MCS devices such as TandemHeart or Impella) for patients with MI and cardiogenic shock refractory to medical therapy. Routine use is discouraged. An expert consensus statement by the Society for Cardiovascular Angiography and Interventions, the American College of Cardiology, the Heart Failure Society of America, and the Society for Thoracic Surgery provides more practical guidance. This statement advocates for use of MCS in the setting of ischemic MR and acutely depressed LV function from a large MI. If a device is to be used, early deployment is encouraged.[1] This statement is intended to provide an expert consensus without formal recommendations with a determined classification and level of evidence.

Clinical severity of cardiogenic shock varies widely (see Chapter 25). There is a spectrum of risk that can be summarized as a progression from pre-shock to shock to severe, refractory shock to cardiac arrest. Patients with continued instability despite maximal medical therapy have severe refractory shock and are at risk for imminent cardiac arrest and death. The principal challenge of MCS device selection is the correct matching of the device to the degree of hemodynamic insult and patient risk.

When to Use Mechanical Circulatory Support

The best available evidence does not support routine use of MCS for patients with MI and pre-shock who are responsive to medical therapy. Instead, clinicians who elect to use MCS should target patients with shock, or refractory shock, at a time when support can be most effective. Patient selection for initiation of MCS is also discussed in Chapter 25 (see Figure 25-6). Consideration of MCS should prompt a discussion with the patient, family, and interdisciplinary care team regarding goals of care and potential adverse events. Clinical providers should recognize that at present the evidence supports that MCS can improve hemodynamic parameters, with advanced MCS options being superior to IABP, but there is insufficient evidence to conclude that this improvement will translate into better clinical outcomes. Nevertheless, the use of MCS, in our experience, is often useful to provide sufficient support to create time for more thorough evaluation of the patient's candidacy for destination therapies and to more thoroughly explore goals of care and expected outcomes with the patient or family and proxies.

How to Select a Mechanical Circulatory Support Device

Few studies have directly compared MCS devices in the setting of MI complications. A meta-analysis identified only three small randomized trials that compared TandemHeart or Impella 2.5 with IABP for treatment of cardiogenic shock.[49] As previously described, TandemHeart and Impella provided superior hemodynamic support with similar clinical outcomes. Therefore, no general recommendation for a specific type of MCS can be made. MCS selection should be determined by (1) institutional experience with each of the MCS devices, (2) the required level of support, (3) whether biventricular support is required, and (4) whether oxygenation is severely compromised. The currently available MCS devices can be placed on a spectrum of increasing hemodynamic support with concomitant increasing risk of complications.

In addition, there are certain device-specific advantages and disadvantages that are outlined in Table 27-3 and ought be considered.[5,6,24,32,50].

Transition to Higher Level of Support

For patients with continued hemodynamic instability despite MCS and optimal medical therapy, options include (1) an alternative percutaneous MCS device, (2) surgically implanted MCS to provide more durable support, and (3) de-escalation of support. In many cases, IABP will be the initial MCS device. Exchanging an IABP for alternative MCS device is technically feasible and reasonable when increased cardiac output support is required. Also, it is possible to use two MCS devices simultaneously (Impella-IABP, ECMO-IABP, ECMO-Impella), but evidence is limited to case reports. Use of surgically implanted VADs can provide excellent long-term hemodynamic support, although these should only be considered if the patient has options for durable VAD or heart transplantation.

TABLE 27-3 Relative Advantages and Disadvantages of Temporary Mechanical Circulatory Support Devices

DEVICE	ADVANTAGES	DISADVANTAGES	DEVICE-SPECIFIC CONTRAINDICATIONS
IABP	Greatest ease of use Rapid insertion Lowest complication rate Widespread availability	Least hemodynamic support Less effective in the setting of tachycardia or arrhythmia	Moderate to severe aortic insufficiency Aortic dissection Large abdominal aortic aneurysm
TandemHeart	Nearly full hemodynamic support Biventricular support possible	Deployment is time-consuming Requires transseptal puncture Cannot be performed easily during CPR High rates of vascular complications	Significant peripheral artery disease
Impella	Support is independent of native LV function Greater ease of insertion than TandemHeart or ECMO Multiple devices permit tailored support	Vascular complications more common than IABP	LV thrombus Mechanical aortic valve Recent stroke or TIA
ECMO	Greatest level or support Biventricular support Provides oxygenation in the setting of pulmonary failure Can be used in the setting of ongoing cardiac arrest	Requires specialized team for ongoing management High rates of vascular complications	

CPR, Cardiopulmonary resuscitation; *ECMO*, extra-corporeal membrane oxygenation; *IABP*, intra-aortic balloon pump; *LV*, left ventricular; *TIA*, transient ischemic attack.

Escalation to devices providing full hemodynamic support (Impella 5.0, TandemHeart, ECMO, or surgical VAD) should be undertaken with careful consideration. Goals of care should be addressed before use. If care is ultimately determined to be futile, withdrawal of these devices may be challenging for family members and the clinical team.

Multidisciplinary Teams

Although patients with cardiogenic shock have traditionally be treated by an interventional cardiologist or a cardiac intensivist, care is now optimally delivered using a "heart team" model (see Chapter 25).[51]

Institutional Experience and Learning Curve

Insertion of MCS devices can be challenging, and ongoing management requires specialized training. A significant learning curve was seen in the PROTECT II trial, which examined the use of Impella for high-risk PCI.[52] The initial patient enrolled at each site had a higher risk of adverse events than subsequent patients. A similar effect has been shown with TandemHeart.[21] Even IABP, which has been in use for four decades and is available at most hospitals, is associated with lower mortality at high-IABP volume hospitals compared with low-IABP volume hospitals.[53] Therefore, the most important factor in selection of MCS devices is institutional and operator experience with the devices. Hospitals can create protocols for device selection, and designate elements of the heart center team (cardiac intensivist, advanced heart disease specialist, interventional cardiology, cardiothoracic surgery) responsible for each device modality.

SUMMARY AND FUTURE CONSIDERATIONS

Despite frequent complications and conflicting clinical trial evidence, MCS devices are commonly used for treatment of patients with MI and cardiogenic shock. The past 40 years have witnessed steady growth in the use of MCS. First, IABP was the dominant technology, based on promising hemodynamic and observational data. Recent studies have cast doubt on the efficacy of IABP. Its use is now declining, with greater reliance on the Impella and TandemHeart devices. These devices provide greater hemodynamic support at the cost of increased complication rates. More recently, VA ECMO has grown in popularity, especially for patients with cardiac arrest or hemodynamic collapse. Definitive efficacy trials for these novel devices have not been performed in the cardiogenic shock setting.

Despite four decades of clinical use, MCS remains a promising but unproven treatment modality for patients with complications of MI. Improving outcomes for these patients requires better understanding of existing technologies. Although large, randomized trials are needed, randomization is challenging in this high-risk population. Relatively rare complications like acute MR or VSD will likely never be studied in a randomized fashion. Increasing use of registries and historical controls could provide evidence where randomized trials are lacking. Simultaneously, development of new MCS technologies may produce a device with an improved risk/benefit ratio, leading to definitive mortality benefits.

In the meantime, MCS devices are available for treatment of patients with severe, refractory cardiogenic shock or mechanical complications in the setting of MI. Clinicians must select and use these devices judiciously, with understanding of their potential benefits and complications.

Classic References

Gurbel PA, et al.: Arterial diastolic pressure augmentation by intra-aortic balloon counterpulsation enhances the onset of coronary artery reperfusion by thrombolytic therapy, *Circulation* 89: 361–365, 1994.

Santa-Cruz RA, Cohen MG, Ohman EM: Aortic counterpulsation: a review of the hemodynamic effects and indications for use, *Catheterization and Cardiovascular Interventions* 67:68–77, 2006.

Stone GW, et al.: Contemporary utilization and outcomes of intra-aortic balloon counterpulsation in acute myocardial infarction: the Benchmark Registry, *Journal of the American College of Cardiology* 41:1940–1945, 2003.

References

1. Rihal CS, et al.: 2015 SCAI/ACC/HFSA/STS clinical expert consensus statement on the use of percutaneous mechanical circulatory support devices in cardiovascular care: endorsed by the American Heart Association, the Cardiological Society of India, and Sociedad Latino Americana de Cardiologia Intervencion; Affirmation of Value by the Canadian Association of Interventional Cardiology-Association Canadienne de Cardiologie d'intervention, *Journal of the American College of Cardiology* 65:e7–e26, 2015.
2. Stretch R, Sauer CM, Yuh DD, Bonde P: National trends in the utilization of short-term mechanical circulatory support: incidence, outcomes, and cost analysis, *Journal of the American College of Cardiology* 64:1407–1415, 2014.
3. Khera R, et al.: Trends in the use of percutaneous ventricular assist devices: analysis of national inpatient sample data, 2007 through 2012, *Journal of the American Medical Association Internal Medicine* 175(6):941–950, 2015.
4. Kolyva C, Pantalos GM, Pepper JR, Khir AW: How much of the intraaortic balloon volume is displaced toward the coronary circulation? *Journal of Thoracic and Cardiovascular Surgery* 140:110–116, 2010.
5. Westaby S, Anastasiadis K, Wieselthaler GM: Cardiogenic shock in ACS. Part 2: Role of mechanical circulatory support, *Nature Reviews Cardiology* 9:195–208, 2012.
6. Myat A, et al.: Percutaneous circulatory assist devices for high-risk coronary intervention, *JACC Cardiovascular Interventions* 8:229–244, 2015.
7. de Waha S, et al.: Intra-aortic balloon counterpulsation - basic principles and clinical evidence, *Vascular Pharmacology* 60:52–56, 2014.

8. Santa-Cruz RA, Cohen MG, Ohman EM: Aortic counterpulsation: a review of the hemodynamic effects and indications for use, *Catheterization and Cardiovascular Interventions* 67:68–77, 2006.
9. Kapur NK, et al.: Hemodynamic effects of standard versus larger-capacity intraaortic balloon counterpulsation pumps, *J Invasive Cardiology* 27:182–188, 2015.
10. Sjauw KD, et al.: A systematic review and meta-analysis of intra-aortic balloon pump therapy in ST-elevation myocardial infarction: should we change the guidelines? *European Heart Journal* 30:459–468, 2009.
11. Holmes Jr DR, et al.: Contemporary reperfusion therapy for cardiogenic shock: the GUSTO-I trial experience. The GUSTO-I Investigators. Global Utilization of Streptokinase and Tissue Plasminogen Activator for Occluded Coronary Arteries, *Journal of the American College of Cardiology* 26:668–674, 1995.
12. Hochman JS, et al.: Early revascularization in acute myocardial infarction complicated by cardiogenic shock. SHOCK Investigators. Should We Emergently Revascularize Occluded Coronaries for Cardiogenic Shock, *New England Journal of Medicine* 341:625–634, 1999.
13. de Waha S, et al.: What is the evidence for IABP in STEMI with and without cardiogenic shock? *Therapeutic Advances in Cardiovascular Disease* 6:123–132, 2012.
14. Prondzinsky R, et al.: Hemodynamic effects of intra-aortic balloon counterpulsation in patients with acute myocardial infarction complicated by cardiogenic shock: the prospective, randomized IABP shock trial, *Shock* 37:378–384, 2012.
15. Thiele H, et al.: Intra-aortic balloon counterpulsation in acute myocardial infarction complicated by cardiogenic shock (IABP-SHOCK II): final 12 month results of a randomised, open-label trial, *Lancet* 382:1638–1645, 2013.
16. Thiele H, et al.: Intraaortic balloon support for myocardial infarction with cardiogenic shock, *New England Journal of Medicine* 367:1287–1296, 2012.
17. Patel MR, et al.: Intra-aortic balloon counterpulsation and infarct size in patients with acute anterior myocardial infarction without shock: the CRISP AMI randomized trial, *Journal of the American Medical Association* 306:1329–1337, 2011.
18. Kettner J, et al.: Utility of intra-aortic balloon pump support for ventricular septal rupture and acute mitral regurgitation complicating acute myocardial infarction, *American Journal of Cardiology* 112:1709–1713, 2013.
19. Kar B, et al.: The percutaneous ventricular assist device in severe refractory cardiogenic shock, *Journal of the American College of Cardiology* 57:688–696, 2011.
20. Unverzagt S, et al.: Intra-aortic balloon pump counterpulsation (IABP) for myocardial infarction complicated by cardiogenic shock, *Cochrane Database of Systematic Reviews* Cd007398, 2011.
21. Alli OO, et al.: Percutaneous left ventricular assist device with TandemHeart for high-risk percutaneous coronary intervention: the Mayo Clinic experience, *Catheterization and Cardiovascular Interventions* 80:728–734, 2012.
22. Kiernan MS, Krishnamurthy B, Kapur NK: Percutaneous right ventricular assist via the internal jugular vein in cardiogenic shock complicating an acute inferior myocardial infarction, *Journal of Invasive Cardiology* 22:E23–E26, 2010.
23. Remmelink M, et al.: Effects of mechanical left ventricular unloading by Impella on left ventricular dynamics in high-risk and primary percutaneous coronary intervention patients, *Catheterization and Cardiovascular Interventions* 75:187–194, 2010.
24. Werdan K, Gielen S, Ebelt H, Hochman JS: Mechanical circulatory support in cardiogenic shock, *European Heart Journal* 35:156–167, 2014.
25. Remmelink M, et al.: Effects of left ventricular unloading by Impella recover LP2.5 on coronary hemodynamics, *Catheterization and Cardiovascular Interventions* 70:532–537, 2007.
26. O'Neill WW, et al.: The current use of Impella 2.5 in acute myocardial infarction complicated by cardiogenic shock: results from the USpella Registry, *Journal of Interventional Cardiology* 27:1–11, 2014.
27. Griffith BP, et al.: The RECOVER I: a multicenter prospective study of Impella 5.0/LD for postcardiotomy circulatory support, *Journal of Thoracic and Cardiovascular Surgery* 145:548–554, 2013.
28. Cheung AW, White CW, Davis MK, Freed DH: Short-term mechanical circulatory support for recovery from acute right ventricular failure: clinical outcomes, *Journal of Heart and Lung Transplantation* 33:794–799, 2014.
29. Lauten A, et al.: Percutaneous left-ventricular support with the Impella-2.5-assist device in acute cardiogenic shock: results of the Impella-EUROSHOCK-registry, *Circulation Heart Failure* 6:23–30, 2013.
30. Engstrom AE, et al.: The Impella 2.5 and 5.0 devices for ST-elevation myocardial infarction patients presenting with severe and profound cardiogenic shock: the Academic Medical Center intensive care unit experience, *Critical Care Medicine* 39:2072–2079, 2011.
31. Manzo-Silberman S, et al.: Percutaneous left ventricular assistance in post cardiac arrest shock: comparison of intra aortic blood pump and IMPELLA Recover LP2.5, *Resuscitation* 84:609–615, 2013.
32. Ouweneel DM, Henriques JP: Percutaneous cardiac support devices for cardiogenic shock: current indications and recommendations, *Heart* 98:1246–1254, 2012.
33. Harmon L, Boccalandro F: Cardiogenic shock secondary to severe acute ischemic mitral regurgitation managed with an Impella 2.5 percutaneous left ventricular assist device, *Catheterization and Cardiovascular Interventions* 79:1129–1134, 2012.
34. La Torre MW, et al.: Posterior ventricular septal defect in presence of cardiogenic shock: early implantation of the Impella recover LP 5.0 as a bridge to surgery, *Texas Heart Institute Journal* 38:42–49, 2011.
35. Allen S, et al.: A review of the fundamental principles and evidence base in the use of extracorporeal membrane oxygenation (ECMO) in critically ill adult patients, *Journal of Intensive Care Medicine* 26:13–26, 2011.
36. Van Herck JL, et al.: Management of cardiogenic shock complicating acute myocardial infarction, *European Heart Journal Acute Cardiovascular Care* 4:278–297, 2015.
37. Lawler PR, et al.: Extracorporeal membrane oxygenation in adults with cardiogenic shock, *Circulation* 131:676–680, 2015.
38. Lafc G, Budak AB, Yener AU, Cicek OF: Use of extracorporeal membrane oxygenation in adults, *Heart, Lung & Circulation* 23:10–23, 2014.
39. Nichol G, et al.: Systematic review of percutaneous cardiopulmonary bypass for cardiac arrest or cardiogenic shock states, *Resuscitation* 70:381–394, 2006.
40. Sheu JJ, et al.: Early extracorporeal membrane oxygenator-assisted primary percutaneous coronary intervention improved 30-day clinical outcomes in patients with ST-segment elevation myocardial infarction complicated with profound cardiogenic shock, *Critical Care Medicine* 38:1810–1817, 2010.
41. Tsao NW, et al.: Extracorporeal membrane oxygenation-assisted primary percutaneous coronary intervention may improve survival of patients with acute myocardial infarction complicated by profound cardiogenic shock, *Journal of Critical Care* 27:530, 2012. e1–11.
42. Kagawa E, et al.: Should we emergently revascularize occluded coronaries for cardiac arrest?: Rapid-response extracorporeal membrane oxygenation and intra-arrest percutaneous coronary intervention, *Circulation* 126:1605–1613, 2012.
43. Bisdas T, et al.: Vascular complications in patients undergoing femoral cannulation for extracorporeal membrane oxygenation support, *Annals of Thoracic Surgery* 92:626–631, 2011.
44. National Institute for Health Care and Excellence: Extracorporeal membrane oxygenation (ECMO) for acute heart failure in adults 2014 [cited 2015 April 24]. http://www.nice.org.uk/guidance/ipg482/resources.
45. Borisenko O, et al.: Thoratec CentriMag for temporary treatment of refractory cardiogenic shock or severe cardiopulmonary insufficiency: a systematic literature review and meta-analysis of observational studies, *ASAIO J* 60:487–497, 2014.
46. Lehr CJ, Zaas DW, Cheifetz IM, Turner DA: Ambulatory extracorporeal membrane oxygenation as a bridge to lung transplantation: walking while waiting, *Chest* 147:1213–1218, 2015.
47. Acharji S, et al.: Have we given up on intra-aortic balloon counterpulsation in post-myocardial infarction cardiogenic shock? *Clinical Cardiology* 36:704–710, 2013.
48. O'Neill WW, et al.: A prospective, randomized clinical trial of hemodynamic support with Impella 2.5 versus intra-aortic balloon pump in patients undergoing high-risk percutaneous coronary intervention: the PROTECT II study, *Circulation* 126:1717–1727, 2012.
49. Cheng JM, et al.: Percutaneous left ventricular assist devices vs. intra-aortic balloon pump counterpulsation for treatment of cardiogenic shock: a meta-analysis of controlled trials, *European Heart Journal* 30:2102–2108, 2009.
50. Kapur NK, Jumean MF: Defining the role for percutaneous mechanical circulatory support devices for medically refractory heart failure, *Current Heart Failure Reports* 10:177–184, 2013.
51. Takayama H, et al.: Clinical outcome of mechanical circulatory support for refractory cardiogenic shock in the current era, *Journal of Heart and Lung Transplantation* 32:106–111, 2013.
52. Henriques JP, et al.: Evaluating the learning curve in the prospective Randomized Clinical Trial of hemodynamic support with Impella 2.5 versus Intra-Aortic Balloon Pump in patients undergoing high-risk percutaneous coronary intervention: a prespecified subanalysis of the PROTECT II study, *American Heart Journal* 167:472–479, 2014. e5.
53. Chen EW, et al.: Relation between hospital intra-aortic balloon counterpulsation volume and mortality in acute myocardial infarction complicated by cardiogenic shock, *Circulation* 108:951–957, 2003.

28 Arrhythmias and Sudden Cardiac Death After Myocardial Infarction

Kalyanam Shivkumar, Jason Bradfield, and Una Buckley

INTRODUCTION

Despite significant advances in the diagnosis and treatment of malignant cardiac arrhythmias, sudden cardiac death (SCD) occurs in 180,000 to 250,000 people annually,[1] mostly in patients with coronary artery disease.[2] Myocardial infarction (MI) remains a vulnerable cardiac pathology that contributes to SCD, and identifying patients with MI who are at heightened risk for SCD continues to be a challenge. Although professional guidelines suggest that patients at risk for SCD after MI often have an impaired left ventricular function (to below 35%), SCD most commonly occurs in those with preserved ejection fraction. Owing to limited or inconclusive data, current professional guidelines simplify SCD risk stratification. However, day-to-day clinical decision making is complex, requiring significant clinical experience and judgment.

The primary difficulty with risk stratification is that it is not clear why some people have ventricular fibrillation (VF) and SCD as a primary manifestation of ischemic heart disease.[3] In view of the fact that a significant number of patients die from out-of-hospital cardiac arrest with no cardiac monitoring at the time, the relationship between ischemia and presumed arrhythmia is difficult to ascertain. Therefore, the current understanding of cardiac arrhythmias in this setting is largely based on experimental models and animal studies, which are imperfect at mimicking the human condition.

PATHOBIOLOGY OF ARRHYTHMIAS IN MYOCARDIAL INFARCTION

Preclinical Experimental Models

Experimental models have evolved in an attempt to fill gaps in knowledge regarding arrhythmias and SCD after MI. Models adopted to help understand different aspects of SCD include (1) in vitro models for cell-cell physiology; (2) ex vivo Langendorff perfusion models; and (3) in vivo small and large animal models. In vitro models were developed because of the difficulty in obtaining microelectrode recordings from the beating heart. Various preparations can be used to examine transmembrane potentials or to detect changes in intracellular ion concentrations caused by ischemia. However, it is difficult to mimic the in vivo effects of ischemia, hypoxia, acidosis, and high potassium concentrations. The Langendorff perfusion model involves isolation of the heart and perfusion through the coronary arteries. The main disadvantage of this preparation is that the heart is disconnected from the neural cardiac hierarchy (central nervous system, extrathoracic, and intrathoracic ganglia), which could alter arrhythmogenicity, similarly to the conditions after cardiac transplantation.

Many hurdles must be overcome in creating large animal models of MI. The method of occlusion of the coronary artery in a large animal model varies. The coronary artery can be ligated by means of a modified thoracotomy, embolized, or injected with ethanol (Figure 28-e1). The duration of the ischemic period and the timing of reperfusion—early versus late versus non-reperfusion—both contribute to differing patterns of ischemia and scar. Some investigators opt for a two-stage occlusion, with initial partial occlusion to create ischemic preconditioning and subsequent complete occlusion. In these studies, immediate lethal ventricular arrhythmias occur less frequently, probably as a result of neural adaptation or memory to ischemia. Commonly, investigators will create a left anterior descending (LAD) infarct after the first diagonal (Figure 28-e2) or a left circumflex artery infarct.

Porcine models have limited or no coronary collaterals, so in such preparations, at the time of infarction, VF due to accelerated cell death is common. Canine coronary artery occlusion results in a predominantly subendocardial infarction, versus a transmural infarction in the porcine model. Differences in collateral development and patterns of infarction can significantly affect the experimental model and how it relates to clinical findings in humans.

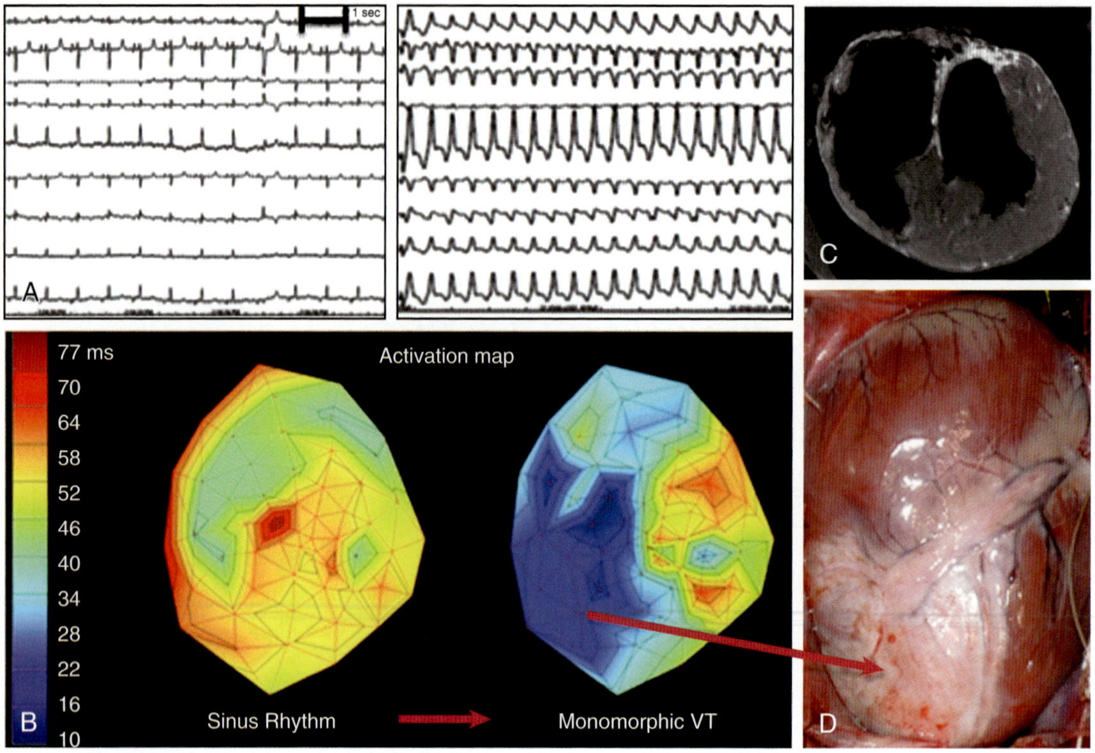

FIGURE 28-1 Left anterior descending artery myocardial infarction in a porcine model with myocardial scar and ventricular tachycardia (VT). (A) A 12-lead electrocardiogram (ECG) shows sinus rhythm and subsequent VT in a porcine MI model **(B)** An example of a polar map of the activation time in sinus rhythm and VT, generated from a unipolar 56-electrode epicardial recording system, showing the earliest activation site in VT originating from the anterior wall of the left ventricle. A photo of the epicardial scar in vivo (**D**) in the same animal and cardiac magnetic resonance image (**C**) show the infarcted region.

After 6 weeks, the substrate for subacute ventricular arrhythmias can be evaluated. However, arrhythmia induction in the terminal procedure is not guaranteed. Ventricular stimulation protocols, with up to three extra stimuli, at two different sites, epicardial and endocardial, are performed to assess for inducibility of ventricular tachyarrhythmia. On occasion, acute ischemia in a different territory can be induced in the setting of an already established chronic infarct to induce more electrical instability. Sympathetic stimulation with isoproterenol infusions or stellate ganglia stimulation also are employed to potentiate electrical instability. Despite these interventions, arrhythmia induction appears to occur in only 30% to 60% of canines and slightly more frequently in porcine models. Cardiac three-dimensional electroanatomic substrate mapping and cardiac imaging modalities such as magnetic resonance imaging (MRI) or echocardiography often are combined to provide additional information on the relationship of scar to ventricular arrhythmia inducibility (Figure 28-1).

Electrophysiological Effects of Myocardial Ischemia

Myocardial ischemia affects the resting membrane potential and inward and outward currents, altering conduction, refractoriness, and automaticity. During ischemia, an initial increase in extracellular K^+ results in a reduction in resting membrane potential.[4] Within the first 15 minutes of ischemia, these changes in resting membrane potential are rapidly reversible and can return to normal. The increase in extracellular K^+ occurs in two phases: After the first 15 minutes, a plateau or slight decrease is seen in extracellular K^+, which then starts to rise again in the second phase, corresponding with irreversible cell death. It is thought that the plateau phase may be related to the release of catecholamines, which pushes K^+ intracellularly owing to enhanced activation of the Na^+-K^+ pump. This pump, which is responsible for K^+ influx into the cell, is energy-consuming. A reduction in available energy in the first 10 to 15 minutes may result in depression of the Na^+-K^+ pump. Efflux of K^+ is due to a complex set of changes that are a result of net inward currents and accumulation of ischemic metabolites.[5] Other elements that contribute to membrane potential alterations, such as Ca^{2+} and magnesium, potentially have some effect on depolarization as a consequence of intracellular accumulation. Additionally, accumulation of the metabolites of phospholipids in the ischemic myocardium may affect the membrane potential.

Myocardial Scar Development Secondary to Ischemia

After 15 to 20 minutes of complete coronary occlusion in a canine model, signs of cell death are evident. The exact timing of cell death with occlusion in humans is not clear. MI can result in transmural necrotic myocardial tissue, but more commonly seen are patchy areas of surviving myocytes. During ischemia, the cells die gradually, and the infarct can increase in size, initially being localized to the subendocardial layer and then spreading to the endocardium and mid- and subepicardium. This pattern evolves because under normal conditions, the coronary blood supply is greatest in the mid- and subepicardial layers, and collaterals are more numerous in the subepicardium. After ischemic injury, necrotic myocardium is replaced by fibrotic tissue that surrounds the surviving myocytes. Ischemia results in

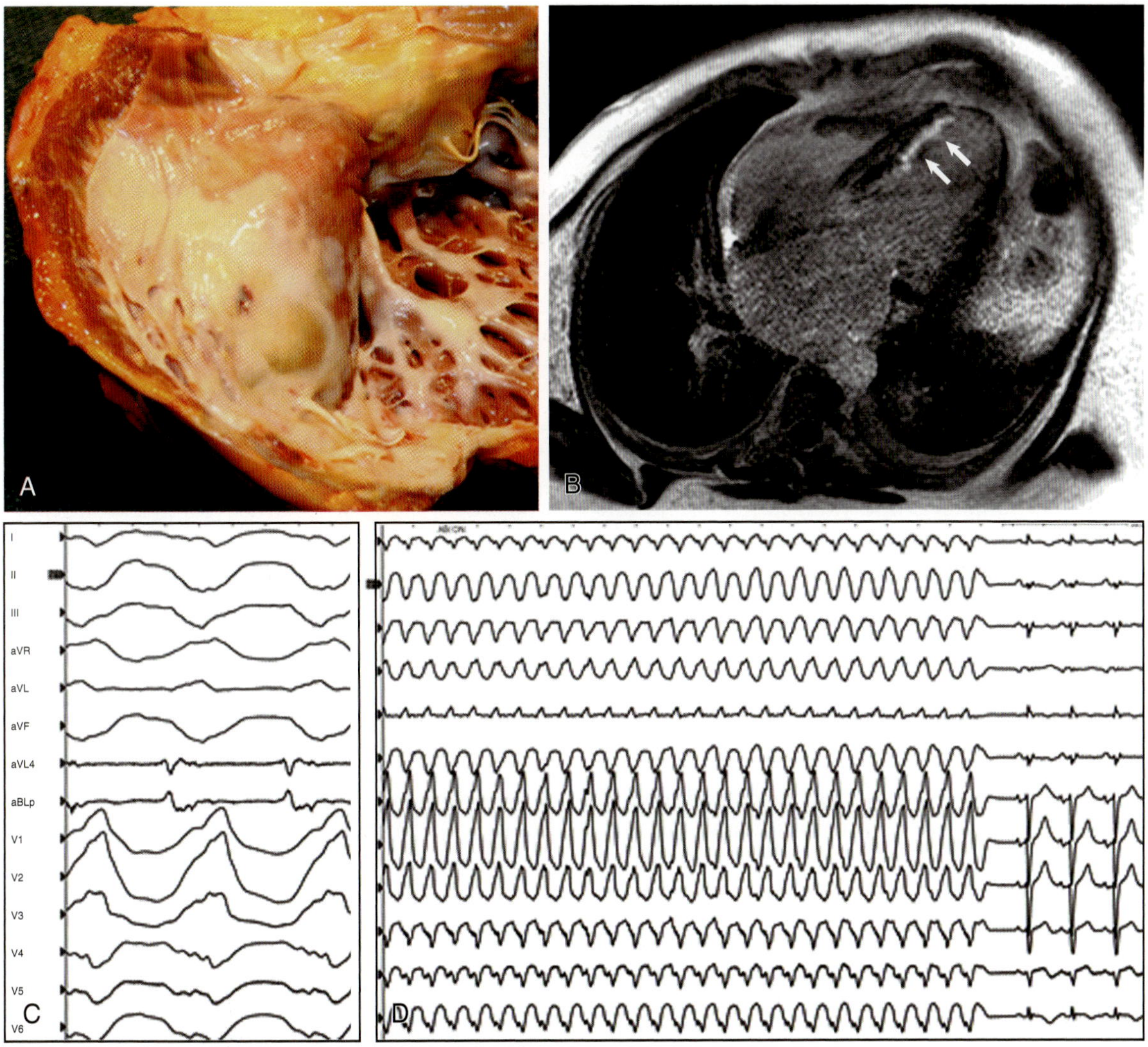

FIGURE 28-2 Ventricular tachycardia originating from a myocardial scar. (A) Histopathologic transverse section through the left ventricle. **(B)** Cardiac magnetic resonance image of a septal hypodense region (*arrows*) indicative of scar. (**C** and **D**) These 12-lead electrocardiogram traces show ventricular tachycardia originating from the left ventricular substrate. *(**A,** From Wallace A: McAlpine collection. UCLA Cardiac Arrhythmia Center.)*

abnormal refractoriness, abnormal conduction velocities, altered excitability, and automaticity, which can facilitate ventricular arrhythmias.[4] Surrounding the infarcted tissue, a "border zone" separates normal myocytes from scar. A border zone region can function as an essential region of slow conduction for reentry or as a site of focal impulse origin (Figure 28-2).

Timing of Ventricular Arrhythmias

Early Ventricular Arrhythmias

Early ventricular arrhythmias occur in two phases in animal models. The first phase, called Harris phase *1a*[6] (made up of so-called immediate ventricular arrhythmias), occurs in the first 2 to 10 minutes after coronary occlusion, with the highest incidence of arrhythmias at approximately 5 to 6 minutes. The second phase, called *1b,* usually occurs from 12 to 30 minutes after coronary occlusion, with a peak at 15 to 20 minutes. This description is based on small and large animal models, and it is unclear if humans have the same two-phase response with early arrhythmias. The mechanism appears to be different for each component.

The *phase 1a arrhythmias* appear to demonstrate conduction slowing and delayed activation of the subepicardial electrograms. The electrograms in these arrhythmias are markedly heterogeneous, with the sharp action potential becoming slurred and biphasic and even spanning diastole (diastolic bridging). Other features include an increase in the refractory period and marked conduction delay. It is thought that phase 1a arrhythmias are caused by reentrant arrhythmias with an appropriately timed trigger, such as a premature ventricular contraction (PVC), along with a heterogeneous electrical activation between the epicardium and the endocardium, and a delay after depolarization, allowing a reentrant circuit to develop.

Phase 1b arrhythmias are thought to be a result of endogenous catecholamine release, which could occur in the 12- to 30-minute period after MI. Information is lacking about whether arrhythmias occur in the same pattern in humans during the first 30 minutes of ischemia. After 3 to 6 hours, arrhythmias are very infrequent and after 8 to 24 hours, PVCs gradually increase in frequency.

Delayed Ventricular Arrhythmias

Delayed ventricular arrhythmias occur 24 to 72 hours after MI, with PVCs, accelerated idioventricular rhythms, and ventricular tachycardia (VT)/VF seen on the electrocardiogram (ECG). The autonomic component of the peripheral nervous system appears to play a critical role in the emergence of delayed ventricular arrhythmias.[7] In fact, autonomic modulation with therapies such as thoracic epidural anesthesia or sympathetic decentralization is recognized to reduce the incidence of ventricular arrhythmias related to MI; however, the timing of these arrhythmias is not well described.[8,9]

Several mechanisms may underlie delayed ventricular arrhythmias. Long cycle lengths with a long coupling interval PVC, late in diastole, may result in abnormal impulse initiation. Normally, sinus rhythm prevents activation of ectopic pacemakers by overdrive suppression, but once the sinus rate slows or has pauses, ectopic pacemaker tissue can become active, generating ectopic ventricular rhythms, through an automatic mechanism. Triggered activity due to early afterdepolarizations can result in reentrant arrhythmias.[4]

As a consequence of the lack of clinical studies, the relevance of comparisons of acute phase arrhythmias between animal models and humans is uncertain. In relation to the delayed ventricular arrhythmias, more data are available to help correlate findings in experimental models and in clinical practice.

Reperfusion Arrhythmias

Experimental models suggest that at least 3 minutes of ischemia is required for the development of reperfusion arrhythmias. In the era of primary percutaneous intervention for MI, reperfusion arrhythmias are commonly seen, ranging from isolated PVCs, accelerated idioventricular rhythms, and VT and VF. In experimental models, phases of arrhythmias related to reperfusion are evident, with none occurring after less than 3 minutes of ischemia. Arrhythmias are more frequent when the ischemic period is increased from 5 minutes to 20 to 30 minutes. Reperfusion arrhythmias are less frequent after 30 to 60 minutes. These arrhythmias are a result of washout of ions such as lactate and potassium and of toxic metabolites from the ischemic zone and also oxidative stress, all of which alter autonomic function.

In humans, the most common rhythm with reperfusion is accelerated idioventricular rhythm, with rates ranging from 70 to 100 beats/min. The absence of reperfusion arrhythmias is thought to be a negative prognostic indicator in that it is suggestive of a longer ischemic period than had been potentially realized. In experimental models, when reperfusion is performed early, a sudden and almost immediate restoration of action potentials to the ischemic area occurs. In the early stages of reperfusion, the action potentials are abnormal, with alternating low to high amplitude. Within the myocardium, marked heterogeneity of action potentials, along with the addition of a trigger, can act as a substrate for arrhythmias. This heterogeneity tends to decrease after the first 30 seconds of reperfusion.

Late or Chronic Ventricular Arrhythmias

Late ventricular arrhythmias occur approximately 1 to 3 weeks after MI, as the infarct evolves and starts to heal. After the early-phase arrhythmias, fewer ventricular arrhythmias typically are seen from 72 hours to 5 days, and then frequent PVCs predominate. The burden of early arrhythmias unfortunately does not predict the frequency of late arrhythmias. The absence of in-hospital or early arrhythmias does not predict the absence of late arrhythmias.

Risk factors predictive of late arrhythmias are the size of the scar, presence of aneurysms, multivessel disease, and anterior location of the MI (Figure 28-3). Before discharge, in the setting of these risk factors, treadmill exercise testing may be helpful in risk stratification (see Chapter 30). The development of arrhythmias during exercise testing is predictive of an increased risk for SCD. Electrophysiology testing for induction of ventricular arrhythmias by programmed stimulation is predominantly helpful for late or chronic ventricular arrhythmias. Chronic ventricular arrhythmias, beyond 3 weeks, tend to be reentrant in nature and result from scarring, with zones of either slow conduction or electrical block facilitating initiation and perpetuation of reentry.

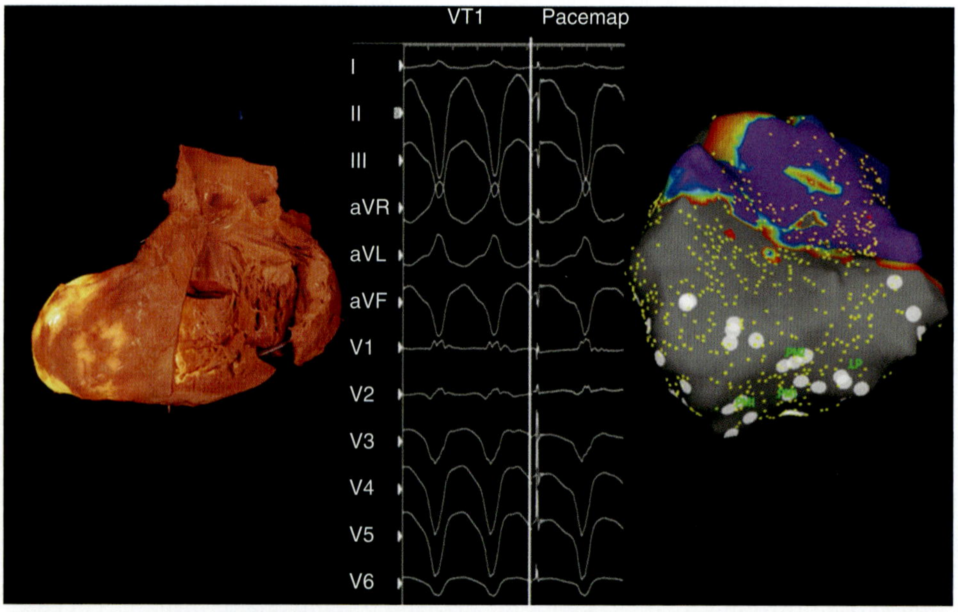

FIGURE 28-3 Anterior myocardial infarction resulting in aneurysmal anteroapical left ventricular (LV) wall. In the example shown, consequent apical thinning is evident on transillumination through the LV apex with a 12-lead electrocardiogram of the ventricular tachycardia (VT) originating from around the scar. A pace map from the critical isthmus shows a pattern identical to the ventricular tachycardia, and an electroanatomic map demonstrates a large anteroapical region of myocardial scar surrounded by a border zone. *(From Wallace A. McAlpine collection, UCLA Cardiac Arrhythmia Center.)*

MECHANISM OF VENTRICULAR ARRHYTHMIAS

Reentrant Arrhythmias

Reentrant tachycardias require a zone of slow conduction and unidirectional block. The longer it takes for the impulse to traverse the area of slow conduction, the more time is required for the impulse to emerge from the zone of reentry, and the longer the coupling interval before onset of tachycardia. Either a single loop or multiple loops may be present within a reentrant circuit (Figure 28-4). Reentrant tachycardias can be terminated by a critically timed premature stimulus that collides with the reentrant circuit, rendering it refractory. Capture of the ventricular electrical activity with pacing that does not affect the tachycardia also is indicative of a reentrant arrhythmia. Resetting of the reentrant arrhythmia to abort the tachycardia also may occur if pacing delivers a premature stimulus within the circuit. In other words, when resetting occurs, the QRS of the tachycardia occurs earlier than expected as a result of the paced stimulus, which advances the QRS. Termination of the tachycardia by overdrive pacing as well as the ability to entrain the arrhythmia is a feature of reentrant tachycardias. Concealed entrainment involves pacing at a faster rate than the tachycardia, whereby the rate of the tachycardia increases to the pacing rate, maintaining the same QRS morphology as for the baseline tachycardia, and fusion no longer occurs, with return of the tachycardia to the previous cycle length on discontinuation of pacing.

Triggered Arrhythmias

Triggered activity is dependent on afterdepolarizations, either early or late, with at least one action potential preceding it. Triggered activity displays features of both automaticity and reentry. If afterdepolarizations are of sufficient magnitude, they can generate another action potential. The action potential can result from either spontaneous leakage of positive ions intracellularly or a premature ventricular beat (Figure 28-5). Two distinct types of triggered activity exist: pause-dependent arrhythmias and catecholamine-dependent arrhythmias. During a pause, if the afterdepolarization reaches the cellular threshold, another action potential can be generated. This circumstance can allow for impulse initiation from the trigger and subsequent sinus node suppression. With catecholamine-dependent triggers, delayed afterdepolarizations lead to the generation of another action potential secondary to an increase in sympathetic activity.

Automaticity

Automaticity can be described as normal or abnormal impulse initiation. *Normal* automaticity, as seen in the sinoatrial node or latent subsidiary pacemaker cells, is responsible for the intrinsic rate at which impulses are initiated. Normal automaticity involves a spontaneous decline in transmembrane potential in diastole called *diastolic depolarization,* followed by a threshold potential, which generates a spontaneous action potential. A subsequent fall in membrane potential alters the membrane currents to a net inward depolarizing current. *Abnormal* automaticity occurs when the resting membrane potential of cells ordinarily responsible for impulse initiation is reduced sufficiently to allow spontaneous diastolic depolarization in other atrial or ventricular cells, causing overdrive suppression of subsidiary latent pacemakers. An example of abnormal automaticity is that of an idioventricular rhythm after MI. Accelerated idioventricular tachycardias demonstrate characteristics suggestive of abnormal automaticity, in how they fail to respond to pharmacologic agents and lack of overdrive suppression with pacing.

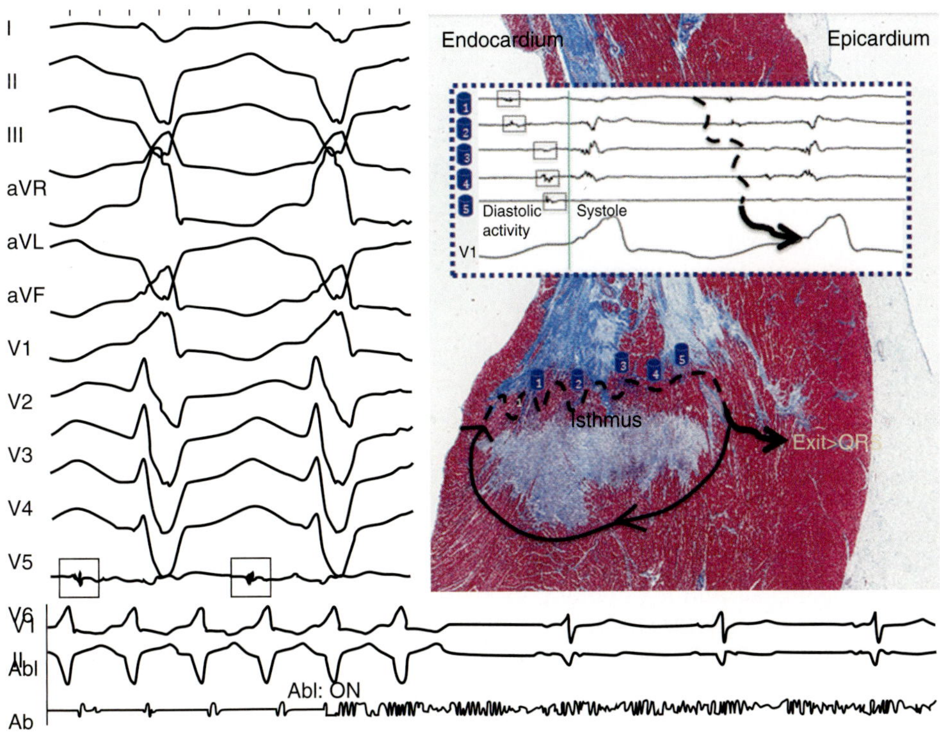

FIGURE 28-4 Histologic scar in ischemic heart disease. *Left,* A 12-lead electrocardiogram from a patient with ventricular tachycardia, with mid- and late diastolic potentials seen by mapping the isthmus of ischemic scar. *Right,* Histologic characterization of the ischemic heart disease substrate shows the ventricular tachycardia originating from the islands of preserved myocardium surrounded by scar tissue. The tachycardia terminates when the radiofrequency ablation (Abl) is turned on.

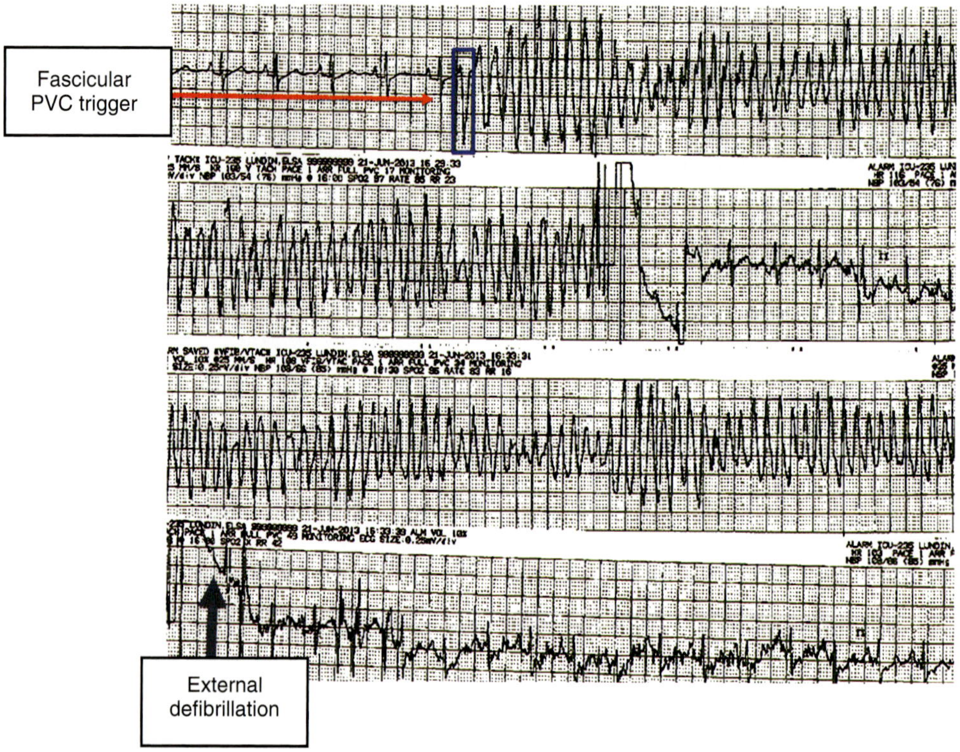

FIGURE 28-5 Fascicular premature ventricular complex (PVC) and ventricular tachycardia (VT). As seen in these electrocardiographic traces, fascicular PVC acts as a trigger (*blue outline*) to initiate polymorphic VT, which is terminated with an external defibrillation.

The Autonomic Nervous System and Ventricular Arrhythmias

It is clear that the autonomic nervous system (ANS) plays a critical role in SCD.[7] This nervous system component modulates all physiologic functions of the heart including chronotropy, dromotropy, lusitropy, and inotropy. The ANS is a finely tuned system regulating sympathetic and parasympathetic response, through a complex neural network between the heart and central cortical structures, and maintaining cardiac stability. The progression of heart disease can result in functional denervation and in cardiac and extracardiac neural remodeling. After MI, an imbalance in the autonomic nervous system, with a relative increase in sympathetic activity and a decrease in parasympathetic activity, is seen (Figure 28-6). This response is vital in the short term to maintain cardiac output but in the long term constitutes a maladaptive process resulting in reorganization of the neural network and precipitation of fatal arrhythmias as a consequence of persistent sympathoexcitation. An increase in sympathetic activity not only affects the Na^+-K^+ pump but also increases Ca^{2+} influx, which is thought to be a mechanism for enhanced automaticity and triggered activity. MI affects the cardiac myocytes but also has a cascade effect on the cardiac neural hierarchy, including the intrinsic cardiac nervous system, intrathoracic extracardiac ganglia (stellate ganglia), extracardiac ganglia (middle cervical ganglia, nodose ganglia, dorsal root ganglia), and the higher centers. Ischemia is the likely mechanism for disruption of the afferent information being transmitted to the central nervous system, with consequent effects on the central drive or reflex efferent parasympathetic input. It is this neural dysregulation that contributes to the pathophysiologic processes responsible for malignant ventricular arrhythmias and heart failure.

Removal of the excessive sympathetic input, such as with the use of beta-blockers, cardiac sympathetic denervation, or thoracic epidural anesthesia for ventricular electrical storm, can help prevent ventricular arrhythmias and reduce mortality[8,9] (Figure 28-7). In the case of cardiac transplantation, when the heart is disconnected from the central nervous system, the intrinsic cardiac nervous system maintains cardiac function, and a low incidence of VT is typical, even with coronary occlusion.[10]

EPIDEMIOLOGY OF VENTRICULAR ARRHYTHMIAS AND SUDDEN CARDIAC DEATH IN ACUTE MYOCARDIAL INFARCTION

Several studies have examined the incidence and timing of sustained ventricular arrhythmias at the time of an acute MI. Despite advances in the treatment of acute MI, the incidence of VT or VF complicating MI does not appear to have declined significantly. A study of 5259 patients with ST-elevation MI (STEMI), 5% of whom had VT/VF, found that 90% of cases of VT/VF occurred within the first 48 hours of STEMI.[11] The 90-day mortality rate in this group was significantly higher (23%) than in patients who did not have VT/VF (3%). The factors contributing to ventricular arrhythmias were identified as no reflow with reperfusion therapy, an inferior MI, total ST-segment deviation, lower systolic blood pressure, decreased creatinine clearance, increased heart rate above70 beats/min, and increased Killip classification.

By contrast, among 3485 patients who underwent primary percutaneous intervention for STEMI, VT/VF, which occurred in 181 of these patients (5.2%), was not associated with increased major adverse events at 3 years. The study population possibly was relatively enriched with lower-risk patients, because the 30-day mortality rate was 2.6%, compared with 4.1% in a contemporary STEMI trial.[12,13]

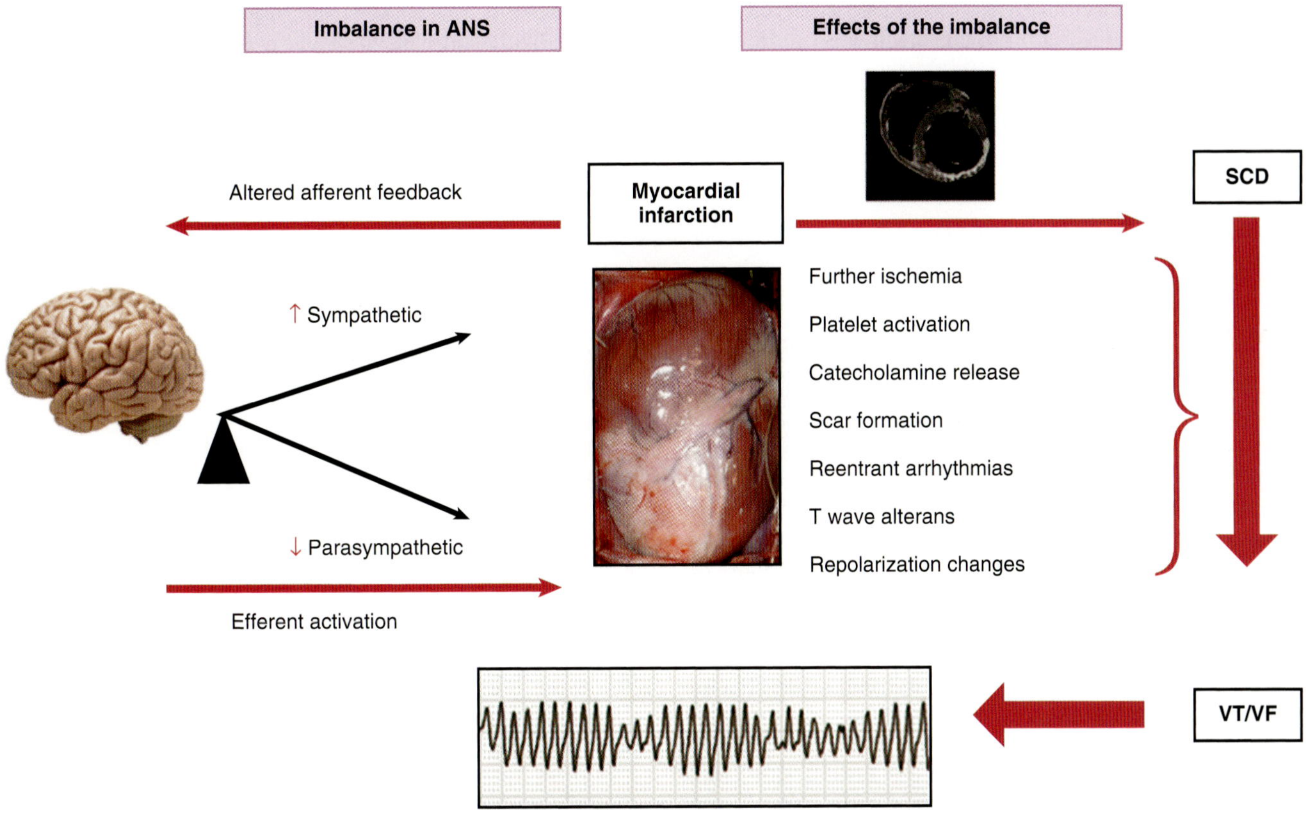

FIGURE 28-6 The autonomic nervous system (ANS) response to ischemic heart disease. After a myocardial infarction, an increase in sympathetic activity and a decrease in parasympathetic activity occur as a result of altered afferent feedback from the myocardium to the central nervous system. This imbalance can precipitate ventricular arrhythmias, potentially resulting in sudden cardiac death (SCD). *VT/VF,* Ventricular tachycardia/ventricular fibrillation.

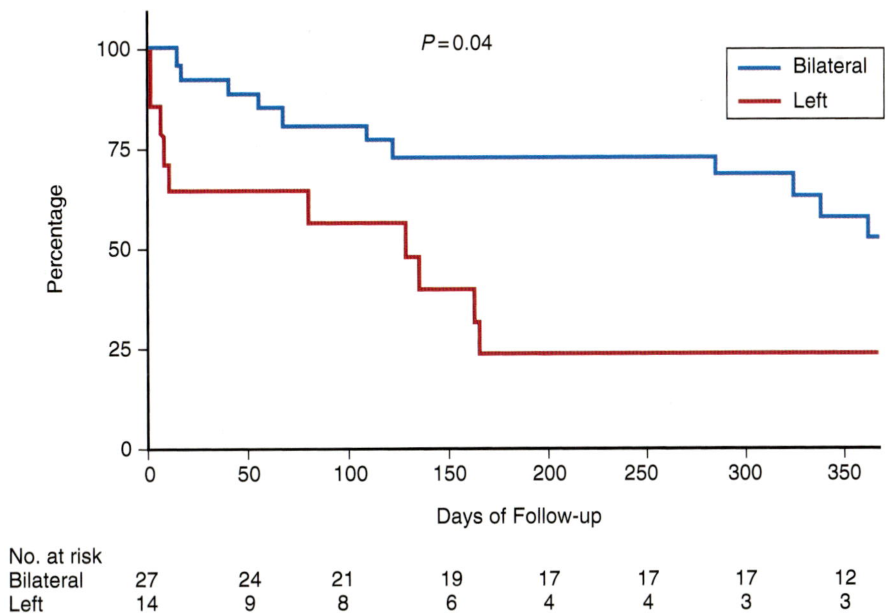

FIGURE 28-7 Analysis of shock-free survival in bilateral versus left cardiac sympathetic denervation (CSD) groups. Kaplan-Meier curves for survival free from implantable cardioverter-defibrillator (ICD) shocks are shown for both bilateral and left CSD subgroups. The 50% median time to shock-free survival was 366 days for patients in the bilateral CSD group and 128 days for those in the left CSD group (P = .04). The longer survival free of ICD shocks in the bilateral CSD group was attributable in part to the higher mortality rate in the left CSD group. *(From Vaseghi M, Gima J, Kanaan C, et al: Cardiac sympathetic denervation in patients with refractory ventricular arrhythmias or electrical storm: intermediate and long-term follow-up.* Heart Rhythm *1[3]:360-366, 2014.)*

In another study investigating the incidence of SCD after VF complicating MI, investigators found that of 3670 patients with MI, 116 had a course complicated by VF. Among survivors to hospital discharge, VF during the acute MI was not associated with increased mortality at 5 years.[14]

Ventricular Fibrillation at Reperfusion

Predictors of VF at the time of reperfusion were presented in a review of data for 3274 patients with STEMI between 2007 and 2012, of whom 71 (1.9%) experienced VF during reperfusion, and the incidence did not change over time.[15] These patients with sustained VF during reperfusion requiring defibrillation were more likely to have a history of a remote MI. The magnitude of ST-segment elevation was predictive of VF during reperfusion. The in-hospital mortality in this group was almost 5 times higher than those without VF, with deaths occurring as a result of heart failure, mechanical complications, or reinfarction.

Resuscitated Cardiac Arrest

The prognosis for those having a resuscitated cardiac arrest in the setting of MI was presented in a registry of 48,749 patients with STEMI, 10% of whom had a cardiac arrest.[16] Previous studies pointed to a higher inpatient mortality among those patients experiencing STEMI complicated by a cardiac arrest. This registry excluded 1557 patients who died at the time of the cardiac arrest or on the same day of hospital admission, so the final number of patients with cardiac arrest and STEMI was 3751. The 30-day mortality was associated with increasing age, lower admission blood pressure, higher admission heart rate, higher admission glucose, and higher admission creatinine clearance. Anterior STEMI was associated with an increased 30-day mortality. Of those having a resuscitated cardiac arrest, 42.6% occurred before arrival at the hospital and 63.4% in the hospital. In this latter group of patients, early cardiac arrest was not associated with increased inpatient mortality; however, the exclusion of patients dying within 1 day of the index cardiac arrest may have affected this observation. Most patients with STEMI and cardiac arrest die within the first 30 days, but if patients live beyond 30 days, survival rates are similar to those for patients who did not experience a cardiac arrest.

In a study of patients with STEMI undergoing primary percutaneous coronary intervention, out-of-hospital cardiac arrest due to VT or VF was associated with poor in-hospital outcomes.[17] Concordant with findings in other studies, if the patient survived to discharge after the initial VT/VF, then the long-term prognosis was similar to that in the absence of cardiac arrest. Out-of-hospital cardiac arrest due to VT/VF was associated with an increased rate of in-hospital deaths secondary to noncardiac causes (e.g., post–anoxic encephalopathy or multiorgan failure). The investigators found that in this group of patients, the left main and/or left anterior descending arteries were the most common culprit arteries.

Specific Considerations

Non–ST-Elevation Myocardial Infarction and Ventricular Tachycardia

In a well-characterized cohort of 6300 patients with non–ST-elevation MI (NSTEMI), the presence of ischemia or ventricular arrhythmias on continuous 7-day electrocardiographic monitoring after the index event was independently associated with poor cardiovascular outcomes, including SCD.[18] Scirica and colleagues observed that the presence of VT or ischemia in the first week was associated with a sixfold increase in the number of such deaths, most of which occurred in the first 90 days. This association was independent of left ventricular function and elevated natriuretic peptides.

Diabetes and Sudden Cardiac Death with Acute Myocardial Infarction

Patients with diabetes have a significantly higher mortality rate secondary to SCD (5.9%) than in those without (1.7%) in this setting.[19] Of interest, the incidence of SCD after MI in patients with diabetes whose EF was above 35% was almost identical to that in nondiabetic patients with EF below 35%.

Atrial Fibrillation and Sudden Cardiac Death

Atrial fibrillation (AF) complicating an acute MI often is disregarded but should be seen as an important clinical entity. A meta-analysis of 43 studies including 278,854 patients demonstrated that AF was associated with increased mortality in patients with MI (mortality odds ratio, 1.46).[20] In fact, for patients with new-onset AF due to MI, mortality was higher than for those without AF, even after adjusting for other risk factors. The reason for this higher mortality is not clear. Hypothesized pathomechanisms include loss of atrial contraction, rapid ventricular rates, loss of atrioventricular synchrony, and variable R–R interval, all resulting in reduced cardiac output, but further studies to clarify this correlation are required. The presence of new AF in the setting of MI also may be a reflection of MI severity.

CLINICAL PRESENTATION AND EVALUATION OF VENTRICULAR ARRHYTHMIAS AFTER MYOCARDAL INFARCTION

The clinical presentation of patients with ventricular arrhythmias attributable to myocardial ischemia is varied. The sole manifestation may in fact be SCD, or the affected person may have relatively mild symptoms such as palpitations, dizziness, chest pain, dyspnea, or syncope. Patients with a previously placed implantable cardioverter-defibrillator (ICD) may receive therapy from the device.

The initial evaluation for ventricular arrhythmias involves blood testing to assess for reversible causes, such as hypoxia, electrolyte disturbance, recurrent ischemia (for which the marker is cardiac troponin), or heart failure (with measurement of natriuretic peptides). Cardiac monitoring should be initiated immediately when arrhythmias are suspected, and a 12-lead ECG should be performed. If the patient has an ICD, interrogation of the device at the earliest possible time is required to identify if therapies were delivered and were appropriate, and if the device settings need to be modified. A transthoracic echocardiogram should be performed to assess left ventricular function, and a coronary angiogram considered if signs or symptoms of coronary ischemia are present. Cardiac MRI may provide assessment of myocardial scar based on evidence of delayed enhancement (see Chapter 33).

Risk Stratification for Sudden Cardiac Death Early After Myocardial Infarction

The current ability to predict SCD is suboptimal. Within the first year after MI, the reported rates of SCD are 3% to 6%. Left ventricular function is the main predictor of the risk of SCD, with LVEF below 35% considered indicative of higher risk. Guidelines recommend ICD implantation in patients with LVEF less than 30% to 40% and New York Heart Association (NYHA) class II or III, and in patients with LVEF less than 30% to 35% and NYHA class I (see later under Treatment Strategies for Ventricular Arrhythmias).[21] However, although LVEF is a good predictor of mortality, it is surprisingly poor at predicting arrhythmic versus nonarrhythmic death.

Two main groups of patients for whom currently available methods fail to predict SCD are (1) patients in the

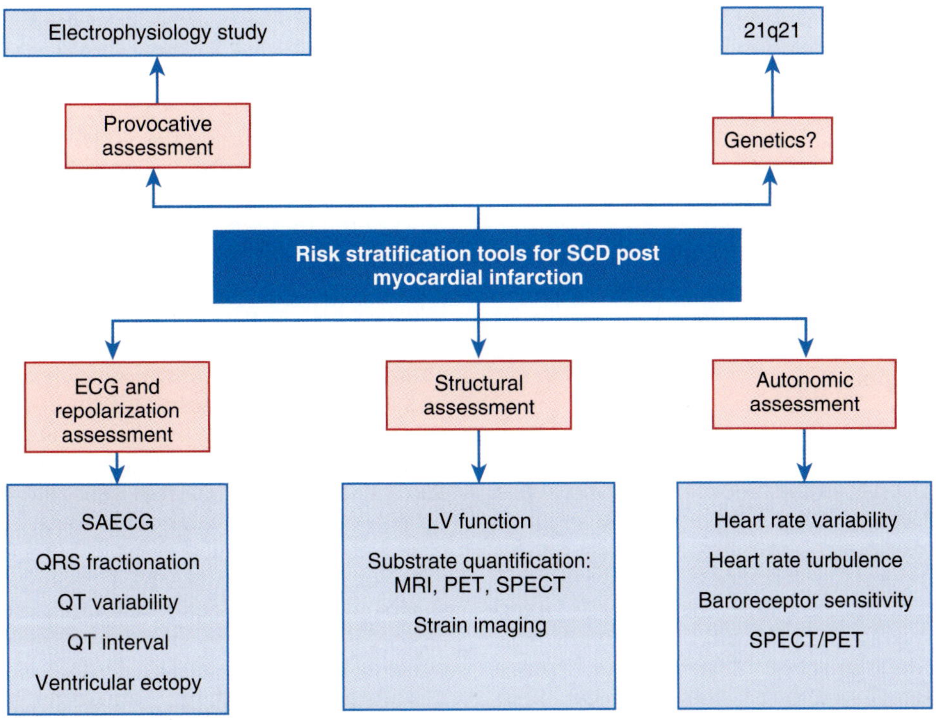

FIGURE 28-8 Approach to stratification of risk for sudden cardiac death (SCD) after myocardial infarction. *ECG,* Electrocardiogram; *LV,* left ventricular; *MRI,* magnetic resonance imaging; *PET,* positron emission tomography; *SAECG,* signal-averaged electrocardiography; *SPECT,* single photon emission computed tomography.

very early stages after an MI and (2) patients with ejection fraction greater than 40%, in whom most SCDs occur. In the VAlsartan In Acute myocardial iNfarcTion (VALIANT) trial, which included 11,256 patients, 83% of SCDs or resuscitated cardiac arrests occurred within the first 30 days after discharge. This staggering finding highlights that a large proportion of this vulnerable population remain unprotected early after MI. The incidence of SCD decreases with time from the index MI and reaches a plateau at 1 year, with reported rates of 1.5% to 2% per year.

The ideal risk stratification tool would identify persons at moderate to high risk for VT/VF but at low risk for nonsudden death. Currently, no single tool is ideal for risk stratification. Combining multiple modalities of risk assessment, along with the clinical history, appears to be the best way of predicting risk (Figure 28-8). It is crucial to recognize that the risk of SCD is dynamic. As the myocardial substrate changes with further ischemic events or with the development of cardiac fibrosis or overt congestive cardiac failure, clinicians need to reassess risk over time. A family history of SCD in a first-degree relative with coronary artery disease is another risk factor. With increasing use of wide genome sequencing, this method may emerge as part of routine clinical screening in the future. Of interest, in a cohort of 972 patients presenting with their first MI, of whom 515 had VF and all of whom underwent wide genome sequencing, an association with VF was identified at chromosomal locus 21q21.[22]

Left Ventricular Ejection Fraction

Left ventricular ejection fraction is one of the best available predictors of SCD after MI.[21] The evidence comes from trials of ICD implantation for primary prevention, such as the Multicenter Automatic Defibrillator Implantation Trial II (MADIT-II) and the Sudden Cardiac Death in Heart Failure Trial (SCD-HeFT) studies. These trials were designed to evaluate ICD benefit in these patients and not to aid with risk stratification. However, prospective studies of risk stratification also have supported a strong relationship between ventricular function and SCD. For example, in the Improved Stratification of Autonomic Regulation trial (ISAR) trial that included 2343 acute MI survivors, LVEF below 30% predicted all-cause mortality, cardiac mortality, and SCD at 5 years.[23]

A majority of patients with MI have preserved or mildly reduced left ventricular function and as a result are considered to be at low risk for SCD; yet SCD occurs most often in those with LVEF greater than 40%. In the Maastricht Circulatory Arrest Registry, 51% of the sudden deaths occurred in those with LVEF greater than 40%. Consequently, additional risk stratification tools are needed. Transthoracic echocardiography is the primary approach for assessment of left ventricular function (see Chapter 31). Alternative imaging methods include radionuclide imaging, cardiac MRI, SPECT (single-photon emission computed tomography), and PET (positron emission tomography). Cardiac MRI is an excellent way to determine the scar density (whether it is heterogeneous or dense), and if the myocardium is hibernating (see Chapter 33). The scar identified on study images correlates well with invasive electroanatomic substrate mapping.[24] Increasing evidence indicates that contrast-enhanced MRI of scar, specifically to establish scar tissue burden and heterogeneity, is an independent predictor of VT/VF.[25] SPECT or PET can clarify if perfusion defects are irreversible and also assess autonomic function by identifying sympathetic denervation (see Chapter 32).[26] Strain rate imaging also is emerging as an even more effective method for risk prediction, especially in patients with LVEF above 35%.[27]

Ventricular Ectopy

Ventricular ectopy initially was identified as a potential predictor of adverse outcome after MI. In the GISSI-2 trial in patients with STEMI, those with more than 10 ventricular ectopic beats per hour were at increased risk for SCD.

The Cardiac Arrhythmia Suppression Trial (CAST) demonstrated that suppression of asymptomatic PVCs with class I agents resulted in successful suppression of ventricular ectopy and VT but was associated with significantly higher mortality. In the setting of primary percutaneous intervention, findings relating ventricular ectopy to outcome are mixed. Therefore, it is not clear that ventricular ectopy is a helpful predictor of SCD. Nevertheless, ventricular ectopy is important to recognize because it can potentially contribute to the development of cardiomyopathy. Catheter ablation can be considered in patients with more than 10,000 PVCs/24 hours, LV dysfunction or ongoing symptoms, and a single or dominant PVC morphology.

Noninvasive Risk Stratification

Many noninvasive strategies have been evaluated with the aim of enhancing SCD risk stratification. These approaches include assesssment of microvolt T wave alternans, signal-averaged electrocardiography, baroreflex sensitivity testing, and measurement of heart rate turbulence and variability.[28]

ECG depolarization abnormalities may provide information. The signal-averaged ECG can help identify late potentials (delayed depolarization of the ventricular myocardium). Signal averaging reduces noise and can help reveal delayed and prolonged activation which can facilitate reentry, so-called late potentials. Additionally fractionation in the QRS or changes in QRS duration (longer than 0.12 msec) have been identified as potential risk stratification tools. A study of 361 ICD recipients with LV dysfunction suggested that QRS fragmentation was a strong predictor of arrhythmic events, whereas prolonged QRS was a predictor of overall mortality.[29] The limitation of depolarization abnormalities is that they can also arise from ventricular dilatation or fibrosis and so have constrained specificity.[30] Increased QT variability after MI with LV dysfunction has been suggested as a marker of repolarization lability and a potential risk factor for VT/VF.

Heart rate variability is a marker of sinus node automaticity, which is modulated by the autonomic nervous system. It has proved to be an effective predictor of mortality when there is a flat chronotropic response. It usually is measured by time domain and frequency domain analysis. *Baroreflex sensitivity* is another marker of autonomic tone, whereby reflex changes in the heart rate are measured in response to blood pressure changes. Both heart rate variability and baroreflex sensitivity were assessed in the Autonomic Tone and Reflexes After Myocardial Infarction (ATRAMI) trial. In this study, impaired responses indicating impaired autonomic function were associated with increased mortality.

Heart rate turbulence is an index of changes in sinus rhythm rate after a PVC, which usually is followed by a compensatory pause. The normal response is for the heart rate to increase and subsequently slow. Impairment of this response also has been associated with increased mortality.

T wave alternans is a marker of electrical heterogeneity or dispersion in ventricular repolarization and has a high negative predictive value. It is not possible to measure T wave alternans in patients with atrial fibrillation, those with frequent PVCs, and patients unable to augment their heart rate, thereby reducing its clinical utility. The REFINE study evaluated all these parameters at 2 to 4 weeks after MI and again at 10 to14 weeks. In this prospective study, early assessment did not predict mortality, but the 10- to 14-week assessment did predict increased risk for SCD or resuscitated cardiac arrest. The combination of impaired heart rate turbulence, abnormal T wave alternans, and left ventricular function below 50% had a low positive predictive value but good negative predictive value of 95%.

Other indicators such as NYHA class and QT dispersion or variability have essentially too low a sensitivity to be useful predictors. Although initial evidence was encouraging, most of the findings have lacked reproducibility among different studies.[1]

Invasive Risk Stratification with Provocative Testing

Findings on electrophysiology (EP) testing immediately after MI as a risk stratification method are mixed. A large body of data suggests that EP studies do not improve outcomes when used to guide ICD implantation. EP testing can be useful in the setting of chronic ventricular arrhythmias and established myocardial substrate or scar. In the early post-infarct period, ventricular stimulation protocols offer poor negative predictive value as a risk stratification tool for SCD. For example, in MADIT I, patients with a negative EP study but with an ejection fraction below 30% were still at risk of SCD. Limitations to several of the key studies were recognized, however. In MADIT II, some of the EP studies were performed through the ICD and as a result may provide less prognostic information. In the CARISMA and ABCD trials, VF and polymorphic VT, which are widely believed to be a nonspecific result, were categorized as a positive study. In these two studies, VT stimulation had specificity and sensitivity similar to those for T wave alternans or heart rate variability.

VT stimulation early after MI, if the result is negative, has been associated with a favorable long-term prognosis in some studies.[31] Of 1910 patients presenting for primary percutaneous coronary intervention, 128 patients had LVEF below 40% and underwent EP testing with up to 4 extra stimuli (i.e., progressively early premature ventricular extra stimulus). EP testing was considered to be positive if stimuli induced monomorphic VT and not VF or polymorphic VT. At 3 years, 93% of the patients with negative EP study findings ($n = 80$) and 63% of those with positive EP study findings ($n = 48$) were free from death or arrhythmia. The investigators stressed the importance of the ventricular stimulation protocol used, the wide variability in stimulation protocols used in different studies, and the criteria considered to define a positive result. Some operator bias toward use of VT stimulation also may exist, in which a more aggressive approach, based on higher operator-perceived likelihood of presence of a ventricular arrhythmia in a specific patient, might be applied.

TREATMENT STRATEGIES FOR VENTRICULAR ARRHYTHMIAS

Treating ventricular arrhythmias associated with acute MI depends on the severity and frequency of the dysrhythmia and on the clinical condition (stability) of the patient (Figure 28-9). Immediate revascularization is the most important initial intervention. General management of ventricular arrhythmias for which revascularization has been feasible involves 24 to 72 hours of telemetry monitoring, when possible in a coronary care unit. PVCs and idioventricular rhythms need not be treated unless the PVCs are a recurrent trigger for VF. It is important to measure serum K^+ and magnesium, with replenishment as appropriate,, and to treat comorbid conditions such as renal failure, diabetes, and hypertension, when present. Early treatment of

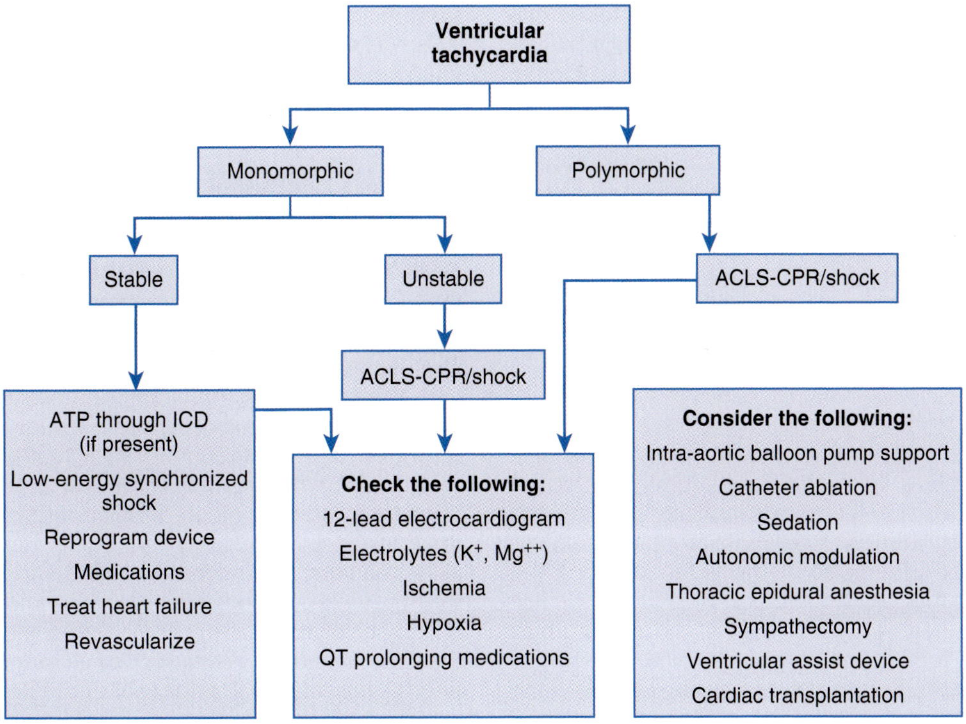

FIGURE 28-9 Treatment of ventricular arrhythmias. *ACLS/CPR,* Advanced cardiac life support/cardiopulmonary resuscitation; *ATP,* antitachycardia pacing; *ICD,* implantable cardioverter-defibrillator.

heart failure and introduction of medications such as beta-blockers, angiotensin-converting enzyme (ACE) inhibitors, and aldosterone receptor blockers (ARBs), as appropriate, if the left ventricular function is depressed will help control or prevent ventricular arrhythmias by reducing substrate formation (see Chapter 13 and Chapter 36).

Implantable Cardioverter-Defibrillator Therapy

Available data from randomized trials indicate that given the chance of improvement in ventricular function as a result of uptitration of medications, reperfusion, and remodeling, it is best to wait at least 40 days after an MI before implantation of an ICD. In the Immediate Risk Stratification Improves Survival (IRIS) trial, in which immediate risk stratification in 898 patients was performed at 5 to 31 days after MI, patients with an ejection fraction below 40% were randomly assigned to receive either medications or medications plus ICD therapy (453 versus 445, respectively). A follow-up study of patients with a mean LVEF of 34% for 37 months found no difference in total mortality at 1, 2, and 3 years, respectively. The benefit of ICD therapy in reducing SCD was negated by the high rates of nonarrhythmic death. These results were very similar to those from the Defibrillator in Acute Myocardial Infarction Trial (DINAMIT).[32]

ICD therapy is effective for reducing mortality later after MI, at which time healed scar is established, and as a result a different substrate compared with the early stages after MI. ICDs and improvements in therapies for acute and chronic MI probably have contributed to a reduced frequency of resuscitation for out-of-hospital cardiac arrest caused by lethal ventricular arrhythmias by 33% in the Netherlands.[33]

The exceptions to waiting 40 days before ICD implantation that should be considered are absence of revascularization options, occurrence of VT in a patient who is already on maximum medical therapy, lack of evidence of myocardial viability, and a previous out-of-hospital cardiac arrest in which no clear culprit lesion for coronary stenosis/occlusion could be identified.

ICDs are considered at 40 days after the acute MI if the left ventricular function is less than 35%. Cardiac resynchronization therapy with or without ICD can be considered after medical therapy has been optimized in patients in whom congestive cardiac failure NYHA class II or III, QRS duration greater than 120 msec, or left bundle morphology with reduced left ventricular function below 35% is still present.[21] Occasionally the decision is made to recommend a wearable defibrillator (e.g., LifeVest, ZOLL, Pittsburgh, Pennsylvania) when the patient is considered at particularly high risk.

Antiarrhythmic Drug Therapy

Prophylactic treatment with antiarrhythmics in patients considered to be at high risk for cardiac events is not recommended. If ventricular arrhythmias occur, despite revascularization and medical therapy as discussed, then antiarrhythmics such as amiodarone or lidocaine may be considered in the acute phase. Class 1C antiarrhythmics are contraindicated in the setting of myocardial ischemia owing to their proarrhythmic potential. If ventricular arrhythmias occur despite all of the foregoing, in the setting of persistent ischemia, then other methods of temporarily optimizing myocardial perfusion, such as with an intra-aortic balloon pump, can be helpful.

Catheter ablation of ventricular arrhythmias tends not to be very effective in the immediate stages after an acute MI but has proven efficacy in established chronic VT (see under Catheter Ablation, next). Thoracic epidural anesthesia or cardiac sympathetic denervation is effective at reducing the frequency of ventricular arrhythmias occurring as a result of electrical storm and mortality in established ischemic cardiomyopathy. Thoracic sympathectomy currently involves surgical removal of the left or bilateral paravertebral sympathetic ganglia from the lower third of the stellate ganglion to T4. Other potential neuromodulation therapy such as spinal cord stimulation has shown promise in reducing ventricular arrhythmias in the setting of myocardial ischemia in preclinical models; clinical studies have proved to be safe but have yet to demonstrate similar efficacy.[34,35] Placement of a ventricular assist device and transplantation are the final options to consider for intractable ventricular arrhythmias refractory to all other therapies.

Catheter Ablation

Catheter ablation for chronic ventricular arrhythmias secondary to scar reduces ventricular arrhythmia recurrence. Catheter ablation involves electroanatomic mapping in sinus or paced rhythm to identify scar. Pace mapping involves pacing at an area considered to be the potential site of the VT and comparing the paced rhythm to the clinical VT pattern. Targets for catheter ablation involve identifying areas prone to slow conduction including areas with late potentials and fractionation. Entrainment mapping can be done if the VT is hemodynamically tolerated. One-year freedom from recurrence of ventricular tachycardia is approximately 72%.[36] High recurrence rates after catheter ablation is associated with lower ejection fraction, advanced heart failure, and multiple VT morphologic patterns.

CONDUCTION DEFECTS ARISING FROM ACUTE MYOCARDIAL INFARCTION

Atrioventricular Conduction Defects

High-degree atrioventricular (AV) block during acute MI occurs infrequently but is associated with a high mortality. The likelihood of developing AV block appears to correlate with the severity of the ischemic insult. AV block tends to occur as a result of occlusion of either the right coronary artery or the LAD secondary to a septal branch occlusion (Figure 28-10). The pathomechanism for high-grade AV block appears to be multifaceted. This conduction defect can be the consequence of direct AV node ischemia, although such ischemia must be severe, because the node itself is relatively well protected by its fibrous capsule and high intracellular glycogen stores. High-grade AV block also may result from the Bezold-Jarisch reflex, in which parasympathetic afferents on the inferoposterior wall of the left ventricle are activated resulting in a reflex bradycardia and AV block.

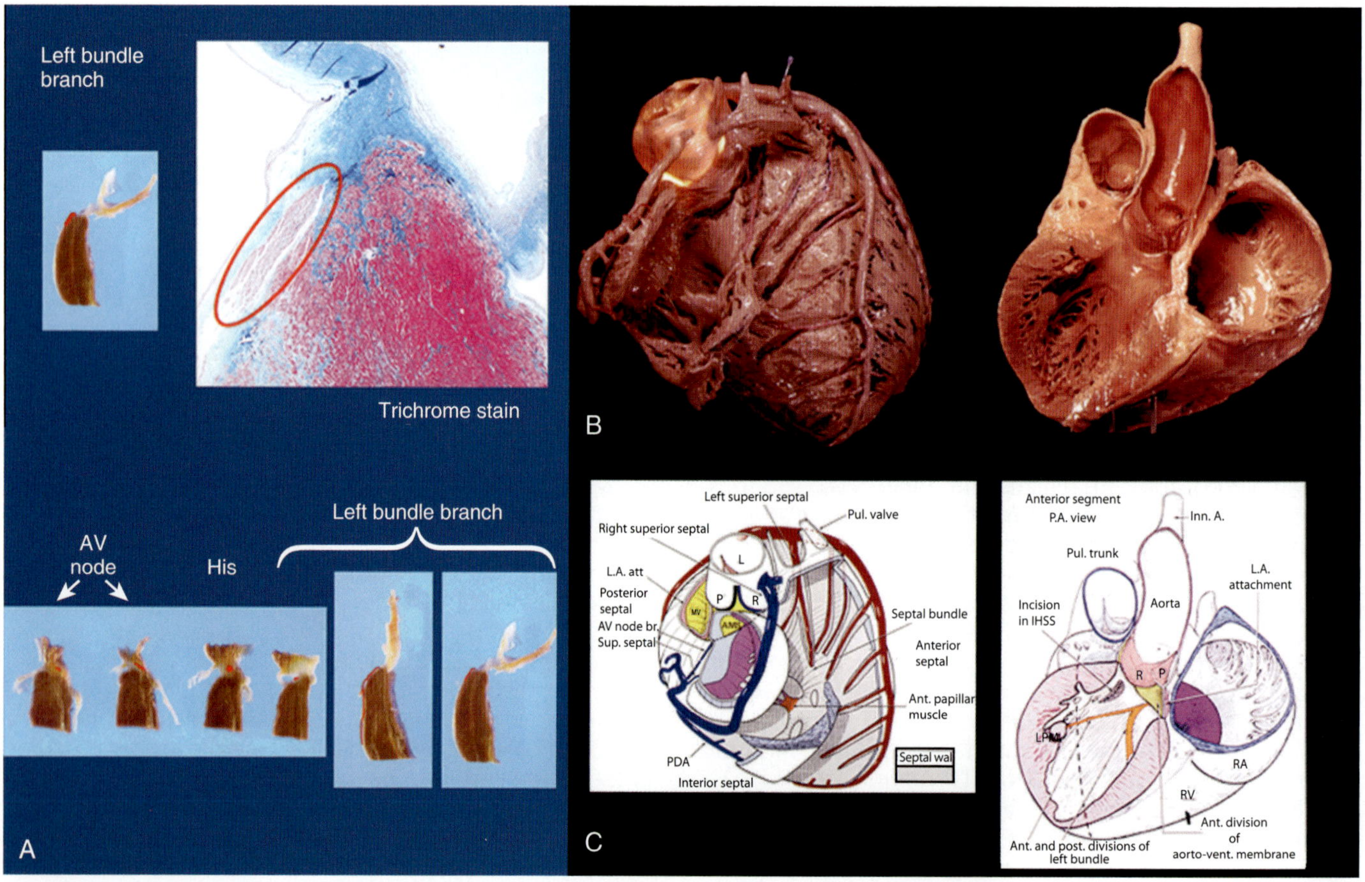

FIGURE 28-10 Atrioventricular (AV) node and coronary artery anatomy. (A) Mason's trichome staining of the left bundle branch as it emerges from below the membranous ventricular septum and the aortic and mitral valve leaflets. Further sectioning of the AV node, His bundle, and left bundle branch. **(B)** Gross section of surgical specimen. The AV node is seen at the base of the atrial septum at the apex of the triangle of Koch. The continuation of the AV node occurs by way of the bundle of His, which penetrates the central fibrous body (CFB). The CFB is formed by the union of the connective tissue of the aortic and mitral valve leaflets and the membranous part of the ventricular septum. It then branches to the right and left bundle branches, where the left branch lies below the junction of the right and noncoronary cusps of the aortic valve, descending then through the subendocardium of the interventricular septum. **(C)** Diagrams of conduction system anatomy with right and left coronary artery anatomy. *AMS,* Aorto-mitral septum; *Ant.,* anterior; *IHSS,* idiopathic hypertrophic subaortic stenosis; *Inn. A,* innominate artery; *L.A.,* left atrium; *LPM,* lateral papillary muscle; *MV,* mitral valve; *PA,* posteroanterior; *PDA,* posterior descending artery; *Post.,* posterior; *RA,* right atrium; *RV,* right ventricle. (**A,** *Images kindly provided with permission from Atsuko Seki, MD, Tokyo Metropolitan Geriatric Hospital and Institute of Gerontology, Japan; and Michael Fishbein, MD, Anatomic Pathology and Clinical Pathology, UCLA Medical Center, Los Angeles, California.* **C,** *From Wallace A: McAlpine collection. UCLA Cardiac Arrhythmia Center.)*

Despite significant advances in acute coronary syndrome (ACS) care, the in-hospital mortality related to high-degree AV block is significant and probably is related to the severity of the infarction. Nevertheless, in the era of primary percutaneous coronary intervention (PCI), mortality for patients who survive to hospital discharge is similar to that in those without AV block. The combined incidence of second-degree Mobitz type II and third-degree AV block ranges anywhere from 2% to 4%. Some studies report a worse outcome for high-degree AV block if it is associated with LAD occlusion. High-degree AV block occurring as a result of LAD occlusion usually results in infra-Hisian block. In a Danish registry of 2073 patients with STEMI treated with primary PCI and followed for three years, high-degree AV block developed in 67 patients, of whom 25 died.[37] In this latter group, the median time to death was 1.5 days, and death occurred after 48 hours in only 9% of those in whom AV block developed. Among patients who survived beyond 30 days, the prognosis was the same as that for patients without AV block. Factors associated with developing AV block include advancing age, hypertension, and diabetes.

Decisions on when to intervene for high-degree AV block can be complex. The block may be transient, and if reperfusion occurs quickly, treatment may not be required. If the patient's clinical status is unstable, with no stable escape rhythm, and if signs of hemodynamic compromise are present, then intervention needs to be considered. Temporary pacing wires are not without complications, such as infection, cardiac tamponade, failure to capture, dislodgement, and ventricular arrhythmia precipitation.

Various groups of investigators have studied the benefits of opting for permanent pacing immediately over inserting a temporary pacing system. This approach may provide a short-term survival benefit in hospital, but it appears that the mortality rate on discharge is similar. If the AV block is a result of increased parasympathetic tone, adenosine release, or potassium fluxes, then the AV block could be transient, such as in the case of a right coronary artery occlusion. It is more likely to be permanent with an LAD occlusion, for reasons described earlier.[37] Presence of a stable escape rhythm eliminates the need to intervene, and telemetry monitoring can be adequate, allowing time for the AV block to potentially resolve. Treating high-degree AV block with inotropic agents or atropine can be problematic, because increasing the heart rate may potentially worsen the AV conduction, resulting in a more profound bradycardia.

Bundle Branch Block

Further defining bundle branch block (BBB) associated with MI may be helpful in relation to prognostic significance, such as left versus right, duration, and time of appearance. BBB can be transiently associated with MI or persistent. One study that examined BBB associated with acute MI included 5570 patients, 964 of whom (17%) had BBB (new and previously identified); 30-day and 7-year all-cause mortality rates were reported.[38] BBB was associated with increasing age and comorbid conditions such as diabetes and heart failure during hospitalization. Compared with those with right BBB (RBBB), patients with left BBB (LBBB) exhibited a higher prevalence of comorbid conditions. Also, if the LBBB was new, it was associated with higher mortality at both 30 days and 7 years. The time of appearance and duration of the bundle branch block have different prognostic significances, and the presence of BBB may help with risk stratification.

SUMMARY

SCD secondary to MI continues to be a major public health problem. Despite substantial advances in the treatment of myocardial ischemia, in a meaningful proportion of patients, MI may be complicated by conducting system disease or ventricular arrhythmias, or precipitate SCD. Continued efforts are needed to identify and optimize risk stratification techniques.

References

1. Priori SG, Blomstrom-Lundqvist C, Mazzanti A, et al.: 2015 ESC guidelines for the management of patients with ventricular arrhythmias and the prevention of sudden cardiac death: The Task Force for the Management of Patients with Ventricular Arrhythmias and the Prevention of Sudden Cardiac Death of the European Society of Cardiology (ESC). Endorsed by: Association for European Paediatric and Congenital Cardiology (AEPC), *Eur Heart J* 36(41):2793–2867, 2015.
2. Subirana MT, Juan-Babot JO, Puig T, et al.: Specific characteristics of sudden death in a Mediterranean Spanish population, *Am J Cardiol* 107:622–627, 2011.
3. Goldberger JJ, Buxton AE, Cain MO, et al.: Risk stratification for arrhythmic sudden cardiac death: Identifying the roadblocks, *Circulation* 123:2423–2430, 2011.
4. Janse MJ, Wit AL: Electrophysiological mechanisms of ventricular arrhythmias resulting from myocardial ischemia and infarction, *Physiol Rev* 69:1049–1169, 1989.
5. Shivkumar K, Deutsch NA, Lamp ST, et al.: Mechanism of hypoxic K loss in rabbit ventricle, *J Clin Invest* 100:1782–1788, 1997.
6. Harris AS, Bisteni A, Russell RA, et al.: Excitatory factors in ventricular tachycardia resulting from myocardial ischemia; potassium a major excitant, *Science* 119:200–203, 1954.
7. Vaseghi M, Shivkumar K: The role of the autonomic nervous system in sudden cardiac death, *Prog Cardiovasc Dis* 50:404–419, 2008.
8. Bourke T, Vaseghi M, Michowitz Y, et al.: Neuraxial modulation for refractory ventricular arrhythmias: Value of thoracic epidural anesthesia and surgical left cardiac sympathetic denervation, *Circulation* 121:2255–2262, 2010.
9. Vaseghi M, Gima J, Kanaan C, et al.: Cardiac sympathetic denervation in patients with refractory ventricular arrhythmias or electrical storm: Intermediate and long-term follow-up, *Heart Rhythm* 11:360–366, 2014.
10. Vaseghi M, Lellouche N, Ritter H, Fonarow GC, et al.: Mode and mechanisms of death after orthotopic heart transplantation, *Heart Rhythm* 6:503–509, 2009.
11. Mehta RH, Starr AZ, Lopes RD, et al.: Incidence of and outcomes associated with ventricular tachycardia or fibrillation in patients undergoing primary percutaneous coronary intervention, *JAMA* 301:1779–1789, 2009.
12. Mehta RH, Yu J, Piccini JP, et al.: Prognostic significance of postprocedural sustained ventricular tachycardia or fibrillation in patients undergoing primary percutaneous coronary intervention (from the HORIZONS-AMI Trial), *Am J Cardiol* 109:805–812, 2012.
13. Mehta RH, Starr AZ, Lopes RD, et al.: Relationship of sustained ventricular tachyarrhythmias to outcomes in patients undergoing primary percutaneous coronary intervention with varying underlying baseline risk, *Am Heart J* 161:782–789, 2011.
14. Bougouin W, Marijon E, Puymirat E, et al.: Incidence of sudden cardiac death after ventricular fibrillation complicating acute myocardial infarction: A 5-year cause-of-death analysis of the FAST-MI 2005 registry, *Eur Heart J* 35:116–122, 2004.
15. Demidova MM, Carlson J, Erlinge D, Platonov PG: Predictors of ventricular fibrillation at reperfusion in patients with acute ST-elevation myocardial infarction treated by primary percutaneous coronary intervention, *Am J Cardiol* 115:417–422, 2015.
16. Alahmar AE, Nelson CP, Snell KI, et al.: Resuscitated cardiac arrest and prognosis following myocardial infarction, *Heart* 100:1125–1132, 2014.
17. Demirel F, Rasoul S, Elvan A, et al.: Impact of out-of-hospital cardiac arrest due to ventricular fibrillation in patients with ST-elevation myocardial infarction admitted for primary percutaneous coronary intervention: Impact of ventricular fibrillation in STEMI patients, *Eur Heart J Acute Cardiovasc Care* 4:16–23, 2015.
18. Scirica BM, Braunwald E, Belardinelli L, et al.: Relationship between nonsustained ventricular tachycardia after non-ST-elevation acute coronary syndrome and sudden cardiac death: Observations from the Metabolic Efficiency with Ranolazine for Less Ischemia in Non-ST-Elevation Acute Coronary Syndrome–Thrombolysis in Myocardial Infarction 36 (MERLIN-TIMI 36) randomized controlled trial, *Circulation* 122:455–462, 2010.
19. Junttila MJ, Barthel P, Myerburg RJ, et al.: Sudden cardiac death after myocardial infarction in patients with type 2 diabetes, *Heart Rhythm* 7:1396–1403, 2010.
20. Jabre P, Roger VL, Murad MH, et al.: Mortality associated with atrial fibrillation in patients with myocardial infarction: A systematic review and meta-analysis, *Circulation* 123:1587–1593, 2011.
21. Epstein AE, DiMarco JP, Ellenbogen KA, et al.: 2012 ACCF/AHA/HRS focused update incorporated into the ACCF/AHA/HRS 2008 guidelines for device-based therapy of cardiac rhythm abnormalities: A report of the American College of Cardiology Foundation/American Heart Association Task Force on Practice Guidelines and the Heart Rhythm Society, *J Am Coll Cardiol* 61:e6–e75, 2013.
22. Bezzina CR, Pazoki R, Bardai A, et al.: Genome-wide association study identifies a susceptibility locus at 21q21 for ventricular fibrillation in acute myocardial infarction, *Nat Genet* 42:688–691, 2010.
23. Bauer A, Barthel P, Schneider R, et al.: Improved Stratification of Autonomic Regulation for risk prediction in post-infarction patients with preserved left ventricular function (ISAR-Risk), *Eur Heart J* 30:576–583, 2009.
24. Perez-David E, Arenal A, Rubio-Guivernau JL, et al.: Noninvasive identification of ventricular tachycardia-related conducting channels using contrast-enhanced magnetic resonance imaging in patients with chronic myocardial infarction: Comparison of signal intensity scar mapping and endocardial voltage mapping, *J Am Coll Cardiol* 57:184–194, 2011.
25. Roes SD, Borleffs CJ, van der Geest RJ, Westenberg JJ, et al.: Infarct tissue heterogeneity assessed with contrast-enhanced MRI predicts spontaneous ventricular arrhythmia in patients with ischemic cardiomyopathy and implantable cardioverter-defibrillator, *Circ Cardiovasc Imaging* 2:183–190, 2009.
26. Bertini M, Schalij MJ, Bax JJ, Delgado V: Emerging role of multimodality imaging to evaluate patients at risk for sudden cardiac death, *Circ Cardiovasc Imaging* 5:525–535, 2012.
27. Haugaa KH, Grenne BL, Eek CH, et al.: Strain echocardiography improves risk prediction of ventricular arrhythmias after myocardial infarction, *JACC Cardiovasc Imaging* 6:841–850, 2013.

28. Dagres N, Hindricks G: Risk stratification after myocardial infarction: Is left ventricular ejection fraction enough to prevent sudden cardiac death? *Eur Heart J* 34:1964–1971, 2013.
29. Das MK, Maskoun W, Shen C, et al.: Fragmented QRS on twelve-lead electrocardiogram predicts arrhythmic events in patients with ischemic and nonischemic cardiomyopathy, *Heart Rhythm* 7:74–80, 2010.
30. Wellens HJ, Schwartz PJ, Lindemans FW, et al.: Risk stratification for sudden cardiac death: Current status and challenges for the future, *Eur Heart J* 35:1642–1651, 2014.
31. Zaman S, Narayan A, Thiagalingam A, et al.: Long-term arrhythmia-free survival in patients with severe left ventricular dysfunction and no inducible ventricular tachycardia after myocardial infarction, *Circulation* 129:848–854, 2014.
32. Dorian P, Hohnloser SH, Thorpe KE, et al.: Mechanisms underlying the lack of effect of implantable cardioverter-defibrillator therapy on mortality in high-risk patients with recent myocardial infarction: Insights from the Defibrillation in Acute Myocardial Infarction Trial (DINAMIT), *Circulation* 122:2645–2652, 2010.
33. Hulleman M, Berdowski J, de Groot JR, et al.: Implantable cardioverter-defibrillators have reduced the incidence of resuscitation for out-of-hospital cardiac arrest caused by lethal arrhythmias, *Circulation* 126:815–821, 2012.
34. Wang S, Zhou X, Huang B, et al.: Spinal cord stimulation protects against ventricular arrhythmias by suppressing left stellate ganglion neural activity in an acute myocardial infarction canine model, *Heart Rhythm* 12(7):1628–1635, 2015.
35. Tse HF, Turner S, Sanders P, et al.: Thoracic Spinal Cord Stimulation for Heart Failure as a Restorative Treatment (SCS HEART study): First-in-man experience, *Heart Rhythm* 12:588–595, 2015.
36. Tung R, Vaseghi M, Frankel DS, et al.: Freedom from recurrent ventricular tachycardia after catheter ablation is associated with improved survival in patients with structural heart disease: An International VT Ablation Center Collaborative Group study, *Heart Rhythm* 12:1997–2007, 2015.
37. Gang UJ, Hvelplund A, Pedersen S, et al.: High-degree atrioventricular block complicating ST-segment elevation myocardial infarction in the era of primary percutaneous coronary intervention, *Europace* 14:1639–1645, 2012.
38. Melgarejo-Moreno A, Galcera-Tomas J, Consuegra-Sanchez L, et al.: Relation of new permanent right or left bundle branch block on short- and long-term mortality in acute myocardial infarction bundle branch block and myocardial infarction, *Am J Cardiol* 116(7):1003–1009, 2015.

29 Epidemiology and Management of Bleeding in Acute Myocardial Infarction

Sunil V. Rao

INTRODUCTION

Clinical outcomes after acute coronary syndrome (ACS) have significantly improved over time. A significant proportion of the reduction in mortality has been the result of development and adoption of potent anticoagulant and antiplatelet therapies coupled with invasive risk stratification in high-risk patients (see Chapter 13). In addition, the use of secondary prevention strategies to control risk factors has further improved long-term outcomes (see Chapter 34). Although antithrombotic medications reduce the risk for recurrent ischemic events, they increase the risk for bleeding and need for blood transfusion. Paradoxically, bleeding events are associated with a subsequent higher risk for myocardial infarction (MI), stroke, stent thrombosis, and death.[1] Randomized trials of "bleeding avoidance strategies" (BAS) in patients with ACS have demonstrated a reduction in adverse events, including mortality.[2] Because of the availability of BAS, use of management strategies that reduce ischemia while minimizing bleeding have the potential to further improve outcomes. This chapter summarizes the epidemiology and management of bleeding events in ACS and MI.

EPIDEMIOLOGY OF BLEEDING

Reported Incidence of Bleeding: Influence of Definitions

The reported incidence of major bleeding events among patients with ACS varies greatly depending on the definition used, the fidelity with which the events are identified, the types of antithrombotic therapies used, and whether invasive risk stratification with revascularization is pursued. Before discussing the incidence of bleeding in ACS, it is important to review how bleeding is defined. Several schemas exist, but a few have been consistently used to identify bleeding events across randomized trials or registries that include ACS patients. Bleeding events as defined by several of these classification systems have also been correlated with other adverse events such as recurrent MI, stroke, stent thrombosis, and death (see section on Bleeding and Outcomes).

Most bleeding definitions are made up of specific data elements that broadly fall into three categories: changes in hemoglobin or hematocrit; clinical events (e.g., gastrointestinal bleeding or intracranial hemorrhage); and consequences (e.g., blood transfusion or fatal bleeding). The extremes of bleeding definitions could focus solely on either changes in hemoglobin or on clinical events, and either could "cast the net" too widely—that is, identify events that would not be considered bleeding events by most clinicians or too narrowly by identifying only the most severe bleeding events and missing other less severe, but clinically important, events. Most definitions include combinations of all three categories. Table 29-1 displays commonly used bleeding definitions across randomized trials and registries.

Established Definitions

Thrombolysis in Myocardial Infarction and Global Use of Strategies to Open Occluded Arteries Definitions

Historically, the most commonly used definitions were the Thrombolysis in Myocardial Infarction (TIMI) and Global Use of Strategies to Open Occluded arteries (GUSTO) bleeding scales. The TIMI definition was developed in the context of fibrinolytic therapy for ST-elevation MI (STEMI) and was generally based on decreases in hemoglobin.[3] The categorization for TIMI bleeding originally consisted of minimal, minor, and major bleeding, defined according to the degree of hemoglobin change. Because intracranial hemorrhage is the most feared complication of fibrinolytic therapy, it was included as part of the TIMI major bleeding definition. Since its original development, the TIMI bleeding definition has evolved to include a qualifier that bases the required decrease in hemoglobin on whether a clinically overt bleeding event has occurred (Table 29-1). The GUSTO definition was also developed in the context of fibrinolytic therapy for STEMI, and was based solely on clinical events. GUSTO bleeding is categorized as mild, moderate, or severe, and again, intracranial hemorrhage is considered severe according to the GUSTO definition. Other definitions listed in Table 29-1 combine elements of the TIMI and GUSTO definitions and add others (e.g., access site hematoma).

The existence of multiple bleeding definitions contributes to the variations in the reported rates of bleeding. When two or more definitions are used in the same study, the assessment of the safety of a management strategy can be confusing. One example of this is the SYNERGY trial, which

TABLE 29-1 Sample Bleeding Definitions in Acute Coronary Syndrome Clinical Trials and Registries

TRIAL/ DEFINITION	PATIENT POPULATION	INTERVENTION	BLEEDING DEFINITION
TIMI	ACS, PCI	N/A	Major • Any intracranial bleeding (excluding microhemorrhages <10 mm evident only on gradient-echo MRI) • Clinically overt signs of hemorrhage associated with a drop in hemoglobin of ≥5 g/dL • Fatal bleeding (bleeding that directly results in death within 7 d)
			Minor • Clinically overt (including imaging), resulting in hemoglobin drop of 3 to <5 g/dL Requiring medical attention • Any overt sign of hemorrhage that meets 1 of the following criteria and does not meet criteria for a major or minor bleeding event, as defined previously: • Requiring intervention (medical practitioner–guided medical or surgical treatment to stop or treat bleeding, including temporarily or permanently discontinuing or changing the dose of a medication or study drug) • Leading to or prolonging hospitalization • Prompting evaluation (leading to an unscheduled visit to a health care professional and diagnostic testing, either laboratory or imaging) Minimal • Any overt bleeding event that does not meet the preceding criteria Bleeding in the setting of CABG • Fatal bleeding (bleeding that directly results in death) • Perioperative intracranial bleeding • Reoperation after closure of the sternotomy incision for the purpose of controlling bleeding • Transfusion of ≥5 U PRBCs or whole blood within a 48-h period; cell saver transfusion will not be counted in calculations of blood products • Chest tube output >2 L within a 24-h period
GUSTO	ACS, PCI	N/A	Severe or life-threatening • Intracerebral hemorrhage • Resulting in substantial hemodynamic compromise requiring treatment Moderate • Requiring blood transfusion, but not resulting in hemodynamic compromise Mild • Bleeding that does not meet previous criteria
SYNERGY	NSTE-ACS	Enoxaparin vs. heparin	TIMI and GUSTO
PURSUIT	NSTE-ACS	Eptifibatide/heparin vs. heparin	TIMI and GUSTO

CURE	NSTE-ACS	Aspirin vs. aspirin + clopidogrel	Major bleeding
			• Life-threatening
			  • Fatal
			  • Intracranial
			  • Requiring surgical intervention
			  • Results in hypotension
			  • Decrease in Hgb ≥5 g/dL
			  • Requires ≥4 U of blood
			• Other major
			  • Requires transfusion of 2 or 3 U
			  • Intraocular

GUSTO IIb	NSTE-ACS	Hirudin vs. heparin	GUSTO
CURRENT-OASIS 7	NSTE-ACS	High-dose aspirin vs. low-dose aspirin; high-dose clopidogrel vs. standard dose clopidogrel	Severe bleeding • Fatal • Requiring transfusion ≥4 U of PRBCs or equivalent whole blood • Resulting in hemoglobin drop ≥ 5 g/dL • Leading to hypotension that requires inotropes • Requiring surgery • Symptomatic intracranial hemorrhage Other major bleeding • Requiring transfusion of 2 to 3 U • Significantly disabling, intraocular bleeding leading to significant loss of vision
OASIS-5	NSTE-ACS	Fondaparinux vs. enoxaparin	Major bleeding • Fatal, intracranial, retroperitoneal, intraocular leading to vision loss • Decrease in Hgb ≥3 g/dL adjusted for transfusion • Transfusion of 2 U of red blood cells
ACUITY and HORIZONS-MI	NSTE-ACS	Bivalirudin alone vs. heparin or enoxaparin + GP IIb/IIIa vs. bivalirudin + GP IIb/IIIa	Major bleeding • Intracranial or intraocular bleeding • Hemorrhage at the access site, requiring intervention • Hematoma with a diameter of ≥5 cm • Reduction in Hgb levels of ≥4 g/dL without an overt bleeding source or ≥3 g/dL with such a source • Reoperation for bleeding • Transfusion of a blood product

TABLE 29-1 Sample Bleeding Definitions in Acute Coronary Syndrome Clinical Trials and Registries—cont'd

TRIAL/ DEFINITION	PATIENT POPULATION	INTERVENTION	BLEEDING DEFINITION
ACTION-GWTG	ACS	N/A	• Absolute Hgb decrease of ≥4 g/dL (baseline to nadir) • Intracranial hemorrhage • Documented or suspected retroperitoneal bleed • Any red cell blood transfusion with baseline Hgb ≥9 g/dL, or any red cell transfusion with Hgb <9 g/dL and a suspected bleeding event
CRUSADE	NSTE-ACS	N/A	Major bleeding • Absolute decrease in hematocrit concentration by 12% from baseline • Intracranial hemorrhage • Retroperitoneal bleeding • Red blood cell transfusion because of bleeding
GRACE	NSTE-ACS		• Life-threatening bleeding requiring a transfusion of >2 U red blood cells • Resulting in a decrease in hematocrit of >10% • Occurring intracerebrally • Resulting in stroke or death
TRITON TIMI 38	NSTE-ACS		TIMI
PLATO	NSTE-ACS		Major life-threatening • Fatal • Intracranial • Intrapericardial with cardiac tamponade • Resulting in hypovolemic shock or severe hypotension that requires pressors or surgery • Clinically overt or apparent bleeding associated with decrease in hemoglobin >5 g/dL • Requiring transfusion of ≥4 U whole blood or PRBCs Other major • Significantly disabling (e.g., intraocular with permanent vision loss) • Associated drop in hemoglobin of 3–5 g/dL • Requiring transfusion of 2–3 U whole blood or PRBCs Any major • Any 1 of the previous criteria

ACS, Acute coronary syndrome; *CABG*, coronary artery bypass grafting; *GP*, glycoprotein; *Hgb*, hemoglobin; *MRI*, magnetic resonance imaging; *NSTE*, non–ST-segment elevation; *PCI*, percutaneous coronary intervention; *PRBC*, packed red blood cell.

compared enoxaparin with unfractionated heparin in 9978 ACS patients without persistent ST-segment elevation who were slated to undergo early invasive risk stratification.[4] The primary efficacy endpoint was 30-day death or MI; the primary safety endpoint was bleeding defined according to both the TIMI and GUSTO scales. There was no significant difference in 30-day death or MI between the two strategies; however, the bleeding data showed disparate findings. There was no significant difference in GUSTO severe bleeding or transfusion rates (i.e., GUSTO moderate bleeding), but there was a significant excess of TIMI major bleeding among patients assigned to enoxaparin. These results challenged any firm conclusion about the relative safety of enoxaparin over unfractionated heparin and underscored the influence of definition on reported bleeding rates.

Capture of Bleeding Events

Another factor that may affect the incidence of bleeding is the methods for detecting events. Clinical trials often use independent clinical events committees that review source documents (medical charts) to detect adverse events. This minimizes the risk of bias at the site level. In contrast, registries generally do not use adjudication and rely on site-identified events. This is particularly true of registries in which the primary purpose is quality improvement rather than comparing the effectiveness of one treatment with another. As such, the rates of bleeding are often higher in clinical trials than in registries, despite the inclusion of higher risk patients in the latter. For example, the rate of postprocedural major bleeding among patients who underwent primary percutaneous coronary intervention (PCI) for STEMI assigned to unfractionated heparin plus glycoprotein IIb/IIIa inhibitors in the HORIZONS-MI trial was 8.4%,[5] whereas the rate of bleeding among patients who underwent primary PCI in the National Cardiovascular Data Registry's Cath-PCI registry was approximately 4% to 5%.[6] Certainly, this difference is driven in part by the differences in definitions, but it is also likely caused by variations in the way the events were identified and reported.

Bleeding Academic Research Consortium Definition

To overcome some of the challenges posed by different bleeding definitions, several groups have attempted to develop a standardized approach to classifying and reporting bleeding events. Rather than developing a new definition, the Academic Research Consortium (ARC) proposed a list of standardized data elements that should be recorded in the case report form for a clinical trial of antithrombotic therapy (or the data collection form of a registry of ACS).[7] These data elements can then either be reported separately or combined to reconstruct other bleeding definitions. The ARC, which originally consisted of members from four academic research organizations that designed and executed pivotal trials of drug-eluting stents, developed a set of standardized definitions for endpoints used in coronary stent trials.[8] Periprocedural bleeding was not considered in their initial deliberations; however, subsequent iterations of ARC have developed definitions for bleeding endpoints for ACS trials, transcatheter valve trials, and peripheral arterial disease trials. The Bleeding Academic Research Consortium (BARC) definition of bleeding for use in ACS trials is shown in Table 29-2.[1]

Bleeding Incidence

After considering the differences in definitions across studies, the estimated incidence of bleeding during acute

TABLE 29-2 Bleeding Academic Research Consortium Definition of Bleeding

Type 0: no bleeding
Type 1: bleeding that is not actionable and does not cause the patient to seek unscheduled performance of studies, hospitalization, or treatment by a health care professional; may include episodes leading to self-discontinuation of medical therapy by the patient without consulting a health care professional
Type 2: any overt, actionable sign of hemorrhage (e.g., more bleeding than would be expected for a clinical circumstance, including bleeding found by imaging alone) that does not fit the criteria for type 3, 4, or 5 but does meet at least 1 of the following criteria: (1) requiring nonsurgical, medical intervention by a health care professional, (2) leading to hospitalization or increased level of care, or (3) prompting evaluation
Type 3
  Type 3a
  - Overt bleeding plus hemoglobin drop of 3 to <5 g/dL (provided hemoglobin drop is related to bleed), corrected for transfusion
  - Any transfusion with overt bleeding

  Type 3b
  - Overt bleeding plus hemoglobin drop ≥5 g/dL (provided hemoglobin drop is related to bleed), corrected for transfusion
  - Cardiac tamponade
  - Bleeding requiring surgical intervention for control (excluding dental/nasal/skin/hemorrhoid)
  - Bleeding requiring intravenous vasoactive agents

  Type 3c
  - Intracranial hemorrhage (does not include microbleeds or hemorrhagic transformation, does include intraspinal)
  - Subcategories confirmed by autopsy or imaging or lumbar puncture
  - Intraocular bleed compromising vision

Type 4: CABG-related bleeding
  Perioperative intracranial bleeding within 48 h
  Reoperation after closure of sternotomy for the purpose of controlling bleeding
  Transfusion of ≥5 U whole blood or packed red blood cells within a 48-h period
  Chest tube output ≥2 L within a 24-h period
Type 5: fatal bleeding
  Type 5a
  - Probable fatal bleeding; no autopsy or imaging confirmation but clinically suspicious

  Type 5b
  - Definite fatal bleeding; overt bleeding or autopsy or imaging confirmation

CABG, coronary artery bypass grafting.

management of ACS is between 1% and 12%; any attempt to report a single number as the rate of ACS-related bleeding complications is likely to be misleading. Moreover, the incidence of bleeding in ACS patients may change with evolution of therapy over time and may be decreasing.[9] One can use either clinical trials or registries to estimate the incidence of bleeding. In the SYNERGY trial, which included ACS patients who underwent an early invasive strategy, the rate of major or severe bleeding ranged between 2.7% (GUSTO severe) to 9.1% (TIMI major) among patients assigned to enoxaparin. Similarly, in the PLATO trial, the rates of TIMI major bleeding and protocol-defined PLATO major bleeding were 7.9% and 11.6%, respectively, among patients assigned to ticagrelor.[10] Another source of information on bleeding complications is registry data. The ACTION–Get With the Guidelines registry is a nationally representative quality improvement registry for ACS that tracks and reports in-hospital bleeding complications (see Table 29-1 for definitions). The incidence of bleeding in this registry is 10.8%.[11] Clinicians should be cognizant of the factors that influence the reporting of bleeding rates, and either use one definition to survey their own practice, or participate in an ACS registry like the ACTION-Get With the Guidelines registry to receive bleeding data on their patients benchmarked against a registry average.

Risk Factors for Bleeding Complications

The presence of numerous clinical trial and registry databases has created a deep knowledge base regarding risk factors and risk indicators associated with hemorrhagic complications in ACS. A major risk for bleeding is the use of invasive procedures, such as cardiac catheterization, percutaneous coronary intervention, and coronary artery bypass grafting (CABG), which compounds the risk for bleeding in patients treated with potent antithrombotic medications. The widespread adoption of these procedures has led to the broad categorization of bleeding into either "access-site related bleeding" and "nonaccess-site related bleeding." This categorization also facilitates the grouping of BAS, which can be directed at the vascular access site or systemically (see the section on Bleeding Avoidance Strategies). The proportion of bleeding related to the vascular access site appears to vary with the patient's clinical presentation. In the context of ACS, patients with non ST-elevation (NSTE)-ACS have a higher proportion of nonaccess-site bleeding. This observation is borne out in registry data and in randomized clinical trials. For example, in the National Cardiovascular Data Registry's Cath-PCI registry, of the bleeding events that occurred in NSTE-ACS patients who underwent PCI, two-thirds of the bleeds were not related to the access site.[12] Similarly, in the RIVAL trial, which compared radial with femoral access in 7021 patients with ACS (>70% of whom had NSTE-ACS), two-thirds of major bleeding was unrelated to the vascular access site.[13] In contrast, patients with STEMI not only have a higher rate of bleeding, but a larger proportion of these patients (~50%) have bleeding related to the vascular access site. These differences are likely related to the much higher use of PCI and its attendant intense antithrombotic therapy among patients with STEMI.

Risk Scores for Bleeding

In addition to clinical presentation, published risk models for bleeding have identified a variety of demographic and clinical features that are associated with a higher risk for bleeding complications. Because most bleeding events in ACS occur early, either during the index hospitalization or within 30 days, most of these models have used in-hospital or 30-day bleeding as the primary outcome. A commonly used bleeding prediction model is one derived from the ACUITY and HORIZONS-MI clinical trials, which examined a bivalirudin strategy in patients with NSTE-ACS or STEMI, respectively, who underwent primary PCI.[14] Both trials used the same definition of bleeding, and the combined trials consisted of 17,421 patients. The overall rate of non-CABG–related major bleeding was 7.4%. Baseline covariates independently associated with bleeding included age, female sex, elevated serum creatinine, elevated white blood cell count, pre-existing anemia, NSTEMI, and STEMI. One treatment covariate—the use of heparin plus a glycoprotein IIb/IIIa inhibitor—was also a significant predictor. The model has reasonable discrimination, with a c-index of 0.74. The goodness-of-fit was evaluated by comparing predicted with observed bleeding. Finally, an integer risk score was developed for use at the bedside (Figure 29-1). Another model was derived from the CRUSADE registry, which is used for risk adjustment in an ACS quality improvement registry.[15] This model included

		Add to score
Gender	Male 0; Female +8	
Age (years)	<50: 0; 50–59: +3; 60–69: +6; 70–79: +9; ≥80: +12	
Serum creatinine (mg/dL)	<1.0: 0; 1.0–: +2; 1.2–: +3; 1.4–: +5; 1.6–: +6; 1.8–: +8; ≥2.0: +10	
White blood cell count (× 10^9)	<10: 0; 10–: +2; 12–: +3; 14–: +5; 16–: +6; 18–: +8; ≥20: +10	
Anemia	No 0; Yes +6	
Presentation	STEMI +6; NSTEMI - Raised biomarkers +2; NSTE-ACS - Normal biomarkers 0	
Antithrombotic medications	Heparin plus a GPI 0; Bivalirudin monotherapy −5	
	Total score*	

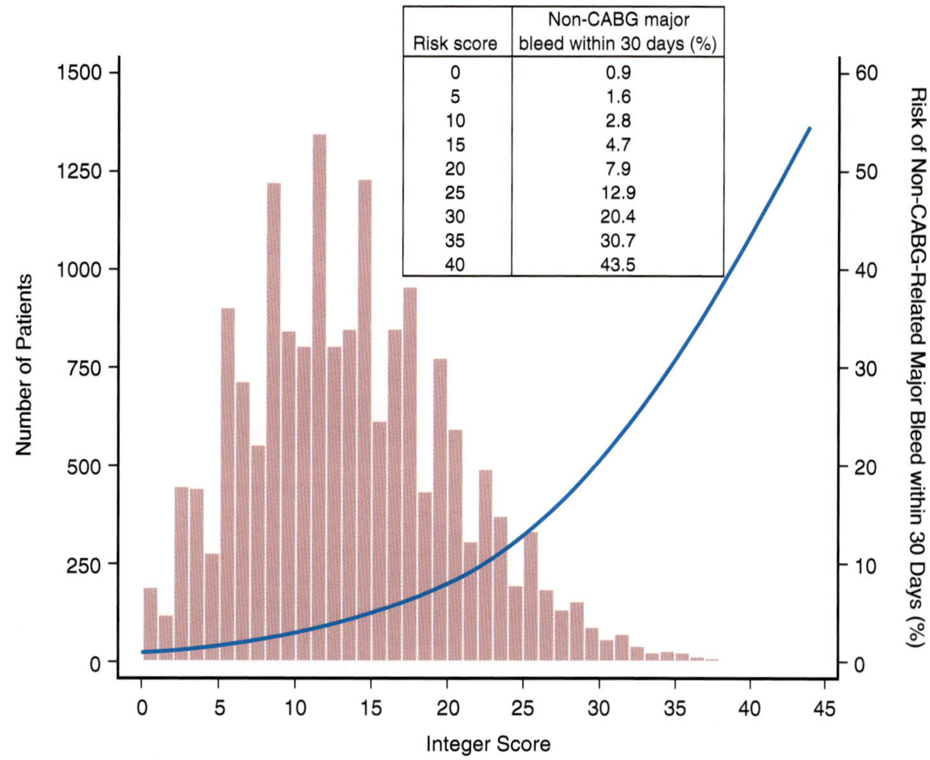

FIGURE 29-1 An integer risk score for non–coronary artery bypass graft (CABG)–related major bleeding within 30 days of patient presentation with acute coronary syndrome (ACS) and distribution of the risk score with subsequent probability of non-CABG—related major bleeding. The study sample includes 17,421 patients from the randomized ACUITY and HORIZONS-AMI clinical trials. *GPI*, Glycoprotein IIb/IIIa receptor inhibitor; *NSTEMI*, non–ST-elevation myocardial infarction; *STEMI*, ST-elevation myocardial infarction. *(From Mehran R, et al: A risk score to predict bleeding in patients with acute coronary syndromes.* J Am Coll Cardiol *55:2556–2566, 2010.)*

only NSTE-ACS patients and did not include treatment variables, so that site-level bleeding outcomes could be benchmarked and allow for process changes to reduce bleeding risk at centers with high bleeding rates. Using 71,277 patients as the development data set and 17,857 patients as the validation data set, the investigators identified eight independent predictors of major bleeding (defined according to the registry; see Table 29-1). These risk indicators included baseline hematocrit, baseline creatinine clearance, baseline heart rate, female sex, heart failure at presentation, baseline systolic blood pressure, previous vascular disease, and diabetes mellitus. The c-indices in the development and validation cohorts were 0.72 and 0.71, respectively. Similar to the ACUITY bedside risk score, the investigators developed the "CRUSADE" bleeding risk score (available at http://www.crusadebleedingscore.org), which showed an increase in the predicted probability as the score increased.

These published models share certain predictors of bleeding, namely, chronic kidney disease, anemia, and female sex (Table 29-3). Chronic kidney disease likely predisposes to bleeding through reduced clearance of antithrombin agents (especially those that are predominantly renally cleared) and platelet dysfunction. Anemia is likely a marker of occult bleeding that may be exacerbated in the setting of aggressive

TABLE 29-3 Predictors of Bleeding from Selected Bleeding Prediction Risk Scores

DATA SOURCE	NCDR CATH-PCI REGISTRY	ACTION-GWTG REGISTRY	ACUITY + HORIZONS MI CLINICAL TRIAL DATA	BLUE CROSS-BLUE SHIELD CONSORTIUM REGISTRY*
Population	PCI	ACS	ACS undergoing PCI	PCI
Risk Factors				
Age	X	X	X	
Sex	X	X	X	
Weight/BMI	BMI	Weight		Height and weight
Renal	Chronic kidney disease	Baseline creatinine	Baseline creatinine	Baseline creatinine
Pre-existing anemia	Baseline hemoglobin	Baseline hemoglobin	Anemia	—
Presentation	• STEMI • Shock • Cardiac arrest within 24 h of PCI	• Systolic blood pressure • Admission heart rate • Heart failure/shock on admission • ECG changes	NSTEMI or STEMI	• CAD presentation • Anginal classification • Heart failure within previous 2 wks • Cardiogenic shock in 24 h before PCI • Pre-procedure cardiac markers (CK-MB, troponin I/T)
History	Previous PCI	• Diabetes mellitus • Peripheral artery disease		• Diabetes mellitus • Chronic lung disease
Interventions	Urgent or emergent/ salvage PCI	—	—	—
Medications	—	Warfarin use	Unfractionated heparin + glycoprotein IIb/IIIa inhibitor	—
Other	—	—	White blood cell count	—

ACS, Acute coronary syndrome; *BMI*, body mass index; *CAD*, coronary artery disease; *CK-MB*, creatine kinase-myocardial band; *ECG*, electrocardiography; *NSTEMI*, non–ST-elevation myocardial infarction; *PCI*, percutaneous coronary intervention.
*Outcome is in-hospital blood transfusion.

antithrombotic therapy. In addition, baseline anemia may increase the likelihood of blood transfusion, which is an element of the bleeding definition in many studies (see Table 29-1). The mechanism underlying the association between female sex and higher bleeding risk has yet to be elucidated. Women presenting with ACS are more likely to be older, to have lower body mass, and to have impaired renal function. As such, overdosing of antithrombotic medications may be responsible for some degree of the increased risk (see the section on Preventive Strategies); however, this does not appear to fully explain the apparent independent association. Further research is needed to understand if there are reversible causes of bleeding in women with ACS.

BLEEDING COMPLICATIONS AND OUTCOMES

Associated Clinical and Nonclinical Outcomes

Clinical Outcomes

Several studies describe an association between bleeding (regardless of definition) in the ACS population and adverse outcomes, including death, MI, stroke, unplanned revascularization, and stent thrombosis. One of the earliest studies in ACS was published by Moscucci and colleagues, who examined the GRACE registry.[16] Of 24,045 patients with ACS (including unstable angina, NSTEMI, and STEMI), 3.9% had a bleeding event (4.8% in STEMI, 4.7% in NSTEMI, and 2.3% in unstable angina). Similar to previous studies, older age, female sex, renal insufficiency, and history of bleeding were associated with an increased risk of bleeding. After adjustment for potential confounders, major bleeding as defined by the GRACE registry was associated with higher in-hospital mortality. Intermediate term outcomes have been examined in a variety of studies using different bleeding definitions. In an analysis by Rao and colleagues that examined 26,452 ACS patients enrolled in the PURSUIT, PARAGON B, and GUSTO IIb trials, there was a stepwise increase in risk between GUSTO bleeding severity and 30-day and 6-month death.[17] Other studies by Eikelboom and colleagues,[18] Manoukian and colleagues,[19] and Segev and colleagues[20] describe a significant association between the OASIS, ACUITY, and the Canadian ACS definitions of major bleeding in ACS patients and adverse short- and long-term outcomes, including stroke and stent thrombosis. With respect to a "standardized" definition, Ndrepepa and colleagues examined the association between BARC-defined bleeding and 1-year mortality and found that BARC type 2 or greater bleeding was associated with a significantly higher 1-year mortality compared with type 0 (no bleeding), with an adjusted hazard ratio of 2.72.[21]

Because of the slight differences in bleeding definitions across studies, it is tempting to compare the prognostic impact of various scales. Rao and colleagues examined 15,898 patients from two ACS clinical trials that used both the GUSTO and TIMI definitions of bleeding to categorize bleeding severity.[22] When applied separately, each scale identified patients as having had bleeding events that were missed by the other scale. In addition, both GUSTO and TIMI bleeding were associated with an increased risk for 30-day death or MI when examined separately. When both definitions were included in the same model, increasing GUSTO bleeding severity was associated with a stepwise increase in the adjusted hazard of death or MI, whereas TIMI bleeding was no longer correlated with outcomes. These data suggest that data elements reflecting clinical events may have more prognostic value than laboratory-based measures; however, this study, as well as others, demonstrated that clinically

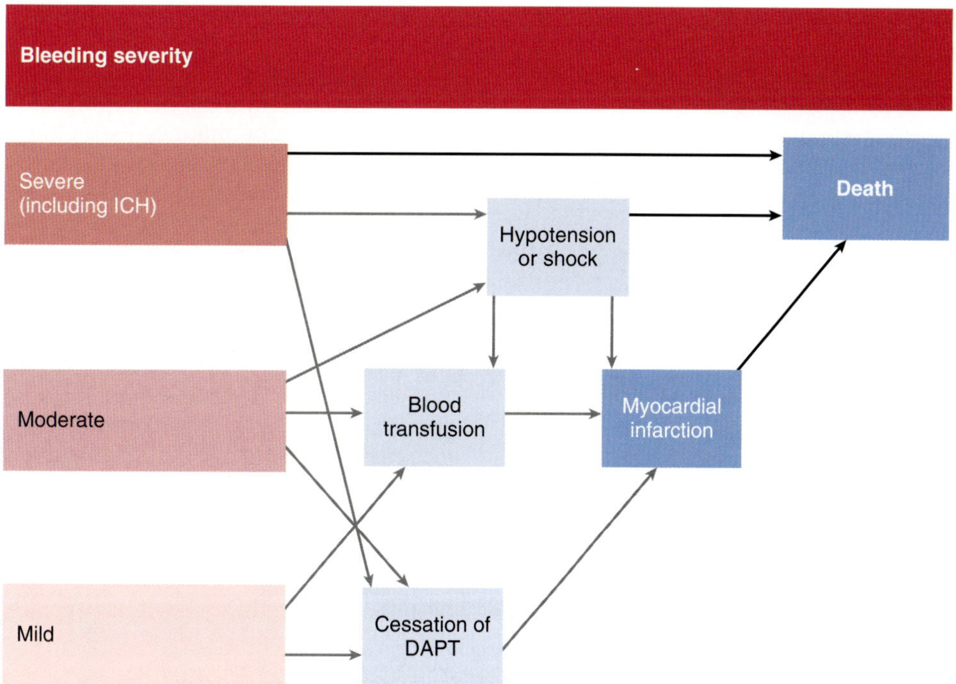

FIGURE 29-2 Potential mechanisms underlying the relationship between bleeding complications and mortality. Blood transfusion is associated with reduced nitric oxide levels, reduced tissue oxygenation, and platelet aggregation and may directly contribute to the risk of adverse outcomes. *DAPT*, Dual antiplatelet therapy. *ICH*, intracerebral hemorrhage. *(From Rao SV: The conundrum of reducing ischemic and bleeding events after PCI.* J Am Coll Cardiol *65:1421–1423, 2015.)*

overt bleeding that results in a decrease in hemoglobin is also associated with adverse outcome.

Cost of Care

In the setting of ACS, bleeding complications are also associated with increased costs of care. Rao and colleagues examined data from the economic substudy of the GUSTO IIb trial, which included 1235 patients from the United States, and found that hospital length of stay and costs increased as bleeding severity increased.[23] After adjustment for baseline differences among patients, each bleeding event was associated with a $3770 increase in costs, and each transfusion event was associated with a $2080 increase. Interestingly, when recurrent MI and bleeding were considered separately, patients who experienced a bleeding event incurred more costs than those who incurred a recurrent MI. Those who experienced both had the highest costs.

Potential Mechanisms of Bleeding and Increased Mortality

It is important to note that the associations between bleeding and outcomes come from post hoc observational analyses of clinical trial data or registry data. As such, assigning causality is problematic. Certainly, intracranial hemorrhage or frank exsanguination can lead directly to death, but such severe bleeding events are exceedingly rare in the contemporary era of ACS management. More commonly, in-hospital bleeding consists of procedure-related bleeding (e.g., access site hematomas), or on occasion, gastrointestinal bleeding. Bruising or ecchymoses generally characterizes bleeding during long-term outpatient therapy with dual antiplatelet therapy. It is difficult to ascribe a direct causal link between these types of bleeding events and subsequent mortality. Therefore, other mechanisms must be involved. Figure 29-2 shows the potential mechanism underlying the association between bleeding and adverse outcomes. First, confounding must be considered; patients in these data sets who develop bleeding complications are fundamentally different from those who do not in both measured and unmeasured ways. Even the most robust statistical adjustment is unlikely to account for these confounders. Second, bleeding complications likely lead to discontinuation of secondary prevention therapies. Third, there may be an independent role of blood transfusion on outcomes that is distinct from bleeding. Finally, chronic blood loss during the post-hospitalization period can result in anemia, which may compromise oxygen delivery to the myocardium, resulting in an increased risk for recurrent myocardial infarction.

Discontinuation of Antithrombotic Therapies

ACS patients who experience bleeding complications are more likely to have secondary prevention therapies discontinued. In an analysis of the GRACE registry, Spencer and colleagues found that patients who developed in-hospital major bleeding were less likely to have received aspirin (ASA), thienopyridines, and parenteral antithrombin therapy.[24] This difference in the use of guideline-directed medical therapies was estimated to account for a significant proportion of the increased risk for in-hospital mortality. Similarly, an analysis of ACS patients enrolled in the PREMIER registry demonstrated an association between in-hospital bleeding and lower use of ASA and thienopyridine at discharge.[25] These patients were less likely to be re-started on therapy up to 1 year after hospitalization, which may account for the correlation between in-hospital bleeding and subsequent stent thrombosis.

Anemia and Transfusions

As described previously, many bleeding definitions include the data element of red blood cell transfusion. The advantage of incorporating transfusions into a definition is that it represents a discrete event that can be recorded with a date and time. The disadvantage is that clinical practice may dictate the use of transfusion even in the absence of clinically overt bleeding. Moreover, there may be an independent association beyond bleeding between transfusion and adverse outcomes among patients with ischemic heart disease. Several observational studies have shown this association,[26,27] and adequately powered prospective randomized trials of transfusion thresholds in the ACS population are lacking. Mechanistically, transfusion may affect myocardial oxygenation by limiting oxygen delivery to already ischemic myocardial tissue. In the setting of hypoxia, oxygen delivery is maintained through compensatory vasodilation. This vasodilatory response may be attenuated in coronary vessels that have significant stenosis, and in response, the heart rate increases as a further compensatory response. Increased heart rate in the setting of ACS increases oxygen demand, and although transfusion may seem to increase oxygen delivery, preclinical studies indicate that stored red blood cells are devoid of nitric oxide and 2,3 diphosphoglycerate, further augment vasoconstriction, and do not increase tissue oxygenation. Two small prospective randomized pilot trials compared transfusion strategies in ACS. Both studies compared a threshold of 8 g/dL (hematocrit 24%) versus 10 g/dL (hematocrit of 30%) and came to different conclusions. The CRIT-Pilot trial randomized 65 patients with ACS and found that a liberal transfusion strategy (i.e., transfusion for a hematocrit ≤30%) resulted in a higher rate of in-hospital death, recurrent MI, or new or worsening heart failure compared with a conservative strategy (liberal 38% vs. restrictive 13%; $P = .046$).[28] In contrast, in the MINT Pilot trial, which randomized 110 patients with ACS and a hemoglobin of less than 10 g/dL, a liberal transfusion strategy resulted in a lower rate of 30-day death, MI, or unplanned revascularization (10.9% vs. 25.5%; $P = .054$).[29] In addition, the rate of 30-day death was lower in those assigned to the liberal strategy (1.8% vs. 17%; $P = .032$). Because of the disparity between the observational and randomized studies, an appropriately powered prospective randomized trial is needed to guide practice. Until then, the mechanistic studies of transfusion and oxygen delivery suggest that red blood cell transfusion should be avoided unless there are symptoms attributable to anemia (see section on Management of Bleeding Complications).

Approximately 15% to 40% of hospitalizations in ACS patients are complicated by anemia.[30] Anemia, which is defined by the World Health Organization as a hemoglobin less than 13 g/dL, is an independent predictor of major adverse cardiovascular events (MACEs) and mortality in patients across the spectrum of ACS. The pathophysiology underlying poor outcomes in anemic ACS patients may be explained by the combination of reduced oxygen delivery to the already hypoxic myocardium and the high myocardial oxygen demand secondary to the compensatory increases in heart rate and stroke volume. These compensatory mechanisms can result in a deleterious disparity between myocardial oxygen supply and demand.

MANAGEMENT OF BLEEDING COMPLICATIONS

Once a bleeding complication develops, management depends on its severity and location. Mild bleeding events like bruising or ecchymoses can be managed conservatively without stopping antithrombotic therapy. For patients who have undergone invasive risk stratification or primary PCI for STEMI, vascular access site bleeding complications can range from superficial hematomas to arteriovenous fistulae and arterial pseudoaneurysms to more severe complications like retroperitoneal hematomas. Superficial access site hematomas can be managed with local compression. Most arteriovenous fistulae formed as a complication of percutaneous femoral arterial access are not hemodynamically significant and close spontaneously. Arterial pseudoaneurysms can occur with either femoral, brachial, or radial artery access, and most will resolve without specific treatment if they are less than 2 cm. For larger pseudoaneurysms, ultrasound-guided compression or ultrasound-guided thrombin injection may be necessary. In rare cases of extremely large pseudoaneurysms, surgical ligation is needed. Radial artery pseudoaneurysms almost always resolve with prolonged compression using a radial hemostatic band. In all of these situations, continuation of dual antiplatelet therapy is appropriate. However, for retroperitoneal hematomas, cessation of antithrombotic therapy may be necessary to reduce persistent bleeding. Although rare, retroperitoneal hematomas are associated with mortality because of the large volume of blood that can accumulate in the retroperitoneal space in an occult fashion.

Nonaccess-site bleeding most commonly occurs from the gastrointestinal tract. For bleeding events that are mild or not associated with hemodynamic compromise, continuation of dual antiplatelet therapy may be appropriate while the source of bleeding is investigated. However, for hemodynamically significant gastrointestinal bleeding, cessation of antithrombotic therapy is reasonable until the bleeding source is identified and definitively treated. Intravenous proton pump inhibitors are useful to minimize bleeding and prevent recurrences.[31] Antithrombotic therapy, especially dual antiplatelet therapy, should be restarted as soon as possible after the bleeding event has resolved.

Bleeding events that occur during ACS hospitalization or during PCI (e.g., coronary artery perforation) when antithrombin agents are being administered may require reversal of the anticoagulant effect. For indirect thrombin inhibitors like unfractionated heparin and enoxaparin, protamine sulfate is useful to reverse the anticoagulation. Protamine fully reverses unfractionated heparin and reverses 60% to 80% of the effect of enoxaparin. The small molecule glycoprotein IIb/IIIa inhibitors epitifbatide and tirofiban have short half-lives of 2.5 to 3 hours and 2 hours, respectively. Abciximab, which is a murine monoclonal antibody against the glycoprotein IIb/IIIa receptor, has a very short initial plasma half-life of only 10 minutes, but its high affinity for binding with platelets causes it to remain platelet-bound in the circulation for up to 15 days. Platelet function recovers over 48 hours after bolus administration. Because abciximab has a short plasma half-life (but a longer biological half-life), platelet transfusion can mitigate its antiplatelet effect because little of the drug is present in plasma.

PREVENTIVE STRATEGIES

Because options for management are limited and rooted in discontinuation of antithrombotic therapy, prevention of bleeding complications is essential to achieving the best outcomes in ACS. Preventive strategies fall broadly into three categories: appropriate dosing and use of antithrombotic therapies; use of targeted anticoagulants; and vascular access strategies (Table 29-4). In many patients,

TABLE 29-4 Strategies to Minimize Bleeding Risk

Pharmacological	Appropriate dosing of antithrombotic medications • Dosing adjusted for renal function if medication is renally cleared • Dosing of unfractionated heparin to maintain aPTT 50–70 sec • Caution with potent antiplatelet agents (prasugrel contraindicated) in patients age ≥75 yrs, body weight <60 kg, previous stroke or TIA • Use of low-dose (≤100 mg) aspirin during long-term therapy with dual antiplatelet therapy Targeted anticoagulants • Fondaparinux* • Bivalirudin
Vascular access	Radial approach Appropriate positioning of femoral arteriotomy

aPTT, Activated partial thrombin time; *TIA*, transient ischemic attack.
*Not approved for treatment of acute coronary syndrome in the United States.

a combination of these approaches may result in the lowest bleeding risk.

Dosing and Selection of Antithrombotic Therapies

In the hospital setting, inappropriate administration and dosing of antithrombotic, antiplatelet, and glycoprotein IIb/IIIa inhibitor therapy has been implicated as a preventable cause of bleeding among ACS patients. An analysis from the CRUSADE registry of ACS patients reported that 42% of patients received at least one excess dose of antithrombotic agent during their hospitalization.[32] Excess dosing of an antithrombotic agent was directly associated with increased rates of bleeding and prolonged length of hospital stay. Risk factors for receiving excessive doses of unfractionated heparin, low–molecular-weight heparin, or glycoprotein IIb/IIIA inhibitors included advanced age, female sex, low body weight, diabetes mellitus, and heart failure. The authors reported that 15% of major bleeding events in ACS patients were preventable with proper bleeding risk assessment and proper administration of anticoagulants. In women, excess dosing may account for up to 25% of the bleeding risk.[33] In this context, it is important to carefully adjust the doses of renally cleared agents, such as eptifibatide and low–molecular-weight heparins, in patients with renal insufficiency; dosing of intravenous unfractionated heparin should be weight-based and apt values should be maintained in the range of 50 to 70 seconds.

In the long-term treatment phase of ACS management, reduction of bleeding risk depends on using low-dose ASA and avoiding more potent $P2Y_{12}$ inhibitors in patients with contraindications. In a post hoc analysis of 12,562 ACS patients enrolled in the CURE trial, Peters and colleagues described an increased incidence in major bleeding directly associated with ASA dose (ASA alone: dose 100 mg; 1.9%, 101 to 199 mg; 2.8%, 200 mg; 3.7%; P = .0001; ASA + clopidogrel: dose 100 mg; 3.0%, 101 to 199 mg; 3.4%, 200 mg; 4.9%; P = .0009).[33a] There was no significant effect of the ASA dose on efficacy. The only randomized trial of ASA dosing in ACS is the CURRENT-OASIS 7 trial.[34] This trial compared high-dose (600 mg, followed by 150 mg/day for 7 days) with standard dose (300 mg followed by 75 mg/day) clopidogrel and high- versus low-dose ASA (300 to 325 mg/day vs. 75 to 100 mg/day). At 30 days, there was no difference in efficacy or safety between the high- and low-dose ASA strategies. The effect of ASA dose on safety after 30 days was not assessed in the CURRENT trial, and until further data are available, it seems reasonable to lower doses of ASA 30 days after an ACS event to minimize the bleeding risk.[35,36]

Antiplatelet Agents and Urgent Coronary Artery Bypass Grafting

A major bleeding risk with clopidogrel use is the risk associated with coronary artery bypass surgery. Because clopidogrel provides irreversible inhibition of the $P2Y_{12}$ receptor, its antiplatelet effect is reversed only when new platelets are generated. Therefore, studies have indicated an increased risk of surgical bleeding if CABG is undertaken within 5 days of clopidogrel therapy.[37] To minimize this risk, it is reasonable to wait 5 to 7 days after clopidogrel discontinuation before proceeding with bypass surgery; importantly, there does not appear to be a risk of increased ischemic events during this waiting period.

More potent $P2Y_{12}$ inhibitors are available for use in ACS patients and lead to greater platelet inhibition than clopidogrel, and consequently, have higher bleeding risk. Prasugrel, a thienopyridine that provides greater inhibition of platelet aggregation compared with clopidogrel, was associated with an increased risk of CABG-related bleeding in the TRITON-TIMI 38 trial (see Chapter 19).[38] Ticagrelor, a $P2Y_{12}$ inhibitor that reversibly binds to the receptor, also provides greater platelet inhibition than clopidogrel. In the PLATO trial, ticagrelor plus ASA was also more efficacious than clopidogrel plus ASA in patients with ACS,[10] with a reported significant reduction in CABG-related bleeding. The pattern of CABG-related bleeding may be caused by the reversible nature of the $P2Y_{12}$ inhibition of ticagrelor, but it is more likely that it is caused by differences in the applied definition of CABG-related bleeding and trial protocol. The PLATO trial mandated discontinuation of the study drug several days before planned CABG, thus minimizing the risk for CABG-related bleeding. Prasugrel requires discontinuation at least 7 days and ticagrelor at least 5 days before CABG to minimize surgical bleeding risk.

Alternative Anticoagulant Strategies

Two anticoagulant agents, bivalirudin and fondaparinux, have been studied in the context of ACS and both have shown reductions in bleeding complications compared with the control strategy. Bivalirudin is a specific and direct inhibitor of thrombin with a half-life of only 25 minutes. With respect to bleeding complications, most of the randomized studies with bivalirudin-based strategies significantly reduced bleeding compared with heparin-based anticoagulation. However, this effect is likely modulated by several factors: the proportion of patients in the control arm who received glycoprotein IIb/IIIa inhibitors, the dosing of heparin, the rate of radial access, and the definition of bleeding (see Chapter 17 and Chapter 18). Consideration may be given to use of bivalirudin and avoidance of glycoprotein inhibitors in patients at high risk of bleeding.

Fondaparinux is an indirect inhibitor of Factor Xa, with a plasma half-life of 17 to 21 hours that has not been approved in the United States for use in ACS, but it has been approved for this use in other countries (see Chapter 18). Fondaparinux reduced bleeding significantly compared with enoxaparin. A survival benefit associated with fondaparinux was evident at the 180-day follow-up period. Patients who experienced bleeding (across both treatment arms) represented most of the mortality difference. These results supported that these pharmacological strategies associated with a reduction in bleeding risk were also associated with improved survival.

Radial Artery Access

Because a large proportion of ACS patients undergo invasive risk stratification and PCI, vascular access management in ACS is an important bleeding avoidance strategy (see also Chapter 17). Careful attention to femoral arteriotomy by using femoral head fluoroscopy can reduce access site complications. An alternative is to use the radial artery approach for PCI, which is associated with a substantial reduction in bleeding and vascular complications. Importantly, this reduction in complications appears to be consistent even compared with a femoral arterial approach with vascular closure devices. A recent meta-analysis of randomized trials that included more than 760,000 patients from both randomized and observational studies demonstrated a strong association between the radial approach and decreased vascular complications.[39] In the setting of ACS, the radial approach has been suggested to reduce mortality in some subsets of patients undergoing PCI. In the RIVAL trial of ACS patients randomized to radial or femoral access, the radial approach did not reduce the primary endpoint of 30-day net adverse cardiovascular events (NACE), which were defined as death, MI, stroke, or major bleeding (defined according to the CURRENT trial definition).[13] However, it did significantly reduce major vascular access site complications and in the subgroup of patients with STEMI, the radial approach was associated with reduced mortality.

The MATRIX Trial randomized 8404 patients with ACS (4394 NSTE-ACS, 4010 STEMI) who were undergoing angiography or PCI to radial or femoral access.[2] There were two primary endpoints: 30-day MACE, which was defined as death, MI, or stroke; and 30-day NACE, which was defined as MACE plus major bleeding (defined as BARC type 3 or 5). The radial approach did not significantly reduce MACE, but did significantly reduce NACE by 17% (P = .0092). In addition, all-cause mortality was significantly lower with the radial approach (1.6% vs. 2.2%; P = .045). The differences in outcomes between RIVAL and MATRIX may be because of differences in the bleeding definitions and potentially improved transradial techniques that improved procedure success in the years between the RIVAL and MATRIX trials. In the setting of primary PCI for STEMI, the RIFLE-STEACS trial randomized 1001 patients to the radial or the femoral approach. Similar to the MATRIX trial, the radial approach significantly reduced 30-day NACE, major bleeding, and mortality.[40]

SUMMARY

Advances in the management of ACS have led to significant improvements in ischemic outcomes. However, this benefit has been balanced by an increased risk for bleeding and blood transfusion. Variability in bleeding definitions across clinical trials makes it difficult to compare the risks of different therapies; however, it is evident that there is an association between bleeding and blood transfusion and an increased risk of adverse events, including death, MI, stroke, and stent thrombosis. Although the mechanisms underlying this association are varied and incompletely understood, it is clear that antithrombotic medications are often discontinued in patients who develop even mild bleeding complications. Therefore, prevention of bleeding is a prudent approach. Patients at high risk for bleeding complications, such as older adults, women, and those with renal dysfunction should be identified as requiring strategies to minimize bleeding risk. When an invasive strategy is employed, consideration should be given to the use of the radial artery approach. In addition, careful dosing of antithrombotic and antiplatelet therapies is essential. Antithrombotic therapy should be selected on the basis of an understanding of the patient's bleeding and thrombotic risk. Bleeding avoidance strategies like these are fundamental to achieving the best outcomes in ACS.

References

1. Mehran R, et al.: Standardized bleeding definitions for cardiovascular clinical trials: a consensus report from the Bleeding Academic Research Consortium, *Circulation* 123:2736–2747, 2011.
2. Valgimigli M, et al.: Radial versus femoral access in patients with acute coronary syndromes undergoing invasive management: a randomised multicentre trial, *Lancet* 385:2465–2476, 2015.
3. Chesebro JH, et al.: Thrombolysis in Myocardial Infarction (TIMI) Trial, Phase I: a comparison between intravenous tissue plasminogen activator and intravenous streptokinase. Clinical findings through hospital discharge, *Circulation* 76:142–154, 1987.
4. Ferguson JJ, et al.: Enoxaparin vs unfractionated heparin in high-risk patients with non-ST-segment elevation acute coronary syndromes managed with an intended early invasive strategy: primary results of the SYNERGY randomized trial, *JAMA* 292:45–54, 2004.
5. Stone GW, et al.: Bivalirudin during primary PCI in acute myocardial infarction, *N Engl J Med* 358:2218–2230, 2008.
6. Subherwal S, et al.: Temporal trends in and factors associated with bleeding complications among patients undergoing percutaneous coronary intervention: a report from the National Cardiovascular Data CathPCI Registry, *J Am Coll Cardiol* 59:1861–1869, 2012.
7. Rao SV, et al.: Standardized reporting of bleeding complications for clinical investigations in acute coronary syndromes: a proposal from the academic bleeding consensus (ABC) multidisciplinary working group, *Am Heart J* 158:881–886 e1, 2009.
8. Cutlip DE, et al.: Clinical end points in coronary stent trials: a case for standardized definitions, *Circulation* 115:2344–2351, 2007.
9. Fox KA, et al.: Has the frequency of bleeding changed over time for patients presenting with an acute coronary syndrome? The Global Registry of Acute Coronary Events, *Eur Heart J* 31: 667–675, 2010.
10. Wallentin L, et al.: Ticagrelor versus clopidogrel in patients with acute coronary syndromes, *N Engl J Med* 361:1045–1057, 2009.
11. Mathews R, et al.: In-hospital major bleeding during ST-elevation and non-ST-elevation myocardial infarction care: derivation and validation of a model from the ACTION Registry(R)-GWTG, *Am J Cardiol* 107:1136–1143, 2011.
12. Rao SV, et al.: The transradial approach to percutaneous coronary intervention: historical perspective, current concepts, and future directions, *J Am Coll Cardiol* 55:2187–2195, 2010.
13. Jolly SS, et al.: Radial versus femoral access for coronary angiography and intervention in patients with acute coronary syndromes (RIVAL): a randomised, parallel group, multicentre trial, *Lancet* 377:1409–1420, 2011.
14. Mehran R, et al.: A risk score to predict bleeding in patients with acute coronary syndromes, *J Am Coll Cardiol* 55:2556–2566, 2010.
15. Subherwal S, et al.: Baseline risk of major bleeding in non-ST-segment-elevation myocardial infarction: the CRUSADE (Can Rapid risk stratification of Unstable angina patients Suppress ADverse outcomes with Early implementation of the ACC/AHA Guidelines) Bleeding Score, *Circulation* 119:1873–1882, 2009.
16. Moscucci M, et al.: Predictors of major bleeding in acute coronary syndromes: the Global Registry of Acute Coronary Events (GRACE), *Eur Heart J* 24:1815–1823, 2003.
17. Rao SV, et al.: Impact of bleeding severity on clinical outcomes among patients with acute coronary syndromes, *Am J Cardiol* 96:1200–1206, 2005.
18. Eikelboom JW, et al.: Adverse impact of bleeding on prognosis in patients with acute coronary syndromes, *Circulation* 114:774–782, 2006.
19. Manoukian SV, et al.: Impact of major bleeding on 30-day mortality and clinical outcomes in patients with acute coronary syndromes: an analysis from the ACUITY Trial, *J Am Coll Cardiol* 49:1362–1368, 2007.
20. Segev A, et al.: Predictors and 1-year outcome of major bleeding in patients with non-ST-elevation acute coronary syndromes: insights from the Canadian Acute Coronary Syndrome Registries, *Am Heart J* 150:690–694, 2005.
21. Ndrepepa G, et al.: Validation of the Bleeding Academic Research Consortium definition of bleeding in patients with coronary artery disease undergoing percutaneous coronary intervention, *Circulation* 125:1424–1431, 2012.
22. Rao SV, et al.: A comparison of the clinical impact of bleeding measured by two different classifications among patients with acute coronary syndromes, *J Am Coll Cardiol* 47:809–816, 2006.
23. Rao SV, et al.: Association between bleeding, blood transfusion, and costs among patients with non-ST-segment elevation acute coronary syndromes, *Am Heart J* 155:369–374, 2008.
24. Spencer FA, et al.: Does comorbidity account for the excess mortality in patients with major bleeding in acute myocardial infarction? *Circulation* 116:2793–2801, 2007.
25. Wang TY, et al.: Antiplatelet therapy use after discharge among acute myocardial infarction patients with in-hospital bleeding, *Circulation* 118:2139–2145, 2008.
26. Rao SV, et al.: The relationship of blood transfusion and clinical outcomes in patients with acute coronary syndromes, *JAMA* 292:1555–1562, 2004.
27. Sherwood MW, Rao SV: Acute coronary syndromes: blood transfusion in patients with acute MI and anaemia, *Nature Reviews Cardiology* 10:186–187, 2013.
28. Cooper HA, et al.: Conservative versus liberal red cell transfusion in acute myocardial infarction (the CRIT Randomized Pilot Study), *Am J Cardiol* 108:1108–1111, 2011.
29. Carson JL, et al.: Liberal versus restrictive transfusion thresholds for patients with symptomatic coronary artery disease, *Am Heart J* 165:964–971 e1, 2013.
30. Sabatine MS, et al.: Association of hemoglobin levels with clinical outcomes in acute coronary syndromes, *Circulation* 111:2042–2049, 2005.
31. Abraham NS, et al.: ACCF/ACG/AHA 2010 expert consensus document on the concomitant use of proton pump inhibitors and thienopyridines: a focused update of the ACCF/ACG/AHA 2008 expert consensus document on reducing the gastrointestinal risks of antiplatelet therapy and NSAID use, *Am J Gastroenterol* 105:2533–2549, 2010.

32. Alexander KP, et al.: Excess dosing of antiplatelet and antithrombin agents in the treatment of non-ST-segment elevation acute coronary syndromes, *JAMA* 294:3108–3116, 2005.
33. Alexander KP, et al.: Sex differences in major bleeding with glycoprotein IIb/IIIa inhibitors: results from the CRUSADE (Can Rapid risk stratification of Unstable angina patients Suppress ADverse outcomes with Early implementation of the ACC/AHA guidelines) initiative, *Circulation* 114:1380–1387, 2006.
33a. Peters RJG, et al.: Effects of aspirin when used alone or in combination with clopidogrel in patients with acute coronary syndromes: observations from the Clopidogrel in Unstable angina to prevent Recurrent Events (CURE) study, *Circulation* 108:1682–1687, 2003.
34. CURRENT-OASIS 7 Investigators, Mehta SR, et al.: Dose comparisons of clopidogrel and aspirin in acute coronary syndromes, *N Engl J Med* 363:930–942, 2010.
35. Campbell CL, Smyth S, Montalescot G, Steinhubl SR: Aspirin dose for the prevention of cardiovascular disease: a systematic review, *JAMA* 297:2018–2024, 2007.
36. Xian Y, et al.: Association of discharge aspirin dose with outcomes after acute myocardial infarction: insights from the Treatment with ADP Receptor Inhibitors: Longitudinal Assessment of Treatment Patterns and Events after Acute Coronary Syndrome (TRANSLATE-ACS) Study, *Circulation* 132:174–181, 2015.
37. Fox KA, et al.: Benefits and risks of the combination of clopidogrel and aspirin in patients undergoing surgical revascularization for non-ST-elevation acute coronary syndrome: the Clopidogrel in Unstable angina to prevent Recurrent ischemic Events (CURE) Trial, *Circulation* 110:1202–1208, 2004.
38. Wiviott SD, et al.: Prasugrel versus clopidogrel in patients with acute coronary syndromes, *N Engl J Med* 357:2001–2015, 2007.
39. Bertrand OF, et al.: Comparison of transradial and femoral approaches for percutaneous coronary interventions: a systematic review and hierarchical Bayesian meta-analysis, *Am Heart J* 163:632–648, 2012.
40. Romagnoli E, et al.: Radial versus femoral randomized investigation in ST-segment elevation acute coronary syndrome: the RIFLE-STEACS (Radial Versus Femoral Randomized Investigation in ST-Elevation Acute Coronary Syndrome) study, *J Am Coll Cardiol* 60:2481–2489, 2012.

30

Clinical Practice/Controversy

Approach to Noninvasive Testing After Presentation with Acute Myocardial Infarction

Todd D. Miller and Nandan S. Anavekar

INTRODUCTION

Noninvasive testing after presentation with acute myocardial infarction (MI) plays an essential role in patient management. Noninvasive testing complements clinical assessment of risk stratification and can be used to aid management decisions. The major purposes of testing are measurement of left ventricular (LV) function in nearly all patients and assessment of ischemic burden, primarily among low-risk patients who are initially treated conservatively, to identify potential candidates for coronary angiography or nonculprit vessel revascularization.[1–4] The most commonly used tests include resting echocardiography, standard stress testing with electrocardiography (ECG) alone, stress imaging with nuclear myocardial perfusion imaging (MPI) or echocardiography, and increasingly, resting and stress cardiac magnetic resonance imaging (CMR). The use of these tests is related to the temporal evolution of the MI. Early imaging (within the first 72 hours) is performed predominantly with resting echocardiography; intermediate testing (day 3 to 6 weeks) uses the standard stress test or stress imaging; and late imaging (beyond 6 weeks) is performed with any of the techniques in selected patient subsets to measure LV ejection fraction (LVEF) after stunning has resolved for assessment of implantable cardiac defibrillator (ICD) consideration and for viability assessment.

In this chapter, we discuss the role of noninvasive testing after MI, patient selection, and considerations for choosing among the alternatives for noninvasive testing. Each modality is discussed in detail elsewhere in the text. Echocardiography is reviewed in Chapter 31, MPI in Chapter 32, and CMR in Chapter 33. Although computed tomographic angiography (CTA) is playing an increasingly important role in the early evaluation of the patient with acute chest pain in the emergency department (see Chapter 9), CTA currently is not widely used in patients with confirmed MI and is not discussed in this chapter.

PATHOPHYSIOLOGY OF MYOCARDIAL INFARCTION AS THE BASIS FOR NONINVASIVE TESTING

The pathophysiology of acute MI is discussed in detail in Chapter 3 and Chapter 4. Understanding the pathophysiology establishes the foundation for appreciating the rationale behind noninvasive testing. The amount of myocardium that is jeopardized by occlusion of a coronary artery is referred to as myocardium at risk (see Chapter 24). This is the amount of myocardium that is expected to become scarred in the absence of spontaneous reperfusion or treatment with reperfusion therapy. The amount of myocardium that ultimately turns into scar is referred to as the final infarct size. The difference between myocardium at risk and final infarct size is labeled myocardial salvage. Both final infarct size and myocardial salvage reflect, in part, the efficacy of reperfusion therapy (see Chapter 13). These measurements can be quantified by nuclear MPI or CMR techniques. This type of imaging has been applied as a surrogate endpoint in numerous research studies that have compared different reperfusion strategies or have examined the efficacy of new MI therapies.[5,6] Measurement of myocardial salvage is somewhat logistically demanding and has not been shown to directly affect patient management; therefore, such measurements are not commonly performed in clinical practice. MI results in worsening wall motion in the infarct zone and commonly compensatory hyperkinesia in noninfarct zones (see Chapter 36). After spontaneous reperfusion or reperfusion therapy, partial or complete recovery may ensue in the motion of these stunned segments. The duration for resolution of stunning and resolution of compensatory hyperkinesia in noninfarct zones is highly variable and occurs within days up to 6 weeks.

Two of the most important prognostic variables in patients with acute MI are global LV function and the extent of coronary artery disease (CAD).[1–4] Measurement of these variables is a primary objective of noninvasive testing after MI. Global LV function is most commonly expressed as the LVEF. Current professional society practice guidelines recommend measurement of LVEF in all patients with ST-elevation MI (STEMI)[1,2] and recognize the relationship with the prognosis among patients with non–ST-elevation MI (NSTEMI).[3,4] LVEF and regional wall motion can be measured in the catheterization laboratory by contrast ventriculography or by noninvasive methods. These measurements are increasingly being obtained noninvasively. Other indices of global LV structure and/or function, including end-diastolic and end-systolic volumes, wall motion score index, and diastolic function can also be measured, but these generally do not provide any incremental knowledge for patient management beyond that provided by LVEF. Because of the effects of stunning, repeated measurement of LVEF beyond 40 days may be required in selected patients, particularly those being considered for ICDs. Some patients with reduced LVEF undergo progressive enlargement of the LV, a process termed remodeling (see Chapter 36). Remodeling is associated with higher mortality and greater risk of future development of heart failure. Angiotensin-converting enzyme (ACE) inhibitors and angiotensin receptor blockers can favorably affect remodeling. An important reason to measure LVEF early in the course of acute MI is to identify patients who are candidates for these medications and aldosterone antagonists.[1,2]

Noninvasive testing can approximate the extent of CAD and its functional significance. In patients with MI who are initially treated conservatively and do not undergo early coronary angiography, stress testing can be performed to identify patients who are candidates for coronary angiography and possible revascularization. Moreover, noninvasive testing may be useful for assessing the functional significance of residual CAD after an initial revascularization of the culprit artery (see Chapter 17).

RATIONAL USE OF NONINVASIVE TESTING

Noninvasive testing should be viewed as an adjunct to clinical assessment for risk stratification and to aid in management decisions. Accurate risk assessment begins with clinical assessment of risk, which can be aided by calculating a clinical risk score (see Chapter 11). Clinical variables and the ECG can also be used to estimate LVEF.[7] This clinical estimate can occasionally suffice for adequate risk assessment in selected patients without the need for further evaluation. In general, testing is least helpful for aiding clinical management at the two ends of the risk spectrum, in patients either at low or at high risk based on prognostic information that is already available. For instance, a young patient who presents early with first MI, and at angiography has single vessel right or circumflex CAD treated with successful PCI followed by an uncomplicated hospital course, also has a very high likelihood of a normal LVEF. Although measurement of LVEF is categorized as a class I indication in STEMI guidelines,[1,2] the measurement reasonably could be avoided in this patient example, because of the high likelihood of normal LVEF on the basis of clinical assessment. At the other end of the risk spectrum, there are an increasing number of patients with end-stage CAD who are living longer and present with multiple MIs during their lifetime. If previous evaluation has demonstrated that coronary anatomy is not amenable to further revascularization, or if LVEF is severely reduced, and the patient is already taking an ACE inhibitor and has an ICD, there is little to be gained from noninvasive testing. Testing should be performed only when the results are likely to affect clinical management and in a cost-effective manner. Redundant testing should be avoided. If a patient undergoes left ventriculography as part of the early catheterization procedure, performance of echocardiography generally is not necessary.

NONINVASIVE TESTING ACCORDING TO TEMPORAL SEQUENCE OF MYOCARDIAL INFARCTION EVOLUTION

The time course of recovery after MI can be separated into three general phases: early (within 72 hours); intermediate (day 3 to week 6); and late (beyond 6 weeks). These phases provide a useful framework in which to consider the goals and alternatives for noninvasive testing (Table 30-1). Resting echocardiography is the most commonly performed test in the early phase (Figure 30-1). The major goal is to provide information on LVEF and regional wall motion. Echocardiography (see Chapter 31) can also identify mechanical complications of MI (see Chapter 26) and aid in the recognition of conditions that mimic MI (see Chapter 6). Early submaximal stress testing (usually performed between days 3 and 5 and before hospital discharge) with or without imaging is performed primarily in the subset of low-risk patients who do not undergo early coronary angiography for risk stratification (Figure 30-2). Delayed symptom-limited stress testing (usually between 3 and 6 weeks) can be helpful to guide additional revascularization decisions in patients who undergo early angiography and have evidence for significant CAD in vessels other than the infarct-related artery (see Figure 30-2). Delayed imaging (beyond 40 days) with any of the imaging techniques can be performed in selected patients primarily for two major purposes: measurement of LVEF to determine eligibility for ICD and assessment of viable myocardium (Figure 30-3).

Early Imaging (Within 72 Hours) After Myocardial Infarction

Resting Echocardiography

The mainstay of early imaging is resting echocardiography.[1,2,8] Echocardiography (see also Chapter 31) possesses

TABLE 30-1 Time Course and Imaging Strategies after Myocardial Infarction

TIME	MAIN MODALITY*	GOAL	IMPACT ON MANAGEMENT
Early (≤2 h)	Resting echo (MUGA or CMR)	Measure global and regional LV function Identify MI complications Identify conditions mimicking MI	Use of ACE inhibitor, ARB, aldosterone antagonist Selection of revascularization strategy Appropriate treatment for identified condition
Intermediate (days 3–5) Intermediate (weeks 3–6)	Submaximal stress test† Symptom limited stress test†	Assess residual ischemic burden Same as submax test (if not performed). Assess ischemia related to the noninfarct artery‡	Identify pts for cor angio Identify pts for cor angio Select pts for additional PCI/CABG
Late (≥40 days)	Echo (MUGA or CMR) Nuclear PET or CMR (echo)	Measure LVEF (after stunning resolves) Assess myocardial viability	Eligibility for ICD Revascularization (usually CABG)

ACE, Angiotensin-converting enzyme; *ARB*, angiotensin receptor blocker; *CABG*, coronary artery bypass graft; *CMR*, cardiac magnetic resonance imaging; *ICD*, implantable cardiac defibrillator; *LV*, left ventricular; *LVEF*, left ventricular ejection fraction; *MI*, myocardial infarction; *MUGA*, multigated analysis; *PCI*, percutaneous coronary intervention; *PET*, positron emission tomography.

*The generally preferred and most commonly applied modality is shown first. Modalities listed in parentheses indicate secondary choices.

†Selection between a standard stress test and stress imaging is based primarily upon ability to exercise and interpretability of the electrocardiogram.

‡If testing is performed to assess ischemia in the noninfarct vessel, stress imaging is recommended over standard stress testing.

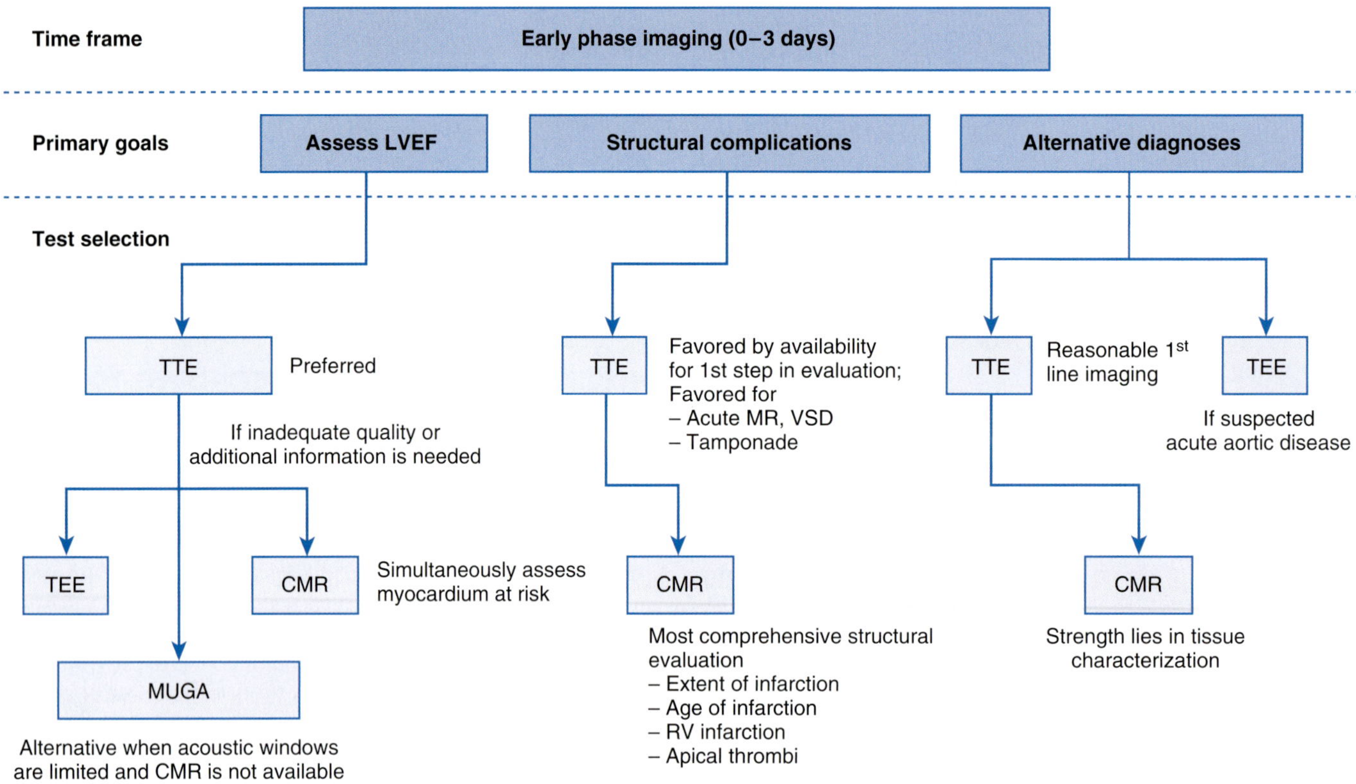

FIGURE 30-1 Imaging options in the acute phase of treatment in the setting of acute coronary syndrome. Echocardiography remains the mainstay. Cardiac MRI (CMR) is an evolving technology that is developing applications in this setting, but it remains limited by availability. Mulitgated analysis (MUGA) is applied in selected patients. *LVEF*, Left ventricular ejection fraction; *MR*, mitral regurgitation; *RV*, right ventricular; *TEE*, transesophageal echocardiography; *TTE*, transthoracic echocardiography; *VSD*, ventral septal defect.

certain advantages over other imaging modalities, including its more widespread availability and portability. There are essentially no contraindications to the performance of an echocardiogram. Transthoracic echocardiography provides a comprehensive cardiac assessment that encompasses global and regional LV systolic function, global right ventricular function, chamber sizes, wall thickness, LV diastolic function, valve status, estimated right ventricular systolic pressure, and pericardial fluid and thickness. Myocardial contrast can be administered to enhance image quality in patients with technically poor images. When clinically necessary, resting echocardiography can be performed at the patient's bedside. Transesophageal echocardiography provides an alternative to transthoracic echocardiography in critically ill patients who may have limited acoustic windows because of chest bandages or for other reasons. Performance of transesophageal echocardiography solely to assess cardiac function is an uncommon indication. Transesophageal echocardiography has particular use in the assessment of the thoracic aorta and main pulmonary arteries to diagnose conditions that can mimic MI. Myocardial strain imaging represents a newer method of assessing systolic function, but its incremental clinical value over routine measurement of LVEF and regional wall motion assessment remains to be determined. Myocardial contrast echocardiography with microbubbles has been used to assess myocardial perfusion, but this technique is not commonly performed clinically.

The major reason for performing resting echocardiography early in the course of MI is measurement of LVEF (see Figure 30-1).[1,2] Knowledge of LVEF can influence medical decision-making. ACE inhibitors and aldosterone antagonists are class I guideline recommendations in patients with reduced LVEF[1,2] (see Chapter 13 and Chapter 25). Knowledge of LVEF may also influence selection of a specific revascularization procedure, particularly in patients with NSTEMI (see Chapter 16). For NSTEMI, or stabilized patients after STEMI, coronary artery bypass grafting (CABG) is preferred instead of multivessel PCI in patients with multivessel CAD if the LVEF is reduced. Assessment of regional wall motion can also provide an estimate of infarct size. Global LV function can also be measured as a wall motion score index, which is determined as the summation of regional wall motion in multiple LV segments. Some studies suggest that this measurement is a more accurate predictor of outcome than LVEF.[8]

A second reason to perform early echocardiography is to aid in the identification of conditions that can mimic acute MI (see Figure 30-1), including pulmonary embolus, aortic dissection, myocarditis and/or pericarditis, and apical ballooning syndrome (see Chapter 6). All of these conditions can present with chest discomfort, ischemic-appearing ECG changes, and elevated troponin. Because these conditions occur much less frequently than MI, there is a higher likelihood that they will be misdiagnosed initially. Echocardiography can provide clues to the presence of these conditions. The echocardiographic findings are not always definitive, and additional imaging procedures are commonly necessary to confirm the alternative diagnosis.

A third major reason to perform early echocardiography is to identify complications of acute MI (see Figure 30-1), including LV thrombus; right ventricular infarction; pericardial effusion, especially when associated with tamponade; rupture of the LV free wall, papillary muscle,

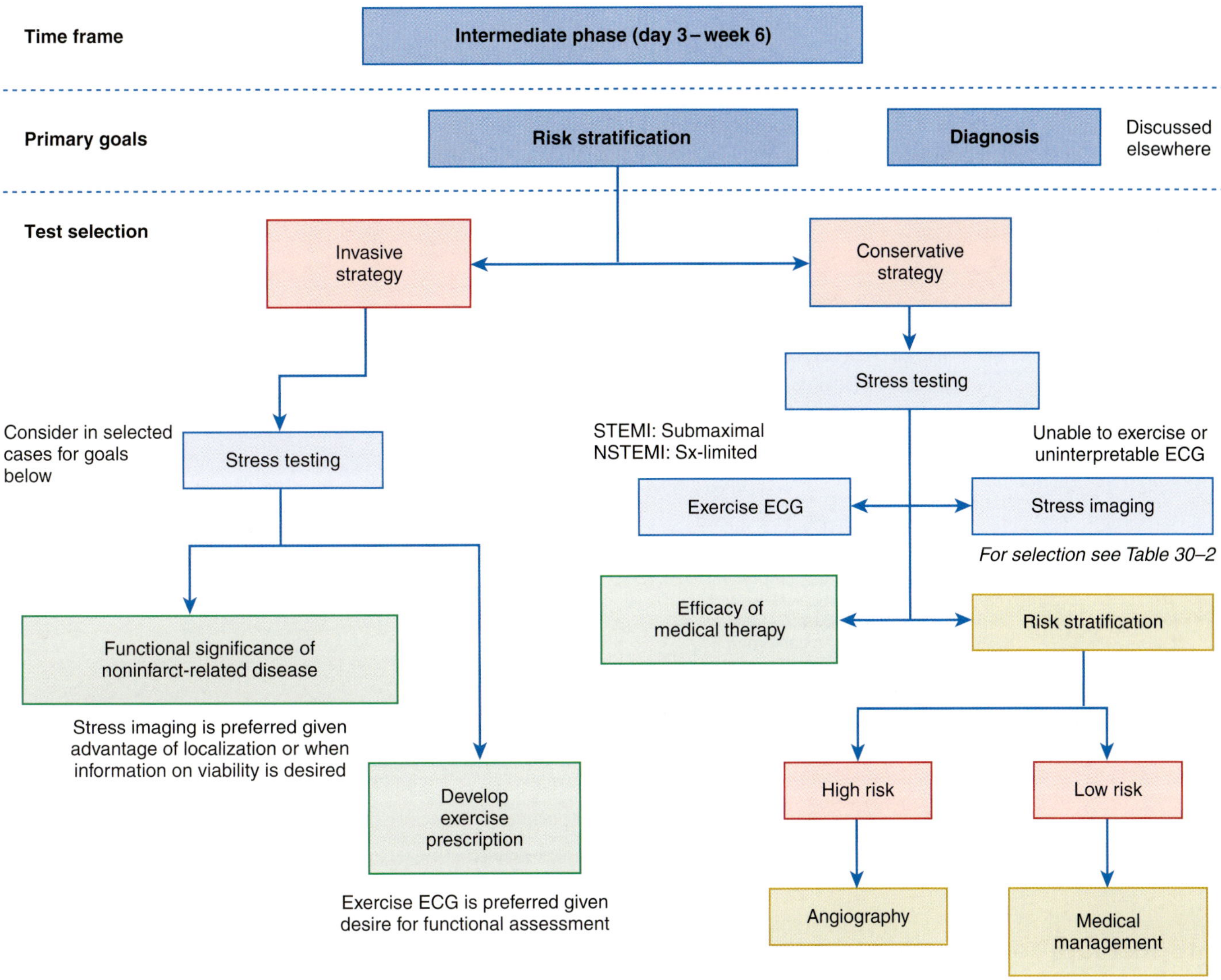

FIGURE 30-2 In the intermediate phase of treatment, functional imaging is the main consideration and can be applied to both early invasive and conservative strategies of care. In the conservative strategy, the role of functional imaging is to further stratify a patient's clinical risk, which may help with further therapeutic decisions. In the invasive arm, functional imaging helps determine the burden of ischemia in the nontreated coronary territories that will affect the timing of further interventions. *ECG*, Electrocardiography; *NSTEMI*, non–ST-segment myocardial infarction.

or interventricular septum; and valvular heart disease, especially new ischemic mitral regurgitation (see Chapter 26). Prompt and accurate identification of these complications can be critical to patient management and outcome.

Cardiac Magnetic Resonance and Nuclear Imaging

CMR (see also Chapter 33) is being increasingly used in the MI setting and possesses certain advantages over other imaging techniques.[9] It provides high spatial resolution and is not limited by acoustic windows as occurs with echocardiography. CMR has been shown to be superior to echocardiography in the assessment of the LV apex, which may have important clinical implications in the setting of anterior infarction, where assessment of apical thrombi may be challenging with echocardiography. CMR can more accurately characterize the anatomy of the right ventricle and provide volumetric measures of right ventricular size and function. Knowledge of these variables may have clinical implications in the care of patients presenting with inferior MI or pure right ventricular infarction. A unique property of CMR is tissue characterization, which helps delineate the presence of inflammation. This property can be very useful to correctly identify the rare patient who presents with myocarditis masquerading as MI.

MPI may be useful in the initial diagnostic evaluation of patients presenting with chest pain suspicious for MI (see Chapter 9). However, there is little role for nuclear MPI (see Chapter 32) in the early setting for patients with confirmed MI. Radionuclide angiography, commonly referred to as multigated analysis (MUGA), can be useful for evaluating LV function when echocardiographic images are limited. This technique provides an accurate quantitative assessment of LVEF. It has the theoretical advantage over other techniques of being geometrically independent and is especially useful for measuring LVEF in patients with distorted LV anatomy, such as an aneurysm. Both CMR and radionuclide angiography apply ECG gating for assessment of LV function. Because accurate measurement of LVEF and regional wall motion by gated techniques depends upon a fairly regular heart rhythm, these techniques generally are not advised in patients with atrial fibrillation or frequent cardiac ectopy.

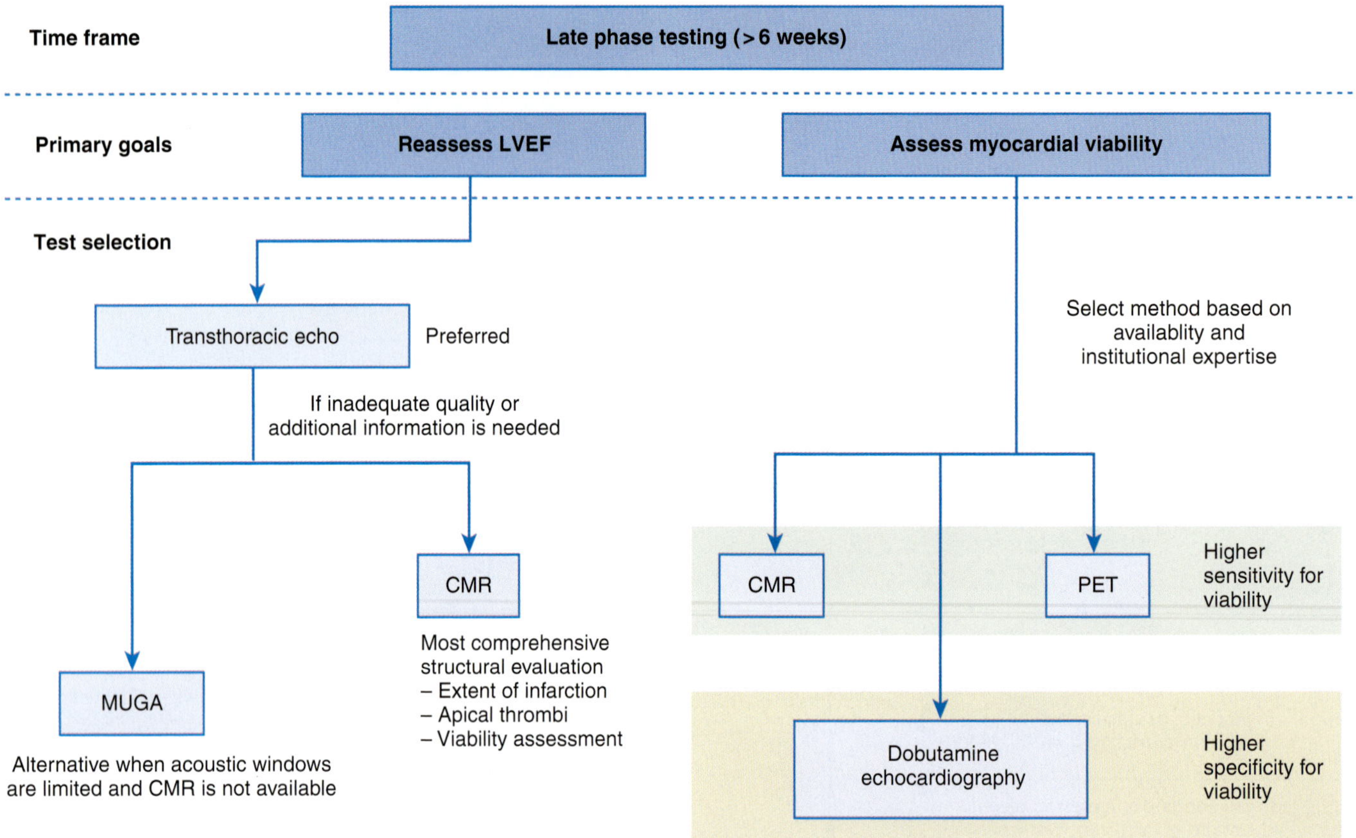

FIGURE 30-3 In the late phase of treatment, decision making is targeted toward two groups. The first are those in whom consideration of an implantable cardiac defibrillator may be warranted. The second group is a high-risk group whose evaluation still remains controversial. In this group of patients, there is moderate to severe ventricular dysfunction coupled with severe coronary artery disease. The decision to pursue further revascularization is challenging. In this setting, viability testing may have a role in this process, but its role is limited by the limited availability of technology and the different aspects of myocardial viability that each technology aims to measure. *CMR*, Cardiac magnetic resonance; *LVEF*, left ventricular ejection fraction; *MUGA*, multigated analysis; *PET*, positron emission tomography.

Intermediate Term Testing (Day 3 to Week 6) After Myocardial Infarction

Traditional Role of Stress Testing

The two most common reasons to perform stress testing are to aid in the diagnosis and prognosis of CAD. In the setting of acute chest pain, stress testing plays a major role as a diagnostic aid to help confirm the presence or absence of underlying CAD when the diagnosis of acute MI has been ruled out by standard emergency department evaluation (see Chapter 6 and Chapter 12).[10] Because most patients with confirmed MI have obstructive CAD, stress testing has no value for diagnostic purposes.

The major goal of stress testing in the setting of acute MI is risk stratification (see Figure 30-2). In contrast to testing for diagnostic purposes, in which medications with antianginal properties are commonly held before testing to enhance test sensitivity, patients with MI are tested on medical therapy. In the pre-reperfusion era, few patients underwent early angiography, because studies demonstrating the benefit of primary PCI and an early invasive strategy had not yet been performed. Stress testing was performed late in the hospital course in most of the population for prognostic purposes to guide decisions regarding the value of coronary angiography. The most important prognostic variables using the standard treadmill test were limited exercise duration and abnormal blood pressure response. ST-segment depression on the exercise ECG was useful to identify increased risk primarily in patients with inferior MI.[11] Studies of MPI reported that delayed redistribution, perfusion defects in more than one vascular region, or increased thallium lung uptake identified high-risk patients.[11] Based on these studies, the clinical paradigm that evolved in the pre-reperfusion era was to perform standard exercise testing or stress imaging to identify patients with poor exercise performance and/or significant ischemia who were candidates for coronary angiography and revascularization.

Stress Testing in the Current Era

Coronary angiography is now performed in most patients with MI as part of primary PCI (see Chapter 17) or delayed invasive management (see Chapter 14) in those with STEMI[1,2] or as part of an early invasive strategy in those with non-STEMI (see Chapter 16).[3,4] As a result, the traditional role of performing stress testing to identify high-risk patients who are candidates for coronary angiography does not apply to patients who undergo immediate or early angiography as part of their treatment. American College of Cardiology Foundation/American Heart Association (ACCF/AHA) guidelines for patients in whom stress testing is recommended are similar for STEMI and non-STEMI, with some minor differences.

Stress Testing in ST-Elevation Myocardial Infarction

Primary PCI or delayed invasive evaluation after fibrinolysis are indicated for most patients with STEMI (see Chapter 13). The sole class I indication for stress testing in the ACCF/AHA

STEMI guideline is limited to the subset of patients without high-risk clinical features who have not undergone early coronary angiography.[1] In addition, it may be reasonable to consider (class IIb indication) stress testing (1) to guide the post-discharge exercise prescription or (2) to evaluate the functional significance of a noninfarcted artery noted on coronary angiography.[1] If stress testing is performed for this purpose, stress imaging is preferred because the exercise ECG cannot localize ischemia.

Stress Testing in ST-Elevation Myocardial Infarction

For patients presenting with NSTEMI, an early invasive approach (between 2 and 72 hours of presentation) is recommended for most patients with ongoing symptoms or indicators of high risk (see Chapter 16).[3] Nevertheless, there are circumstances in which patient preferences are for a noninvasive course of evaluation or the risks of the comorbid conditions and/or the revascularization procedure outweigh the benefits of revascularization. Similar to STEMI, stress testing in patients with NSTEMI is performed primarily in the small subset who are at low to intermediate risk on the basis of clinical risk score (Thrombolysis In Myocardial Infarction [TIMI] score 0 or 1 or Global Registry of Acute Coronary Events [GRACE] score <109), with a stable clinical course, or in whom a noninvasive management strategy is selected for the previously identified reasons. Initial noninvasive evaluation with stress testing may also be preferable in patients with troponin elevation that is suspected to be on the basis of demand ischemia (type 2 MI; see Chapter 1 and Chapter 6) in the clinical setting of other significant comorbidities, such as sepsis or acute renal failure. This approach mitigates against the immediate performance of coronary angiography in such patients. After recovery from the acute illness, stress testing can help guide the decision to proceed with coronary angiography.

Justification for an Ischemia-Guided Approach in Patients with Acute Myocardial Infarction

The rationale supporting current recommendations for stress testing in acute MI is based in large part upon the results of studies from the pre-reperfusion era and the results of studies of stress testing performed in the setting of chronic CAD. The evidence base addressing stress testing in these domains is much more extensive than the relatively small number of studies performed in acute MI in the reperfusion era. The goal of the stress test is to identify potentially high-risk patients among a generally low-risk population on the basis of significant ischemia that develops at a low workload. These patients are then referred for angiography, based upon the assumption that revascularization will result in improved clinical outcome. Although this approach appears logical and is a class I guideline recommendation, there is little evidence to indicate that this approach results in lower mortality or lower risk of re-infarction.

Studies from the pre-reperfusion era upon which this paradigm is partially based involved performing stress testing in most of the acute MI population, which generally was a "sicker" population at high risk.[11] The current subset of MI patients for whom stress testing is recommended represents a very different population. In the setting of chronic CAD, the presence of ischemia has long been regarded as an important variable that influences patient management. However, three stress imaging substudies that were performed as part of recent large randomized trials comparing medical therapy with revascularization, COURAGE (Clinical Outcomes Using Revascularization),[12] BARI-2D (Bypass Angioplasty Revascularization Investigation 2 Diabetes),[13] and STICH (Surgical Treatment for Ischemic Heart Failure),[14] reported that ischemia had no value as a prognostic variable and failed to identify patients who experienced better outcomes if treated with revascularization.[15–17] A common explanation for this observation is that optimal medical therapy is associated with such a low event rate that the rate cannot be lowered further with revascularization.[18] This issue is continuing to be evaluated in the ongoing International Study of Comparative Health Effectiveness with Medical and Invasive Approaches (ISCHEMIA) trial.[19]

There are even less data that address this issue in patients with acute MI. In a subset of the GISSI-2 (Gruppo Italiano per lo Studio della Sopravvivenza nell'Infarto Miocardico 2) trial, the prognostic value of three exercise test scores that incorporated multiple variables was demonstrated in 6251 patients who presented with STEMI and who were treated with thrombolysis. Six-month mortality rates calculated from a modified version of the Duke treadmill score, the most widely applied score, were low risk 0.6%, moderate risk 1.8%, and high risk 3.4% (P <.0001).[20] The SWISSI II (Swiss International Study on Silent Ischemia Type II) trial studied a selected population of patients with recent (<3 months) MI; silent ischemia demonstrated by exercise ECG, which was confirmed by nuclear or echocardiographic imaging; and one- or two-vessel CAD at coronary angiography. Patients were randomized to PCI (n = 96) or medical therapy (n = 105). At a mean follow-up of 10.2 years, the primary endpoint (a composite of cardiac death, nonfatal recurrent MI, or symptom-driven revascularization) was significantly lower in the PCI group (adjusted hazard ratio, 0.33; P <.001).[21] The main limitation of applying the results of this study to broader patient populations relates to the restricted entry criteria (performance of early coronary angiography, one- or two-vessel CAD, and silent ischemia). At the present time, stress testing in the MI setting is performed primarily in low-risk patients who are treated with optimal medical therapy. The ability of stress testing to accurately further risk stratify this generally low-risk patient subset and to identify those who benefit from revascularization remains to be demonstrated.

Types of Stress Testing

Standard Treadmill Testing

Exercise testing can be performed using a treadmill or cycle ergometer. In the United States, the most common modality is the treadmill. Other exercise modalities such as hand crank ergometry are not widely available and are rarely used. The hallmark of an ischemic response is ST-segment depression, defined as ≥1.0 mm horizontal or downsloping ST-segment depression 60 to 80 msec after the J point.[22] ST-segment depression most commonly occurs in the lateral precordial leads. ST-segment depression does not localize the site of myocardial ischemia. ST-segment elevation in leads without Q waves occurs infrequently, but, when it does occur, it can identify the site of myocardial ischemia and usually indicates a high-grade stenosis in the coronary artery that supplies the myocardium in those leads where the ST-segment elevation occurs. In the post-MI patient, ST-segment elevation can occur in leads with Q waves and is considered a nonspecific response. In the pre-reperfusion era, exercise duration and abnormal blood pressure response (defined in various studies as a failure of systolic blood pressure to increase or a decrease with exercise) were the most important prognostic variables.[11] Exercise scores that combine variables can be applied for risk stratification.[22] The most commonly used score is the Duke treadmill score, which can be calculated as:

exercise duration (estimated metabolic equivalents) − maximum ST depression (in millimeters) − angina index

where 0 = no angina; 1 = nonlimiting; and 2 = limiting.

This score was originally developed in patients with chronic CAD and has been extensively validated in this population. There are few data validating its relationship with prognosis post-MI.

Stress Imaging

The two most commonly used types of stress imaging are MPI by single-photon emission computed tomography (SPECT) or positron emission tomography (PET) and stress echocardiography. Stress CMR is also being increasingly performed for post-MI risk stratification. Each of these modalities provides information on LVEF and infarct size. The major role of the stress component of the test is for assessment of the presence and extent of inducible ischemia. The extent and severity of ischemia on nuclear MPI can be expressed as the summed difference score, reflecting the difference between the extent and severity of the perfusion defect on the stress images (summed stress score) and the extent and severity of the perfusion defect on the resting images (summed rest score).[23] The extent and severity of ischemia on stress echocardiography can be expressed as the wall motion score index.[8] With stress, CMR ischemia can be assessed by vasodilator perfusion imaging or dobutamine-induced wall motion abnormality.[24] Stress SPECT and echocardiography can be performed with exercise stress or pharmacologic stress. Sometimes, stress SPECT applies a combination of the two.[25]

Exercise stress is the preferred modality in most patients who are capable of performing adequate exercise, which is generally defined as a minimum workload of 5 to 6 metabolic equivalents (METs). Advantages of exercise over pharmacologic stress include measurement of exercise duration and blood pressure response, both of which are important prognostic variables. Exercise stress also mimics the physical demands that the patient is likely to experience after discharge and can be used as a guide for formulating the exercise prescription for cardiac rehabilitation purposes (see Chapter 34). Pharmacologic stress is usually reserved for patients unable to exercise or those with selected abnormalities on the resting ECG, including left bundle branch block (LBBB) or ventricular pacing. For SPECT, pharmacologic stress has been shown to be more specific in patients with these conduction abnormalities because of the frequent development of false-positive perfusion defects, especially in the septum, that occur as a result of the greater increase in heart rate with exercise.[26] Exercise stress is technically possible with PET and CMR, but it is highly demanding. In practice, stress PET and stress CMR are usually performed with pharmacologic agents.

Vasodilator Myocardial Perfusion Imaging Stress Testing

Most pharmacologic MPI stress testing is performed with agents that activate adenosine receptors. There are multiple adenosine receptor types.[27] Stimulation of the adenosine A2A receptor causes coronary vasodilation, primarily through production of cyclic adenosine monophosphate. The vasodilation results in up to a fourfold increase in myocardial blood flow. In the presence of obstructive CAD, the increase in blood flow is impaired, resulting in heterogeneous increases in flow. Stimulation of adenosine A1 receptors promotes conduction delay through the atrioventricular node and can result in heart block. Stimulation of adenosine A2B, A3, and A4 receptors enhances mast cell degranulation and can result in bronchospasm. Available agents include dipyridamole, adenosine, and regadenoson. Dipyridamole is an indirect coronary vasodilator that inhibits intracellular reuptake and deamination of adenosine. Adenosine is a nonspecific adenosine receptor agonist. Regadenoson is a more specific adenosine A2A receptor agonist, with weak affinity for the A2B and A3 receptors. Currently, regadenoson is the most widely used agent in the United States. Logistically, it is easier to administer, given at a standard dose of 0.4 mg as an intravenous bolus over 10 seconds. Both dipyridamole and adenosine require weight-based dosing and are administered as continuous intravenous infusions over 4 to 6 minutes through an infusion pump. These agents usually cause modest hemodynamic changes, with an average decrease in blood pressure of 10 to 20 mm Hg and a reflex-mediated average increase in heart rate of 10 to 30 beats/min. Approximately 5% of patients experience more severe hemodynamic changes with decreases in systolic blood pressure of ≥35 mm Hg and increases in heart rate of ≥40 beats/min. Methyl xanthines (aminophylline, caffeine) can block or attenuate the effects of these agents and should be held for a minimum of 24 hours before testing. Oral dipyridamole can exaggerate the physiologic effects of regadenoson and adenosine, resulting in significant hypotension and/or heart block, and represents a contraindication to the use of these agents. Other contraindications include significant cardiac conduction system disease (sick sinus syndrome or second- or third-degree heart block, in the absence of a pacemaker), significant obstructive airways disease (active asthma or severe obstructive pulmonary disease, especially if wheezing is present), and hypotension (systolic blood pressure <90 mm Hg). Side effects can occur with all of the agents and may include flushing, light-headedness, headache, dyspnea, chest discomfort, and abdominal discomfort or cramping. Regadenoson causes fewer and less severe side effects than adenosine.[28] A relative advantage of adenosine is its short half-life (<10 seconds), with prompt resolution of side effects, usually within 2 to 3 minutes by simple termination of the infusion. Aminophylline can be administered as an antidote for patients with severe and/or prolonged side effects. Dobutamine can also be used with pharmacologic stress MPI, but it is used much less frequently, being reserved primarily for patients with contraindications to vasodilator agents.

Dobutamine Echocardiography Stress Testing

This test is used mostly outside of the acute MI setting; inotropic stimulation with dobutamine is the most common form of pharmacologic stress echocardiography performed in the United States. Vasodilator stress echocardiography is more commonly performed in parts of Europe and elsewhere. Dobutamine is a synthetic catecholamine that directly stimulates β-1 and β-2 receptors.[29] Stimulation of the β-1 receptors results in an increase in cardiac contractility and heart rate. Stimulation of the β-2 receptors causes vasodilation. Dobutamine also results in mild stimulation of α-1 receptors, which causes vasoconstriction. The vasodilating effects usually dominate over the vasoconstricting effects. Dobutamine is administered intravenously with an infusion pump in increasing incremental doses, starting at 5 to 10 μg/kg per minute and increasing by 10 μg/kg per minute every 3 minutes up to a maximal dose of 40 μg/kg per minute. Dobutamine results in dose-related increases in myocardial contractility and heart rate. The blood pressure response is variable, with a continuous increase in systolic blood pressure in some patients and with an initial increase followed by a decrease in others. Beta-blockers attenuate the physiologic actions of dobutamine. In patients who do not reach the target heart rate (generally 85% of age-predicted maximal heart rate), atropine in doses of 0.25 to 0.50 mg, up to a maximal dose of 2 mg, is commonly administered. Testing can be labor-intensive in some patients. Dobutamine has the potential to cause significant hemodynamic shifts and may be arrhythmogenic. Contraindications include uncontrolled hypertension, atrial tachyarrhythmia with uncontrolled ventricular response rate, history of ventricular tachycardia, or significant LV outflow tract obstruction. Side effects include chest discomfort, dyspnea, palpitations, headache, nausea, and discomfort at the injection site. The plasma half-life is 2 minutes, but the physiologic effects can last for several minutes. The effects can be reversed by administering an intravenous beta-blocker.

Safety and Timing of Stress Testing After Myocardial Infarction

Contraindications to stress testing include acute coronary syndromes that have not been stabilized, uncontrolled significant arrhythmias, severe symptomatic aortic stenosis, acute myocarditis/pericarditis, aortic dissection, and pulmonary embolus.[22] The major concern with performing stress testing in the acute MI setting relates to precipitating a complication, including infarct extension caused by provocation of ischemia or myocardial rupture caused by increased wall stress. The ventricle is also more arrhythmogenic in the acute versus chronic CAD setting, with a greater potential to precipitate a life-threatening ventricular arrhythmia. These concerns are more theoretical and anecdotal than evidence-based. There are limited data addressing stress test complications in the MI setting from the current era.[30,31]

The optimal timing of performing the stress test and the intensity of exercise that should be achieved in terms of maximizing the yield of the test while at the same time minimizing risk are uncertain. The two traditional approaches that have been applied are low-level testing at days 2 to 5 or symptom-limited testing, which is sometimes performed as early as day 5, but is commonly delayed to between 3 and 6 weeks. Low-level testing is usually terminated at a workload of 5 to 6 METs or a heart rate of 120 beats/min. For STEMI patients, U.S. practice guidelines favor pre-discharge low-level testing over delayed symptom-limited testing.[1] Advantages include: (1) potentially identifying high-risk patients who could experience an event before the delayed performance of symptom-limited testing; (2) acquiring information useful for formulating the cardiac rehabilitation exercise prescription; and (3) psychological benefit for the patient. For the specific subset of patients who have undergone successful PCI of the infarct artery and who have significant CAD in other locations, this guideline recommends symptom-limited stress imaging at 3 to 6 weeks. In patients with NSTEMI, practice guidelines recommend symptom-limited testing for low- to intermediate-risk patients with stable clinical courses at 12 to 24 hours for those with unstable angina and at 2 to 5 days for those with NSTEMI.[3]

The timing of performing a pharmacologic stress test is essentially the same as an exercise test. The INSPIRE (Adenosine Sestamibi Post-Infarction Evaluation) trial[31] evaluated the accuracy of adenosine MPI for risk stratification in 728 clinically stable survivors of MI. Median time to testing at the U.S. sites was 2 days, and patients were tested as early as 12 hours. Early administration of regadenoson in the MI setting has not been systematically evaluated, but its use should be similar to adenosine. Both agents should be used with appropriate caution in the MI setting. The Food and Drug Administration (FDA) performed a review of the FDA Adverse Event Reporting System database and identified 26 MI cases and 29 deaths after regadenoson administration between June 2008 and April 2013, and 6 MI cases and 27 deaths after adenosine administration between May 1995 and April 2013.[32] This review prompted the FDA to require changes to the drug labels specifically to recommend against the use of these agents in patients with evidence for acute myocardial ischemia (e.g., unstable angina or cardiovascular instability). The package inserts for both agents also note that seizures have been reported following their administration. Dobutamine is not an FDA-approved agent for cardiac stress testing. Nonetheless, it is commonly used off-label for this purpose. Dobutamine theoretically may be associated with higher risk than vasodilator stress agents, because it stimulates the adrenergic nervous system. Its effects, especially tachycardia when administered with atropine, may be prolonged and challenging to reverse in individual patients. Various sources recommend delaying MI dobutamine stress testing at least until day 3.[8] Clinical experience suggests that all types of stress testing in the acute chest pain population are generally safe when performed at experienced centers with careful supervision.

Selection Between the Standard Treadmill Test and a Stress Imaging Procedure

The major decision influencing selection of a specific stress test most commonly involves the standard exercise treadmill test versus a stress imaging procedure. Stress imaging is more sensitive than the standard treadmill test for diagnostic purposes. However, for prognostic purposes in patients with a normal or a near-normal resting ECG, the standard treadmill test is nearly as accurate as stress imaging for predicting clinical outcome.[33,34] The WOMEN (What is the Optimal Method for Ischemia Evaluation in Women) trial also reported that in middle-aged women at intermediate risk for CAD, the standard treadmill provided results comparable to exercise MPI for purposes of risk stratification.[35] Advantages of the standard treadmill test include lower cost, wider availability, and simplicity. U.S. practice guidelines recommend the standard treadmill test as the "most reasonable" option in patients capable of adequate exercise who have an interpretable resting ECG.[3] Stress imaging is recommended for patients unable to exercise or in those with an uninterpretable ECG, which is defined as baseline ST-segment abnormalities, LV hypertrophy with secondary ST-T changes, paced rhythm, pre-excitation, and digoxin use.[33,34] Patients with LBBB represent a unique subset. Patients who present with acute chest pain and new LBBB are considered to have a variant of STEMI and generally undergo early angiography. Patients with chronic LBBB or paced ventricular rhythm who are at low to intermediate risk are candidates for stress imaging. Exercise MPI in these patients has been shown to have more frequent false-positive perfusion defects, especially in the septum.[26] These patients are preferentially stressed with a vasodilator agent. Stress imaging is also recommended over the standard treadmill test in patients who undergo early coronary angiography and have significant CAD in vessels other than the infarct-related artery. The standard treadmill test cannot localize ischemia. In this setting, a symptom-limited imaging test delayed to 3 to 6 weeks is preferred.[1]

Selection Between Stress Imaging Procedures

There is little direct comparative data that evaluates the different stress imaging modalities. In the setting of chronic CAD, a large meta-analysis reported that outcome of patients with either normal stress MPI or a normal stress echocardiogram is excellent.[36] For most patients, any of the imaging techniques can be used to address the relevant clinical issues. Two of the most practical considerations for selecting between modalities include availability and cost/reimbursement. In institutions where multiple imaging modalities are available, a common recommendation for deciding among them is "local expertise." However, this recommendation generally is of little value because institutions performing multiple modalities usually consider themselves to be "expert" in each modality that they perform. The cost issue is complex and is related to different charges applied in Medicare versus non-Medicare patients and the inpatient versus outpatient setting. Characteristics of the individual patient can be helpful for conferring relative advantages of one technique over another. These advantages for some common clinical characteristics are listed in Table 30-2. The advantages listed for individual techniques for a specific characteristic should be viewed as relative advantages and not absolute recommendations. Contraindications to the use of pharmacologic stress agents also factor into test selection.

Patient age is a consideration for test selection primarily because of the potential impact of radiation exposure.[37,38] Although the minimal radiation exposure associated with increased cancer risk is unknown, there generally is not great concern in performing a single imaging procedure that exposes an older adult patient to ionizing radiation. However, most young MI patients are potentially facing a lifetime of multiple imaging procedures associated with ionizing radiation, including coronary angiography and possible nuclear and CT imaging. For this reason, echocardiography and CMR are advantageous over nuclear techniques in young patients.

As stated earlier, exercise is generally preferred when possible over pharmacologic stress testing. Most laboratories are not capable of performing exercise PET or exercise CMR. Patients with LBBB or paced ventricular rhythm are preferentially studied with vasodilator MPI or CMR. Worsening wall motion in the septum in the presence of LBBB or pacing is less specific because of the conduction abnormality. An analogous situation occurs in patients who have extensive (multiple) regional wall motion abnormalities at rest. Ischemia in this setting is generally more accurately determined by MPI or perfusion CMR. Echocardiographic image quality in patients with obesity or chronic obstructive pulmonary disease can be highly variable, but, in general, is more likely to be technically challenging in these patient subsets.[39] In some patients, quality remains significantly compromised even after contrast administration. Obesity can compromise image quality with any technique, but nuclear MPI or CMR usually are not affected to the same degree as echocardiography. In patients with severe obesity, image quality with the newer SPECT ultrafast camera systems[40,41] or with PET[42] (which has built-in attenuation correction) or CMR[43] is often excellent. Patients with significant renal failure or cardiac devices generally are not candidates for CMR, although technical advances will likely result in changes to these relative contraindications in the future.

TABLE 30-2 Patient Characteristics That Influence Test Selection

PATIENT CHARACTERISTIC	FAVORED TECHNIQUE
Young age	Echo, MRI
Stress modality exercise	Nuclear SPECT, Echo
ECG LBBB or paced ventricular rhythm	Vasodilator SPECT or PET, MRI perfusion
Multiple regional wall motion abnormalities	Nuclear MPI, MRI perfusion
Obesity	Nuclear SPECT or PET, MRI
COPD	Nuclear SPECT or PET, MRI
Renal failure	Echo, Nuclear MPI
Pacemaker or ICD	Echo, Nuclear MPI

COPD, Chronic obstructive pulmonary disease; *ECG*, electrocardiography; *ICD*, implantable cardiac defibrillator; *LBBB*, left bundle branch block; *MPI*, myocardial perfusion imaging; *MRI*, magnetic resonance imaging; *PET*, positron emission tomography; *SPECT*, single-photon emission tomography.

Late Testing (Beyond 6 Weeks) After Myocardial Infarction

Evaluation of Left Ventricular Ejection Fraction for Implantable Cardiac Defibrillator Candidacy

Re-evaluation of LVEF more than 40 days after hospital discharge in patients with initially reduced LVEF $\leq 40\%$ is useful for application of current practice guidelines for implantation of an ICD for primary prevention of sudden death after MI (see Figure 30-3; see also Chapter 28).[1] The rationale to delay the measurement beyond 40 days is to allow the effects of stunning to resolve. As with early assessment of LVEF, any of the techniques can be applied to perform this measurement. In practice, the measurement is most commonly performed with echocardiography. Nuclear techniques or CMR are usually reserved for cases in which the echocardiographic images are technically suboptimal, and sometimes, when the patient and/or cardiologist are equivocal to proceed with ICD implantation and a confirmatory measurement of the LVEF adds more certainty to the decision-making.

Viability Testing

In contemporary cardiovascular medicine there have been great advances in both fields of pharmacotherapeutics and cardiovascular surgical techniques. This progress has led to the development of a challenging clinical scenario—the patient with severe ischemic cardiomyopathy who is receiving optimal medical therapy and is carrying significant surgical risk for complete revascularization. Despite a large volume of available literature in the field, the role for viability testing to help in the decision process remains in question.

Both myocardial stunning and hibernating myocardium represent conditions with reduced myocardial function (see Chapter 24). Myocardial stunning results from acute coronary occlusion.[44] The reduction in blood flow initially causes contractile dysfunction that persists after blood flow is restored. Stunning resolves by 6 weeks. Hibernating myocardium has been described as a myocardial adaptation to a reduction in blood flow; it is significant enough to impair function but not to the extent to produce infarction.[44–46] However, the pathogenesis of myocardial hibernation may be more complex, with examples of reductions in coronary blood flow that follow LV dysfunction rather than preceding it. Ultrastructurally, there are phenotypic changes characterized by loss of sarcomeres and myofibrils that are coupled with changes in the extracellular milieu that typically involve an increase in the deposition of collagenous material in the extracellular matrix. The extent of extracellular fibrosis may predict reversibility of hibernation, with areas of reduced or absent fibrosis that are predictive of functional recovery after revascularization. Recovery of the hibernating myocardium is variable, depending upon the duration and extent of these ultrastructural changes. The time of recovery can be as little as 10 days when there are few structural abnormalities to 6 months and beyond when there is severe ultra-structural derangement. Patients with persistently severely reduced LVEF may be candidates for viability testing. The different imaging modalities rely upon different mechanisms to demonstrate viable myocardium.[47]

Dobutamine echocardiography and CMR depend upon contractile reserve. The classic viability response is initial improvement in wall motion with low-dose dobutamine in a region with reduced function at rest followed by worsening function at higher dose dobutamine as the region becomes ischemic (biphasic response).

Nuclear SPECT MPI with thallium or technetium requires cellular membrane integrity. The myocardial uptake of thallium depends upon an active sodium–potassium adenosine triphosphatase process. Standard stress thallium imaging includes redistribution imaging performed at 3 to 4 hours after stress imaging. Detection of viable myocardium can be enhanced by performing thallium re-injection before obtaining the redistribution images or by performing late imaging delayed to 18 to 24 hours. In contrast to thallium, the cellular uptake of technetium occurs by passive diffusion. This process relies upon intact mitochondrial membranes. Detection of viable myocardium using technetium can be enhanced by administering nitroglycerin before acquiring the resting images.

Nuclear PET requires preserved metabolism to demonstrate myocardial viability. Hibernating myocardium preferentially uses glucose over free fatty acids as the major fuel source. The classic finding is an area of mismatch consisting of reduced perfusion but preserved fluorodeoxyglucose (FDG) uptake.

Perfusion CMR depends upon demonstrating the absence of scar formation to identify viable myocardium. Gadolinium slowly diffuses into the extracellular space in the regions of myocardium scarring. The absence of gadolinium uptake on delayed imaging is consistent with viable myocardium. Literature reviews indicate that among these modalities, the perfusion techniques have higher sensitivity, whereas the dobutamine techniques have a higher specificity for identifying viable myocardium (applied primarily to recovery of regional function after revascularization as the endpoint).[48,49]

Viability Assessment and Coronary Revascularization

Revascularization in patients with significant viability has been shown to improve cardiac function and clinical outcome.[45–49] The evidence supporting these observations is based primarily upon small, observational studies from single centers. The studies in the field have been challenging from a design standpoint, resulting in issues with generalizability and applicability of their results. These challenges arise secondarily to: (1) differences in definition of viability and cutoffs for clinical endpoints used as outcome measures; (2) differences in inclusion criteria for these studies, which culminate in the inability to directly compare studies of viability testing with reasonable validity; (3) heterogeneity in the imaging modalities used in these studies; and (4) lack of description of completeness of revascularization in those patients selected for aggressive revascularization based upon the results of viability testing.

A nonrandomized substudy of STICH trial[14] (see Chapter 25) examined the role of myocardial viability assessment in identifying patients in whom there may be a survival benefit with CABG.[50] Viability testing included SPECT or dobutamine echocardiography. Of the 1212 patients enrolled into STITCH, only 601 underwent viability testing. Unadjusted analysis suggested that the presence of substantial myocardial viability portended a survival benefit, with 63% survival of patients with viability versus 49% survival of patients without viability (P = .003). However, this difference did not persist after adjustment for baseline variables (P = .21). There was no demonstrable interaction between viability, treatment allocation, and survival (P = .53). The results of the STICH viability substudy have been controversial.[46,48,49] There are several limitations to this study. Less than 50% of patients enrolled into STICH underwent viability testing. Viability testing was limited to SPECT or dobutamine echocardiography, and did not include FDG-PET or cardiac CMR. The presence of myocardial viability was measured in a binary fashion, whereas the available evidence suggests that the concept of viability is more of a continuous, progressive process rather than an all or none phenomenon. Finally, integral parameters of ventricular function were not reported, such as ventricular geometry, volumes, wall thickness, and ejection fraction.

The decision to proceed with revascularization, especially CABG, in patients with significantly depressed ventricular function represents a clinical challenge, balancing the risks of the procedure against the potential benefit. Despite the negative results of the STICH viability study, many clinicians find that viability testing can be helpful in this setting. FDG-PET and perfusion CMR predominate as the most favored techniques. In institutions where both modalities are available, either technique can be selected. PET-CMR cameras are becoming increasingly available. Hybrid PET-CMR imaging will likely emerge as the preferred method of viability assessment in the future.

SUMMARY

Noninvasive testing after presentation with MI plays a prominent role in patient management. The specific tests that can be applied include resting and stress echocardiography, standard treadmill testing, stress nuclear imaging using SPECT or PET, and resting and stress MRI. The specific test or tests that are selected in individual patients depends upon the clinical question being addressed, the time course of the acute MI, and specific characteristics of the patient.

References

1. O'Gara PT, et al.: 2013 ACCF/AHA guideline for the management of ST-elevation myocardial infarction: a report of the American College of Cardiology Foundation/American Heart Association Task Force on Practice Guidelines, *Journal of the American College of Cardiology* 61:e78–e140, 2013.
2. Steg PG, et al.: ESC guidelines for the management of acute myocardial infarction in patients presenting with ST-segment elevation, *European Heart Journal* 33:2569–2619, 2012.
3. Amsterdam EA, et al.: 2014 AHA/ACC guideline for the management of patients with non–ST-elevation acute coronary syndromes: a report of the American College of Cardiology/American Heart Association Task Force on Practice Guidelines, *Journal of the American College of Cardiology* 64:e139–e228, 2014.
4. Hamm CW, et al.: ESC guidelines for the management of acute coronary syndromes in patients presenting without persistent ST-segment elevation, *European Heart Journal* 32:2999–3054, 2011.
5. Miller TD, Sciagra R, Gibbons RJ: Application of technetium-99m sestamibi single photon emission computed tomography in acute myocardial infarction: measuring the effect of therapy, *The Quarterly Journal of Nuclear Medicine and Molecular Imaging* 54:213–229, 2010.
6. Botker HE, Kaltoft AK, Pedersen SF, Kim WY: Measuring myocardial salvage, *Cardiovascular Research* 94:266–275, 2012.
7. Silver MT, et al.: A clinical rule to predict preserved left ventricular ejection fraction in patients after myocardial infarction, *Annals of Internal Medicine* 121:750–756, 1994.
8. Flachskampf FA, et al.: Cardiac imaging after myocardial infarction, *European Heart Journal* 32:272–283, 2011.
9. Marra MP, Lima JAC, Iliceto S: MRI in acute myocardial infarction, *European Heart Journal* 32:284–293, 2011.
10. Amsterdam EA, et al.: Testing of low-risk patients presenting to the emergency department with chest pain: a scientific statement from the American Heart Association, *Circulation* 122:1756–1776, 2010.
11. Shaw LJ, et al.: A metaanalysis of predischarge risk stratification after acute myocardial infarction with stress electrocardiographic, myocardial perfusion, and ventricular function imaging, *American Journal of Cardiology* 78:1327–1337, 1996.
12. Boden WE, et al.: Optimal medical therapy with or without PCI for stable coronary disease, *New England Journal of Medicine* 356:1503–1516, 2007.
13. The BARI 2D Study Group: A randomized trial of therapies for type 2 diabetes and coronary artery disease, *New England Journal of Medicine* 360:2503–2515, 2009.
14. Velazquez EJ, et al.: Coronary-artery bypass surgery in patients with left ventricular dysfunction, *New England Journal of Medicine* 364:1607–1616, 2011.
15. Shaw LJ, et al.: Baseline stress myocardial perfusion imaging results and outcomes in patients with stable ischemic heart disease randomized to optimal medical therapy with or without percutaneous coronary intervention, *American Heart Journal* 164:243–250, 2012.
16. Shaw L, et al.: Impact of left ventricular function and the extent of ischemia and scar by stress myocardial perfusion imaging on prognosis and therapeutic risk reduction in diabetic patients with coronary artery disease: results from the Bypass Angioplasty Revascularization Investigation 2 Diabetes (BARI 2D) trial, *Journal of Nuclear Cardiology* 19:658–669, 2012.
17. Panza JA, et al.: Inducible myocardial ischemia and outcomes in patients with coronary artery disease and left ventricular dysfunction, *Journal of the American College of Cardiology* 61:1860–1870, 2013.
18. Fang JC: Underestimating medical therapy for coronary disease, *Again. New England Journal of Medicine* 364:1671–1673, 2011.
19. ClinicalTrials.gov. International Study of Comparative Health Effectiveness with Medical and Invasive Approaches (ISCHEMIA). https://clinicaltrials.gov/ct2/show/NCT01471522.
20. Villella M, et al.: Ergometric score systems after myocardial infarction: prognostic performance of the Duke Treadmill Score, Veterans Administration Medical Center Score, and of a novel score system, GISSI-2 index, in a cohort of survivors of acute myocardial infarction, *American Heart Journal* 145:475–483, 2003.
21. Erne P, et al.: Effects of percutaneous coronary interventions in silent ischemia after myocardial infarction: the SWISSI II randomized controlled trial, *JAMA* 297:1985–1991, 2007.
22. Fletcher GF, et al.: Exercise standards for testing and training: a scientific statement from the American Heart Association, *Circulation* 128:873–934, 2013.
23. Shaw L, et al.: Prognosis in the era of comparative effectiveness research: where is nuclear cardiology now and where should it be? *Journal of Nuclear Cardiology* 19:1026–1043, 2012.
24. Heydari B,Y, Kwong R: Cardiac magnetic resonance imaging for ischemic heart disease: update on diagnosis and prognosis, *Topics in Magnetic Resonance Imaging* 23:21–31, 2014.
25. Elhendy AA, Gregory SA, Holly TA, Vitola JV: ASNC clinical update. Combined pharmacologic and low-level exercise stress protocols for radionuclide myocardial perfusion imaging, *Journal of Nuclear Cardiology* 16:163–166, 2009.
26. Henzlova MJ, et al.: ASNC imaging guidelines for nuclear cardiology procedures. Stress protocols and tracers, *Journal of Nuclear Cardiology* 16:331–343, 2009.
27. Chen J-F, Eltzschig HK, Fredholm BB: Adenosine receptors as drug targets–what are the challenges? *Nature Reviews Drug Discovery* 12:265–286, 2013.
28. Iskandrian AE, et al.: Adenosine versus regadenoson comparative evaluation in myocardial perfusion imaging: Results of the ADVANCE Phase 3 Multicenter International Trial, *Journal of Nuclear Cardiology* 14:645–658, 2007.
29. Gilstrap LG, Bhatia RS, Weiner RB, Dudzinski DM: Dobutamine stress echocardiography: a review and update, *Research Reports in Clinical Cardiology* 5:69–81, 2014.
30. Karha J, et al.: Safety of stress testing during the evolution of unstable angina pectoris or non–ST-elevation myocardial infarction, *The American Journal of Cardiology* 94:1537–1539, 2004.
31. Mahmarian JJ, et al.: A multinational study to establish the value of early adenosine technetium-99m sestamibi myocardial perfusion imaging in identifying a low-risk group for early hospital discharge after acute myocardial infarction, *Journal of the American College of Cardiology* 48:2448–2457, 2006.
32. US Food and Drug Administration: FDA warns of rare but serious risk of heart attack and death with cardiac nuclear stress test drugs Lexiscan (regadenoson) and Adenosan (adenosine). http://www.fda.gov/downloads/Drugs/DrugSafety/UCM375668.pdf.
33. Fihn SD, et al.: 2012 ACCF/AHA/ACP/AATS/PCNA/SCAI/STS guideline for the diagnosis and management of patients with stable ischemic heart disease: a report of the American College of Cardiology Foundation/American Heart Association Task Force on Practice Guidelines, and the American College of Physicians, American Association for Thoracic Surgery, Preventive Cardiovascular Nurses Association, Society for Cardiovascular Angiography and Interventions, and Society of Thoracic Surgeons, *Circulation* 126:e354–e471, 2012.
34. Wolk MJ, et al.: ACCF/AHA/ASE/ASNC/HFSA/HRS/SCAI/SCCT/SCMR/STS 2013 multimodality appropriate use criteria for the detection and risk assessment of stable ischemic heart disease: a report of the American College of Cardiology Foundation Appropriate Use Criteria Task Force, American Heart Association, American Society of Echocardiography, American Society of Nuclear Cardiology, Heart Failure Society of America, Heart Rhythm Society, Society for Cardiovascular Angiography and Interventions, Society of Cardiovascular Computed Tomography, Society for Cardiovascular Magnetic Resonance, and Society of Thoracic Surgeons, *Journal of the American College of Cardiology* 63:380–406, 2014.
35. Shaw LJ, et al.: Comparative effectiveness of exercise electrocardiography with or without myocardial perfusion single photon emission computed tomography in women with suspected coronary artery disease: results from the What Is the Optimal Method for Ischemia Evaluation in Women (WOMEN) Trial, *Circulation* 124:1239–1249, 2011.
36. Metz LD, et al.: The prognostic value of normal exercise myocardial perfusion imaging and exercise echocardiography: a meta-analysis, *Journal of the American College of Cardiology* 49:227–237, 2007.
37. Mark DB, et al.: ACC/AHA/ASE/ASNC/HRS/IAC/Mended Hearts/NASCI/RSNA/SAIP/SCAI/SCCT/SCMR/SNMMI 2014 health policy statement on use of noninvasive cardiovascular imaging: a report of the American College of Cardiology Clinical Quality Committee, *Journal of the American College of Cardiology* 63:698–721, 2014.
38. Fazel R, et al.: Approaches to enhancing radiation safety in cardiovascular imaging: a scientific statement from the American Heart Association, *Circulation* 130:1730–1748, 2014.
39. Supariwala A, et al.: Feasibility and prognostic value of stress echocardiography in obese, morbidly obese, and super obese patients referred for bariatric surgery, *Echocardiography* 31:879–885, 2014.
40. Gimelli A, et al.: Evaluation of ischaemia in obese patients: feasibility and accuracy of a low-dose protocol with a cadmium-zinc Telluride camera, *European Journal of Nuclear Medicine and Molecular Imaging* 39:1254–1261, 2012.
41. Nakazato R, et al.: Quantitative high-efficiency cadmium-zinc-Telluride SPECT with dedicated parallel-hole collimation system in obese patients: results of a multi-center study, *Journal of Nuclear Cardiology* 22:266–275, 2015.
42. Chow BJW, et al.: Prognostic value of PET myocardial perfusion imaging in obese patients, *JACC: Cardiovascular Imaging* 7:278–287, 2014.
43. Shah RV, et al.: Vasodilator stress perfusion CMR imaging is feasible and prognostic in obese patients, *JACC: Cardiovascular Imaging* 7:462–472, 2014.
44. Canty Jr JM, Suzuki G: Myocardial perfusion and contraction in acute ischemia and chronic ischemic heart disease, *Journal of Molecular and Cellular Cardiology* 52:822–831, 2012.
45. Lim SP, McArdle BA, Beanlands RS, Hessian RC: Myocardial viability: it is still alive, *Seminars in Nuclear Medicine* 44:358–374, 2014.
46. Shah BN, Khattar RS, Senior R: The hibernating myocardium: current concepts, diagnostic dilemmas, and clinical challenges in the post-STICH Era, *European Heart Journal* 34:1323–1336, 2013.
47. Arrighi J, Dilsizian V: Multimodality imaging for assessment of myocardial viability: nuclear, echocardiography, MR, and CT, *Current Cardiology Reports* 14:234–243, 2012.
48. Bax J, Delgado V: Myocardial viability as integral part of the diagnostic and therapeutic approach to ischemic heart failure, *Journal of Nuclear Cardiology* 22:229–245, 2015.
49. Allman K: Noninvasive assessment myocardial viability: current status and future directions, *Journal of Nuclear Cardiology* 20:618–637, 2013.
50. Bonow RO, et al.: Myocardial viability and survival in ischemic left ventricular dysfunction, *New England Journal of Medicine* 364:1617–1625, 2011.

31 Echocardiography in Patients with Myocardial Infarction

Anique Ducharme and Jean-Claude Tardif

INTRODUCTION

Echocardiography is a rapid, noninvasive, portable, and inexpensive imaging modality, making it the preferred technique for the assessment of patients with myocardial infarction (MI).[1] The echocardiographic evaluation focuses on the functional outcome of coronary artery disease (CAD), evaluation of global and segmental wall motion, and the complications of MI.[2]

This chapter focuses on the role of echocardiography in patients with MI, for its assessment, the diagnosis of complications, and risk stratification. The use of echocardiography for the evaluation of chest pain in the emergency department is discussed elsewhere in this book (see Chapter 9). Selection from among echocardiography and other alternative imaging approaches for structural and ischemic evaluation after MI is addressed in Chapter 30.

Ischemia results from an abnormal myocardial oxygen supply-to-demand ratio. The first physiologic abnormalities to emerge (Figure 31-1) are cellular biochemical changes, followed by a perfusion defect and then diastolic dysfunction and, shortly afterward, impairment of regional systolic wall thickening and motion. The ischemic electrocardiographic changes and clinical symptoms of angina (if they appear) are late manifestations of ischemia. In light of this sequence of events, echocardiography represents a unique and sensitive tool for early detection of myocardial ischemia.[2] It may be difficult to discriminate regional wall motion abnormalities (RWMAs) caused by acute ischemia from those due to a previous MI, but the preservation of normal wall thickness and echogenicity suggests an acute event, whereas a thin akinetic, reflective segment is associated with chronicity. Furthermore, the presence of reversible RWMAs and changes on the electrocardiogram (ECG) suggests reversible ischemia; recovery of segmental wall function after disappearance of chest pain may take from several minutes for ischemic episodes of short duration (10 minutes or less) to days in patients with prolonged ischemia, a phenomenon called *myocardial stunning* (see Chapter 4).

INFARCT SIZE AND LOCALIZATION

Wall Motion and Electrocardiographic Infarct Location

ECG changes do not always correlate with the quantity of damaged myocardium, and the extent of the dysfunction often is considerably greater than expected relative to the size of the necrotic area, because it encompasses not only the zone of the actual infarct but also stunned and hibernating segments and dysfunction from previous coronary events. Consequently, echocardiography is a better predictor of the extent and location of the MI and associated ventricular dysfunction than the ECG. This observation is especially true in inferior MI, because the septum is not assessed well by electrocardiographic modalities.[3] When an anterior MI is identified on the ECG, at least one of the anterior segments will exhibit RWMA on echocardiography, with the extent of the dysfunction being determined by the level at which the obstruction occurs in the left anterior descending coronary artery. If the obstruction is located proximal to the first septal perforator, all of the segments of the anterior septum, the anterior wall, and the apex will be affected, whereas obstruction distal to the first septal perforator usually spares the basal segments of the anterior septum and anterior wall. The sensitivity and specificity of the 12-lead ECG for the detection of an apical MI are low despite meeting several well-characterized ECG criteria, whereas apical involvement is clearly identified and quantified by echocardiography.[2] The presence of Q waves is associated with a larger area and more severe degree of apical dysfunction, and persistent ST-segment elevation may be associated with a left ventricular aneurysm on the echocardiogram.[4]

Echocardiography and Coronary Anatomy

Using correlative studies with coronary angiography and echocardiography in patients with acute MI, the specific coronary artery perfusing each segment of the left ventricle was determined (Figure 31-2).

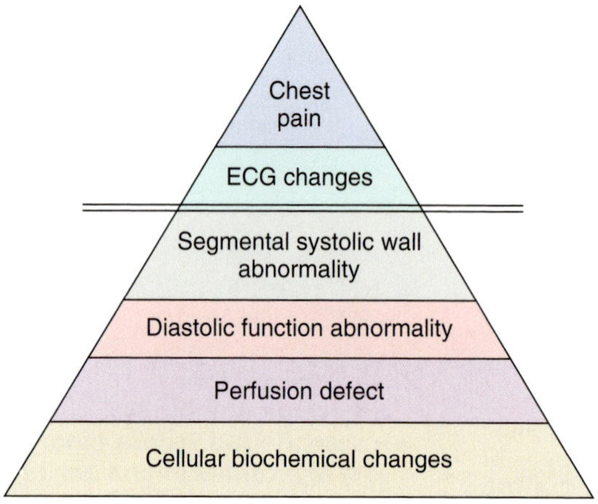

FIGURE 31-1 The sequence of events during myocardial ischemia. *ECG,* Electrocardiogram. *(From Diaz A, Ducharme A, Tardif JC: Echocardiography in acute coronary syndromes. In Théroux P, editor:* Acute coronary syndromes, *Saunders, Philadelphia, 2011.)*

The early stage of a nonrevascularized acute MI is characterized on echocardiography by decreased amplitude of regional endocardial excursion with normal wall thickness, followed in 4 to 6 weeks by wall thinning in the affected region and often increased echogenicity secondary to a fibrotic response. Studies have found good correlation between histologic evidence of infarction and the presence of segmental dysfunction on echocardiography in more than 90% of cases.[5] Experimentally, necrosis of 20% or less of the wall thickness results in a decrease in systolic thickening of approximately 50%, whereas necrosis of more than 20% of the thickness is uniformly associated with systolic thinning, with the extent of RWMAs shown by echocardiography shortly after coronary occlusion (up to 2 days) correlating well with actual infarct size. Echocardiography can overestimate infarct size, however, because of contractile abnormalities ("tethering") in the noninfarcted myocardium immediately adjacent to the severely ischemic regions. Accordingly, transthoracic imaging (i.e., transthoracic echocardiography [TTE]) can identify the location and extent of myocardial infarction (Videos 31-1, 31-2, 31-3, 31-4, and 31-5).

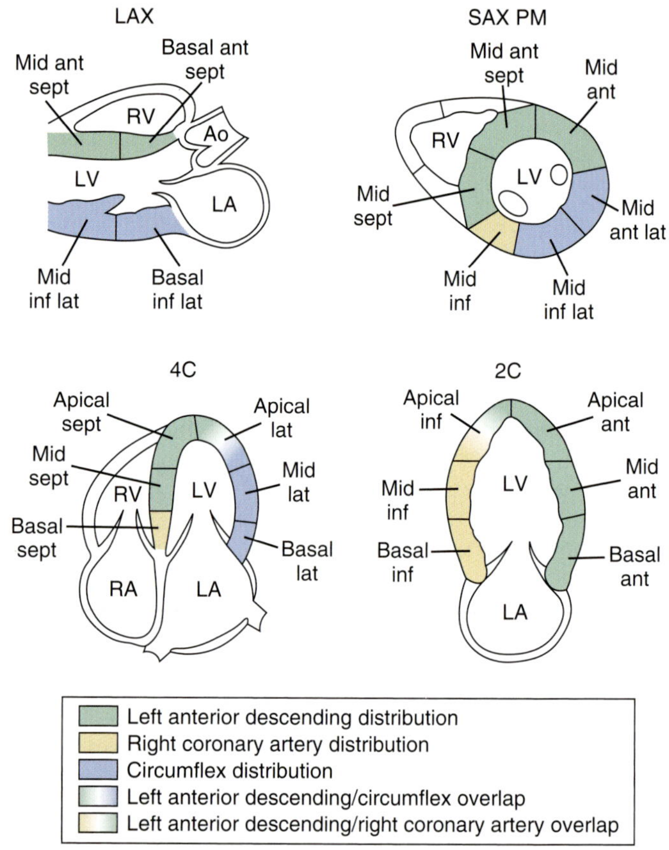

FIGURE 31-2 Diagrammatic representation of coronary perfusion of the 16 left ventricular segments. In the *parasternal long-axis view* (LAX), the anterior interventricular septum is perfused by the left anterior descending artery (LAD), the first 1 to 2 cm being perfused by the first septal perforator, allowing determination of whether the obstruction is proximal or distal to this LAD branch. The inferolateral wall usually is perfused by the circumflex artery. In the *parasternal short-axis view* (SAX), the LAD supplies the anterior wall and the anterior septum, the circumflex artery supplies the lateral wall, and the right coronary artery (RCA) supplies the inferior septum and inferior wall. In the *apical two-chamber view* (2C), the anterior wall is perfused by the LAD, the inferior wall is supplied by the RCA, and the apex often has a dual coronary supply. In the *apical four-chamber view* (4C), the mid-septum is perfused by the LAD, the basal septum usually is part of the RCA, and the apex usually is perfused by the LAD, with the basal and mid-lateral walls being supplied by the circumflex artery. *SAX PM,* Parasternal short-axis view at the papillary muscle level. *(From Diaz A, Ducharme A, Tardif JC: Echocardiography in acute coronary syndromes. In Théroux P, editor:* Acute coronary syndromes, *Saunders, Philadelphia, 2011.)*

Echocardiography After Reperfusion Therapy

Restoration of antegrade flow after pharmacologic or mechanical reperfusion usually is associated with improved wall motion, fewer complications, and decreased mortality. The extent of functional recovery is related to the duration of the occlusion, the extent of the ischemic zone, and the success of reperfusion. Recovery usually occurs 24 hours to 10 days after reperfusion but may take up to 6 weeks if stunning is present (see Chapter 4 and Chapter 32).[5] The stunned myocardium has had, by definition, flow restored (by angioplasty or thrombolysis or spontaneously) yet remains temporarily dysfunctional. Echocardiography combined with low-dose inotropic stimulation with dobutamine (5 to 10 μg/kg/min) can be used to distinguish stunned myocardium after revascularization from nonviable myocardium (see Stress Echocardiography).[6] Patency of the infarct-related coronary artery, as seen within days of the acute MI, has been associated with an improvement in regional function and attenuation of left ventricular dilation 1 to 6 months after the initial event; by contrast, adverse remodeling of the left ventricular wall will continue to increase in patients without successful reperfusion.[7]

Angiographic restoration of flow in an epicardial artery does not accurately reflect perfusion at the microvascular level.[8] The lack of myocardial reperfusion despite restored epicardial flow is referred to as the "no-reflow" phenomenon (see Chapter 24).[8] Adequacy of myocardial blood flow after either pharmacologic or mechanical revascularization can be assessed using contrast echocardiography of the myocardium, in addition to the classic clinical and ECG parameters. Myocardial contrast techniques have shown good correlation with angiographic methods of assessing microvascular reperfusion in patients with acute MI, such as the corrected Thrombolysis In Myocardial Infarction (TIMI) frame count (cTFC), TIMI myocardial perfusion grade (TMPG), and TIMI myocardial blush grade.[9]

ASSESSMENT OF LEFT VENTRICULAR FUNCTION

Evaluation of Systolic Left Ventricular Function

A reduced left ventricular ejection fraction (LVEF) after MI is a strong predictor of poor outcome. An immediate decline in left ventricular systolic function may be observed with onset of necrosis, but further adverse remodeling of the left ventricle due to infarct expansion also can occur (see Chapter 4 and Chapter 36). Such remodeling is characterized by the enlargement of the primary hypokinetic/akinetic zone and left ventricular dilation, potentially leading to the development of heart failure. Initially enlarged left ventricular volumes are suggestive of extensive myocardial injury, but sequential echocardiograms may be required for detection of adverse left ventricular remodeling; left ventricular systolic function also can improve over time after a reperfused MI. In patients with at least moderate ventricular dysfunction early after MI, reevaluation of LVEF approximately 40 days later is needed to determine whether implantation of a cardiac defibrillator is warranted (see Chapter 28).[10]

Qualitative and Semiquantitative Evaluation of Left Ventricular Systolic Function

Global and regional ventricular function can be evaluated with echocardiography. A few seconds after coronary occlusion, decreases in the amplitude of endocardial excursion and wall thickening become apparent in the area supplied by the obstructed artery; the abnormality is defined as *hypokinesis* when contraction normally is directed but reduced in magnitude, *akinesis* when it is absent, or *dyskinesis* when systolic bulging is present.

Wall Motion Score Index

Semiquantitative assessment of regional left ventricular contraction is provided by the wall motion score index (WMSI). The American Heart Association (AHA), as part of an effort to unify wall motion analysis among various imaging modalities, recommended a 17-segment model when perfusion is assessed, but the 16-segment model (Figure 31-2) remains clinically recommended for functional imaging, because the apical cap does not contract.[11] The various echocardiographic views permit visualization of regions of the myocardium perfused by the different coronary artery branches (Figure 31-3). Professional society recommendations[11] suggest that a score be assigned to each segment according to its contractility, as follows: (1) normal or hyperkinetic, (2) hypokinetic, (3) akinetic (absent or negligible thickening), and (4) dyskinetic (systolic thinning or stretching, e.g., aneurysm). In contrast with previous recommendations, clinicians should refrain from assigning a separate wall motion score for aneurysm; furthermore, no specific score has been designated for compensatory hyperkinesis. The WMSI is equal to the sum of the regional scores divided by the number of evaluable segments and can range between 1 (for normal ventricular contraction) and 3.9 (for severe systolic dysfunction) (Figure 31-4). A good correlation exists between the echocardiographic WMSI and the LVEF measured by radionuclide ventriculography. A WMSI of 1.7 or higher usually suggests dysfunction involving greater than 20% of the left ventricle after acute MI. In addition, the WMSI has important prognostic value, with a significantly higher mortality rate in the group with the most abnormal score than in patients with favorable ones (61% versus 3%).[2]

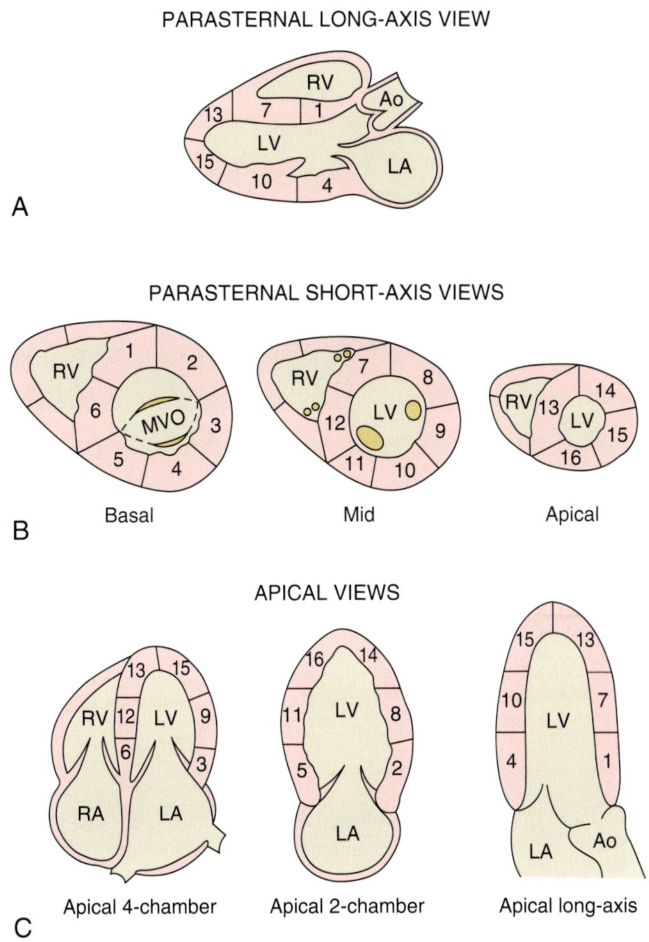

FIGURE 31-3 Schematic of the 16 segments of the left ventricle (LV), as described by the American Society of Echocardiography. (A) Parasternal long-axis view. **(B)** Parasternal short-axis views. **(C)** Apical views. The numbers in the diagram correspond to the following segments: *1,* basal anteroseptum; *2,* basal anterior wall; *3,* basal anterolateral wall; *4,* basal inferolateral wall; *5,* basal inferior wall; *6,* basal inferior septum; *7,* mid-anterior septum; *8,* mid-anterior wall; *9,* mid-anterolateral wall; *10,* mid-inferolateral wall; *11,* mid-inferior wall; *12,* mid-inferior septum; *13,* septal apex; *14,* anterior apex; *15,* lateral apex; *16,* inferior apex. *Ao,* Aorta; *LA,* left atrium; *MVO,* mitral valve orifice; *RA,* right atrium; *RV,* right ventricle. *(From Diaz A, Ducharme A, Tardif JC: Echocardiography in acute coronary syndromes. In Théroux P, editor:* Acute coronary syndromes, *Saunders, Philadelphia, 2011.)*

Because CAD causes segmental dysfunction, which can be accompanied by compensatory hyperkinesis of nonischemic segments, regional assessment of systolic function is more sensitive than global approaches. Nevertheless, determination of the LVEF is part of a standard examination. The correlation between the visual echocardiographic estimation and the radionuclide determination of LVEF is good, but *visual assessment* requires experience, and clinicians should validate their own performance with quantitative methods.

Quantitative Evaluation of Global Left Ventricular Systolic Function

Global quantitative evaluation is based on endocardial border tracing, with or without epicardial border tracing, at end diastole and end systole in several views. Assessment is based on either analysis of wall motion (endocardial excursion) or wall thickening (interface separation). Evaluation of regional wall thickening is not influenced by cardiac

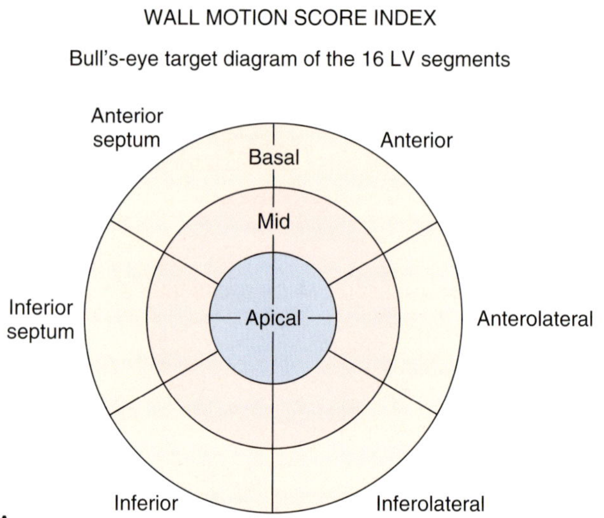

A

Wall motion score

1. Normal/hyperkinesia
2. Hypokinesia
3. Akinesia
4. Dyskinesia

B

$$\text{WMSI} = \frac{\text{Sum of wall motion scores}}{\text{Number of segments evaluated}}$$

C

FIGURE 31-4 (**A**) The 16 segments of the left ventricle displayed in a bull's-eye diagram. (**B**) The wall motion score, which assigns a number according to the contractile function of each segment. (**C**) The wall motion score index (WMSI) is obtained by dividing the sum of the scores for evaluable segments by the number of segments evaluated. *LV,* Left ventricular. *(From Diaz A, Ducharme A, Tardif JC: Echocardiography in acute coronary syndromes. In Théroux P, editor:* Acute coronary syndromes, *Saunders, Philadelphia, 2011.)*

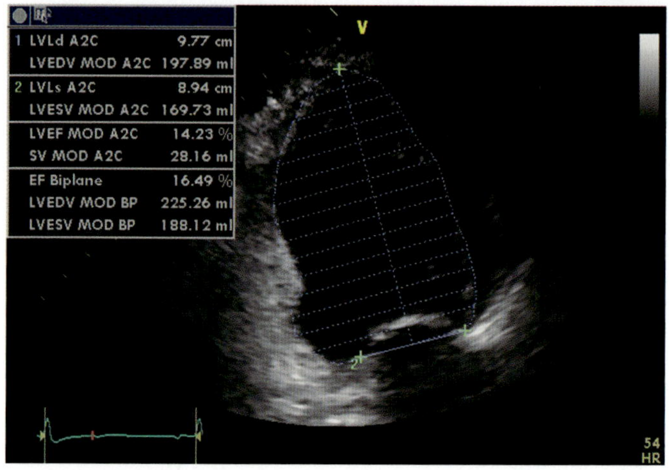

FIGURE 31-5 Evaluation of left ventricular (LV) volumes and systolic function using the Simpson's method of disks. The LV endocardial borders are traced at end systole and end diastole in two orthogonal views, the apical four- and two-chamber views, and the LV ejection fraction (LVEF) is derived.

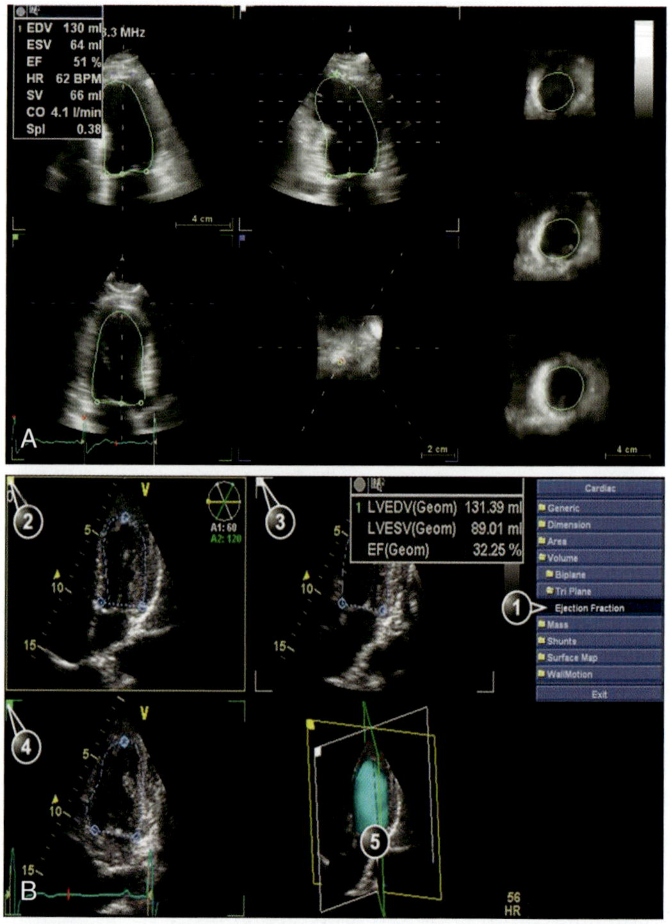

FIGURE 31-6 Three-dimensional model of left ventricular (LV) function. (**A**) Automated determination of LV ejection fraction (LVEF) using volumetric assessment and multislice (5 to 12) short-axis volumes. (**B**) Three-dimensional full volume of the left ventricle can be processed from apical four-chamber, two-chamber, and long-axis views with special analytical software to create a dynamic three-dimensional cast.

translation or rotation, as opposed to wall motion, but requires excellent definition of the endocardial and epicardial borders, which constitutes its major limitation.

Determination of left ventricular cavity dimensions is an important component of evaluation of wall thickening. Volume estimations are based on geometric assumptions about ventricular shape, which range from a simple ellipsoid to a complex hemicylindrical, hemiellipsoid shape. Descriptions of each geometric shape and the corresponding formula and requirements are beyond the scope of this chapter. The American Society of Echocardiography (ASE) recommendations for chamber quantification favor the *modified Simpson's biplane* method of disks for left ventricular volumes and LVEF.[11] This method involves tracing of the endocardial borders in the apical four-chamber and two-chamber views, at end systole and end diastole (Figure 31-5 and Videos 31-6, 31-7, 31-8, and 31-9). Determination of the left ventricular end-diastolic (EDV) and end-systolic (ESV) volumes allows calculation of the stroke volume (EDV – ESV = SV), cardiac output (SV × heart rate), and ejection fraction ([SV/EDV] × 100). In patients whose echograms have good image quality, three-dimensional echocardiography–based measurements are accurate and reproducible and should be used when available and feasible[12] (Figures 31-6 and 31-7 and Videos 31-10, 31-11, 31-12, and 31-13). Three-dimensional echocardiography has been shown to be superior to standard two-dimensional echocardiography for determination of left ventricular volumes and mass, using cardiac magnetic resonance imaging (MRI) as the gold standard.[21] In patients with LVEF less than 40%, three-dimensional echocardiography–derived EDV, ESV, and LVEF gave excellent correlation with MRI (r = 0.98 for EDV, 0.99 for ESV, and 0.97 for LVEF; $P < .0001$)—better than with two-dimensional echocardiography.[22]

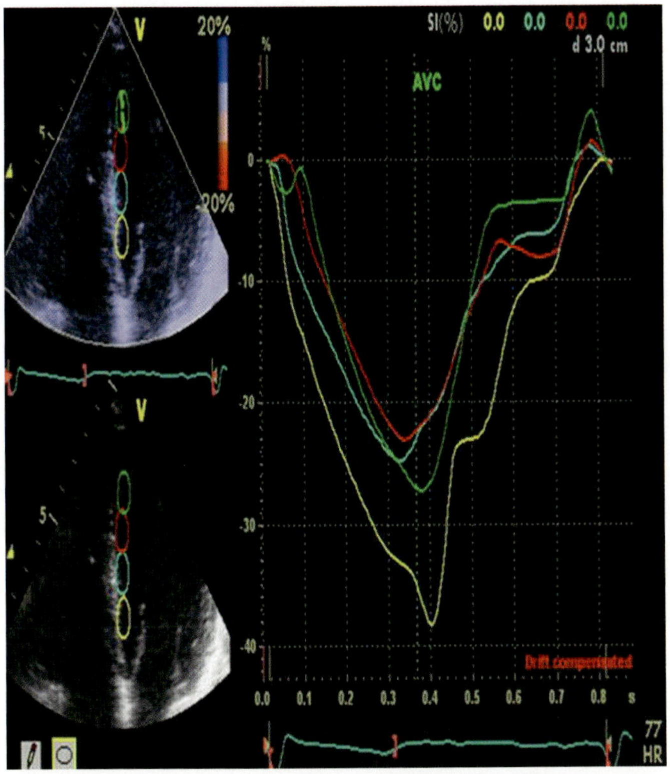

FIGURE 31-7 Assessment of myocardial mechanics using myocardial tissue Doppler imaging (TDI). Apical four-chamber view from echocardiogram in a normal patient showing myocardial TDI and the derived velocity profiles from four septal segments. TDI uses the pulsed-wave Doppler method, modified to record the low-velocity and high-amplitude signals from tissue, to measure the velocity and timing of myocardial motion. Different velocity profiles are obtained, called peak systolic filling (S_{1m}, S_{2m}; negative deflection), peak diastolic rapid filling (E_m), and atrial contraction (A_m; positive deflection). Curve color corresponds to sample volume location (*color ovals*). *AVC,* Aortic valve closure.

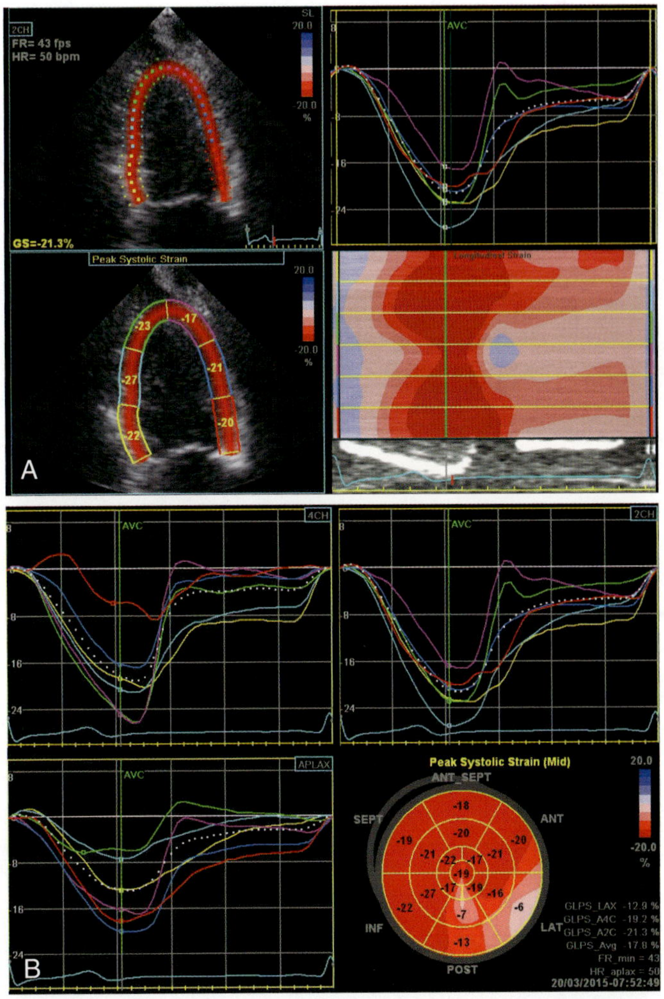

FIGURE 31-8 Assessment of myocardial mechanics using speckle-tracking echocardiography (SPE) techniques. (**A**) Normal peak longitudinal strain measured by SPE, two-dimensional strain (GE Healthcare, Milwaukee, Wisc.); the tracking and parametric images results are on the *left* and the results curves in the *upper right panel*. (**B**) Peak longitudinal strain measured by SPE, two-dimensional strain, from the apical four-chamber (4CH, *upper left panel*), two-chamber (2CH, *upper right panel*), and three-chamber (*lower left panel*) views, with bull's-eye representation of the midwall peak systolic strain (*lower right panel*). The *dotted white lines* show a reduced global longitudinal (peak) strain (GLPS) averaged from the inferoseptal (*red line,* 4CH) and inferolateral (*yellow, blue,* and *green curves,* APLAX) walls (global strain = −12.9% in LAX). The *bull's-eye* demonstrates RWMAs of the lateral and posterior walls (*light pink*). *APLAX,* Apical long-axis view; *AVC,* aortic valve closure (for event timing); *bpm,* beats/min; *FR,* frame rate; *HR,* heart rate; *RWMAs,* regional wall motion abnormalities.

Quantification of Regional Wall Motion using Doppler and Speckle-Tracking Echocardiography

Quantification of regional myocardial function currently is based on myocardial tissue Doppler imaging (TDI) or speckle-tracking echocardiography (STE) techniques. TDI uses pulsed-wave Doppler methods (modified to record the low-velocity, high-amplitude signals from tissue) to measure the velocity and timing of myocardial motion. Because Doppler signals are angle-dependent, the apical views usually are chosen. Different velocity profiles are obtained, called peak systolic velocity (S_1m, S_2m), peak diastolic rapid filling (E_m), and atrial contraction (A_m) (Figure 31-7). Although reasonably well correlated with global left ventricular function, these measures are limited by preload and afterload dependence[13] and are sensitive to inotropic stimulation and ischemia.[24] Because velocity and motion are measured relative to the transducer, measurements may be influenced by tethering or overall heart motion. Accordingly, the use of deformation parameters such as strain and strain rate is preferable.

Global Longitudinal Strain and Strain Rate[14]

Strain describes the deformation of an object normalized to its original shape and size. *Strain rate* reflects the speed of myocardial deformation. Strain is a dimensionless entity, reported as a percentage that represents the movement of one tissue site relative to another and permits differentiaton between movement caused by tethering of adjacent tissues and normal motion, which is crucial in dealing with CAD. The most commonly used strain-based measure of left ventricular long-axis systolic function is the *global longitudinal strain* (GLS), usually assessed by STE.[14] On two-dimensional echocardiography, peak GLS describes the relative length change of the left ventricular myocardium between end diastole and end systole.

Strain (%) = $(L_t - L_0)/L_0$, where L_t = length at time t and L_0 = initial length at time 0, usually taken at end diastole.

$$\textit{Strain Rate} = \frac{(L_t - L_0)/L_0}{\Delta t},$$ where Δt = time required for the change in length.

GLS (%) = $(ML_s - ML_d)/ML_d$, where MLs = myocardial length at end systole and ML_d = myocardial length at end diastole.

After optimizing image quality, maximizing frame rate, and minimizing foreshortening, which all are critical to reduce measurement variability, GLS measurements should be made in the three standard apical views and averaged[15] (Figure 31-8 and Videos 31-14 and 31-15).

Midwall GLS is a sensitive measure of myocardial injury and correlates better with infarct size than LVEF.[16,17] In addition, ischemia may lead to inhomogeneous ventricular electrical conduction and contraction, a phenomenon called *mechanical dispersion,* which can be detected by strain; it is measured as the standard deviation of the time from the peak R-wave to peak negative strain and is predictor of arrhythmic events late after MI (beyond 40 days), independently of LVEF.[18] This parameter may be particularly interesting in patients with relatively preserved LVEF, for whom a cardiac defibrillator is not indicated (in accordance with accepted guidelines).[10] Because GLS offers incremental predictive value in patients undergoing echocardiography after MI, it should be measured clinically, in view of the ease of obtaining this additional information.[19,20]

Regional (Longitudinal and Radial) Strain and Strain Rate Imaging

Similar to global strain, regional deformation measurements may differ in amplitude depending on not only the myocardial region being evaluated but also the system and method used and sample volume definition.[14] Independent of strain magnitude, characteristic changes in temporal pattern of myocardial deformation can be assessed as well (Figure 31-9).

Longitudinal shortening or radial thickening of the myocardium after aortic valve closure (polysystolic shortening or thickening, sometimes referred to as *tardokinesis*) of more than 20% of the total deformation during the cardiac cycle is a consistent sign of regional functional inhomogeneity (e.g., ischemia, scar).[4,14] Furthermore, during angioplasty, strain decreased considerably in 94% of the patients,[27] suggesting a good sensitivity to ischemia. One of the most interesting aspects of strain and strain rate is their independence from tethering,[11] with close correlation with cardiac magnetic resonance tissue tagging for GLS ($r = -0.87$) and global radial strain ($r = -0.92$) on strain rate imaging (SRI) studies.[13]

Contrast Echocardiography

Despite improved ultrasound imaging, up to 20% of patients have suboptimal endocardial border definition for quantitative assessment of LVEF.[21] Contrast echocardiography can be used to improve the delineation of the endocardial borders, using lipid-shelled, gas-filled encapsulated microbubbles (Figure 31-10 and Videos 31-8 and 31-9). Such microspheres are clinically available in most echocardiographic laboratories for left ventricular cavity opacification or diagnosis of mural thrombus or left ventricular aneurysm.[22] In the acute coronary syndrome (ACS) setting, left ventricular opacification also offers the advantage of better assessment of left ventricular RWMAs, by increasing the number of interpretable segments.

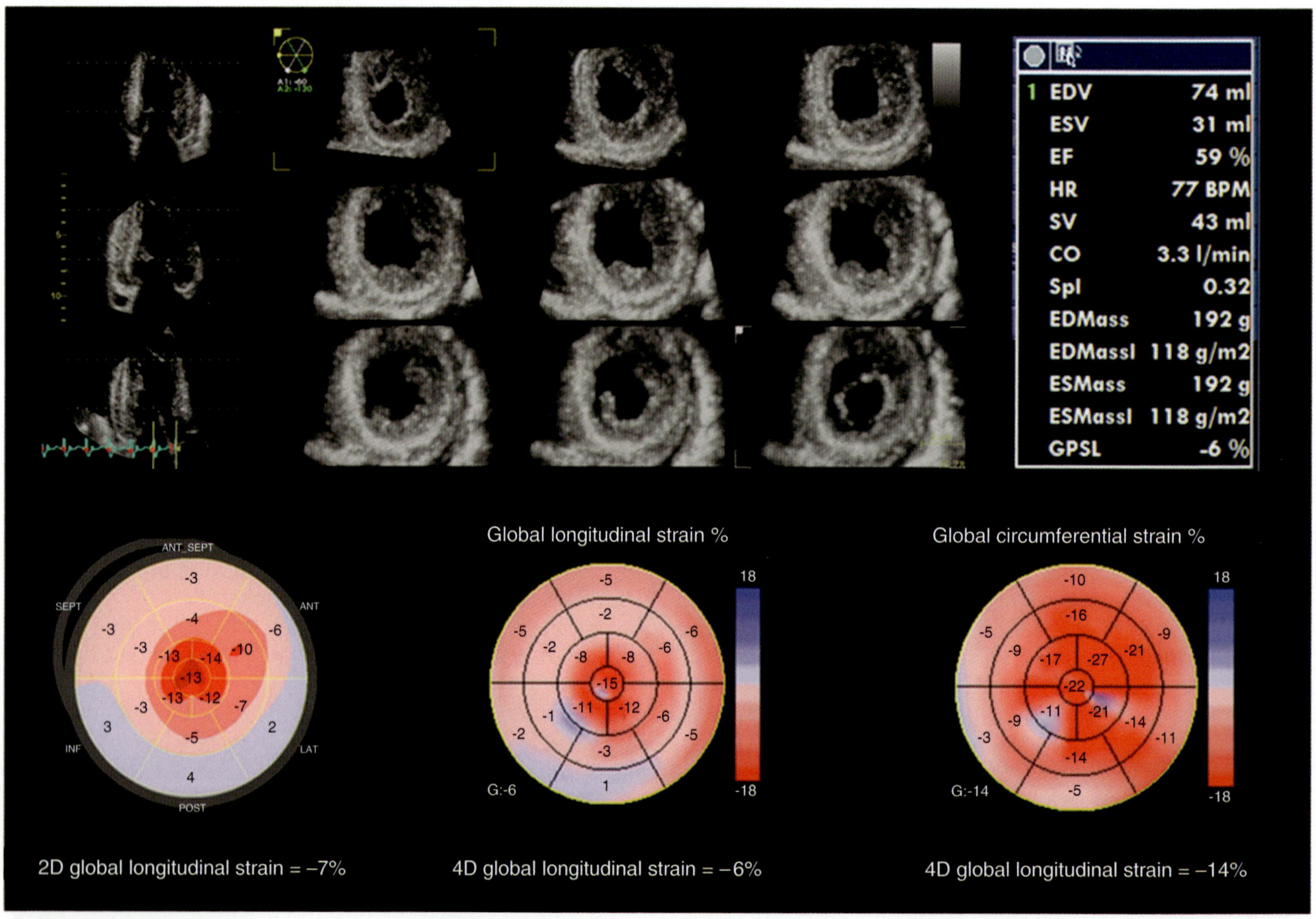

FIGURE 31-9 Assessment of myocardial mechanics: two-dimensional (2D), and four-dimensional (4D) longitudinal and radial strain. Representative example of normal strain patterns obtained by speckle-tracking echocardiography, two- and three-dimensional strain (GE Healthcare, Milwaukee, Wisc.). In this example, a good correlation is found for global longitudinal strain between two- and three-dimensional echocardiography. *CO,* Cardiac output; *EDMassI,* EDmass indexed; *EDV,* end-diastolic volume; *EF,* ejection fraction; *ESMassI,* ESmass indexed; *ESV,* end-systolic volume; *GPSL,* global peak longitudinal strain; *HR,* heart rate.

Hemodynamic Assessment and Diastolic Function

Changes in the transmitral flow profile for pulsed-wave Doppler during coronary occlusion have been shown to be secondary to impaired left ventricular relaxation. Such changes include a decrease in the peak rate of early filling (E wave) resulting in a reduced proportion of total left ventricular filling during the rapid filling phase, an increased rate of filling secondary to atrial contraction (A wave), and a reduced E/A ratio (i.e., peak mitral early to late inflow velocity) with a prolonged deceleration time (DT) (Figure 31-11). These changes parallel the diastolic function measured invasively (–dP/dt, LV end-diastolic pressure, and

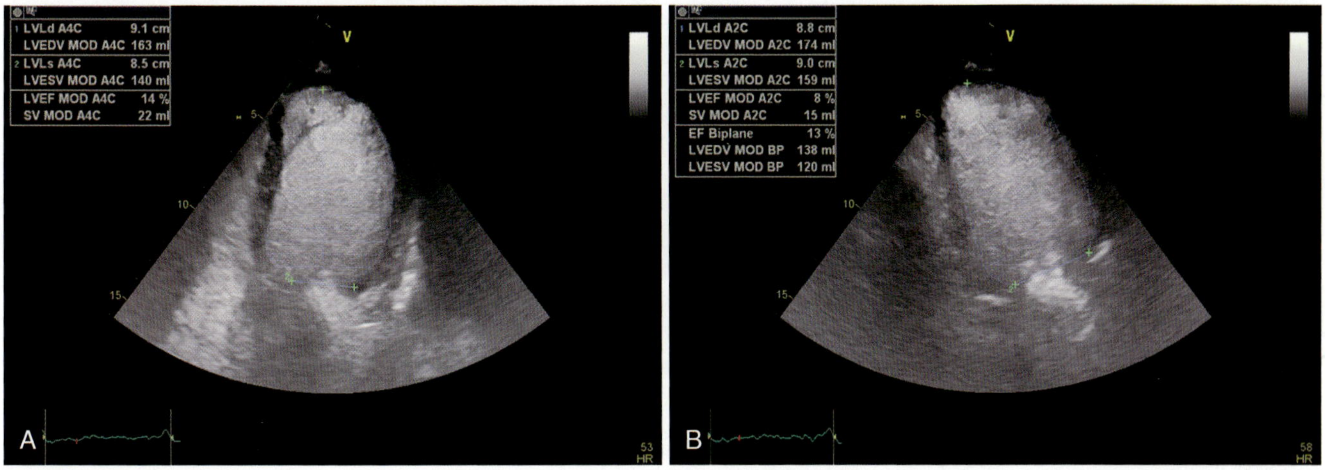

FIGURE 31-10 Left ventricular (LV) opacification using contrast ultrasound agent. Evaluation of LV volumes and systolic function using the Simpson's method of disks after injection of lipid-shelled, gas-filled encapsulated microbubbles (echocardiographic contrast agent, Definity). The LV endocardial borders are traced at end systole and end diastole in two orthogonal views: the apical four-chamber (**A**) and two-chamber (**B**) views. The LV end-diastolic and end-systolic volumes (LVEDV, LVESV) and the LV ejection fraction (LVEF) are derived. *V*, Xxxxxxxxxxx.

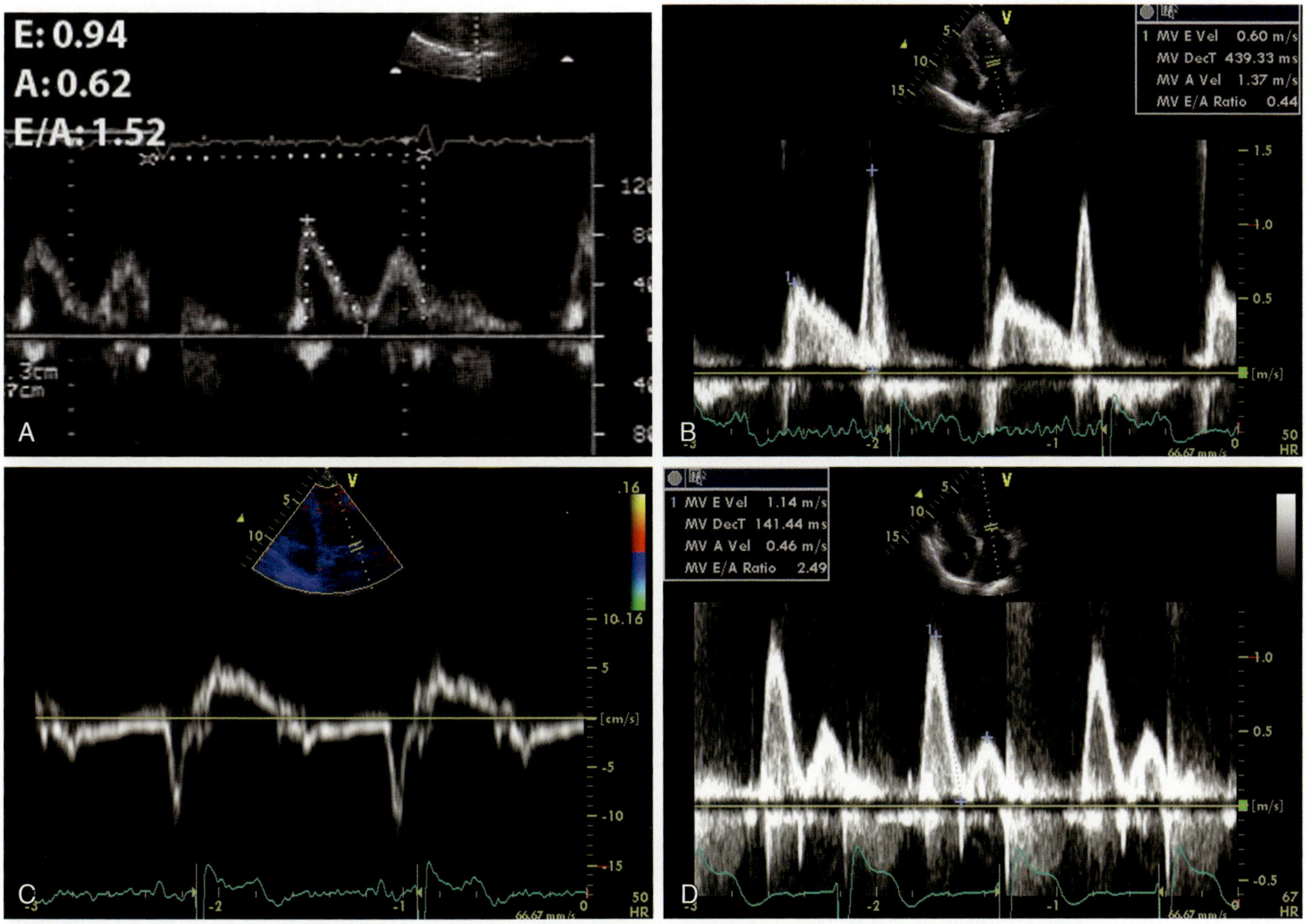

FIGURE 31-11 Evaluation of left ventricular (LV) diastolic dysfunction (see also Table 31-1). (**A**) Example of a normal pulsed-wave Doppler mitral valve (MV) profile: E wave is 94 cm/sec, deceleration time (DecT) is 174 msec, and E/A ratio is 1.52. (**B**) Mitral flow velocity recording shows abnormal relaxation: E/A ratio is 0.44, and DecT is prolonged (439 msec). (**C**) Pseudonormal pattern: Myocardial tissue Doppler imaging (TDI) of the mitral annulus at the lateral level depicts inversion of the normal pattern, with E_m less than A_m. (**D**) Restrictive MV flow pattern with short DecT (141 msec) and E/A of 2.5.

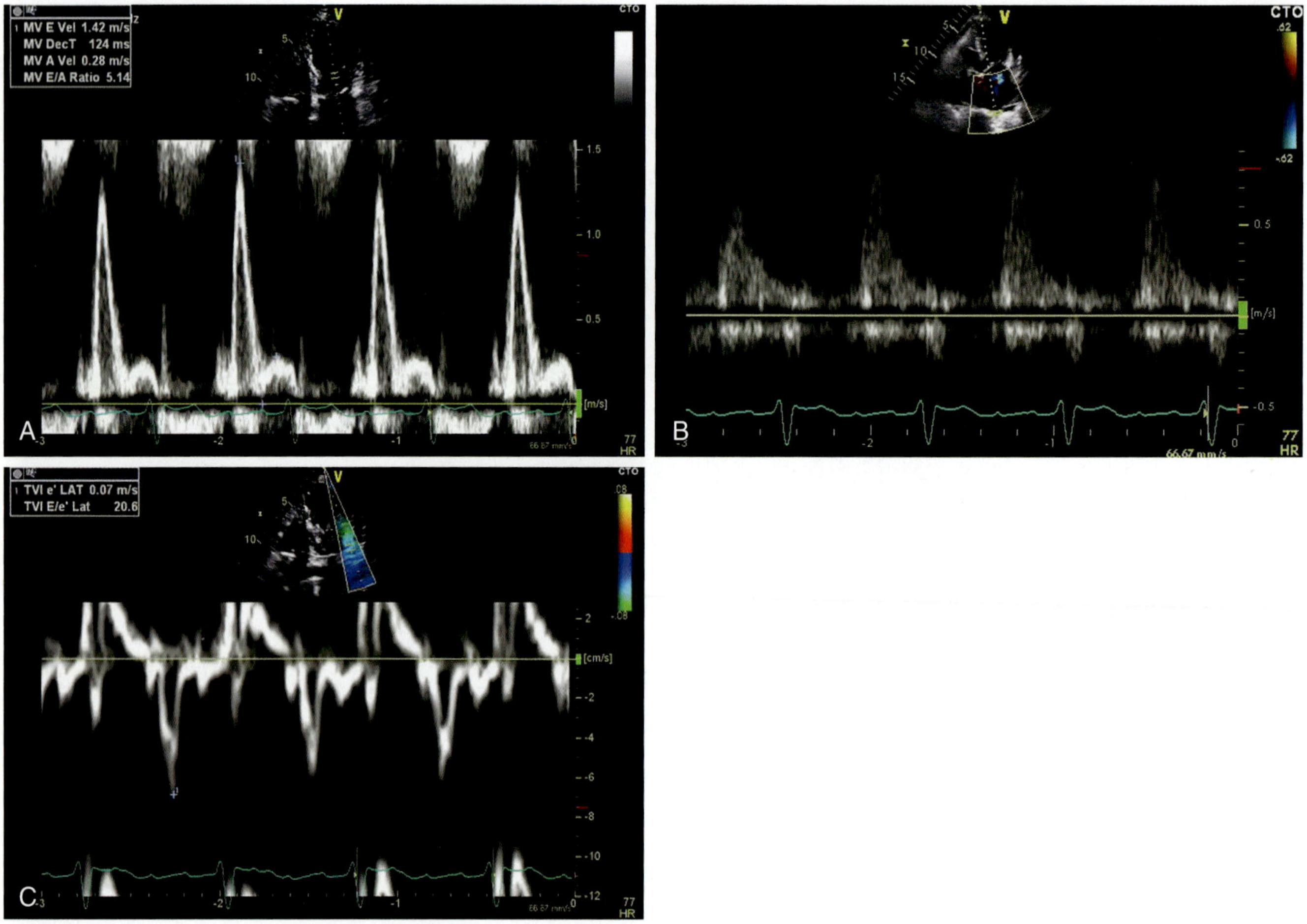

FIGURE 31-12 Severe left ventricular (LV) diastolic dysfunction after myocardial infarction (MI). Restrictive LV filling after MI demonstrated by pulsed-wave Doppler interrogation of the transmitral flow (**A**) and pulmonary venous flow (**B**), and by tissue Doppler imaging of the lateral mitral annulus (**C**). *A,* Peak late diastolic transmitral flow velocity; A_m, peak late diastolic mitral annulus velocity; *D,* peak diastolic pulmonary venous flow velocity; *DecT,* deceleration time; E_m, peak early diastolic mitral annulus velocity; *MAV,* mitral annulus velocity; *MV,* mitral valve; *S,* peak systolic velocity; *Sm,* systolic MAV; *TVI,* time velocity integral.

the time constant of isovolumic relaxation, tau) and may be present even when systolic function remains normal. Most patients with ACS demonstrate the typical abnormal relaxation pattern (E/A ratio less than 1 and prolonged DT to more than 250 msec). A large infarct size or severe systolic dysfunction, however, can result in a restrictive pattern (high peak E wave velocity, E/A greater than 2, and DT below 150 msec), which reflects abnormal ventricular compliance with elevated filling pressures. A third intermediate or pseudonormal Doppler pattern also can be seen, with E/A ratio between 1 and 2 and a DT between 150 and 250 msec, which can be unmasked by the Valsalva maneuver, in that it decreases venous return and results in an inversion of the E/A ratio and prolongation of the DT in patients with abnormal diastolic dysfunction. This pseudonormal pattern also can be differentiated from a truly normal Doppler profile by determining the isovolumic relaxation time using the mitral and aortic Doppler profiles, analyzing the TDI pattern at the mitral annulus (inverted E_m to A_m ratio) and/or by examining pulmonary venous flow.[23,24]

TDI is a useful adjunct to pulsed-wave Doppler in the assessment of diastolic function. The pattern of mitral annulus motion during diastole by TDI is similar to that of the pulsed-wave Doppler transmitral flow, but lower in velocity. Doppler signals of early diastolic (E_m), atrial contraction (A_m) and E_m/A_m ratio can be derived and seems less dependent on preload than the transmitral profile; hence the E_m/A_m pattern on TDI helps to distinguish normal left ventricular filling from the pseudonormal pattern (in which this ratio is less than 1 on TDI) seen in patients with moderate to severe diastolic dysfunction (Figure 31-12). It is important to recognize that in the context of an ACS, nearly all Doppler-derived indices are influenced by several physiologic factors (e.g., heart rate) and may not consistently reflect left ventricular filling. Nevertheless, these quantifiable measures of left ventricular filling have been shown to have predictive value,[25] but interrogation of multiple Doppler parameters is required for reliable results[24,26] (Table 31-1).

Transthoracic echocardiography provides important information to determine the *hemodynamic profile* of a patient, by allowing noninvasive measurement of the cardiac output and estimation of pulmonary capillary wedge pressure (PCWP). After MI, a mitral DT below 120 msec is considered highly predictive of a PCWP greater than 20 mm Hg. Likewise, the DT of the diastolic component of the pulmonary venous flow (less than 160 msec) or a decreased systolic fraction of the pulmonary venous flow (less than 45%) correlated well with a PCWP above 18 mm Hg. The left ventricular filling pressure also can be estimated using the mitral regurgitant jet with a continuous-wave Doppler technique (Figure 31-13). Finally, a novel predictor called the *kinetics-tracing index,* using a combination of left atrial volume and function, has been recently proposed[27] but will require further confirmation,

TABLE 31-1 Grading of Diastolic Dysfunction Using a Combination of Multiple Echocardiographic Parameters

PARAMETER	NORMAL (ADULT)	DELAYED RELAXATION	PSEUDONORMAL FILLING	RESTRICTIVE FILLING
E/A (cm/sec)	>1	<1	1-2	>2
DT (msec)	<220	>220	150-200	<150
IVRT (msec)	<100	>100	60-100	<60
E′ (cm/sec)	>8	<8	<6	<6

DT, Deceleration time; *E′,* peak diastolic myocardial velocity; *E/A,* peak mitral early to late inflow velocity; *IVRT,* isovolumetric relaxation time.
Modified from Jons C, Joergensen RM, Hassager C, et al: Diastolic dysfunction predicts new-onset atrial fibrillation and cardiovascular events in patients with acute myocardial infarction and depressed left ventricular systolic function: A CARISMA substudy. Eur J Echocardiogr *11(7):602-607, 2010.*

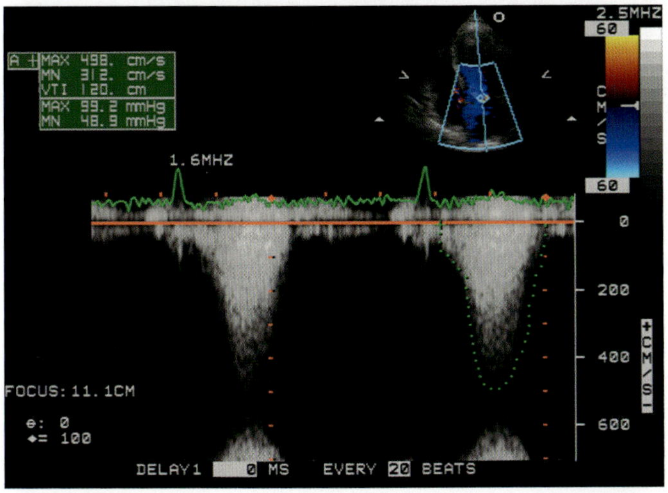

FIGURE 31-13 Hemodynamic evaluation of left ventricular (LV) filling pressure. Left atrial pressure (LAP) can be estimated from the mitral regurgitation signal. In this patient, the maximal pressure gradient between the left ventricle and the left atrium was 99 mm Hg; the systolic arterial pressure was measured at 125 mm Hg by cuff and is assumed to be equal to the LV systolic pressure. Hence the estimated maximum LAP is (125 − 99) = 26 mm Hg.

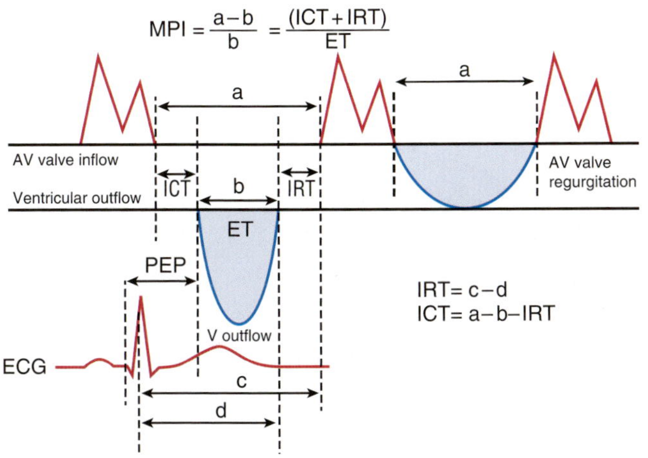

FIGURE 31-14 Doppler-derived myocardial performance index (MPI), or Tei index. *a,* Interval between end and onset of the atrioventricular (AV) inflow. *b,* Ejection time (ET). Isovolumetric relaxation time (IRT) is the interval between the end of ventricular ejection (V) and onset of AV inflow. Isovolumetric contraction time (ICT) is obtained by subtracting IRT from the quantity (a − b). *ECG,* Electrocardiogram.

especially in patients with mitral regurgitation (MR) or atrial fibrillation.

The *myocardial performance index* (MPI), or Tei index, is a Doppler-derived parameter combining assessment of systolic and diastolic function; it is defined as the sum of the isovolumic contraction and relaxation times divided by the ejection time (Figure 31-14). After MI, a left ventricular MPI of 0.60 or more can diagnose impaired hemodynamics (PCWP of 18 mm Hg or greater and/or cardiac index of 2.2 L/min/m^2 or less) with sensitivity, specificity, and accuracy of 86%, 82%, and 83%, respectively. Furthermore, an index greater than 0.66 is an independent predictor of heart failure or cardiac death.[28]

Finally, pulmonary artery hypertension has been shown to be associated with higher mortality after MI. Echocardiography remains the mainstay for the noninvasive evaluation of pulmonary artery pressure.[29] Continuous-wave Doppler can estimate systolic right ventricular pressure (and systolic pulmonary artery pressure), using tricuspid regurgitation flow and the Bernouilli equation to determine the trans-tricuspid gradient to which right atrial pressure should be added; the latter is estimated either clinically or as based on the diameter of the inferior vena cava and its variation with respiration determined with two-dimensional echocardiography (Figure 31-15).

RIGHT VENTRICULAR INFARCTION

The diagnosis of a right ventricular infarction requires a high level of suspicion because the sensitivity and specificity of clinical and electrocardiographic signs are low.[30] Nevertheless, diagnosis of right-sided involvement in the setting of an acute MI can significantly change the clinical management of these patients, because "intractable cardiogenic shock" may become easily reversible with fluid infusion (see Chapter 26). Furthermore, the presence of right ventricular dysfunction has an adverse impact after MI, increasing threefold the risk of death, cardiogenic shock, sustained ventricular arrhythmias, and advanced atrioventricular block, even in the current era and despite successful percutaneous coronary intervention (PCI).[3]

Echocardiographically, the right ventricle is divided into four segments: the infundibulum (or outflow tract), anterior free wall, lateral wall, and inferior wall[30] (Figure 31-16). The dual blood supply (from the right coronary and left anterior descending arteries) of the infundibulum and the anterior wall makes these segments most resistant to ischemia, whereas the inferior wall is the most vulnerable, with intermediate susceptibility for the lateral wall.

Echocardiographic Assessment of Right Ventricular Function

Transthoracic echocardiography is an excellent modality to identify right ventricular infarction, with findings including right ventricular regional or global dysfunction usually with left ventricular inferior wall involvement. Because right ventricular infarction sometimes may be revealed only by dysfunction of its inferior wall, attention should be paid to this region in optimized parasternal short-axis views. Indirect signs such as right ventricular dilation, tricuspid

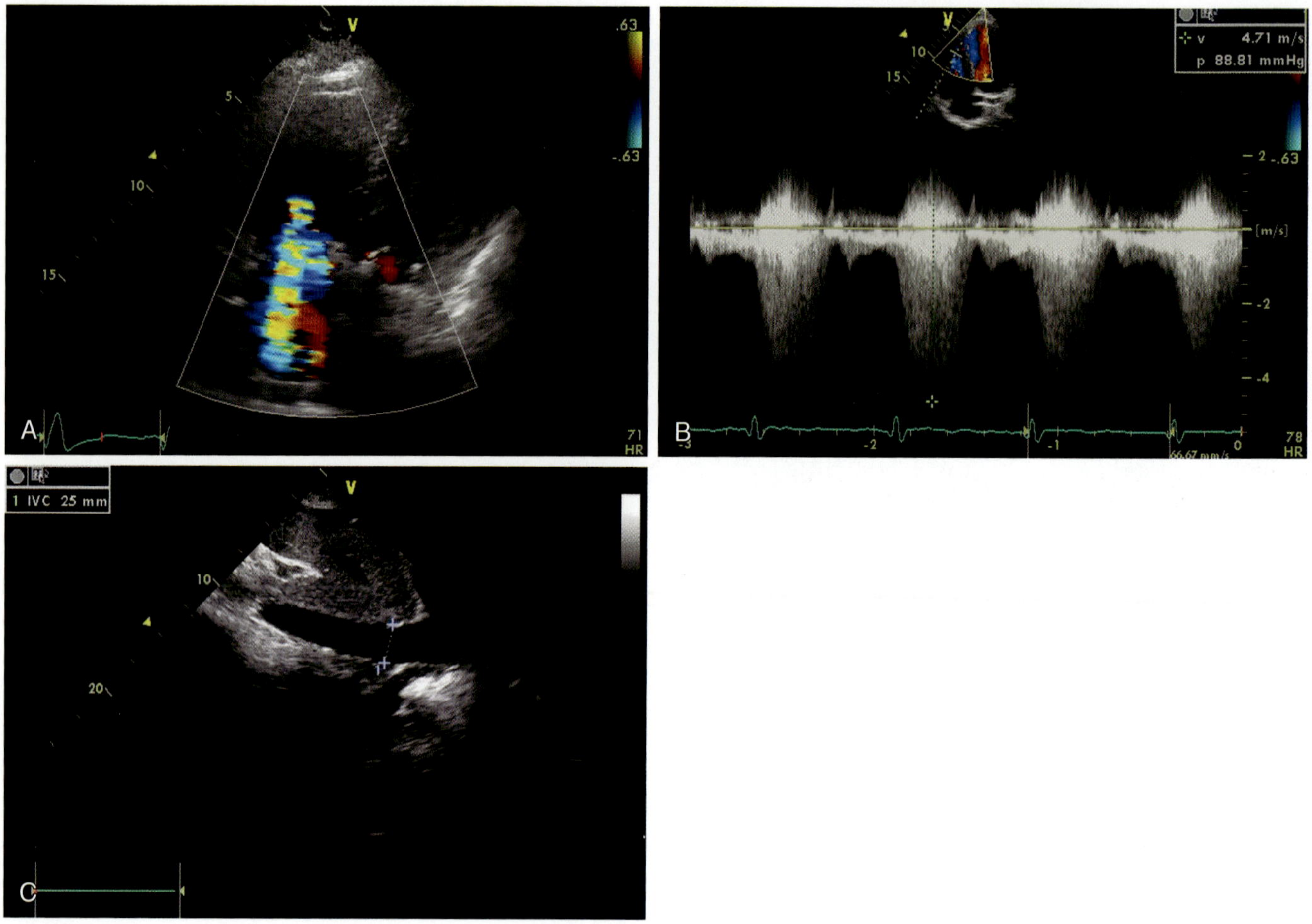

FIGURE 31-15 Tricuspid regurgitation (TR). (**A**) Transthoracic echocardiography apical four-chamber view showing severe TR associated with right ventricular (RV) dysfunction. (**B**) The TR maximum pressure gradient was 88 mm Hg. (**C**) The inferior vena cava (IVC) is dilated, for estimated right atrial pressure of 10 mm Hg and RV systolic pressure of 98 mm Hg.

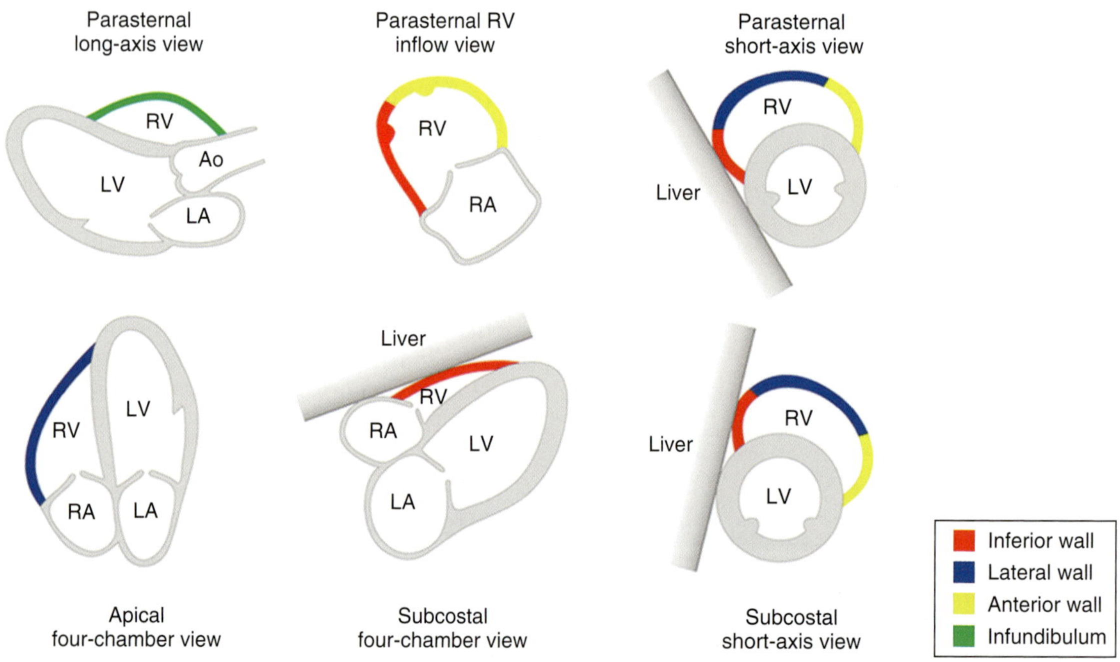

FIGURE 31-16 Echocardiographic analysis of the right ventricle (RV). The RV is divided into four segments: the infundibulum, anterior wall, lateral wall, and inferior wall. The most useful projections for assessing right ventricular function are shown. *Ao,* Aorta; *LA,* left atrium; *LV,* left ventricle; *RA,* right atrium. *(From Rallidis LS, Makavos G, Nihoyannopoulos P: Right ventricular involvement in coronary artery disease: Role of echocardiography for diagnosis and prognosis.* J Am Soc Echocardiogr *27(3):223-229, 2014.)*

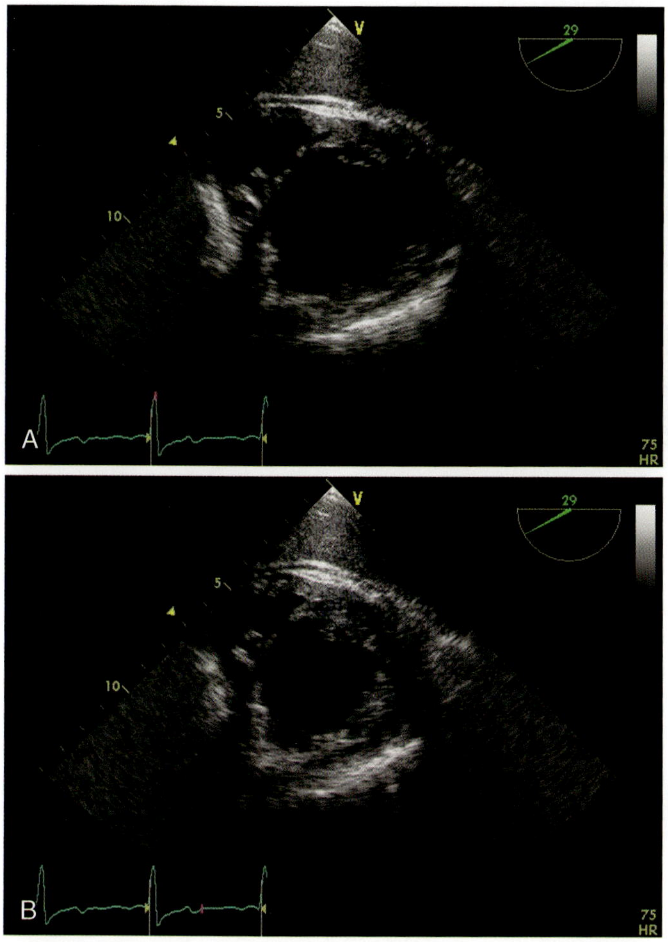

FIGURE 31-17 Right ventricular (RV) infarction. Transesophageal echocardiography (TEE) short-axis view at the midpapillary level showing akinesia of the left ventricular (LV) inferoseptal and inferior walls, together with RV inferior wall in diastole (**A**) and systole (**B**). A ventricular septal defect also is seen (see Video 31-24). Echocardiographic findings also may include RV regional or global dysfunction, usually with LV inferior wall involvement. Because infarction of the right ventricle sometimes may be manifested only as dysfunction of its inferior wall, attention should be paid to this region, with modified views obtained if needed.

regurgitation, reduced excursion of the tricuspid annulus, and dilation of the inferior vena cavae also often can be found (Figure 31-17).

Many methods have been developed to quantify right ventricular systolic function, with good correlation with MRI (see Chapter 33) and radionuclide ventriculography.[31] Fractional area change expresses the percentage change of right ventricular area at end systole in comparison with right ventricular end-diastolic area from the four-chamber view and has a good correlation with right ventricular ejection fraction (RVEF) estimated by MRI[31]; it is therefore the recommended echocardiographic method to quantify right ventricular dysfunction in the presence of a right ventricular MI. In addition, strain-derived parameters can be used to assess the degree of myocardial deformation (longitudinal strain) and the rate of deformation (strain rate) (Figure 31-18A), which are lower in patients with inferior MI and right ventricular involvement when measured at the basal and middle segments.[32]

To overcome the limitations of the right ventricle's complex geometry, three-dimensional echocardiography (Figure 31-18B and Videos 31-16, 31-17, 31-18, and 31-19) recently has been shown to have good correlations with MRI measurements of right ventricular volumes and ejection fraction, even if three-dimensional echocardiography–derived volumes were slightly smaller. In the setting of an acute inferior MI, an RVEF less than 51% assessed by three-dimensional echocardiography had sensitivity of 91% and specificity of 80% for the diagnosis of right ventricular MI.[33]

Other methods have been developed for assessment of the right ventricle (Table 31-2). Displacement of the right ventricular base during systole and diastole in apical four-chamber view, also called tricuspid annular plane systolic excursion (TAPSE), is an indirect measurement of right ventricular systolic function that can be performed using M-mode or TDI techniques. An excursion of less than 1.5 cm by M-mode or less than 10 cm/sec by TDI is very specific for the detection of an RVEF less than 50%. A right ventricular MPI (see earlier) of 0.70 or greater results in the best combination of sensitivity and specificity for the diagnosis of right ventricular infarction in the context of left ventricular inferior wall infarction.[34] Table 31-2 summarizes the recommended echocardiographic measurements for assessment of right ventricular function.[11]

COMPLICATIONS OF MYOCARDIAL INFARCTION

Despite a marked improvement in outcomes after MI in the past few decades with early reperfusion and improved medical therapy, in-hospital mortality rates remain significant as a consequence of refractory cardiogenic shock or mechanical complications of MI (see Chapter 26). Mechanical complications include septal rupture with ventricular septal defect, rupture of the left ventricular free wall, and acute MR due to papillary muscle infarction and rupture. Although these complications are infrequent, they carry a poor prognosis. Early detection of mechanical complications with echocardiography is crucial to plan the most appropriate management.

Left Ventricular Aneurysm

Left ventricular aneurysms are classified as true or false aneurysms. *True aneurysms* are the most common type, historically occurring in approximately one fifth of all cases of transmural MI before routine use of reperfusion therapy. The aneurysm results from expansion of the infarct area and thinning of the myocardium and contains all three layers of the ventricular wall. Echocardiographically, the aneurysmal segments are dyskinetic or akinetic, and cause distortion of left ventricular shape (with a wide neck) that persists in diastole (Figure 31-19A). Almost 90% of true left ventricular aneurysms involve the apex, and in the remaining cases, the lesion generally is localized to the inferobasal region. Detection of an aneurysm within the first 5 days of hospitalization has been associated with high mortality rates at 3 months and 1 year after MI, probably reflecting the larger infarct size and the more depressed global systolic function. Aneurysm also can be a site of predilection for thrombus formation.[2]

Left ventricular pseudoaneurysm is a rare and potentially life-threatening entity that results from a rupture through the myocardium, the extravasated blood being contained by the parietal pericardium. Pathologic examination shows a small channel connecting the left ventricle with a large blood- and thrombus-filled cavity lined by fibrous pericardial tissue, with a tear evident in the myocardium.

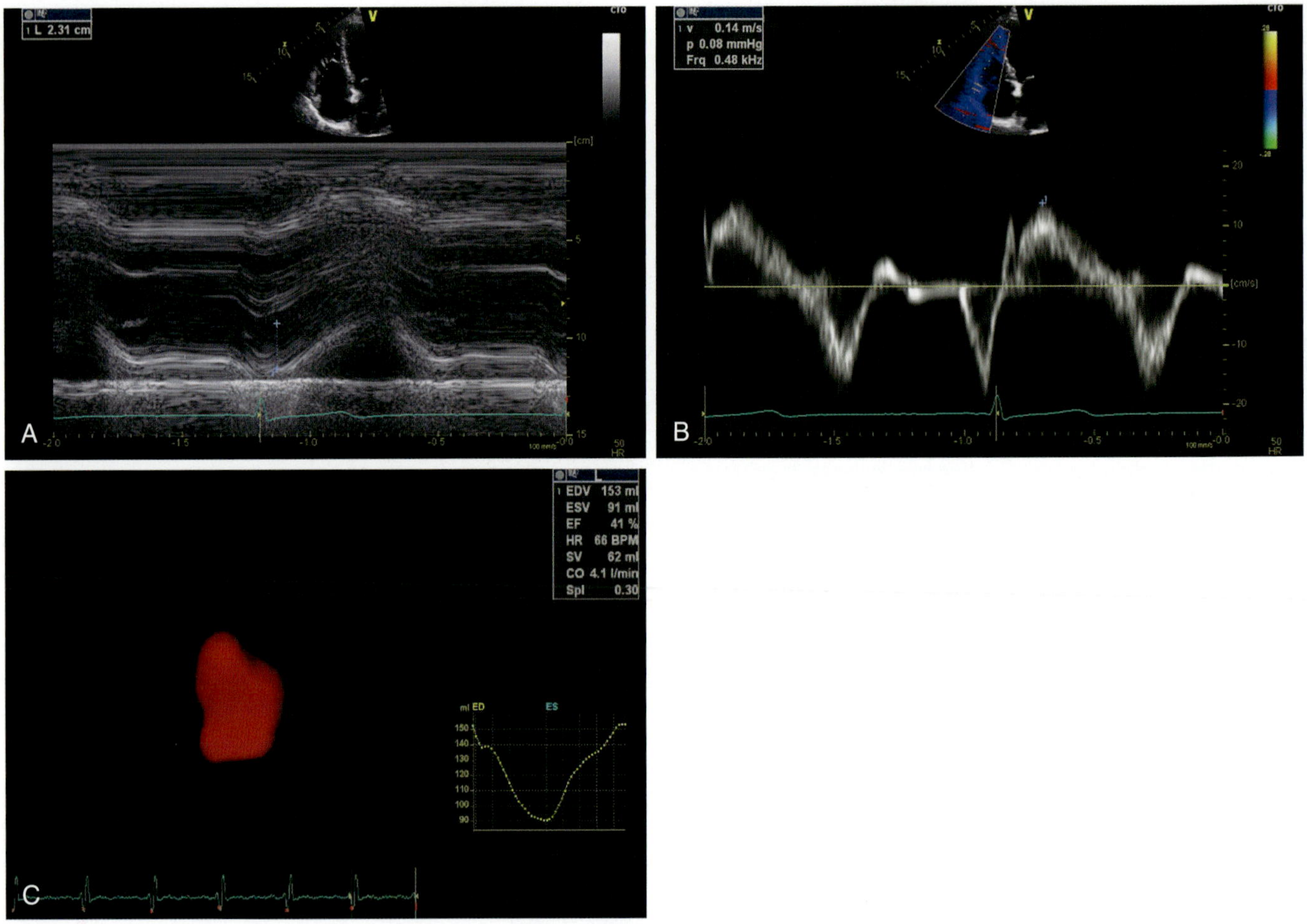

FIGURE 31-18 Methods to quantify right ventricular (RV) systolic function. (**A**) In this example, RV systolic function estimated using the tricuspid annular systolic plane excursion (TAPSE) assessed by M-mode is normal. (**B**) Myocardial tissue Doppler imaging (TDI) of the RV lateral annulus (RV-TDI) showing a systolic velocity (SV) of the right ventricle of 14 cm/sec. (**C**) To overcome the imaging difficulties posed by the complex geometry of the ventricle, three-dimensional echocardiography may be useful. *CO,* Cardiac output; *EDV,* end-diastolic volume; *EF,* ejection fraction; *ESV,* end-systolic volume; *HR,* heart rate.

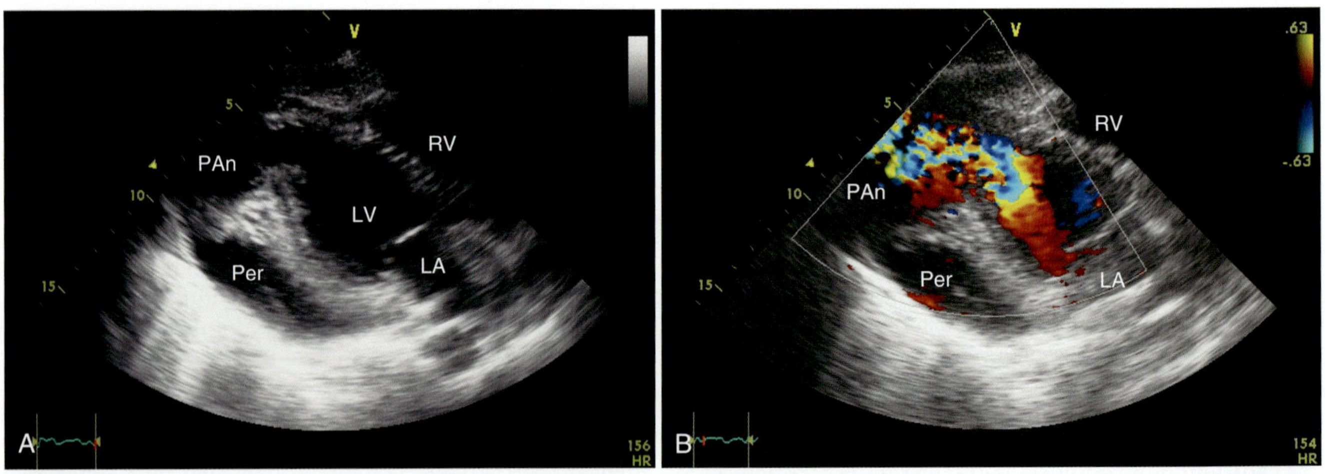

FIGURE 31-19 Free-wall rupture and left ventricular pseudoaneurysm. (**A**) Apical long-axis view, slightly off-axis, showing abrupt discontinuity of the inferolateral wall resulting in a communication between the left ventricle (LV) and a large cavity that appears to be a pseudoaneurysm. The cavity was pulsatile during real-time imaging (see Videos 31-20 and 31-21). (**B**) Using color flow Doppler, flow is seen from the LV toward the pericardial cavity (*arrow*). *LA,* Left atrium; *PAn,* pseudoaneurysm; *Per,* pericardial effusion; *RV,* right ventricle.

On echocardiography, an echo-free area outside the left ventricular cavity is seen connected to it by a narrow neck, with an abrupt interruption in the ventricular wall.[2] Bulging also can be observed in the false aneurysm during each systole (Figure 31-19B and Videos 31-20 and 31-21). Because a ventricular pseudoaneurysm is a contained rupture, mortality is high, and urgent surgery is warranted as soon as the diagnosis is made with echocardiography (see Chapter 26).

Myocardial Rupture

Cardiac rupture complicating MI, although infrequent, has a dramatic presentation and often is rapidly fatal. It can

TABLE 31-2 Normal Values and Threshold for Echocardiographic Parameters of Right Ventricular Function

PARAMETER	MEAN ± SD	ABNORMALITY THRESHOLD
TAPSE (mm)	24 ± 3.5	<17
Pulsed Doppler S wave (cm/sec)	14.1 ± 2.3	<9.5
Color Doppler S wave (cm/sec)	9.7 ± 1.85	<6.0
RV fractional area change (%)	49 ± 7	<35
RV free wall two-dimensional strain (%)*	−29 ± 4.5	>−20
RV three-dimensional EF (%)	58 ± 6.5	<45
Pulsed Doppler MPI	0.26 ± 0.085	>0.43
Tissue Doppler MPI	0.38 ± 0.08	>0.54
E wave deceleration time (msec)	180 ± 31	<119 or >242
E/A	1.4 ± 0.3	<0.8 or >2.0
e′/a′	1.18 ± 0.33	<0.52
e′	14.0 ± 3.1	<7.8
E/e′	4.0 ± 1.0	>6.0

e′, Early wave at the mitral annulus by TDI;; *E/A,* peak mitral early to late inflow velocity; *e′/a′,* ratio of e′ to the atrial contraction wave (a′) at the mitral annulus by TDI; *E/e′*, ratio of the early wave at mitral inflow by PWD to e′; *EF,* ejection fraction; *MPI*, myocardial performance index; *RV,* right ventricular; *TAPSE,* tricuspid annular systolic plane excursion.
**Limited data; values may vary depending on vendor and software version.*
From Lang RM, Badano LP, Mor-Avi V, et al: Recommendations for cardiac chamber quantification by echocardiography in adults: An update from the American Society of Echocardiography and the European Association of Cardiovascular Imaging. J Am Soc Echocardiogr *28(1):1-39, 2015.*

involve the left ventricular free wall, the ventricular septum, or papillary muscle (see Chapter 26).

Ventricular Free Wall Rupture

Rupture of the left ventricular free wall usually is a sudden event and accounts for 10% to 15% of all in-hospital deaths after MI. Echocardiographic recognition of free-wall rupture, although unusual because of rapid hemodynamic deterioration, occasionally has been possible, allowing rapid intervention.[35]

Ventricular Septal Defect

In the reperfusion era, a ventricular septal defect (VSD) is an uncommon complication of MI (with a frequency of less than 1%) but is associated with high mortality rates.[36] Rupture of the interventricular septum is more common with anterior than with inferior infarcts. The perforation may be a direct through-and-through hole or may be more irregular and serpiginous, with a variable defect size but usually less than 4 cm in diameter. Echocardiography often directly detects the septal defect as an interruption in the myocardium in an akinetic region, often at the junction with normal or hyperkinetic tissue (Figure 31-20A and Videos 31-22, 31-23, 31-24, 31-25, and 31-26). As a complication of anterior infarction, the septal defect usually is located distally near the apex, in association with anterior akinesis. Careful two-dimensional and color Doppler scanning of the ventricular septum is required, particularly in the apical four-chamber and five-chamber views. When a VSD occurs with an inferior infarction, the apex typically is spared, and the defect is in the basal septum, generally associated with an extensive area of inferior wall dyskinesis. Commonly the VSD in the basal inferior septum is identified using an off-axis position, with an intermediate rotation between the apical four-chamber and two-chamber views. Pulsed-wave, continuous-wave, and color Doppler studies confirm the left-to-right shunt across the septal defect. The defect size determined by color Doppler echocardiography has been shown to correlate closely with that determined at surgery or autopsy and with the pulmonic artery–to–systemic flow ratio measured at cardiac catheterization. Transesophageal echocardiography (TEE) is useful in guiding percutaneous VSD closure (Figure 31-20B).[36]

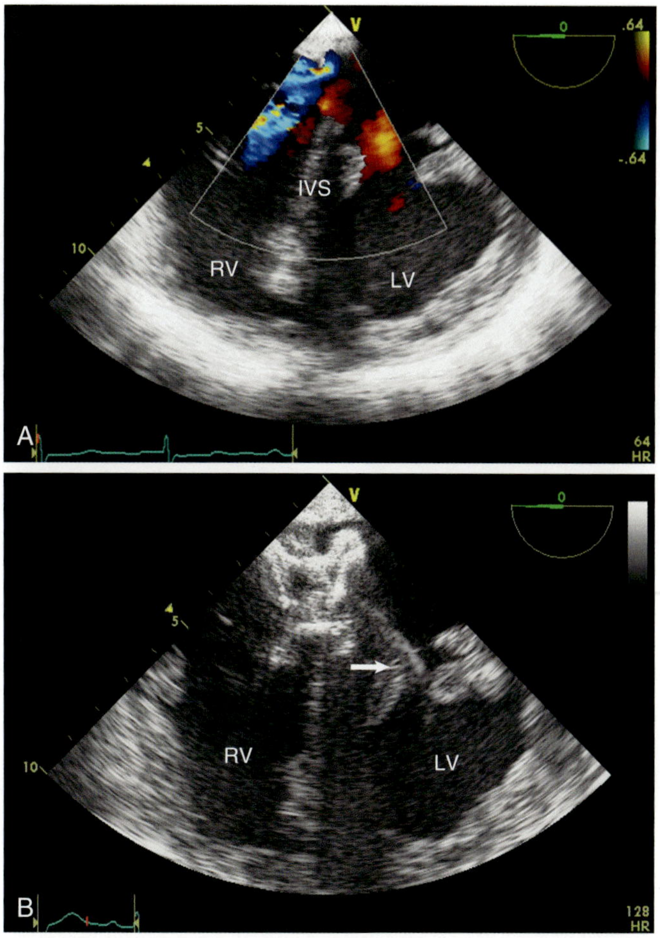

FIGURE 31-20 Ventricular septal defects (VSDs). Three days after an acute inferior myocardial infarction, the patient exhibited clinical deterioration, and a new systolic murmur was heard. (**A**) Transesophageal echocardiography (TEE) transgastric view at 0 degrees with color Doppler showed a shunt from the left to the right ventricle (*LV, RV*), typical of a VSD. (**B**) TEE guidance (*arrow,* delivering catheter) for percutaneous closure of the VSD, achieved using an Amplatzer device. *IVS,* Interventricular septum.

Mitral Regurgitation and Papillary Muscle Rupture

In a majority of the cases, MR develops as a result of impaired mitral leaflet coaptation in the absence of structural mitral valve disease,[37] as seen with papillary muscle displacement, left ventricular dilation, left ventricular wall remodeling, and/or dyssynergy of the left ventricular wall adjacent to the papillary muscle (Figure 31-21 and Video 31-27); in this setting, increased mitral tenting is an independent predictor of progression of MR after MI. Although left ventricular remodeling itself and left ventricular sphericity contribute to ischemic MR, this influence seems directly dependent on alterations in mitral geometry. By contrast, ischemic rupture of the mitral apparatus (chordae tendinae, a papillary muscle, or a muscle head) is a rare (occurring in 1% to 3% of the cases) but dramatic complication of acute MI.[38] Because its blood supply is dependent on a single coronary artery, the posteromedial papillary muscle is more

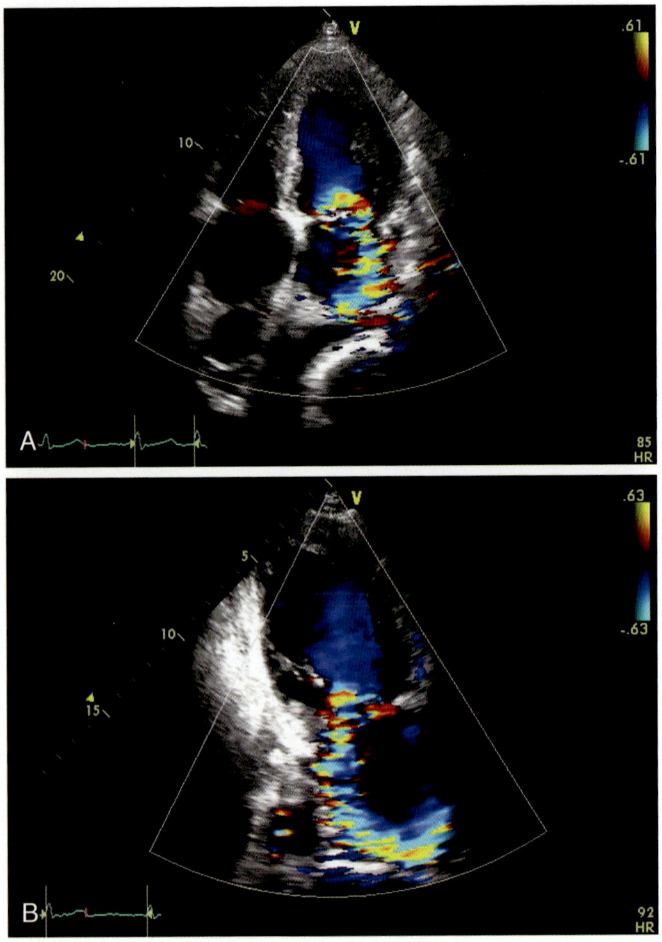

FIGURE 31-21 Mitral regurgitation (MR). MR due to impaired mitral leaflet coaptation with relatively normal mitral apparatus (leaflets and chordae). Apical four-chamber (**A**) and three-chamber (**B**) views show left ventricular (LV) dilation and akinesia of the inferolateral LV wall involving the posteromedial papillary muscle.

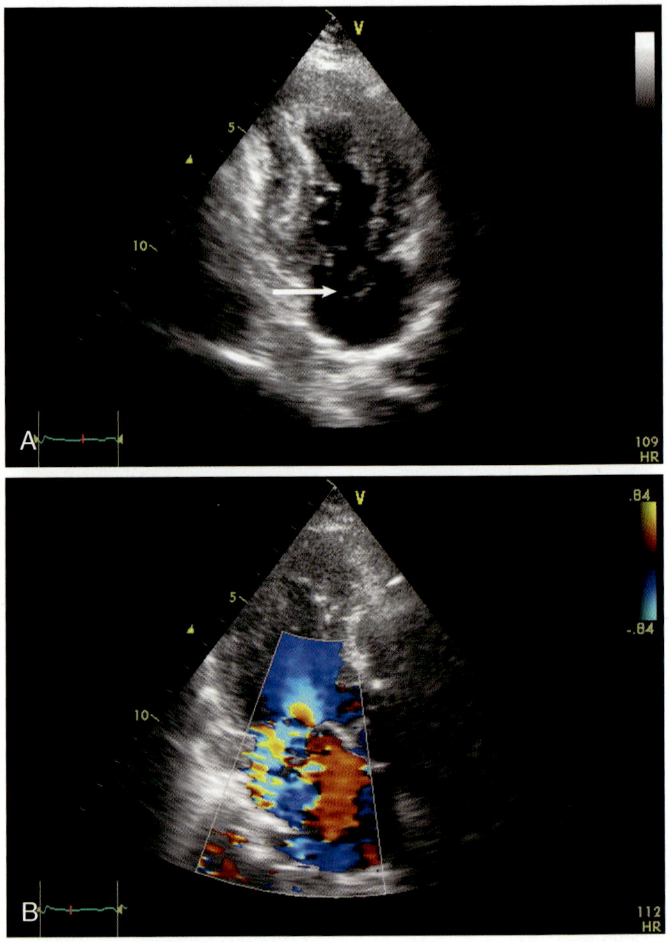

FIGURE 31-22 Papillary muscle rupture. Transthoracic echocardiography (TTE) in a patient in cardiogenic shock 24 hours after an anterior myocardial infarction. (**A**) Apical two-chamber view shows rupture of the anterolateral papillary muscle, which has moved freely into the left atrium (*arrow*). (**B**) Apical long-axis view shows severe mitral regurgitation in the same patient.

frequently affected. For that reason, papillary muscle rupture occurs more commonly in the setting of an inferior MI. In clinical settings, partial rupture of a papillary muscle head is seen more frequently, because complete rupture generally is rapidly fatal. Two-dimensional echocardiography can show accurately the structural abnormality of the mitral apparatus, which usually includes a flail leaflet or prolapse and partial or complete rupture of one of the papillary muscle heads (Figure 31-22 and Videos 31-28 and 31-29). Because chordae tendinae originating from the posteromedial papillary muscle are connected to both mitral leaflets, a flail anterior leaflet can also complicate an acute inferior wall infarct. The left ventricle often is hyperdynamic in the presence of papillary muscle rupture and severe MR, and this activity frequently renders difficult the identification of an RWMA in the inferior wall. The addition of color flow Doppler permits the identification of MR and assessment of its severity in nearly all patients.[38] In the presence of an eccentric jet or a noncompliant left atrium (as commonly encountered in this setting), color Doppler occasionally may underestimate the severity of MR, however, and a thorough echocardiographic assessment is required, using TEE when needed (Videos 31-30 and 31-31).

Left Ventricular Thrombus

A relatively frequent complication before the era of thrombolytic therapy, left ventricular thrombi are still found in 4% to 15% of cases of anterior STEMI treated with PCI, more often with large infarcts and/or severely depressed left ventricular systolic function with longer time to reperfusion[39]; in addition, however, they can be found with small apical infarctions and preserved LVEF. Thrombus is always located in the akinetic/dyskinetic zone and typically appears as a homogeneous, mildly echogenic mass on the endocardial contour. It may be fixed or pedunculated and freely mobile, or it may have a fixed base with a mobile filament extending from its surface (Figure 31-23 and Video 31-32). The echogenicity can increase, however, and calcification may be found within an organized thrombus. Because most left ventricular thrombi are in the apical region, standard and off-axis apical views (with optimized imaging of the region of interest) often are required to confirm their presence and to distinguish them from a near-field artifact or a fibrous band (false tendon).[2] The use of contrast agents may be necessary in this situation.

PROGNOSIS AFTER MYOCARDIAL INFARCTION

The prognosis after MI is determined in part by the severity of systolic dysfunction (infarct size) and the presence and extent of ischemic myocardium (see Chapter 11 and Chapter 30).[40] Echocardiographically determined left ventricular end-systolic area, WMSI, and LVEF are strong predictors of

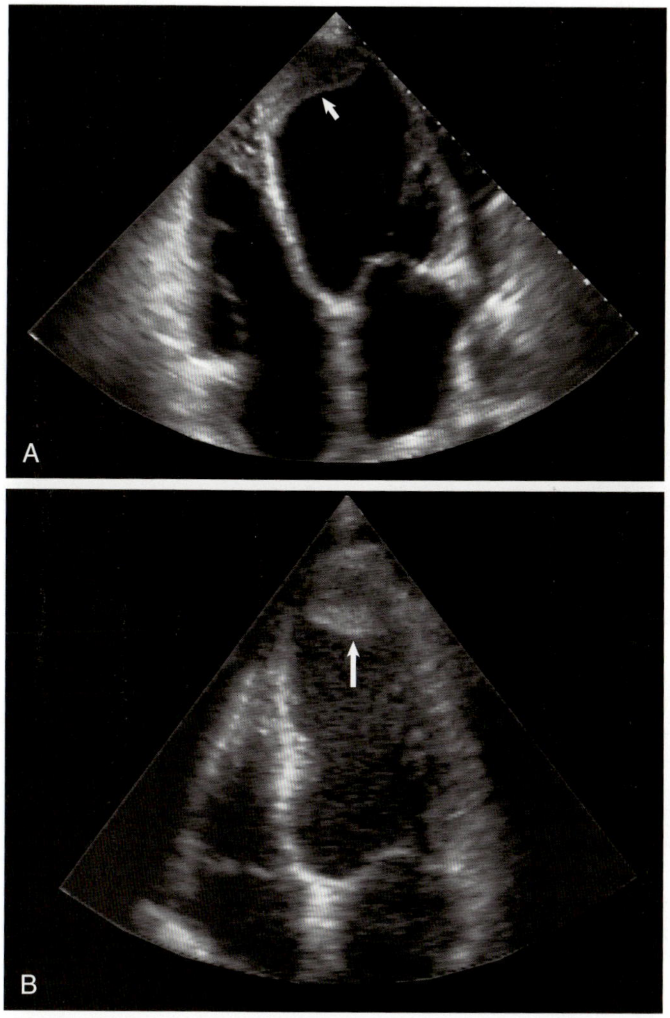

FLGURE 31-23 Left ventricular (LV) thrombus. (**A** and **B**) LV thrombi in the apical four-chamber view from echocardiograms for two different patients. (**A**) An organized and nonmobile thrombus is detected in the first patient (*arrow*). (**B**) In the second patient, a mobile thrombus (*arrow*) is seen in a region of akinesia and apical aneurysm. *(From Diaz A, Ducharme A, Tardif JC: Echocardiography in acute coronary syndromes. In Théroux P, editor:* Acute coronary syndromes, *Saunders, Philadelphia, 2011.)*

adverse outcome after an MI. For patients with LVEF less than 40% and end-systolic volume (ESV) greater than 130 cc, 5-year survival rates were 65% and 52%, respectively. By contrast, a low WMSI can prospectively identify patients at low risk for cardiac events after MI. Furthermore, the echocardiogram may help to distinguish infarct extension from recurrent ischemia and to quantify the amount of myocardium at risk. Indeed, during MI, the nonaffected ventricular segments usually are hyperdynamic as a compensatory mechanism. The absence of such compensatory hyperkinesis suggests multivessel coronary disease and is associated with worse outcome.[2] Echocardiography is therefore a useful tool in establishing prognosis in patients with MI, larger infarcts being associated with left ventricular shape distortion and predicting progressive left ventricular dilation; the lower the LVEF and the larger the volumes, the higher the mortality and the worse the morbidity will be.

ISCHEMIA AND VIABILITY ASSESSMENT: STRESS ECHOCARDIOGRAPHY

Stress echocardiography can be used for risk stratification in patients after MI, in an effort to identify a subset of patients at high risk for recurrent ischemia, MI, and death.[41] Stress echocardiography techniques increase the sensitivity of a standard exercise stress test, and both exercise and pharmacologic stress can be used; the choice of one modality over the other depends on the patient's ability to perform an exercise, the presence of baseline electrocardiographic abnormalities, and the goal of the examination (e.g., pharmacologic stress testing is required to assess myocardial viability) (see Chapter 30).

Exercise Stress Echocardiography

For exercise stress echocardiography (ESE) testing, either treadmill or bicycle exercise may be used, but the workload and maximum heart rate achieved usually are higher with treadmill, whereas blood pressure is higher with bicycle. Hence, if the aim of the exam is the assessment of RWMAs only, treadmill exercise usually is preferred; if additional Doppler information is needed (e.g., assessment of mitral regurgitation or pulmonary artery pressure during exercise), bicycle exercise allows assessment of both RWMAs and Doppler-derived parameters during exercise (as opposed to only *immediately after* exercise for treadmill testing).[42] The prognostic value of ESE after MI is well established, with exercise-induced new or worsened RWMA being associated with a fivefold increase in cardiac events (MI, revascularization, or death) over the next 12 months; of interest, development of stress-induced RWMA remote from the MI area is predictive of multivessel CAD and identifies a population with a worse prognosis. ESE's sensitivity is similar to that for exercise SPECT imaging (85% versus 87%), but the specificity is higher (77% versus 65%). Furthermore, a normal ESE result is associated with an annual event rate of cardiac death and nonfatal MI of less than 1%, equivalent to that for an age- and sex-matched population.[42] In addition to its diagnostic value, stress echocardiography offers the advantages of low cost and avoidance of exposure to radiation.[43]

Pharmacologic Stress Echocardiography

Pharmacologic stress echocardiography (PSE) may be used for evaluation of both *myocardial viability* and *ischemia*. PSE reveals the so-called inotropic reserve of the dysfunctional but viable myocardium through the administration of an inotropic agent, usually dobutamine (DSE), which has a positive inotropic effect at low doses (5 to 10 μg/kg/min) and additional inotropic and chronotropic effects at higher doses (ischemia). In response to inotropic stimulation, the viable but dysfunctional myocardium exhibits improved contractile function (inotropic reserve) (Figure 31-24 and Video 31-33), suggesting that at least 50% of the myocytes in the responsive segment are viable, predicting improvement in global left ventricular systolic function after revascularization. However, its prognostic value has been recently challenged.[44] This relationship may not be correct if the infarct-related artery is severely stenotic. In this situation, viable myocardium can be identified by a biphasic response (improvement of contractility at low dose, suggesting viability) and worsening at high dose (indicating ischemia).

The second indication for DSE in MI is for the assessment of the presence, severity and extent of residual myocardial ischemia, using high-dose dobutamine (see Chapter 30).[41,45] An abnormal DSE after an uncomplicated MI is an independent predictor of outcome and is associated with

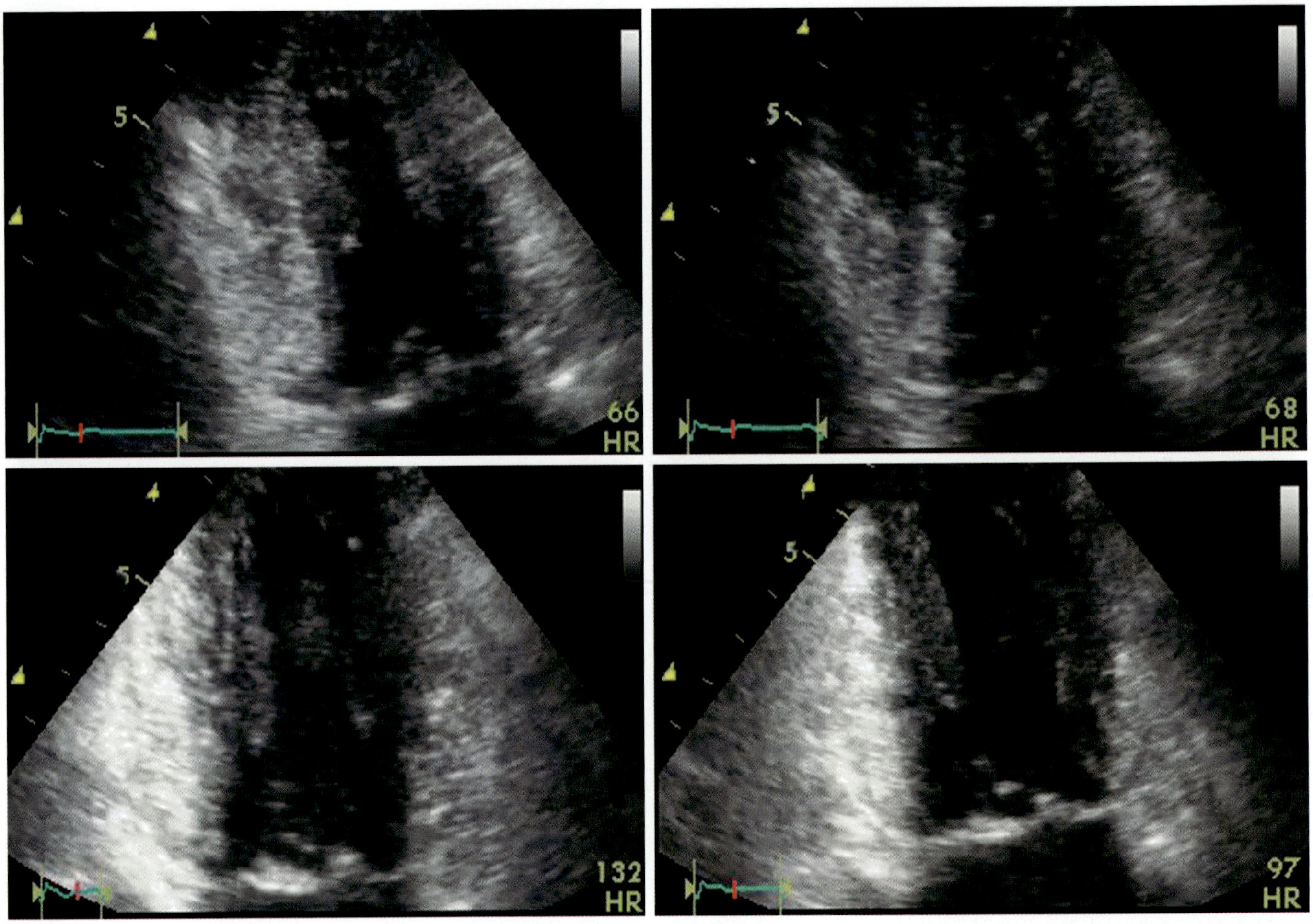

FIGURE 31-24 Dobutamine stress echocardiography (DSE). *Upper left panel,* DSE in apical two-chamber view demonstrating three-vessel disease. A biphasic response is shown, with improvement of contraction in the inferior and anterior walls at low dose of dobutamine (10 µg/kg/min, *right upper panel*), akinesia of the inferior and anterior walls with dyskinesia of the apex at higher dose (40 µg/kg/min, *left lower panel*), showing myocardial viability and ischemia, respectively. These changes persisted during recovery (*right lower panel*). *(Courtesy of Dr. François Marcotte, Montreal Heart Institute.)*

a fivefold increase in cardiac events after 17 months. The overall sensitivity and specificity are higher for the detection of multivessel or left main coronary artery disease than single-vessel disease, similar to thallium-201 perfusion imaging.[41] However, the accuracy of DSE is markedly reduced if the target heart rate is not achieved.[46]

Myocardial TDI during DSE also may be used to improve its diagnostic accuracy for viability, with an increment of peak velocity greater than 1 cm/sec being a predictor of functional recovery 5 months after MI, with improved sensitivity from 75% to 87%, without any change in specificity compared with ^{18}FDG positron emission tomography.[41] Furthermore, TDI may improve DSE accuracy in the presence of left bundle branch block, with failure to increase by more than 2.5 cm/sec the peak systolic and peak early diastolic velocities identifying CAD with 88% sensitivity (for both) and 90% and 87% specificity, respectively. Finally, *strain rate* (SR) increases with increasing doses of dobutamine, with stunned myocardium, ischemic segments, and nontransmural infarction associated with higher strain, SR, and postsystolic thickening than transmural necrosis. SR during DSE improves sensitivity (83%) and specificity (84%) compared with DSE alone and PET.[47]

Myocardial contrast echocardiography (MCE) also can be performed during stress echocardiography,[22] with good concordance between dipyridamole stress MCE and SPECT for detection of coronary artery disease. Recently, real-time myocardial contrast perfusion imaging has been shown to improve the detection of CAD during stress echocardiography, and to identify patients more likely to undergo revascularization after an abnormal study, when compared with conventional stress echocardiography,[48] but loses some of its predictive value in women.[49]

Stress echocardiography, although less well validated, also can detect *right ventricular ischemia*,[3] but the ischemic threshold is higher, and usually only the inferior wall of the ventricle is affected. In patients with three-vessel CAD undergoing DSE, failure to increase TAPSE by more than 2 mm identified ischemic right ventricular dysfunction with sensitivity of 79% and specificity of 88%. Additional studies, particularly with the use of speckle-tracking and three-dimensional echocardiography, are needed to increase the diagnostic and prognostic information on right ventricular ischemia.

Transesophageal Echocardiography and Myocardial Infarction

Transesophageal echocardiography (TEE) is a useful alternative when the transthoracic approach is technically difficult and provides suboptimal or nondiagnostic images, as may be the case in obese persons, people with lung disease, or patients who have had recent cardiothoracic surgery. Assessment of regional and global ventricular function can be performed with TEE at rest or with stress, using either dobutamine infusion of cardiac pacing. Detection and detailed evaluation of mechanical complications of an acute MI, such as a ruptured papillary muscle or a VSD (see Figure 31-20), also is possible with TEE.[2] MR secondary to ischemia or infarction is a frequent finding in patients with MI, but it is occasionally difficult to determine precisely its severity or mechanism with transthoracic echocardiography. TEE provides additional information, with important therapeutic implications, especially if mitral valve repair is being considered. TEE also can be useful in patients with MI and atrial fibrillation, particularly if the duration of the latter is unknown. TEE is indeed a reliable and safe method to evaluate for the presence of an intracardiac thrombus before cardioversion is performed in this setting. Occasionally a suspected embolus during the course of an MI may represent an indication for TEE.

SUMMARY

Rest and stress echocardiography studies provide important information on systolic and diastolic ventricular function in patients after MI. Evaluation of residual ischemia and of myocardial viability after MI can be done with stress echocardiography incorporating newer technologies such as three-dimensional echocardiographic techniques, TDI, and SRI. Assessment of myocardial viability and perfusion with MCE is another emerging approach with excellent correlation with radionuclide imaging, which has the potential to expand further the use of cardiac ultrasound modalities. These techniques also are available for better quantitative evaluation of global and regional left ventricular function after MI. Echocardiography is a valuable part of the evaluation of most patients with MI.

ACKNOWLEDGMENTS

The authors are grateful to Celine Pitre, chief sonographer at the Montreal Heart Institute, for her contribution to the figures and videos, and to Dr François Marcotte for kindly providing the dobutamine stress echocardiography videos.

Classic References

Labovitz AJ, Lewen MK, Kern M, et al.: Evaluation of left ventricular systolic and diastolic dysfunction during transient myocardial ischemia produced by angioplasty, *J Am Coll Cardiol* 10(4):748–755, 1987.

Levine RA, Thomas JD: Insights into the physiologic significance of the mitral inflow velocity pattern, *J Am Coll Cardiol* 14(7):1718–1720, 1989.

Pandian NG, Koyanagi S, Skorton DJ, et al.: Relations between 2-dimensional echocardiographic wall thickening abnormalities, myocardial infarct size and coronary risk area in normal and hypertrophied myocardium in dogs, *Am J Cardiol* 52(10):1318–1325, 1983.

Theroux P, Ross Jr J, Franklin D, et al.: Regional myocardial function and dimensions early and late after myocardial infarction in the unanesthetized dog, *Circ Res* 40:158–165, 1977.

References

1. Douglas PS, Garcia MJ, Haines DE, et al.: ACCF/ASE/AHA/ASNC/HFSA/HRS/SCAI/SCCM/SCCT/SCMR 2011 appropriate use criteria for echocardiography. A report of the American College of Cardiology Foundation Appropriate Use Criteria Task Force, American Society of Echocardiography, American Heart Association, American Society of Nuclear Cardiology, Heart Failure Society of America, Heart Rhythm Society, Society for Cardiovascular Angiography and Interventions, Society of Critical Care Medicine, Society of Cardiovascular Computed Tomography, and Society for Cardiovascular Magnetic Resonance. Endorsed by the American College of Chest Physicians, *J Am Coll Cardiol* 57(9):1126–1166, 2011.
2. Sia YT, O'Meara E, Ducharme A: Role of echocardiography in acute myocardial infarction, *Curr Heart Fail Rep* 5(4):189–196, 2008.
3. Rallidis LS, Makavos G, Nihoyannopoulos P: Right ventricular involvement in coronary artery disease: Role of echocardiography for diagnosis and prognosis, *J Am Soc Echocardiogr* 27(3):223–229, 2014.
4. Voigt JU, Schneider TM, Korder S, et al.: Apical transverse motion as surrogate parameter to determine regional left ventricular function inhomogeneities: A new, integrative approach to left ventricular asynchrony assessment, *Eur Heart J* 30(8):959–968, 2009.
5. Solomon SD, Shin SH, Shah A, et al.: Effect of the direct renin inhibitor aliskiren on left ventricular remodelling following myocardial infarction with systolic dysfunction, *Eur Heart J* 32(10):1227–1234, 2011.
6. Innocenti F, Caldi F, Tassinari I, et al.: Prognostic value of exercise stress test and dobutamine stress echo in patients with known coronary artery disease, *Echocardiography* 26(1):1–9, 2009.
7. Solomon SD, Skali H, Anavekar NS, et al.: Changes in ventricular size and function in patients treated with valsartan, captopril, or both after myocardial infarction, *Circulation* 111(25):3411–3419, 2005.
8. Kaul S: The "no reflow" phenomenon following acute myocardial infarction: Mechanisms and treatment options, *J Cardiol* 64(2):77–85, 2014.
9. Funaro S, Galiuto L, Boccalini F, et al.: Determinants of microvascular damage recovery after acute myocardial infarction: Results from the Acute Myocardial Infarction Contrast Imaging (AMICI) multi-centre study, *Eur J Echocardiogr* 12(4):306–312, 2011.
10. Russo AM, Stainback RF, Bailey SR, et al.: ACCF/HRS/AHA/ASE/HFSA/SCAI/SCCT/SCMR 2013 appropriate use criteria for implantable cardioverter-defibrillators and cardiac resynchronization therapy: A report of the American College of Cardiology Foundation Appropriate Use Criteria Task Force, Heart Rhythm Society, American Heart Association, American Society of Echocardiography, Heart Failure Society of America, Society for Cardiovascular Angiography and Interventions, Society of Cardiovascular Computed Tomography, and Society for Cardiovascular Magnetic Resonance, *J Am Coll Cardiol* 61(12):1318–1368, 2013.
11. Lang RM, Badano LP, Mor-Avi V, et al.: Recommendations for cardiac chamber quantification by echocardiography in adults: An update from the American Society of Echocardiography and the European Association of Cardiovascular Imaging, *J Am Soc Echocardiogr* 28(1):1–39, 2015.
12. Muraru D, Badano LP, Piccoli G, et al.: Validation of a novel automated border-detection algorithm for rapid and accurate quantitation of left ventricular volumes based on three-dimensional echocardiography, *Eur J Echocardiogr* 11(4):359–368, 2010.
13. Onishi T, Saha SK, Delgado-Montero A, et al.: Global longitudinal strain and global circumferential strain by speckle-tracking echocardiography and feature-tracking cardiac magnetic resonance imaging: Comparison with left ventricular ejection fraction, *J Am Soc Echocardiogr* 28(5):587–596, 2015.
14. Voigt JU, Pedrizzetti G, Lysyansky P, et al.: Definitions for a common standard for 2D speckle tracking echocardiography: Consensus Document of the EACVI/ASE/Industry Task Force to Standardize Deformation Imaging, *J Am Soc Echocardiogr* 28(2):183–193, 2015.
15. Mor-Avi V, Lang RM, Badano LP, et al.: Current and evolving echocardiographic techniques for the quantitative evaluation of cardiac mechanics: ASE/EAE consensus statement on methodology and indications endorsed by the Japanese Society of Echocardiography, *J Am Soc Echocardiogr* 24(3):277–313, 2011.
16. Mignot A, Donal E, Zaroui A, et al.: Global longitudinal strain as a major predictor of cardiac events in patients with depressed left ventricular function: A multicenter study, *J Am Soc Echocardiogr* 23(10):1019–1024, 2010.
17. Stanton T, Leano R, Marwick TH: Prediction of all-cause mortality from global longitudinal speckle strain: Comparison with ejection fraction and wall motion scoring, *Circ Cardiovasc Imaging* 2(5):356–364, 2009.
18. Haugaa KH, Grenne BL, Eek CH, et al.: Strain echocardiography improves risk prediction of ventricular arrhythmias after myocardial infarction, *JACC Cardiovasc Imaging* 6(8):841–885, 2013.
19. Popovic ZB: The uncertainties of certainty: Using LV function to predict arrhythmic event after AMI, *JACC Cardiovasc Imaging* 6(8):861–863, 2013.
20. Edvardsen T, Haugaa KH: The thorny way of 3D strain from research to clinical use: Are we getting closer? *JACC Cardiovasc Imaging* 8(3):246–247, 2015.
21. Hu K, Liu D, Niemann M, et al.: Methods for assessment of left ventricular systolic function in technically difficult patients with poor imaging quality, *J Am Soc Echocardiogr* 26(2):105–113, 2013.
22. Ito H: Myocardial contrast echocardiography after myocardial infarction, *Curr Cardiol Rep* 14(3):350–358, 2012.
23. Little WC, Oh JK: Echocardiographic evaluation of diastolic function can be used to guide clinical care, *Circulation* 120(9):802–809, 2009.
24. Tschope C, Paulus WJ: Is echocardiographic evaluation of diastolic function useful in determining clinical care? Doppler echocardiography yields dubious estimates of left ventricular diastolic pressures, *Circulation* 120(9):810–820, 2009.
25. Gharacholou SM, Scott CG, Takahashi PY, et al.: Left ventricular diastolic function and long-term outcomes in patients with normal exercise echocardiographic findings, *Am J Cardiol* 112(2):200–207, 2013.
26. Jons C, Joergensen RM, Hassager C, et al.: Diastolic dysfunction predicts new-onset atrial fibrillation and cardiovascular events in patients with acute myocardial infarction and depressed left ventricular systolic function: A CARISMA substudy, *Eur J Echocardiogr* 11(7):602–607, 2010.
27. Kawasaki M, Tanaka R, Ono K, et al.: A novel ultrasound predictor of pulmonary capillary wedge pressure assessed by the combination of left atrial volume and function: A speckle tracking echocardiography study, *J Cardiol* 66(3):253–262, 2015.
28. Rahman N, Kazmi KA, Yousaf M: Non-invasive prediction of ST elevation myocardial infarction complications by left ventricular Tei index, *J Pak Med Assoc* 59(2):75–78, 2009.
29. Vonk NA, Haddad F, Bogaard HJ, Hassoun PM: Noninvasive imaging in the assessment of the cardiopulmonary vascular unit, *Circulation* 131(10):899–913, 2015.
30. Rudski LG, Lai WW, Afilalo J, et al.: Guidelines for the echocardiographic assessment of the right heart in adults: A report from the American Society of Echocardiography endorsed by the European Association of Echocardiography, a registered branch of the European Society of Cardiology, and the Canadian Society of Echocardiography, *J Am Soc Echocardiogr* 23(7):685–713, 2010.
31. Anderson K, Prylutska H, Ducharme A, et al.: Evaluation of the right ventricle: Comparison of gated blood-pool single photon electron computed tomography and echocardiography with cardiac magnetic resonance, *Int J Cardiol* 171(1):1–8, 2014.
32. Leibundgut G, Rohner A, Grize L, et al.: Dynamic assessment of right ventricular volumes and function by real-time three-dimensional echocardiography: A comparison study with magnetic resonance imaging in 100 adult patients, *J Am Soc Echocardiogr* 23(2):116–126, 2013.
33. Kidawa M, Chizynski K, Zielinska M, et al.: Real-time 3D echocardiography and tissue Doppler echocardiography in the assessment of right ventricle systolic function in patients with right ventricular myocardial infarction, *Eur Heart J Cardiovasc Imaging* 14(10):1002–1009, 2013.
34. Hsu SY, Lin JF, Chang SH: Right ventricular function in patients with different infarction sites after a first acute myocardial infarction, *Am J Med Sci* 342(6):474–479, 2011.
35. Roberts WC, Burks KH, Ko JM, et al.: Commonalities of cardiac rupture (left ventricular free wall or ventricular septum or papillary muscle) during acute myocardial infarction secondary to atherosclerotic coronary artery disease, *Am J Cardiol* 115(1):125–140, 2015.
36. Calvert PA, Cockburn J, Wynne D, et al.: Percutaneous closure of postinfarction ventricular septal defect: In-hospital outcomes and long-term follow-up of UK experience, *Circulation* 129(23):2395–2402, 2014.
37. Enriquez-Sarano M, Akins CW, Vahanian A: Mitral regurgitation, *Lancet* 373(9672):1382–1394, 2009.
38. Culp Jr WC, Knight WL: Echo rounds: Three-dimensional transesophageal echocardiography of papillary muscle rupture, *Anesth Analg* 111(2):358–360, 2010.
39. Shacham Y, Leshem-Rubinow E, Ben AE, et al.: Frequency and correlates of early left ventricular thrombus formation following anterior wall acute myocardial infarction treated with primary percutaneous coronary intervention, *Am J Cardiol* 111(5):667–670, 2013.
40. Solomon SD, Anavekar N, Skali H, et al.: Influence of ejection fraction on cardiovascular outcomes in a broad spectrum of heart failure patients, *Circulation* 112(24):3738–3744, 2005.

41. Shaw LJ, Berman DS, Picard MH, et al.: Comparative definitions for moderate-severe ischemia in stress nuclear, echocardiography, and magnetic resonance imaging, *JACC Cardiovasc Imaging* 7(6):593–604, 2014.
42. Douglas PS, Khandheria B, Stainback RF, et al.: ACCF/ASE/ACEP/AHA/ASNC/SCAI/SCCT/SCMR 2008 appropriateness criteria for stress echocardiography: A report of the American College of Cardiology Foundation Appropriateness Criteria Task Force, American Society of Echocardiography, American College of Emergency Physicians, American Heart Association, American Society of Nuclear Cardiology, Society for Cardiovascular Angiography and Interventions, Society of Cardiovascular Computed Tomography, and Society for Cardiovascular Magnetic Resonance. Endorsed by the Heart Rhythm Society and the Society of Critical Care Medicine, *J Am Coll Cardiol* 51(11):1127–1147, 2008.
43. Douglas PS, Hoffmann U, Patel MR, et al.: Outcomes of anatomical versus functional testing for coronary artery disease, *N Engl J Med* 372(14):1291–1300, 2015.
44. Bonow RO, Maurer G, Lee KL, et al.: Myocardial viability and survival in ischemic left ventricular dysfunction, *N Engl J Med* 364(17):1617–1625, 2011.
45. Bernheim AM, Kittipovanonth M, Takahashi PY, et al.: Does the prognostic value of dobutamine stress echocardiography differ among different age groups? *Am Heart J* 161(4):740–745, 2011.
46. Sadeghian H, Majd-Ardakani J, Lotfi-Tokaldany M, et al.: Comparison between dobutamine stress echocardiography and myocardial perfusion scan to detect viable myocardium in patients with coronary artery disease and low ejection fraction, *Hellenic J Cardiol* 50(1):45–51, 2009.
47. Vitarelli A, Montesano T, Gaudio C, et al.: Strain rate dobutamine echocardiography for prediction of recovery after revascularization in patients with ischemic left ventricular dysfunction, *J Card Fail* 12(4):268–275, 2006.
48. Porter TR, Smith LM, Wu J, et al.: Patient outcome following 2 different stress imaging approaches: A prospective randomized comparison, *J Am Coll Cardiol* 61(24):2446–2455, 2013.
49. Laiq Z, Smith LM, Xie F, et al.: Differences in patient outcomes after conventional versus real time perfusion stress echocardiography in men versus women: A prospective randomised trial, *Heart* 101(7):559–564, 2015.

32 Nuclear Cardiology Techniques After Myocardial Infarction

Marcelo F. Di Carli and Róisín Morgan

INTRODUCTION

Cardiovascular nuclear medicine imaging techniques are part of the ever-growing clinical noninvasive imaging armamentarium for the evaluation of suspected or known coronary artery disease (CAD). These techniques provide valuable information regarding diagnosis and clinical risk, and consequently have established a role in the management of this disease. In this chapter, we will provide a concise summary of contemporary nuclear cardiology techniques, and then use a case-based approach to illustrate their practical utility in the evaluation and management of patients after myocardial infarction (MI). The role of nuclear cardiology techniques in the initial assessment of patients with chest pain suspicious for MI is discussed in Chapter 9. The use of echocardiography and use of cardiac magnetic resonance imaging (MRI) after MI are addressed in Chapter 31 and Chapter 33, respectively.

TECHNICAL CONSIDERATIONS FOR RADIONUCLIDE IMAGING

Fundamentals of Single Photon Emission Computed Tomography and Positron Emission Tomography Imaging

Radionuclide imaging techniques are commonly used for the evaluation of patients with known or suspected CAD, including those presenting with acute coronary syndromes (ACS). These techniques use radiolabeled drugs, or radiopharmaceuticals[1] (Table 32-1), which are injected intravenously and trapped in myocardial tissue. Radioactivity within the heart decays by emitting gamma rays. The interaction between these gamma rays and the detectors in specialized scanners—single photon emission computed tomography (SPECT) and positron emission tomography (PET)—creates a scintillation event or light output, which can be captured by digital recording equipment to form an image of the heart. Like computed tomography (CT) (see Chapter 9) and MRI (see Chapter 33), radionuclide imaging also can generate tomographic (three-dimensional) views of the heart.

Protocols for Myocardial Perfusion and Viability Imaging

Imaging protocols are tailored to the individual patient based on the clinical question and on patient-specific risk, ability to exercise, and body mass index, among other factors. Electrocardiogram (ECG)-triggered gated rest and stress images are acquired after intravenous injection of the radiopharmaceutical and used to define the extent and severity of myocardial ischemia and scar, as well as regional and global cardiac function and remodeling. The choice between exercise versus pharmacologic stress with vasodilators (adenosine, dipyridamole, or regadenoson) and direct chronotropic/inotropic stimulation with dobutamine is based on well-defined guidelines depending on the patient's condition, the clinical question, and safety considerations, especially in the post-MI patient (see Chapter 30).[1,2]

For SPECT imaging, technetium-99m (^{99m}Tc)-labeled tracers are the most commonly used imaging agents because they are associated with the best image quality and the lowest radiation dose to the patient. After intravenous injection, myocardial uptake of ^{99m}Tc-labeled tracers is rapid (1 to 2 minutes). After uptake, these tracers become trapped intracellularly in mitochondria and show minimal change over time. Because of these kinetics, ^{99m}Tc tracers can be helpful in the investigation of chest pain occurring at rest, in that the tracer can be injected while the patient is having chest pain and images obtained some time later after symptoms subside (within 6 hours after injection). Because the radiotracer is trapped at the time of injection, the images provide a snapshot of myocardial perfusion at that moment, even if the acquisition was delayed. This property is a key requirement for the use of ^{99m}Tc SPECT in the quantification of myocardium

TABLE 32-1 Radiopharmaceuticals for Clinical Radionuclide Imaging

RADIOPHARMACEUTICAL	IMAGING TECHNIQUE	PHYSICAL HALF-LIFE	APPLICATION
^{99m}Tc agents (sestamibi, tetrofosmin)	SPECT	6 hours	Myocardial perfusion and viability imaging
^{201}Tl	SPECT	72 hours	Myocardial perfusion and viability imaging
^{123}I-mIBG	SPECT	13 hours	Cardiac sympathetic neuronal imaging
^{82}Rb	PET	76 seconds	Myocardial perfusion imaging
^{13}N-ammonia	PET	10 minutes	Myocardial perfusion imaging
^{18}F-FDG	PET	120 minutes	Myocardial viability imaging

FDG, Fluorodeoxyglucose; *mIBG,* metaiodobenzylguanidine; *PET,* positron emission tomography; *SPECT,* single photon emission computed tomography.

at risk and salvage in patients with acute MI (see later under Quantification of Myocardium at Risk, Infarct Size, and Myocardial Salvage). Indeed, a normal myocardial perfusion study after a rest injection in a patient with active chest pain effectively excludes myocardial ischemia as the cause of chest pain (high negative predictive value) (see Chapter 9). Although commonly used in the past for perfusion imaging, thallium-201 (^{201}Tl) protocols are now rarely used because they are associated with a higher radiation dose to the patient.

PET myocardial perfusion imaging is an alternative to SPECT and is associated with improved diagnostic accuracy and lower radiation dose to the patient, owing to the fact that radiotracers typically are short-lived (Table 32-1). The ultrashort half-life of some PET radiopharmaceuticals in clinical use, such as rubidium-82 (^{82}Rb), is the primary reason that PET imaging generally is combined with pharmacologic stress, as opposed to exercise, because pharmacologic stress allows for faster imaging of these rapidly decaying tracers. However, use of exercise is possible with relatively longer-lived radiotracers (e.g., ^{13}N-ammonia). For myocardial perfusion imaging, ^{82}Rb does not require an onsite medical cyclotron (it is available from a strontium-82 [^{82}Sr]/^{82}Rb generator), so it is the most commonly used radiopharmaceutical. ^{13}N-ammonia has better flow characteristics (higher myocardial extraction) and imaging properties than ^{82}Rb, but use of this agent does require access to a medical cyclotron. In comparison with SPECT, PET gives improved spatial and contrast resolution, and it provides absolute measures of myocardial perfusion (in mL/min/g of tissue), thereby providing a quantitative measure of regional and global coronary flow reserve. As discussed later on, quantitative measures of myocardial blood flow and flow reserve help improve diagnostic accuracy and risk stratification.

Contemporary PET and SPECT scanners frequently are combined with a CT scanner, for so-called hybrid PET-CT and SPECT-CT. CT is used primarily to guide patient positioning in the field of view and for correcting inhomogeneities in radiotracer distribution from attenuation by soft tissues (so-called attenuation correction). However, it also can be used to obtain diagnostic data including coronary artery calcium score and/or CT coronary angiography (see Chapter 9), although the usefulness of combined studies in the post-MI patient is more limited.

For the evaluation of myocardial viability in patients after MI, myocardial perfusion imaging with SPECT or PET usually is combined with metabolic imaging—specifically, ^{18}F-fluorodeoxyglucose (FDG) PET. In hospital settings lacking access to PET scanning, ^{201}Tl SPECT imaging is a useful alternative.[1]

Evaluation of Myocardial Ischemia, Viability, and Function

The presence of a reversible myocardial perfusion defect is indicative of ischemia (Figure 32-1, top), whereas a fixed perfusion defect generally reflects scarred myocardium from previous infarction (Figure 32-1, bottom). Regional myocardial perfusion usually is assessed by semiquantitative visual analysis of the rest and stress images.[3] The regional scores are then summed into global scores that reflect the total burden of ischemia and scar in the left ventricle. Objective quantitative image analysis is a helpful tool for a more accurate and reproducible estimation of total defect size and severity and generally is used in combination with semiquantitative visual analysis. The semiquantitative and quantitative scores for ischemia and scar are linearly related to the risk of adverse cardiovascular events and are most useful in guiding patient management, especially the need for revascularization, and for assessing response to medical therapy.

Quantification of Myocardial Ischemia and Viability

Myocardial perfusion and metabolic imaging are commonly used to evaluate the patient after MI, especially when the question of revascularization is being considered. The protocols are tailored to the clinical question and provide important quantitative information: (1) myocardial infarct size; (2) extent of stunning and hibernating myocardium; (3) magnitude of inducible myocardial ischemia within the infarct-related territory and in remote myocardium, the latter reflecting multivessel CAD; and (4) left ventricular function and volumes.

Both ^{201}Tl-labeled and, especially, ^{99m}Tc-labeled agents provide accurate and reproducible measurements of regional and global myocardial infarct size (Figure 32-2). The use of metabolic imaging with PET has been extensively validated and is commonly used for assessing myocardial viability. ^{18}F-FDG is used to assess regional myocardial glucose utilization (an index of tissue viability) and compared to perfusion images to define metabolic abnormalities associated with infarction and hibernation.[4,5] Myocardial regions showing reduced perfusion and increased FDG uptake at rest (so-called *perfusion-FDG mismatch*) identify areas of viable but hibernating myocardium, whereas regions showing reduced perfusion and reduced FDG uptake at rest (so-called *perfusion-FDG match*) are consistent with myocardial

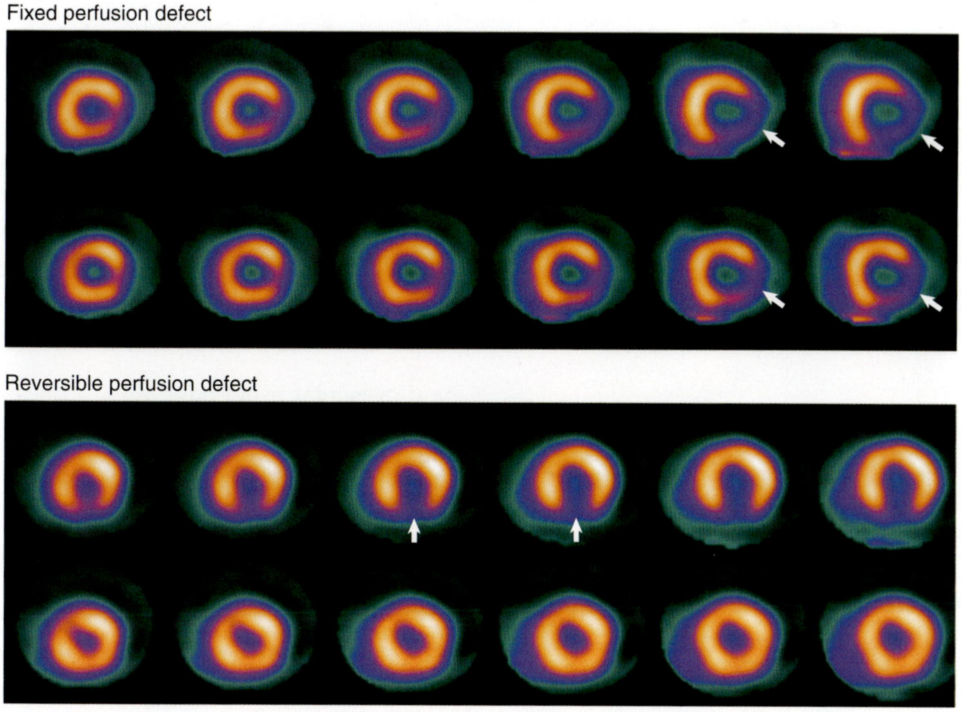

FIGURE 32-1 **Stress *(top row)* and rest *(bottom row)* short-axis myocardial perfusion images demonstrating the presence of fixed and reversible perfusion defects *(arrows)*.**

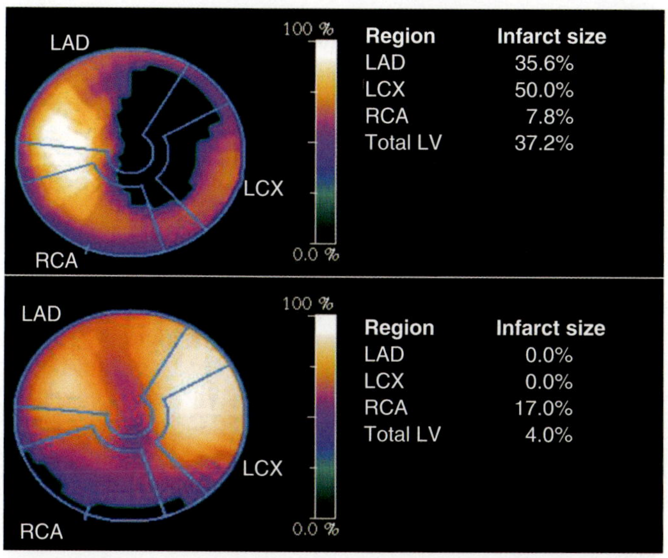

FIGURE 32-2 **Two-dimensional bull's-eye display *(polar map)* of regional count profiles at rest for two patients with a large *(top)* and a small *(bottom)* myocardial infarction *(blackout defect)*.** The total infarct size typically is calculated by adding the number of pixels in the polar map showing less than 50% or 60% of the peak myocardial counts. *LAD,* Left anterior descending artery; *LCx,* left circumflex artery; *LV,* left ventricle; *RCA,* right coronary artery.

scar (Figure 32-3). These metabolic patterns have important implications for selection of patients for revascularization (see later under Evaluation of Patients with Heart Failure after Myocardial Infarction).

Quantification of Myocardial Blood Flow and Coronary Flow Reserve

Myocardial blood flow (in mL/min/g of myocardium) and coronary flow reserve (CFR)—defined as the ratio between peak stress and rest myocardial blood flow)—are important physiologic parameters that can be measured by routine postprocessing of myocardial perfusion PET images. These absolute measurements of tissue perfusion are accurate and reproducible.[6] Pathophysiologically, CFR estimates provide a measure of the integrated effects of epicardial coronary stenoses, diffuse atherosclerosis and vessel remodeling, and microvascular dysfunction on myocardial perfusion; accordingly, the value obtained is a more sensitive measure of myocardial ischemia. In the setting of increased oxygen demand, a reduced CFR can upset the supply-demand relationship and lead to myocardial ischemia, subclinical left ventricular dysfunction (diastolic and systolic), symptoms, and death. One of the practical applications of CFR measurements is in the evaluation of flow-limiting stenosis, especially useful in the context of multivessel CAD (Figure 32-4). Indeed, a relatively normal CFR (above 1.9) virtually excludes the possibility of significant stenosis.[7]

Furthermore, consistent evidence indicates that CFR measurements by PET can identify subgroups of patients with different clinical risk across a wide spectrum of ischemic burden[8,9] (Figure 32-5). Indeed, the presence of relatively preserved CFR identifies patients with CAD at a significantly lower risk for cardiac death, regardless of the semiquantitative extent of stress-induced ischemia.[8,9] Conversely, a reduced CFR identifies patients at significantly higher risk for cardiac death, even among those in whom the semiquantitative extent of ischemia is mild to moderate. These data suggest that the traditional (semiquantitative) measures of ischemia alone may be insufficient to identify potential prognostic benefit from myocardial revascularization.

Quantification of Myocardium at Risk, Infarct Size, and Myocardial Salvage

Radionuclide imaging has been extensively validated and used to quantify myocardium at risk, infarct size, and

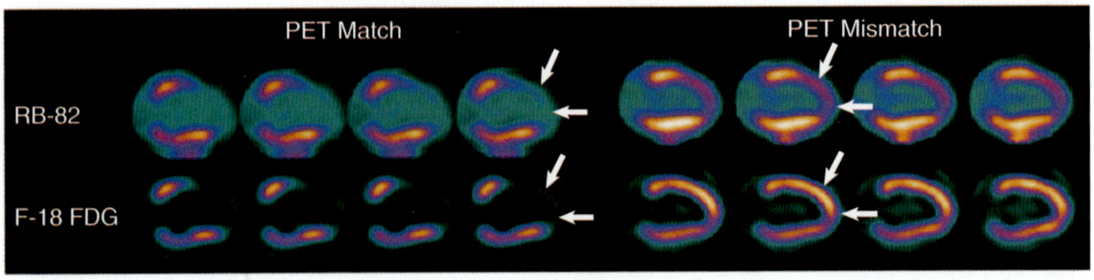

FIGURE 32-3 Examples of myocardial viability patterns assessed by integrating perfusion and metabolic imaging with positron emission tomography (PET) imaging. *Left,* Concordant reduction in perfusion (RB-82) and glucose uptake as labeled with ^{18}F-fluorodeoxyglucose (FDG) *(arrows)* throughout the anterior wall and apex, consistent with nonviable myocardium from previous infarction. *Right,* Increase in FDG uptake relative to perfusion in the anterior wall and apex, consistent with viable but hibernating myocardium. *(From Di Carli MF, Hachamovitch R: New technology for noninvasive evaluation of coronary artery disease.* Circulation *115:1464-1480, 2007.)*

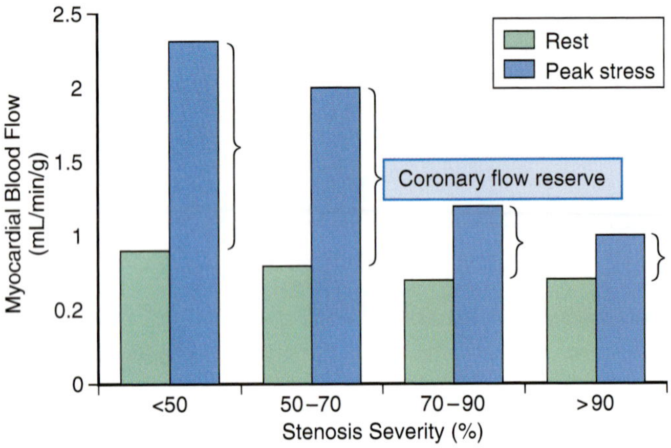

FIGURE 32-4 Bar graph illustrating the relationship between myocardial blood flow and flow reserve as quantified by positron emission tomography (PET) imaging and angiographic coronary stenosis assessed by quantitative coronary angiography. Peak myocardial blood flow and coronary flow reserve are significantly reduced with increasing percent stenosis. *(Data from Di Carli M, Czernin J, Hoh CK, et al: Relation among stenosis severity, myocardial blood flow, and flow reserve in patients with coronary artery disease.* Circulation *91[7]:1944-1951, 1995.)*

myocardial salvage after reperfusion therapy for acute MI.[10] Both ^{201}Tl and ^{99m}Tc agents have been used for this purpose. However, ^{99m}Tc agents have been the most widely used and validated. The fact that after intravenous injection and initial myocardial uptake, tissue retention of ^{99m}Tc agents remains relatively constant is especially important in the setting of acute MI. Consequently, these agents can be injected intravenously when a patient with acute MI first presents to the emergency department. Imaging can be delayed while the patient undergoes acute care and still reflect myocardial tissue perfusion at the time of initial presentation (i.e., myocardium at risk). Final infarct size is then assessed by a second injection of ^{99m}Tc agents and imaging 5 to 7 days after reperfusion therapy. The quantitative difference between the total perfusion defect size in the initial and late images reflects myocardial salvage (Figure 32-6). This protocol has been widely used in clinical trials evaluating the effect of therapies designed to limit infarct size. FDG PET also provides accurate quantification of infarct size.[11] Clinically, the measurement of infarct size with radionuclide imaging is widely used, especially for evaluating myocardial viability.

Quantification of Left Ventricular Function and Volumes

The acquisition of ECG-gated myocardial perfusion images allows quantification of regional and global systolic function, and left ventricular volumes. ECG-gated images typically are collected at rest and after stress (SPECT) or during stress (PET). Rest left ventricular ejection fraction (LVEF) measurements are helpful to define the patient's risk for a cardiovascular event after MI. A drop in LVEF after or during stress testing can be helpful to identify high-risk patients with multivessel CAD.[6]

Accuracy of Radionuclide Imaging for Identification of Flow-Limiting Coronary Artery Disease

The most relevant clinical issue in post-MI patients is not the diagnosis of CAD, which is already established, but rather the identification of residual flow-limiting stenosis in the infarct-related artery and/or non–culprit coronary arteries. Traditionally, diagnostic accuracy of physiologic imaging methods for CAD assessment has been defined using a threshold of 50% or 70% stenosis on coronary angiography. This traditional measure, however, has limited clinical applicability, because it is now clear that more than two thirds of angiographic stenoses are not flow-limiting when assessed by a physiologic gold standard such as fractional flow reserve (FFR). A recent meta-analysis has evaluated the relative accuracy of myocardial perfusion imaging techniques including radionuclide imaging (SPECT and PET), echocardiography, MRI, and CT for identifying flow-limiting stenosis as assessed by FFR.[12] Thirty-seven studies reporting on 4721 vessels and 2048 patients were included. On a patient-based level, PET, MRI, and CT had higher sensitivity and negative predictive value compared with SPECT and echocardiography. Similar results were observed on a vessel-based analysis (Table 32-2).

Beyond detection of angiographic stenosis, an extensive literature supports the role of radionuclide imaging for risk assessment, including in the post-MI patient. Well-recognized markers of higher clinical risk with radionuclide perfusion imaging are (1) large perfusion defects, often involving multiple coronary territories; (2) presence of transient cavity dilation with stress; (3) transient increase in radiotracer uptake in the right ventricular free wall during stress; and (4) increased pulmonary uptake (Figure 32-7). All of these markers identify patients with extensive multivessel myocardial ischemia at higher risk for adverse cardiovascular events, including death.

Radiation Dose

Radionuclide imaging studies expose patients to ionizing radiation. Several recent publications have raised concern regarding the potential harmful effects of ionizing radiation associated with cardiac imaging. The so-called *effective dose* is a measure used to estimate the biologic effects of radiation and expressed in millisieverts (mSv). However, measuring the radiation effective dose associated with diagnostic imaging is complex and imprecise, often resulting in variable estimates, even among experts. The effective dose from a typical myocardial

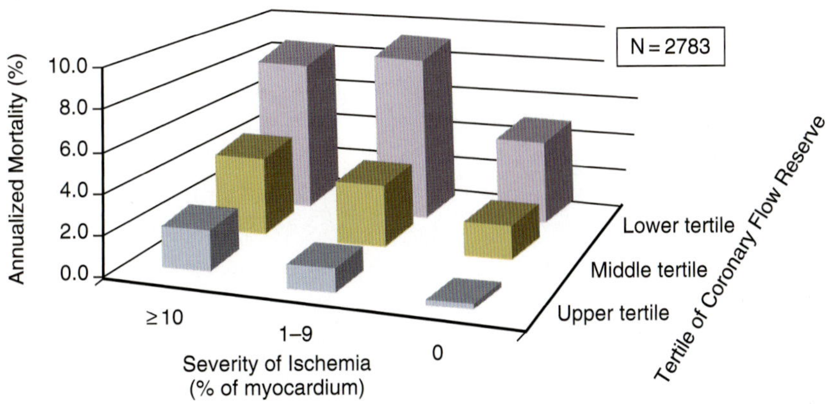

	≥10%	(n)	1–9%	(n)	0%	(n)
Upper tertile	2.2%	(50)	1.1%	(197)	0.1%	(681)
Middle tertile	4.2%	(119)	3.3%	(234)	1.8%	(575)
Lower tertile	8.5%	(232)	9.1%	(298)	4.5%	(397)

FIGURE 32-5 Unadjusted annualized cardiac mortality by tertiles of coronary flow reserve (CFR) and categories of myocardial ischemia. The annual rate of cardiac death increased with increasing extent and severity of ischemia. Lower CFR consistently identified higher-risk patients at every level of myocardial ischemia, including among those with normal-appearing positron emission tomography (PET) scans. *(From Ziadi MC, Dekemp RA, Williams KA, et al: Impaired myocardial flow reserve on rubidium-82 positron emission tomography imaging predicts adverse outcomes in patients assessed for myocardial ischemia.* J Am Coll Cardiol *58:740-748, 2011.)*

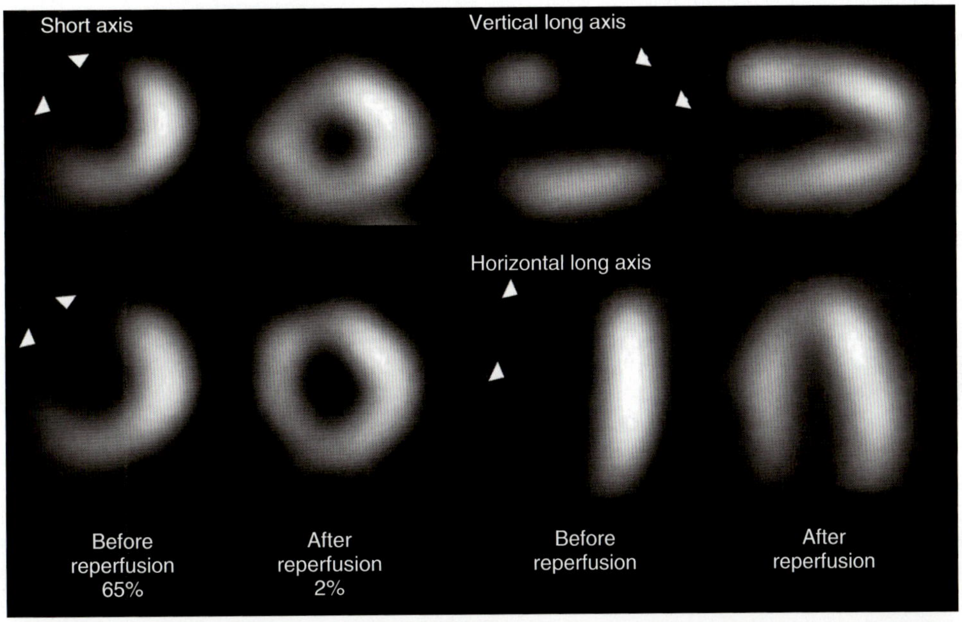

FIGURE 32-6 Representative short, vertical long-axis, and horizontal long-axis images obtained with ^{99m}Tc- sestamibi single positron emission computed tomography (SPECT) in a patient with anterior myocardial infarction. The initial sestamibi injection image (obtained before reperfusion) shows a large and severe perfusion defect *(arrowheads)* throughout the left anterior descending artery (LAD) territory, reflecting the total territory of myocardium at risk. Image obtained after a second dose of sestamibi a week later reflects the final infarct size *(arrowheads)* after reperfusion. The percentage difference between the initial and final images reflects the magnitude of salvaged myocardium after reperfusion. *(Courtesy of Dr. Todd Miller, Mayo Clinic, Rochester, Minnesota.)*

TABLE 32-2 Diagnostic Accuracy of Noninvasive Imaging Techniques for Identification of Flow-Limiting Coronary Artery Disease*

MODALITY	SENSITIVITY	SPECIFICITY	PLR	NLR	AUC
SPECT	0.74 (0.67-0.70)	0.79 (0.74-0.83)	3.1 (2.1-4.7)	0.39 (0.27-0.55)	0.82 (0.73-0.91)
PET	0.84 (0.75-0.91)	0.87 (0.8-0.92)	6.53 (2.83-15.1)	0.14 (0.02-0.87)	0.93 (NA)
Echocardiography	0.69 (0.56-0.79)	0.84 (0.75-0.9)	3.68 (1.89-7.15)	0.42 (0.3-0.59)	0.83 (0.74-0.93)
MRI	0.89 (0.86-0.92)	0.87 (0.83-0.9)	6.29 (4.88-8.12)	0.14 (0.1-0.18)	0.94 (0.92-0.96)
CT	0.88 (0.82-0.92)	0.8 (0.73-0.86)	3.79 (1.94-7.4)	0.12 (0.04-0.33)	0.93 (0.89-0.97)

*As assessed by coronary angiography with fractional flow reserve.
AUC, Area under the (receiver operating characteristic) curve; *CT,* computed tomography; *MRI,* magnetic resonance imaging; *NLR,* negative likelihood ratio; *PET,* positron emission tomography; *PLR,* positive likelihood ratio; *SPECT,* single photon emission computed tomography.

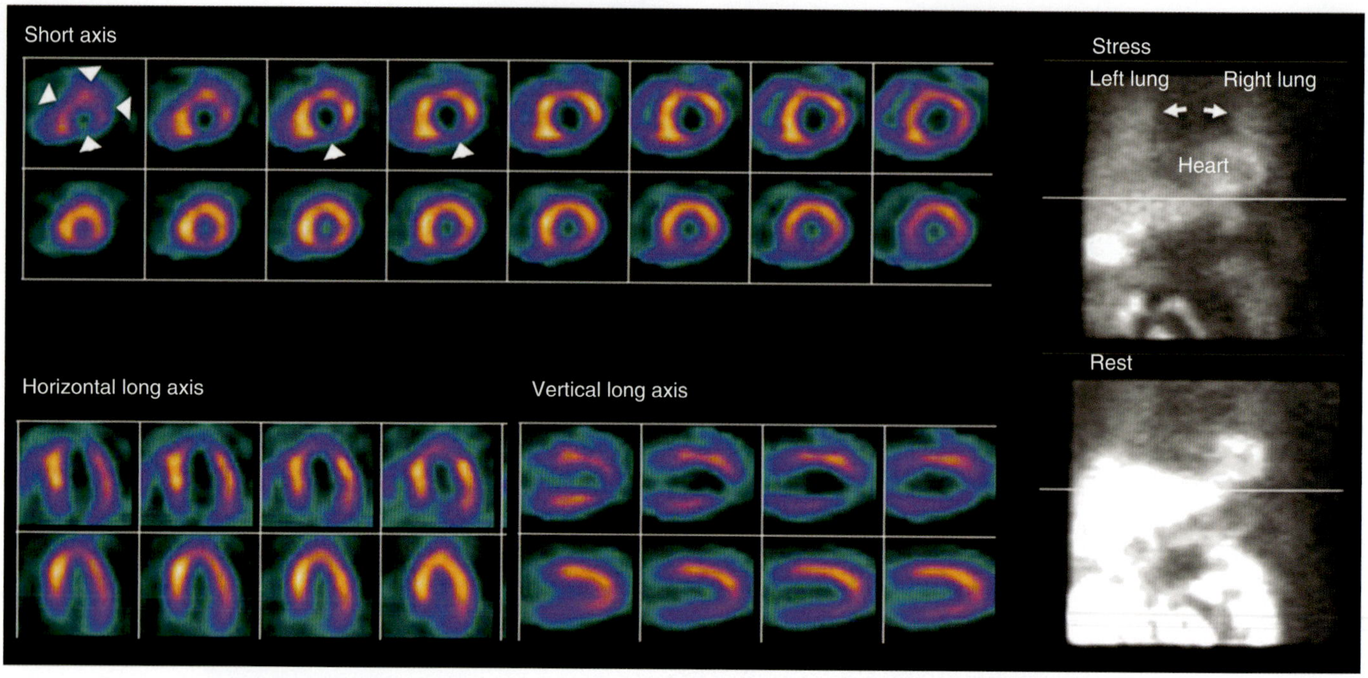

FIGURE 32-7 Exercise stress and rest myocardial perfusion single positron emission computed tomography (SPECT) images in a patient with atypical angina. The study shows transient cavity dilation during stress (so-called transient ischemic dilation [TID]), transient increased tracer uptake in the right ventricular free wall, extensive multiterritory defects *(arrowheads)*, and increased pulmonary retention of the radiotracer after stress *(arrows)*. Taken together, these findings are consistent with multivessel coronary artery disease (CAD) and are associated with clinical risk for adverse events.

perfusion SPECT scan ranges between approximately 4 and 11 mSv, depending on the protocol and type of scanner that is used.[13] The effective dose from a typical myocardial perfusion PET scan is lower, at approximately 2.5 to 4 mSv.

Imaging laboratories follow the ALARA principle ("As Low As Reasonably Achievable") when balancing the clinical need and imaging approach. By comparison, exposure to radiation from natural sources in the United States amounts to approximately 3 mSv annually. The risk of a fatal malignancy from medical imaging–related radiation is difficult to estimate precisely but is likely to be small and difficult to discriminate from the background risk of natural malignancies. The small but potential radiation risks from imaging mandates an assessment of the risk-versus-benefit ratio in the individual patient. In this context, it is essential to take into account the risks of missing important diagnostic information by not performing a test (which could potentially influence near-term management and outcomes) for a theoretical concern regarding long-term small risk of malignancy. Before ordering any test, especially one associated with ionizing radiation, the clinician must ensure the appropriateness of the study and decide whether the potential benefits outweigh the risks. The likelihood that the study being considered will affect clinical management of the patient should be addressed before testing is performed. It also is important that "routine" follow-up scans in asymptomatic persons be avoided.

PATIENT-CENTERED CLINICAL APPLICATIONS

Evaluation of Patients with Nondiagnostic Electrocardiogram and Troponin Elevation

Case Vignette 1

The patient was a 49-year-old man with a history of hypertension, active cigarette smoking, and alcohol dependence who presented with chest pain and evidence of supraventricular tachycardia (SVT) on ECG monitoring. The SVT was terminated with adenosine. His initial cardiac troponin level was elevated at 0.12 ng/mL, rising to a peak of 0.44 ng/mL. In view of his cardiovascular risk factors, an exercise myocardial perfusion SPECT study was requested to rule out underlying obstructive CAD. Exercise capacity was limited, with a peak of only 6.9 METs (metabolic equivalents [of task]) attained; accordingly, intravenous regadenoson was given to achieve maximal hyperemia.

The SPECT images demonstrate normal regional myocardial perfusion (Figure 32-8). The ECG-gated images demonstrated a borderline-normal LVEF of 46% at rest that rose to 58% after stress (Video 32-1). In the context of the normal SPECT imaging findings, the mildly elevated troponin was attributed to the SVT event, and no further coronary evaluation was undertaken.

Normal radionuclide perfusion imaging in patients with low-level cardiac troponin elevation without typical symptoms or ECG changes and at low-intermediate risk (TIMI risk score less than 5) is associated with very low short-term cardiac mortality. Conversely, an abnormal perfusion study identifies patients at significantly higher clinical risk. In such patients, the magnitude of stress-induced ischemia quantified by perfusion imaging helps guide the subsequent need of referral to cardiac catheterization and revascularization.

The pathophysiology of minimally elevated levels of serum cardiac troponin in the absence of an ACS is heterogeneous (see Chapter 7). In one study, impaired global coronary flow reserve in the absence of obstructive CAD as measured by PET was independently associated with troponin elevation, suggesting an association between chronic microvascular ischemia and myocardial injury.[14] More important, this quantitative imaging marker provides prognostic information incremental to other clinical markers of risk. Indeed, patients with positive troponin and impaired CFR have a higher annualized event rate compared to those

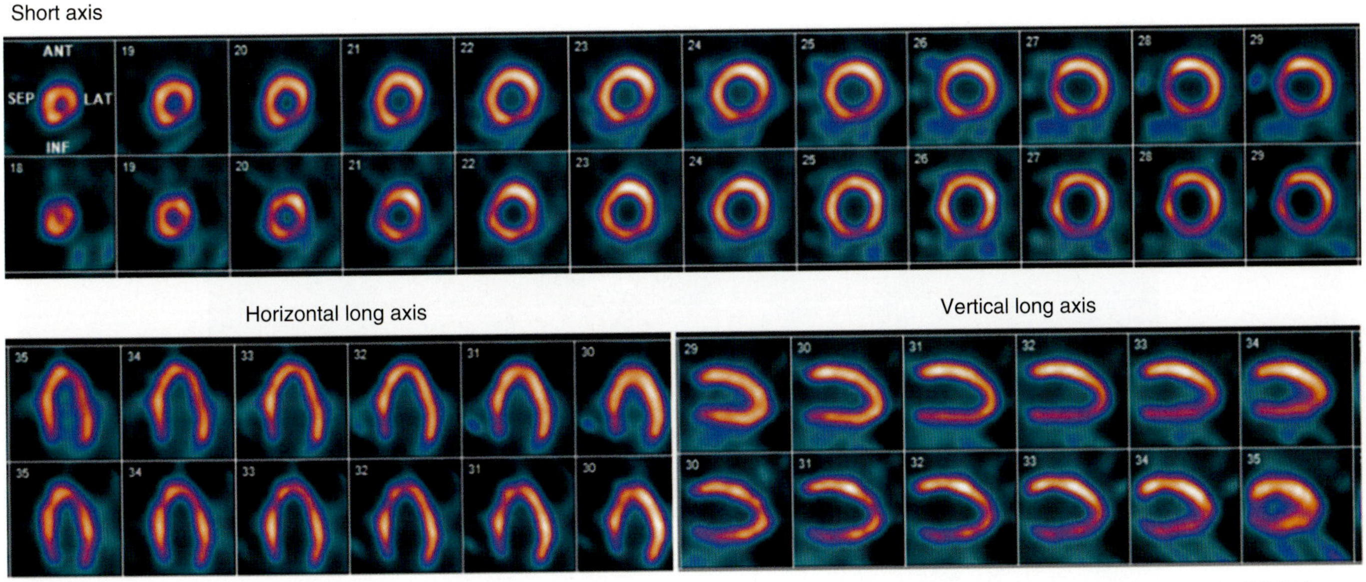

FIGURE 32-8 Images for Case Vignette 1. Stress and rest technetium-99m (^{99m}Tc) myocardial perfusion single positron emission computed tomography (SPECT) images. See text for details.

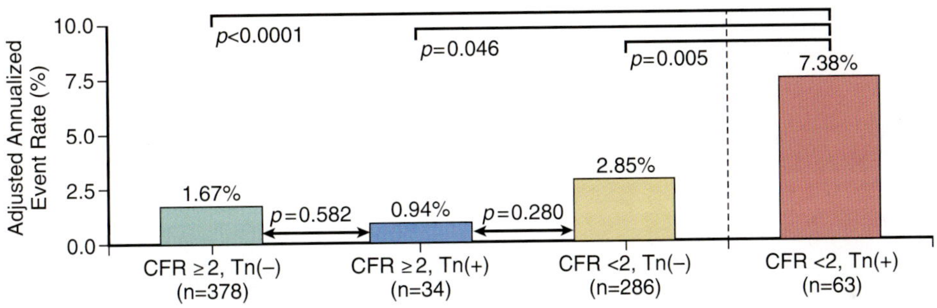

FIGURE 32-9 Adjusted annualized rates of major adverse cardiovascular events among patients by coronary flow reserve (CFR) and troponin (Tn) strata. Patients with a low CFR and positive Tn *(red)* had significantly higher event rates than in any other subgroups. Annualized event rates were adjusted for pretest clinical score, left ventricular ejection fraction, and estimated glomerular filtration rate. *(From Shaw LJ, Hage FG, Berman DS, et al: Prognosis in the era of comparative effectiveness research: where is nuclear cardiology now and where should it be?* J Nucl Cardiol *19:1026-1043, 2012.)*

with a positive troponin but preserved CFR[14] (Figure 32-9). Therefore, in intermediate- to high-risk patients with low-level elevation of cardiac troponin, quantitative stress PET perfusion imaging may offer an advantage over SPECT and may be preferable if available.

Evaluation of Patients with Non–ST-Elevation Myocardial Infarction

Case Vignette 2

The patient was a 76-year-old woman with a history of CAD and previous PCI, type 2 diabetes, hypertension, and stroke. She presented with chest discomfort, ST-segment depressions on the ECG, and a cardiac troponin T level of 5.67 ng/mL. Coronary angiography revealed three-vessel CAD (Videos 32-2, 32-3, and 32-4). Vasodilator stress myocardial perfusion PET was performed to evaluate ischemic burden, an approach that is supported by current American Heart Association/American College of Cardiology (AHA/ACC) guidelines (see Chapter 30).

The myocardial perfusion images show a dilated left ventricle, with a large and severe perfusion defect throughout the inferolateral, inferior, and inferoseptal walls showing moderate reversibility *(arrowheads)*, consistent with previous MI with moderate residual stress-induced peri-infarct ischemia in the right coronary artery (RCA) territory (Figure 32-10A). ECG-gated images revealed a rest LVEF of 34%, which fell to 32% after stress (Video 32-5). The polar maps confirmed the presence of moderate reversibility (*hatched area* in Figure 32-10A) in the RCA territory. However, the quantitative blood flow data are consistent with significant flow-limiting disease in the left anterior descending artery (LAD) and moderate in the left circumflex artery (LCx) territories (CFR less than 1.5 is severely reduced, and CFR of 1.5 to 2.0 is moderately reduced) (Figure 32-10B). The patient was deemed to be at prohibitively high risk for surgical revascularization and underwent multivessel PCI to open the LAD and RCA.

The goals of noninvasive testing in patients with non–ST-elevation ACS who did not have an early revascularization strategy are to detect ischemia and assess prognosis. This information guides further diagnostic steps and therapeutic measures (see Chapter 11 and Chapter 16).[15] The standard exercise electrocardiographic stress test may be reasonable for lower-risk patients with interpretable rest ECGs. For higher-risk patients, especially those with abnormal rest ECGs as in Case Vignette 2, stress imaging is more appropriate (see also Chapter 30).

The power of radionuclide myocardial perfusion imaging (SPECT and PET) for risk stratification is based on the fact that the major determinants of prognosis in patients with CAD are readily available from gated myocardial perfusion imaging. These risk indicators include the scintigraphic

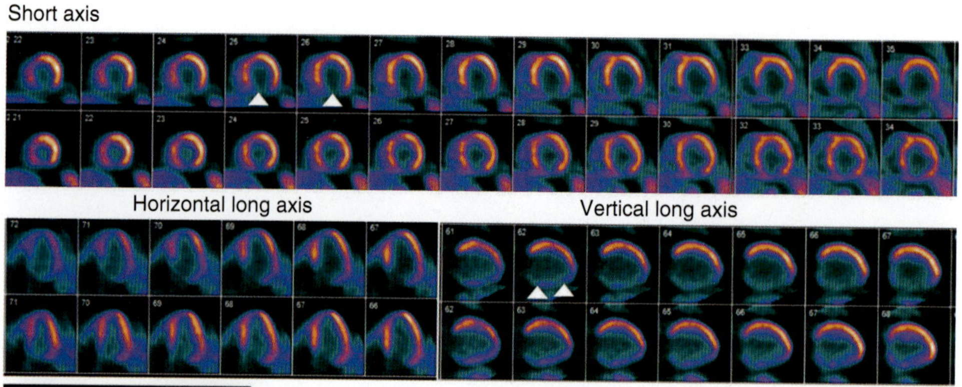

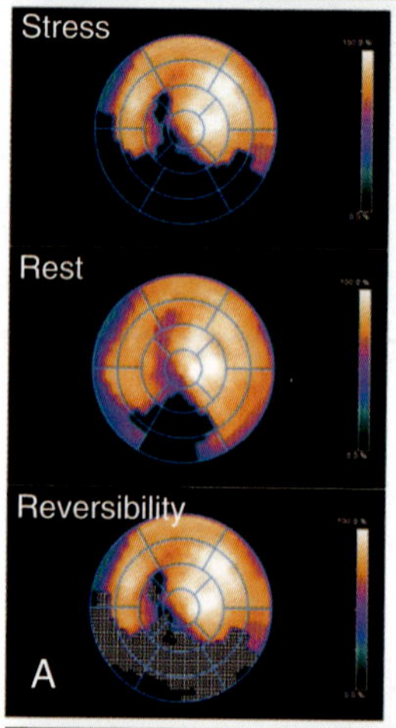

Quantitative myocardial blood flow

	Rest (mL/min/g)	Stress (mL/min/g)	CFR (stress/rest)
LAD	0.84	1.20	1.43
LCX	1.03	1.56	1.50
RCA	0.68	0.69	1.01
Global LV	0.85	1.14	1.35

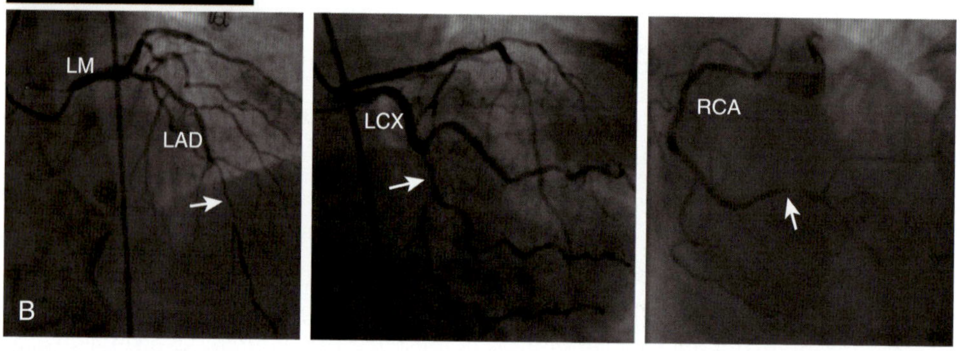

FIGURE 32-10 Images for Case Vignette 2. (**A**) Stress and rest ^{13}N-ammonia myocardial perfusion positron emission tomography (PET) images. (**B**) Corresponding coronary angiographic images demonstrating severe three-vessel obstructive coronary artery disease (CAD). *Arrows* indicate sites of potential targets for multivessel PCI. *CFR,* Coronary flow reserve; *LAD,* left anterior descending artery; *LCx,* left circumflex artery; *LM,* left main artery; *LV,* left ventricle; *RCA,* right coronary artery. See text for details.

infarct size, the extent and severity of residual stress-induced ischemia, measurements of left ventricular volumes, and LVEF. Extensive evidence in stable patients after MI supports the application of radionuclide perfusion imaging for risk assessment.[16] Exercise stress testing is a useful approach to risk stratification after MI (see Chapter 30). Indeed, poor exercise effort (less than 4 METs), exercise-induced angina, ST-segment depression, ventricular arrhythmias, and hypotension during exercise identify high-risk patients. However, the frequency of such markers of risk is greatly diminished in the era of emergent coronary angiography and primary PCI, because most high-risk patients (e.g., left main artery and/or multivessel CAD) are identified and treated before stress testing. Because most high-risk patients have been triaged at the time of presentation, noninvasive testing after MI most often is used for identification of residual stress-induced ischemia. In this regard, radionuclide imaging has improved sensitivity over that for stress ECG alone for identification of ischemia/viability with the infarct-related territory or in remote myocardium. Indeed, the data indicate that risk increases with the extent and severity of perfusion abnormalities and scintigraphic ischemia. For any given LVEF, a greater degree of scintigraphic ischemia identifies patients at higher clinical risk. This concept applies to all patient demographics and types of stress testing (exercise and pharmacologic stress). Data also support a potential role for perfusion imaging in guiding revascularization. Propensity-matched observational data have supported an apparent benefit from revascularization for patients with a considerable extent of inducible ischemia (involving greater than 10% of left ventricular mass).[17]

As discussed in this chapter, CFR is a sensitive measure of myocardial ischemia and overall vascular health that is emerging as a unique and robust marker of clinical risk. As shown in Figure 32-5, a severely reduced CFR (less than 1.5) is associated with a six-fold increased risk of cardiac death.

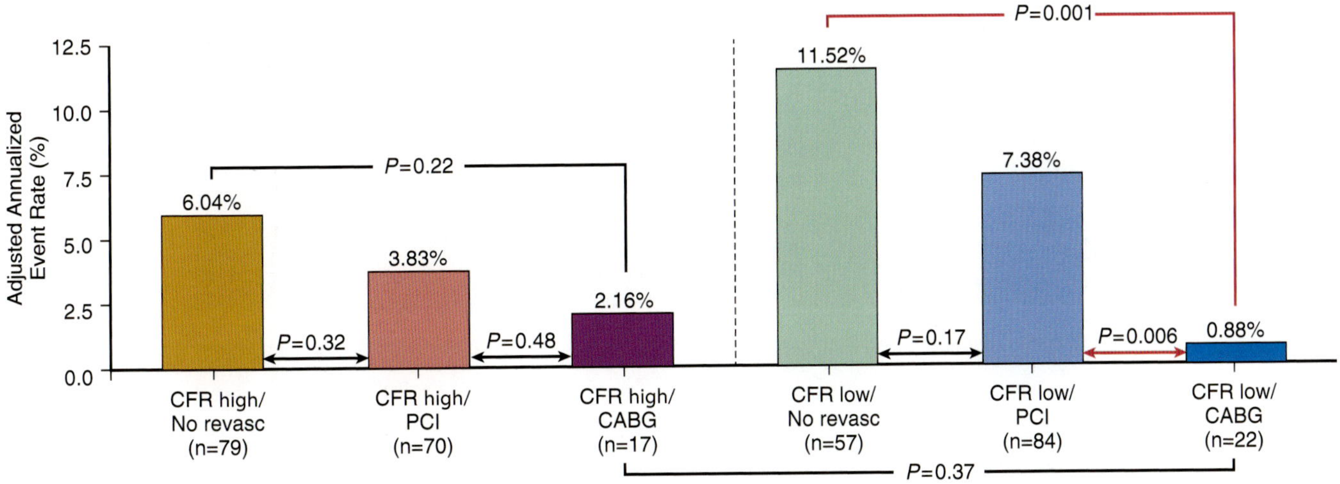

FIGURE 32-11 Adjusted annualized rates of cardiovascular death and heart failure admission among patients referred for coronary angiography by coronary flow reserve (CFR) and early revascularization (Revasc) strategy—either coronary artery bypass grafting (CABG), percutaneous coronary intervention (PCI), or neither. No difference in event rates was seen in patients with high CFR *(orange, red, maroon)*, regardless of revascularization strategy pursued. Among patients with low CFR, those who underwent CABG *(dark blue)* had lower event rates than those who underwent PCI *(light blue)* or no revascularization *(green)* and had event rates similar to those with high CFR who underwent CABG *(maroon)*. Annualized event rates were adjusted for pretest clinical score, left ventricular ejection fraction, left ventricular ischemia, and coronary artery disease (CAD) prognostic index as assessed by coronary angiography. *(From Tonino PA, Fearon WF, De Bruyne B, et al: Angiographic versus functional severity of coronary artery stenoses in the FAME study fractional flow reserve versus angiography in multivessel evaluation.* J Am Coll Cardiol *55:2816-2821, 2010.)*

Of importance, this information is incremental to other markers of clinical risk, and to semiquantitative measures of myocardial ischemia, and thus can refine risk estimates and potentially guide revascularization. Indeed, data suggest that global CFR may be able to modify the effect of revascularization, such that only patients with low global CFR may benefit from revascularization[18] (Figure 32-11). These data also raise the possibility that revascularization in patients with relatively preserved CFR may not be associated with improved outcomes, which is consistent with the results observed in the FAME (FFR vs. Angiography for Multivessel Evaluation, NCT00267774) trial.[19,20]

Assessment of Non-Culprit Vessels After Primary Percutaneous Coronary Intervention

Case Vignette 3

The patient was a 53-year-old man with a history of hypertension, dyslipidemia, diabetes, and tobacco use who presented with an anterior ST-elevation myocardial infarction (STEMI). Initial coronary angiography showed a 100% occluded LAD, 80% stenosis in a diagonal branch, and 80% stenosis in the RCA (Figure 32-12A and Videos 32-6 and 32-7). At the time of the initial event he underwent successful PCI to open the LAD (Video 32-8). His non-culprit coronary artery disease was managed medically (see also Chapter 17). One month later, he presented with recurrent chest pain. An exercise myocardial perfusion SPECT was performed to quantify residual ischemia, to direct further management. He exercised for 7 minutes of a modified Bruce protocol, achieving 87% of age-predicted maximal heart rate. The symptomatic response to this regimen was chest heaviness with exercise. The ECG response to exercise indicated no significant ST-T changes.

The myocardial perfusion SPECT images show a severely dilated left ventricle with a large and severe perfusion defect throughout the LAD territory, without evidence of residual exercise-induced ischemia *(arrowheads)* (Figure 32-12B). The polar maps confirm the presence of a large area of scar throughout the LAD territory, with minimal evidence of ischemia. Increased radiotracer uptake also is evident in the right ventricular free wall, consistent with elevated pulmonary artery pressures. The ECG-gated images showed akinesis of the anterior, septal and apical walls, and an LVEF of 25% (Video 32-9). On the basis of these findings, the patient was managed conservatively, because there was no objective evidence of significant ischemia to justify repeat angiography and revascularization.

This stepwise approach is particularly useful in symptomatic patients with residual angiographic disease in non-culprit coronary arteries, especially those in higher-risk groups (e.g., elderly persons or those with diabetes or renal disease) and patients with recurrent symptoms, as in Case Vignette 3, and is considered reasonable by current guidelines[21] (see Chapter 30).

Evaluation of Patients with Heart Failure After Myocardial Infarction

Case Vignette 4

The patient was a 61-year-old man who presented with an MI at 3 days after onset of chest pain complicated by heart failure. Coronary angiography revealed significant two-vessel disease with an occluded LCx and moderate disease in the LAD and diagonal territories (Figure 32-13A and Videos 32-10 and 32-11). He underwent PET scanning to evaluate residual myocardial viability for potential revascularization.

The PET images show mild left ventricular dilation with a large and severe perfusion defect at rest throughout the anterolateral and inferolateral walls (Figure 32-13B, top). On the FDG images (Figure 32-13B, bottom), significant glucose uptake is evident in all hypoperfused segments (perfusion-FDG mismatch), except at the base of the left ventricle, where perfusion and FDG are matched. This pattern is consistent with a large area of predominantly viable but hibernating myocardium throughout the LCx territory, which was confirmed by quantitative analysis. The rest LVEF was 49% (Video 32-12). On the basis of these findings, the patient underwent successful revascularization of the LCx coronary artery.

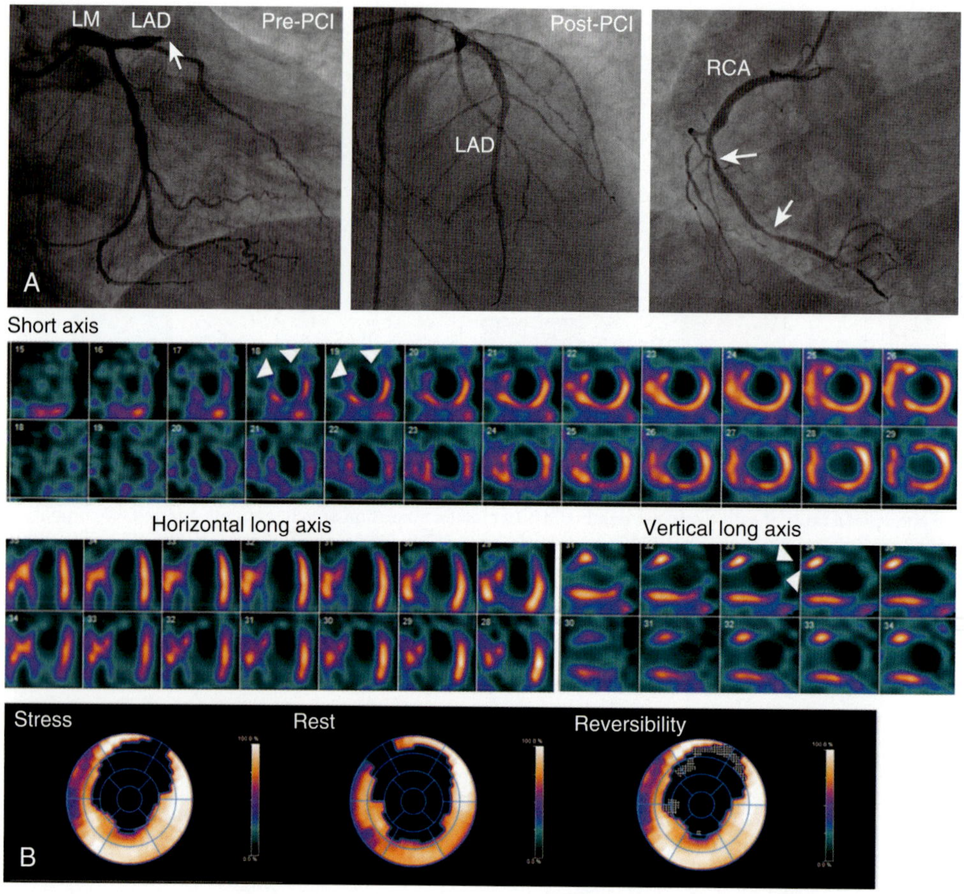

FIGURE 32-12 Images for Case Vignette 3. (**A**) Coronary angiographic images. *Arrows* identify occluded LAD and serial 80% stenoses in the RCA. (**B**) Corresponding stress and rest ^{13}N-ammonia myocardial perfusion positron emission tomography (PET) images. See text for details. *LAD,* Left anterior descending artery; *LM,* left main artery; *PCI,* percutaneous coronary intervention; *RCA,* right coronary artery.

Metabolic imaging with PET has an established role in the evaluation of myocardial viability (see also Chapter 30). As discussed previously, specific abnormalities in myocardial metabolism reflecting viable and scarred myocardium have been described (see Figure 32-3). Contractile dysfunction is predicted to be reversible after revascularization in regions with increased FDG uptake, or *perfusion-FDG mismatch,* and irreversible in those with reduced FDG uptake, or *perfusion-FDG match* pattern. Using these criteria, the average positive predictive value for predicting improved segmental function after revascularization is 76 (range, 52% to 100%), whereas the average negative predictive value is 82% (range, 67% to 100%). A clinically meaningful improvement in global left ventricular function can be expected after revascularization in patients with relatively large areas of hibernating and/or stunned myocardium (approximately 20% of the left ventricular mass). There is evidence that delineation of myocardial viability with FDG-PET is largely concordant with cardiac MRI but is more sensitive than dobutamine echocardiography and radionuclide perfusion SPECT imaging (see Figure 30-3). Other relative advantages of radionuclide imaging over MRI relate to its improved ability to quantify peri-infarct ischemia, as well as its relative safety in patients with impaired renal function and cardiac devices (defibrillators and pacemakers).

The use of viability imaging also plays a role in determining size and extent of scar in planning optimal implantable cardioverter-defibrillator (ICD)/cardiac resynchronization therapy (CRT) lead position in patients with ischemic cardiomyopathy. Studies have shown that cardiac resynchronization plus defibrillator therapy (CRT-D) devices are more successful when lead position is in an area of viable myocardium, with improved left ventricular systolic function and outcomes.[22]

EMERGING APPLICATIONS OF NUCLEAR IMAGING TECHNIQUES

Neuronal Imaging and Risk Stratification for Sudden Cardiac Death

Both experimental and clinical evidence support the concept that sympathetic activation plays an important role as a potential trigger of ventricular arrhythmias after MI (see also Chapter 28).[23] Indeed, MI and ischemia can lead to sympathetic denervation in both the infarct and the peri-infarct zone[24] (Figure 32-14). Viable but denervated myocardial regions show supersensitive shortening of effective refractory period in response to the infusion of norepinephrine and are more vulnerable to ventricular arrhythmias. These observations suggest that direct imaging of cardiac sympathetic innervation may have an important clinical role in risk stratification of patients after MI.

The PAREPET (Prediction of ARrhythmic Events with Positron Emission Tomography) study was designed to test the hypothesis that the extent of inhomogeneity in myocardial sympathetic innervation and/or hibernating myocardium increased the risk of arrhythmic death independently of left ventricular function in patients with ischemic cardiomyopathy (LVEF of 35% or less).[24] The study included

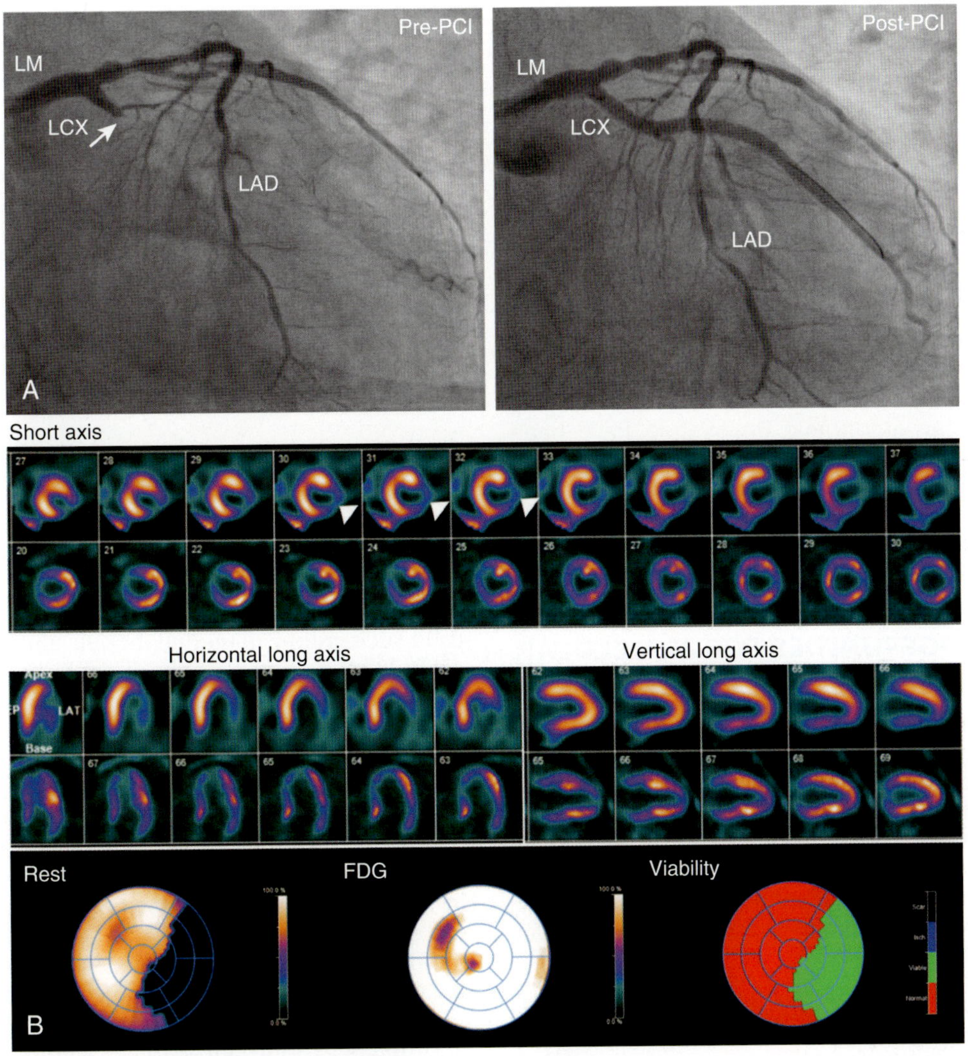

FIGURE 32-13 Images for Case Vignette 4. (**A**) Coronary angiographic images. (**B**) Corresponding rest perfusion and fluorodeoxyglucose-uptake positron emission tomography (FDG-PET) images. See text for details. *LAD,* Left anterior descending artery; *LCx,* left circumflex artery; *LM,* left main artery; *PCI,* percutaneous coronary intervention.

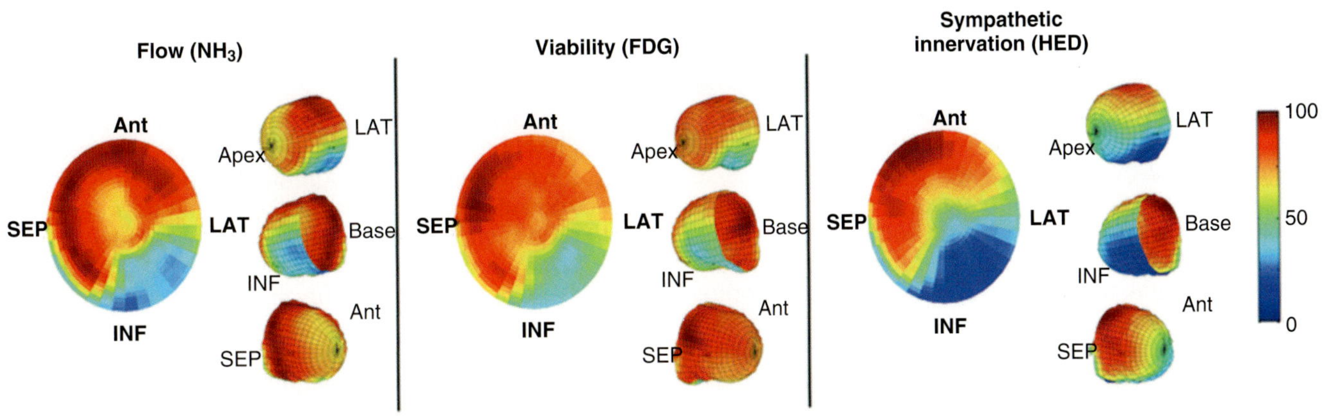

FIGURE 32-14 Bull's-eye maps of myocardial perfusion evidenced by 13N-ammonia uptake (NH_3) reflecting regional blood flow (*left panel*), fluorodeoxyglucose (FDG)-labeled areas of viability (*middle panel*), and sympathetic innervation (*right panel*) in a patient who experienced sudden cardiac arrest (SCA). Color scale to the right indicates increasing amount of uptake. A large matched perfusion-metabolic defect involving the inferior and inferolateral walls is evident, consistent with previous myocardial infarction. The hydroxyephedrine (HED)-labeled images demonstrate a larger myocardial volume of sympathetic denervation (i.e., reduced HED uptake) compared with the scarred area. This mismatch between infarct size (i.e., reduced FDG uptake) and the volume of sympathetic denervation (larger HED defect) has been identified as an imaging marker for ventricular arrhythmias. *Ant,* Anterior; *INF,* inferior; *LAT,* lateral; *SEP,* septum. *(Courtesy of Dr. James A. Fallavollita, University of Buffalo, Buffalo, New York.)*

204 patients who were eligible for primary-prevention ICDs. PET imaging was used to quantify myocardial sympathetic denervation (with carbon-11 [^{11}C]-labeled hydroxyephedrine [HED]), perfusion, and metabolism. The primary endpoint was sudden cardiac arrest, defined as arrhythmia-related death or ICD discharge for ventricular fibrillation or ventricular tachycardia at a rate higher than 240 beats/min. Compared with patients in the lowest tertile of cardiac

sympathetic denervation assessed by HED PET, patients in the highest tertile showed a greater than six-fold increase in the risk of sudden cardiac arrest. In multivariable analysis, the extent of PET-defined sympathetic denervation, left ventricular end-diastolic volume index, and serum creatinine were significantly associated with the risk of sudden cardiac arrest. Similar findings were reported in the ADMIRE-HF (ADreView Myocardial Imaging for Risk Evaluation in Heart Failure) study using iodine-123 metaiodobenzylguanidine (^{123}I-mIBG) imaging, in a more heterogeneous cohort of patients with ischemic and nonischemic heart failure.[25] In this study, patients with a heart-to-mediastinum (H/M) count ratio below1.6 had a relatively lower risk of death or of ventricular arrhythmias. Although none of the imaging approaches assessing autonomic innervation have been linked to therapeutics, including implantation of ICDs, the results of these clinical studies support the hypothesis that these techniques may be helpful in the identification of patients with sufficiently low risk of sudden cardiac death to guide subsequent therapy.

POTENTIAL OPPORTUNITIES FOR MOLECULAR IMAGING

Targeted molecular imaging offers unique insights into the biology of ischemia-reperfusion injury after MI in vivo. In some cases, molecular imaging techniques have the potential to identify useful diagnostic targets. However, these techniques offer their greatest promise for assessing the response to novel therapies and/or preventive strategies in vivo, especially during research and development. Reviewed next are potential applications of molecular imaging in the setting of acute and/or chronic MI.

Myocardial Injury and Remodeling After Acute Myocardial Infarction

Acute myocardial ischemia and injury results in a marked inflammatory response characterized by acute leukocytosis. Neutrophils and pro-inflammatory monocytes infiltrate the myocardium within the first few hours after ischemic injury.[26] The neutrophil response dissipates quickly. However, inflammatory monocytes supplied initially by the spleen and later by the bone marrow continue to infiltrate the site of myocardial injury at high rates for the first week after ischemia (see Chapter 4). Initially, monocytes differentiate to highly inflammatory macrophages. These cells induce proteolysis of extracellular matrix and help with phagocytosis of dying cells and debris. After a few days, infarct-bound monocytes undergo transition to an anti-inflammatory phenotype, which supports tissue repair, including the formation of scar and new extracellular matrix. A decrease or exaggerated inflammatory response can affect infarct healing and affect LV remodeling. This process can be quantified noninvasively using targeted molecular imaging. For example, metabolic imaging with ^{18}F-FDG PET was used to assess inflammation after MI in humans and experimental animals.[27,28] These studies have shown increased FDG uptake in the infarcted territory within 2 weeks after reperfusion. In animals, the increased FDG signal correlated with the degree of inflammation and density of monocyte/macrophage presence in infarcted tissue.[27] Activated macrophages also enhance neoangiogenesis and are a major source of proteases that regulate the turnover of the extracellular matrix.[26] Consequently, targeted imaging of angiogenesis[29] and matrix metalloproteinases[30] also has been used to characterize inflammation and healing post-MI. In animal models of MI, enhanced angiogenesis has been associated with a lower likelihood of adverse LV remodeling, while increase MMP activation has been linked to adverse remodeling and LV dilatation. Although it is unlikely that these highly technical imaging approaches will develop into diagnostic/prognostic applications, such applications have the potential to be extremely useful in early-phase clinical trials to evaluate the efficacy of novel therapies to modulate inflammation after MI and to potentially prevent adverse left ventricular remodeling (see Chapter 36).

Cell Therapy

Molecular imaging techniques also can provide information beyond the functional outcome (i.e., LVEF) of cell therapy. Such techniques have the potential to guide advances in cell therapy protocols to enhance homing, engraftment, and cell survival (see Chapter 22). Several techniques have been used successfully in animal models and in early clinical trials in humans. For example, direct radionuclide labeling of human bone marrow cells with FDG has been used to demonstrate accumulation of cells in infarcted myocardium after intracoronary cell administration using PET.[31] Likewise, indium-111 oxyquinolone (^{111}In oxine) also has been used to label circulating progenitor cells isolated from peripheral blood in subjects with MI. Upon reinjection of labeled cells, SPECT imaging demonstrated differential cell engraftment in acute versus chronic infarcts.[31] Although these imaging techniques can provide valuable information early after cell administration, radioactivity decay results in loss of the signal within hours or days. Imaging of perfusion and/or metabolic activity after cell therapy also can provide quantitative information about cell viability within areas of infarcted myocardium.

SUMMARY

Cardiovascular nuclear medicine techniques have an established clinical role in risk stratification of patients after MI. Indeed, quantification of the burden of myocardial ischemia and/or viability in this setting is very effective for identification of low- and high-risk patients, and to guide the potential need for revascularization. Although more detailed discussion is outside the scope of this chapter, an important point is that the high sensitivity and versatility of nuclear medicine based imaging present new opportunities for targeted molecular imaging approaches that can help identify new biology and potentially direct novel therapies (e.g., stem cells, anti-inflammatory therapies) targeting myocardial healing and post-MI remodeling. These molecular imaging markers may open an exciting opportunity for precision medicine in this patient population.

Classic References

Di Carli MF, Hachamovitch R: New technology for noninvasive evaluation of coronary artery disease, *Circulation* 115:1464–1480, 2007.

Dorbala S, Giugliano RP, Logsetty G, et al.: Prognostic value of SPECT myocardial perfusion imaging in patients with elevated cardiac troponin I levels and atypical clinical presentation, *J Nucl Cardiol* 14:53–58, 2007.

Kuhl HP, Beek AM, van der Weerdt AP, et al.: Myocardial viability in chronic ischemic heart disease: comparison of contrast-enhanced magnetic resonance imaging with (18)F-fluorodeoxyglucose positron emission tomography, *J Am Coll Cardiol* 41:1341–1348, 2003.

Udelson JE, Beshansky JR, Ballin DS, et al.: Myocardial perfusion imaging for evaluation and triage of patients with suspected acute cardiac ischemia: a randomized controlled trial, *JAMA* 288:2693–2700, 2002.

References

1. Henzlova MJ, Cerqueira MD, Hansen CL, et al: ASNC imaging guidelines for nuclear cardiology procedures. Stress protocols and tracers. American Society of Nuclear Cardiology. http://www.asnc.org/files/Stress%20Protocols%20and%20Tracers%202009.pdf.
2. Klocke FJ, Baird MG, Lorell BH, et al.: ACC/AHA/ASNC guidelines for the clinical use of cardiac radionuclide imaging—executive summary: a report of the American College of Cardiology/American Heart Association Task Force on Practice Guidelines (ACC/AHA/ASNC Committee to Revise the 1995 Guidelines for the Clinical Use of Cardiac Radionuclide Imaging), *J Am Coll Cardiol* 42:1318–1333, 2003.
3. Tilkemeier PL, Cook CD, Grossman GB, et al: ASNC imaging guidelines for nuclear cardiology procedures. Standardized reporting of radionuclide myocardial perfusion and function. American Society of Nuclear Cardiology. http://www.asnc.org/files/Radionuclide%20MP%20&%20Function.pdf.
4. Di Carli MF, Hachamovitch R: New technology for noninvasive evaluation of coronary artery disease, *Circulation* 115:1464–1480, 2007.
5. Bengel FM, Higuchi T, Javadi MS, Lautamaki R: Cardiac positron emission tomography, *J Am Coll Cardiol* 54:1–15, 2009.
6. Dorbala S, Di Carli MF: Cardiac PET perfusion: prognosis, risk stratification, and clinical management, *Semin Nucl Med* 44:344–357, 2004.
7. Naya M, Murthy VL, Taqueti VR, et al.: Preserved coronary flow reserve effectively excludes high-risk coronary artery disease on angiography, *J Nucl Med* 55:248–255, 2014.
8. Murthy VL, Naya M, Foster CR, et al.: Improved cardiac risk assessment with noninvasive measures of coronary flow reserve, *Circulation* 124:2215–2224, 2011.
9. Ziadi MC, Dekemp RA, Williams KA, et al.: Impaired myocardial flow reserve on rubidium-82 positron emission tomography imaging predicts adverse outcomes in patients assessed for myocardial ischemia, *J Am Coll Cardiol* 58:740–748, 2011.
10. Gibbons RJ, Valeti US, Araoz PA, Jaffe AS: The quantification of infarct size, *J Am Coll Cardiol* 44:1533–1542, 2004.
11. Klein C, Nekolla SG, Bengel FM, et al.: Assessment of myocardial viability with contrast-enhanced magnetic resonance imaging: comparison with positron emission tomography, *Circulation* 105:162–167, 2002.
12. Takx RA, Blomberg BA, El Aidi H, et al.: Diagnostic accuracy of stress myocardial perfusion imaging compared to invasive coronary angiography with fractional flow reserve meta-analysis, *Circ Cardiovasc Imaging* 8(1):e002666, 2015.
13. Dey D, Slomka PJ, Berman DS: Achieving very-low-dose radiation exposure in cardiac computed tomography, single-photon emission computed tomography, and positron emission tomography, *Circ Cardiovasc Imaging* 7:723–734, 2014.
14. Taqueti VR, Everett BM, Murthy VL, et al.: Interaction of impaired coronary flow reserve and cardiomyocyte injury on adverse cardiovascular outcomes in patients without overt coronary artery disease, *Circulation* 131:528–535, 2015.
15. Amsterdam EA, Wenger NK, Brindis RG, et al.: 2014 AHA/ACC guideline for the management of patients with non-ST-elevation acute coronary syndromes: executive summary: a report of the American College of Cardiology/American Heart Association Task Force on Practice Guidelines, *Circulation* 130:2354–2394, 2014.
16. Shaw LJ, Hage FG, Berman DS, et al.: Prognosis in the era of comparative effectiveness research: where is nuclear cardiology now and where should it be? *J Nucl Cardiol* 19:1026–1043, 2012.
17. Hachamovitch R, Hayes SW, Friedman JD, et al.: Comparison of the short-term survival benefit associated with revascularization compared with medical therapy in patients with no prior coronary artery disease undergoing stress myocardial perfusion single photon emission computed tomography, *Circulation* 107:2900–2907, 2003.
18. Taqueti VR, Hachamovitch R, Murthy VL, et al.: Global coronary flow reserve is associated with adverse cardiovascular events independently of luminal angiographic severity and modifies the effect of early revascularization, *Circulation* 131:19–27, 2015.
19. De Bruyne B, Fearon WF, Pijls NH, et al.: Fractional flow reserve-guided PCI for stable coronary artery disease, *N Engl J Med* 371:1208–1217, 2014.
20. Tonino PA, Fearon WF, De Bruyne B, et al.: Angiographic versus functional severity of coronary artery stenoses in the FAME study fractional flow reserve versus angiography in multivessel evaluation, *J Am Coll Cardiol* 55:2816–2821, 2010.
21. O'Gara PT, Kushner FG, Ascheim DD, et al.: 2013 ACCF/AHA guideline for the management of ST-elevation myocardial infarction: executive summary: a report of the American College of Cardiology Foundation/American Heart Association Task Force on Practice Guidelines: developed in collaboration with the American College of Emergency Physicians and Society for Cardiovascular Angiography and Interventions, *Catheter Cardiovasc Interv* 82:E1–E27, 2013.
22. Bax JJ, Delgado V, et al.: Myocardial viability as integral part of the diagnostic and therapeutic approach to ischemic heart failure, *J Nucl Cardiol* 22:229–245, 2015.
23. Wellens HJ, Schwartz PJ, Lindemans FW, et al.: Risk stratification for sudden cardiac death: current status and challenges for the future, *Eur Heart J* 35:1642–1651, 2014.
24. Fallavollita JA, Heavey BM, Luisi Jr AJ, et al.: Regional myocardial sympathetic denervation predicts the risk of sudden cardiac arrest in ischemic cardiomyopathy, *J Am Coll Cardiol* 63:141–149, 2014.
25. Jacobson AF, Senior R, Cerqueira MD, et al.: Myocardial iodine-123 meta-iodobenzylguanidine imaging and cardiac events in heart failure. Results of the prospective ADMIRE-HF (AdreView Myocardial Imaging for Risk Evaluation in Heart Failure) study, *J Am Coll Cardiol* 55:2212–2221, 2012.
26. Nahrendorf M, Frantz S, Swirski FK, et al.: Imaging systemic inflammatory networks in ischemic heart disease, *J Am Coll Cardiol* 65:1583–1591, 2015.
27. Lee WW, Marinelli B, van der Laan AM, et al.: PET/MRI of inflammation in myocardial infarction, *J Am Coll Cardiol* 59:153–163, 2012.
28. Wollenweber T, Roentgen P, Schafer A, et al.: Characterizing the inflammatory tissue response to acute myocardial infarction by clinical multimodality noninvasive imaging, *Circ Cardiovasc Imaging* 7:811–818, 2014.
29. Sherif HM, Saraste A, Nekolla SG, et al.: Molecular imaging of early alphavbeta3 integrin expression predicts long-term left-ventricle remodeling after myocardial infarction in rats, *J Nucl Med* 53:318–323, 2012.
30. Sahul ZH, Mukherjee R, Song J, et al.: Targeted imaging of the spatial and temporal variation of matrix metalloproteinase activity in a porcine model of postinfarct remodeling: relationship to myocardial dysfunction, *Circ Cardiovasc Imaging* 4:381–391, 2011.
31. Bengel FM: Noninvasive stem cell tracking, *J Nucl Cardiol* 18:966–973, 2011.

33 Cardiac Magnetic Resonance Imaging After Myocardial Infarction

John D. Grizzard and Raymond J. Kim

INTRODUCTION

The use of sensitive biomarkers has significantly improved the diagnosis of myocardial infarction (MI), and has been incorporated into the "Universal Definition" of MI (see Chapter 1).[1] However, the diagnosis of MI can still be difficult. There is significant overlap with other disorders that result in myocardial injury (see Chapter 6). For instance, disorders such as Takotsubo cardiomyopathy and myocarditis are associated with elevation of cardiac biomarkers, and their clinical differentiation from acute MI can be problematic and can often result in invasive diagnostic procedures (see Chapter 7). In other instances, patients may present late, after cardiac biomarkers have normalized, resulting in an "unrecognized" MI. Recognizing the value of cardiac imaging in such circumstances, the Universal Definition of MI incorporates imaging findings of a new loss of viable myocardium or new wall motion abnormality in conjunction with other clinical criteria (see Chapter 9). Because of its capacity for state-of-the-art imaging of both myocardial structure and wall motion, cardiac magnetic resonance (CMR) has emerged as an important method to confirm the diagnosis in suspected cases, as well as to differentiate MI from other conditions.

Complementing its usefulness in the diagnosis of MI, CMR can provide substantial additional information in the patient with known or suspected MI, including the determination of the infarct-related artery, particularly in non–ST-elevation MI (NSTEMI), the detection of inducible ischemia, and the determination of residual viability (see Chapter 30). In addition, CMR can accurately assess various complications of MI such as thrombus formation, or the development of a ventricular aneurysm (see also Chapter 26). Lastly, because of its accuracy and precision in determining infarct size, CMR is increasingly used as a research tool in population studies of MI and as a surrogate endpoint in randomized trials of investigational MI therapies. In this chapter, we examine the application of CMR in patients with known or suspected MI, with an emphasis on demonstrating modality-specific aspects and the possible implications for patient care.

CARDIAC MAGNETIC RESONANCE TECHNIQUE

CMR has undergone rapid evolution, and technical advances in scanner hardware and coil technology and the development of new pulse sequences have resulted in progressive expansion of clinical applications (Figure 33-1).[2] In particular, new pulse sequences have leveraged the inherently superior soft tissue contrast provided by MR to improve anatomic definition and the delineation of diseased tissue from normal tissue. Overall, these advances have led to the recognition of CMR as the reference standard for the assessment of regional and global systolic function, imaging of MI and viability,[3] and the evaluation of pericardial disease and cardiac masses. In addition, the pattern and distribution of scar as demonstrated by CMR can forewarn of the presence of nonischemic disorders and may be helpful in determining the specific cause of cardiomyopathy. Although previously CMR examinations were lengthy (~1 hour), and many patients were not capable of completing a standard examination, accelerated imaging techniques are now sufficiently robust such that useful diagnostic information can be provided for patients with arrhythmias and/or limited ability to cooperate in 30 minutes or less. The multiplicity of techniques and the variety of information that can be obtained in a CMR examination can be exhaustive, but increasingly there has been a move toward standardization of imaging protocols tailored to specific indications, an effort spearheaded by the Society of Cardiovascular Magnetic Resonance.[4] Our suggested implementation and a timeline (Figure 33-2) of a CMR protocol for a standard CMR examination is as follows.

Standard Cardiac Magnetic Resonance Examination

Cine Images

Cine images are typically acquired in the short-axis plane from above the mitral valve through the left ventricular (LV) apex, together with standard two-, three-, and four-chamber

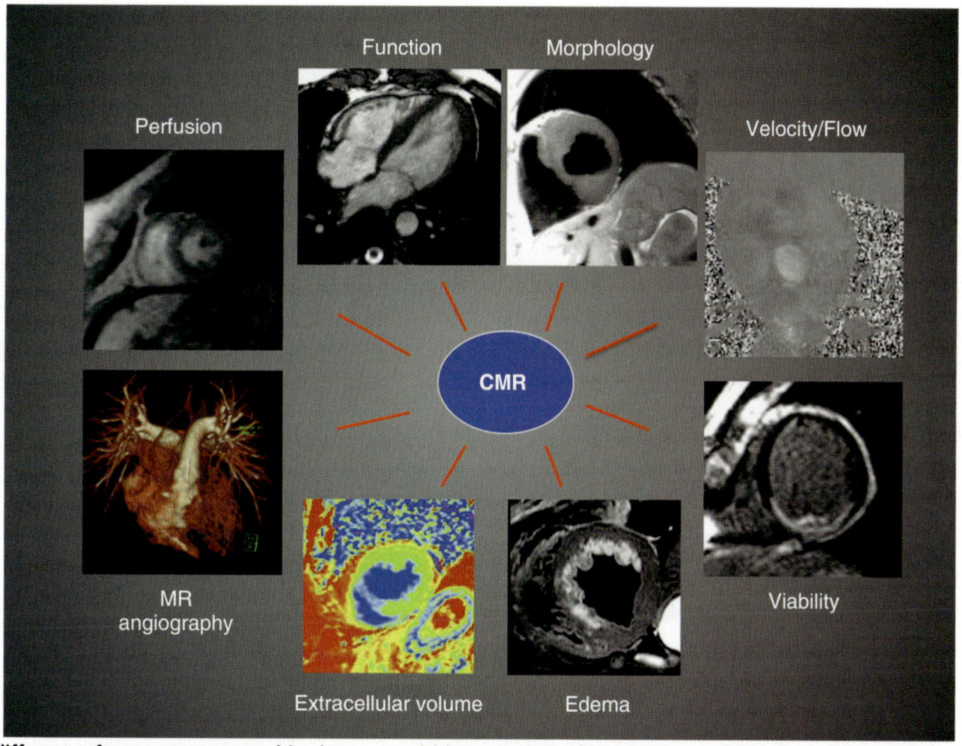

FIGURE 33-1 Using different software programs to drive image acquisition, a variety of imaging is possible using a magnetic resonance (MR) scanner. As a result of innovations in pulse sequences, multiple parameters of cardiovascular structure and function can now be evaluated with cardiac (CMR).

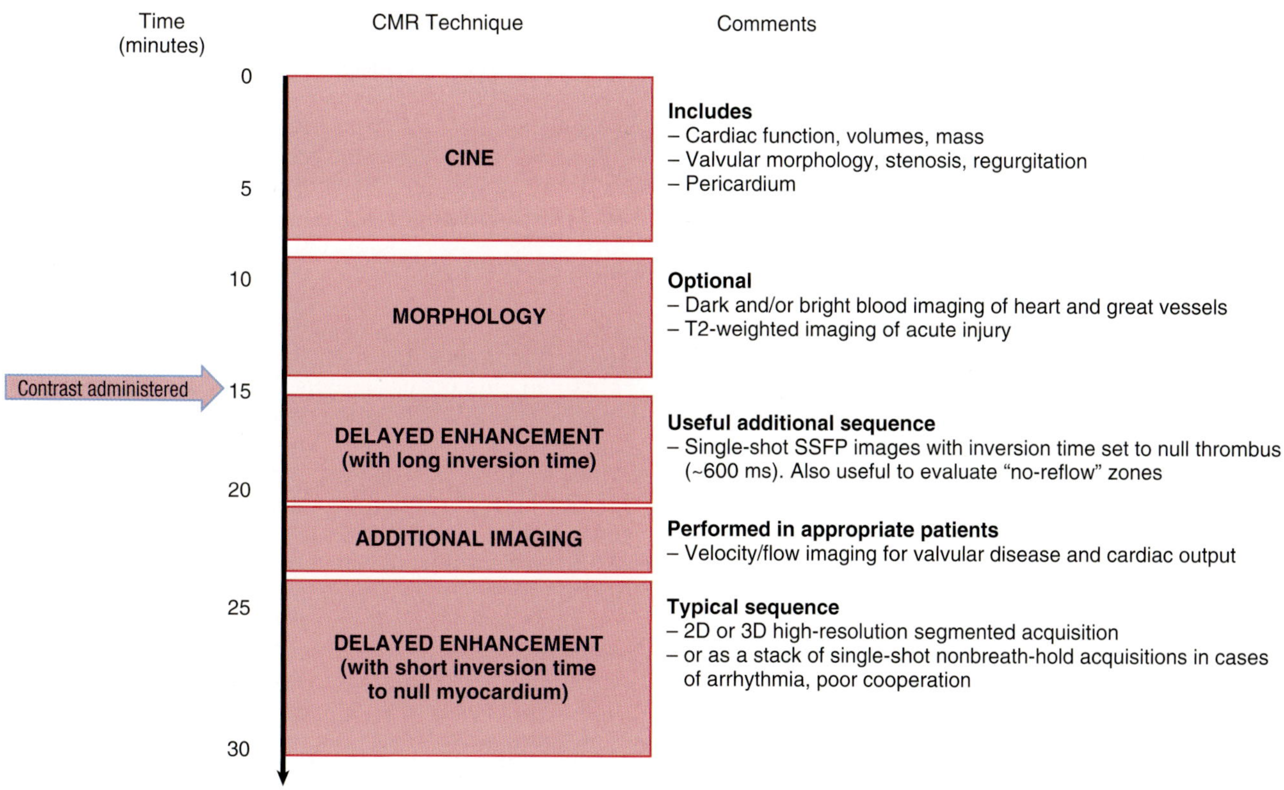

FIGURE 33-2 Timeline of a standard cardiac magnetic resonance (CMR) examination. Note that the entire examination can be performed within 30 minutes. In cases in which the patient is unable to cooperate, the cine examination can be performed with real-time imaging and delayed enhancement with single-shot techniques. This technique will reduce artifacts in patients unable to perform a breath-hold, and total examination time will be shortened further. *SSFP*, Steady-state free-precession; *3D*, three-dimensional; *2D*, two-dimensional.

TABLE 33-1 Sequences and Imaging Parameters Used in a Typical Cardiac Magnetic Resonance Examination

IMAGING	SEQUENCE TYPE	LOCATION	IMAGING PARAMETERS	RESOLUTION	NOTES
Localizers	Single-shot SSFP images	Axial, sagittal, coronal	400-mm FOV	Low resolution	Allows scan planning for cardiac imaging
Cine SSFP (standard)	Segmented SSFP images obtained with retrospective gating	Short-axis images from base to apex; 2-, 3-, and 4-chamber long-axis views	FOV ≈ 360 × 290 mm Matrix ≈ 256 × 168 pixels; slice thickness, 6–8 mm	Pixel size ≈ 1.7 × 1.4 × 6 mm Temporal res. ≈ 40 ms	6–10 s breath-hold required
DE-CMR (standard)	Segmented gradient echo inversion recovery images with data obtained every other heartbeat	Exactly matched to cines	FOV ≈ 360 × 290 mm Matrix ≈ 256 × 168 pixels; slice thickness, 6–8 mm	Pixel size ≈ 1.7 × 1.4 × 6 mm Temporal res. ≈ 160–200 ms	Inversion time chosen to null signal from myocardium
Modifications					
Cine SSFP (real-time)	Real-time images where each cine frame is obtained in single-shot fashion	Short-axis images from base to apex; 2-, 3-, and 4-chamber images	FOV ≈ 380 × 260 mm Matrix ≈ 192 × 84 pixels; slice thickness, 10 mm	Pixel size ≈ 3.1 × 2.0 × 10 mm Temporal res. ≈ 70 ms	Useful in uncooperative or severely arrhythmic patients
DE-CMR (single-shot)	Single-shot SSFP inversion recovery images	Short-axis stack from base to apex; long-axis stack(s) can also be obtained	FOV ≈ 360 × 290 mm Matrix ≈ 208 × 128 pixels; slice thickness, 8 mm	Pixel size ≈ 2.3 × 1.7 × 8 mm Temporal res. ≈ 160–200 ms	Useful in uncooperative or severely arrhythmic patients
Optional Sequences					
Morphologic images	Bright-blood imaging performed with single-shot SSFP; dark-blood imaging performed with HASTE	Stack of images obtained usually in the axial plane; can also obtain sagittal and coronal stacks	FOV ≈ 380 × 315 mm Matrix ≈ 256 × 152 pixels; slice thickness, 8 mm	Pixel size ≈ 2.0 × 1.5 × 8 mm Temporal res. ≈ 60–100 ms	Survey of heart and great vessels; aortic abnormalities, congenital defects
T2-weighted images	Gated T2 FSE or STIR images	Matched to short-axis cine and DE-MR images	FOV ≈ 360 × 290 mm Matrix ≈ 256 × 168 pixels; slice thickness, 6–8 mm	Pixel size ≈ 1.7 × 1.4 × 6 mm Temporal res. ≈ 60–80 ms	To evaluate for edema seen with acute disorders (AMI, myocarditis)
Flow sensitive images	Velocity-encoded gated images	Typically obtained through stenotic valves or proximal great vessels	FOV ≈ 360 × 240 mm Matrix ≈ 256 × 116 pixels; slice thickness, 6–8 mm	Pixel size ≈ 2.0 × 1.4 × 6 mm Temporal res. ≈ 45 ms	Used to measure peak gradients and flow
Perfusion imaging	Saturation recovery (T1-weighted) images to evaluate the transit of contrast through the myocardium	Typically obtained as a stack of 4 short-axis images to cover the LV	FOV ≈ 340 × 255 mm Matrix ≈ 208 × 98 pixels; slice thickness, 8 mm	Pixel size ≈ 2.6 × 1.6 × 8 mm Temporal res. ≈ 120 ms	Can be performed with pharmacologic stress to evaluate for inducible ischemia

AMI, Acute myocardial infarction; *DE-CMR*, delayed-enhancement cardiac magnetic resonance; *FOV*, field of view; *FSE*, fast spin echo; *HASTE*, half-acquisition turbo spin-echo; *LV*, left ventricular; *res*, resolution; *SSFP*, steady-state free-precession; *STIR*, short T1 inversion recovery.

long-axis views (Figure 33-e1). Typical parameters are shown in Table 33-1. The cine images have excellent spatial and temporal resolution, and are not limited by acoustic windows. Therefore, they allow comprehensive evaluation of regional and global ventricular function and overall cardiac morphology. Visual evaluation of valvular function and morphology is also performed using these images.

Inter- and intra-observer reproducibility of cine CMR imaging for the quantification of LV volumes and function has been shown in multiple studies to be excellent, predominantly because of its high spatial and temporal resolution and its capacity for complete LV coverage. The improvement in reproducibility relative to echocardiography allows a significant reduction in the sample sizes required for research studies to demonstrate meaningful changes as a result of experimental therapies. This feature has led to increasing use of CMR in research studies that use cardiac morphology and/or function as an efficacy endpoint.[5]

Delayed-Enhancement Images

These images are obtained 5 to 10 minutes after intravenous (IV) administration of gadolinium-based contrast with 6- to 8-mm slices that are spatially matched to the previously obtained cine images (Figure 33-e2). The delayed-enhancement CMR (DE-CMR) sequence has been shown to be the most sensitive noninvasive imaging test for the detection of MI. It can accurately depict the presence, location, and extent of MI with high spatial resolution irrespective of infarct age. In animal models, DE-CMR has been shown to demonstrate acute and chronic MI with a near-exact spatial match to histopathology specimens (Figure 33-3). In addition, these studies show that DE-CMR can distinguish between reversible and irreversible injury independent of wall motion, infarct age, and reperfusion status.[6] Studies in humans have shown that infarct size measured by DE-CMR and by positron emission tomography (see Chapter 32) is associated with peak cardiac biomarker release (see Chapter 7). Compared with single-photon emission computed tomography (SPECT) imaging, the DE-CMR technique is significantly more sensitive for the detection of subendocardial infarction, of which more than 40% are missed with SPECT (Figure 33-4). With standard imaging parameters, DE-CMR is capable of demonstrating infarcts involving as little as one one-thousandth of total LV mass, which are undetectable by techniques that

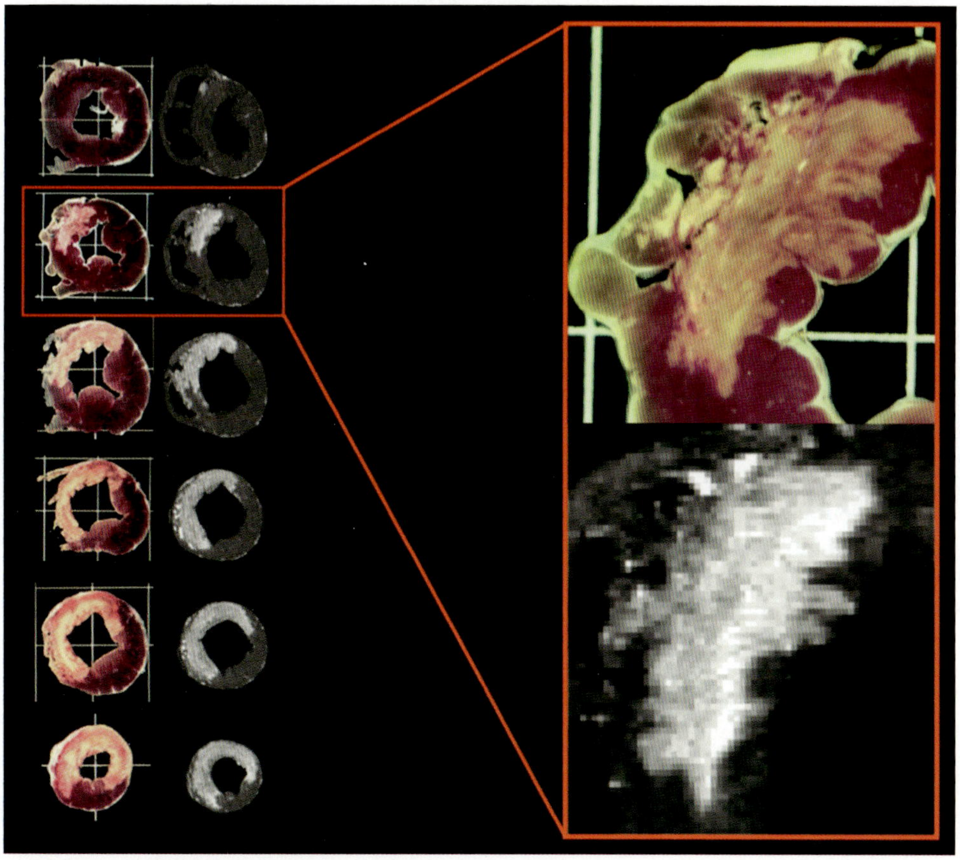

FIGURE 33-3 Comparison of high-resolution ex vivo delayed-enhancement cardiac magnetic resonance (*right*) with acute myocyte necrosis defined by histopathology (*left*). The size and shape of the infarcted region (*yellowish-white region*) defined histologically by triphenyltetrazolium chloride (TTC) stain is nearly exactly matched by the size and shape of the hyperenhanced (*bright*) region of delayed-enhancement cardiac magnetic resonance. *(Adapted from Kim RJ, Fieno DS, Parrish TB, et al: Relationship of MRI delayed contrast enhancement to irreversible injury, infarct age, and contractile function.* Circulation *100:1992–2002, 1999.)*

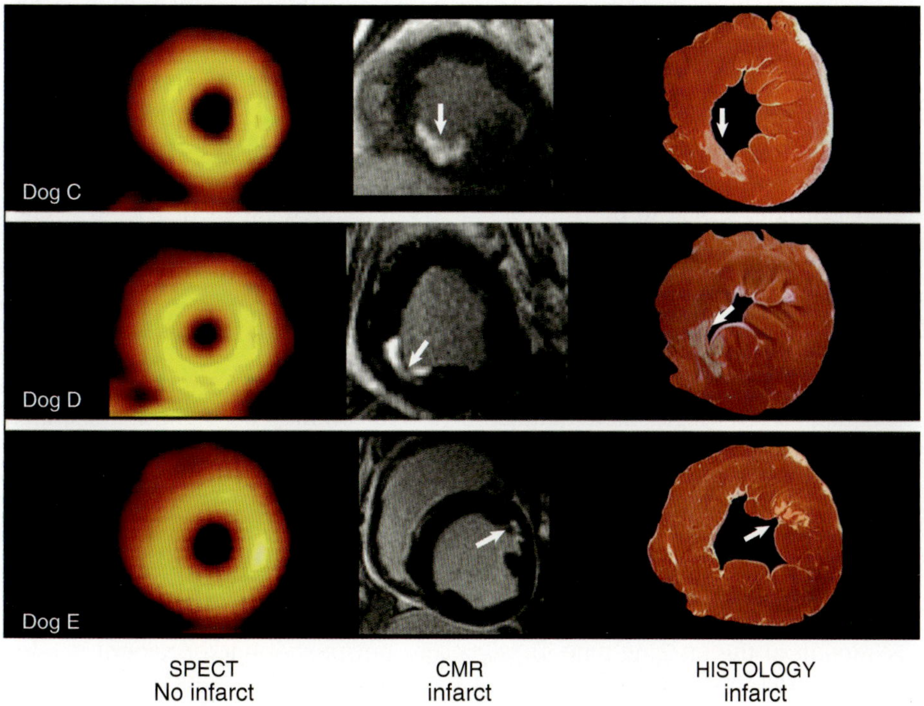

FIGURE 33-4 Short-axis views from three dogs that had subendocardial infarctions. Unlike the single-photon emission computed tomography (SPECT) images, delayed-enhancement cardiac magnetic resonance (CMR) readily demonstrates the infarcted regions *(arrows)*. *(Adapted from Wagner A, Mahrholdt H, Holly TA, et al: Contrast-enhanced MRI and routine single photon emission computed tomography [SPECT] perfusion imaging for detection of subendocardial myocardial infarcts: an imaging study.* Lancet *361:374–379, 2003.)*

assess myocardial perfusion or contractile function. The high spatial resolution of DE-CMR has been used to visualize microinfarctions, involving as little as 1 g of tissue, which may occur during otherwise successful percutaneous coronary intervention.

The technique of DE-CMR has been extensively validated. Its ability to delineate viable from nonviable myocardium is based on the differential distribution of gadolinium contrast in diseased tissue compared with normal tissue. It is important to note that all myocardium—normal, infarcted, or scarred—will demonstrate some contrast enhancement. However, conventional gadolinium contrast agents localize to the extracellular space because they are inert, and intact sarcolemmal membranes prevent them from entering the intracellular space. Normal myocardium, in which the myocytes are densely packed, thus has a limited extracellular volume of distribution (20%) and can be thought of as excluding the contrast agent. With acute necrosis (e.g., acute MI, myocarditis), there is membrane rupture that allows gadolinium to diffuse into myocytes. This diffusion results in increased gadolinium concentration, shortened T1 relaxation, and thus, hyperenhancement. In the chronic setting, scar has replaced necrotic tissue, and the interstitial space is expanded, leading to increased gadolinium concentration and hyperenhancement. In both acute and chronic settings (and all stages in between), viable myocytes are considered as actively excluding gadolinium. Thus, the unifying mechanism of hyperenhancement appears to be the absence of viable myocytes rather than any inherent properties that are specific for acute necrosis, collagenous scar, or other forms of nonviable myocardium (Figure 33-e3).

The standard DE imaging sequence is a heavily T1-weighted segmented gradient echo sequence, in which an inversion pulse has been applied. The inversion pulse serves to flip the magnetization 180 degrees. The recovery of magnetization back to baseline by areas that have a higher gadolinium concentration (e.g., infarcts or scar tissue) will be more rapid (because they have a lower T1 value) than those with a lesser concentration of gadolinium, such as normal myocardium. The time after the inversion pulse at which the magnetization of normal myocardium is at the zero-crossing line will result in maximum suppression of signal from normal myocardium (the myocardium is said to be "nulled"), and will result in maximum conspicuity of the area of infarction (Figure 33-e4). Because the magnetization of infarcted regions, by virtue of their increased contrast content, will recover above the baseline more rapidly (the contrast will accelerate the recovery back to baseline magnetization), infarctions will appear to be bright on these images.

The standard DE sequences are segmented acquisitions, acquired at every other heartbeat to allow recovery of longitudinal magnetization in normal myocardium before the next inversion pulse is applied. They typically take approximately 8 to 12 seconds to acquire. For patients with significant arrhythmia or difficulty with breath-holding, single-shot DE images using a steady-state free-precession (SSFP) inversion recovery readout can provide comparable data in a fraction of the imaging time. These images have slightly worse spatial resolution and contrast-to-noise ratio, but provide a satisfactory alternative in these circumstances.[7]

The DE single-shot inversion recovery images may also be obtained with a long inversion time (550 to 600 ms at 1.5 T) and are quite useful in the detection of thrombi.[8]

In these images with a long inversion time, thrombi will appear dark in contrast to normal and infarcted myocardium, which will be medium to high in signal intensity. Because these do not require "washout" of contrast from the myocardium, these can be performed shortly after contrast administration, while waiting for the appropriate delay for standard DE-CMR imaging (see Figure 33-2).

Optional Sequences

Morphologic Static Images

In many cases, an overview of cardiac and great vessel anatomy is desirable and can be rapidly performed using single-shot dark blood and/or single-shot bright blood techniques such as half-acquisition turbo spin-echo and SSFP sequences, respectively. These result in a stack of still-frame images and are usually acquired in the standard orthogonal imaging planes (axial, sagittal, or coronal). The rapidity of acquisition is such that breath-holding is not required. These produce excellent depiction of the overall myocardial structure and the relationships of the great vessels (Figure 33-e5).

T2-Weighted Images

In cases in which the acuity of an infarction is uncertain, or in cases of suspected acute myocarditis, T2-weighted imaging may be useful in demonstrating the edema characteristically seen in the acute phase of these disorders. These sequences are performed before the administration of IV contrast, because the presence of contrast may complicate image interpretation. These can be obtained via a double or triple inversion fast spin-echo black-blood sequence or with a T2-preparation SSFP bright-blood sequence. The T2-prep bright-blood sequence is far more resistant to artifacts than the black-blood sequence. However, the bright-blood sequence may be less sensitive for detecting regions with more moderate levels of edema, particularly if limited to the subendocardium.[9]

Perfusion Imaging

Increasingly, stress and rest CMR perfusion imaging are being used to detect ischemia in patients with known or suspected coronary disease, and multiple studies have demonstrated excellent sensitivity and specificity, similar to or exceeding those of SPECT imaging.[10,11] Combined with the superior delineation of infarction provided by DE-CMR relative to SPECT, it is not surprising that some centers are now using stress perfusion CMR as a first-line test, particularly in the United Kingdom, where cardiac imaging is not reimbursed according to a "fee per procedure" structure. A modification of the standard examination to include stress and rest perfusion imaging is shown in Figure 33-e6. Unlike vasodilator radionuclide imaging in which adenosine is typically infused for 6 minutes (tracer injection at 3 minutes), stress perfusion MR imaging is performed using an abbreviated adenosine protocol (~3 minutes) because vasodilation needs to be maintained only for the initial first-pass through the myocardium. Although severe reactions to adenosine are rare, a shortened protocol is relevant because moderate reactions that affect patient tolerability are relatively commonplace.

Other Optional Sequences

Velocity-encoded flow studies can be performed as necessary in cases of complicating known or suspected valvular pathology. These sequences can be used to quantify peak gradients through stenotic valves and to measure regurgitant flow.

T1 and T2 mapping techniques are increasingly being investigated in studies of infarction and other myocardial disorders, and can be performed before and/or after the administration of IV contrast. These sequences provide a quantitative assessment of regional myocardial T1 and T2 values and are not subject to surface coil sensitivity profiles that can result in variable image intensity for different regions of the heart. In the absence of gadolinium contrast, T1 and T2 values are increased in the setting of acute necrosis-related edema, and thus, these sequences allow the depiction of edema and provide a metric that may be useful for purposes of quantification and serial assessment. A parametric map of extracellular volume fraction can be made by combining precontrast ("native") and postcontrast T1 mapping values (see Figure 33-1).[12] Extracellular volume fraction will be increased both in the setting of acute necrosis and chronic collagenous scar.

TYPICAL IMAGING FINDINGS IN MYOCARDIAL INFARCTION

Acute Ischemic Injury

Cine Imaging

Acute ischemic injury of the myocardium usually results in myocardial dysfunction, with reduction of systolic wall thickening evident on cine images. Such dysfunction may occur even in the absence of infarction. Acute infarction may result in transient swelling of the affected segment, with increased signal often apparent on SSFP cine images, reflecting the partial T2 weighting of SSFP sequences and the presence of edema (Figure 33-5).

Delayed-Enhancement Cardiac Magnetic Resonance

Acute ischemic injury that does not cause infarction will not result in hyperenhancement. Acute infarctions are recognized as focal areas of subendocardial hyperenhancement on DE-CMR, and may extend transmurally toward the epicardium for a variable distance, depending on the duration and severity of the ischemia (see Figure 33-5C). They characteristically follow a vascular territory. More severe and long-standing ischemic episodes will usually result in a greater transmural extent of infarction, because necrosis proceeds in a "wavefront" from the subendocardium toward the epicardium. If ischemia is sufficiently severe, it may result in the development of a "no-reflow zone," as evidenced on DE-CMR as a dark, nonenhancing core at the center of an extensive infarction (see Figure 33-5C). These regions (see the section on Characterization of Myocardial Infarction) are the DE-CMR correlates of microvascular damage from an ischemic injury that is sufficiently severe as to cause endothelial damage in the core of the infarct.[13] DE caused by MI is thus recognized as an area of subendocardial or transmural hyperenhancement that follows a vascular perfusion territory (Figure 33-e7).

Native T2 and T1 Imaging/Mapping

In the setting of acute myocardial injury, increased signal may be seen in areas of infarction, reflecting the presence of edema and increased tissue T2 values (see Figure 33-5D). It has also been reported that the entire myocardial region that becomes ischemic after occlusion of its supplying coronary artery—the so-called "area at risk"—may be discerned as an edematous region on T2-weighted images and T2 maps. This method has garnered much interest, because in combination with DE-CMR, which delineates the infarcted region, it could represent an approach to noninvasively identify "salvaged" myocardium.[14] However, there is remaining uncertainty regarding the ability of T2 imaging and/or T2 maps to depict the area at risk, and therefore, this issue is controversial.[15] T1 maps obtained without contrast in patients with acute MI will also show increased T1 values, indicating the presence of edema in areas of acute infarction.[12]

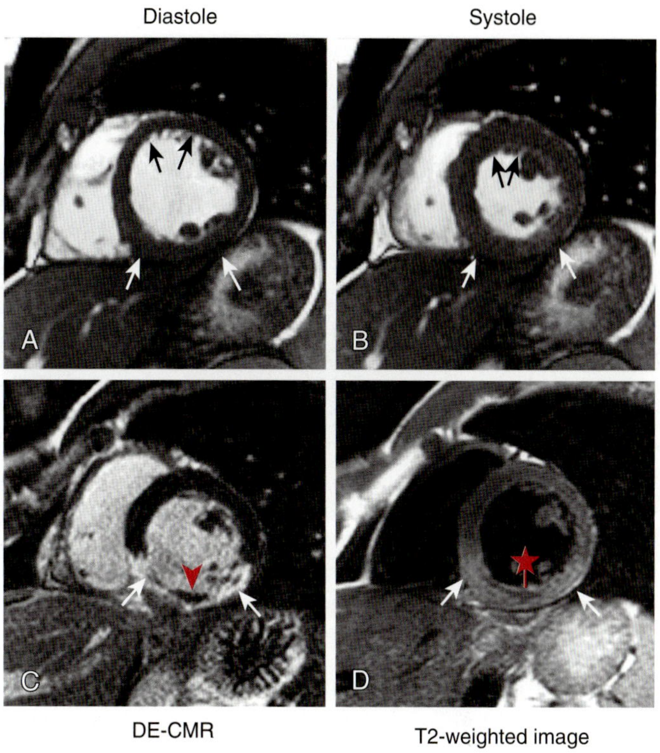

FIGURE 33-5 Cine steady-state free-precession images in (**A**) diastole and (**B**) systole from a patient with an acute inferior myocardial infarction. The inferior, inferoseptal, and inferolateral segments, although thicker in diastole, do not show normal thickening (*white arrows*) compared with the noninfarcted anterior wall (*black arrows*), which demonstrates normal systolic thickening. (**C**) The spatially matched delayed-enhancement cardiac magnetic resonance (DE-CMR) image shows a transmural infarction of the inferior wall and the inferoseptal segment (*arrow*). The small dark area in the center of the hyperenhanced inferior wall on the DE-CMR image is a no-reflow zone (*red arrowhead*) reflecting microvascular damage and the absence of gadolinium contrast uptake. (**D**) A T2-weighted image (precontrast) at the same location shows a high signal consistent with edema (*arrows*) and a low signal centrally in the infarct that corresponds to the no-reflow zone and represents coexisting intramural hemorrhage (*red star*), which results in lower myocardial T2 values.

Chronic Ischemic Injury

Cine Imaging

Chronic ischemic injury may result in impaired function, with regional or global hypokinesia, or even akinesia. Wall thinning may also occur in the affected segments, which may be caused by previous infarction, but can also be seen with "hibernation," a potentially reversible form of dysfunction. Cine imaging (without dobutamine stimulation) cannot differentiate these possibilities (Figure 33-6).

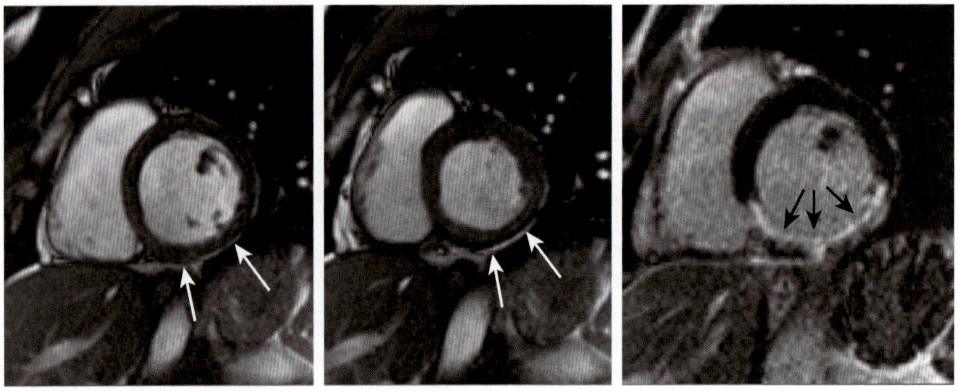

FIGURE 33-6 **Images 3 months later from the patient shown in Figure 33-5.** The inferior and inferolateral walls (*white arrows*) show thinning in diastole, and no significant thickening in systole. The delayed-enhancement cardiac magnetic resonance (DE-CMR) image shows transmural enhancement of the inferior wall (*black arrows*). Note the absence of the previously seen no-reflow zone evident on the acute phase images.

Delayed-Enhancement Cardiac Magnetic Resonance

Similar to acute infarctions, chronic infarctions will hyperenhance while areas of hibernation will not, allowing their differentiation, as discussed in detail later in the chapter.

Native T2 and T1 Imaging/Mapping

Chronic infarctions (>3 to 6 months in age) lacking edema will not show increased T2-weighted signal or increased T2 values, potentially allowing distinction from an acute MI, a distinction that is often not possible with DE-CMR alone (Figure 33-e8). Recently, some studies suggest that native T1 values are increased in the setting of chronic infarction, and could be used to identify chronic MI; however, there may be significant overlap with normal values.

Clinical Reporting

For general clinical reporting, we use the 17-segment model recommended by the American Heart Association. This model divides the basal and mid-cavity levels into six segments each, an apical level into four segments, and the true apex into one segment (Figure 33-e9). For each segment, LV systolic function is graded visually using a five-point scale ranging from normal wall thickening to systolic thinning and dyskinesis. The LV ejection fraction (LVEF) is also provided and estimated from visual inspection of all the short- and long-axis views. Occasionally, LVEF is quantitatively measured by planimetry, such as in patients who are undergoing chemotherapy with potentially cardiotoxic agents. The DE images are also interpreted using a five-point scale. For each segment, the average transmural extent of hyperenhanced tissue is graded visually. Examples of myocardial segments with various transmural extents of hyperenhancement are shown in Figure 33-e10. It is important that the DE images are interpreted with the cine images immediately adjacent. The cine images can provide a reference of the diastolic wall thickness of each region. Use of cine imaging in this manner will be helpful if DE imaging is performed before there is significant contrast washout from the LV cavity, and there is difficulty in differentiating the bright signal from the LV cavity from hyperenhanced myocardium, as seen in Figure 33-e11.

APPLICATIONS OF CARDIAC MAGNETIC RESONANCE IN MYOCARDIAL INFARCTION

Diagnosis of Myocardial Infarction

Because of late timing, patients with MI may present without diagnostic biomarker elevation of electrocardiographic (ECG) abnormalities (see Chapter 6). Moreover, wall motion abnormalities on cardiac imaging may not occur unless the infarcted region exceeds 20% to 50% of the myocardial wall thickness. Similarly, scintigraphic defects may not be apparent until greater than 10 g of tissue is infarcted. Thus, because a sizable threshold of damage is required, echocardiography or SPECT may miss the MI, particularly when it is small or subendocardial. Wall motion abnormalities may also occur in entities other than MI, such as Takotsubo cardiomyopathy, which indicates a lack of specificity. In these instances, where the diagnosis of MI is difficult, DE-CMR may prove helpful. The performance of DE-CMR for the detection of MI was tested in an international multicenter trial.[16] In that study, 282 patients with acute and 284 with chronic first-time MI were scanned, using commercially available scanners and sequences from a variety of different manufacturers, in 26 centers throughout the United States, Europe, and South America. The sensitivity of DE-CMR increased with an increasing gadolinium dose, reaching 99% and 94% in acute and chronic MI, respectively, with the 0.3-mmol/kg dose. Furthermore, with doses of 0.2 mmol/kg or higher, when MI was identified, the location of hyperenhancement matched the perfusion territory of the infarct-related artery in more than 97% of patients. It should be emphasized that the study demonstrated high sensitivity for the detection of chronic MIs, although they are often more difficult to detect than acute MI because substantial infarct shrinkage may occur during healing.

Detection of Unrecognized Myocardial Infarction

Because of its high sensitivity, DE-CMR has been used in population studies to evaluate the prevalence of unrecognized MI. In patients who underwent clinically indicated CMR, Kwong and colleagues demonstrated that the prevalence of unrecognized MI by DE-CMR was 76% higher than by ECG criteria.[17] In a research cohort with suspected coronary artery disease (CAD) but that did not have a history of MI, Kim and colleagues observed that the prevalence of unrecognized MI was 313% higher than that found by ECG.[18] A study of 670 subjects of the ICELAND MI study of 70-year-old residents of Sweden demonstrated a 340% increase in detection.[19] From a public health standpoint, the implications of these studies may be considerable. It has been estimated that 190,000 patients in the United States and perhaps as many as 300,000 in Europe experience an unrecognized MI annually. Because these estimates reflect only patients identified by ECG, the DE-CMR studies suggest that the actual incidence may be threefold higher.

One might postulate that the MIs not recognized by standard criteria are likely small and of uncertain significance. However, in the report by Kwong, the presence of unrecognized MI detected by DE-CMR was associated with a greater than sixfold higher risk of major adverse cardiac events compared with the absence of such an MI. Importantly, the information from DE-CMR was a stronger predictor of outcome than standard clinical risk factors and even catheterization data.[17] Similarly, the study by Kim and colleagues reported that the presence of unrecognized MI by DE-CMR predicted an 11-fold higher risk of all-cause mortality than those without MI.

Use in Non–ST-Elevation Myocardial Infarction

In many patients with NSTEMI, the culprit artery may not be apparent from the x-ray angiogram, particularly if there has been intervening clot dissolution; the affected artery is a branch vessel that is flush occluded at its origin, or there is multivessel disease. The overall rate in which the infarct-related artery cannot be identified in the setting of NSTEMI is as high as 50% in some studies. In this setting, the performance of CMR will often allow a definitive localization of the infarct-related artery (Figure 33-7).

Discrimination of Myocardial Injury Other Than Infarction

Many entities other than MI can cause acute chest pain syndromes accompanied by increases in cardiac biomarkers, particularly sensitive assays for troponin (see Chapter 7). Multiple studies have evaluated the role of CMR in patients with chest pain, elevated troponin, and unobstructed coronary arteries. In this clinical setting, DE-CMR was reported to provide a new diagnosis in up to 65% of patients, with myocarditis being the most common identifiable cause (60%).[20] Similarly, in a large study of patients with ST-elevation MI (STEMI) who underwent coronary angiography, it was reported that 14% had no culprit artery detected, and 9.5% did not have significant CAD. In the group without a clear culprit artery, CMR established that the most common diagnoses were myocarditis (31%), Takotsubo cardiomyopathy (31%), and STEMI without an angiographic lesion (28%)[21] (see Chapter 6).

Similar to troponin, the detection of injury by DE-CMR is specific for irreversible myocardial damage, but it is not specific for MI. One potential advantage of DE-CMR is that the pattern of hyperenhancement, rather than simply the presence or extent, may offer important information regarding the cause of myocardial damage. For this purpose, the concept that ischemic myonecrosis proceeds as a wavefront from the subendocardium to the epicardium with increasing coronary occlusion time is crucial. Correspondingly, hyperenhancement patterns that spare the subendocardium and are limited to the middle or epicardial portion of the LV wall are invariably nonischemic in origin because damage in the setting of CAD almost always involves the subendocardium. Moreover, certain nonischemic disorders, such as myocarditis, have characteristic hyperenhancement patterns that suggest specific diagnoses, and a systematic approach to interpreting DE-CMR images in patients with cardiomyopathy has been proposed.[22] Figure 33-e12 shows representative examples of how DE-CMR may be clinically useful in three patients presenting with chest discomfort, ST-segment elevation, and elevated troponin. In all three, the initial diagnosis was STEMI, but insignificant CAD was found at coronary angiography. DE-CMR was performed because the diagnosis was uncertain, and in each case, it provided information to clarify the diagnosis. Figure 33-e13 shows an algorithm demonstrating the possible uses of CMR in cases of suspected STEMI.

Characterization of Myocardial Infarction

DE-CMR may also allow assessment of gradations of injury within acute MI. Rather than simply identifying a region of acute infarction as nonviable, DE-CMR can distinguish acute infarcts with only necrotic myocytes from acute infarcts with necrotic myocytes and damaged microvasculature. The presence of a dark, nonenhancing central area contained within an area of hyperenhancement on DE-CMR is termed a no-reflow zone, and represents an area of markedly delayed diffusion of contrast into the central core of what is usually an extensive infarction (see Figure 33-5C). These regions represent myocardium with compromised perfusion at the tissue level even after patency of the epicardial coronary artery has been restored. They are usually seen in the setting of transmural infarctions, and are transient phenomena, because they are usually not visualized after 4 to 6 weeks. Within a given examination, they are also transient phenomena, because after contrast administration, the spatial extent is greater at earlier time points, and it may disappear as contrast diffuses into the area of injury over time (Figure 33-e14). The presence of microvascular obstruction has been associated with worse outcomes, including adverse ventricular remodeling, ventricular arrhythmias, and major adverse cardiac events (see Chapter 24 and Chapter 36).[23] Occasionally, circumstances arise in which the patient may have more than one infarction, and the acuity of each is uncertain. As noted previously, DE imaging will demonstrate hyperenhancement in both acute and chronic MI, and thus by itself cannot distinguish between these possibilities. However, the presence of microvascular obstruction indicates an acute MI, and additional findings that suggest an area of hyperenhancement is likely acute include increased focal wall thickness on cine imaging and the presence of edema on T2-weighted imaging. The absence of all three features is suggestive but not specific for a chronic MI, because in the setting of acute MI these features may also be absent if the infarct is small and subendocardial.

Imaging of Acute Complications of Myocardial Infarction

Right Ventricular Myocardial Infarction

In patients with acute inferior MI, it has been shown that even when physical examination, ECG with right precordial leads, and echocardiography are negative, DE-CMR could

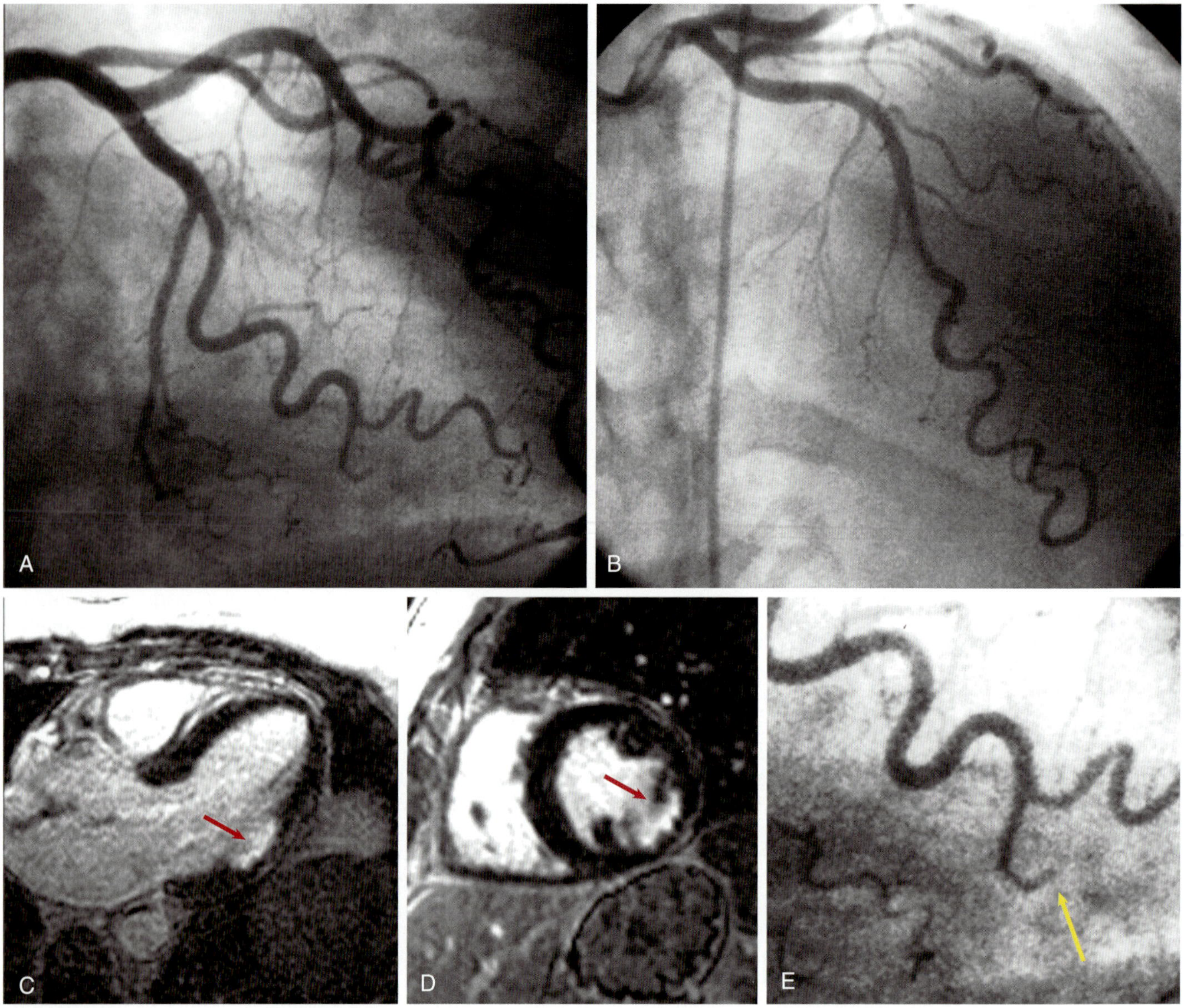

FIGURE 33-7 Images from a patient with a non–ST-elevation myocardial infarction. The initial diagnostic coronary angiogram was interpreted as negative (images **A** and **B** are selected still frames), and the patient was referred for cardiac resonance imaging. (**C** and **D**) Delayed-enhancement cardiac magnetic resonance images show a focus of hyperenhancement in the inferolateral wall (*red arrows*), consistent with a circumflex territory myocardial infarction. Upon review of the angiogram (**E**, which is a magnified image from the series shown in **A**), a subtle occlusion of a small obtuse marginal branch is noted (*yellow arrow* in **E**).

detect right ventricular (RV) involvement in nearly 25% of patients (see Chapter 26). DE-CMR typically shows an extensive LV wall inferior MI with extension to involve the RV inferior wall and a variable portion of the RV free wall (Figure 33-e15).[24]

Cardiac Rupture

Few patients come to imaging, and those who do often have contained ruptures, but cine MR can demonstrate the focal loss of contractility in the affected segment, and the presence of intrapericardial fluid and blood products. DE-CMR demonstrates the causative infarction as an area of transmural enhancement (see Chapter 26).

Interventricular Septal Defects

Although usually assessed adequately by echo, MR can demonstrate the septal defect, the transseptal flow, and the underlying MI (Figure 33-e16) (see Chapter 26). Importantly, MR can also noninvasively measure the pulmonary to systemic flow ratio (Qp/Qs), a parameter that may be useful on follow-up imaging of smaller defects or in those treated with septal occlusion devices.

Pericarditis/Pericardial Effusion

Up to 31% of acute STEMI patients have evidence of pericardial inflammation on CMR, manifested by pericardial effusions or abnormal enhancement on DE-CMR (see Chapter 26).[25] Effusions are easily recognized as high-signal fluid in the pericardial space, and are readily depicted with cine MR. Complicating hemorrhage is usually identifiable because of the increased complexity of the pericardial fluid (Figure 33-e17). Thickening of the pericardium can also clearly be seen. Post-contrast imaging can be helpful in assessing for the presence of enhancement, signifying inflammatory pericarditis, and distinguishing it from chronic fibrous thickening, which often does not enhance.

Imaging of Chronic Complications of Myocardial Infarction

Thrombus

DE-CMR is the most sensitive imaging technique for detection of LV thrombus, and picks up approximately twice as many ventricular thrombi as cine CMR and transthoracic echocardiography (see Chapter 26). Clinically, it is frequently noted that ventricular thrombi are found adherent to sites of previous infarction, where wall motion abnormalities and possibly denudation of the endothelium produced by previous infarction result in a nidus for thrombus formation. The latter mechanism is suggested because CMR data demonstrate that patients with ischemic cardiomyopathy have an approximately fivefold increased risk relative to those with nonischemic systolic dysfunction of similar extent, and the presence of regions with more than 50% transmural infarction appears to be an additional risk factor for thrombus development (Figure 33-8).[26] In particular, thrombi are often noted along the endocavitary aspect of ventricular aneurysms (see Figures 33-8C and 8D).

Thrombus is recognized on cine imaging when it presents as an intracavitary filling defect that is discernible from adjacent trabeculations and papillary muscles. However, recognition of mural thrombus can be quite difficult on noncontrast cine images, and likely accounts for the lower sensitivity (40%) of cine CMR relative to contrast-enhanced CMR.

The ability of DE-CMR to identify thrombus based on tissue characteristics rather than just anatomical appearance likely explains its improved performance compared with cine CMR or echocardiography. The basic underlying principle is that thrombi are avascular and have essentially no gadolinium uptake. Thus, thrombus can be identified as a nonenhancing defect surrounded by bright ventricular blood and contrast-enhanced myocardium. Image intensity differences between normal myocardium and thrombus can be accentuated by using a DE-CMR sequence in which the inversion time is increased to null avascular tissue such as thrombus (500 to 600 ms).[8] With long-inversion time imaging, regions with contrast uptake such as viable myocardium increase in image intensity, whereas thrombus appears homogeneously black, and there is improved delineation, particularly of mural thrombus (see Figures 33-8C and 33-8D). This long-inversion recovery variation of DE-CMR can be acquired using a single-shot inversion-recovery SSFP sequence in multiple planes to rapidly screen for thrombus, even in patients with arrhythmias or who are uncooperative.

Ventricular Aneurysms

Certain imaging characteristics have been noted to provide differentiation in most cases between true aneurysms (intact thinned myocardium) and false aneurysms (contained rupture) (see Figures 33-8C and 33-8D) (see Chapter 26). True aneurysms are said to have a wide neck that is similar in diameter to the base of the aneurysm, whereas false aneurysms, which represent a contained rupture, typically have a narrow neck with a broad base (Figure 33-e18). Ultimately, however, the real distinction between the two is the presence of residual myocardium forming the boundary of the lesion in the case of a true aneurysm or the lack thereof in a false aneurysm. Visualization of the wall of the aneurysm as separate and distinct from the pericardium is usually possible with cine MR imaging. Conversely, if the pericardium appears to make up the boundary of the aneurysm without residual myocardium, the lesion should be deemed a false aneurysm. DE imaging is also helpful, in that pericardial enhancement has been described as occurring frequently in false aneurysms with a lower incidence in true aneurysms. Both may have associated mural thrombus.

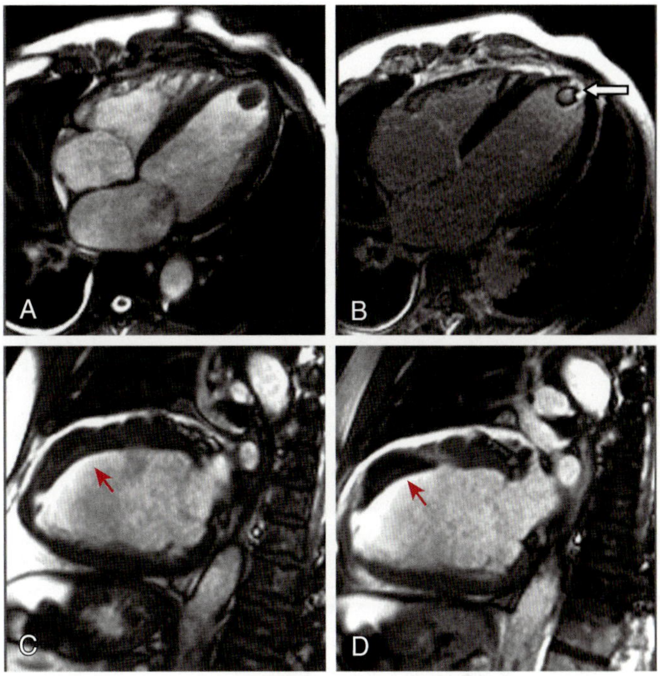

FIGURE 33-8 Intracavitary thrombus is recognized as a filling defect separate from papillary muscles and trabeculae on the four-chamber cine view (**A**) and is noted on the delayed enhancement image (**B**) to be adherent to a site of previous apical infarction (*white arrow*). Thrombus may sometimes have an "etched" appearance on delayed-enhancement cardiac magnetic resonance images obtained with a standard inversion time, but will be homogenously dark on images with a long inversion time (550 to 600 ms). In another patient with a mural thrombus lining a true aneurysm of the anterior wall, the precontrast two-chamber cine steady-state free-precession image (**C**) does not clearly differentiate the thrombus (*red arrow*) from the myocardium, because their signal intensities are similar. (**D**) The postcontrast inversion-recovery steady-state free-precession image with a long inversion time (600 ms) allows clear differentiation of thrombus from myocardium. Echocardiography did not detect this thrombus.

PREDICTING FUNCTIONAL RECOVERY AND OUTCOMES

Predicting Left Ventricular Recovery

In the setting of acute MI, prompt restoration of coronary blood flow has been shown to result in salvage of viable myocardium, improvement in LVEF, and long-term improvement in survival (see Chapter 13). However, early after successful coronary reperfusion, myocardial dysfunction may persist, and it is important to distinguish whether it is caused by myocardial necrosis or stunning (see Chapter 24). In the setting of acute MI, the transmural extent of infarction (TEI) as measured on DE-CMR has been shown by multiple studies to be highly predictive of later improvement in wall motion (Figure 33-e19). That is, the greater the TEI in a given segment, the lower the likelihood of recovery of function.

In one representative study, almost 80% of segments without infarction showed improvement, whereas only 5% of segments with greater than 75% TEI showed improvement. Areas of intermediate TEI demonstrated intermediate levels of recovery. In addition to predicting segmental functional

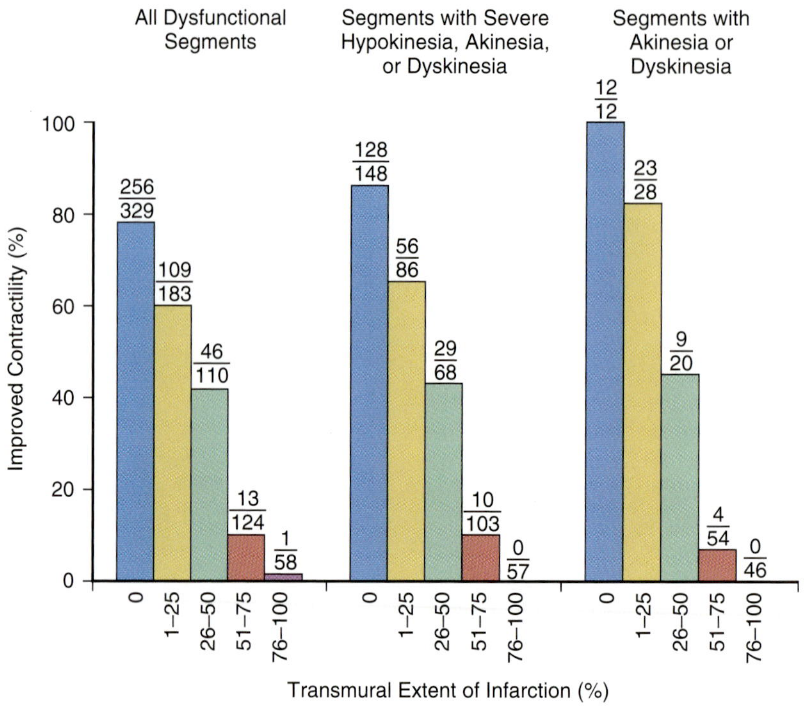

FIGURE 33-9 The likelihood of recovery of wall motion following revascularization is inversely related to the transmural extent of infarction (hyperenhancement) on delayed enhancement imaging, even in severely hypokinetic, akinetic, or dyskinetic segments. *(From Kim RJ, et al: The use of contrast-enhanced magnetic resonance imaging to identify reversible myocardial dysfunction.* N Engl J Med *343:1445–1453, 2000.)*

recovery, DE-CMR also predicted improvement in global function. On a per patient basis, the total number of segments that were dysfunctional but viable (<25% TEI) was directly related to a change in LVEF. Multiple other studies have subsequently confirmed that the transmural extent of enhancement on DE-CMR predicts functional improvement after MI.

Predicting the Impact of Revascularization

In patients who have severe myocardial dysfunction after MI and are incompletely revascularized or not yet revascularized, a common clinical question centers on whether to proceed with coronary revascularization. In this setting, improvement in LVEF after revascularization will likely improve symptoms and outcome, but such recovery requires viable myocardium. Multiple studies have demonstrated that among patients with chronic CAD, the likelihood of functional improvement is inversely related in a progressive stepwise fashion to the TEI as depicted by DE-CMR. That is, the greater the TEI, the lower the likelihood of recovery of wall motion in any given segment. Alternatively, minimal or no enhancement is associated with a high probability of improvement after revascularization (Figure 33-9). This observation is true even in segments that are akinetic or dyskinetic before revascularization.

When interpreting the information that DE-CMR can provide in this setting, it is important to take advantage of the high spatial resolution it affords; DE-CMR allows the visualization of the transmural extent of viability and/or infarction, and thus changes the assessment of viability from a binary "yes/no" characterization to that of a continuum, which better reflects reality. This ability to grade myocardial viability along a continuum is one of the great strengths of DE-CMR. As such, the use of a single cutoff value on which to base predictions of functional improvement would not have a physiologic basis and would be suboptimal.

Other Aspects of Viability Assessment

DE imaging provides significantly better spatial resolution than the competing modality of SPECT imaging. However, even if SPECT imaging had similar spatial resolution, DE-CMR would still have a significant advantage in that it allows the assessment of the amount of viability and the amount of infarction simultaneously. This property of DE-CMR is particularly important in the differentiation of possibly hibernating myocardium from myocardium that is significantly thinned as a result of extensive scar. As an example of this principle, consider the evaluation of a patient with a region of thinned (<5.5 mm in diastole) dysfunctional myocardium (Figure 33-e20). Classic echo teaching would infer that such areas are invariably reflective of transmural infarction, and nuclear perfusion imaging would indicate that such areas are nonviable, simply based on the significant reduction of counts in the thinned area relative to remote, normal myocardium. However, CMR provides evidence that this assertion is not always the case. Shah and colleagues found that 19% of a group of 1055 patients who underwent CMR had regional wall thinning (≤5.5 mm) that involved an average of 34% of the LV.[27] Of those regions with thinning, 18% were found to have a limited scar burden (defined as <50% hyperenhancement), and such patients who underwent revascularization uniformly demonstrated significant improvement in contractile function (Figure 33-10). It was also notable that in regions with limited scar burden, there was substantial reverse remodeling of the myocardial wall and disappearance of thinned regions because diastolic wall thickness increased from a mean of 4.4 mm to a mean of 7.5 mm (see Figure 33-10). Hence, it appears for a given

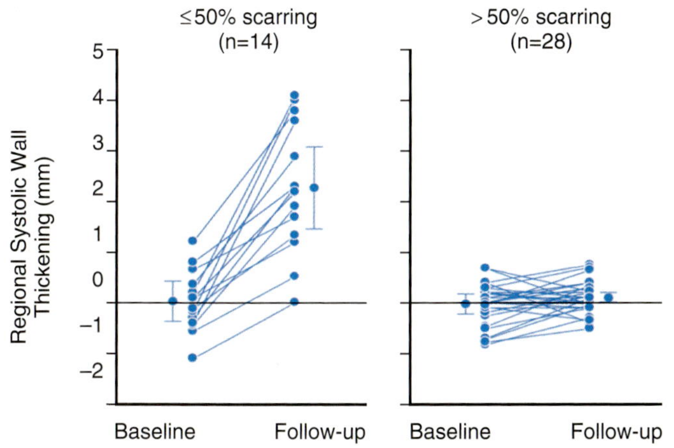

FIGURE 33-10 In patients with regional left ventricular wall thinning and akinesis, significant improvement in contractile function can be seen post-revascularization. However, contractile function (e.g., systolic wall thickening) improved only in those with limited scarring (<50% transmural scar). *(Modified from Shah DJ, et al: Prevalence of regional myocardial thinning and relationship with myocardial scarring in patients with coronary artery disease.* JAMA *309:909–918, 2013.)*

myocardial region that the amount of scar in relation to the amount of viability is more important than just the absolute amount of viability in predicting contractile improvement and reverse remodeling after revascularization.

USE IN CLINICAL TRIALS

The ultimate goal of a new therapy for acute MI is a reduction in mortality. In the current era, treatment of acute MI is quite effective; therefore, demonstrating a further reduction in mortality with novel treatments is increasingly difficult and necessitates studies with large sample sizes with corresponding logistical and financial barriers. As such, there is considerable interest in using surrogate endpoints to assess the efficacy of acute MI therapies. Infarct size is a particularly attractive surrogate endpoint for several reasons. First, it is useful in early screening studies to test whether a new therapy is biologically active. Second, it can serve as an endpoint for phase II dose-ranging studies to test efficacy and/or safety. Third, it may indicate a late mortality benefit, and thus rationale for performing a longer term study, even if an early benefit is not seen. For instance, a reduction in infarct size may lead to a long-term improvement in ventricular remodeling, a benefit that may not be manifest on 30-day mortality rates. Fourth, it can provide a mechanism for improvement in outcome, because prognosis after acute MI is strongly determined by infarct size. Several investigations have reported that infarct size measured by DE-CMR is a stronger predictor of outcome than that of LVEF and LV volumes.[28,29]

Care should be taken in planning the timing of the CMR acquisition, because MIs are known to demonstrate what Reimer and Jennings have termed "a changing anatomic reference base." That is, the size of infarction can show dramatic changes over time, with edema and swelling resulting in a near-doubling of infarct size in the acute phase and significant shrinkage (up to 75% reduction of infarct size) occurring in the chronic phase as necrosis is replaced by collagenous scar. These findings have been confirmed in CMR studies of the evolution of infarct size over time. Fieno and colleagues demonstrated that terminal infarct size at 4 to 8 weeks in a canine model averaged 24% of that found at 3 days. Moreover, the mass of viable myocardium increased systematically with time, although the time course of hypertrophy was different from that of infarct resorption. Importantly, measurements of total LV mass did not reflect the changes that occurred separately in infarcted and viable regions. These results highlight the capability of DE-CMR to improve the assessment of post-infarction ventricular remodeling by allowing evaluation of concurrent changes, such as resorption of infarcted tissue and hypertrophy of viable myocardium, at an early time point before measurements of ventricular volumes and mass change.

Another important implication of the "changing anatomic reference base" is that a reduction in hyperenhancement size from an acute scan to a chronic scan should not lead to confusion regarding the interpretation of hyperenhancement zones. Some previous studies have suggested that hyperenhancement in the acute phase represents both infarcted myocardium and a rim of surrounding viable myocardium, whereas hyperenhancement in the chronic phase solely represents infarcted myocardium in an effort to explain the differences in hyperenhancement size. This interpretation is incorrect. In both acute and chronic settings, hyperenhancement depicts infarction; however, the infarct size itself is dynamic (see Chapter 4 and Chapter 24).

Several studies have shown that the measurement of infarct size by DE-CMR is highly reproducible. The implication of high reproducibility is that DE-CMR may enable robust detection of small changes in infarct size, and potentially allow substantial reduction in sample size for clinical trials using infarct size as an efficacy endpoint. Few studies have directly compared infarct size measurements by DE-CMR with those by technetium-99m SPECT, although the latter is considered one of the best available techniques for the quantification of infarct size. An early study by Mahrholdt and colleagues reported that the SD of infarct size was 6% by DE-CMR and 7.5% by SPECT in a population with chronic MI. Because DE-CMR led to a 20% reduction in variability (1.5 of 7.5), the improved precision would result in a nearly 40% reduction in sample size. Similarly, Lunde and colleagues evaluated infarct size in STEMI patients who were randomized to intracoronary injection of mononuclear bone marrow cells at both acute and chronic time points. In the control group, both early and late after MI, the SD of infarct size was lower by DE-CMR than by SPECT (14.0 vs. 21.1 and 12.5 vs. 20.9, respectively).[3] Although the variability of infarct size will change with the population being studied (e.g., cohorts with a high prevalence of anterior MI will have larger mean infarct size and a larger SD), these data suggest that the total variability is smaller when using DE-CMR and will lead to appreciable differences in sample size. As a result, interest in DE-CMR for infarct size quantification is rapidly growing. General strengths and weaknesses of CMR for clinical trials are shown in Table 33-e1.

SUMMARY

In patients with known or suspected MI, CMR provides a comprehensive, multifaceted view of the heart. The data, including those from a multicenter clinical trial, indicate that DE-CMR is a well-validated, robust technique that can be easily implemented on scanners that are commonly available worldwide, with an effectiveness that rivals the best available imaging techniques for the detection and assessment of acute and chronic MI. CMR may be especially useful when patients present outside the diagnostic window of cardiac biomarkers. Moreover, because CMR can uniquely differentiate between ischemic and various nonischemic forms of injury, it may be helpful in cases of diagnostic uncertainty, such as in patients with classical features of MI in whom coronary angiography does not show a culprit lesion. Even after the diagnosis of MI has been made, CMR can provide clinically relevant information with regard to identification of post-MI sequelae and further infarct characterization. The high accuracy and reproducibility of DE-CMR has led to the increasing use of this technique as the preferred method for quantification of infarct size in many clinical trials.

Classic References

Choi KM, et al.: Transmural extent of acute myocardial infarction predicts long-term improvement in contractile function, *Circulation* 104:1101–1107, 2001.

Fieno DS, et al.: Contrast-enhanced magnetic resonance imaging of myocardium at risk: distinction between reversible and irreversible injury throughout infarct healing, *J Am Coll Cardiol* 36:1985–1991, 2000.

Kim RJ, et al.: The use of contrast-enhanced magnetic resonance imaging to identify reversible myocardial dysfunction, *N Engl J Med* 343:1445–1453, 2000.

Simonetti OP, et al.: An improved MR imaging technique for the visualization of myocardial infarction, *Radiology* 218:215–223, 2001.

Wagner A, et al.: Contrast-enhanced MRI and routine single photon emission computed tomography (SPECT) perfusion imaging for detection of subendocardial myocardial infarcts: an imaging study, *Lancet* 361:374–379, 2003.

References

1. Thygesen K, et al.: Third universal definition of myocardial infarction, *J Am Coll Cardiol* 60:1581–1598, 2012.
2. Ghosn MG, Shah DJ: Important advances in technology and unique applications related to cardiac magnetic resonance imaging, *Methodist Debakey Cardiovasc J* 10:159–162, 2014.
3. Kim HW, Farzaneh-Far A, Kim RJ: Cardiovascular magnetic resonance in patients with myocardial infarction: current and emerging applications, *J Am Coll Cardiol* 55:1–16, 2009.
4. Kramer CM, et al.: Standardized cardiovascular magnetic resonance (CMR) protocols 2013 update, *J Cardiovasc Magn Reson* 15:91, 2013.
5. Grothues F, Braun-Dullaeus R: Serial assessment of ventricular morphology and function, *Heart Fail Clin* 5:301–314, 2009.
6. Van Assche LM, Kim HW, Kim RJ: Cardiac MR for the assessment of myocardial viability, *Methodist Debakey Cardiovasc J* 9:163–168, 2013.
7. Wildgruber M, et al.: Inversion-recovery single-shot cardiac MRI for the assessment of myocardial infarction at 1.5 T with a dedicated cardiac coil, *Br J Radiol* 85:e709–e715, 2012.
8. Weinsaft JW, et al.: Contrast-enhanced anatomic imaging as compared to contrast-enhanced tissue characterization for detection of left ventricular thrombus, *JACC Cardiovasc Imaging* 2:969–979, 2009.
9. Viallon M, et al.: T2-weighted cardiac MR assessment of the myocardial area-at-risk and salvage area in acute reperfused myocardial infarction: comparison of state-of-the-art dark blood and bright blood T2-weighted sequences, *J Magn Reson Imaging* 35:328–339, 2012.
10. Schwitter J, et al.: MR-IMPACT II: Magnetic Resonance Imaging for Myocardial Perfusion Assessment in Coronary Artery Disease trial: perfusion-cardiac magnetic resonance vs. single-photon emission computed tomography for the detection of coronary artery disease: a comparative multicentre, multivendor trial, *Eur Heart J* 34:775–781, 2013.
11. Greenwood JP, et al.: Cardiovascular magnetic resonance and single-photon emission computed tomography for diagnosis of coronary heart disease (CE-MARC): a prospective trial, *Lancet* 379:453–460, 2012.
12. Salerno M, Kramer CM: Advances in parametric mapping with CMR imaging, *JACC Cardiovasc Imaging* 6:806–622, 2013.
13. Wu KC: CMR of microvascular obstruction and hemorrhage in myocardial infarction, *J Cardiovasc Magn Reson* 14:68, 2012.
14. Arai AE, Leung S, Kellman P: Controversies in cardiovascular MR imaging: reasons why imaging myocardial T2 has clinical and pathophysiologic value in acute myocardial infarction, *Radiology* 265:23–32, 2012.
15. Croisille P, Kim HW, Kim RJ: Controversies in cardiovascular MR imaging: T2-weighted imaging should not be used to delineate the area at risk in ischemic myocardial injury, *Radiology* 265:12–22, 2012.
16. Kim RJ, et al.: Performance of delayed-enhancement magnetic resonance imaging with gadoversetamide contrast for the detection and assessment of myocardial infarction: an international, multicenter, double-blinded, randomized trial, *Circulation* 117:629–637, 2008.
17. Kwong RY, et al.: Impact of unrecognized myocardial scar detected by cardiac magnetic resonance imaging on event-free survival in patients presenting with signs or symptoms of coronary artery disease, *Circulation* 113:2733–2743, 2006.
18. Kim HW, et al.: Unrecognized non-Q-wave myocardial infarction: prevalence and prognostic significance in patients with suspected coronary disease, *PLoS Med* 6:e1000057, 2009.
19. Schelbert EB, et al.: Prevalence and prognosis of unrecognized myocardial infarction determined by cardiac magnetic resonance in older adults, *JAMA* 308:890–896, 2012.
20. Leurent G, et al.: Diagnostic contributions of cardiac magnetic resonance imaging in patients presenting with elevated troponin, acute chest pain syndrome and unobstructed coronary arteries, *Arch Cardiovasc Dis* 104:161–170, 2011.
21. Larson DM, et al.: False-positive cardiac catheterization laboratory activation among patients with suspected ST-segment elevation myocardial infarction, *JAMA* 298:2754–2760, 2007.
22. Senthilkumar A, et al.: Identifying the etiology: a systematic approach using delayed-enhancement cardiovascular magnetic resonance, *Heart Fail Clin* 5:349–367, 2009. vi.
23. Klug G, et al.: Prognostic value at 5 years of microvascular obstruction after acute myocardial infarction assessed by cardiovascular magnetic resonance, *J Cardiovasc Magn Reson* 14:46, 2012.
24. Jensen CJ, et al.: Right ventricular involvement in acute left ventricular myocardial infarction: prognostic implications of MRI findings, *AJR Am J Roentgenol* 194:592–598, 2010.
25. Doulaptsis C, et al.: Assessment of early post-infarction pericardial injury by CMR, *JACC Cardiovasc Imaging* 6:411–413, 2013.
26. Weinsaft JW, et al.: LV thrombus detection by routine echocardiography: insights into performance characteristics using delayed enhancement CMR, *JACC Cardiovasc Imaging* 4:702–712, 2011.
27. Shah DJ, et al.: Prevalence of regional myocardial thinning and relationship with myocardial scarring in patients with coronary artery disease, *JAMA* 309:909–918, 2013.
28. Lonborg J, et al.: Final infarct size measured by cardiovascular magnetic resonance in patients with ST elevation myocardial infarction predicts long-term clinical outcome: an observational study, *Eur Heart J Cardiovasc Imaging* 14:387–395, 2013.
29. Klem I, et al.: Prognostic value of routine cardiac magnetic resonance assessment of left ventricular ejection fraction and myocardial damage: an international, multicenter study, *Circ Cardiovasc Imaging* 4:610–619, 2011.

SECTION V

DISCHARGE AND BEYOND

34 New Concepts in Cardiac Rehabilitation and Secondary Prevention After Myocardial Infarction

Rod S. Taylor and Ann-Dorthe Olsen Zwisler

INTRODUCTION

Evidence-based treatments for patients with myocardial infarction (MI) have improved outcomes, with substantive reductions in mortality rates (Chapter 2). Nevertheless, patients who survive an acute MI remain at increased risk for recurrent MI and death and also suffer from clinical symptoms and loss of physical, psychological, or social functioning after discharge that can lead to impaired health-related quality of life.[1] The effectiveness and accessibility of cardiac rehabilitation and secondary prevention services after MI have therefore never been more important. Current international clinical guidelines, including those of the American Heart Association, the American College of Cardiology, and the European Society of Cardiology, endorse rehabilitation and secondary prevention as key elements of standard post-MI management.[2-5]

Our approach to post-MI rehabilitation has changed radically in the last 80 or so years. In the 1930s, restriction of physical activity and prolonged bed rest were standard of care for patients suffering from an MI. Subsequent evolution of practices such as chair therapy (1940s), brief daily walks of 3 to 5 minutes (1950s), and structured inpatient cardiac rehabilitation programs for early ambulation after MI (1960s) led to the development of today's multidisciplinary, comprehensive cardiac rehabilitation and secondary prevention programs for a broad group of patients with atherosclerotic cardiovascular disease.[6]

The following definition from the Agency for Health Care Policy and Research encompasses these contemporary concepts:

> Cardiac rehabilitation [and secondary prevention] services are comprehensive, long-term programs involving medical evaluation, prescribed exercise, cardiac risk factor modification, education, and counselling. These programs are designed to limit the physiologic and psychological effects of cardiac illness, reduce the risk for sudden death or re-infarction, control cardiac symptoms, stabilize or reverse the atherosclerotic process, and enhance the psychosocial and vocational status of selected patients.[6a]

Although exercise training remains a cornerstone of intervention, current practice guidelines consistently recommend "comprehensive rehabilitation" programs that should contain the necessary core components to optimize cardiovascular risk reduction, foster healthy behaviors and compliance with these behaviors, reduce disability, and promote an active lifestyle.[2]

Cardiac rehabilitation and secondary prevention services should begin in the inpatient setting for patients who have survived an acute MI and continue into the early-outpatient and late-outpatient phases of follow-up (Figure 34-1). Although in many countries this inpatient and early-outpatient care is covered by health care providers and insurers,

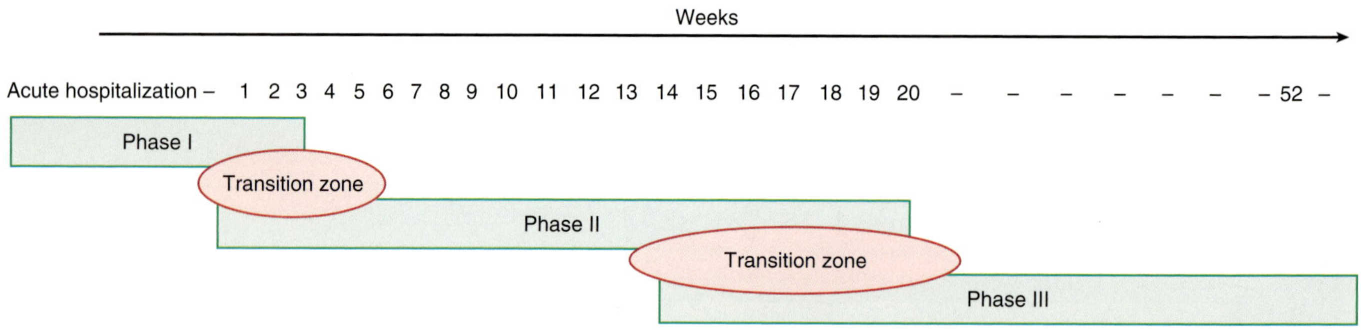

Phase I (in-hospital)	Phase II (early follow-up period)	Phase III (long-term follow-up and maintenance)
Early intervention during the stay in acute hospital, including early mobilization and prevention of complications. Most importantly phase I today includes assessment and referral to phase II rehabilitation.	Promotes and delivers rehabilitative and preventive services to patients following an index event with the aim of clinical stabilization, risk stratification, and promotion of long-term intervention. It may be performed in inpatient as well as in outpatient settings. The components and activities of phase II rehabilitation and secondary prevention are similar across mode of delivery.	Long-term outpatient follow-up, which seeks to provide sustained delivery of preventive and rehabilitative services. It takes place in an outpatient setting and/or in the community and is often delivered in collaboration with primary health care provider/primay physicians.
Transition zone – needs special attention	Risk of loss of information Risk of loss of gained outcomes	Risk of loss of information Risk of loss of gained outcomes

FIGURE 34-1 The trajectory of cardiac rehabilitation and secondary prevention after acute coronary syndrome.

the costs of late-outpatient or "maintenance" programs often need to be met by the patients themselves.

This chapter presents the evidence for cardiac rehabilitation and secondary prevention after MI, focusing on the findings of systematic reviews and meta-analyses; details the components of cardiac rehabilitation and secondary prevention delivery using current high-profile international practice and policy statements; and finally, considers current and future key challenges facing rehabilitation and secondary prevention services.

EVIDENCE FOR CARDIAC REHABILITATION AND SECONDARY PREVENTION

The first systematic reviews and meta-analyses of cardiac rehabilitation were published more than 20 years ago and reported a 20% to 25% reduction in all-cause and cardiovascular mortality in pooled data from 22 randomized controlled trials (RCTs) in more than 4300 post-MI patients, comparing exercise-based cardiac rehabilitation with a no-exercise rehabilitation approach in the control group. A number of updated versions of this systematic review/meta-analysis of cardiac rehabilitation and secondary prevention have since been published.[7]

The 2016 Cochrane systematic review and meta-analysis "Exercise-based cardiac rehabilitation for coronary heart disease" provides a useful summary of the available evidence.[8] The inclusion and exclusion criteria for the 2016 Cochrane review are summarized in Table 34-1. Bibliographic databases of Cochrane Central Register of Controlled Trials, MEDLINE, EMBASE, CINAHL, and Science Citation Index Expanded were searched to July 2014. The study authors identified a total of 63 RCTs (Table 34-e1). Although this update included a total of 14,486 patients, most trials were relatively small in size (median number of patients, 126; range, 28 to 2304). Greater than 80% of the trial populations were post-MI patients, with the remainder consisting of patients who had undergone coronary artery bypass grafting (CABG) or percutaneous coronary intervention (PCI); in more than one half of the patients in these cohorts, previous MI was the exclusive diagnosis. The median follow-up period was 12 months. Programs typically were conducted in a supervised outpatient hospital/center-based setting, either exclusively or in combination with

TABLE 34-1 Inclusion and Exclusion Criteria for 2016 Cochrane Review

Inclusion
• *Study design*: RCTs of exercise-based CR with a follow-up period of at least 6 months post randomisation • *Population*: Patients of all gender or ages who have had an MI, or who have undergone revascularization (coronary artery bypass grafting [CABG], percutaneous coronary intervention [PCI]) or who have angina pectoris or coronary heart disease defined by angiography • *Intervention*: Exercise-based CR, defined as a supervised or unsupervised inpatient, outpatient, or community- or home-based intervention that includes some form of exercise training, either alone or in addition to psychosocial and/or educational interventions • *Control*: Standard medical care, such as drug therapy, but without any form of structured exercise training program • *Outcomes*: One or more of the following outcomes: death (total and cardiovascular-related); MI (fatal and nonfatal); revascularizations (CABG and PCI); hospitalizations; health-related quality of life assessed using validated instruments (e.g., Short-Form-36, EQ-5D); or costs and cost-effectiveness
Exclusion
Studies exclusively recruiting patients with heart failure, with atrial fibrillation, after heart valve surgery, with heart transplants, or implanted with cardiac resynchronization device or with implantable cardioverter-defibrillator; or patients who completed a cardiac rehabilitation program before randomization

CR, Cardiac rehabilitation; *MI*, myocardial infarction; *RCTs*, randomized controlled trials.
From Anderson L, Thompson DR, Oldridge N, et al: Exercise-based cardiac rehabilitation for coronary heart disease: Cochrane systematic review and meta-analysis. J Am Coll Cardiol 67:1-12, 2016.

TABLE 34-2 Summary of Meta-analysis of Effects of Exercise-Based Cardiac Rehabilitation on Clinical Event Outcomes

OUTCOME	NO. OF PARTICIPANTS (WITH NO. OF STUDIES)	NO. OF EVENTS/ PARTICIPANTS		RELATIVE RISK (WITH 95% CI)	STATISTICAL HETEROGENEITY[2]/ STATISTIC CHI-SQUARE TEST (WITH *P* VALUE)	GRADE/ QUALITY OF EVIDENCE
		Intervention	Comparator			
All-cause mortality (all studies)	12,455 (47)	838/6424	865/6031	0.94 (0.87-1.02)	0% (0.58)	+ + + – Moderate*
CV mortality (all studies)	7469 (27)	292/3850	375/3619	0.74 (0.64-0.85)	0% (0.70)	+ + + – Moderate*
Fatal and/or nonfatal MI (all studies)	971 (36)	356/4951	387/4766	0.89 (0.78-1.02)	0% (0.48)	+ + – – Low*†
CABG (all studies)	5891 (29)	208/3021	212/2870	0.94 (0.78-1.12)	0% (0.86)	+ + + – Moderate*
PCI (all studies)	4012 (16)	171/2013	197/1999	0.86 (0.71-1.04)	0% (0.59)	+ + + – Moderate*
Hospital admissions (all studies)	3030 (15)	407/1556	453/1474	0.86 (0.77-0.95)	34.5% (0.10)	+ + – – Low*†

CABG, Coronary artery bypass grafting; *CV,* cardiovascular; *GRADE,* Grades of Recommendation, Assessment, Development and Evaluation [with plus or minus assigned for each of the four grading categories]; *MI,* myocardial infarction; *PCI,* percutaneous coronary intervention.
*Random sequence generation, allocation concealment, and blinding of outcome assessors were poorly described in greater than 50% of included studies; bias likely.
†Funnel plots and/or Egger test suggest evidence of asymmetry.

Grade Working Group Quality of Evidence

High quality: Further research is very unlikely to change our confidence in the estimate of effect.
Moderate quality: Further research is likely to have an important impact on our confidence in the estimate of effect and may change the estimate.
Low quality: Further research is very likely to have an important impact on our confidence in the estimate of effect and is likely to change the estimate.
Very low quality: We are very uncertain about the estimate.
Adapted from Anderson L, Thompson DR, Oldridge N, et al: Exercise-based cardiac rehabilitation for coronary heart disease. Cochrane Database Syst Rev (1):CD001800, 2016.

some maintenance home exercise sessions. Although it was noted that the quality of reporting had improved in more recently published RCTs, overall, the authors judged the various individual categories of study risk of bias as either high or unclear.

Meta-analyses showed that cardiac rehabilitation had no effect on total mortality compared with that for the control group but led to a reduction in cardiovascular mortality (relative risk, 0.74; 95% CI, 0.64 to 0.86) (Table 34-2 and Figure 34-2). Exercise-based rehabilitation reduced the risk of hospital admissions (relative risk, 0.82; 95% CI, 0.70 to 0.96) (Figure 34-e1). No significant impact on either the risk of recurrent MI or revascularization was noted. In view of the variation in health-related quality of life outcome measures across trials, meta-analysis for this aspect of outcomes was not possible. Of 20 studies that reported quality of life, however, a majority (13 trials, 65%) showed higher outcome levels in one or more quality of life domains after rehabilitation compared with those for control groups. With data from multiple RCTs and meta-analyses of RCTs, the efficacy of cardiac rehabilitation fulfills grade A/level I evidence.[3]

In addition to efficacy, two key additional key evidence considerations for rehabilitation and secondary prevention are safety and cost-effectiveness. Exercise-based rehabilitation appears to be very safe. An observational study of more than 25,000 patients in a French registry of rehabilitation-related complications reported one cardiac event for 50,000 hours of exercise training—equivalent to 1.3 cardiac arrests per 1 million patient-hours.[9] An earlier American study reported only one case of ventricular fibrillation per 111,996 patient-hours of exercise and one MI per 294,118 patient-hours. A systematic review of economic evaluations of cardiac rehabilitation and secondary prevention reported a cost per life-year gained ranging from US$2193 to US$28,193.[10] In 2007, the National Institute of Health and Care Excellence (NICE) in the United Kingdom estimated the incremental cost-effectiveness ratio for rehabilitation after MI at approximately £7860 and £8360 per quality-adjusted life-year (QALY) gained for men and women, respectively.[11] NICE's current funding threshold is £20,000/QALY, indicating the provision of cardiac rehabilitation and secondary prevention to be cost-effective.

COMPONENTS OF CARDIAC REHABILITATION AND SECONDARY PREVENTION

Systematic Referral

All eligible patients with acute MI and all patients in the immediate postoperative period after CABG or PCI should be referred to a comprehensive outpatient rehabilitation and secondary prevention program either before hospital discharge or during the first immediate follow-up visit.[3] The services should be instituted as soon as possible after hospital admission. Cardiac rehabilitation and secondary prevention generally are considered most beneficial when delivered soon after the index hospitalization. In certain situations, however, clinical, social, and logistic reasons can delay enrollment in a structured program. To ensure effective access to rehabilitation and preventive services, referral should be considered by all health care practitioners with responsibility for the care of post-MI patients in the 12 months after their acute event or cardiac surgery.[5]

Despite the substantive evidence for the benefits of such services, implementation of and patient enrollment in cardiac rehabilitation and secondary prevention programs remain below desired levels.[12-14] Studies in Europe, North America, and Australia have reported participation rates

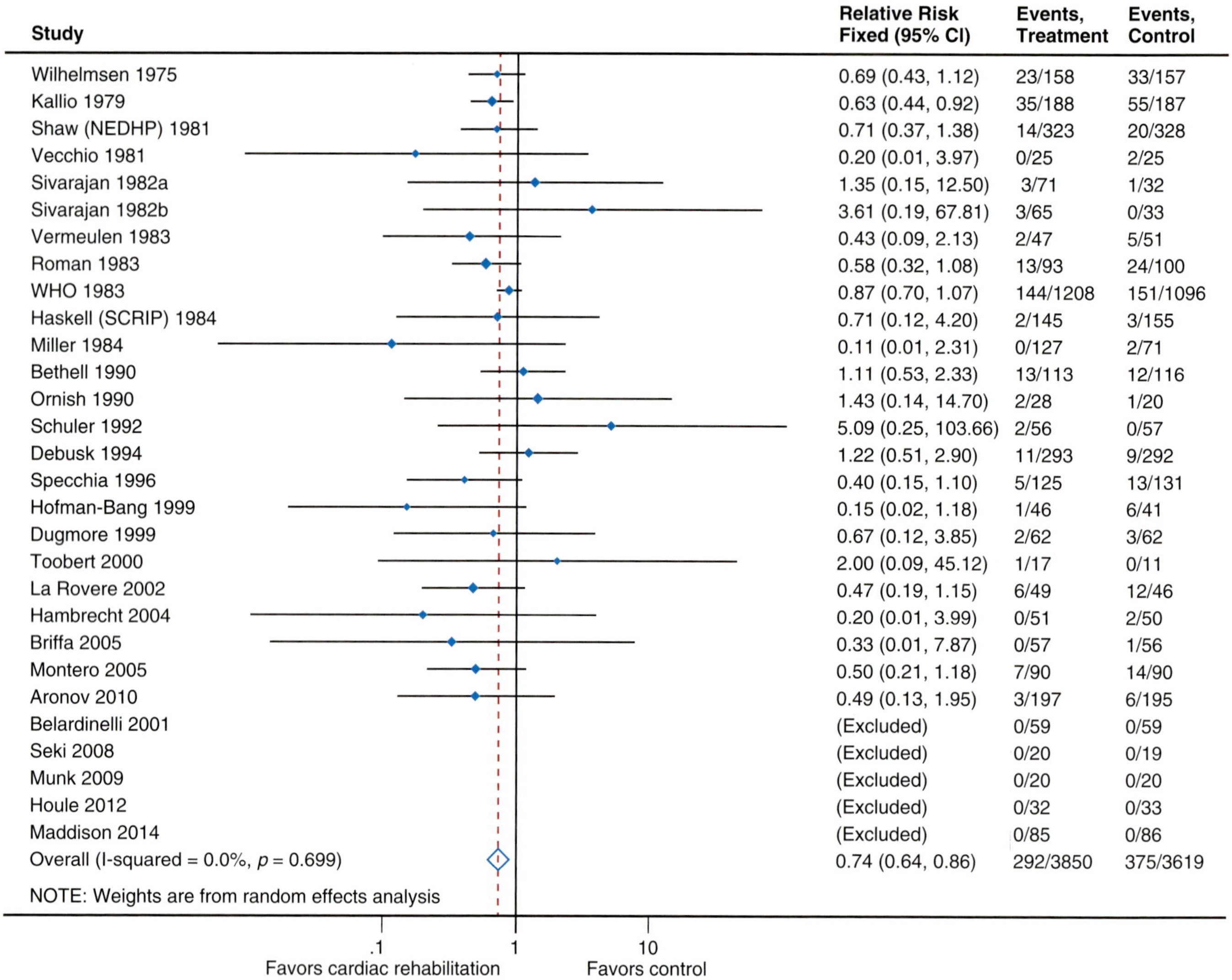

FIGURE 34-2 Meta-analysis of cardiovascular mortality. *(From Anderson L, Thompson DR, Oldridge N, et al: Exercise-based cardiac rehabilitation for coronary heart disease: Cochrane systematic review and meta-analysis.* J Am Coll Cardiol *67:1-12, 2016.)*

of 20% to 50%.[15] The gap in delivery is especially large in older patients, women, and members of ethnic minorities. Reasons behind these gaps in participation are generally classified into three categories: (1) patient-based, especially lack of sufficient financial resources and/or health care insurance coverage to participate or lack of interest in participating in the program; (2) provider-based, especially lack of physician referral of patients; and (3) system-based barriers, especially lack of resources to fund rehabilitation/preventive services or lack of services within close proximity to a patient's home.[16] A Cochrane systematic review assessed the efficacy of interventions to improve uptake of and adherence to cardiac rehabilitation and secondary prevention.[17] However, this review found only weak evidence (11 RCTs) supporting specific interventions to increase uptake. Systematic referral procedures and interventions targeting patient-identified barriers may increase the likelihood of success. At referral, clinicians need to be aware of potential patient barriers (Table 34-3). Some particular approaches to overcoming these barriers are presented later under Innovative and Models of Rehabilitation and Prevention (in the section on maintaining long-term behavioral changes).

TABLE 34-3 Barriers to Participation in Cardiac Rehabilitation and Secondary Prevention

PATIENT-RELATED BARRIERS	PROVIDER- AND SYSTEM-RELATED BARRIERS
Older age, female sex	Lack of services
Smoking	Distance to services
Depression	Lack of systematic referral
Social isolation	Lack of physician endorsement
Family obligations	
Limited finances	
Lack of transportation	
Patient refusal	

Patient Risk Assessment and Tailored Planning

Formulation of an individually tailored, patient-specific plan for cardiac rehabilitation and secondary prevention should be based on a careful risk assessment at discharge or as soon as possible after hospital admission and before initiation of the program. This risk assessment should systematically collect and document the clinical information as listed in Table 34-4.

TABLE 34-4 Patient Risk Assessment and Clinical Data Collection

ASSESSMENT COMPONENT	DESCRIPTION
Clinical history	Screening for cardiovascular risk factors, comorbid conditions and disabilities, psychological stress, vocational situation
Symptoms	Cardiovascular disease—NYHA functional class for dyspnea and Canadian Cardiovascular Society (CCS) class for symptoms of angina
Medication	Including dose, frequency, side effects
Adherence	To medical regimen and self-monitoring (weight, BP, symptoms)
Physical examination	General health status, body mass index (BMI), waist circumference, heart failure signs, cardiac and carotid murmurs, pulse, BP control, extremities for presence of arterial pulses and orthopedic pathology, neurological abnormalities
ECG	Heart rate and rhythm, repolarization
Cardiac imaging	2D and Doppler echocardiography when appropriate—in particular, ventricular function, valvular heart disease, presence of effusion
Blood testing	For routine biochemical assay: including full blood count, electrolytes, renal and liver function, fasting blood glucose (HbA_{1C} if fasting blood glucose is elevated or with known diabetes), total cholesterol, LDL-C, HDL-C, triglycerides
Physical activity level by history	Domestic, occupational, and recreational needs; activities relevant to age, gender, and daily life; readiness to change behavior; self-confidence; barriers to increased physical activity; and social support in making positive changes
Peak exercise capacity	Symptom-limited exercise testing, either on bicycle ergometer or on treadmill. If this is not feasible (e.g., because of recent surgery), submaximal exercise evaluation and/or six-minute walk test should be considered.
Education	Clear, comprehensible information on the basic purpose of the CR program and the role of each component (including optimal medical therapy compliance) Education on self-monitoring protocols (weight, blood pressure, warning symptoms and signs of instability, e.g., angina, dyspnea) and self-management

BP, Blood pressure; *CR*, cardiac rehabilitation; *2D*, two-dimensional; *ECG*, electrocardiogram; *HbA_{1C}*, A_{1C} hemoglobin (glycosylated); *HDL-C*, high-density lipoprotein cholesterol; *LDL-C*, low-density lipoprotein cholesterol; *NYHA*, New York Heart Association.

Adapted from Balady GJ, Williams MA, Ades PA, et al: Core components of cardiac rehabilitation/secondary prevention programs: 2007 update: a scientific statement from the American Heart Association Exercise, Cardiac Rehabilitation, and Prevention Committee, the Council on Clinical Cardiology; the Councils on Cardiovascular Nursing, Epidemiology and Prevention, and Nutrition, Physical Activity, and Metabolism; and the American Association of Cardiovascular and Pulmonary Rehabilitation. Circulation *115:2675-2682, 2007; and Piepoli MF, Corra U, Adamopoulos S, et al: Secondary prevention in the clinical management of patients with cardiovascular diseases. Core components, standards and outcome measures for referral and delivery: a policy statement from the cardiac rehabilitation section of the European Association for Cardiovascular Prevention & Rehabilitation. Endorsed by the Committee for Practice Guidelines of the European Society of Cardiology.* Eur J Prev Cardiol *21:664-681, 2014.*

Exercise Testing and Training

Symptom-limited exercise testing before participation in an exercise-based cardiac rehabilitation program is strongly recommended (see also Chapter 30).[2] Exercise test parameters should include assessment of heart rate and rhythm, signs and symptoms, ST-segment changes, hemodynamics, perceived exertion, and exercise capacity. On the basis of this exercise test, patients can then be risk-stratified to select the appropriate level of supervision and monitoring required during their exercise-based rehabilitation program. Exercise training should incorporate an individualized exercise prescription for aerobic training that should be regularly reviewed by the program team and modified if necessary. Current recommendations for exercise prescription are as follows:

- Frequency: 3 to 5 sessions per week
- Intensity: 50% to 80% of maximal exercise capacity
- Duration: 20 to 60 minutes per session
- Modality: walking, treadmill, cycling, rowing, stair climbing, arm/leg ergometry, and other modalities, using continuous or interval training as appropriate

Exercise-based rehabilitation programs also can include resistance exercise.

Education

A Cochrane review[18] identified 13 RCTs examining patient education interventions among 68,556 subjects with coronary heart disease, with a follow-up period of 6 to 60 months. The meta-analysis from this review showed weak evidence of an effect of education compared with usual care on all-cause mortality (relative risk [RR], 0.79; 95% CI, 0.55 to 1.13) and cardiac morbidity (recurrent MI: RR, 0.63; 95% CI, 0.26 to 1.48; revascularization: RR, 0.58; 95% CI, 0.19 to 1.71; and hospitalization: RR, 0.83; 95% CI, 0.65 to 1.07). After education, some evidence indicates that quality of life scores were higher than those in control groups. These findings generally are supportive of cardiac rehabilitation and secondary prevention, including some form of education, either in groups or as individual consultations. Further research into different models of education is needed, however, to inform future more specific recommendations on the nature and content of this education delivery.

Current guidelines[2-5] for education include its role in providing a positive impact on healthy behavior (Table 34-5), risk factor modification (Table 34-6) and improving adherence to cardioprotective medications (Table 34-7), as well as psychosocial support including vocational guidance and sexual functioning (Table 34-8).

Several principles of behavior change and validated educational theories are helpful in improving the patient's motivation as well as individual ability to comprehend and digest a broad array of information. None of these principles (i.e., stages of change, self-efficacy concepts, outcome models, biofeedback) should be regarded as mutually exclusive, often the principles are combined, depending on patients' needs and staff competences. Table 34-9 lists "ten strategic steps" to enhance counseling on behavioral change.[4]

Psychosocial Support

The relationship between psychosocial and cardiac health is complex, and both direct (e.g., psychological effects on immunologic function) and indirect (e.g., behaviorally mediated) mechanisms are thought to play a role.[19] Consequently, patients may be offered a wide variety of psychological therapies to treat depression, anxiety, stress, or maladaptive behaviors, and these treatments aim to improve both psychological and cardiac health. Underpinning all psychosocial therapies for cardiac patients is some combination of the following

TABLE 34-5 Assessment, Clinical Interventions, and Expected Outcomes for Behavioral Interventions after Acute Myocardial Infarction

AREA OF INTEREST, WITH TREATMENT GOALS*	EVALUATION/ASSESSMENT	INTERVENTION	EXPECTED OUTCOMES
Physical activity counseling • *E: Moderate aerobic activity,* minimum 2.5 hours/week, in multiple bouts each lasting ≥10 minutes • *U: Moderate aerobic activity,* 30 minutes/day, 5-7 days/week • *U: Complementary resistance training,* 2 days/week	Assess current physical activity level and determine domestic, occupational, and recreational needs. Assess readiness to change behavior, self-confidence, and barriers.	*Recommend* gradual increases in daily lifestyle activities over time, and how to incorporate it into daily routine and evenly spread throughout the week, i.e., minimum 5 days a week. *Emphasize* sedentary lifestyle as risk factor and the benefits of physical activity: Any increase in activity has a positive health benefit. *Advise*: Individualize physical activity according to patient's age, past habits, comorbid conditions, preferences, and goals. *Reassure* regarding the safety of the recommended protocol. *Encourage* involvement in leisure activities that are enjoyable. *Forewarn*: Inform patients on the risk of relapses; education should underline how benefits may be achieved and the need for lifelong continuation. If physical activity interruption has occurred, physical, social, and psychological barriers should be explored, and alternative approaches suggested.	Increased participation physical activities. Improved psychosocial well-being Prevention of disability Improved aerobic fitness and body composition
Smoking cessation • *Nonsmoker status*	Smoking status and use of other tobacco products Amount of smoking (per day) (number of years) Determine readiness to change; if ready, choose a date for quitting.	All smokers should be encouraged professionally to stop smoking all forms of tobacco permanently. *Follow-up*: Referral to special programs and/ or pharmacotherapy (including nicotine replacement) are recommended, as is a stepwise strategy for smoking cessation. Provide structured follow-up. Offer behavioral advice and group or individual counseling. *Consider nicotine replacement therapy,* combined with bupropion or varenicline if not contraindicated.	Long-term abstinence from smoking
Nutritional counseling • *Heart-healthy diet*	Daily caloric intake and dietary content of fat, saturated fat, sodium, and other nutrients Assess eating habits.	*Education* regarding dietary goals and how to attain them • Healthy food choices: Wide variety of foods; low-salt foods Mediterranean diet: fruits, vegetables, wholegrain cereals and bread, fish (especially oily), lean meat, low fat dairy products Replace saturated fat with the above foods and with monounsaturated and polyunsaturated fats from vegetable (oleic acid as in olive oil and rapeseed oil) and marine sources to reduce total fat to <30% of energy, of which less than 1/3 is saturated *Avoid*: beverages and foods with added sugars and salty food • *Integrate* behavior-change models and compliance strategies into counseling sessions.	Patient understands basic principles of dietary content. Patient adheres to prescribed diet.
Weight control management • *Body mass index (BMI)*: 18.5-24.9 kg/m^2 • *Waist circumference*: 80 cm in women, 94 cm in men	Measure weight, height, and waist circumference. Calculate BMI.	*BMI*: It is useful to consistently encourage weight control through an appropriate balance of physical activity, caloric intake, and formal behavioral programs when indicated. *Waist circumference*: It is beneficial to initiate lifestyle changes and consider treatment strategies for metabolic syndrome as indicated.	To lose 5%-10% of body weight in 6 months. Consider referring patient to specialist obesity clinic if goal not reached.

**E*, Europe[5]; *U*, United States of America.[3]

Adapted from Smith SC Jr, Benjamin EJ, Bonow RO, et al: AHA/ACCF secondary prevention and risk reduction therapy for patients with coronary and other atherosclerotic vascular disease: 2011 update: a guideline from the American Heart Association and American College of Cardiology Foundation. Circulation *124:2458-2473, 2011; Balady GJ, Williams MA, Ades PA, et al: Core components of cardiac rehabilitation/secondary prevention programs: 2007 update: a scientific statement from the American Heart Association Exercise, Cardiac Rehabilitation, and Prevention Committee, the Council on Clinical Cardiology; the Councils on Cardiovascular Nursing, Epidemiology and Prevention, and Nutrition, Physical Activity, and Metabolism; and the American Association of Cardiovascular and Pulmonary Rehabilitation.* Circulation *115:2675-2682, 2007; and Piepoli MF, Corra U, Adamopoulos S, et al: Secondary prevention in the clinical management of patients with cardiovascular diseases. Core components, standards and outcome measures for referral and delivery: a policy statement from the cardiac rehabilitation section of the European Association for Cardiovascular Prevention & Rehabilitation. Endorsed by the Committee for Practice Guidelines of the European Society of Cardiology.* Eur J Prev Cardiol *21:664-681, 2014.*

TABLE 34-6 Assessment, Clinical Interventions, and Expected Outcomes with Risk Factor Control after Acute Myocardial Infarction

AREA OF INTEREST, WITH TREATMENT GOAL	EVALUATION AND ASSESSMENT	INTERVENTION	EXPECTED OUTCOMES
Blood pressure management • *For hypertensive patients*: ≤140/≤90 mm Hg • *For patients with diabetes, heart failure, or chronic kidney disease*: ≤130/≤80 mm Hg	Measure seated resting blood pressure on at least two visits. Measure blood pressure in both arms at program entry. To rule out orthostatic hypotension, measure lying, seated, and standing blood pressure at program entry and after adjustments in antihypertensive drug therapy. Assess current treatment and compliance. Assess use of nonprescription drugs that may adversely affect blood pressure.	Provide and/or monitor drug therapy in concert with primary HCP as follows: *For blood pressure 120-139 mm Hg systolic or 80-89 mm Hg diastolic*: Provide counseling on lifestyle modifications, including regular physical activity/exercise; weight management; moderate sodium restriction and increased consumption of fresh fruits, vegetables, and low-fat dairy products; alcohol moderation; and smoking cessation. Provide drug therapy for patients with chronic kidney disease, heart failure, or diabetes if blood pressure is >130/>80 mm Hg after lifestyle modification. *For blood pressure >140/>90 mm Hg*: Provide counseling on lifestyle modifications and drug therapy according to current guidelines on hypertension.	*Short-term*: Continue to assess and modify intervention until normalization of blood pressure in prehypertensive patients. *Long-term*: Maintain blood pressure at goal levels.
Lipid management	Obtain fasting measures of total cholesterol, HDL-C, LDL-C, and triglycerides. In patients with abnormalities, obtain a detailed history to determine whether diet, drug, and/or other conditions that may affect lipid levels can be altered. Assess current treatment and compliance.	*Nutritional counseling*: Provide guidance consistent with the Therapeutic Lifestyle Change diet, such as the recommendation to add plant stanol/sterols and viscous fiber and the encouragement to consume more omega-3 fatty acids, as well as weight management counseling, as needed, in all patients. Add or intensify drug treatment in those with LDL-C <100 mg/dL; consider adding drug treatment in those with LDL-C <70 mg/dL. Provide interventions directed toward management of triglycerides to attain non–HDL-C <130 mg/dL. These include nutritional counseling; guidance and support in weight management, exercise, smoking cessation, and alcohol moderation; and drug therapy. Monitor treatment in collaboration with primary health care provider. Repeat lipid profiles at 4-6 weeks after hospitalization and at 2 months after initiation or change in lipid-lowering medications. Assess creatine kinase levels and liver function in patients taking lipid-lowering medications as recommended by drug manufacturer.	*Short-term*: Continue to assess and modify intervention until LDL-C is <100 mg/dL (further reduction to a goal of <70 mg/dL is considered reasonable) and non–HDL-C is <130 mg/dL (further reduction to a goal of <100 mg/dL is considered reasonable). *Long-term*: LDL-C <100 mg/dL is recommended goal (further reduction to <70 mg/dL is considered reasonable). Non–HDL-C <130 mg/dL is recommended goal (further reduction to <100 mg/dL is considered reasonable).

HCP, Health care provider; *HDL-C*, high-density lipoprotein cholesterol; *LDL-C*, low-density lipoprotein cholesterol.
Adapted from Smith SC Jr, Benjamin EJ, Bonow RO, et al: AHA/ACCF secondary prevention and risk reduction therapy for patients with coronary and other atherosclerotic vascular disease: 2011 update: a guideline from the American Heart Association and American College of Cardiology Foundation. Circulation *124:2458-2473, 2011; Balady GJ, Williams MA, Ades PA, et al: Core components of cardiac rehabilitation/secondary prevention programs: 2007 update: a scientific statement from the American Heart Association Exercise, Cardiac Rehabilitation, and Prevention Committee, the Council on Clinical Cardiology; the Councils on Cardiovascular Nursing, Epidemiology and Prevention, and Nutrition, Physical Activity, and Metabolism; and the American Association of Cardiovascular and Pulmonary Rehabilitation.* Circulation *115:2675-2682, 2007; and Piepoli MF, Corra U, Adamopoulos S, et al: Secondary prevention in the clinical management of patients with cardiovascular diseases. Core components, standards and outcome measures for referral and delivery: a policy statement from the cardiac rehabilitation section of the European Association for Cardiovascular Prevention & Rehabilitation. Endorsed by the Committee for Practice Guidelines of the European Society of Cardiology.* Eur J Prev Cardiol *21:664-681, 2014.*

four hypotheses: (1) that coronary heart disease and associated medical or surgical treatments may cause psychological distress; (2) that psychological symptoms may cause or exacerbate cardiac disease; (3) that unhealthy behaviors may be increased when people experience psychological distress; and (4) that psychological techniques may be useful in modifying risky behaviors.

Major depressive disorder is present in approximately 20% of patients with ischemic heart disease,[20] which makes depression the most important psychosocial target in the clinical practice of cardiology.[21] Depression and ischemic heart disease have a bidirectional relationship—that is, ischemic heart disease can cause depression, and depression is an independent risk factor for ischemic heart disease and its complications.[22] Depression among people with established ischemic heart disease is clinically important in that it is associated with worse medical outcomes including poorer health-related quality of life, greater morbidity (odds ratio [OR], 2.0) and mortality (OR, 1.8 to 2.6), and greater use of routine and unscheduled health care.[23,24]

The impact of psychological interventions for patients with a coronary heart disease has been the subject of a Cochrane review.[19] The review included 24 RCTs comparing psychological interventions with usual care in 9296 participants who were predominantly at low risk for adverse outcomes after an MI or PCI procedure. The evidence showed of a trend toward a reduction in all-cause mortality (RR, 0.89; 95% CI, 0.75 to 1.05) and fewer cardiac deaths with psychological intervention (RR, 0.80; 95% CI, 0.64 to 1.00). No significant effects were observed in terms of the risk of

TABLE 34-7 Recommendations for Cardioprotective Medication after Acute Myocardial Infarction

DRUG CATEGORY	RECOMMENDATIONS
Antiplatelet agents/anticoagulants	See Chapter 35.
Renin-angiotensin-aldosterone system blockers	
ACE inhibitors	ACE inhibitors should be started and continued indefinitely in all patients with left ventricular ejection fraction ≤40% and in those with hypertension, diabetes, or chronic kidney disease, unless contraindicated. It is reasonable to use ACE inhibitors in all other patients.
ARBs	The use of ARBs is recommended in patients who have heart failure or who have had a myocardial infarction with left ventricular ejection fraction ≤40% and who are ACE inhibitor–intolerant. It is reasonable to use ARBs in other patients who are ACE inhibitor–intolerant. The use of ARBs in combination with an ACE inhibitor is *not* well established in patients with systolic heart failure.
Aldosterone-blocking agents	Use of aldosterone blockade in post–myocardial infarction patients *without* significant renal dysfunction (creatinine clearance >30 mL/min) *or* hyperkalemia (potassium should be <5.0 mEq/L) is recommended in patients who are already receiving therapeutic doses of an ACE inhibitor and a β-blocker, who have a left ventricular ejection fraction of 40% or less, and who have either diabetes or heart failure.
β-Adrenergic blockers (β-blockers)	1. β-Blocker therapy should be used in all patients with previous myocardial infarction or with left ventricular systolic dysfunction (as indicated by ejection fraction of 40% or less) unless contraindicated. (Use should be limited to carvedilol, metoprolol succinate, or bisoprolol.) 2. β-Blocker therapy should be started and continued for 3 years in all patients with normal left ventricular function who have had a myocardial infarction or an ACS. 3. It is reasonable to continue β-blockers beyond 3 years as chronic therapy in all patients with normal left ventricular function who have had a myocardial infarction or an ACS. 4. It is reasonable to use β-blocker therapy in patients with left ventricular systolic dysfunction (as indicated by ejection fraction of 40% or less) without heart failure or previous myocardial infarction.
Influenza vaccine	Patients should have an annual influenza vaccination.

ACE, Angiotensin-converting enzyme; *ACS,* Acute cardiac syndrome; *ARBs,* angiotensin receptor blockers.
Adapted from Smith SC Jr, Benjamin EJ, Bonow RO, et al: AHA/ACCF secondary prevention and risk reduction therapy for patients with coronary and other atherosclerotic vascular disease: 2011 update: a guideline from the American Heart Association and American College of Cardiology Foundation. Circulation *124:2458-2473, 2011.*

TABLE 34-8 Assessment, Clinical Interventions, and Expected Outcomes for Psychosocial Management and Vocational Advice after Myocardial Infarction

AREA OF INTEREST, WITH TREATMENT GOAL	EVALUATION AND ASSESSMENT	INTERVENTION	EXPECTED OUTCOMES
Psychosocial management • *Absence of clinically significant depression and psychosocial problems*	Screen for psychological distress using interview and/or other standardized measurement tools. Screen for substance abuse of alcohol and/or other psychotropic agents.	Offer individual and/or small group education and counseling on adjustment to heart disease, stress management, and health-related lifestyle change (e.g., profession, car driving, sexual activities), relaxation techniques. Whenever possible, offer spouses and other family members, domestic partners, and/or significant others access to information sessions. Teach and support self-help strategies and ways of obtaining effective social support. Provide vocational counseling in case of work-related stress. *Treatment of depression* in collaboration with mental health specialist and primary care provider	Emotional well-being Absence of clinically significant psychosocial problems and acquisition of stress management skills Improved health-related quality of life
Vocational advice • *Return to previous activities unless contraindications*	Before discharge, return to previous activities must be discussed with the patients and their partners and return to previous activities must be promoted, unless there is a medical contraindication. The presence of any barriers to return to work (RTW) after illness should be assessed.	All procedures to help patients to overcome barriers to RTW and thereby remain in, return to, or gain access to employment; e.g., retraining and capacity building, reasonable adjustments and control measures, disability awareness, condition management, and medical treatment	Return to previous activities
Sexual functioning • *Return to previous activities unless contraindicated*		Offer individual and/or small group education and counseling on sexual functioning and sexual activities.	Return to previous activities unless contraindicated.

Adapted from Smith SC Jr, Benjamin EJ, Bonow RO, et al: AHA/ACCF Secondary prevention and risk reduction therapy for patients with coronary and other atherosclerotic vascular disease: 2011 update: a guideline from the American Heart Association and American College of Cardiology Foundation. Circulation *124:2458-2473, 2011; Balady GJ, Williams MA, Ades PA, et al: Core components of cardiac rehabilitation/secondary prevention programs: 2007 update: a scientific statement from the American Heart Association Exercise, Cardiac Rehabilitation, and Prevention Committee, the Council on Clinical Cardiology; the Councils on Cardiovascular Nursing, Epidemiology and Prevention, and Nutrition, Physical Activity, and Metabolism; and the American Association of Cardiovascular and Pulmonary Rehabilitation.* Circulation *115:2675-2682, 2007; and Piepoli MF, Corra U, Adamopoulos S, et al: Secondary prevention in the clinical management of patients with cardiovascular diseases. Core components, standards and outcome measures for referral and delivery: a policy statement from the cardiac rehabilitation section of the European Association for Cardiovascular Prevention & Rehabilitation. Endorsed by the Committee for Practice Guidelines of the European Society of Cardiology.* Eur J Prev Cardiol *21:664-681, 2014.*

TABLE 34-9 Ten Strategic Steps to Enhance Counseling on Behavioral Change

1. Develop a therapeutic alliance.
2. Provide counseling for all patients at risk for or with manifest cardiovascular disease.
3. Assist patients to understand the relationship between their behavior and health.
4. Help patients assess the barriers to behavior change.
5. Gain commitments from patients to own their behavior change.
6. Involve patients in identifying and selecting the risk factors to change.
7. Use a combination of strategies including reinforcement of the person's capacity for change.
8. Design a lifestyle modification plan.
9. Involve other health care staff whenever possible.
10. Monitor progress through follow-up contact.

From Perk J, De Backer G, Gohlke H, et al: European guidelines on cardiovascular disease prevention in clinical practice (version 2012). The Fifth Joint Task Force of the European Society of Cardiology and Other Societies on Cardiovascular Disease Prevention in Clinical Practice (constituted by representatives of nine societies and by invited experts). Eur Heart J *33*:1635-1701, 2012.

revascularization (RR, 0.95; 95% CI, 0.80 to 1.13) and nonfatal reinfarction (RR, 0.87; 95% CI, 0.67 to 1.13). One of seven trials reported superiority in health-related quality of life after a psychological intervention compared with that in the control group.

A possible explanation for the fact that this analysis does not provide more unequivocal evidence for support of psychological interventions in terms of reductions in mortality and morbidity is that a majority of trials included all cardiac patients, regardless of their psychological symptoms. A plausible theory is that patient psychological screening after an acute event and then targeting interventions to those meeting a clinical threshold for psychological symptoms, depression or anxiety may be important to discerning efficacy of these interventions. The clinical value and cost-effectiveness of a strategy of targeting psychological interventions after an MI in those patients with diagnosed depression are being addressed in an ongoing RCT (CADENCE, ISRCTN 34701576). Under the umbrella of psychosocial support, current guidelines also advocate the integration of vocational advice on return to work and advice on resuming normal sexual functioning (see Table 34-8).

Comprehensive Risk Factor Management

As summarized in Table 34-6, risk factor management is a pivotal part of comprehensive cardiac rehabilitation and secondary prevention.

Physical Activity Counseling

Participation in an exercise training program as part of cardiac rehabilitation and secondary prevention, as described previously, is considered an important tool to increase long-term physical activity level in post-MI patients.[3,5] Regular physical activity is associated with a reduced risk of fatal and nonfatal coronary events in healthy people, persons with coronary risk factors, and cardiac patients over a wide age range. A sedentary lifestyle is one of the major risk factors for cardiovascular diseases. Engaging in regular physical activity is therefore suggested by guidelines as a very important nonpharmacologic component of risk factor control in primary as well as secondary prevention (see Table 34-5).[4]

After an acute MI, a regimen of 30 to 60 minutes of moderate-intensity aerobic activity, such as brisk walking, at least 5 days and preferably 7 days per week, supplemented by an increase in daily lifestyle activity to improve cardiorespiratory fitness, should be encouraged. The basic goal in this context is to move patients out of the least-fit, least-active high-risk cohort.[3]

Smoking Cessation

Smoking is associated with an increased risk of all types of cardiovascular and coronary artery diseases. The risk associated with smoking is primarily related to the amount of tobacco smoked daily and shows a clear dose–response relationship, with no lower limit for deleterious effects.

Although the exact mechanisms by which smoking increases the risk of atherosclerotic disease are not fully understood, it is clear that smoking enhances both the development of atherosclerosis and the occurrence of superimposed thrombotic phenomena.[4] Stopping smoking after an MI is considered one of the most effective preventive initiatives. The Cochrane review of 20 cohort studies of smoking cessation after MI showed a substantive mortality benefit (RR, 0.64; 95% CI, 0.58 to 0.71) compared with continued smokers.[25] Further evidence points toward a risk of cardiovascular disease approaching that for never-smokers within 10 to 15 years.[4]

Based on existing evidence, professional guidelines recommend complete cessation of smoking among patients following an acute coronary event.[3,4] Furthermore, it is recommended that patients who have had an acute coronary event should avoid environmental exposure to tobacco smoke (see Table 34-5). Stopping smoking is a complex and difficult process, because the habit is strongly addictive both pharmacologically and psychologically. The most important predictor of successful quitting is motivation, which can be increased by professional assistance. The period after an acute coronary event or revascularization procedure is an ideal time to encourage patients to stop smoking.[3,4] The physician's firm and explicit advice that the person should stop smoking completely is important in starting the smoking cessation process and increases the odds of success. Pooled data from the Cochrane review of 17 RCTs of brief advice versus no advice showed an increase in the rate of quitting for the former (RR, 1.66; 95% CI, 1.42 to 1.94).[26] Figure 34-3 shows the World Health Organization (WHO) smoking cessation algorithm recommended by American and European guidelines.

Among patients with coronary heart disease, psychosocial smoking cessation interventions are effective in promoting abstinence for up to 12 months, provided that they are of sufficient duration, making systematic smoking cessation interventions an important part of cardiac rehabilitation and secondary prevention.[27] Pharmacologic aids can further improve quit rates among patients with coronary heart disease. Consequently, in addition to advice and encouragement, as well as psychosocial smoking cessation nicotine replacement therapy,[26] and, in some cases, bupropion or varenicline can be offered to assist cessation.[28] No associated increase in adverse cardiac events for bupropion was found,[26] but concerns have been raised about adverse cardiac events caused by varenicline.[29] Nicotine replacement therapy, varenicline, or bupropion normally should be prescribed as part of an abstinent-contingent treatment, in which the smoker makes a commitment to stop smoking on a particular date.[4] NICE in the United Kingdom offers detailed advice on stopping smoking services (https://www.nice.org.uk/guidance/ph10).[30]

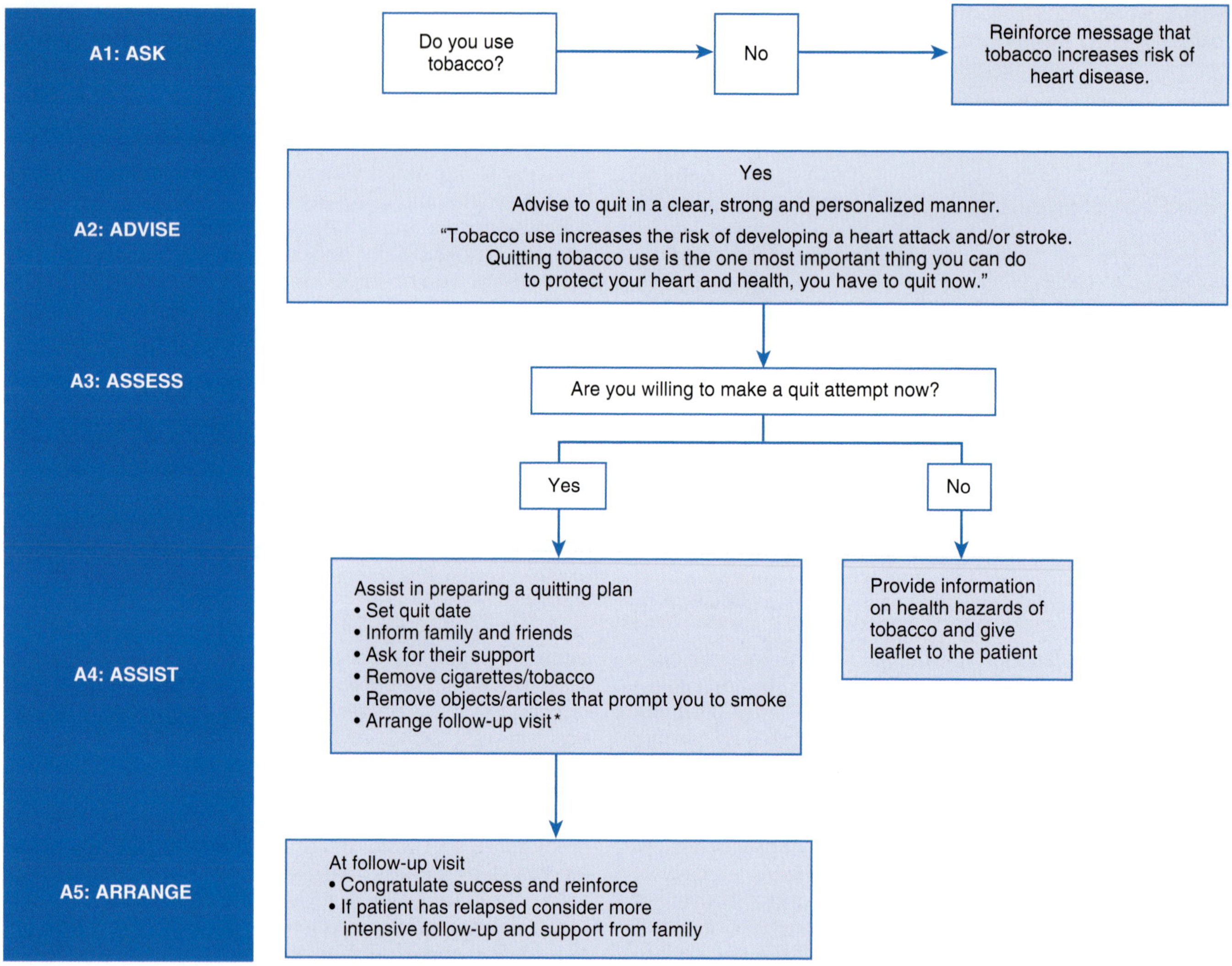

*Ideally second follow-up visit is recommended within the same month and every month thereafter for 4 months and evaluation after one year. If not feasible, reinforce counseling whenever the patient is seen for blood pressure monitoring.

FIGURE 34-3 World Health Organization (WHO) smoking cessation algorithm. *(From Perk J, De Backer G, Gohlke H, et al: European guidelines on cardiovascular disease prevention in clinical practice (version 2012). The Fifth Joint Task Force of the European Society of Cardiology and Other Societies on Cardiovascular Disease Prevention in Clinical Practice (constituted by representatives of nine societies and by invited experts).* Eur Heart J *33:1635-1701, 2012.)*

Nutritional Counseling and Weight Management

Dietary behavior has direct effects on weight, serum lipids, blood pressure, blood sugar and insulin sensitivity, cardiac rhythm, endothelial function, and oxidative stress—all factors associated with cardiovascular health and disease. Poor diet may therefore increase the risk of coronary events, and healthy eating is expected to decrease the risk. Observational studies support this correlation between nutrition and risk of coronary events.[4] Two more recent RCTs have provided evidence for the importance of nutritional counseling (Table 34-e2) in primary and secondary prevention after MI.[31]

At the population level, obesity is associated with increased cardiovascular disease incidence and mortality. Among persons with established coronary artery disease, the evidence is contradictory. Systematic reviews of data for patients with coronary artery disease or undergoing PCI have suggested an "obesity paradox," whereby obesity appears to be protective against an adverse prognosis. Based on this evidence, current guidelines agree that clinicians should encourage weight maintenance/reduction through an appropriate balance of lifestyle physical activity, structured exercise, and caloric intake and a formal behavioral program when indicated to achieve or maintain a body mass index between 18.5 and 24.9 km/m^2 (quality and level of evidence: class I, level B).[3] NICE in the United Kingdom provides detailed guidance on managing overweight and obesity in adults (https://www.nice.org.uk/guidance/ph53).[32]

Hyperlipidemia and Lipid Control

Genetic and histopathologic studies, as well as observational and interventional studies, have established the crucial role of dyslipidemia, especially hypercholesterolemia, in the development of cardiovascular disease and coronary heart disease (see Chapter 2). The evidence that reducing plasma levels of low-density lipoprotein (LDL) cholesterol decreases cardiovascular disease risk is unequivocal. Meta-analyses of RCTs across a variety of LDL-lowering therapies show a clear dose-dependent relative reduction in cardiovascular disease with effective lowering of LDL cholesterol.[4]

Guidelines recommend that statin treatment using a high-intensity regimen (Table 34-e3) should be initiated in all post-MI patients as early as possible, before hospital discharge (see Table 34-7).[3,4] European guidelines recommend that the target LDL cholesterol level should be below 70 mg/dL (less than 1.8 mmol/L) for high-risk patients, whereas the 2014 ACCF/AHA guidelines removed specific LDL targets in favor of recommending the intensity of statin therapy based on patient risk irrespective of LDL concentration.[33] Of importance, early drug treatment should be combined with effective lifestyle changes and dietary counseling after hospital discharge. We advise that blood lipids be checked 4 to 6 weeks after the MI to determine whether the target level has been reached and that the treatment be continued with the same dose, or the dose adapted accordingly.[3,4]

Although these secondary prevention guidelines for lipid-lowering therapy are built on the observation that high-intensity statin therapy is superior to low-intensity statin therapy in lowering LDL cholesterol levels and rates of nonfatal cardiovascular events, it had been uncertain whether a nonstatin lipid-lowering therapy would confer similar improvement in cardiovascular outcomes. The Improved Reduction of Outcomes: Vytorin Efficacy International Trial (IMPROVE-IT) evaluated the effect of ezetimibe combined with simvastatin, compared with that of simvastatin alone, in stable patients with a recent acute coronary syndrome (ACS) and whose LDL cholesterol values were within guideline recommendations.[34] The addition of ezetimibe, which reduces the absorption of cholesterol from the gastrointestinal tract, lowered LDL cholesterol by approximately 24%, to an average of 53.2 mg/dL (1.4 mmol/L), and lowered the risk of cardiovascular events from that achieved with statin monotherapy (hazard ratio [HR], 0.936), a magnitude of clinical benefit that was consistent with the degree of LDL cholesterol lowering as predicted by the Cholesterol Treatment Trialists' meta-analysis. The observation that a nonstatin lipid-lowering agent also reduces cardiovascular risk was an important one. In addition, the trial demonstrated that further reduction from an average LDL cholesterol of 70 mg/dL is associated with an improvement in outcomes.

Management of Hypertension

Elevated blood pressure is a major risk factor for coronary disease heart, heart failure, cerebrovascular disease, peripheral arterial disease, renal failure, and atrial fibrillation (see Chapter 2). Patients with an elevated blood pressure (Table 34-e4) more commonly have other risk factors for cardiovascular disease (i.e., diabetes, insulin resistance, dyslipidemia) and target organ damage. Because risk factors may interact, the overall risk for cardiovascular-related disease in hypertensive patients is increased, even in those with only mild or moderate blood pressure elevation.[4]

Blood pressure should be measured several times, on several separate occasions. Post-MI patients with a blood pressure of 140/90 mm Hg or higher should be treated, as tolerated, with appropriate medication, initially β-blockers and/or ACE inhibitors, with addition of other drugs as needed to achieve a goal blood pressure of less than 140/90 mm Hg (see Table 34-6).[35]

Cardioprotective Medications and Adherence

Patients who have had an acute MI should be prescribed disease-modifying medications for secondary prevention, as listed in Table 34-7.[3]

Antiplatelet Therapy

Decisions regarding antiplatelet therapy for long-term secondary prevention are discussed in Chapter 35.

Inhibitors of the Renin-Angiotensin-Aldosterone System

The use of angiotensin-converting enzyme (ACE) inhibitors in patients with heart failure and impaired ventricular function is discussed in Chapter 25 and Chapter 36, respectively. The rationale for inhibition of the renin-angiotensin-aldosterone system (RAAS) in post–acute MI patients includes experimental and clinical evidence of a favorable impact on ventricular remodeling, improvement in hemodynamics, and reductions in congestive heart failure (see Chapter 13). Large RCTs have demonstrated that ACE inhibitors improve survival in patients who have had an acute MI.[36] Trials of ACE inhibitors in patients with MI and indicators of increased mortality risk, including left ventricular ejection fraction <40%, signs and symptoms of congestive heart failure, or anterior location of infarction, generally maintained therapy for 1 to 4 years, with 42 to 76 lives saved per 1000 patients treated. The mortality reduction with ACE inhibitors adds to that conferred by aspirin and β-blockers. The benefits achieved with ACE inhibitors appear to be a class effect. To replicate these benefits in clinical practice, however, physicians should select a specific agent and adhere as closely as possible to the dosing protocols used in the successful clinical trials.

Inhibition of the RAAS may also be achieved by administration of angiotensin II receptor blockers (ARBs), which may be used as an alternative in patients who do not tolerate ACE inhibitors. Aldosterone blockade is another pharmacologic alternative for inhibition of the RAAS. The EPHESUS trial assigned 6642 patients with acute MI complicated by left ventricular dysfunction and heart failure or diabetes mellitus to receive either the selective aldosterone blocker eplerenone or placebo.[36] During a mean follow-up period of 16 months, eplerenone reduced the post-MI mortality rate by 15%. Serious hyperkalemia (serum potassium concentration of 6 mmol/L or higher) occurred in 5.5% of patients in the eplerenone group, compared with 3.9% of patients in the placebo group.

Patients with MI complicated by heart failure or impaired ventricular function should receive life-long treatment with ACE inhibitors.[3,36,37] In addition, patients with MI who also have hypertension, diabetes, or chronic kidney disease should be treated with an ACE inhibitor for long-term secondary prevention unless contraindicated (see Table 34-7). It is reasonable to use ACE inhibitors in all other patients with MI. ARBs are a clinically effective alternative to ACE inhibitors. The choice between ACE inhibition and an ARB after an MI should be based on provider experience with the agents, patient tolerability, safety, convenience, and cost. Long-term aldosterone blockade should be administered for high-risk patients after MI (ejection fraction of 40% or less, in association with clinical heart failure or diabetes mellitus) who are already receiving an ACE inhibitor and a β-blocker and do not have contraindications. Periodic monitoring of the serum potassium level is necessary.

β-Adrenergic Blockers

The administration of β-adrenergic blockers for the initial management of MI is addressed in Chapter 13. The collective data from five trials providing information on long-term follow-up with use of β-blockers after infarction indicate a benefit through at least 2 to 3 years of therapy. Several

TABLE 34-10 Indicators of Poor Adherence to a Medication Regimen

NONADHERENCE CATEGORY	COMMON CONTRIBUTING FACTORS
Health system	Poor quality of provider-patient relationship; poor knowledge on medication and/ or low acceptance of guidelines; poor communication (e.g., limited, complex, or confusing advice); lack of access to health care; lack of continuity of care
Condition	Asymptomatic chronic disease (lack of physical cues); comorbid mental health disorders (e.g., depression)
Patient	Physical impairments (e.g., vision problems or impaired dexterity); cognitive impairment; psychological/behavioral factors (e.g., lack of motivation, low self-efficacy, impulsivity); younger age
Therapy	Complexity of regimen; side effects
Socioeconomic	Low literacy; high medication costs; poor social support

From Perk J, De Backer G, Gohlke H, et al: European guidelines on cardiovascular disease prevention in clinical practice (version 2012). The Fifth Joint Task Force of the European Society of Cardiology and Other Societies on Cardiovascular Disease Prevention in Clinical Practice (constituted by representatives of nine societies and by invited experts). Eur Heart J *33:1635-1701, 2012.*

nonrandomized studies of the long-term use of β-blockers in patients with a previous MI have failed to demonstrate a benefit.[38,39] These and similar data have raised questions regarding the benefit of β-blockers late after an MI and brought attention to the lack of definitive data for patients surviving beyond 3 years after an MI. Nevertheless, on the basis of the early survival advantage of patients treated with β-blockers in randomized trials, these agents remain a first-line option for lifelong secondary preventive therapy in patients with persistent hypertension, tachyarrhythmias, or reduced left ventricular function after an MI. Moreover, if a β-blocker initiated after an MI is well tolerated and if there is no reason to discontinue therapy, such therapy probably should be continued in most patients who have had an MI.

Adherence to Therapy

Despite the strong evidence for each of these therapies, the rates of prescriptions for and adherence to cardioprotective medications are suboptimal.[40] Although nearly 90% of patients are discharged with appropriate medications after an acute MI, a steady decline in medication adherence is seen over a period of 5 years, and most prescribed doses were substantially below those with proven efficacy in clinical trials.[41] Two studies have found a significant short-term improvement (3 years) of adherence to cardioprotective medications with participation in a cardiac rehabilitation program,[42] but the effect on long-term (10 years) outcome remains unknown. Thus clinical follow-up evaluation with a focus on medication dosing and nonadherence is an important component of cardiac rehabilitation and secondary prevention programs.[4,5]

At baseline assessment and every clinical follow-up examination, a medication history should be taken. It is important to ensure that patients are actually taking the medication as prescribed, and to pay attention to potential side effects. Physicians should ask patients nonjudgmentally how often they miss doses. Recognition of indicators of poor adherence to a medication regimen, summarized in Table 34-10, is important for clinicians to help identify patients who are most in need of interventions to improve adherence. A list of simple strategies for improving adherence to medication regimen is presented in Table 34-11. It is expected that a focus on medication adherence will have a positive impact on outcomes for post-MI patients.[6]

TABLE 34-11 Simple Strategies for Improving Adherence to Medication Regimen

- Provide clear advice regarding the benefits and possible adverse effects of the medication, and on the duration and timing of dosing.
- Consider the patient's habits and preferences.
- Reduce dosage demands to the lowest feasible level.
- Ask patients in a nonjudgmental way how the medication works for them and discuss possible reasons for nonadherence (e.g., side effects, worries) and their perceived acceptability.
- Implement repetitive monitoring and feedback.
- In the case of lack of time, introduce physician assistants and/or nurse practitioners whenever necessary and feasible.
- In the case of persistent nonadherence, offer multisession or combined behavioral interventions.

From Perk J, De Backer G, Gohlke H, et al: European Guidelines on cardiovascular disease prevention in clinical practice (version 2012). The Fifth Joint Task Force of the European Society of Cardiology and Other Societies on Cardiovascular Disease Prevention in Clinical Practice (constituted by representatives of nine societies and by invited experts). Eur Heart J *33:1635-1701, 2012.*

CURRENT CHALLENGES IN CARDIAC REHABILITATION AND SECONDARY PREVENTION

Patient Subgroups with Specific Needs

Although the benefits of cardiac rehabilitation and secondary prevention appear to be consistent across post-MI patients, including gender and age, certain subgroups merit special consideration.

Heart Failure

Chronic systolic heart failure is a common complication of ACS. A Cochrane review of 33 RCTs with 4740 participants has shown that patients with established chronic heart failure, with or without an implantable cardioverter-defibrillator and with or without cardiac resynchronization therapy device, will benefit from exercise-based cardiac rehabilitation.[43] International guidelines recommend supervised cardiac rehabilitation as a safe and beneficial intervention for patients with clinically stable heart failure (quality and level of evidence: class I, level A).[44]

Inpatient rehabilitation could begin as soon as possible after hospital admission. As the length of stay for acute decompensation and intervention procedures continues to decrease, a structured outpatient program is crucial for the development of a lifelong approach to prevention. This may be provided in a variety of settings, such as heart failure clinics, nonclinic settings (community health centers and general medical practices), or a combination of these. Outpatient cardiac rehabilitation also may be provided on an individual basis at home, including a combination of home visits, telephone support, telemedicine, or specially developed self-education materials.[45]

Diabetes

Diabetes increases the risk of cardiovascular disease two- to four-fold, and cardiovascular disease contributes to approximately 70% of deaths among persons with diabetes. Diabetes is very common among patients who have experienced an ACS (15% to 20%). It is recommended that the presence or absence of diabetes be confirmed in all patients with atherosclerotic vascular disease.[3]

Lifestyle modifications including daily physical activity, weight management, blood pressure control, and lipid management are recommended for all patients with diabetes. Metformin is an effective first-line pharmacotherapy agent and can be useful if not contraindicated. It is reasonable to individualize the intensity of blood sugar–lowering interventions based on the individual patient's risk of hypoglycemia during treatment. Initiation of pharmacotherapy interventions to achieve target glycosylated hemoglobin may be a reasonable approach. A target glycosylated hemoglobin of 7% or below may be considered. Less stringent glycosylated hemoglobin goals may be considered for patients with a history of severe hypoglycemia, limited life expectancy, advanced microvascular or macrovascular complications, or extensive comorbidity, or for those in whom the goal is difficult to attain despite intensive therapeutic interventions.

The two trials of oral hypoglycemics with the longest follow-up are the EXAMINE and SAVOR-TIMI trials.[46,47] EXAMINE enrolled approximately 5500 patients who had recently suffered an ACS and received either alogliptin or placebo, and the study found no difference in terms of the cardiovascular outcomes. The SAVOR-TIMI trial compared saxagliptin and placebo in approximately 16,500 subjects who were at high risk for cardiovascular events but who had not recently experienced any such events. SAVOR-TIMI showed no difference in rates of cardiovascular endpoints, but it did find an increased risk for congestive heart failure necessitating hospitalization.

Elderly Persons

Older cardiac patients often are excluded from cardiac rehabilitation and secondary prevention programs.[14] However, benefits of cardiac rehabilitation and secondary prevention have been shown in older patients, even in those with a high level of clinical severity and multiple comorbid conditions.[8] Particular program goals in the older patient include the preservation of mobility, independence and mental function, prevention/treatment of anxiety and depression, improving quality of life, encouragement of social adaptation and reintegration, and a return to the same or similar lifestyle as before their acute event.[45]

Planning and implementation of cardiac rehabilitation and secondary prevention programs in older groups require a high level of individual care and support, with a careful clinical evaluation beyond cardiovascular function, including psychosocial assessment and evaluation of comorbid conditions. Residential cardiac rehabilitation and secondary prevention programs may be an appropriate option in this age group.

Women

Women benefit from comprehensive cardiac rehabilitation and secondary prevention programs as much as men.[8] In the planning and implementation of cardiac rehabilitation and secondary prevention programs, the following considerations are important. Women are more likely to be older, and to have hypertension, diabetes, hypercholesterolemia, obesity, and heart failure, as well as lower exercise and functional capacity, compared with male patients and may therefore be at higher cardiac risk. Beyond the impact of the cardiac disease, older women are more likely to experience physical activity limitations and other exercise-limiting comorbid conditions such as arthritis, osteoporosis, and urinary incontinence. At recruitment to cardiac rehabilitation and secondary prevention programs, women typically score lower in health-related quality of life, and they are more likely to be diagnosed with depressive disorders and higher scores of anxiety.[45]

Maintaining Long-Term Behavior Change

Of all patients referred to cardiac rehabilitation and prevention, relatively few complete the program, and less than 50% maintain an exercise regimen for as long as 6 months after completion.[17] Factors reported to predict attendance and adherence include illness perception, geographic location, presence or absence of financial and work constraints, gender, age, and social support. Depression and a dislike of group-based rehabilitation sessions are specifically associated with less favorable compliance.[48] A Cochrane review of interventions for improving adherence found only eight RCTs that had addressed this issue.[17] Effective interventions included daily self-monitoring of activity, action planning, and adherence facilitation by cardiac rehabilitation staff. Interventions that are multifaceted are likely to be more effective. Further research to identify effective interventions is needed, particularly in underrepresented groups including women, ethnic minorities, elderly persons, higher-risk populations, and patients with comorbid conditions.

Quality Assurance

Despite recommendations, less than one half of eligible cardiac patients benefit from rehabilitation and prevention.[14,49,50] Systematic monitoring of the process of delivery and outcomes has been recommended to address this challenge.[5,51] Accreditation of rehabilitation and prevention programs with the use of clinical quality databases has been pointed out as an important tool to improve clinical practice and clinical follow-up care (Figure 34-4).[52] It is proposed that accreditation and quality assurance be conducted at the patient level as well as the program and provider levels. In the United States, referral to cardiac rehabilitation has been added to the performance measures after percutaneous intervention.[53] In the United Kingdom, the introduction of the National Audit of Cardiac Rehabilitation has resulted in steady increase in the rates of referrals to and enrollment in rehabilitation programs.[54] In the drive to increase quality assurance, this national audit program has introduced reporting performance on key service indicators and benchmarking services against evidence-based guidelines.

Inadequate reporting of cardiac rehabilitation and secondary prevention interventions in research studies is a substantial problem, with essential information frequently missing and, for almost one half of all interventions, unobtainable after publication. A conscientious effort to address this problem could facilitate an improvement in the quality of cardiac rehabilitation interventions delivered in clinical practice.[55]

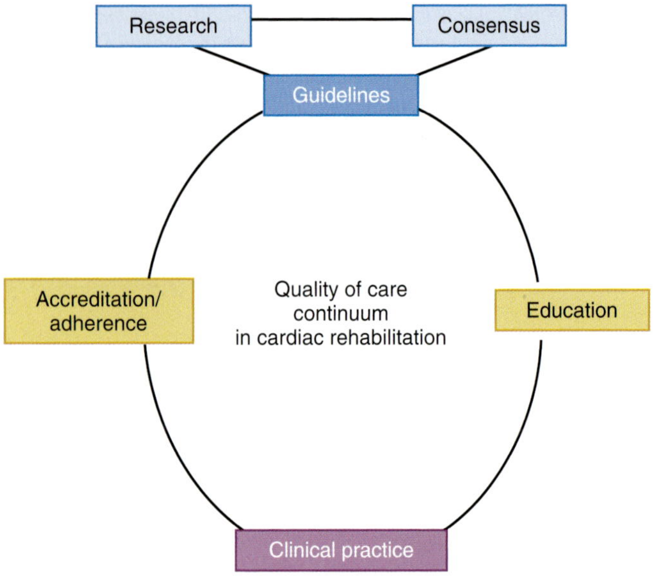

FIGURE 34-4 Quality care continuum in cardiac rehabilitation and secondary prevention. *(From Zwisler AD, Bjarnason-Wehrens B, McGee H, et al: Can level of education, accreditation and use of databases in cardiac rehabilitation be improved? Results from the European Cardiac Rehabilitation Inventory Survey.* Eur J Prev Cardiol *19:143-150, 2012.)*

The Role of the Cardiologist

Jelinek and colleagues have criticized cardiologists for not taking a leadership role in the provision of cardiac rehabilitation and secondary prevention services.[15] These investigators argue that cardiologists traditionally have not been actively involved in the delivery of such services or in the ongoing quality assurance process for assessment of their efficacy. Furthermore, cardiologists were neither consulted about nor involved with decisions regarding their patients' return to work. Most patients who have had an acute cardiac event receive clinical follow-up with a cardiologist once at 6 weeks after discharge from the hospital. Jellinek's group makes the call for cardiologists to "re-engage" with the recovery process after an MI-related hospitalization, inasmuch as hospital discharge equates to cutting of the "umbilical cord" of security regarding perceived clinical support—when patients are at their most anxious and depressed. Such re-engagement, most usefully at approximately 2 weeks after hospital discharge, could initially consist of inquiries about the patient's fears and expectations for the future, with rationales and recommendations regarding resumption of driving, sexual activity, and work, as appropriate.

In the United Kingdom, one of the seven core national standards for the delivery of rehabilitation and prevention services is "an integrated multidisciplinary team consisting of qualified and competent practitioners, led by a clinical coordinator," which should include a hospital or community-based cardiologist.

Innovative Models of Rehabilitation and Prevention

Cardiac rehabilitation and secondary prevention programs need to innovate and offer patients an alternative to the traditional, center-based model of rehabilitation.[6,15] When post-MI patients are offered a choice of home-based rehabilitation or hospital-based classes, almost two thirds choose the home-based option. A Cochrane systematic review of 18 RCTs in 1938 participants showed that home-based cardiac rehabilitation was as effective as center-based rehabilitation in reducing mortality and cardiac morbidity and improving coronary risk and health-related quality of life.[56]

With increasing access to mobile phones and the Internet, programs using such technology have the potential to expand both the capacity and capability of delivery and reduce costs. A meta-analysis of data on use of home-based programs provided through telemedicine and other models has confirmed the potential of such benefits.[57] Although use of mobile technologies is feasible, more robust evidence showing that Internet-based interventions can improve uptake and clinical outcomes in cardiac rehabilitation is needed before they are adopted more widely. A recent systematic review of alternative models of rehabilitation reported that in view of the costs and difficulties in accessing center-based rehabilitation, patients should be offered community- and home-based programs so that they can choose the model that best fits their needs and preferences.[58] Alternative models are likely to be of particular value in hard-to-reach post-MI populations that are more rural, remote, or culturally and linguistically diverse.

SUMMARY

Patients who have had an acute MI should be offered a program of comprehensive cardiac rehabilitation and secondary prevention that comprises of exercise training/physical activity promotion, education including risk factor management and medication adherence, and psychosocial interventions including stress management and behavioral change techniques. Meta-analysis of RCTs show rehabilitation and prevention measures for post-MI patients provides important health benefits that include reductions in the rates of cardiovascular mortality and rehospitalization and improvements in health-related quality of life.

Despite the proven benefits of cardiac rehabilitation and secondary prevention services, only a minority of eligible patients receive these services. Strategies to improve the delivery of services are bearing fruit, but the capacity of current delivery models for rehabilitation and preventions services is insufficient to provide such services to all eligible patients. New delivery strategies are needed that will supplement traditional, center-based rehabilitation and prevention programs and expand the reach of these important services.

Classic References

Oldridge NB, Guyatt GH, Fischer ME, Rimm AA: Cardiac rehabilitation after myocardial infarction. Combined experience of randomized clinical trials, *JAMA* 260:945–950, 1988.

O'Connor GT, Buring JE, Yusuf S, et al.: An overview of randomized trials of rehabilitation with exercise after myocardial infarction, *Circulation* 80:234–244, 1989.

Van Camp SP, Peterson RA: Cardiovascular complications of outpatient cardiac rehabilitation programs, *JAMA* 256:1160–1163, 1986.

Wenger N, Froelicher E, Smith L, et al.: Cardiac rehabilitation as secondary prevention. Agency for Health Care Policy and Research and National Heart, Lung, and Blood Institute, *Clin Pract Guideline Quick Ref Guide Clin* 1–23, 1995.

References

1. Alphin S, Kjøller M, Davidsen M, et al.: Self-reported ischemic heart disease: prevalence, sociodemographics, health behavior, health-care utilization, and quality of life, *Open J Prev Med* 2:240–248, 2012.
2. Balady GJ, Williams MA, Ades PA, et al.: Core components of cardiac rehabilitation/secondary prevention programs: 2007 update: a scientific statement from the American Heart Association Exercise, Cardiac Rehabilitation, and Prevention Committee, the Council on Clinical Cardiology; the Councils on Cardiovascular Nursing, Epidemiology and Prevention, and Nutrition, Physical Activity, and Metabolism; and the American Association of Cardiovascular and Pulmonary Rehabilitation, *Circulation* 115:2675–2682, 2007.

3. Smith Jr SC, Benjamin EJ, Bonow RO, et al.: AHA/ACCF secondary prevention and risk reduction therapy for patients with coronary and other atherosclerotic vascular disease: 2011 update: a guideline from the American Heart Association and American College of Cardiology Foundation, *Circulation* 124:2458–2473, 2011.
4. Perk J, De Backer G, Gohlke H, et al.: European guidelines on cardiovascular disease prevention in clinical practice (version 2012). The Fifth Joint Task Force of the European Society of Cardiology and Other Societies on Cardiovascular Disease Prevention in Clinical Practice (constituted by representatives of nine societies and by invited experts), *Eur Heart J* 33:1635–1701, 2012.
5. Piepoli MF, Corra U, Adamopoulos S, et al.: Secondary prevention in the clinical management of patients with cardiovascular diseases. Core components, standards and outcome measures for referral and delivery: a policy statement from the cardiac rehabilitation section of the European Association for Cardiovascular Prevention & Rehabilitation. Endorsed by the Committee for Practice Guidelines of the European Society of Cardiology, *Eur J Prev Cardiol* 21:664–681, 2014.
6. Sandesara PB, Lambert CT, Gordon NF, et al.: Cardiac rehabilitation and risk reduction: time to "rebrand and reinvigorate.", *J Am Coll Cardiol* 65:389–395, 2015.
6a. Wenger N, Froelicher E, Smith L, et al.: Cardiac rehabilitation as secondary prevention. Agency for Health Care Policy and Research and National Heart, Lung, and Blood Institute, *Clin Pract Guideline Quick Ref Guide Clin* 1–23, 1995.
7. Lawler PR, Filion KB, Eisenberg MJ: Efficacy of exercise-based cardiac rehabilitation post-myocardial infarction: a systematic review and meta-analysis of randomized controlled trials, *Am Heart J* 162:571–584.e2, 2011.
8. Anderson L, Thompson DR, Oldridge N, et al.: Exercise-based cardiac rehabilitation for coronary heart disease: Cochrane systematic review and meta-analysis, *J Am Coll Cardiol* 67:1–12, 2016.
9. Pavy B, Iliou MC, Meurin P, et al.: Safety of exercise training for cardiac patients: results of the French registry of complications during cardiac rehabilitation, *Arch Intern Med* 166:2329–2334, 2006.
10. Wong WP, Feng J, Pwee KH, et al.: A systematic review of economic evaluations of cardiac rehabilitation, *BMC Health Serv Res* 12:243, 2012.
11. Bethell H, Lewin R, Dalal H: Cardiac rehabilitation in the United Kingdom, *Heart* 95:271–275, 2009.
12. Kotseva K, Wood D: The challenge for preventive cardiology, *Eur J Cardiovasc Prev Rehabil* 16(Suppl 2):S19–S23, 2009.
13. Kotseva K, Wood D, De Backer G, et al.: Cardiovascular prevention guidelines in daily practice: a comparison of EUROASPIRE I, II, and III surveys in eight European countries, *Lancet* 373: 929–940, 2009.
14. Bjarnason-Wehrens B, McGee H, Zwisler AD, et al.: Cardiac rehabilitation in Europe: results from the European Cardiac Rehabilitation Inventory Survey, *Eur J Cardiovasc Prev Rehabil* 17:410–418, 2010.
15. Jelinek MV, Thompson DR, Ski C, et al.: 40 years of cardiac rehabilitation and secondary prevention in post-cardiac ischaemic patients. Are we still in the wilderness? *Int J Cardiol* 179:153–159, 2015.
16. Dunlay SM, Witt BJ, Allison TG, et al.: Barriers to participation in cardiac rehabilitation, *Am Heart J* 158:852–859, 2009.
17. Karmali KN, Davies P, Taylor F, et al.: Promoting patient uptake and adherence in cardiac rehabilitation, *Cochrane Database Syst Rev*(6), 2014. CD007131.
18. Brown JP, Clark AM, Dalal H, et al.: Patient education in the management of coronary heart disease, *Cochrane DatabaseSyst Rev*(12), 2011. CD008895.
19. Whalley B, Rees K, Davies P, et al.: Psychological interventions for coronary heart disease, *Cochrane Database Syst Rev*(8), 2011. CD002902.
20. Thombs BD, Ziegelstein RC, Pilote L, et al.: Somatic symptom overlap in Beck Depression Inventory-II scores following myocardial infarction, *Br J Psychiatry* 197:61–66, 2010.
21. Rutledge T, Reis VA, Linke SE, et al.: Depression in heart failure a meta-analytic review of prevalence, intervention effects, and associations with clinical outcomes, *J Am Coll Cardiol* 48:1527–1537, 2006.
22. Khawaja IS, Westermeyer JJ, Gajwani P, et al.: Depression and coronary artery disease: the association, mechanisms, and therapeutic implications, *Psychiatry (Edgmont)* 6:38–51, 2009.
23. Dickens C, Cherrington A, McGowan L: Depression and health-related quality of life in people with coronary heart disease: a systematic review, *Eur J Cardiovasc Nurs* 11:265–275, 2012.
24. Dickens C, Katon W, Blakemore A, et al.: Does depression predict the use of urgent and unscheduled care by people with long term conditions? A systematic review with meta-analysis, *J Psychosom Res* 73:334–342, 2012.
25. Critchley JA, Capewell S: WITHDRAWN: Smoking cessation for the secondary prevention of coronary heart disease, *Cochrane Database Syst Rev*(2), 2012. CD003041.
26. Stead LF, Buitrago D, Preciado N, et al.: Physician advice for smoking cessation, *Cochrane Database Syst Rev*(5), 2013. CD000165.
27. Barth J, Jacob T, Daha I, et al.: Psychosocial interventions for smoking cessation in patients with coronary heart disease, *Cochrane Database Syst Rev*(7), 2015. CD006886.
28. Cahill K, Stevens S, Perera R, et al.: Pharmacological interventions for smoking cessation: an overview and network meta-analysis, *Cochrane Database Systc Rev*(5), 2013. CD009329.
29. Singh S, Loke YK, Spangler JG, et al.: Risk of serious adverse cardiovascular events associated with varenicline: a systematic review and meta-analysis, *CMAJ* 183:1359–1366, 2011.
30. NICE: Stop smoking services: National Institute for Health and Care Excellence. https://www.nice.org.uk/guidance/ph10, 2008.
31. Estruch R, Ros E, Martinez-Gonzalez MA: Mediterranean diet for primary prevention of cardiovascular disease, *N Engl J Med* 369:676–677, 2013.
32. NICE: Weight management: lifestyle services for overweight or obese adults, *National Institute for Health and Care Excellence*, 2014. https://www.nice.org.uk/guidance/ph53.
33. Stone NJ, Robinson JG, Lichtenstein AH, et al.: 2013 ACC/AHA guideline on the treatment of blood cholesterol to reduce atherosclerotic cardiovascular risk in adults: a report of the American College of Cardiology/American Heart Association Task Force on Practice Guidelines, *J Am Coll Cardiol* 63:2889–2934, 2014.
34. Cannon CP, Blazing MA, Giugliano RP, et al.: Ezetimibe added to statin therapy after acute coronary syndromes, *N Engl J Med* 372:2387–2397, 2015.
35. Rosendorff C, Lackland DT, Allison M, et al.: Treatment of hypertension in patients with coronary artery disease: a scientific statement from the American Heart Association, American College of Cardiology, and American Society of Hypertension, *J Am Coll Cardiol* 65:1998–2038, 2015.
36. O'Gara PT, Kushner FG, Ascheim DD, et al.: 2013 ACCF/AHA guideline for the management of ST-elevation myocardial infarction: a report of the American College of Cardiology Foundation/American Heart Association Task Force on Practice Guidelines, *J Am Coll Cardiol* 61:e78–e140, 2013.
37. Fihn SD, Blankenship JC, Alexander KP, et al.: 2014 ACC/AHA/AATS/PCNA/SCAI/STS focused update of the guideline for the diagnosis and management of patients with stable ischemic heart disease: a report of the American College of Cardiology/American Heart Association Task Force on Practice Guidelines, and the American Association for Thoracic Surgery, Preventive Cardiovascular Nurses Association, Society for Cardiovascular Angiography and Interventions, and Society of Thoracic Surgeons, *J Am Coll Cardiol* 64:1929–1949, 2014.
38. Bangalore S, Bhatt DL, Steg PG, et al.: Beta-blockers and cardiovascular events in patients with and without myocardial infarction: post hoc analysis from the CHARISMA trial, *Circ Cardiovasc Qual Outcomes* 7:872–881, 2014.
39. Huang BT, Huang FY, Zuo ZL, et al.: Meta-analysis of relation between oral beta-blocker therapy and outcomes in patients with acute myocardial infarction who underwent percutaneous coronary intervention, *Am J Cardiol* 115:1529–1538, 2015.
40. Naderi SH, Bestwick JP, Wald DS: Adherence to drugs that prevent cardiovascular disease: meta-analysis on 376,162 patients, *Am J Med* 125:882–887.e1, 2012.
41. Arnold SV, Spertus JA, Masoudi FA, et al.: Beyond medication prescription as performance measures: optimal secondary prevention medication dosing after acute myocardial infarction, *J Am Coll Cardiol* 62:1791–1801, 2013.
42. Shah ND, Dunlay SM, Ting HH, et al.: Long-term medication adherence after myocardial infarction: experience of a community, *Am J Med* 122(961), 2009. e967-e913.
43. Taylor RS, Sagar VA, Davies EJ, et al.: Exercise-based rehabilitation for heart failure, *Cochrane Database Syst Rev*(4), 2014. CD003331.
44. McMurray JJ, Adamopoulos S, Anker SD, et al.: ESC guidelines for the diagnosis and treatment of acute and chronic heart failure 2012: the Task Force for the Diagnosis and Treatment of Acute and Chronic Heart Failure 2012 of the European Society of Cardiology. Developed in collaboration with the Heart Failure Association (HFA) of the ESC, *Eur J Heart Fail* 14:803–869, 2012.
45. Piepoli MF, Corra U, Benzer W, et al.: Secondary prevention through cardiac rehabilitation: from knowledge to implementation. A position paper from the Cardiac Rehabilitation Section of the European Association of Cardiovascular Prevention and Rehabilitation, *Eur J Cardiovasc Prev Rehabil* 17:1–17, 2010.
46. Zannad F, Cannon CP, Cushman WC, et al.: Heart failure and mortality outcomes in patients with type 2 diabetes taking alogliptin versus placebo in EXAMINE: a multicentre, randomised, double-blind trial, *Lancet* 385:2067–2076, 2015.
47. Scirica BM, Braunwald E, Raz I, et al.: Heart failure, saxagliptin, and diabetes mellitus: observations from the SAVOR-TIMI 53 randomized trial, *Circulation* 130:1579–1588, 2014.
48. Turk-Adawi KI, Oldridge NB, Tarima SS, et al.: Cardiac rehabilitation patient and organizational factors: what keeps patients in programs? *J Am Heart Assoc* 2:e000418, 2013.
49. Aragam KG, Dai D, Neely ML, et al.: Gaps in referral to cardiac rehabilitation of patients undergoing percutaneous coronary intervention in the United States, *J Am Coll Cardiol* 65:2079–2088, 2015.
50. Thomas RJ: The gap in cardiac rehabilitation referral: a system-based problem with system-based solutions, *J Am Coll Cardiol* 65:2089–2090, 2015.
51. Thomas RJ, King M, Lui K, et al.: AACVPR/ACCF/AHA 2010 update: performance measures on cardiac rehabilitation for referral to cardiac rehabilitation/secondary prevention services endorsed by the American College of Chest Physicians, the American College of Sports Medicine, the American Physical Therapy Association, the Canadian Association of Cardiac Rehabilitation, the Clinical Exercise Physiology Association, the European Association for Cardiovascular Prevention and Rehabilitation, the Inter-American Heart Foundation, the National Association of Clinical Nurse Specialists, the Preventive Cardiovascular Nurses Association, and the Society of Thoracic Surgeons, *J Am Coll Cardiol* 56:1159–1167, 2010.
52. Zwisler AD, Bjarnason-Wehrens B, McGee H, et al.: Can level of education, accreditation and use of databases in cardiac rehabilitation be improved? Results from the European Cardiac Rehabilitation Inventory Survey, *Eur J Prev Cardiol* 19:143–150, 2012.
53. Nallamothu BK, Tommaso CL, Anderson HV, et al.: ACC/AHA/SCAI/AMA-convened PCPI/NCQA 2013 performance measures for adults undergoing percutaneous coronary intervention: a report of the American College of Cardiology/American Heart Association Task Force on Performance Measures, the Society for Cardiovascular Angiography and Interventions, the American Medical Association-Convened Physician Consortium for Performance Improvement, and the National Committee for Quality Assurance, *J Am Coll Cardiol* 63:722–745, 2014.
54. Dalal H, Doherty P, Taylor RS: Cardiac rehabilitation, *BMJ* 351:h5000, 2015.
55. Abell B, Glasziou P, Hoffmann T: Reporting and replicating trials of exercise-based cardiac rehabilitation: do we know what the researchers actually did? *Circ Cardiovasc Qual Outcomes* 8:187–194, 2015.
56. Taylor RS, Dalal H, Jolly K, et al.: Home-based versus centre-based cardiac rehabilitation, *Cochrane Database Syst Rev*(8), 2010. CD007130.
57. Neubeck L, Redfern J, Fernandez R, et al.: Telehealth interventions for the secondary prevention of coronary heart disease: a systematic review, *Eur J Cardiovasc Prev Rehabil* 16:281–289, 2009.
58. Clark RA, Conway A, Poulsen V, et al.: Alternative models of cardiac rehabilitation: a systematic review, *Eur J Prev Cardiol* 22:35–74, 2015.

35 Clinical Practice/Controversy

Antiplatelet Therapy After Myocardial Infarction

Marc P. Bonaca, Marc S. Sabatine, and David A. Morrow

INTRODUCTION

Myocardial infarction (MI) is caused by atherothrombosis (see Chapter 3), with platelets playing a pivotal role in the initial onset of MI and its recurrence. Antiplatelet therapy targets this key element in the pathobiology of cardiovascular ischemic events. Patients who have suffered an MI have a sustained heightened risk for recurrent ischemic events and therefore have the potential to benefit from long-term antiplatelet therapy as part of secondary preventive management (Figures 35-1 and 35-2). Antiplatelet therapy, however, also increases the risk of bleeding. Accordingly, the type, intensity, and duration of antiplatelet therapy after MI should be tailored in accordance with the patient's risk of subsequent ischemic events and of bleeding. This chapter considers the rationale for antiplatelet therapy for long-term secondary prevention in patients with MI, reviews trials of specific agents and strategies, and describes the application of clinical trial evidence in real-world practice.

EPIDEMIOLOGY OF RECURRENT ATHEROTHROMBOSIS

Myocardial Infarction as a Marker of Long-Term Atherothrombotic Risk

Atherothrombotic events, including MI and ischemic stroke, remain a primary contributor to morbidity and mortality worldwide (see Chapter 2). Among patients with established atherosclerosis, those who have suffered a previous acute thrombotic ischemic event have sustained activation of coagulation (Figure 35-3) and are at higher risk than those with no history of such an event.[1] Thus a history of previous spontaneous (type 1) MI marks the presence of an underlying disease state predisposing the patient to recurrent spontaneous atherothrombotic ischemic events.

Several modern observational data sets have characterized long-term ischemic risk in patients with previous atherothrombosis. An analysis of data for 64,977 stable outpatients enrolled in the REduction of Atherothrombosis for Continued Health (REACH) Registry evaluated the risk of cardiovascular death, MI, and stroke over a 4-year period based on a clinical history of either cardiovascular risk factors only, known atherosclerosis but no previous ischemic event, or a previous ischemic event (Figure 35-4).[2] Patients with a previous ischemic event had the highest risk of cardiovascular death, MI, or stroke at 4 years (18.3%) compared with patients with stable atherosclerosis (12.2%) or risk factors alone (9.1%). Although this risk was higher for those within 1 year of their event (21.1%), it remained heightened for those patients who had survived more than a year from their most recent event (17.2%).[2]

The long-term risk of recurrent major cardiovascular events after MI was characterized in a Swedish Registry including 97,254 patients surviving after hospitalization for an MI.[3] Within the first year, the rate of recurrent MI, stroke, or cardiovascular death was 18.3%, with a majority of these events being recurrent MI (56%), followed by cardiovascular death (31.0%) and ischemic stroke (13.4%). An additional 4.2% of patients died from noncardiovascular causes—approximately one-third the rate of death from cardiovascular causes. For those patients who survived 1 year after their MI without a recurrent event, the rate of subsequent cardiovascular death, MI, or stroke was 20% over 3 years. Although recurrent MI was the most frequent event (40.8% of the population), the relative proportions of cardiovascular death (40.6%) and stroke (18.6%) were higher than those within the first year.[3] Independent predictors of recurrent events included age, previous MI, previous stroke, and diabetes. Other national registries have estimated similar adjusted rates of subsequent recurrent MI, stroke, or death, ranging

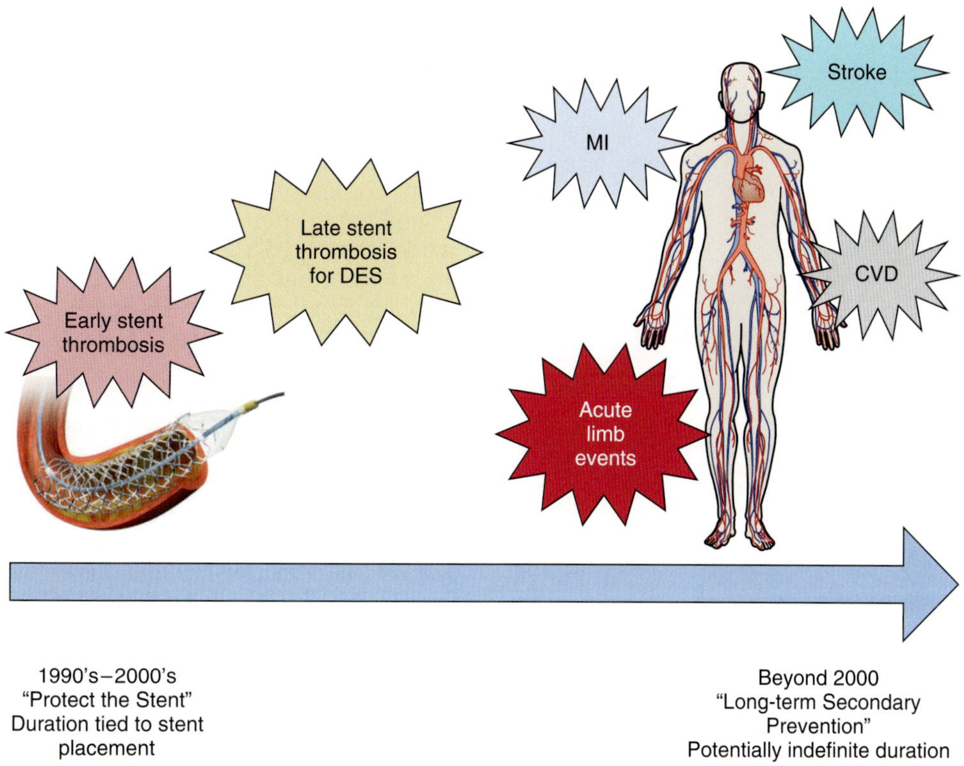

FIGURE 35-1 **Evolution in the role of $P2Y_{12}$ inhibition added to aspirin in patients with previous myocardial infarction (MI).** *CVD,* Cardiovascular disease; *DES,* drug-eluting stent.

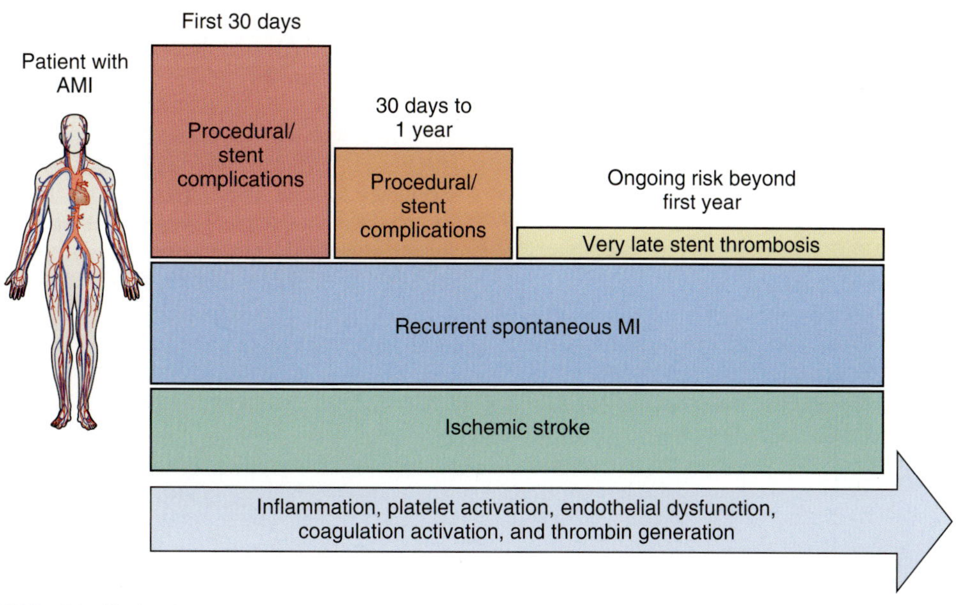

FIGURE 35-2 **Risk of ischemic events over time in patients presenting with spontaneous myocardial infarction (MI).** *AMI,* Acute MI.

from 16.7% to 21.3% at 3 years in patients who had survived 1 year from MI.[4]

Types of Atherothrombotic Events in Stable Patients with Previous Myocardial Infarction

Because atherosclerosis is a systemic condition, patients with symptomatic disease in any vascular bed are at heightened risk for systemic atherothrombotic events. In the REACH registry, when stratified by symptomatic vascular bed compared with patients with risk factors alone, patients with established atherosclerosis were at higher risk for cardiovascular death, MI, stroke, or hospitalization for atherothrombosis regardless of the symptomatic vascular bed and were at the highest risk when multiple vascular beds were symptomatic.[5]

In patients presenting with acute MI, the risk of early ischemic complications generally is related to the culprit coronary lesion or associated coronary interventions.[6-9] More potent antiplatelet strategies reduce the risk of periprocedural MI (type 4a MI) occurring in the setting of

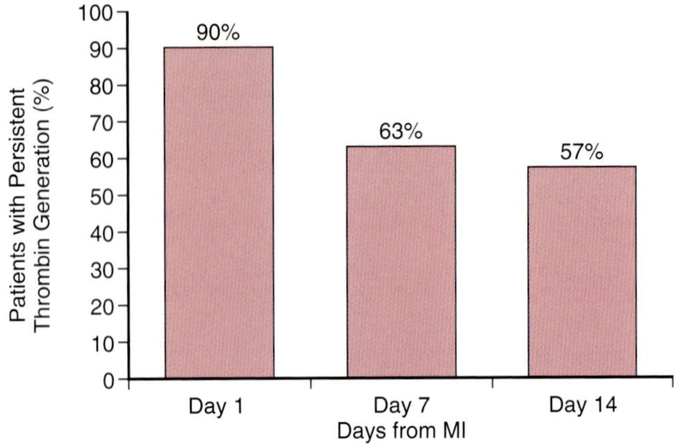

FIGURE 35-3 Serial blood samples obtained after acute myocardial infarction (MI) in 100 patients over a period of 14 days demonstrate that thrombin generation extends beyond the acute phase of MI in more than one half of the patients. *(Adapted from Szczeklik A, Dropinski J, Radwan J, Krzanowski M: Persistent generation of thrombin after acute myocardial infarction.* Arterioscler Thromb *12:548-553, 1992.)*

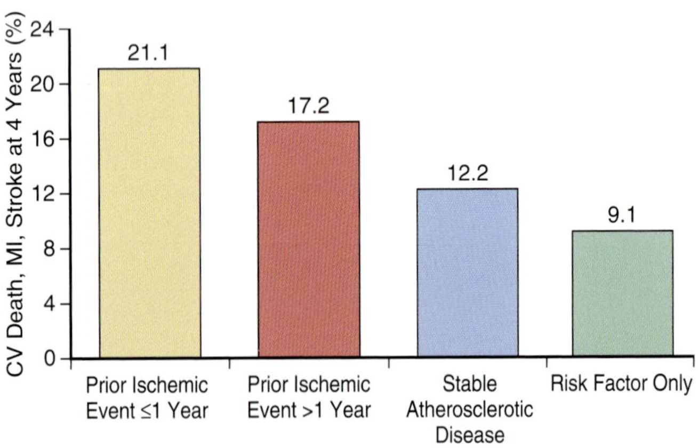

FIGURE 35-4 Rate of cardiovascular (CV) death, myocardial infarction (MI), or stroke at 4 years by history of previous ischemic event, stable atherosclerotic disease, or risk factors only. *(Adapted from Bhatt DL, Eagle KA, Ohman EM, et al: Comparative determinants of 4-year cardiovascular event rates in stable outpatients at risk of or with atherothrombosis.* JAMA *304:1350-1357, 2010.)*

percutaneous coronary intervention (PCI), as well as stent thrombosis (type 4b MI).[10] After discharge, however, the risk of stent-related complications decreases, whereas the risk of recurrent spontaneous events remains relatively constant[11] (see Figure 35-2). Moreover, in a study of cardiovascular events occurring after successful PCI in 697 patients with acute coronary syndrome (ACS), rates of recurrent events related to the culprit lesion and to non-culprit lesions were similar (Figure 35-5).[12] In addition, non-culprit lesions leading to recurrent atherothrombosis frequently were angiographically mild at initial angiography but were associated with markers of instability, including thin-cap fibroatheroma (see Chapter 10).[12]

Clinical trials enrolling stable patients with previous MI have prospectively adjudicated recurrent MI and applied the Universal Definition of MI classification system to categorize events according to their etiology (see Chapter 1). In such cohorts of stable patients, recurrent MIs are predominantly new spontaneous events (type 1 MI, 78%), with lower relative frequencies of demand ischemia (type 2 MI, 10%), PCI-related MI, or stent thrombosis (type 4 MI, 12%).[13] These data indicate that as patients stabilize from an acute MI, the type of recurrent coronary event for which they are at risk switches from events primarily related to the culprit lesion and coronary intervention to those primarily occurring in the setting of de novo plaque rupture elsewhere in the coronary tree (see Figure 35-2). This pattern is likely to persist in coming years, particularly as procedural risk and stent-related complications continue to decrease with improvements in technology.

In addition to their risk of spontaneous MI, patients with previous MI are at higher long-term risk for ischemic stroke. As patients survive beyond their first year after MI, the proportion of recurrent cardiovascular events that are ischemic strokes remains similar or increases; for example, in the REACH registry, the proportion of events that were ischemic strokes was 13.4% within 1 year after MI, increasing to 18.6% beyond 1 year after MI.[2] Although the risk of an incident ischemic stroke is greatest in patients who have suffered a previous stroke, at a population level a majority

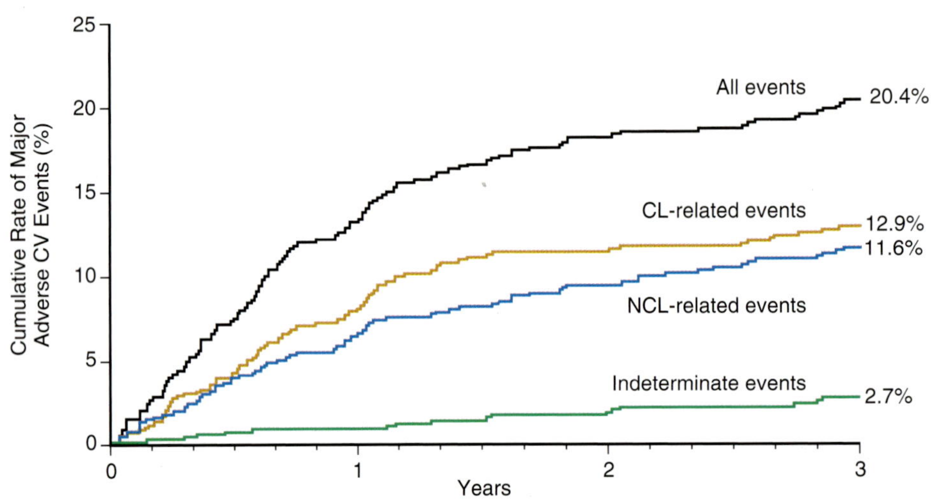

FIGURE 35-5 Rates of cardiovascular (CV) death, cardiac arrest, myocardial infarction, or rehospitalization for unstable or progressive angina (major adverse CV events) related to culprit lesions (CL), non-culprit lesions (NCL), and events of indeterminate origin. CL-related events were those adjudicated to be recurrent disease at the sites of originally treated culprit lesions; NCL-related events were adjudicated to be at sites of non-culprit lesions. Some patients had both CL-related and NCL-related events, and some patients had multiple CL-related events, multiple NCL-related events, or both at different times (in which case the first event is represented in the time-to-event curve). *(Adapted from Stone GW, Maehara A, Lansky AJ, et al: A prospective natural-history study of coronary atherosclerosis.* N Engl J Med *364:226-235, 2011.)*

of incident strokes occur as first strokes in patients with atherosclerosis.[14,15]

Rationale for Antiplatelet Therapy for Long-Term Secondary Prevention

Because atherosclerosis is a systemic disease and patients with a history of MI are at heightened long-term risk for spontaneous atherothrombotic events across vascular territories, strategies using systemic preventive therapies are necessary to reduce this risk. Components of medical secondary prevention target specific processes involved in the pathobiology of atherothrombosis, including dyslipidemia and inflammation, and activation of both the coagulation cascade and platelets (see Chapter 13).

Secondary prevention strategies to reduce atherothrombotic risk include lifestyle interventions, lipid lowering, blood pressure lowering, and antithrombotic therapy (see Chapter 34). Although both oral antiplatelet and anticoagulant strategies have been studied for secondary prevention, anticoagulants at traditional therapeutic doses have generally resulted in excessive bleeding and are currently not used routinely for this purpose. Trials evaluating very-low-dose anticoagulants, however, have shown efficacy when such agents are added to antiplatelet therapy in patients with ACS, and future trials in stable populations may expand the use of this strategy to long-term secondary prevention (see Chapter 21).[16] Several antiplatelet agents targeting differing mechanisms used alone or in combination are currently used for the first year after an MI and are now supported by evidence showing benefits for long-term secondary prevention.

CLINICAL TRIALS OF ANTIPLATELET THERAPY FOR SECONDARY PREVENTION AFTER MYOCARDIAL INFARCTION

Aspirin

Aspirin has been studied for ischemic risk reduction in multiple randomized trials and analyzed in a meta-analysis conducted by the Antithrombotic Trialists' Collaborative. In early iterations of the meta-analysis, a total of 287 randomized, controlled studies involving 135,000 patients in trials of a variety of antiplatelet agents were combined and showed a reduction in 36 serious vascular events prevented per 1000 patients with prevous MI treated for 2 years (Figure 35-6A).[17] A more recent analysis that focused specifically on the efficacy and safety of aspirin for primary and secondary prevention included 6 trials in patients with previous MI and 10 trials in patients with previous stroke or transient ischemic attack (TIA).[18] In the secondary prevention population, aspirin reduced the risk of any serious vascular event by 19% (hazard ratio [HR], 0.81; 95% confidence interval [CI], 0.75 to 0.87), with an absolute risk reduction of 1.49% per year versus placebo. There were consistent reductions in coronary mortality, myocardial infarction, and ischemic stroke.[18]

In a study considering the safety of antiplatelet therapy, aspirin increased the risk of major extracranial bleeding, primarily gastrointestinal (absolute risk increase of 0.4% per year[19]) and hemorrhagic stroke (absolute risk increase of 0.01% per year).[18] Overall, the study investigators concluded that a net benefit was achieved with aspirin for secondary prevention due to the ischemic risk in that population.[18]

Although the optimal dose of aspirin for long-term secondary prevention has not been definitively established, the aggregate evidence favors aspirin doses of 75 to 162 mg daily. The CURRENT-OASIS 7 trial evaluated whether high-dose (300 to 325 mg daily) aspirin is superior to low-dose aspirin (75 to 100 mg daily) for 30 days in patients presenting with ACS (see Figure 35-6B).[20] In this acute setting, in which potent platelet inhibition might be expected to be most beneficial, there was no difference in the composite of cardiovascular death, MI, or stroke with high- versus low-dose aspirin (HR, 0.97; 95% CI, 0.86 to 1.09; P = .61); however, the rates of major gastrointestinal bleeding (P = .04) and minor bleeding (P = .04) were higher.[20] These data indicate that the ischemic benefit from aspirin is achieved at a low dose (100 mg or less daily) and that higher doses result in more bleeding.

$P2Y_{12}$ Inhibitors

Oral therapies to inhibit the platelet $P2Y_{12}$ adenosine diphosphate (ADP) receptor are available. Each of the available oral agents (clopidogrel, prasugrel, and ticagrelor) are described in Chapter 19 (see Figure 19-2 and Table 19-1). The second-generation thienopyridine clopidogrel was studied head-to-head against aspirin as monotherapy for secondary prevention in the Clopidogrel versus Aspirin in Patients at Risk of Ischemic Events (CAPRIE) trial.[21] A total of 19,185 patients with stable atherosclerotic vascular disease (6302 in the MI subgroup and 8446 with previous MI) were randomly assigned to receive either clopidogrel 75 mg daily or aspirin 325 mg daily, with follow-up periods ranging from 1 to 3 years. At a mean of 1.91 years of follow-up, clopidogrel was superior to aspirin for reducing the composite of cardiovascular death, MI, or stroke (relative risk reduction, 8.7%; P = .043), with a modest absolute risk reduction (ARR) of 0.51%. When subgroups were evaluated on the basis of their symptomatic vascular bed (peripheral arterial disease, previous MI, cerebrovascular disease), the benefit appeared to be most robust in patients with peripheral arterial disease, although statistical heterogeneity between groups was lacking.[21] When studied in patients with ACS, the addition of clopidogrel to aspirin reduced the rate of recurrence of major cardiovascular events in the first 30 days and through 12 months by 20%, depending on the endpoint and whether the population had non–ST-elevation (NSTE) or ST-elevation ACS (see Chapter 19).[8,9] Although the treatment duration was for 3 to 12 months after NSTE-ACS, the survival curves demonstrated continued separation over the course of follow-up, suggesting continued benefit over time.[22] Subsequent trials evaluating more potent, less variable $P2Y_{12}$ inhibitors against clopidogrel in patients presenting with ACS have published consistent landmark analyses showing benefits of the more potent regimens even when landmarked at later timepoints.[23,24]

CHARISMA Trial

The benefits of adding a $P2Y_{12}$ inhibitor to aspirin in ACS raised the hypothesis that such a strategy also may be beneficial in stable patients with risk factors for either long-term secondary prevention or primary prevention. This hypothesis was tested in the Clopidogrel and Aspirin versus Aspirin Alone for the Prevention of Atherothrombotic Events (CHARISMA) trial.[25] A total of 15,603 patients were randomly assigned to receive clopidogrel 75 mg daily or

PEGASUS-TIMI 54 Trial

The Prevention of Cardiovascular Events in Patients with Prior Heart Attack Using Ticagrelor Compared to Placebo on a Background of Aspirin–Thrombolysis in Myocardial Infarction 54 (PEGASUS-TIMI 54) trial was designed to address the hypothesis that prolonged dual-antiplatelet therapy is beneficial in patients with previous MI regardless of previous coronary stenting.[29] The study subjects were selected with the primary criterion of a history of a spontaneous MI 1 to 3 years before enrollment. In addition, patients needed to have at least one high-risk feature for ischemic complications (age 65 years or older, diabetes mellitus requiring medication, a second previous MI, multivessel coronary disease, or non–end-stage renal dysfunction) and be without specific risk factors for bleeding (history of ischemic stroke or intracranial bleeding, central nervous system tumor, or an intracranial vascular abnormality; gastrointestinal bleeding within the previous 6 months; or major surgery within the previous 30 days). Patients were randomly assigned to receive one of two doses of the non-thienopyridine $P2Y_{12}$ antagonist ticagrelor or a matching placebo, with all patients receiving low-dose aspirin. The two doses studied were a 90-mg dose, which was shown to be superior to clopidogrel in the ACS setting,[24] and a 60-mg dose, which had not previously been studied in humans and was anticipated to provide a better tolerability profile compared with the 90-mg dose. At a median of 33 months, both doses of ticagrelor significantly reduced the composite of cardiovascular death, MI, or stroke (60-mg dose: HR, 0.84; 95% CI, 0.74 to 0.95; $P = .004$; 90-mg dose: HR, 0.85; 95% CI, 0.75 to 0.96; $P = .008$) (Figure 35-9).[30] The efficacy of ticagrelor was consistent for all components of the primary endpoint including stroke and cardiovascular death as well as MI.[30] Both doses significantly increased TIMI major bleeding (60-mg dose: HR, 2.32; $P < .001$; 90-mg dose: HR, 2.69; $P < .001$), with no significant excess of fatal or intracranial bleeds.[30] Based on the data from this trial, for every 10,000 patients who began treatment, 40 primary endpoint events would be prevented with the 90-mg dose and 42 with the 60-mg dose. This efficacy would come at a cost of 41 TIMI major bleeds with the 90-mg dose and 31 with the 60-mg dose.

Pooled Analysis of $P2Y_{12}$ Trials

The results of the CHARISMA previous-MI subgroup, the DAPT previous-MI subgroup, and PEGASUS-TIMI 54 were pooled together with those for the MI subgroups in several other trials in a meta-analysis evaluating prolonged DAPT ($N = 20{,}203$) with a $P2Y_{12}$ inhibitor plus aspirin versus aspirin alone ($N = 13{,}232$) for secondary prevention.[31] Consistent with the individual trials, the pooled analysis showed a significant reduction in the composite of cardiovascular death, MI, or stroke with prolonged DAPT (Figure 35-10). Of importance, in this pooled analysis with greater statistical power, the addition of a $P2Y_{12}$ inhibitor to aspirin significantly reduced rates for each of the individual components of the endpoint including MI, stroke, as well as CV death alone ($P = .03$) (Figure 35-e2). Safety was consistent with that in the individual trials, with the details presented in a subsequent section (Figure 35-11).

Protease-Activated Receptor Antagonists

The protease-activated receptor 1 (PAR-1), which is the primary receptor for thrombin on human platelets, has also been tested as a target for secondary prevention.[32] Vorapaxar, an oral competitive antagonist of PAR-1, has been studied in both the ACS and secondary prevention settings.[33,34] The Thrombin Receptor Antagonist in Secondary Prevention of Atherothrombotic Ischemic Events (TRA 2P)–Thrombolysis in Myocardial Infarction (TIMI) 50 trial randomly assigned a broad population of patients with atherosclerotic vascular disease (previous MI, symptomatic peripheral arterial disease, or ischemic stroke) to receive vorapaxar sulfate 2.5 mg daily or a matching placebo.[33] Background antithrombotic therapy in the trial was at the discretion of the treating physicians and included antiplatelet monotherapy as well as DAPT with aspirin and clopidogrel.

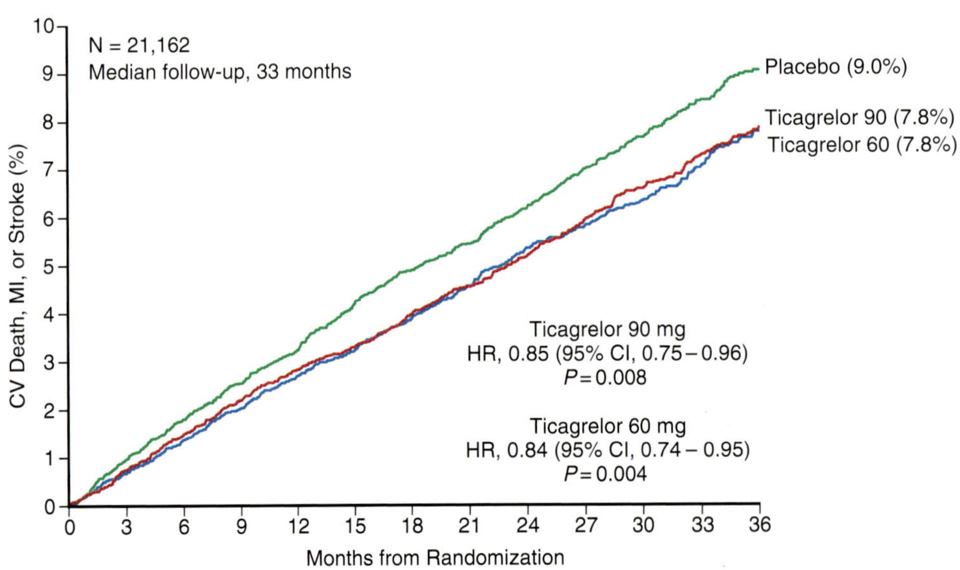

FIGURE 35-9 **Cardiovascular (CV) death, myocardial infarction (MI), or stroke at 2 years in patients with history of MI (1 to 3 years previously) randomly assigned to a regimen of ticagrelor 60 mg twice daily (*blue*), ticagrelor 90 mg twice daily (*red*), or placebo (*green*).** All patients received low-dose aspirin. *(Adapted from Bonaca MP, Bhatt DL, Cohen M, et al: Long-term use of ticagrelor in patients with prior myocardial infarction.* N Engl J Med *372:1791-1800, 2015.)*

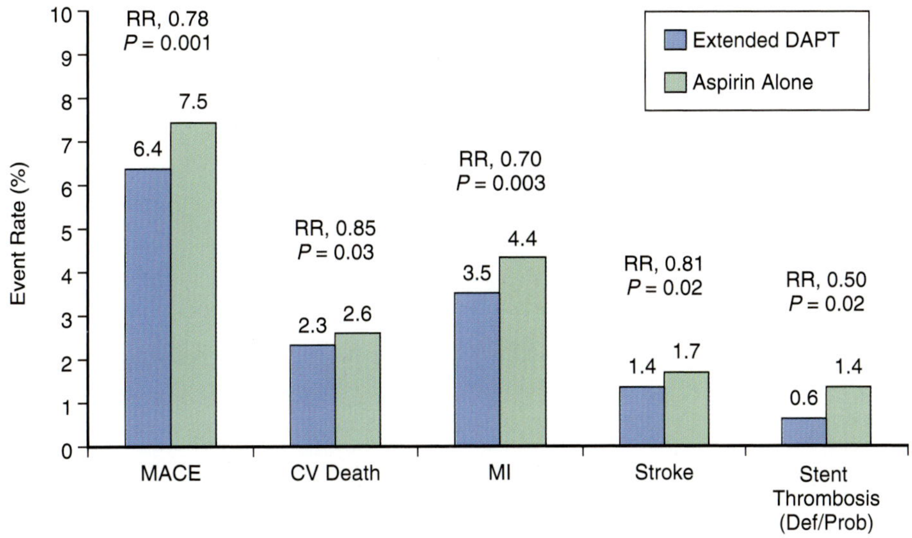

FIGURE 35-10 Rates of ischemic outcomes with extended dual-antiplatelet therapy with aspirin and a P2Y$_{12}$ inhibitor (*blue*) versus aspirin alone (*green*) for long-term secondary prevention after myocardial infarction. *CV,* Cardiovascular; *MACE,* major adverse cardiac event; *RR,* risk ratio.

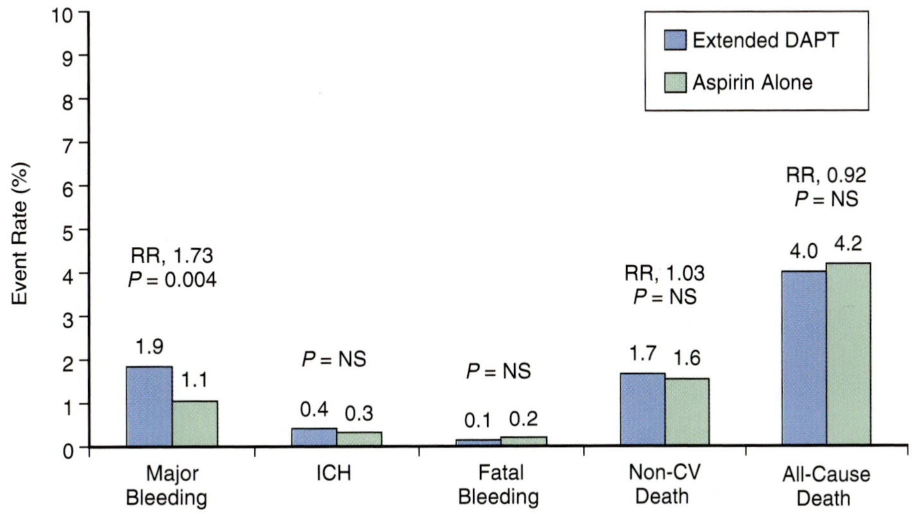

FIGURE 35-11 Rates of safety outcomes with extended dual-antiplatelet therapy with aspirin and a P2Y$_{12}$ inhibitor (*blue*) versus aspirin alone (*green*) for long-term secondary prevention after myocardial infarction. *CV,* Cardiovascular; *ICH,* intracranial hemorrhage; *NS,* not significant; *RR,* relative risk.

Overall, vorapaxar significantly reduced the primary endpoint of cardiovascular death, MI, or stroke (HR, 0.87; 95% CI, 0.80 to 0.94; $P < .001$) at 3 years. Vorapaxar increased the rate of bleeding, including GUSTO-defined moderate or severe bleeding, with an ARI of 1.7% (0.57% per year) (HR, 1.66; 95% CI, 1.43 to 1.93; $P < .001$) and intracranial hemorrhage (HR, 1.94; 95% CI, 1.39 to 2.70; $P < .001$). There was heterogeneity in the risk of intracranial hemorrhage with vorapaxar by symptomatic vascular bed, with the highest risk in those with a history of stroke (ARI, 1.5%; 2.4% with vorapaxar versus 0.9% with placebo; $P < .001$) relative to those without a history of stroke (ARI, 0.2%; 0.6% with vorapaxar group versus 0.4% with placebo; $P = .049$).[33] As a result, the drug was subsequently approved for clinical use on the basis of its overall efficacy; however, vorapaxar is contraindicated in patients with previous stroke or TIA owing to the increased risk of intracranial hemorrhage in that population.[35]

In the subgroup of 17,779 patients with previous MI (including those with previous stroke/TIA), vorapaxar reduced the primary endpoint rate by 20%, translating to an ARR of 1.6% at 3 years (0.53% per year) (Figure 35-12) in the composite of cardiovascular death, MI, or stroke when added to aspirin (98%) and clopidogrel (78%).[36] Vorapaxar also reduced the incidence of first ischemic stroke and stent thrombosis.[37,38] GUSTO-defined moderate or severe bleeding was increased with vorapaxar, with an ARI of 1.3% at 3 years (0.43% per year; HR, 1.61; 95% CI, 1.31 to 1.97; $P < .001$). As in the DAPT trials, the rates of intracranial hemorrhage (0.6% versus 0.4%; HR, 1.54; 95% CI, 0.96 to 2.48; $P = .076$) and fatal bleeds (0.2% versus 0.1%; HR, 1.56; 95% CI, 0.67 to 3.60; $P = .30$) were low and not significantly different between the randomized treatment groups.[36] The net outcome all-cause mortality, MI, stroke, or GUSTO-defined severe bleeding at 3 years was significantly reduced with vorapaxar in the post-MI population (ARR, 1.3%; HR, 0.86; 95% CI, 0.78 to 0.95; $P = .003$). Of note, vorapaxar had consistent efficacy in reducing cardiovascular death, MI, or stroke in patients planned for aspirin

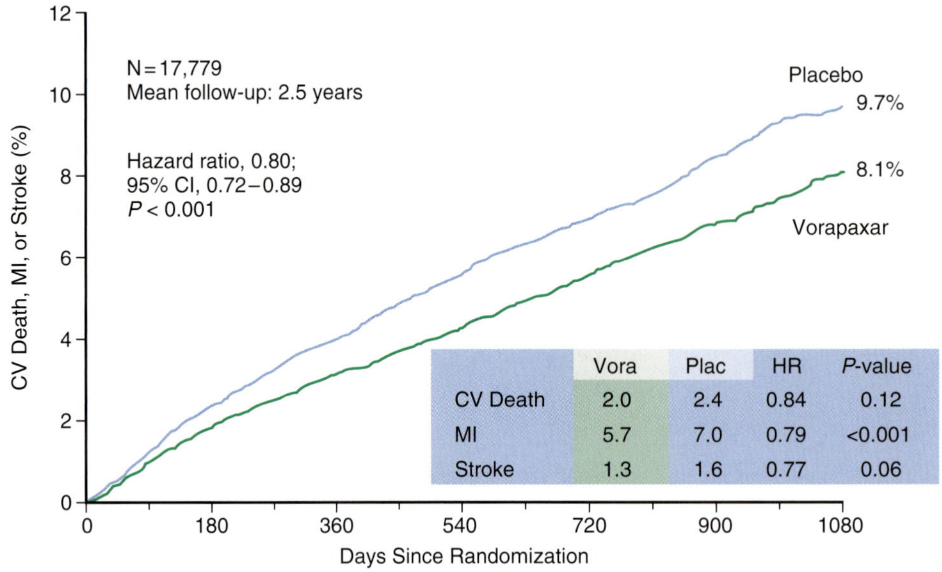

	Vora	Plac	HR	*P*-value
CV Death	2.0	2.4	0.84	0.12
MI	5.7	7.0	0.79	<0.001
Stroke	1.3	1.6	0.77	0.06

FIGURE 35-12 Cardiovascular (CV) death, myocardial infarction (MI), or stroke at 3 years with vorapaxar versus placebo in patients with a history of MI. The table shows event rates at 3 years, hazard ratios (HRs), and *P*-values. *(Adapted from Scirica BM, Bonaca MP, Braunwald E, et al: Vorapaxar for secondary prevention of thrombotic events for patients with previous myocardial infarction: a prespecified subgroup analysis of the TRA 2°P-TIMI 50 trial.* Lancet *380:1317-1324, 2012.)*

monotherapy (HR, 0.75; 95% CI, 0.60 to 0.94; *P* = .011) and those planned for DAPT with aspirin and clopidogrel (HR, 0.80; 95% CI, 0.70 to 0.91; *P* < .001).[39] The risk for bleeding with vorapaxar also was similar regardless of background thienopyridine use (*P*-interaction, .37). This analysis confirmed that PAR-1 antagonism was efficacious for secondary prevention after MI when added to aspirin alone or DAPT with aspirin and clopidogrel.[39] Insufficient experience with coadministration of vorapaxar with prasugrel or ticagrelor has accumulated to permit conclusions regarding efficacy or safety.

Bleeding with Long-Term Antiplatelet Therapy

Aspirin monotherapy increases the risk of bleeding, primarily gastrointestinal bleeding but also intracranial hemorrhage. Although rates vary in secondary prevention studies, in dedicated analyses, it is estimated that aspirin causes an excess of 4 major GI bleeds per 1000 patients per year of therapy.[19] The increase in hemorrhagic stroke has been estimated to be 1 in 2500 patients per year of therapy.[40]

The addition of clopidogrel to aspirin in stable patients treated in the CHARISMA trial resulted in increased GUSTO moderate or severe bleeding, with an ARI of 1.2% at a median of 28 months (0.51% per year; 3.7% versus 2.5%; HR, 1.48; 95% CI, 1.24 to 1.78; *P* < .001). This increase was driven primarily by moderate bleeding (HR, 1.63; 95% CI, 1.27 to 2.09; *P* < .001), with consistent trends in severe bleeding (HR, 1.25; 95% CI, 0.97 to 1.62; *P* = .087) and fatal bleeding (HR, 1.53; 95% CI, 0.83 to 2.82; *P* = .17).[41] Although the DAPT trial included patients with stable coronary disease and no history of ACS as well as a secondary prevention group of patients, the safety with prolonged DAPT was similar to that seen in CHARISMA (Figure 35-13). At 18 months an excess of GUSTO moderate or severe bleeding was seen, with an ARI of 1.0% (0.66% per year; 2.5% versus 1.6%; HR, 1.61; 95% CI, 1.21 to 2.16; *P* = .001), driven primarily by moderate bleeding (ARI of 0.7% at 18 months; *P* = .004). There were numerically more GUSTO severe (38 versus 26) and fatal bleeds (7 versus 4) with clopidogrel, but the differences were not statistically significant.[27] The absolute increase in bleeding risk was similar in patients with and those without previous MI.[28]

A similar pattern of bleeding risk was present in PEGASUS-TIMI 54. An ARI in TIMI major bleeding at 3 years of 1.24% was noted for the 60-mg dose (0.41% per year) and 1.54% for the 90-mg dose (0.51%).[30] TIMI-defined minor bleeding also was significantly increased, with an ARI of 0.82% for the 60-mg dose (0.27% per year) and 0.95% for the 90-mg dose (0.32%).[30] The composite of fatal bleeding or intracranial hemorrhage was numerically higher for both the 60-mg (33 [0.72%]) and the 90-mg (32 [0.63%]) doses relative to placebo (30 [0.60%]), but differences were not statistically significant.[30]

A meta-analysis of trials evaluating DAPT with aspirin and a $P2Y_{12}$ inhibitor versus aspirin monotherapy showed findings for bleeding similar to those in the individual trials.[31] The absolute excess in major bleeding was 0.8% (HR, 1.73; *P* = .004), but even with more than 33,000 patients, there was no statistically significant difference in the rate of intracranial hemorrhage or fatal bleeding[31] (see Figure 35-11).

Among patients without a history of stroke or TIA, vorapaxar increases the risk of GUSTO moderate or severe bleeding, with an ARI of 1.3% at 3 years (0.43% per year; *P* < .001). As seen with antiplatelet agents with other mechanisms of action in this population, there were more intracranial hemorrhages with vorapaxar than with placebo (0.6% versus 0.4%; HR, 1.46; 95% CI, 0.92 to 2.31; *P* = .10), but this finding did not reach statistical significance. When patients were stratified by intended background therapy, the absolute increases in GUSTO moderate or severe bleeding were similar in patients on background aspirin only (ARI, 0.5% per year) and in patients on background aspirin and clopidogrel (ARI, 0.3% per year).

Summary Across Trials

Overall, the risk of bleeding with these antiplatelet therapies in outpatients with previous MI at low bleeding risk (e.g.,

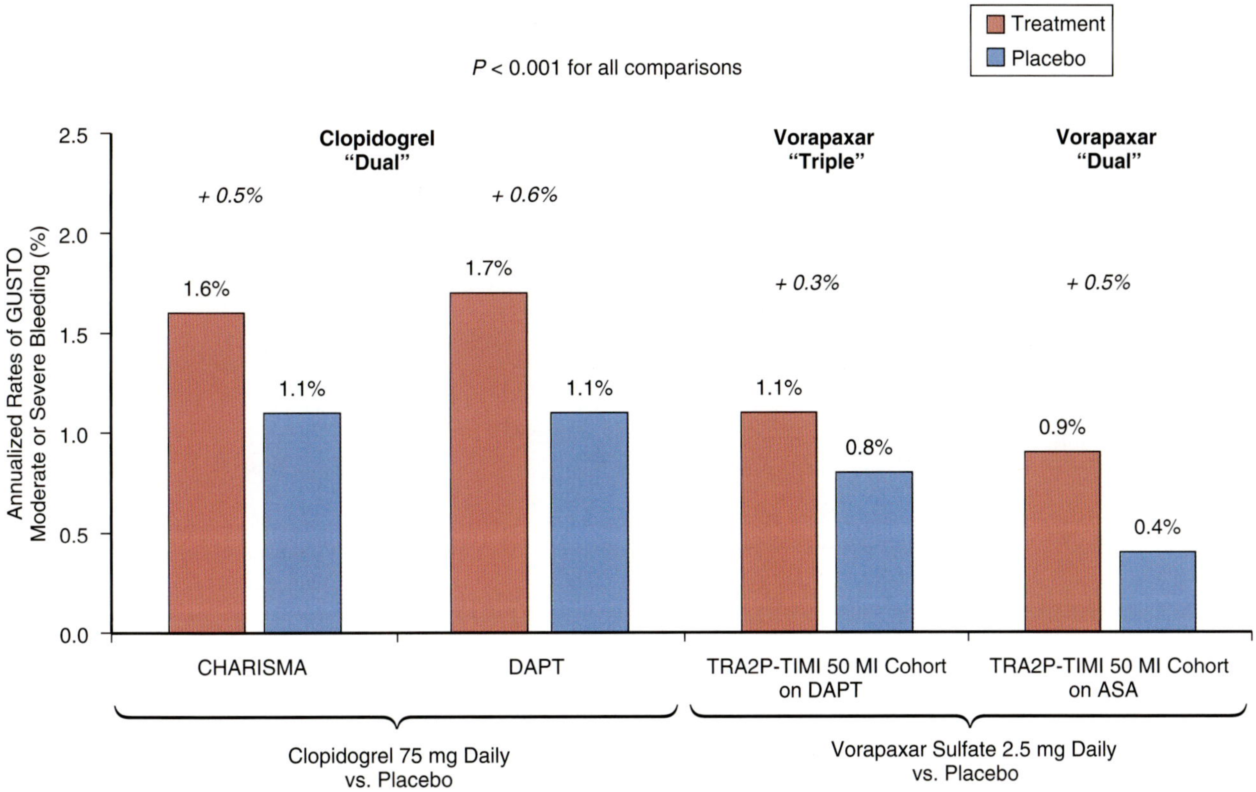

FIGURE 35-13 **GUSTO-defined moderate or severe bleeding at 1 year with clopidogrel (*red*) versus placebo (*blue*) added to aspirin in the CHARISMA trial[41] (*first from left*) and the DAPT trial[27] (*second from left*) as well as with vorapaxar versus placebo in TRA2P-TIMI 50 added to aspirin and clopidogrel[39] (*third from left*) and aspirin monotherapy[39] (*far right*).** See text for details. *ASA,* Acetylsalicylic acid; *MI,* myocardial infarction.

selected for trials, no history of stroke) generally is consistent and on the order of 0.5% per year (see Figure 35-13). Aspirin increases the risk of ICH (approximately 0.04% per year increase) compared with placebo. The addition of a $P2Y_{12}$ inhibitor to aspirin, or a PAR-1 antagonist to either aspirin or aspirin plus clopidogrel, does not appear to result in statistically significant further increases in the risk of ICH or fatal bleeding in selected patients without previous stroke/TIA. These are, however, rare safety events, and none of the individual trials has been powered to solely detect differences in fatal bleeding or intracranial hemorrhage in the MI subgroups.

Withdrawal of Antiplatelet Therapy in Patients with Previous Myocardial Infarction

Duration of $P2Y_{12}$ inhibitor therapy has generally been tied to the most recent unstable coronary event and/or the type of stent used, with the perspective that withdrawal of therapy in the stable phase generally is benign. This practice has been supported by findings from ACS trials that show the greatest divergence in treatment groups early on, when patients are at highest risk.[42] However, observations from registries and in the DAPT trial raise the hypothesis that withdrawal of $P2Y_{12}$ inhibition may result in heightened short- and long-term ischemic risk. In DAPT, there appeared to be a heightened ischemic risk in the $P2Y_{12}$ withdrawal group (see Figure 35-8) within the first 3 months of randomization (12 months after coronary stenting). In addition, this risk appeared in the continuation group at 30 months when $P2Y_{12}$ inhibition was stopped (see Figure 35-8).[27] In a subsequent analysis in the PEGASUS-TIMI 54 trial, patients were grouped by the time from their last dose of a $P2Y_{12}$ inhibitor to the point of randomization.[43] Patients randomly assigned to receive placebo (a median of 1.7 years from their most recent MI) who were withdrawn from a $P2Y_{12}$ inhibitor recently (within 30 days) had the highest risk, followed by those who stopped between 30 days and 1 year, and then patients who had been stable on aspirin monotherapy for more than a year (Figure 35-e3).[43] Although these populations were different at baseline, even after adjustment, the withdrawal of a $P2Y_{12}$ inhibitor within 30 days was associated with a more than two-fold increase in the rate of cardiovascular death, MI, or stroke at 90 days and a significantly increased hazard ratio (adjusted HR, 1.47; 95% CI, 1.12 to 1.93).[43] Furthermore, the efficacy of ticagrelor was greater (*P*-interaction = .0097) in patients who continued or restarted within 30 days (27% relative risk reduction in cardiovascular death, MI, or stroke) than in those who were withdrawn from therapy (7.7% versus 9.9% at 3 years) (Figure 35-14).[43]

These data fit with the notion introduced earlier that patients with previous MI have an underlying disease state associated with an increased risk of atherothrombotic complications that persists well after their initial ischemic event, and that is independent of whether or not they have been treated with a coronary stent. Withdrawal of antithrombotic therapy, even more than a year from MI, may unmask this thrombotic potential, resulting in ischemic complications. In addition, patients who survive on aspirin alone without ischemic complications for an extended period (beyond 1 year) may represent a de facto lower risk group.

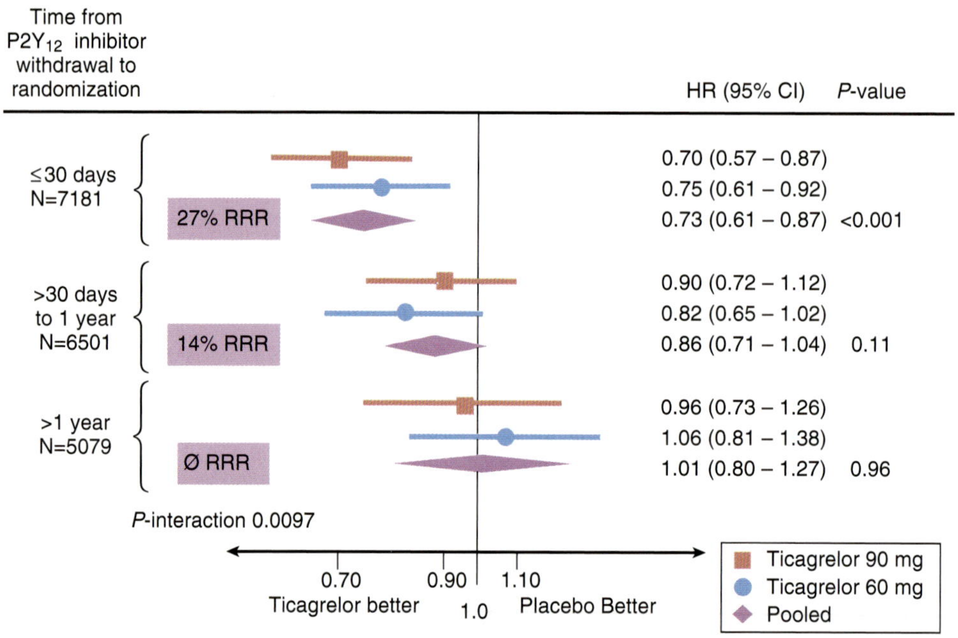

FIGURE 35-14 **The reduction in cardiovascular (CV) death, myocardial infarction (MI), and stroke with ticagrelor 60 mg twice daily (*blue*), ticagrelor 90 mg twice daily (*red*), and both ticagrelor doses pooled (*purple*) stratified by time from last dose of a $P2Y_{12}$ inhibitor to institution of ticagrel regimen or placebo in PEGASUS-TIMI 54 trial.** *HR,* Hazard ratio; *RRR,* relative risk reduction. *(Adapted from Bonaca MP, Bhatt DL, Steg PG, et al: Ischaemic risk and efficacy of ticagrelor in relation to time from P2Y12 inhibitor withdrawal in patients with prior myocardial infarction: insights from PEGASUS-TIMI 54.* Eur Heart J *2015 Oct 21. pii: ehv531. Epub ahead of print.)*

Patient Selection: Subgroups and Risk Stratification

As described earlier, among the full spectrum of persons with atherosclerotic vascular disease, patients with previous MI are at increased long-term risk for recurrent atherothrombosis and have the clearest benefit with more intensive antiplatelet regimens.[36,44,45] By contrast, patients with previous stroke have unfavorable net clinical outcomes with long-term intensive antiplatelet therapy, owing to an increase in intracranial bleeding.[10,46-49] Because bleeding is the primary side effect of potent antiplatelet regimens, particularly with prolonged exposure, patients with clear indicators of heightened risk generally have been excluded from trials (e.g., recent bleeding or surgery, history of intracranial bleeding, known bleeding diathesis).[30] Although trial populations generally are highly selected, and the risk reduction with more potent antiplatelet regimens relative to placebo generally is consistent across subgroups of patients with previous MI, differences in absolute risk may translate to greater or lesser absolute risk reductions. These differences in absolute risk may have significant impact on net outcomes.

In the TRA2°P-TIMI 50 trial, patients with diabetes mellitus at enrollment had approximately twice the risk of cardiovascular death, MI, or stroke at 3 years relative to that in patients without diabetes (15.7% versus 7.9%).[50] Although the relative effect of vorapaxar on the primary endpoint was similar in patients with and those without diabetes (*P*-interaction = .51), by nature of their greater absolute risk, patients with diabetes had a robust ARR of 3.1% at 3 years (1.0% per year), with a resulting number needed to treat (NNT) of 30, as compared with patients without diabetes, with an ARR of 1.1% at 3 years and NNT of 76.[50] This benefit translated to a significant reduction in the net outcome of all-cause mortality, MI, stroke, or GUSTO-defined severe bleeding (HR, 0.77; 95% CI, 0.65 to 0.93; *P* = .006) in the diabetic population.[50] Therefore diabetics with previous MI are at heightened risk, and the addition of vorapaxar to either aspirin or aspirin and clopidogrel for long-term secondary prevention appears to result in significant net benefit. Other subgroups of patients who share this heightened absolute risk and greater absolute benefit include those with previous MI and a history of coronary artery bypass grafting surgery (with a predominance of multivessel coronary disease).

In the PEGASUS-TIMI 54 trial, patients with previous MI and non–end-stage renal dysfunction, manifesting as an estimated glomerular filtration rate (eGFR) of less than 60 mL/min, had approximately twice the rate of cardiovascular death, MI, or stroke at 3 years reported for patients with eGFR of 60 or greater (13.99% versus 7.43%).[51] Although no statistical interaction was found in the relative efficacy of ticagrelor with baseline renal function, by nature of their higher absolute risk, patients with eGFR below 60 had an ARR of 2.7% (0.9% per year), resulting in an NNT of 37.[51] Although patients with impaired renal function were at heightened risk for bleeding overall, this did not translate to excessively higher rates of TIMI-defined major bleeding with ticagrelor versus placebo.

Risk Scores

Because patients may have several risk characteristics (e.g., age, diabetes, renal dysfunction), individual subgroup estimates from trials may reflect only one dimension of risk. Risk scores provide a mechanism to assess an individual's risk by assessing all of their risk factors in an integrated model. Although risk scores have been developed to assess individual risk in stable ischemic heart disease, not all have been demonstrated to differentiate the benefit of antiplatelet therapy.[52]

A risk score developed among patients enrolled in the TRA2°P-TIMI 50 trial demonstrated a significant gradient of risk in the placebo arm.[39] The benefit and risk of vorapaxar was then assessed by number of risk elements (i.e., 0, 1-2, 3 or more). Classifying patients into low-, intermediate-, or high-risk categories also identified a gradient in the benefit

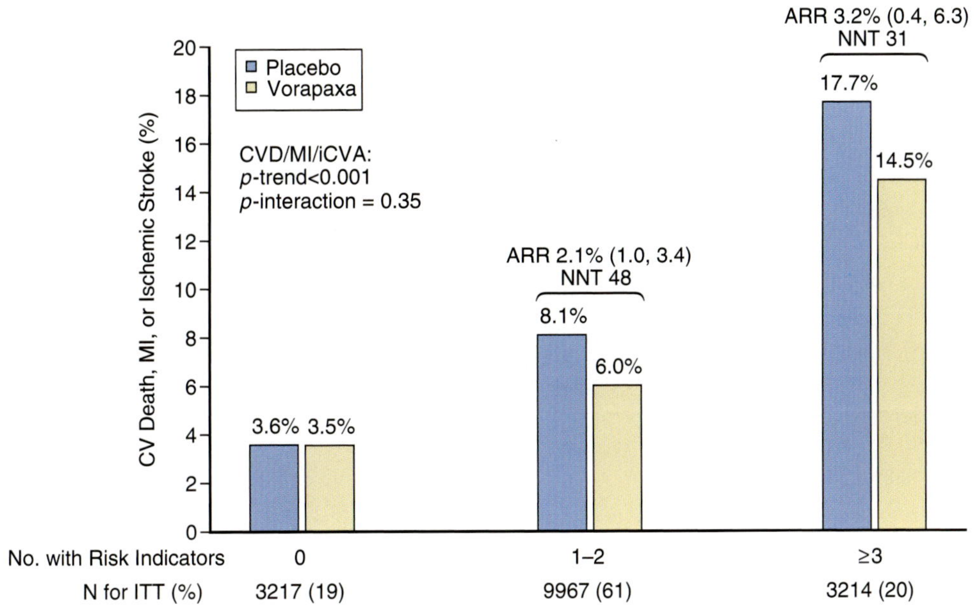

FIGURE 35-15 The absolute risk difference in the composite of cardiovascular (CV) death, myocardial infarction (MI), or stroke with vorapaxar versus placebo in patients with previous MI and no history of stroke or transient ischemic attack (TIA) by risk score category (0, *left*; 1-2, *middle*; ≥3, *right*). *ARR*, Absolute risk reduction; *ITT*, Intention-to-treat analysis *NNT*, number needed to treat.

of vorapaxar, with no benefit in patients with a risk score of 0, an ARR of 2.1% (NNT = 48) in those with 1 or 2 risk elements, and an ARR of 3.2% (NNT = 31) in those with 3 or more risk factors (Figure 35-15). Conversely, the risk of bleeding with vorapaxar was greatest in patients with a score of 0 (ARI 0.6%) as compared with those with 1 or 2 risk elements (ARI 0.1%) or those with 3 or more risk elements (ARI 0.0%).

Similarly, a score to predict the net benefit of prolonged DAPT after coronary stenting was derived from the DAPT trial.[28] The derivation of this score differed from that in TRA2°P-TIMI 50 in that instead of predicting absolute ischemic risk and then looking at the efficacy and safety of therapy, the DAPT score was derived to predict the magnitude of net benefit directly. Several patient and angiographic characteristics were independently associated with the benefit of prolonged DAPT and assigned an integer weight. When stratified at a score of 2, patients with a score below 2 had a smaller ARR in MI or stent thrombosis at 18 months (ARR, 0.52%) relative to patients with a DAPT score of 2 or higher (ARR, 1.90%) (Figure 35-16). At the same time, patients with a DAPT score below 2 had more bleeding with DAPT (ARI, 1.44%) at 18 months relative to those who had a DAPT score of 2 or higher (ARI, 0.38%) (see Figure 35-16).

Although such risk scores require validation in other data sets and with other agents, they represent a potential mechanism for individualizing the ischemic risk of a post-MI patient and evaluating their benefit and risk with more long-term potent secondary prevention with antiplatelet therapy.

PRACTICAL APPROACH TO ANTIPLATELET THERAPY AFTER MYOCARDIAL INFARCTION

Although the evidence from large randomized, controlled trials supports the efficacy of antiplatelet therapy for long-term secondary prevention of adverse events after MI, the multiple options for selection of individual agents and their combinations as well as the need to balance bleeding risk have complicated application of these findings in clinical practice. This section outlines our strategy for treatment with antiplatelet agents for secondary prevention after MI (Figure 35-17).

On the basis of the design of the supporting clinical trials and possible heterogeneity in the benefit of therapy based both on time and stability after MI, we structure our decision making by first considering whether the patient is within 1 year of the most recent ACS. Patients whose most recent ischemic event is more distant in time (e.g., 2 years ago) and who have been event-free on aspirin monotherapy for more than a year have shown themselves to be more stable and, broadly considered, appear to derive less benefit from additional antiplatelet therapy. Nevertheless, risk stratification in this latter population may identify individuals at persistent higher atherothrombotic risk who would benefit from the addition of a $P2Y_{12}$ inhibitor and/or a PAR-1 antagonist.

Patients Within 1 Year from the Most Recent Myocardial Infarction

The risk of recurrent atherothrombosis is highest during the first year after an MI, and net clinical outcomes are clearly improved by adding another antiplatelet agent to aspirin during this period, with the exception of subgroups of patients with contraindications to antithrombotic therapy or at particularly high risk for serious bleeding. In patients without a history of previous stroke or TIA, very low body weight, or advanced age, we adhere to current professional society guidelines and use a third-generation $P2Y_{12}$ inhibitor (ticagrelor or prasugrel). Among patients receiving clopidogrel as the $P2Y_{12}$ inhibitor, vorapaxar provides further reduction in major cardiovascular events. Insufficient experience has accumulated to allow assessment of the efficacy and safety of vorapaxar on top of ticagrelor or prasugrel. In counterbalancing the risk of bleeding and considerations of cost of therapy, it appears reasonable to be selective in choosing

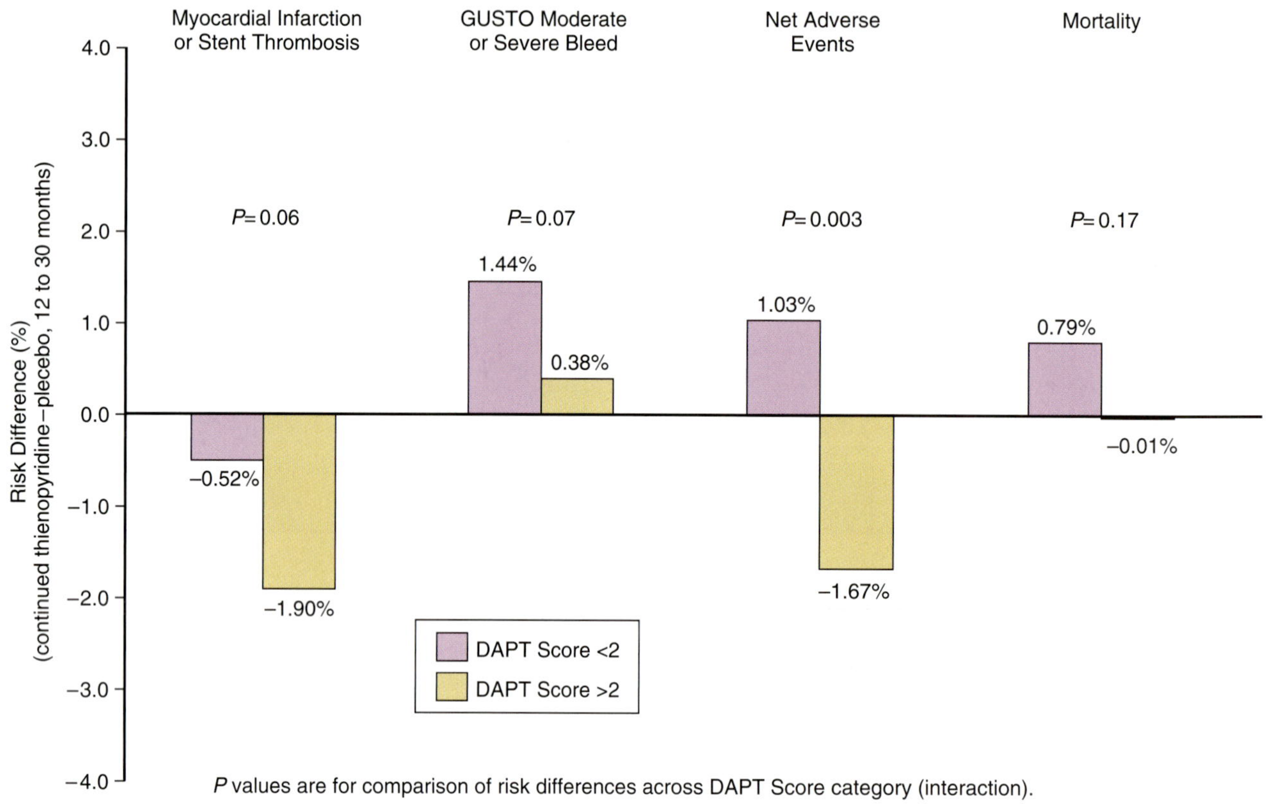

FIGURE 35-16 The absolute risk difference in efficacy and safety events with extended-duration clopidogrel versus placebo on a background of aspirin, stratified by DAPT risk score (<2 in *purple*, >2 in *yellow*). *(From Yeh RW, Secemsky E, Kereiakes DJ, et al: LBCT 03: individualizing treatment duration of dual antiplatelet therapy after percutaneous coronary intervention: an analysis from the DAPT study.* JAMA *315:1735-1749, 2016.)*

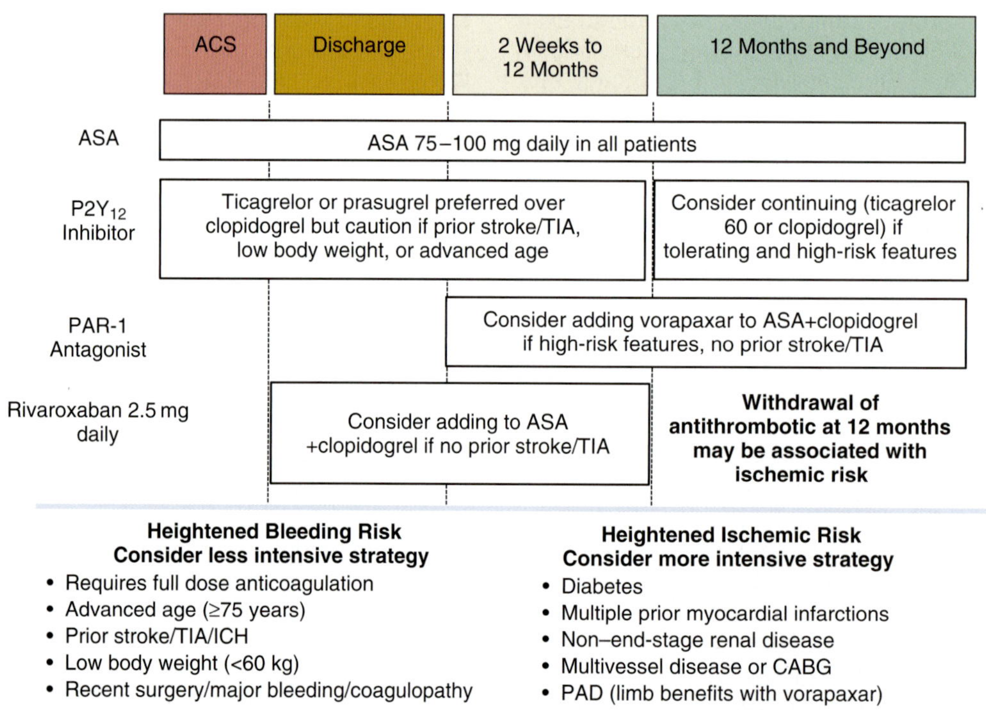

FIGURE 35-17 A schema for considering antiplatelet and anticoagulant therapies as secondary prevention after myocardial infarction. *ACS,* Acute coronary syndrome; *ASA,* acetylsalicylic acid [aspirin]; *CABG,* coronary artery bypass grafting; *ICH,* intracranial hemorrhage; *PAD,* peripheral arterial disease; *PAR-1,* protease-activated receptor 1; *TIA,* transient ischemic attack.

candidates for "triple" antiplatelet therapy. Net clinical outcomes with the addition of vorapaxar are most favorable in patients with high-risk features (e.g., diabetes mellitus, previous bypass surgery, heightened risk as indicated by a clinical risk score). An alternative strategy that has shown efficacy in this setting, started early after stabilization from ACS, is the addition of rivaroxaban 2.5 mg (a very-low-dose anticoagulant); however, this therapy is not currently approved for this indication in the United States (see Chapter 21).

Patients at 1 Year from Myocardial Infarction

At 1 year from MI, patients should be evaluated for a long-term antiplatelet strategy. Important considerations include assessing their ischemic risk versus their bleeding risk (e.g., previous stroke/TIA, low body weight, known bleeding diathesis) and their demonstrated ability to tolerate antiplatelet therapy. We generally continue the $P2Y_{12}$ inhibitor in patients with high-risk ischemic features as studied in clinical trials (e.g., age of 65 years or older, non–end-stage renal dysfunction, diabetes mellitus [treated], multiple previous MIs, or multivessel coronary disease) who are tolerating the combination of aspirin and a $P2Y_{12}$ inhibitor. Patients receiving clopidogrel as their $P2Y_{12}$ inhibitor also may benefit from the addition or continuation of vorapaxar for long-term secondary prevention. As already described, risk stratification for recurrent atherothrombosis is useful in identifying candidates for the addition of vorapaxar.

For patients who are being treated with ticagrelor 90 mg twice daily and will continue the $P2Y_{12}$ inhibitor, the ticagrelor dose should be down-titrated to 60 mg twice daily, because this regimen has been shown to have similar efficacy and better tolerability in the setting of long-term secondary prevention. Patients who are withdrawn from therapy may be at heightened risk for ischemic events, particularly in the ensuing 3 months. This risk is apparent even beyond 1 year from MI.

Patients Beyond 1 Year from Myocardial Infarction

In patients who are tolerating DAPT with aspirin and a $P2Y_{12}$ inhibitor or vorapaxar, we generally continue therapy for long-term secondary prevention unless new concerns for increased bleeding risk have emerged. Patients receiving aspirin monotherapy who last took a $P2Y_{12}$ inhibitor within the past year may benefit from adding ticagrelor 60 mg twice daily, clopidogrel, or vorapaxar, particularly if they have indicators of high atherothrombotic risk. Selected patients who have done well for more than a year on aspirin alone and had no ischemic complications were unlikely to benefit from the addition of ticagrelor 60 mg twice daily or vorapaxar; however, subgroups within this stable population may still be at high ischemic risk (e.g., those with diabetes, polyvascular disease, or multiple previous MIs). Additional data from clinical risk scores, biomarkers, and genetics are likely to continue to improve risk stratification in this population.

When to Stop $P2Y_{12}$ Inhibitor or Protease-Activated Receptor 1 Antagonist Therapy

Currently only limited data are available for reliably predicting bleeding risk within populations of patients with previous MI. Patients with previous stroke or TIA, previous intracranial bleeding, low body weight, bleeding diathesis, or history of spontaneous bleeding are likely to be at heightened bleeding risk and generally should be considered for shorter durations of intensive regimens. Patients without these factors who are tolerating therapy generally should continue. Persons who are unable to tolerate therapy on account of bleeding or other adverse effects may choose to stop. It should be recognized that in trials of antiplatelet therapy, patients most often stop for adverse events, including bleeding episodes, that generally are categorized as "nonserious" by clinical trial standards. Patients whose management plan includes frequent procedures requiring treatment cessation also may choose to stop. Future risk scores may identify additional characteristics or dynamic factors that improve prediction of bleeding risk.

SUMMARY

In addition to its near-term complications, MI reflects an underlying diffuse and chronic condition with a natural history marked by a "stuttering" clinical course and by a substantial risk of recurrent atherothrombosis that extends for years beyond the initial acute event. This disease state is characterized by a risk not only of recurrent MI but also of future stroke and complications of peripheral arterial disease; events that lead to permanent disability and shorten lifespan. The history of MI, therefore, is an indication to the clinician of an underlying condition that warrants chronic treatment.

Antiplatelet therapy not only is effective in managing the acute event but also mitigates the long-term risk of recurrence. As with anticoagulant therapy for atrial fibrillation, an inherent risk of bleeding must be balanced against the potential prevention of irreversible harm such as ischemic stroke or MI, with this tradeoff warranted in selected patients. In the coming years, more sophisticated strategies for assessing this risk-benefit balance, including clinical risk models, genetics, and biomarkers, are likely to become available to facilitate such therapeutic risk stratification with increasing greater precision.

A number of open questions remain regarding the optimal type and duration of antiplatelet therapy after MI. The efficacy and safety of aspirin in the setting of third-generation $P2Y_{12}$ inhibitors are being evaluated in trials in patients with a history of ACS. The removal of aspirin offers the potential to simplify treatment regimens and reduce bleeding risk. Additionally, the efficacy and safety of vorapaxar when added to prasugrel or ticagrelor (with or without aspirin) are unknown. The optimal approach to antiplatelet therapy in patients with previous MI who require anticoagulation is unknown and under investigation.

References

1. Szczeklik A, Dropinski J, Radwan J, Krzanowski M: Persistent generation of thrombin after acute myocardial infarction, *Arterioscler Thromb* 12:548–553, 1992.
2. Bhatt DL, Eagle KA, Ohman EM, et al.: Comparative determinants of 4-year cardiovascular event rates in stable outpatients at risk of or with atherothrombosis, *JAMA* 304:1350–1357, 2010.
3. Jernberg T, Hasvold P, Henriksson M, et al.: Cardiovascular risk in post-myocardial infarction patients: nationwide real world data demonstrate the importance of a long-term perspective, *Eur Heart J* 36(19):1163–1170, 2015.
4. Rapsomaniki E, Stogiannis D, Emmas C, et al.: Health outcomes in patients with stable coronary artery disease following myocardial infarction; construction of a PEGASUS-TIMI-54 like population in UK linked electronic health records, *Eur Heart J* 35:363, 2014.
5. Steg PG, Bhatt DL, Wilson PW, et al.: One-year cardiovascular event rates in outpatients with atherothrombosis, *JAMA* 297:1197–1206, 2007.
6. Sabatine MS, Cannon CP, Gibson CM, et al.: Effect of clopidogrel pretreatment before percutaneous coronary intervention in patients with ST-elevation myocardial infarction treated with fibrinolytics: the PCI-CLARITY study, *JAMA* 294:1224–1232, 2005.

7. Bertrand ME, Rupprecht HJ, Urban P, et al.: Double-blind study of the safety of clopidogrel with and without a loading dose in combination with aspirin compared with ticlopidine in combination with aspirin after coronary stenting: the Clopidogrel Aspirin Stent International Cooperative Study (CLASSICS), *Circulation* 102:624–629, 2000.
8. Yusuf S, Zhao F, Mehta SR, et al.: Effects of clopidogrel in addition to aspirin in patients with acute coronary syndromes without ST-segment elevation, *N Engl J Med* 345:494–502, 2001.
9. Sabatine MS, Cannon CP, Gibson CM, et al.: Addition of clopidogrel to aspirin and fibrinolytic therapy for myocardial infarction with ST-segment elevation, *N Engl J Med* 352:1179–1189, 2005.
10. Wiviott SD, Braunwald E, McCabe CH, et al.: Prasugrel versus clopidogrel in patients with acute coronary syndromes, *N Engl J Med* 357:2001–2015, 2007.
11. Scirica B, Morrow D, Antman E, et al.: Timing and clinical setting of cardiovascular death or myocardial infarction following PCI for ACS—observations from the TRITON-TIMI 38 trial, *J Am Coll Cardiol* 59(13s1):E340, 2012.
12. Stone GW, Maehara A, Lansky AJ, et al.: A prospective natural-history study of coronary atherosclerosis, *N Engl J Med* 364:226–235, 2011.
13. Kidd S, Bonaca M, Scirica B, et al.: Universal classification system type of incident myocardial infarction in patients with stable atherosclerosis: observations from TRA 2°P-TIMI 50, *J Am Coll Cardiol* 63(12S), 2014.
14. Mozaffarian D, Benjamin EJ, Go AS, et al.: Heart disease and stroke statistics—2015 update: a report from the American Heart Association, *Circulation* 131(4):e29–e322, 2015.
15. Mozaffarian D, Benjamin EJ, Go AS, et al.: Heart disease and stroke statistics—2016 update: a report from the American Heart Association, *Circulation* 133(4):e38–e360, 2016.
16. Mega JL, Braunwald E, Wiviott SD, et al.: Rivaroxaban in patients with a recent acute coronary syndrome, *N Engl J Med* 366:9–19, 2012.
17. Antithrombotic Trialists' Collaboration: Collaborative meta-analysis of randomised trials of antiplatelet therapy for prevention of death, myocardial infarction, and stroke in high risk patients, *BMJ* 324:71–86, 2002.
18. Antithrombotic Trialists' (ATT) Collaboration, Baigent C, Blackwell L, et al.: Aspirin in the primary and secondary prevention of vascular disease: collaborative meta-analysis of individual participant data from randomised trials, *Lancet* 373:1849–1860, 2009.
19. Derry S, Loke YK: Risk of gastrointestinal haemorrhage with long term use of aspirin: meta-analysis, *BMJ* 321:1183–1187, 2000.
20. CURRENT-OASIS 7 Investigators, Mehta SR, Bassand JP, et al.: Dose comparisons of clopidogrel and aspirin in acute coronary syndromes, *N Engl J Med* 363:930–942, 2010.
21. CAPRIE Investigators: A randomised, blinded, trial of clopidogrel versus aspirin in patients at risk of ischaemic events (CAPRIE). CAPRIE steering committee, *Lancet* 348:1329–1339, 1996.
22. Yusuf S, Mehta SR, Zhao F, et al.: Early and late effects of clopidogrel in patients with acute coronary syndromes, *Circulation* 107:966–972, 2003.
23. Antman EM, Wiviott SD, Murphy SA, et al.: Early and late benefits of prasugrel in patients with acute coronary syndromes undergoing percutaneous coronary intervention: a TRITON-TIMI 38 (TRial to assess improvement in therapeutic outcomes by optimizing platelet InhibitioN with prasugrel-thrombolysis in myocardial infarction) analysis, *J Am Coll Cardiol* 51:2028–2033, 2008.
24. Wallentin L, Becker RC, Budaj A, et al.: Ticagrelor versus clopidogrel in patients with acute coronary syndromes, *N Engl J Med* 361:1045–1057, 2009.
25. Bhatt DL, Fox KA, Hacke W, et al.: Clopidogrel and aspirin versus aspirin alone for the prevention of atherothrombotic events, *N Engl J Med* 354:1706–1717, 2006.
26. Bhatt DL, Flather MD, Hacke W, et al.: Patients with prior myocardial infarction, stroke, or symptomatic peripheral arterial disease in the CHARISMA trial, *J Am Coll Cardiol* 49:1982–1988, 2007.
27. Mauri L, Kereiakes DJ, Yeh RW, et al.: Twelve or 30 months of dual antiplatelet therapy after drug-eluting stents, *N Engl J Med* 371:2155–2166, 2014.
28. Yeh RW, Secemsky E, Kereiakes DJ, et al.: LBCT 03: individualizing treatment duration of dual antiplatelet therapy after percutaneous coronary intervention: an analysis from the DAPT study, *JAMA* 315:1735–1749, 2016.
29. Bonaca MP, Bhatt DL, Braunwald E, et al.: Design and rationale for the Prevention of Cardiovascular Events in Patients With Prior Heart Attack Using Ticagrelor Compared to Placebo on a Background of Aspirin–Thrombolysis in Myocardial Infarction 54 (PEGASUS-TIMI 54) trial, *Am Heart J* 167:437–444.e5, 2014.
30. Bonaca MP, Bhatt DL, Cohen M, et al.: Long-term use of ticagrelor in patients with prior myocardial infarction, *N Engl J Med* 372:1791–1800, 2015.
31. Udell JA, Bonaca MP, Collet JP, et al.: Long-term dual antiplatelet therapy for secondary prevention of cardiovascular events in the subgroup of patients with previous myocardial infarction: a collaborative meta-analysis of randomized trials, *Eur Heart J* 37(4):390–399, 2016.
32. Bonaca MP, Morrow DA: SCH 530348: a novel oral thrombin receptor antagonist, *Future Cardiol* 5:435–442, 2009.
33. Morrow DA, Alberts MJ, Mohr JP, et al.: Efficacy and safety of vorapaxar in patients with prior ischemic stroke, *Stroke* 44:691–698, 2013.
34. Tricoci P, Huang Z, Held C, et al.: Thrombin-receptor antagonist vorapaxar in acute coronary syndromes, *N Engl J Med* 366:20–33, 2012.
35. Magnani G, Bonaca MP, Braunwald E, et al.: Efficacy and safety of vorapaxar as approved for clinical use in the United States, *J Am Heart Assoc* 4:e001505, 2015.
36. Scirica BM, Bonaca MP, Braunwald E, et al.: Vorapaxar for secondary prevention of thrombotic events for patients with previous myocardial infarction: A prespecified subgroup analysis of the TRA 2°P-TIMI 50 trial, *Lancet* 380:1317–1324, 2012.
37. Bonaca MP, Scirica BM, Braunwald E, et al.: New ischemic stroke and outcomes with vorapaxar versus placebo: Results from the TRA 2 degrees P-TIMI 50 trial, *J Am Coll Cardiol* 64:2318–2326, 2014.
38. Bonaca MP, Scirica BM, Braunwald E, et al.: Coronary stent thrombosis with vorapaxar versus placebo: Results from the TRA 2 degrees P-TIMI 50 trial, *J Am Coll Cardiol* 64:2309–2317, 2014.
39. Bohula EA, Bonaca MP, Aylward PE, et al.: Development of a TIMI risk score for stable ischemic heart disease. Abstract 17338, *Circulation* 132:A17338, 2015.
40. He J, Whelton PK, Vu B, Klag MJ: Aspirin and risk of hemorrhagic stroke: a meta-analysis of randomized controlled trials, *JAMA* 280:1930–1935, 1998.
41. Berger PB, Bhatt DL, Fuster V, et al.: Bleeding complications with dual antiplatelet therapy among patients with stable vascular disease or risk factors for vascular disease: results from the clopidogrel for high atherothrombotic risk and ischemic stabilization, management, and avoidance (CHARISMA) trial, *Circulation* 121:2575–2583, 2010.
42. Mehta SR, Yusuf S: Clopidogrel in Unstable angina to prevent Recurrent Events (CURE) Study Investigators: The Clopidogrel in Unstable angina to prevent Recurrent Events (CURE) trial programme; rationale, design and baseline characteristics including a meta-analysis of the effects of thienopyridines in vascular disease, *Eur Heart J* 21:2033–2041, 2000.
43. Bonaca MP, Bhatt DL, Steg PG, et al.: Ischaemic risk and efficacy of ticagrelor in relation to time from P2Y12 inhibitor withdrawal in patients with prior myocardial infarction: insights from PEGASUS-TIMI 54, *Eur Heart J*, 2015 Oct 21. pii: ehv531. [Epub ahead of print].
44. Bhatt DL, Flather MD, Hacke W, et al.: Patients with prior myocardial infarction, stroke, or symptomatic peripheral arterial disease in the CHARISMA trial, *J Am Coll Cardiol* 49:1982–1988, 2007.
45. Yeh RW, Kereiakes DJ, Steg PG, et al.: Benefits and risks of extended duration dual antiplatelet therapy after PCI in patients with and without acute myocardial infarction, *J Am Coll Cardiol* 65:2211–2221, 2015.
46. Morrow DA, Braunwald E, Bonaca MP, et al.: Vorapaxar in the secondary prevention of atherothrombotic events, *N Engl J Med* 366:1404–1413, 2012.
47. Sacco RL, Diener HC, Yusuf S, et al.: Aspirin and extended-release dipyridamole versus clopidogrel for recurrent stroke, *N Engl J Med* 359:1238–1251, 2008.
48. Diener HC, Sacco RL, Yusuf S, et al.: Effects of aspirin plus extended-release dipyridamole versus clopidogrel and telmisartan on disability and cognitive function after recurrent stroke in patients with ischaemic stroke in the prevention regimen for effectively avoiding second strokes (PRoFESS) trial: a double-blind, active and placebo-controlled study, *Lancet Neurol* 7:875–884, 2008.
49. Diener HC, Bogousslavsky J, Brass LM, et al.: Aspirin and clopidogrel compared with clopidogrel alone after recent ischaemic stroke or transient ischaemic attack in high-risk patients (MATCH): randomised, double-blind, placebo-controlled trial, *Lancet* 364:331–337, 2004.
50. Cavender MA, Scirica BM, Bonaca MP, et al.: Vorapaxar in patients with diabetes mellitus and previous myocardial infarction: findings from the thrombin receptor antagonist in secondary prevention of atherothrombotic ischemic events-TIMI 50 trial, *Circulation* 131:1047–1053, 2015.
51. Magnani G, Storey RF, Steg G, et al.: Efficacy and safety of ticagrelor for long-term secondary prevention of atherothrombotic events in relation to renal function: insights from the PEGASUS-TIMI 54 trial, *Eur Heart J* 37:400–408, 2016.
52. Ducrocq G, Wallace JS, Baron G, et al.: Risk score to predict serious bleeding in stable outpatients with or at risk of atherothrombosis, *Eur Heart J* 31:1257–1265, 2010.

36 Tackling the Problem of Adverse Ventricular Remodeling After Myocardial Infarction

Antonio Abbate

INTRODUCTION

Improvement in the acute treatment of myocardial infarction (MI) has made it possible for many patients to survive an initial MI and subsequently be exposed to the risk of recurrent MI and/or of heart failure (HF). The acute ischemic and reperfusion myocardial injury (see Chapter 24), as well as the acute hemodynamic effects of MI (see Chapter 25) and the potential complications of MI (see Chapter 26), are described elsewhere in this book (see also Chapter 13). The chronic consequences of MI leading to global structural and functional changes to the heart are summarized in a process known as *adverse ventricular remodeling*. The designation "adverse" refers both to the disadvantageous changes from a hemodynamic standpoint and to the negative prognostic implications of the process. This chapter reviews the definition of ventricular remodeling, its macroscopic and microscopic characteristics, and the therapeutic approaches to mitigation of adverse remodeling. The role of stem cell therapy in MI is, however, treated separately (see Chapter 22).

DEFINITION OF ADVERSE VENTRICULAR REMODELING

Experimental animal models and longitudinal follow-up studies in patients with large non-reperfused MI have led to the identification of a dynamic process involving the heart muscle occurring after the MI, yet separate and largely independent from the initial ischemic changes. The definition of ventricular (or cardiac) remodeling refers to changes in size, shape, thickness, and elastance of the left and/or right ventricles involving both the infarcted and noninfarcted myocardial segments, and leading to impairment of regional or global systolic contractility and of diastolic function (Table 36-1). The changes may progress for weeks and months after MI and lead to worsening left ventricular dilation and systolic dysfunction, HF symptoms, need for hospitalization, and premature death (Figure 36-1). Quantitative evaluation of ventricular remodeling can therefore be used to predict clinical outcome and the therapeutic effects of a drug or device intervention.[1]

Larger infarct size, greater extent of initial wall motion abnormalities, and greater initial reduction in global systolic function are all independent predictors of adverse ventricular remodeling (Table 36-2). Ventricular dilation, indeed, begets further dilation. Accordingly, in the pre-reperfusion era, adverse ventricular remodeling—defined as a significant increase in left ventricular end-diastolic volume (relative increase greater than 25%) or a reduction in left ventricular ejection fraction (LVEF) (decreasing to below 45%)—was seen in more than one half of MI survivors. The degree of adverse remodeling was associated with mortality, and despite close follow-up, the mortality rates in MI survivors after hospital discharge exceeded 5% and 10% at 1 and 12 months, respectively. The advent of reperfusion strategies has changed the treatment and revolutionized the natural history of MI (see Chapter 2 and Chapter 13). In the current reperfusion era with primary percutaneous coronary intervention (PCI), not only has acute in-hospital MI mortality significantly decreased, but a majority of MI survivors have preserved left ventricular systolic function (at discharge and at 1-year follow-up evaluation), and correspondingly, the 1-year survival rate for MI survivors generally is excellent (greater than 97%). Despite the marked improvement in survival, the incidence of HF after MI is rising.[2] This shifting incidence probably reflects multiple concurrent influences: (1) Higher-risk patients with MI are surviving the acute MI yet remain at risk for HF; (2) patients presenting with MI constitute an older age group than before and thus may have survived a previous MI, have more comorbid illnesses, and be at risk for preexisting HF; and (3) among today's physicians, recognition of HF symptoms has improved. Of note, not all patients with HF after MI have systolic dysfunction. Indeed, the incidence and prevalence of HF with preserved LVEF—"diastolic HF"[3]—are rising, reflecting that impairment in diastolic function can occur independently of changes in

TABLE 36-1 Structural and Functional Changes in Adverse Left Ventricular Remodeling

Infarct Segment	Edema Scar formation Contractile dysfunction Wall thinning → aneurysm formation
Border Zone Segment	Increased wall stress → infarct expansion Hypertrophy
Non-Infarct Segments	Increased wall stress Hypertrophy
Global Dimensions	Eccentric hypertrophy Dilation
Systolic Function	Regional → global dysfunction
Diastolic Function	Impaired relaxation Elevated filling pressures
Dimensions and Function of the Atria	Atrial enlargement Atrial fibrillation
Valvular Function	Functional mitral regurgitation Functional tricuspidal regurgigation
Electrical Function	Conduction block (AV block, BB block) Increased automaticity Reentrant tachycardia
Neuroautonomic Function	Increased sympathetic tone Decreased parasympathetic tone
Systemic Vascular Function	Increased systemic vascular resistance Systemic venous hypertension Reduced venous capacitance
Pulmonary Vascular Function	Pulmonary venous congestion Post-capillary arterial hypertension Reactive precapillary arterial hypertension

AV, Atrioventricular; *BB,* bundle branch.

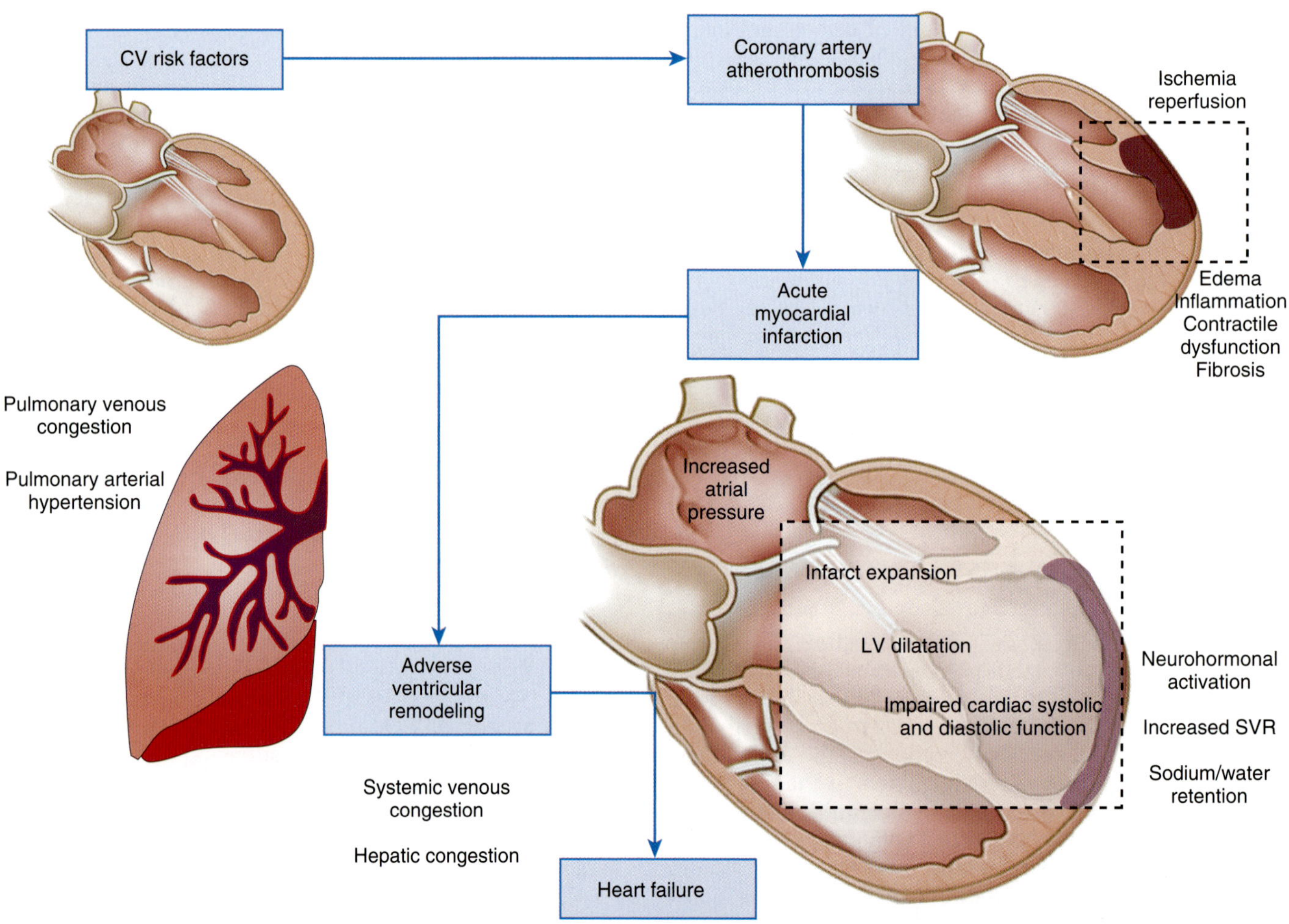

FIGURE 36-1 Adverse ventricular remodeling after acute myocardial infarction (MI). Acute coronary artery atherothrombosis is the most common cause of acute MI. The ensuing ischemia induces an acute injury to the myocardium and initiates an intense inflammatory response. The acute hemodynamic effects of MI are amplified by structural and functional changes in the infarct border zone and remote myocardium, and by a systemic neurohormonal and inflammatory response. Impaired cardiac systolic and diastolic function and increased filling pressures with pulmonary and systemic venous congestion lead to the syndrome of heart failure. *CV,* Cardiovascular; *LV,* left ventricular; *SVR,* systemic vascular resistance.

TABLE 36-2 Predictors of Adverse Left Ventricular Remodeling

Infarct Size	Length, mass, or volume Transmurality Microvascular obstruction (no reflow) Previous infarct in other segment(s) Anterior location
Wall Motion Abnormalities	Number of segment(s)
Systolic Function	Left ventricular ejection fraction Systolic strain pattern
Diastolic Function	Diastolic pattern (I-IV) Impaired LV filling (elevated E/E′ ratio) Diastolic strain pattern Filling pressures Natriuretic peptides
Cardiac Dimensions	End-diastolic and end-systolic diameter and volume Left ventricular mass
Valvular Function	Mitral regurgitation Aortic valvular regurgitation or stenosis
Clinical Conditions	Male sex Advanced age or other conditions of senescence Systemic arterial hypertension Diabetes mellitus Chronic glucocorticoid use
Biomarkers	Biomarkers of myocardial necrosis Leukocyte count with neutrophilia Red blood cell distribution width (RDW) C-reactive protein Galectin-3 Soluble ST2 Natriuretic peptides—brain natriuretic peptide (BNP), N-terminal pro-BNP (NT-proBNP)

E/E′ ratio, Ratio of transmitral E wave velocity to mitral annulus tissue Doppler velocity E′.

	Cardiomyocyte	Endothelial cell	Fibroblast	Leukocyte
Ischemic core/ infarct zone	Necrosis Apoptosis/necroptosis Stunning	Necrosis/apoptosis Loss of cell-cell contact Chemiotaxis	Necrosis/ apoptosis	Cytokine release Phagocytosis Release of proteases Cytotoxicity
Infarct border zone	Hibernation/hypertrophy Degeneration/vacuolization Apoptosis/pyroptosis	Neo-angiogenesis (granulation tissue)	Myofibroblast Collagen synthesis (scar formation)	Cytokine release Proteases Cytoxicity
Noninfarcted remote myocardium	Hypertrophy Apoptosis		Collagen synthesis (interstitial fibrosis)	
Role in promoting adverse ventricular remodeling	Loss of contractile myocardium Impaired diastolic function	Impaired tissue perfusion Inflammation	Scar formation Increased cardiac stiffness	Inflammatory injury

FIGURE 36-2 Contribution of the different cellular components in ventricular remodeling. The ventricular remodeling after acute myocardial infarction involves all the different cellular components. The cardiomyocyte represents the contractile structure of the heart, a loss of viable cells and/or an impairment in contractility or relaxation represent the central events in the progression toward adverse ventricular remodeling and heart failure. The entire myocardial structure needs to be preserved, however, for the cardiomyocytes to exert their contractile function resulting in cardiac systole. The myocardium has a very well-developed capillary structure. Endothelial cell dysfunction and/or injury undermine the tissue perfusion during acute myocardial infarction and infarct healing. The heart is rich in fibroblasts, responsible for creating and maintaining a strong interstitial connective tissue able to support the intense forces associated with cardiac systole. The fibroblasts are also responsible for creating a thick infarct scar opposing the tendency of the infarct area to deform and dilate (aneurysm). Leukocytes are recruited to the heart after ischemic injury, and while inflammation is necessary for infarct healing and debris clearance, an exaggerated inflammatory response can promote further injury and delay infarct healing.

global systolic function, and it is common in the general population, as well as in the post-MI population. In a recent study in patients with ST-elevation myocardial infarction (STEMI) a restrictive diastolic filling pattern at echocardiography was associated with a five-fold increased risk of HF or cardiogenic shock, even in those patients with preserved left ventricular systolic function, whereas the association of restrictive diastolic pattern and depressed left ventricular systolic function (LVEF less than 45%) was associated with greater than an eight-fold increased risk.

CELLULAR AND MOLECULAR MECHANISMS

Although the original description of adverse remodeling refers to macroscopic changes, research over the past decades has identified a cellular and molecular remodeling process that precedes and causes the macroscopic changes of ventricular remodeling. The myocardium is composed of cardiomyocytes, endothelial cells, fibroblasts, and resident and infiltrating leukocytes (see also Chapter 4). Each of these cellular components plays a role in preventing or promoting adverse ventricular remodeling (Figure 36-2).

Cardiomyocytes

Cardiomyocyte death is the hallmark of MI, and the release of sarcomere proteins (i.e., troponins) in the bloodstream is used to diagnose acute MI (see Chapter 6 and Chapter 7). The acute phase of cardiomyocyte death by oncosis or necrosis, referring to cell death with swelling and rupture, peaks within 24 to 48 hours of the onset of ischemia. Reperfusion provides rescue of the injured-but-salvageable cardiomyocytes but accelerates the demise of the nonsalvageable cardiomyocytes (see Chapter 24). Morphologic and molecular studies in acute MI have shown that multiple overlapping modalities of cell death contribute to the infarct core. Although the exact nature and nomenclature of cell death in MI is a subject of debate, apoptosis generally refers to a "silent"' form of cell death, and all these forms of cell death are characterized and differentiated from oncosis, by the fact that they are mediated by active, energy-dependent, signaling processes. Necroptosis also is referred to programmed cell death but while it is an energy-dependent, coordinated process, it shares morphologic features of necrosis (i.e., cell rupture). Loss of cardiomyocytes continues for days to weeks after MI, occurring mainly in the myocardium bordering the infarct (border zone), and promoting progression toward adverse ventricular remodeling and HF.[4]

The surviving cardiomyocytes in the border zone display structural and functional changes. These cells often are described as "degenerated," "myofibrillarlytic," "vacuolized," or "autophagic" cardiomyocytes and exist in a delicate balance between death and survival.[4] These changes lead to impaired contraction, with increased risk of infarct expansion and of arrhythmogenesis. Cardiomyocytes in the remote myocardium, by contrast, are subject to prohypertrophic stimuli such as increased wall stress (stretch) and locally or systemically released neurohormones—such as angiotensin II, aldosterone, and norepinephrine—or inflammatory mediators—such as interleukin-1β (IL-1β) and tumor necrosis factor-α (TNF-α). Increases in the cardiomyocyte cross-sectional area or volume (hypertrophy) and development of interstitial fibrosis without a parallel growth in the capillary bed lead to an imbalance between perfusion and demand as a consequence primarily of an impaired diffusion (increased distance between the capillary oxygen content and the cardiomyocyte mitochondria) and an impaired diastolic relaxation and increased intracavitary filling pressures, thereby further reducing the subendocardial perfusion gradient.

The imbalance in perfusion-versus-demand and the neurohormonal and proinflammatory milieu promote cardiomyocyte diastolic and systolic dysfunction and transition from prohypertrophy to proapoptosis signaling. This process results in further loss of viable myocardium, further stimulation of the compensatory mechanisms, in a vicious circle, leading to progressive ventricular remodeling and HF.[4] Loss of contractile function and impaired relaxation in cardiomyocytes are, therefore, major contributors to adverse ventricular remodeling and HF after MI (see Chapter 25).

Endothelial Cells

The endothelium regulates the transit of oxygen and nutrients between the blood and the cardiomyocytes. Endothelial cells are exquisitely sensitive to ischemia. Death of endothelial cells precedes and promotes cardiomyocyte death in ischemia, through the release of proapoptotic factors. There is no *restitutio ad integrum* (restoration to original condition) after infarction in the heart—largely owing to the fact that once the vascular integrity is compromised, the microvasculature is not reestablished in a functional way.[5] The capillary network in the infarct area resembles the granulation tissue in a wound with short, ectatic, and chaotically distributed capillaries. The endothelium also regulates adhesion and migration of the leukocytes during the repair phase. Proinflammatory changes in endothelial cells occur within minutes of onset of ischemia and persist for weeks. Loss of microvascular integrity is considered to be responsible for the lack of tissue level reperfusion despite the epicardial coronary revascularization that is occasionally seen in MI ("no reflow" phenomenon) and portends greater myocardium loss and adverse remodeling changes (see Chapter 24).[5]

Fibroblasts

The heart contains a large number of fibroblasts.[6] The interstitial collagen matrix in the myocardium is essential to maintain the myocardial structure compact during systole, when intense tension forces are applied. If the connective tissue was not present or if it had reduced tensile strength, the heart would "break" during systole by "leaking" at the points of least resistance. This matrix is carefully maintained by the resident fibroblasts. When the pressure in the heart increases, such as with systemic arterial hypertension or aortic valve stenosis, the collagen content increases in parallel. During acute MI, the infarct area undergoes a necrotic process that significantly reduces the tensile strength. Leukocyte-derived collagenases further weaken the infarct area by breaking up connective tissue. As a compensatory mechanism to the increased wall stress (stretch), fibroblasts proliferate and differentiate into myofibroblasts, which align along the ventricular wall, providing a partial contraction during systole and producing large amounts of collagen. These changes provide an opposing resistance to the systolic forces that would promote outward excursion of the infarct zone and rupture.[6] Inflammatory cytokines, however, inhibit fibroblast proliferation and collagen synthesis, so unresolved inflammation delays infarct healing and repair (see also Chapter 4).

In the pre-reperfusion era, when infarcts were larger and more likely to be fully transmural, the incidence of cardiac rupture 3 to 5 days after MI was not negligible, with reported rates of 1% to 2%. With prompt reperfusion, the wavefront phenomenon of ischemic death is aborted, and the infarct more often involves 25% to 75% of the ventricular wall, leaving an epicardial rim of viable myocardium, and making cardiac rupture rather rare (less than 0.1%).

Another critical role of the fibroblast is the synthesis of collagen to progressively substitute the infarct area with a fibrotic scar. Although impairment in collagen deposition reduces tensile strength and promotes dilation and aneurysm formation, excessive collagen deposition may promote HF by increasing ventricular stiffness, leading to diastolic dysfunction and impaired filling.

Leukocytes

Leukocytes occupy a central role in the tissue response to injury (see also Chapter 4).[7] During MI, myocardial inflammation peaks between 24 and 96 hours and then gradually resolves within 2 to 4 weeks. Injury is associated with the release of danger-associated molecular patterns triggering the formation of a macromolecular structure, the inflammasome, which initiates and amplifies the inflammatory response by releasing large amounts of IL-1β and IL-18. Although some degree of inflammation probably is necessary for normal healing, an exuberant inflammatory response promotes myocardial dysfunction, edema, infarct expansion, cell death in cardiomyocytes in the border zone, and worsening systolic and diastolic function. Resolution of the inflammatory response is a physiologic response that limits unnecessary edema, stiffness, and dysfunction. A delay in inflammation resolution, therefore, represents an additional potential pathogenetic mechanism of adverse ventricular remodeling.

Elevated levels of C-reactive protein (CRP) and other inflammatory biomarkers measured at hospital admission, during the first 2 to 5 days, or at discharge consistently predict adverse ventricular remodeling and HF.[8] Elevated CRP levels independently predict impaired diastolic function in patients with acute MI, independent of impaired systolic function.

DETERMINANTS OF ADVERSE VENTRICULAR REMODELING

Timely Reperfusion and "No Reflow"

Infarct size is the single most important predictor of adverse remodeling, and it is linearly dependent on the amount of myocardial salvage by reperfusion ("time is muscle"). As such, lack of timely reperfusion due to ineffective treatment or delayed presentation portends an unfavorable prognosis. Impaired tissue-level reperfusion, or "no reflow," relates to persistence of microvascular obstruction despite epicardial coronary artery patency.[5] Reduction of time to reperfusion—including initiation of treatment before hospital arrival and optimization of antiplateletet and anticoagulant therapies—appears to favor more complete reperfusion, to prevent no-reflow, and to combat adverse remodeling changes (see Chapter 13). The exact duration of the myocardial salvage window in patients with MI is not established (Figure 36-3). In the early fibrinolysis trials, the benefits of reperfusion were largest within the first 6 hours and minimal between 13 and 24 hours (see Chapter 15). By contrast, in a study in which primary PCI for MI was performed between 12 and 48 hours, primary PCI led to measurable myocardial salvage as compared with medical therapy and a subsequent survival benefit at 4-year follow-up versus medical therapy alone.[9]

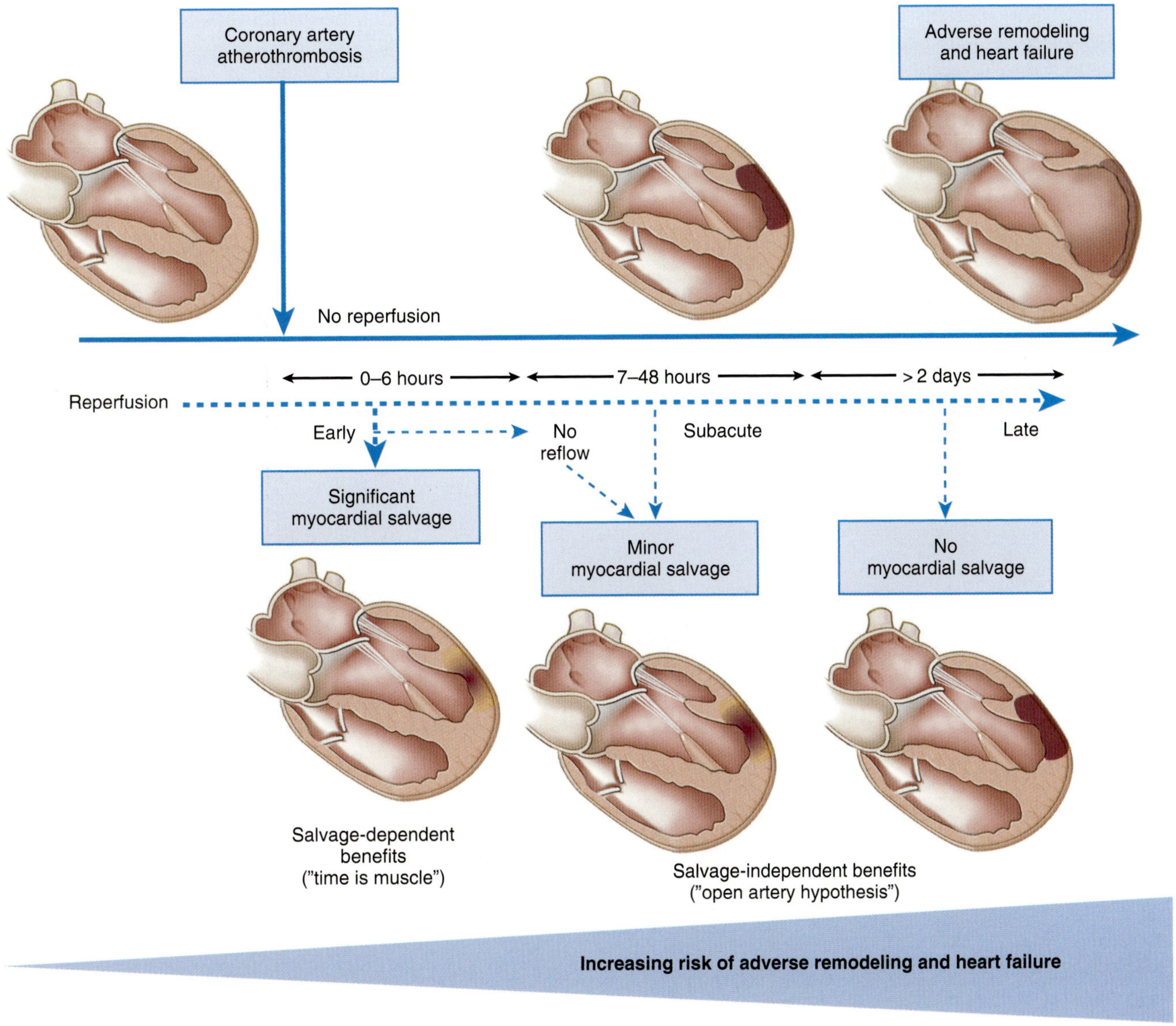

FIGURE 36-3 Effect of reperfusion on adverse remodeling and heart failure. Prompt reperfusion during acute myocardial infarction prevents adverse ventricular remodeling and heart failure by providing significant, time-dependent myocardial salvage. In the pre-reperfusion era, large transmural infarcts were associated with early cardiac dilation, wall rupture, heart failure, and cardiac death. Impaired tissue reperfusion despite epicardial coronary artery patency ("no reflow") or delayed reperfusion leads to a significantly smaller extent of myocardial damage, with improved clinical outcomes, compared with no reperfusion. Late reperfusion, beyond the window of opportunity for myocardial salvage, is considered to be potentially beneficial in selected patients, providing time- and salvage-independent protection ("open artery hypothesis").

Delayed Reperfusion and the "Open Artery Hypothesis"

Patients who have not received early reperfusion are at significantly higher risk for adverse remodeling, HF, and death. The "open artery hypothesis" postulates that compared with no reperfusion, a delayed reperfusion of the infarct-related artery provides a benefit that is independent of infarct sparing and, at least in part, time-independent. This hypothesis was largely based on longitudinal analysis of data from reperfusion trials in which it was apparent that patients with a patent infarct-related artery had a survival advantage after hospital discharge that remained highly statistically significant even after correction for infarct size and baseline left ventricular ejection fraction. The results of prospective randomized clinical trials, however, only partially support this hypothesis. The largest clinical trial randomly assigned more than 2000 patients 3 to 21 days after MI to undergo PCI or receive medical therapy and failed to show any advantage of late revascularization of a totally occluded artery. However, a meta-analysis of 5 studies, including an echocardiographic substudy within the largest trial, showed a beneficial effect of late revascularization of a totally occluded artery on left ventricular remodeling.[10] The benefits of late revascularization were enhanced when the meta-analysis included studies also enrolling patients with significant yet non–totally occlusive disease of the infarct-related artery,[9] suggesting that recurrent ischemia of the infarct border zone may jeopardize infarct healing and/or ventricular remodeling, and/or promote arrhythmias.

Hypertrophic Response

Compensatory hypertrophy of the noninfarcted myocardium segments is, at least in part, protective. The ratio of the left ventricular diameter to wall thickness reflects the progression of the hypertrophic response relative to the magnitude of dilation. When the dilation prevails, it is referred to as *eccentric hypertrophy*, which is characterized by initially preserved cardiac output but also is linked to progressive dilation and systolic dysfunction (Figure 36-4). This pattern is seen more commonly in males.[11] When the hypertrophy prevails, the pattern is called *concentric hypertrophy*, which is protected from progressive dilation but also is associated with more significant acute hemodynamic compromise, with significantly elevated filling pressures and reduced cardiac output. This pattern is seen more commonly in females[11] (see Figure 36-4).

Cell Death, Senescence, and Regeneration

Postmortem studies in patients with recent MI and animal experimental studies show that cardiomyocyte death in the infarct, border zone, and remote myocardium continues for days and weeks after the initial insult, promoting adverse ventricular remodeling.[4] The roles of senescence and regeneration in MI and HF are not fully established. Advanced age and other conditions promoting senescence and/or impairing regeneration ability (i.e., cancer, chemotherapy, chronic inflammatory or autoimmune disease, immunosuppressive therapies) are associated with significantly worse ventricular remodeling.

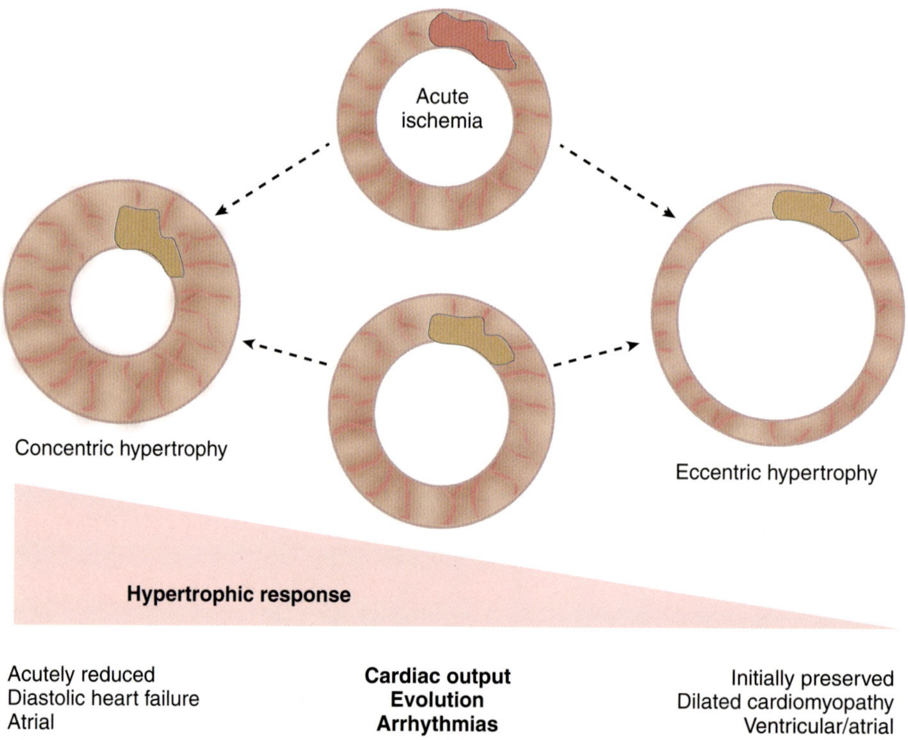

FIGURE 36-4 Role of the hypertrophic response in ventricular remodeling. The loss of viable contractile myocardium induces an increased stress on the surviving myocardium which, in turn, triggers a hypertrophic response. The intensity of the hypertrophic response varies among individuals. It is affected by sex, cavitary dimensions, and afterload. The compensatory hypertrophic response may be sufficient to normalize wall stress without providing any negative effects. An insufficient hypertrophic response is associated with ventricular dilation (eccentric hypertrophy), which serves well to initially preserve cardiac output by allowing for an increased end-diastolic volume but ultimately generates more wall stress and promotes evolution toward a dilated cardiomyopathy, with increased risk for ventricular and atrial arrhythmias. An exuberant hypertrophic response may impair the initial compensatory increase in end-diastolic volume, leading to acutely reduced cardiac output and increased cardiac filling pressures (diastolic heart failure), while maintaining normal systolic function and preventing evolution toward dilated cardiomyopathy (concentric hypertrophy). Patients with concentric hypertrophy are at lower risk for ventricular arrhythmias yet remain at increased risk for atrial arrhythmias.

Fibrotic Response

As discussed earlier, impaired collagen synthesis may promote ventricular dilation and aneurysm formation; however, an exuberant response may make the ventricle excessively stiff with consequent impairment of left ventricular filling (Figure 36-5). Biomarkers of collagen synthesis and turnover predict adverse ventricular remodeling.[12]

Afterload, Preload, and Wall Stress

Increased wall stress (stretch) induces prohypertrophic, profibrotic, and proapoptotic signals in the heart. Preexisting systemic arterial hypertension is common in patients with MI and predicts unfavorable ventricular remodeling. This increased risk often is related to the presence of left ventricular hypertrophy, which makes the myocardium more sensitive to ischemia and to changes in preload and afterload. Elevated ventricular filling pressures during MI, secondary to impaired relaxation and/or fluid retention, reflect more severe hemodynamic compromise and predict worse outcome. Accordingly, patients with significant aortic valvular stenosis have a similar unfavorable profile during MI. Aortic or mitral valvular insufficiency, leading to increased preload, generally are better tolerated but also provide an increased wall stress and stimulate ventricular dilation. Markers of abnormal wall stress—that is, natriuretic peptides—predict adverse cardiac remodeling and HF after MI.

Neurohormonal Activation

The translation of results of preclinical studies of neurohormonal blockade to clinical trials in MI has been one of the greatest scientific and clinical successes in cardiology. In experimental models, large unreperfused MI induces an intense activation of the renin-angiotensin-aldosterone and sympathetic adrenergic systems. These systems respond to injury and hypoperfusion and are highly conserved through evolution. During acute MI, as a consequence of ischemia and injury, contractility drops and filling pressures rise, leading to a reduction in stroke volume and reflex vasoconstriction and tachycardia in an attempt to maintain an adequate perfusion of vital organs. Although these mechanisms are essential for the immediate survival during large MI, they also promote adverse ventricular remodeling and HF by favoring extension of the infarct size secondary to increased demand, infarct expansion from increased wall stress, and compensatory eccentric hypertrophy in response to increased afterload (Figure 36-6). The larger the infarct size and the initial hemodynamic compromise, the greater the degree of neurohormonal activation and more likely the progression toward adverse ventricular remodeling. In keeping with these observations, inhibitors of the angiotensin-converting enzyme (ACE) (or blockers of the angiotensin receptor), β-adrenergic receptor blockers, and aldosterone antagonists all reduce the likelihood and severity of adverse ventricular remodeling in high-risk MI (i.e., large-infarct and MI associated with depressed LVEF or HF symptoms).

Inflammation

More than a century ago, physicians noted that a low-grade fever during MI portended a poor prognosis. A long list of inflammatory biomarkers (see Chapter 8) have been shown to predict cardiac rupture, worse ventricular remodeling, HF,

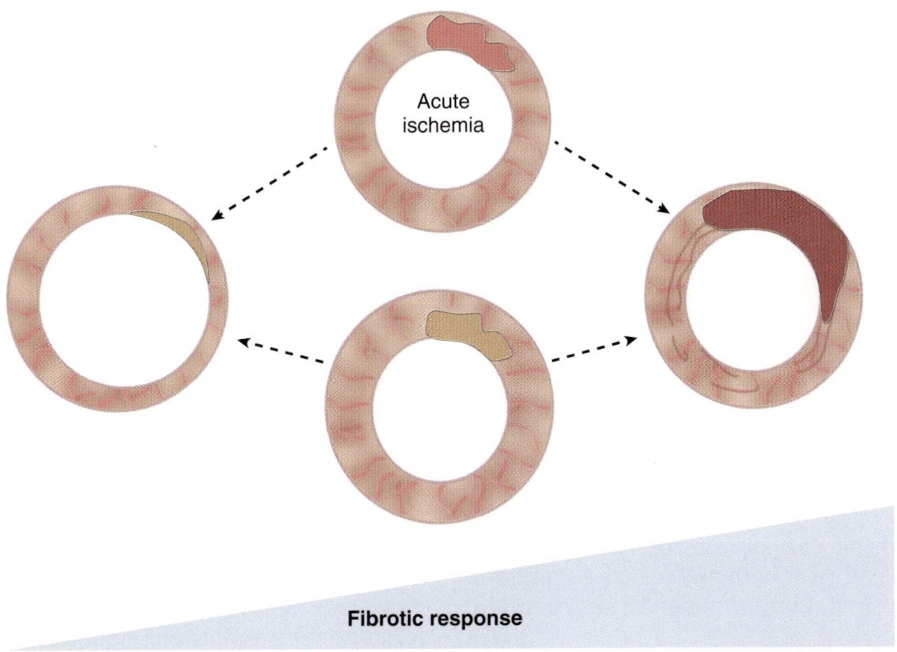

Increased risk	**Cardiac rupture**	Reduced risk
Increased risk	**Aneurysm formation**	Reduced risk
Reduced	**Cardiac stiffness**	Increased
Dilated cardiomyopathy	**Evolution**	Diastolic heart failure

FIGURE 36-5 Role of the fibrotic response in ventricular remodeling. The infarcted myocardium is substituted by a fibrotic scar. Interstitial fibrosis also is increased in the noninfarcted myocardium in response to the increased wall stress. If a strong scar fails to form and the tensile strength of the cardiac wall is reduced, the risk of cardiac rupture and aneurysm formation is increased, in association with evolution toward dilated cardiomyopathy. On the other hand, if the fibrotic response is exuberant, then the cardiac stiffness is overly increased, and although the risk of rupture and aneurysm formation is reduced, filling pressures are markedly increased (leading to diastolic heart failure).

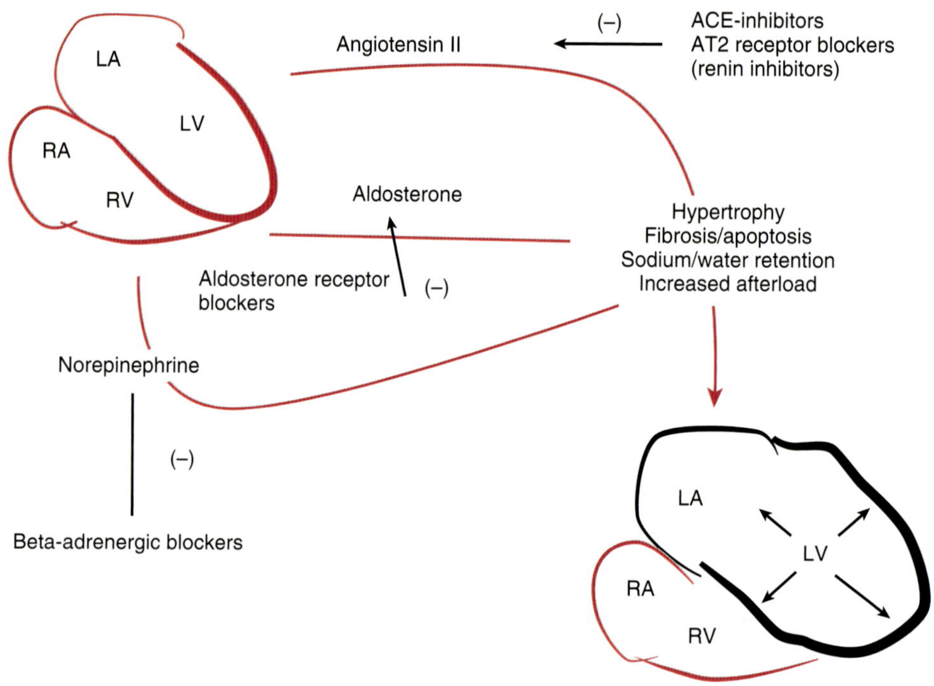

FIGURE 36-6 Neurohormonal activation and ventricular remodeling. The initial tissue injury and the hemodynamic consequences initiate a systemic neurohormonal activation characterized by the activation of the renin-angiotensin-aldosterone system and the neuroadrenergic sympathetic nervous system. Although these responses have been evolutionarily conserved to preserve mean arterial pressure during hypotension and may therefore be, in part, necessary for immediate survival in patients with acute cardiogenic shock, the same neurohormones promote the adverse ventricular remodeling and heart failure by directly promoting further cardiomyocyte loss and increased cardiac stiffness, and indirectly by promoting sodium and water retention by the kidneys and increasing afterload acting on the systemic vascular resistance. Neurohormonal blockade in patients with acute myocardial infarction is shown to prevent adverse remodeling, prevent heart failure, and prolong survival. *ACE,* Angiotensin-converting enzyme; *AT2,* angiotensin II; *LA,* left atrium; *LV,* left ventricle; *RA,* right atrium; *RV,* right ventricle.

and death after MI independently of other variables such as infarct size or left ventricular systolic function, suggesting that an overzealous inflammatory response may promote further injury and adverse remodeling.[7]

In light of the enhanced ability of mankind to reduce microbial infection (due to improved hygiene conditions) and to fight them (with antimicrobials), the biology of the inflammatory response to injury now appears redundant. Toll-like and Nod-like receptors (TLR and NLR) and other sensors are essential to detect microbial infection, activate the inflammasome, and initiate the inflammatory response. The TLR and NLR receptors and the inflammasome, however, also are activated in sterile injury such as acute MI (see also Chapter 4).[13] In the absence of a microbial factor, the inflammatory response generally is excessive in relation to the extent of injury. Although some degree of response is necessary to recruit leukocytes and clear the tissue debris, inflammation becomes itself a mechanism of disease. The mechanisms by which inflammation promotes further injury are related to promotion of cardiomyocyte death (by apoptosis or pyroptosis), impaired contractile function of the surviving cardiomyocytes, destruction of the interstitial tissue leading to reduced tensile strength of the myocardium, and impaired formation of a structured infarct scar (Figure 36-7).

Cardiac Electrical and Neuroautonomic Remodeling

Ventricular and atrial arrhythmias are significantly more common in patients with HF. The structural changes in heart muscle, primarily dilation and fibrosis, promote reentry and other arrhythmogenic mechanisms. In parallel with the changes in structure, the electrical function of the cardiomyocyte also is altered, and these changes too are considered to promote arrhythmias. Such functional changes are not the passive result of injury but rather energy-requiring adaptations known as cardiac electrical remodeling.[14] The exact mechanisms and the clinical implications of electrical remodeling are not well understood to date. The heart is innervated by the sympathetic and parasympathetic nervous systems. HF is characterized by an imbalance in sympathetic/parasympathetic tone, with increased sympathetic tone and blunted parasympathetic tone, which is considered to be another mechanism by which adverse remodeling promotes arrhythmias (see Chapter 28).[15]

TACKLING ADVERSE VENTRICULAR REMODELING IN CLINICAL PRACTICE

Ventricular remodeling is an established surrogate marker for disease severity after MI.[1] Using the HF classification from the American College of Cardiology/American Heart Association (ACC/AHA), ventricular enlargement or dysfunction is referred to as "HF stage B"—structural heart disease predisposing to HF. Indeed, more extensive remodeling predicts HF symptoms, need for hospitalization for HF, and premature death due to HF or arrhythmias. Moreover, treatments that have shown to combat adverse ventricular remodeling also reduce late mortality related to MI. It is therefore a standard of care to assess cardiac dimensions and systolic function during the initial hospitalization in patients with acute MI, and then again within 6 months to identify high-risk subjects (see Chapter 13 and Chapter 30).

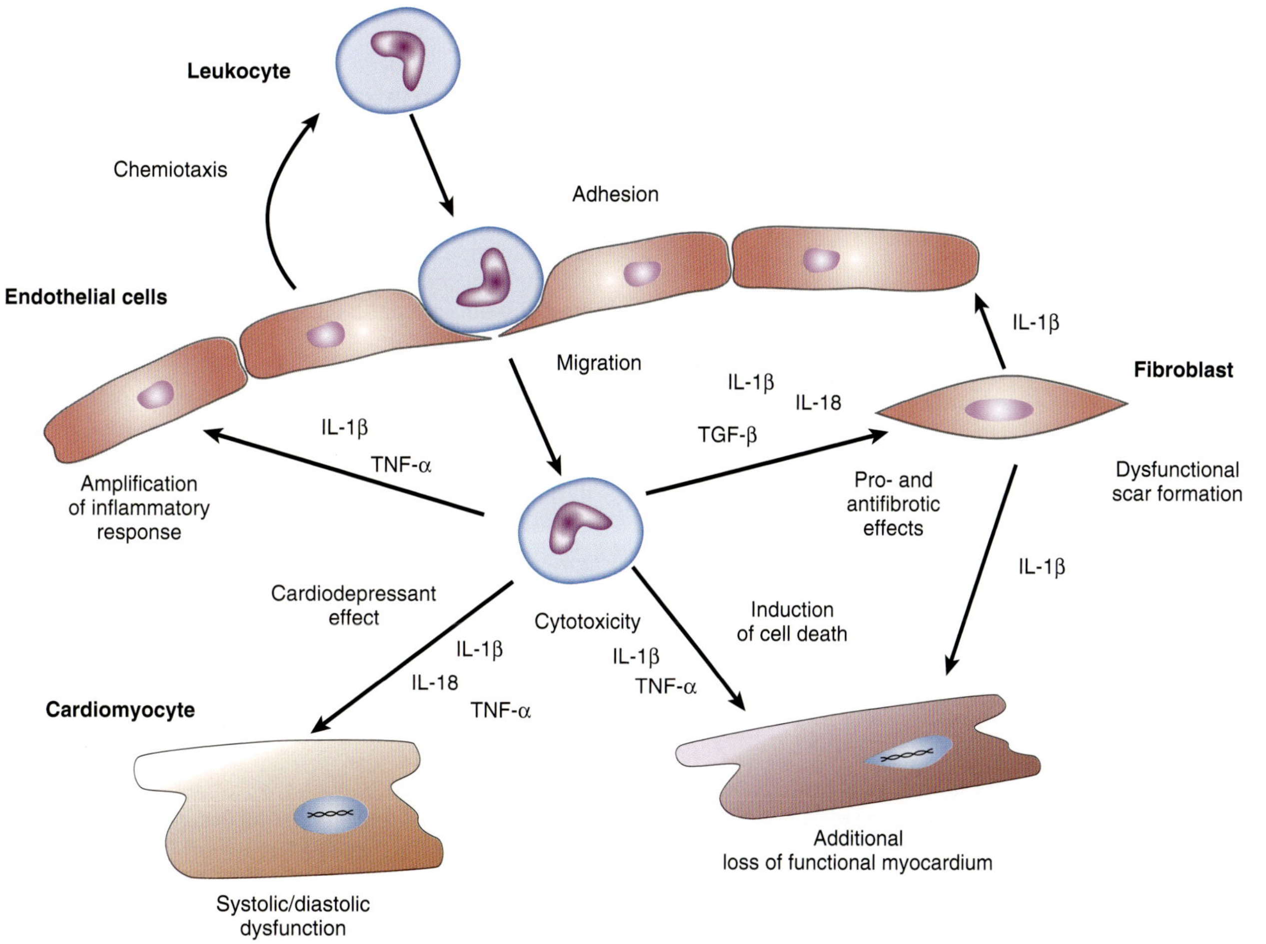

FIGURE 36-7 Role of the leukocyte in the postinfarction inflammatory response. Leukocytes are recruited to the infarct area through the release of chemokines and the expression of adhesion molecules by endothelial cells. Activated leukocytes amplify the inflammatory response and promote further myocardial injury and dysfunction through the release of pro-inflammatory cytokines (interleukin-1β [IL-1β], interleukin-18 [IL-18], tumor necrosis factor-α [TNF-α], and transforming growth factor-β [TGF-β]) and through direct cytotoxicity.

Guideline-Recommended Medical Therapy

As discussed previously, timely reperfusion during MI is the mainstay of MI therapy and the first step in limiting infarct size and decreasing the likelihood of adverse remodeling. Once reperfusion and/or stabilization have been achieved, adjunctive medical therapy is indicated for the prevention of adverse ventricular remodeling (Table 36-3). Moreover, the ACC/AHA guidelines recommend stratification for the risk of HF in the patient with MI.

Angiotensin and Aldosterone Blockers

The use of ACE inhibitors in patients with AMI represents one of most illustrious successes of translational research. Research in animals with AMI had shown activation of systemic and regional activation of the renin-angiotensin system and identified in the ACE a limiting step in cascade. Reduction of angiotensin II levels with ACE inhibitors significantly improved the ventricular remodeling process, preventing adverse remodeling. The benefits on remodeling and HF were reproduced in phase II and III clinical trials and contributed to a significant reduction in AMI mortality in the pre-reperfusion era. Those clinical trials, however, showed that the benefits that accrued for the different blockers of the renin-angiotensin-aldosterone system were mostly limited to those patients already showing signs of adverse remodeling before initiation of therapy (i.e., left ventricular enlargement or systolic dysfunction). Those patients with small infarct sizes or small areas of wall motion abnormalities and preserved global systolic function tended to do well, independently of treatment. With the advent of prompt reperfusion, infarct size tends

TABLE 36-3 Medical Therapy to Prevent or Treat Adverse Ventricular Remodeling

MEDICATION	RECOMMENDATIONS IN PATIENTS WITH ACUTE MI (IN ABSENCE OF CONTRAINDICATIONS)
β-Adrenergic receptor blocker(s)	• All patients (class I, LOE B)
Angiotensin-converting enzyme (ACE) inhibitor(s)	• All patients (class IIa, LOE A) • Symptomatic heart failure (class I, LOE A) • LVEF <40% (class I, LOE A) • Anterior location (class I, LOE A)
Angiotensin receptor blocker(s)	As an alternative to ACE inhibitor(s) (class I, LOE B)
Aldosterone antagonist(s)	In addition to ACE inhibitor(s) if LVEF <40% and: • Symptomatic heart failure (class I, LOE B) • Diabetes mellitus (class I, LOE B)

LOE, Level of evidence; *LVEF*, left ventricular ejection fraction; *MI*, myocardial infarction.

to be smaller and the initial hemodynamic effects tend to be less pronounced. The efficacy of these inhibitors in the setting of reperfused AMI with preserved left ventricular systolic function is not established, so treatment with angiotensin or aldosterone blockers is recommended for those patients with MI and either reduced global systolic function, symptoms of HF, anterior infarct location in STEMI, or diabetes (see also Chapter 25).

β-Adrenergic Blockers

β-Adrenergic blockers (β-blockers), on the other hand, are recommended for oral therapy, to be started at low doses, primarily to reduce the arrhythmic and ischemic risk in all patients with MI (see Chapter 13). Whether β-blockers also prevent adverse remodeling in all circumstances is controversial, and systematic use of higher doses of β-blockers during MI increases the risk of hypotension and cardiogenic shock.

Other Pharmacologic Therapies

Whether adjunctive treatments for MI, such as 3-hydroxy-3-methylglutaryl–coenzyme A (CoA) reductase inhibitors, statins, and antiplatelet therapies, have any effect on adverse remodeling is not established.

ONGOING CLINICAL AND TRANSLATIONAL RESEARCH

Anti-Inflammatory Therapies

An intense organized inflammatory response is triggered after myocardial ischemia and necrosis and involves all components of innate immunity, affecting both cardiomyocytes and noncardiomyocyte cells. Inflammation is triggered by tissue injury. The inflammatory response mediates wound healing and scar formation and affects ventricular remodeling. Despite a wealth of preclinical research, many therapeutic attempts aimed at reducing inflammation in acute MI during the past several decades have failed to translate to the clinical setting owing to impaired healing, increased risk of cardiac rupture, or lack of additional benefit in addition to standard therapies (Table 36-4).[16] To date, therefore, there are no targeted anti-inflammatory therapies proven to prevent or treat adverse left ventricular remodeling.[16]

Nonspecific Anti-Inflammatory Agents

Steroids

Glucocorticoids are powerful anti-inflammatory agents acting on genomic and nongenomic pathways and are

TABLE 36-4 Overview of Clinical Trials with Anti-Inflammatory Therapies

INTERVENTION	PRECLINICAL RESEARCH	PHASE II CLINICAL TRIALS	PHASE III CLINICAL TRIALS	NOTES/COMMENTS
Glucorticoids (methylprednisolone, prednisone, hydrocortisone)	Mixed results, depending on ischemic model and species used	Conflicting results in the many phase II clinical trials	No large phase III trial completed Meta-analysis of phase II trials shows no harm, and a trend toward a small beneficial effect in terms of recurrent MI.	Glucocorticoids have many undesired effects such as sodium/ volume retention, hyperglycemia, and impaired healing.
NSAIDs (diclofenac, ibuprofen, aspirin [high-dose])	Mixed results, depending on ischemic model and species used	Conflicting results in the many phase II clinical trials	None available	NSAIDs increase risk of gastrointestinal bleeding, increase blood pressure, and increase risk of thrombotic events.
Integrin-targeted blockers (recombinant human antibody against CD18, Hu23F2G, inclacumab)	Favorable results in animal models of myocardial ischemia-reperfusion injury	Phase II clinical trials, including between 394 and 544 patients each, showed no beneficial effects or effects inconsistent across endpoints.	None available	None of these drugs are currently used in clinical practice.
Inhibitors of the complement cascade (pexelizumab)	Favorable results in animal models of myocardial ischemia- reperfusion injury	Phase II clinical trials negative for the primary endpoint of infarct size reduction, but reduced 90-day mortality with pexelizumab with bolus and infusion	Phase III clinical failed to confirm the beneficial effects of pexelizumab.	Beneficial effects of pexelizumab have been reported in patients undergoing cardiac surgery.
Interleukin-1 blocker (anakinra)	Favorable results in animal models of myocardial ischemia-reperfusion and of ischemic cardiomyopathy without reperfusion	Two very small pilot studies suggest a beneficial effect of anakinra on the incidence of heart failure after STEMI. A third phase II study is ongoing.	None available. A secondary prevention trial is ongoing.	Anakinra is widely used to treat rheumatoid arthritis and other autoinflammatory disease. Anakinra has an established safety profile.
Plasma derived alpha-1 antitrypsin (Prolastin C)	Favorable results in animal models of myocardial ischemia-reperfusion and of ischemic cardiomyopathy without reperfusion	A small pilot study showed safety of Prolastin C infusion in patients with STEMI.	None available	Used as replacement therapy for patients with genetic deficiency. Prolastin C has an established safety profile.
Metalloproteinase inhibitors (PG-116800, doxycycline)	Favorable results in animal models of myocardial ischemia-reperfusion and of ischemic cardiomyopathy without reperfusion	Doxycycline showed a significant improvement in ventricular remodeling versus placebo at 6 months in patients with STEMI and LVEF <40%.	None available	Doxycycline is widely available and has an established safety profile.

LVEF, Left ventricular ejection fraction; *MI*, myocardial infarction; *NSAIDs*, nonsteroidal anti-inflammatory drugs.

commonly used in a variety of clinical conditions. The clinical trials of glucocorticoids in patients with MI have shown conflicting results. Early concerns regarding impaired infarct healing—arising seen in the pre-reperfusion era—are not supported by findings in the more recent clinical trials, and such impairment either is only seen in some subset of patients (e.g., those with long-term steroid use, first MI, or transmural MI without reperfusion) or is more of a perceived rather than a real effect. However, glucocorticoids also have an effect on water retention, edema, hyperglycemia, and muscular atrophy. Therefore current guidelines advise against the use of glucocorticoids in acute MI.[16]

Nonsteroidal Anti-Inflammatory Drugs

Nonsteroidal anti-inflammatory drugs (NSAIDs) also are broad anti-inflammatory agents inhibiting the production of prostanoids. Observational studies in MI in the pre-reperfusion era showed an association between NSAID use and worse clinical outcomes and an association with ventricular rupture. NSAIDs also led to a significant increase in blood pressure values, reduced renal blood flow, increased platelet aggregation, and increased risk of gastrointestinal bleeding. Therefore current clinical guidelines recommend against NSAID treatment and actively recommend NSAID discontinuation at the time of STEMI.[16]

Inhibition of Targeted Inflammatory Processes

Leukocyte Adhesion and Migration

A more targeted approach, inhibiting leukocyte adhesion and migration, has been tested with antibody-derived technologies blocking integrins, which are contact molecules expressed on the cell surface of neutrophils, platelets, or endothelial cells. Clinical trials blocking the key integrins, such as CD11, CD18, and P-selectin, failed to show clear improvement in infarct healing or clinical outcomes.[16] A possible explanation for negative results with these agents is that the duration of ischemia observed in trials is longer than that in experimental models of ischemia-reperfusion, leading to irreversible endothelial cell barrier damage and thus limiting the efficacy of the proposed intervention.

Complement Cascade

The complement cascade is activated early during acute MI and actively participates in ischemia-reperfusion injury, activating leukocytes and endothelial cells, increasing proinflammatory cytokine release, and causing cardiomyocyte cell death. Despite promising preclinical research, favorable safety/tolerability studies, and positive signals from phase II studies, the phase III clinical trials with complement cascade inhibitors failed to show the proposed clinical benefit.[16]

Cytokines

More recent strategies aimed at selectively blocking cytokines acting upstream in the cascade rather than globally suppressing the response downstream have shown some promising results in preclinical research and pilot clinical trials.[16] IL-1β is an apical cytokine in the cascade, released at the site of injury after activation of the inflammasome, and amplifying the local and systemic inflammatory response.[17] Small pilot clinical trials have shown acceptable safety and tolerability of IL-1β blockade in patients with STEMI, and initial evidence suggests a clinical benefit in preventing HF after MI.[17] A large phase III secondary prevention clinical trial of IL-1β blockade in patients with previous MI is currently ongoing (Clinicaltrials.gov NCT 0127846). Plasma-derived α_1-antitrypsin (AAT) exerts an anti-inflammatory effect independent of the serine protease–inhibiting activity, leading to reduced IL-1β release. A small pilot study of plasma-derived AAT recently has been completed in acute MI.[16]

Tumor necrosis factor (TNF)-α is another proinflammatory cytokine. TNF-α is upregulated early in MI, promoting cardiac dysfunction. Blockade of the TNF-α system in experimental AMI, however, led to conflicting results. A recent small clinical trial with etanercept, a TNF-α blocker acting as a circulating trap, in 26 patients with acute MI showed reduced neutrophil count and plasma IL-6 concentrations at 24 hours but unexpectedly increased platelet-monocyte aggregation.[16] No other clinical trials to date have tested the effects of TNF-α blockade in patients with acute MI. However, TNF-α blockers (etanercept and infliximab) have given disappointing results in patients with chronic HF, with a dose-dependent increase in adverse cardiac events. Therefore TNF-α–blocking drugs are considered to be contraindicated in patients with or at risk for HF.[16]

Metalloproteinases

Metalloproteinases (MMPs) degrade collagen, contributing to scar thinning, aneurysm formation and rupture in the infarcted area, and to adverse ventricular remodeling in remote areas. Preclinical research suggested that inhibition of MMP-2 and -9 would lead to more favorable remodeling and prevent HF. Clinical trials with a targeted MMP inhibitor, however, failed to show benefits in a phase II clinical trial, whereas doxycycline, a tetracycline antimicrobial, which also inhibits MMP-2 and -9, was shown in a phase II clinical trial to reduce ventricular dilation at 6 months in patients with STEMI and left ventricular systolic dysfunction.[18]

Immunoglobulin Therapy

Intravenous immunoglobulin (IVIG) is made by pooling of human immunoglobulin antibodies from donors, with anti-inflammatory effects occurring through several mechanisms. A recent small phase II study in patients with MI showed no effect on ventricular remodeling.[16]

Growth Factors

Infarct healing is characterized by an increase in endogenous growth factors that act by concomitantly protecting cardiomyocytes and endothelial cells from the ischemic and inflammatory injury, promoting neoangiogenesis, and possibly promoting cardiomyocyte regeneration. Despite a significant number of preclinical studies showing beneficial effects of erythropoietin (EPO) and derivatives, granulocyte colony-stimulating factor (G-CSF), and granulocyte-monocyte colony-stimulating factor (GM-CSF), the results of clinical trials in patients in STEMI are not sufficiently clear to justify use of these agents in clinical practice (Table 36-5).[19,20] Administration of EPO has been studied in several single- and multi-center trials that have reported conflicting results regarding its efficacy and safety, with concerns inherent to increased infarct size, microvascular obstruction, or thrombotic complications. G-CSF also has been studied in several rather small clinical trials, showing a potential small beneficial effect of G-CSF on left ventricular remodeling but accompanied

TABLE 36-5 Overview of Clinical Trials with Growth Factors

INTERVENTION	PRECLINICAL RESEARCH	PHASE II CLINICAL TRIALS	PHASE III CLINICAL TRIALS	NOTES/COMMENTS
Erythropoietin (EPO)	Favorable results in animal models of myocardial ischemia-reperfusion and of ischemic cardiomyopathy without reperfusion	Conflicting results of the phase II clinical trials	Conflicting results of phase III clinical trials	Concerns raised regarding thrombotic complications
Granulocyte colony-stimulating factor (G-CSF)	Favorable results in animal models of myocardial ischemia-reperfusion and of ischemic cardiomyopathy without reperfusion	Favorable results of multiple phase II clinical trials	There have been no large phase III clinical trials. A meta-analysis of all studies showed no significant effects on clinical endpoints and a small potential benefit on ventricular remodeling.	G-CSF is clinically used to treat febrile neutropenia, and as an adjunct to cancer chemotherapy regimens.
Granulocyte- monocyte colony-stimulating factor (GM-CSF)	Favorable results in animal models of myocardial ischemia-reperfusion and of ischemic cardiomyopathy without reperfusion	One pilot clinical trial in patients with STEMI not eligible for early reperfusion showed promising results in terms of remodeling and outcomes.	None available	GM-CSF is clinically used to treat febrile neutropenia, and as an adjunct to cancer chemotherapy regimens.

MI, Myocardial infarction.

by a signal-to-noise ratio insufficient to derive conclusive results. GM-CSF was studied in a small single-center study of patients with STEMI considered to be ineligible for early reperfusion, and showed beneficial effects on left ventricular remodeling. To date, therefore, no targeted growth factor therapies have been proved to prevent or treat adverse left ventricular remodeling in large randomized clinical trials.

Cardiac Regeneration

The regeneration of cardiomyocytes in the adult heart occurs physiologically at an extremely low rate, which led scientists in the past to consider the heart a postmitotic organ. An increase in this regeneration is seen after MI in the myocardium bordering the infarct. Although it is clear that the physiologic regeneration process is insufficient to restore the integrity of the heart, preclinical research and pilot clinical trials have suggested that augmentation of the process can be used to prevent adverse cardiac remodeling. This topic is treated separately in Chapter 22.

Cardiac Diastolic Constraining Devices

The loss of contractile myocardium during MI leads to changes in regional and global strain. The stretch of the infarct and border zone not only is mechanically inefficient but also induces biologic changes in the entire heart, promoting hypertrophy, apoptosis, and fibrosis. In a model of large anterior wall MI in the sheep, the border zone progressively enlarges (infarct expansion) and loses contractility despite presence of normal coronary perfusion. To counter the strain, several diastolic constraining devices have been developed.[21] After an initial interest in using a chest wall muscle, latissimus dorsi, to wrap the left ventricle and have it contract at optimal frequency (dynamic cardiomyoplasty), phase I and II clinical trials in patients with dilated cardiomyopathy have led to reduced enthusiasm in the field owing to concerns regarding the long-term viability of the procedure.

Devices also have been developed for a similar purpose. The most widely studied device of this kind, the CorCap cardiac support device (CSD) (Acorn Cardiovascular, St. Paul, Minnesota), is a polyester mesh device that has undergone extensive preclinical testing and phase I-II clinical testing in patients with dilated cardiomyopathy. The preclinical studies in the sheep MI model showed preservation in the border zone contractility and global systolic function. Phase I and II clinical studies have followed in patients with established dilated valvular and nonvalvular cardiomyopathy, showing a significant improvement in ventricular remodeling, with "reverse remodeling"—reduction in end-diastolic and end-systolic volumes—seen in many cases. These improvements were associated with a mild subjective decrease in HF symptoms and a reduced need for advanced HF support, without any effects on LVEF or on 5-year survival. Experience with the CorCap cardiac support device in patients with acute or recent MI, however, is lacking, and the CorCap device is not approved for clinical use at present.

The HeartNet cardiac restraint device (Paracor Medical Inc., Sunnyvale, California) is a device made of flexible and elastic nitinol mesh that is inserted to fit over both ventricles, leaving the apex uncovered. Experimental data in sheep with ischemic cardiomyopathy were promising. A phase I-II clinical trial in 39 patients was completed but showed only a mild abatement of subjective HF symptoms and failed to show significant change in cardiac dimensions and function. Clinical experience with the HeartNet device in acute or recent MI also is lacking.

The Coapsys device (Myocor, Maple Grove, Minnesota) is a system composed of two pads connected with a transventricular cord. This device has been tested mainly to reduce the severity of functional mitral regurgitation associated with ischemic and nonischemic cardiomyopathy. The RESTOR-MV phase II trial showed promising results in patients with ischemic cardiomyopathy and severe functional mitral regurgitation. Clinical experience with the Coapsys device in acute or recent MI also is lacking.

The Parachute device is a percutaneous ventricular restoration device inserted in the left ventricular apex. In a phase I-II feasibility study of 31 patients with ischemic cardiomyopathy and HF, device implantation appeared to be safe and resulted in effective left ventricular apical